Quick Consult Manual of Evidence-Based Medicine

Quick Consult Manual of Evidence-Based Medicine

Editors

Burton W. Lee, M.D.
Fellow in Pulmonary and Critical Care Medicine
Pulmonary and Critical Care Unit
Massachusetts General Hospital
Boston, Massachusetts

Stephen I. Hsu, M.D., Ph.D.
Fellow in Nephrology
Renal Unit
Massachusetts General Hospital
Boston, Massachusetts

David S. Stasior, M.D., M.P.P.
Fellow in Department of Medicine
Massachusetts General Hospital
Boston, Massachusetts
Director of Wellness Management Services
Strategic Health Solutions
KPMG Peat Marwick
Boston, Massachusetts

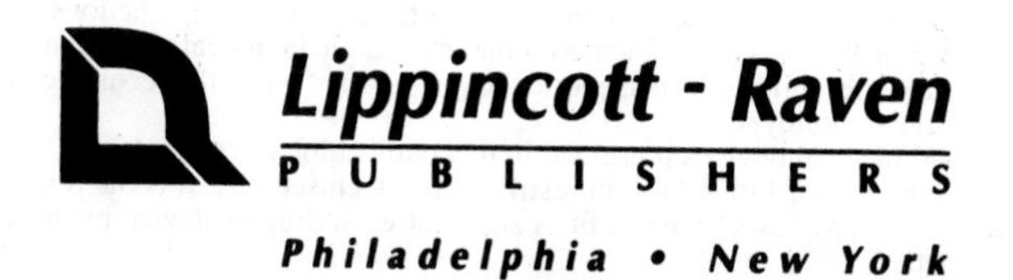

Developmental Editor: Brian Brown
Manufacturing Manager: Dennis Teston
Production Manager: Maxine Langweil
Production Editor: Mary Ann McLaughlin
Cover Designer: Patricia Gast
Indexer: Gerry Lynn Messner
Compositor: Compset, Inc.
Printer: Donnelley, Crawfordville

Printed in the United States of America

9 8 7 6 5 4 3 2 1

Library of Congress Cataloging-in-Publication Data

Quick consult manual of evidence-based medicine / editors, Burton W. Lee, Stephen I. Hsu, David S. Stasior.
p. cm.
Includes bibliographical references and index.
ISBN 0-316-51887-5
1. Internal medicine—Handbooks, manuals, etc. I. Lee, Burton W. II. Hsu, Stephen I. III. Stasior, David S.
[DNLM: 1. Evidence-Based Medicine—handbooks. 2. Decision Support Techniques—handbooks. WB 39 Q4 1997]
RC55.Q53 1997
616—DC21
DNLM/DLC
for Library of Congress 97-3306
CIP

Care has been taken to confirm the accuracy of the information presented and to describe generally accepted practices. However, the authors, editor, and publisher are not responsible for errors or omissions or for any consequences from application of the information in this book and make no warranty, express or implied, with respect to the contents of the publication.

The authors, editor, and publisher have exerted every effort to ensure that drug selection and dosage set forth in this text are in accordance with current recommendations and practice at the time of publication. However, in view of ongoing research, changes in government regulations, and the constant flow of information relating to drug therapy and drug reactions, the reader is urged to check the package insert for each drug for any change in indications and dosage and for added warnings and precautions. This is particularly important when the recommended agent is a new or infrequently employed drug.

Some drugs and medical devices presented in this publication have Food and Drug Administration (FDA) clearance for limited use in restricted research settings. It is the responsibility of the health care provider to ascertain the FDA status of each drug or device planned for use in their clinical practice.

Contents

Contributing Authors

Jonathan S. Bogan, M.D.
Clinical and Research Fellow in Medicine
Department of Medicine (Endocrinology)
Massachusetts General Hospital
14 Fruit Street
Boston, Massachusetts 02114

Joseph V. Bonventre, M.D., Ph.D.
Associate Professor of Medicine
Department of Medicine
Harvard University/Massachusetts General Hospital
Building 149, 13th Street, Room 4002
Charlestown, Massachusetts 02129

Marc L. Boom, M.D., M.B.A.
Assistant Professor of Medicine
Department of Medicine
Baylor College of Medicine
One Baylor Plaza
Houston, Texas 77030

Daniel C. Chung, M.D.
Instructor in Medicine
Gastrointestinal Unit
Massachusetts General Hospital and Harvard Medical School
32 Fruit Street
Boston, Massachusetts 02114

Cecil H. Coggins, M.D.
Associate Professor of Medicine
Department of Renal Medicine
Massachusetts General Hospital
Boston, Massachusetts 02114

Stephanie A. Coulter, M.D.
Clinical and Research Fellow in Cardiology
Department of Medicine
Massachusetts General Hospital
55 Fruit Street
Boston, Massachusetts 02114

Robert B. Fogel, M.D.
Clinical and Research Fellow in Medicine
Department of Pulmonary and Critical Care Medicine
Massachusetts General Hospital
55 Fruit Street, Bulfinch 148
Boston, Massachusetts 02114

Lawrence S. Friedman, M.D.
Associate Professor of Medicine
Harvard Medical School
Associate Physician, Gastrointestinal Unit
Massachusetts General Hospital
32 Fruit Street
Boston, Massachusetts 02114

R. Scott Harris, M.D.
Fellow, Pulmonary/Critical Care Medicine
Department of Pulmonary/Critical Care
Massachusetts General Hospital
55 Fruit Street
Boston, Massachusetts 02114

Stephen I. Hsu, M.D., Ph.D.
Fellow in Nephrology
Renal Unit
Massachusetts General Hospital
5 Fruit Street
Boston, Massachusetts 02114

Gordon S. Huggins, M.D.
Fellow, Cardiology Division
Massachusetts General Hospital
Fruit Street
Boston, Massachusetts 02114

Walter J. Koroshetz, M.D.
Assistant Professor of Neurology and Medicine
Department of Neurology
Massachusetts General Hospital
Harvard Medical School
Fruit Street
Boston, Massachusetts 02114

Burton W. Lee, M.D.
Fellow in Pulmonary and Critical Care Medicine
Pulmonary and Critical Care Unit
Massachusetts General Hospital
Fruit Street
Boston, Massachusetts 02114

John J. Lepore, M.D.
Cardiology Fellow
Cardiac Unit, Department of Medicine
Massachusetts General Hospital
Fruit Street
Boston, Massachusetts 02114

Donald M. Lloyd-Jones, M.D.
Fellow in Cardiology, Research Fellow in Medicine
Cardiac Unit
Massachusetts General Hospital, Harvard University
Fruit Street
Boston, Massachusetts 02114

David G. Morris, M.D.
Division of Pulmonary and Critical Care Medicine
University of California, San Francisco
405 Parnassus Avenue
Room 1087M
San Francisco, California 94143

Laura A. Napolitano, M.D.
Fellow in Infectious Diseases
Department of Medicine
University of California, San Francisco
Room C443, Box 0654
Division of Infectious Diseases, UCSF
San Francisco, California 94143

Patrick T. O'Gara, M.D.
Assistant Professor of Medicine
Department of Medicine, Cardiovascular Division
Harvard Medical School/Brigham and Women's Hospital
75 Francis Street, Tower 3
Boston, Massachusetts 02115

Will P. Schmitt, M.D.
Instructor in Medicine
Department of Medicine
Massachusetts General Hospital
Fruit Street
Boston, Massachusetts 02114

Albert C. Shaw, M.D., Ph.D.
Research Fellow in Medicine
Infectious Disease Unit
Massachusetts General Hospital/Harvard Medical School
Fruit Street
Boston, Massachusetts 02114

David S. Stasior, M.D., M.P.P.
Fellow in Department of Medicine
Massachusetts General Hospital
Fruit Street
Boston, Massachusetts 02114
Director of Wellness Management Services
Strategic Health Solutions
KPMG Peat Marwick
Boston, Massachusetts 02110

Morton N. Swartz, M.D.
Professor of Medicine
Department of Medicine
Harvard Medical School/Massachusetts General Hospital
Fruit Street
Boston, Massachusetts 02114

Les A. Szekely, M.D.
Fellow in Pulmonary and Critical Care
Department of Pulmonary and Critical Care

Massachusetts General Hospital
55 Fruit Street, Bulfinch 148
Boston, Massachusetts 02114

Ravi I. Thadhani, M.D., M.P.H.
Instructor of Medicine
Department of Medicine
Massachusetts General Hospital
55 Fruit Street, Founders 036
Boston, Massachusetts 02114

B. Taylor Thompson, M.D.
Associate Professor of Medicine, Harvard Medical School;
Director of the Medical Intensive Care Unit, Massachusetts General Hospital;
Department of Pulmonary and Critical Care Medicine
55 Fruit Street
Boston, Massachusetts 02114

Preface

During the first few months of our internal medicine residencies at Massachusetts General Hospital in Boston, we often asked many of the staff and senior residents specific questions about how they practiced medicine. Should we administer theophylline to asthma patients during an acute flare? Should we use a β-adrenergic receptor antagonist or an angiotensin-converting-enzyme inhibitor for patients who have suffered a myocardial infarction? Sometimes, senior physicians would answer by citing a study or quoting a reference. Not infrequently, however, they would explain that they had learned these practice habits earlier in their careers from someone still more senior. When we turned to textbooks for answers, these references usually gave standard advice about how to practice, often describing many of the same habits adopted by our mentors. Sometimes, we found that the advice in one text disagreed with that in other texts or with what one of our mentors had told us verbally. In general, these textbooks rarely distinguished between those parts of their advice based on sound research and those aspects simply handed down from earlier generations of physicians.

Because we were troubled by the uncertainty of the data underlying our practice patterns, we began conducting literature searches of our own. We selected topics that we encountered daily in the hospital or in clinic. We pulled the relevant original articles, summarized the key points from each reference, including the primary data which we reproduced in table form, and noted the faults or limits of each study. We kept the printed summaries in a notebook that we carried with us daily. During our training period, many fellow residents expressed how much they appreciated our summaries. Because of their persistence and our belief that these summaries really differ from any available reference book, we decided to publish them as a portable handbook.

Consistent with our original plan, we have tried to provide an in-depth discussion and summary of the relevant literature for each selected topic. The goal of this book is to give the reader a degree of familiarity and expertise on a given topic that would generally be expected of a subspecialist in that field. However, this book concentrates on only the very common topics that an internist is likely to face regularly, such as management of myocardial infarction, asthma, gastrointestinal bleeding, HIV infection, renal failure, or stroke. Thus, the list of topics covered in this book is, by design, incomplete. We have purposefully avoided relatively uncommon topics, such as management of carcinoid syndromes, or topics that are relevant only for subspecialists, such as specific chemotherapeutic regimens for various cancers.

Based on our own experience, this book can be utilized in a number of ways. We believe that having the important information at the fingertips allows for better patient care. For example, when confronted with a patient with pleuritic chest pain and dyspnea, the text could be used to readily look up the critical data on the role of V/Q scans for diagnosis of pulmonary embolism. During attending rounds, work rounds, or discussions in the corridor, this book could be used to easily review the primary data on the role of aspirin versus warfarin for prevention of stroke in patients with atrial fibrillation. We have found these summaries to be helpful for informal discussion, as well as for structured didactic talks. In addition, when a new article appears in a medical journal, this book can provide a quick overview of the literature and facilitate the reader's evaluation of new information in light of prior knowledge.

To some degree, the practice of medicine will always involve making decisions in the absence of complete certainty. However, a literature-based or evidence-based approach to clinical practice can help to reduce the element of uncertainty to within the limits of current knowledge, and thereby promote the best possible care of each patient. We hope that this portable handbook will prove to be as valuable to others as it has been for us and encourages all students and practitioners of medicine to be more critical thinkers, as well as better clinicians.

Acknowledgments

We would like to thank the internal medicine residency classes of 1994 and 1995 at Massachusetts General Hospital for making the residency experience truly enjoyable. Many class members directly or indirectly contributed to the writing of this book. We would also like to thank the many staff physicians of the Medicine Service at Massachusetts General Hospital who have tirelessly dedicated their time and energy to teaching residents. In particular, we are especially grateful to Morton Swartz, Leslie Fang, Lloyd Axelrod, John Mills, Patrick O'Gara, Cecil Coggins, Joseph Bonventre, B. Taylor Thompson, Lawrence Friedman, and Walter Koroshetz. They have inspired us to think critically throughout our residency and many have been enthusiastic contributors and/or advisors for this book. Most of all, we would like to thank our spouses and children: Sandy, Kyle, Bianca, Janine, and Elizabeth. This book could not have been completed without their love, support, and encouragement.

Quick Consult Manual of Evidence-Based Medicine

1

Atrial Fibrillation

Burton W. Lee and
Patrick T. O'Gara

A. Introduction

1. Atrial fibrillation (AF) is a common disorder affecting about 2% of adults (≥30 years) in the general population. Of the 5209 individuals in the Framingham Heart Study, the cumulative incidence of AF during a 22-year follow-up period was 21.5 per 1000 men and 17.1 per 1000 women (86). This risk increased sharply with age so that the lifetime prevalence of AF was 0.5% for 50- to 59-year-old subjects compared with almost 9% for 80- to 89-year-old subjects (163).
2. **Risk Factors for Development of AF**
   a. The major risk factors that have been linked to the development of AF are summarized in Table 1 (1,15,113,136). Although the distinction may not be exact, some of these factors cause or precipitate AF and others may only predispose the patient (see Table 1-1).
   b. In a multivariate analysis of the data from the Framingham Heart Study, six clinical variables were identified as independent predictors for development of AF: increasing age, diabetes mellitus, hypertension, congestive heart failure (CHF), valvular heart disease, and myocardial infarction (MI). MI was a significant risk factor only for men. Men were about 1.5 times more likely to develop AF than women (15) (see Table 1-2).

Table 1-1 Major risk factors for AF (1,15,113,136)

Cardiac Conditions	Pulmonary Conditions	Other Conditions
Coronary artery disease	Pneumonia	Fever
Myocarditis	Pulmonary embolism	Surgery
Cardiomyopathy	Lung cancer	Hypertension
Congestive heart failure	Other chronic lung disease	Diabetes mellitus
Hypertensive heart disease		Thyrotoxicosis
Valvular heart disease		Alcoholism
Congential heart disease		Severe infections
Wolff-Parkinson-White syndrome		
Pericarditis		

Table 1-2 Predictors for development of AF in multivariate analysis (15)

	Men		Women	
Independent Risk Factors	Odds Ratio	*P*	Odds Ratio	*P*
Myocardial infarction	1.4	<0.05	1.2	NS
Diabetes mellitus	1.4	<0.05	1.6	<0.01
Hypertension	1.5	<0.01	1.4	<0.05
Valvular heart disease	1.8	<0.01	3.4	<0.01
Age	2.1 per decade	<0.0001	2.2 per decade	<0.0001
Congestive heart failure	4.5	<0.0001	5.9	<0.0001

3. The major clinical manifestations of AF can be related to three features of the arrhythmia: rapid and irregular ventricular response, loss of atrioventricular (AV) synchrony, and formation of intracardiac thrombus. Exceedingly rapid, irregular ventricular response may cause palpitations, hemodynamic deterioration, CHF, syncope, or chest pain. The loss of AV synchrony and the lack of atrial contribution to ventricular filling may cause decreased exercise tolerance, CHF, or dyspnea. Finally, the formation of intracardiac thrombus increases the risk of systemic embolization. In the Framingham Heart Study, the risk of stroke was five times higher in patients with AF after adjusting for the presence of other risk factors for stroke (163). In addition, chronic AF was associated with an almost twofold increase in the rate of all-cause mortality, compared with the rate in patients without AF, during 22 years of follow-up (86). The strategies for management of AF are aimed primarily at attaining control of these three features of the arrhythmia. The management goals of ventricular rate control, restoration and maintenance of sinus rhythm, and prevention of thromboembolism are discussed in ensuing sections.

B. Ventricular Rate Control

1. Chronic AF

a. Cardiac Glycosides—Digoxin is a time-honored therapy for ventricular rate control in patients with chronic AF. It decreases the ventricular rate primarily by enhancing the vagal activity on the AV node (61,128). Because the resting autonomic tone of the heart is predominantly vagal, digoxin further enhances this tone and effectively controls the ventricular rate at rest. However, under conditions of exercise or stress, the dominance of vagal tone is removed and digoxin becomes less effective (36,47,94,98,165). A study by Lang best illustrates this point (98). In a multiphasic crossover design, the heart rate response to exercise was tested in 24 patients with chronic AF under five different treatment conditions: (a) "No Therapy"; (b) "Low-Dose Digoxin" (0.25 mg/day with mean serum concentration of 0.81 ng/ml); (c) "High-Dose Digoxin" (0.5 mg/day with mean serum concentration of 1.71 ng/ml); (d) "Verapamil" (80 mg TID); and (e) "Combination Therapy" (verapamil 80 mg TID plus digoxin 0.25 mg/day with mean serum digoxin concentration of 1.52 ng/ml) (see Table 1-3).

(1) With "No Therapy," the ventricular rate increased from 109 bpm at rest to 160 bpm during exercise. Therapy with "Low-Dose Digoxin" significantly decreased the resting ventricular rate to 95 bpm but failed to reduce the ventricular rate during exercise.

(2) Therapy with "High-Dose Digoxin" significantly decreased the ventricular rate both at rest and during exercise but these effects were only modest. With exercise, the ventricular rate increased to 147 bpm, only an 8% reduction compared with "No Therapy." Therefore, despite adequate serum levels, digoxin could not effectively control the ventricular rate during exercise.

b. Calcium Channel Blockers—Numerous studies have demonstrated the superiority of calcium channel blockers over digoxin for ventricular rate control in chronic AF (12,94,97–99,105,108,134,143,144). Unlike digoxin, verapamil and diltiazem significantly decrease the ventricular rate both at

Table 1-3 Digoxin for chronic ventricular rate control (98)

	No Therapy	Low-Dose Digoxin	High-Dose Digoxin
Ventricular rate at rest	109 bpm	95 bpm	88 bpm
P (vs. "No Therapy" at rest)	—	<0.01	<0.01
Ventricular rate during exercise	160 bpm	155 bpm	147 bpm
P (vs. "No Therapy" during exercise)	—	NS	<0.025

rest and exercise. Again, the previously described study by Lang best illustrates this point (98). The design of this study has already been summarized (see Table 1-4).

(1) With "Verapamil," the ventricular rate increased from 86 bpm at rest to 122 bpm during exercise, a 23% decrease compared with "No Therapy."

(2) With "Combination Therapy," the ventricular rate increased from 75 bpm at rest to 114 bpm during exercise. This represents a 29% reduction compared with "No Therapy" and a 26% reduction compared with "Low-Dose Digoxin."

(3) The combination of verapamil and digoxin was more effective than verapamil alone for 11 of the 24 patients. For the remaining 13 patients, verapamil alone was as effective as the combination.

c. β-Blockers—The superiority of β-blockers over digoxin for ventricular rate control in chronic AF has also been demonstrated in a number of studies (8,13,47,49,164). As with calcium channel blockers, β-blockers decrease the ventricular rate both at rest and during exercise. A study by David illustrates this point (47). In a multiphasic crossover design, the heart rate response to exercise was tested in 28 patients with chronic AF under five different treatment conditions: (a) "Low-Dose Digoxin" (mean serum concentration of 0.6 ng/ml); (b) "High-Dose Digoxin" (mean serum concentration of 1.8 ng/ml); (c) "Low-Dose Combination" (timolol plus low-dose digoxin with mean serum concentration of 0.6 ng/ml); (d) "High-Dose Combination" (timolol plus high-dose digoxin with mean serum concentration of 1.8 ng/ml); and (e) "Timolol" (mean daily dose of 30 mg) (see Table 1-5).

(1) As before, digoxin was largely ineffective for ventricular rate control during exercise. With "Low-Dose Digoxin," the ventricular rate increased from 91 bpm at rest to 135 bpm during exercise. Therapy with "High-Dose Digoxin" was not significantly better than therapy with

Table 1-4 Calcium channel blockers for chronic ventricular rate control (98)

	No Therapy	Verapamil	Combination
Ventricular rate at rest	109 bpm	86 bpm	75 bpm
P (vs. "No Therapy" at rest)	—	<0.0005	<0.0005
Ventricular rate during exercise	160 bpm	122	114 bpm
P (vs. "No Therapy" during exercise)	—	<0.0005	<0.0005

Table 1-5 β-blockers for chronic ventricular rate control (47)

	Low-Dose Digoxin	High-Dose Digoxin	Timolol	Low-Dose Combination	High-Dose Combination
Ventricular rate at rest	91 bpm	98 bpm	76 bpm	68 bpm	67 bpm
P (vs. "Low-dose Digoxin" at rest)	—	NS	<0.05	<0.001	<0.001
Ventricular rate during exercise	155 bpm	139 bpm	110 bpm	94 bpm	92 bpm
P (vs. "Low-dose Digoxin" during exercise)	—	NS	<0.01	<0.001	<0.001

"Low-Dose Digoxin." Similarly, "High-Dose Combination" was not superior to "Low-Dose Combination."

(2) In comparison with "Low-Dose Digoxin," timolol, alone or in combination with digoxin, significantly decreased the ventricular rate both at rest and during exercise. However, 5 patients were excluded from the study because timolol caused fatigue or CHF.

2. Paroxysmal AF

a. Cardiac Glycosides—Digoxin is often administered to patients with paroxysmal AF in an attempt to control the ventricular rate during an attack. However, it does not appear to be effective for this purpose (65,130). The study by Rawles is described for illustration (130). Seventy-two consecutive patients with paroxysmal AF documented on a 48-hour Holter monitor recording were selected for the study. The frequency of attacks, the ventricular rate during AF, and the duration of paroxysms were compared among 31 patients receiving digoxin versus 43 patients not receiving digoxin at the time of the recording. Prolonged episodes were defined as attacks of AF lasting >30 minutes.

(1) Digoxin did not reduce either the frequency of attacks or the ventricular rate during AF. The mean ventricular rate during AF was 140 bpm for those receiving digoxin compared with 134 bpm for those not receiving digoxin. There were too few patients receiving β-blockers or calcium channel blockers to make meaningful comparisons.

(2) Instead, patients receiving digoxin were more likely to experience prolonged episodes of AF. Forty-two percent of patients receiving digoxin had one or more prolonged episodes of AF during the 48-hour period, compared with 10% of those not receiving digoxin. However, because digoxin was not randomly assigned, it is possible that digoxin may have been given preferentially to patients with more frequent, more prolonged, or more rapid episodes of AF. Therefore, the study may have been biased against digoxin (128).

b. β-Blockers and Calcium Channel Blockers—It is generally assumed that β-blockers and calcium channel blockers are as effective for patients with paroxysmal AF as they are for those with chronic AF. However, the efficacy of these agents specifically for paroxysmal AF has not adequately been evaluated.

3. Intravenous Medications for Acute Ventricular Rate Control

a. Cardiac Glycosides—Traditionally, digoxin has also been used for acute rate control in patients with rapid AF. In a prospective randomized comparison, digoxin was superior to placebo for acute rate control but a statistically significant reduction in the ventricular rate did not occur until 5.5 hours after the first dose of digoxin (60). Not surprisingly, IV calcium channel blockers and β-blockers are favored over digoxin because of their more rapid onset of action (128).

b. Calcium Channel Blockers—Several randomized controlled trials have demonstrated the efficacy of diltiazem (55,79,135) and verapamil (82,153, 158) for treatment of rapid AF.

(1) The largest of these trials was reported by Salerno (135). In a double-blind fashion, 113 patients with spontaneously occurring rapid AF or atrial flutter were randomly assigned to receive either IV diltiazem (0.25 mg/kg over 2 minutes) or placebo. Seventy-nine percent of patients had AF and 21% had atrial flutter. Therapeutic end points were (a) conversion to sinus rhythm, (b) decrease in the ventricular rate to <100 bpm, or (c) 20% reduction in the ventricular rate compared with baseline. If a therapeutic end point was not achieved within 15 minutes of the initial dose, 0.35 mg/kg of diltiazem or an equivalent volume of placebo was administered. Placebo patients who failed to improve were subsequently treated with diltiazem on an open-label basis.

(a) Overall, 94% of patients were treated effectively with diltiazem. In the double-blind portion of the study, a therapeutic end point was achieved in 93% of patients with diltiazem and 12% with placebo. In the open-label portion of the study, diltiazem successfully treated 96% of the 49 patients who did not initially respond to placebo.

(b) Among the 99 patients who responded favorably to diltiazem, 2% converted to sinus rhythm, 38% had a decrease in the heart rate to <100 bpm, and 60% had a heart rate >100 bpm that was 20% slower than baseline.

(c) The median time from the start of treatment to maximal ventricular rate control was 4.3 minutes for diltiazem. When atrial flutter and AF were analyzed separately, diltiazem was effective for both conditions.

(2) Typical doses of IV verapamil or diltiazem used in these studies are shown in Table 1-6. Diltiazem is favored over verapamil by some authors because it may have less negative inotropic effect (21,55,135). Whether this advantage translates into fewer episodes of CHF, however, is unclear (see Table 1-6).

c. β-Blockers—Intravenously administered esmolol, metoprolol, or propranolol has been touted as a good alternative to calcium channel blockers for acute rate control of rapid AF (126,139). In the event that bronchospasm, bradycardia, or hypotension develops as an adverse reaction to therapy, esmolol's short half-life of 9 minutes makes it attractive. In one study, 50% of esmolol-treated patients with new-onset atrial flutter or AF converted to sinus rhythm, compared with 12% of verapamil-treated patients (126). However, because esmolol requires continuous infusion and multiple dose adjustments, it is more cumbersome to use than other agents (128).

4. Adverse Consequences of Rate Control

a. Although calcium channel blockers and β-blockers are effective in ventricular rate control of AF, their negative chronotropic and inotropic activity may cause fatigue, heart failure, hypotension, or bradycardia. In addition, β-blockers may induce bronchospasm. Almost all of the trials demonstrating the efficacy of these agents have excluded patients with significant CHF, chronic obstructive pulmonary disease, asthma, or cardiac conduction system disease.

b. For patients with exercise-induced tachycardia but bradycardia at rest, cardioselective β-blockers with partial agonist activity may be helpful in avoiding excessive bradycardia or prolonged ventricular pauses (8,105). Patients who cannot tolerate rate-controlling drugs because of excessive bradycardia may require insertion of a pacemaker to allow therapy with these agents.

c. The impact of calcium channel blockers on patients' exercise performance is controversial. The exercise capacity of patients with chronic AF was improved by calcium channel blockade in some studies (97,105), adversely affected in one study (103), and not significantly changed in others (12,143). Reports of the effect of β-blockers on the exercise capacity of pa-

Table 1-6 Calcium channel blockers for acute ventricular rate control

	Typical Dose	References
Verapamil bolus injection	0.075 mg/kg IV over 1 min (5 mg maximum)	82,153,158
Diltiazem bolus injection	0.25–0.35 mg/kg IV over 2 min	79,135
Diltiazem continuous infusion	Initial bolus of 20 mg IV followed by continuous infusion of 10–15 mg/h. An additional bolus of 25 mg was necessary for some patients.	55

tients with AF have been similarly mixed (29,49,118,165). In theory, cardioselective β-blockers with partial agonist activity, such as xamoterol or celiprolol, may minimize the negative effect on exercise performance, but convincing advantage has not been demonstrated in clinical trials (13,103).

d. Finally, both digoxin and calcium channel blockers have been implicated in prolonging the duration of attack in patients with paroxysmal AF. In a nonrandomized study involving 72 patients with paroxysmal AF, 42% of digoxin-treated patients experienced one or more prolonged episodes (>30 minutes) of AF, compared with 10% of those patients not receiving digoxin (130). In another study involving 18 patients with paroxysmal AF and 17 patients with no prior history of AF, the duration of induced AF with programmed electrical stimulation was significantly longer when patients were given calcium channel blockers (138).

C. Cardioversion

1. Electrical Cardioversion

a. Synchronized direct current (DC) cardioversion is useful for patients for whom rapid AF causes CHF, hypotension, or cardiac ischemia. Restoration of sinus rhythm may also be helpful for those who experience palpitations, fatigue, decreased exercise tolerance, or systemic embolization due to chronic AF. Electrical cardioversion is a rapid and highly successful method for restoration of sinus rhythm, although most patients revert to AF with time (2,46,89,104,117,119,152). For example, in one study involving 181 patients with AF, DC cardioversion was successful in 81.2% of patients. However, despite maintenance therapy with quinidine, only 22% remained in sinus rhythm at 1 year (2).

b. For patients who are refractory to DC cardioversion, pretreatment with quinidine or disopyramide may increase the likelihood of conversion to sinus rhythm. In Lundstrom's study of 100 consecutive patients with chronic AF, 86% were successfully converted to sinus rhythm by the first attempt at cardioversion without antiarrhythmic therapy. After pretreatment with class Ia antiarrhythmic agents, another 8 of the remaining 14 patients were successfully converted to sinus rhythm (104).

c. Complications of Electrical Cardioversion—In a review of the literature, Morris reported the risk of complications associated with DC cardioversion to be 2.9% among 784 patients included in eight studies (119). The most common complications were sustained ventricular arrhythmias and systemic embolization. Sustained ventricular arrhythmia was observed in 0.8% of patients in the study. Half of these patients probably experienced ventricular fibrillation in association with digitalis intoxication. Therefore, digoxin toxicity should be carefully excluded before electrical cardioversion. Systemic embolization was observed in 1.1% of patients in the study.

2. Chemical Cardioversion

a. Class Ia Agents—Chemical cardioversion of AF has most often been tried with class Ia antiarrhythmic drugs. If restoration of sinus rhythm is not urgent, oral quinidine is the most popular choice, but more rapid cardioversion can be achieved with IV procainamide or disopyramide (24,33,63,72). Nevertheless, these drugs have not been rigorously compared with placebo in well-designed trials (128).

(1) Procainamide—In two uncontrolled series involving patients with recent-onset AF, infusion of procainamide (15 to 30 mg/minute to a maximum dose of 20 mg/kg) resulted in conversion of 43% to 58% of patients (63,72).

(2) Disopyramide—In a study comparing sotalol with disopyramide among 40 patients with postoperative AF or atrial flutter, the combination of IV digoxin (0.75 mg) and disopyramide (2 mg/kg bolus 2 hours after the digoxin dose, followed by 0.4 mg/kg/hour for 10 hours) successfully cardioverted 85% of patients. This rate was identical to the conversion rate for sotalol (33).

(3) **Quinidine**—In a study comparing flecainide with quinidine in 60 consecutive patients with AF, orally administered quinidine sulfate (200 mg q 2 hours up to a maximum dose of 1200 mg in 12 hours, followed by 200 mg TID of quinidine bisulfate) successfully converted 60% of patients. This rate was statistically similar to the conversion rate of 67% for flecainide. The mean time to conversion was 8.2 hours with quinidine versus 1.4 hours with flecainide (24).

b. **Class Ic Agents**—Recently, flecainide and propafenone have been proposed as alternatives to class Ia agents for chemical cardioversion of AF (24,34,52,92,149,150,160). These agents have been shown to be superior to placebo or verapamil (34,52,92,149,150,160) and equivalent to quinidine (24). Flecainide may be more effective than propafenone although the latter is less likely to cause side effects (92,149). Representative studies are described for illustration.

(1) **Flecainide Compared With Placebo**—Donovan compared flecainide (2 mg/kg over 30 minutes) versus placebo in 102 consecutive patients with recent-onset AF. The duration of AF was >30 minutes but <72 hours in all patients. Those with significant CHF, hypotension, or conduction system disease were excluded (52) (see Table 1-7).

(a) Flecainide was significantly more effective than placebo. By 6 hours, conversion to sinus rhythm had occurred in 67% of flecainide-treated patients and 35% of placebo-treated patients. The mean time to conversion was 53 minutes with flecainide.

(b) On the other hand, adverse reactions were much more common with flecainide. Significant hypotension was observed in 22% of flecainide-treated patients compared with 6% of placebo-treated patients. Five deaths were observed with flecainide and two with placebo. One patient in the flecainide group experienced torsades de pointes.

(2) **Propafenone Compared With Verapamil**—Weiner compared propafenone (150 mg q 4 hours up to 48 hours or until conversion to sinus rhythm) versus verapamil (40 mg PO q 4 hours up to 48 hours or until conversion to sinus rhythm) in 50 patients with AF of <2 weeks' duration. Patients with CHF were excluded from the study. After randomization, 4 patients were excluded because of refusal to continue in the study or because of CHF (160) (see Table 1-8).

(a) Cardioversion occurred in 87% of propafenone-treated patients compared with 41% of verapamil-treated patients.

(b) There were no episodes of proarrhythmia with propafenone, and it was generally well tolerated without major side effects. Two patients receiving verapamil developed CHF, and 1 other patient suffered an embolic stroke.

Table 1-7 Flecainide vs. placebo for cardioversion of AF (52).

	Flecainide (n=51)	Placebo (n=51)	*P*
Sinus rhythm at 6 h	67%	35%	0.000013
Mean time to conversion	53 min	150 min	0.04
Hypotension	22%	6%	?

Table 1-8 Propafenone vs. verapamil for cardioversion of AF (160).

	Propafenone (n=24)	Verapamil (n=22)	*P*
Sinus rhythm by 48 h	87%	41%	<0.001

(3) Flecainide Compared With Quinidine—Borgeat compared flecainide (up to 2 mg/kg IV bolus followed by 100 mg BID to TID) versus quinidine (200 mg PO q 2 hours up to 1.2 g in 12 hours, followed by quinidine bisulfate 200 mg PO TID) in 60 consecutive patients with AF. Patients with AF of >3 days' duration were anticoagulated for 15 days before enrollment. Patients with ischemic heart disease, conduction system disease, or uncompensated CHF were excluded (24) (see Table 1-9).

(a) The rate of conversion was similar in the two groups. Sixty percent of the patients taking quinidine converted to sinus rhythm, compared with 67% of those taking flecainide. However, conversion to sinus rhythm occurred significantly earlier with flecainide. The mean time to conversion was 81 minutes with flecainide and 493 minutes with quinidine.

(b) The risk of adverse reaction was higher with quinidine, but flecainide tended to cause more serious reactions, such as conduction disturbances and severe bradycardia.

c. Class III Agents—Class III antiarrhythmic agents, such as amiodarone and sotalol, have also been proposed as alternatives to class Ia agents for chemical cardioversion of AF (33,122,166). These agents appear to be more effective than verapamil (122) but comparable to class Ia agents (33,166). Representative studies are described here.

(1) Amiodarone Compared With Verapamil—Noc compared amiodarone (5 mg/kg IV over 3 minutes) versus verapamil (0.075 mg/kg IV over 1 minute, repeated after 10 minutes) in 24 consecutive patients with paroxysmal AF. The duration of AF was 20 minutes to 48 hours. Patients with significant conduction system disease, preexcitation, CHF, or hypotension were excluded, as were those receiving concomitant antiarrhythmic medications (122) (see Table 1-10).

(a) Amiodarone was significantly better than verapamil for conversion of AF to sinus rhythm. None of the 11 patients initially randomly assigned to receive verapamil, but 77% of those assigned to amiodarone, converted to sinus rhythm.

(b) One patient treated with verapamil experienced marked bradycardia and hypotension. One patient treated with amiodarone developed significant hypotension without bradycardia.

(2) Amiodarone Compared With Quinidine—Zehender compared amiodarone versus quinidine plus verapamil in 40 consecutive patients with AF lasting from 4 weeks to 2 years. Amiodarone was given as follows: 200 mg IV over 3 hours initially, followed by 50 mg/hour IV for 3 days, then 200 mg PO QID for 11 days. Patients responding to amiodarone were continued on 200 mg/day for 3 months and then

Table 1-9 Flecainide vs. quinidine for cardioversion of AF (24)

	Flecainide (n=30)	Quinidine (n=30)	*P*
Sinus rhythm	67%	60%	NS
Mean time to conversion	81 min	493 min	<0.001
Adverse reaction	7%	27%	?

Table 1-10 Amiodarone vs. verapamil for cardioversion of AF (122)

	Amiodarone (n=13)	Verapamil (n=11)	*P*
Sinus rhythm	77%	0%	<0.001

given fixed doses of quinidine (160 mg TID) plus verapamil (80 mg TID) for 2 years. Quinidine and verapamil were given as follows: quinidine 500 mg PO TID for 6 days, with the addition of verapamil 80 mg PO TID on days 4 through 6. Patients responding to quinidine plus verapamil were continued on lower doses for 2 years. All patients had therapeutic digoxin levels, but other drugs used for treatment of AF were not permitted (166) (see Table 1-11).

(a) The conversion rates were similar in the two treatment groups. With amiodarone, 60% of patients converted to sinus rhythm after a mean of 7.1 days. With quinidine plus verapamil, 55% converted after a mean of 3.5 days.

(b) In addition to its antiarrhythmic effect, amiodarone also slowed the mean ventricular rate by 28%. However, it caused severe bradycardia in 15% of patients. No significant rate reduction was observed with quinidine plus verapamil.

(c) Among those who were successfully cardioverted with either regimen, 60% remained in sinus rhythm for 2 years while receiving quinidine plus verapamil.

(d) Side effects were common with both drugs but the need for discontinuation of the drug was uncommon. Only 5% of patients in each group were intolerant of the respective drugs.

d. Digoxin—In an uncontrolled study, digoxin converted 85% of patients with acute AF to sinus rhythm (159). However, in a controlled study, digoxin was no more effective than placebo. Falk described a double-blind randomized comparison of digoxin versus placebo in 36 patients with recent-onset AF. All patients had ventricular rates of 85 to 175 bpm at the time of randomization. Patients with CHF, preexcitation, acute MI, or unstable angina were excluded (60) (see Table 1-12).

(1) There was no significant difference in the rate of conversion with digoxin versus placebo. About half of the patients converted to sinus rhythm with either regimen.

(2) Digoxin did slow the ventricular rate but only after an average of 5.5 hours from the first digoxin dose.

e. Calcium Channel Blockers—Although controlled studies have clearly demonstrated their efficacy for ventricular rate control in AF, calcium channel blockers appear to play a minimal role in conversion of AF to sinus rhythm (55,82,128,135,153,158). For example, in Salerno's study of 113 patients with spontaneous AF or atrial flutter, 4% converted to sinus rhythm after diltiazem therapy and 10% after placebo (135). In Hwang's study of 14 patients with AF or atrial flutter, 29% converted to sinus rhythm

Table 1-11 Amiodarone vs. quinidine & verapamil for cardioversion of AF (166)

	Amiodarone (n=20)	Quinidine Plus Verapamil (n=20)	*P*
Sinus rhythm	60%	55%	NS
Transient side effects	40%	25%	NS
Drug withdrawn due to intolerance	5%	5%	NS

Table 1-12 Digoxin vs. placebo for cardioversion of AF (60)

	Digoxin (n=18)	Placebo (n=18)	*P*
Sinus rhythm	50%	44%	NS

with verapamil and 0% with placebo (82). This difference was not statistically analyzed in the study.

f. β-Blockers—As with calcium channel blockers, β-blockers are more effective for rate reduction than for conversion of AF to sinus rhythm (128). In a double-blind placebo-controlled study involving 71 patients with atrial tachyarrhythmias (61% with AF, 21% with atrial flutter, and 18% with other atrial arrhythmias), only 6% of esmolol-treated patients converted to sinus rhythm (7). On the other hand, in an open-label comparison involving 45 patients with AF or atrial flutter, 50% of esmolol-treated patients converted to sinus rhythm, compared with 12% of verapamil-treated patients (126). Additional studies are needed to clarify this discrepancy.

g. Summary of Chemical Cardioversion for AF—Chemical cardioversion can be achieved with class Ia agents (quinidine, disopyramide, or procainamide) with an efficacy of 40% to 60%. Class Ic agents (flecainide, encainide, or propafenone) and class III agents (amiodarone, sotalol) are comparable to class Ia agents in efficacy. Patients who have been in AF for longer than 1 year and those with enlarged left atria are less likely to convert. Digoxin, calcium channel blockers, and β-blockers are no more effective than placebo for conversion of AF to sinus rhythm.

3. Decreasing the Risk of Embolization During Cardioversion—Morris estimated the risk of embolization during cardioversion for AF to be about 1.1% (119). Currently, there are two major strategies that are aimed at decreasing this risk: prophylactic anticoagulation and exclusion of thrombus by echocardiography.

a. Anticoagulation Before Cardioversion—Before elective cardioversion, it is now common practice to anticoagulate patients who have been in AF for >2 days. Generally, anticoagulation is recommended for 2 to 4 weeks before cardioversion to decrease the risk of acute thromboembolism (128) and is continued for at least 3 to 4 weeks after cardioversion to decrease the the risk of delayed thromboembolism from sluggish atrial mechanical recovery.

(1) This practice is supported by Bjerkelund's observational study of 228 patients who were anticoagulated versus 209 patients who were not anticoagulated at the time of successful electrical cardioversion of various atrial arrhythmias. The assignment to anticoagulation was not randomized. In fact, those with rheumatic heart disease and those with prior history of embolic disease were more likely to be on anticoagulation at the time of cardioversion. Despite this bias against anticoagulation, the risk of thromboembolic events was substantially lower for those receiving this therapy (17) (see Table 1-13).

(2) In a similar retrospective study by Arnold, the risk of embolic complications during elective cardioversion of AF was 3.4% among 179 nonanticoagulated patients compared with 0% among 153 anticoagulated patients. The duration of AF in patients with embolic complications ranged from 3 to 19 days. Incidentally, no patient with atrial flutter had an embolic complication regardless of anticoagulation status (10) (see Table 1-14).

Table 1-13 Effect of anticoagulation for cardioversion of AF (17)

	Anticoagulation (n=228)	No Anticoagulation (n=209)	*P*
Rheumatic heart disease	82%	41%	—
Prior history of embolization	29%	7%	—
Risk of embolization	0.8%	5.3%	0.016

Table 1-14 Effect of anticoagulation for cardioversion of AF and flutter (10)

	AF		Atrial Flutter	
	Anticoagulation (n=153)	No Anticoagulation (n=179)	Anticoagulation (n=32)	No Anticoagulation (n=90)
Embolism	0%	3.4%	0%	0%
P	.026		NS	

b. **Exclusion of Thrombus by Transesophageal Echocardiography**—Although prophylactic anticoagulation appears to decrease the risk of embolization, it can be associated with bleeding complications, additional costs, and delays in cardioversion. To avoid these disadvantages, transesophageal echocardiography has been used to exclude patients with atrial thrombi before cardioversion. Among 94 non-anticoagulated patients with AF in one study, transesophageal echocardiography identified 12 patients with atrial thrombi. These patients were anticoagulated in the traditional manner before delayed cardioversion. The remaining 82 patients underwent electrical or chemical cardioversion without anticoagulation. Ninety-five percent of these 82 patients were successfully cardioverted and none experienced a thromboembolic complication (106). However, a subsequent study reported a 2.4% rate of embolism among 712 cardioversions without anticoagulation after negative transesophageal echocardiography. It is unclear whether these failures were caused by insensitivity of the echocardiogram or *de novo* formation of atrial thrombus at the time of cardioversion (18).

4. **Predictors of Successful Cardioversion**—Numerous clinical and echocardiographic variables have been proposed as useful predictors of successful cardioversion. These factors include the duration of AF, left atrial size, presence of absence of CHF, left ventricular function, underlying heart disease, and the age of the patient (2,24,46,51,72,78,89,155,166). Among these factors, short duration of AF and normal left atrial size have been the most consistently identified predictors of success. For example, in Borgeat's study involving 40 patients with AF, 67% of those with AF for <12 months converted to sinus rhythm, compared with 30% of those with longer duration of AF. Similarly, 71% of patients with left atrial size <55 mm converted to sinus rhythm, compared with 25% of those with larger left atrial size (24).

D. **Maintenance of Sinus Rhythm**—Although electrical or chemical cardioversion can restore sinus rhythm in most patients with AF, reversion to AF with time is very common (2,24,33,34,46,52,63,72,89,92,104,117,119,122,149,150,166). Therefore, antiarrhythmic agents have been recommended for maintenance of sinus rhythm after cardioversion. Class Ia agents have been most commonly used for this purpose (22,31,75,76,80,88,102,142), but class Ic agents (6, 39, 125, 127, 129, 154) and class III agents (5,9,19,28,45,50,67,81,85,91,116,123,131,140,141,157,166) have also been used. Although these agents appear to be effective for maintenance of sinus rhythm, their overall safety for long-term use is controversial (40,41,54).

1. **Class Ia Agents**—Although disopyramide, procainamide, and quinidine are probably all effective for prevention of recurrence of AF, quinidine remains the best studied and the most commonly used agent. Coplen conducted a meta-analysis of all major studies that have evaluated the efficacy of quinidine for this role (40,41). Among 52 studies that addressed quinidine's effectiveness for suppression of AF, six trials met the following criteria: (a) a randomized controlled study comparing quinidine to placebo or to no therapy, (b) exclusion of patients in AF for <72 hours, (c) minimal follow-up period of 3 months, and (d) use of no other antiarrhythmic medication except digoxin (22,31,76,80,

102,142). Kaplan–Meier life-table estimates of the probability of being in sinus rhythm at 3, 6, and 12 months after cardioversion were calculated with the use of an intention-to-treat method. Patients who withdrew from the study or died during the study were considered to have reverted to AF unless they were specifically known to be in sinus rhythm before death or withdrawal (40,41) (see Table 1-15).

a. Five of the six studies found quinidine to be superior to placebo (22, 31,76,80,142), and one study found no significant difference (102). In pooled analysis, the percentages of patients in sinus rhythm with quinidine were 69.4%, 57.7%, and 50.2% at 3, 6, and 12 months after cardioversion, respectively. With placebo or no treatment, 45.1%, 33.3%, and 24.7% of patients were in sinus rhythm at 3, 6, and 12 months, respectively. Therefore, quinidine was significantly better than control at all time points. On the other hand, because about 25% of patients remained in sinus rhythm at 1 year without quinidine, not all patients required maintenance antiarrhythmic therapy after cardioversion.

b. About 9% of patients required discontinuation of quinidine because of adverse reaction. Furthermore, because class Ia agents decrease the refractoriness of the AV node, they can increase the ventricular rate during AF, and for this reason they should be combined with digoxin, calcium channel blockers, or β-blockers.

c. More importantly, as determined by the odds ratio, the risk of dying among patients receiving quinidine was almost three times as high as the risk among patients receiving placebo. The unadjusted mortality rate was 2.9% for the quinidine group and 0.8% for the control group. At least four fatal and one nonfatal cardiac arrests occurred among patients assigned to quinidine.

d. Relatively fewer patients with AF have rheumatic heart disease today than at the time of these studies, and ischemic heart disease is more common than before. Therefore, the efficacy as well as the safety of quinidine in the modern population is less certain. Furthermore, the fact that quinidine can increase the concentration of digoxin was not as widely appreciated at the time of these studies as it is today. It is possible that the excess number of deaths associated with quinidine resulted in part from digoxin toxicity. If so, quinidine may be safer under modern practice settings (128). Nevertheless, based on current evidence, quinidine appears to be effective for suppression of AF but this advantage may be balanced by an increase in the risk of death.

2. Class Ic Agents—In randomized controlled trials, both flecainide and propafenone have been shown to be effective in prevention of AF (6,39, 125,129,154). Unlike class Ia agents, these drugs increase the refractoriness of the AV node. In one study, propafenone was effective even in patients who were refractory to other antiarrhythmic drugs (9). However, as with class Ia drugs, the long-term safety of these drugs is controversial (54,58,59). Representative studies are described here.

a. Flecainide Compared With Placebo—Anderson compared flecainide versus placebo for prevention of paroxysmal AF in a randomized double-blind crossover study using transtelephonic monitoring. All patients had

Table 1-15 Quinidine vs. control for maintenance of sinus rhythm (40,41)

	Quinidine (n=373)	Control (n=354)	*P*
% in sinus rhythm at 3 mo	69.4%	45.1%	<0.001
% in sinus rhythm at 6 mo	57.7%	33.3%	<0.001
% in sinus rhythm at 12 mo	50.2%	24.7%	<0.001
Unadjusted mortality rate	2.9%	0.8%	<0.05

symptomatic paroxysmal AF occurring two or more times during a 4-week observation period. Patients with a history of syncope, significant CHF, angina, conduction system disease, or recent MI were excluded. Other antiarrhythmic medications including β-blockers and calcium channel blockers were not permitted. Sixty-four patients entered an open-label dose titration phase of the study to determine the maximal dose that would not cause limiting side effects for each patient. Fifty-five patients entered the double-blind phase of the study, which compared flecainide (previously determined optimal dose) versus placebo for 8 weeks. Two patients on flecainide dropped out of this phase of the study because of side effects. The remaining patients were then crossed over to the alternate therapy for 8 additional weeks. Five of these 53 patients were excluded from the analysis because of protocol violations. Symptoms and episodes of AF were documented by transtelephonic monitoring, diary, and periodic interview. Four outcome measures were studied: (a) time to first episode of paroxysmal AF, (b) average interval between attacks, (c) percentage of patients free of AF, and (d) average ventricular rate during AF (6) (see Table 1-16).

(1) Flecainide significantly improved all four outcome measures compared with placebo. The median time to first episode of AF and the average interval between attacks were 3 days and 6.2 days, respectively, with placebo, compared with 14.5 days and 27 days with flecainide. Thirty-one percent of patients receiving flecainide were free of symptomatic AF, compared with 8% of those receiving placebo. The average ventricular rate during an attack of AF was 118 bpm with flecainide and 123 bpm with placebo.

(2) Symptomatic side effects were significantly more common with flecainide than with placebo (58% versus 38%, respectively), but only 2 patients required discontinuation of the drug. Visual disturbance and dizziness were frequently observed, and 7 patients experienced proarrhythmia, conduction disturbance, or increased automaticity with flecainide. One of these patients underwent a cardiac arrest in the setting of subendocardial ischemia.

b. Propafenone Compared With Placebo—Pritchett compared propafenone versus placebo for prevention of paroxysmal supraventricular arrhythmia in a randomized double-blind crossover study using transtelephonic monitoring. Patients were excluded if the paroxysm of arrhythmia precipitated angina, CHF, or neurologic symptoms. Other antiarrhythmic medications including β-blockers and calcium channel blockers were not permitted. Thirty-three patients entered an open-label dose titration phase of the study to determine the maximal dose that would not cause limiting side effects for each patient. Sixteen patients had supraventricular tachycardia and 17 had AF. Twenty-three patients entered the double-blind phase of the study, which compared propafenone (previously determined optimal dose) versus placebo. Patients were observed for 60 days or until the first recurrence of arrhythmia. Patients were then crossed over to the alternate therapy for 60 days or until the first recurrence of arrhythmia. Symptoms and episodes of AF were documented by transtelephonic moni-

Table 1-16 Flecainide vs. placebo for maintenance of sinus rhythm (6)

	Flecainide (n=48)	Placebo (n=48)	*P*
Median time to first attack	14.5 d	3 d	<0.001
Average interval between attacks	27 d	6.2 d	<0.001
Free of AF	31%	8%	0.013
Ventricular rate during AF	118	123	0.017
Symptomatic side effects	58%	38%	<0.05

toring and periodic interview. Three outcome measures were studied: (a) median time to first recurrence of arrhythmia, (b) average ventricular rate during arrhythmia, and (c) rate of adverse effects (129).

(1) Propafenone significantly increased the time to first recurrence of arrhythmia compared with placebo (*P*=0.004). Based on a proportional hazards model, the rate of recurrence of arrhythmia among patients receiving propafenone was about one fifth the rate among those receiving placebo. Subgroup analysis of patients with AF yielded similar results but the benefit was no longer statistically significant.

(2) There was no statistically significant difference in the average ventricular rate during an arrhythmia between propafenone-treated and placebo-treated patients.

(3) Adverse reaction to propafenone caused one-third of patients to discontinue participation in the trial. Nevertheless, in patients who tolerated propafenone, it effectively suppressed the recurrence of supraventricular arrhythmia.

c. Although propafenone and flecainide appear to be effective in suppressing the recurrence of AF, the long-term safety of these agents is controversial. As with quinidine, the risk of sudden cardiac death may be increased by long-term use of these agents. The Cardiac Arrhythmia Suppression Trial (CAST) suggested that class Ic agents may increase the risk of death in patients with premature ventricular ectopy after MI. (54) Sudden cardiac deaths associated with flecainide have also been reported in patients with AF who did not have traditional risk factors for ventricular arrhythmia (58,59).

3. Class III Agents—Because class Ia and Ic drugs are often poorly tolerated and have been associated with a possible increase in mortality, class III agents such as amiodarone or sotalol have been advocated for suppression of AF (9,19,28,67,68,81,85,109,131,140,157). In nonrandomized studies, low-dose amiodarone (200 to 600 mg/day) maintained sinus rhythm in 53% to 79% of patients with refractory AF who had previously failed therapy with two to eight other antiarrhythmic drugs (19,28,67,68,81,116). Similarly, 50% of patients with AF or atrial flutter who had been refractory to other antiarrhythmic drugs were maintained in sinus rhythm for 6 months with sotalol (9). In randomized studies, amiodarone was more effective than quinidine (157) or disopyramide (109), but only the advantage over quinidine was statistically significant. Similarly, sotalol was equally effective and better tolerated than quinidine (85) or propafenone (131). Representative studies are described here.

a. Amiodarone Compared With Quinidine—In a prospective, randomized controlled trial, Vitolo compared amiodarone (400 mg QD for 15 days then for 5 days each week) versus quinidine polygalacturonate (400 mg TID) in 54 patients who were in sinus rhythm after reversion of AF. Minimum follow-up was 6 months. Treatment was deemed successful if patients were maintained in sinus rhythm for at least 6 months (157) (see Table 1-17).

(1) Amiodarone was significantly more effective than quinidine. With amiodarone, therapy was successful in 78.5% of patients, compared with 46.1% with quinidine.

(2) Side effects requiring discontinuation of therapy occurred in 4 patients receiving quinidine and 1 patient receiving amiodarone. However, 3 patients required lowering of the amiodarone dose because of

Table 1-17 Amiodarone vs. quinidine for maintenance of sinus rhythm (157)

	Amiodarone (n=28)	Quinidine (n=26)	*P*
Maintenance of sinus rhythm for 6 mo	78.5%	46.1%	0.014

bradycardia or electrocardiographic abnormalities. Abnormalities in thyroid function tests were observed in 60% of patients treated with amiodarone, but no clinical signs of thyroid disease were found in any patient.

b. Toxicity of Amiodarone

(1) Despite the effectiveness of amiodarone, its well known toxicity limits the utility of this drug. Its major side effects include pulmonary fibrosis, thyroid dysfunction, tremor, nausea, hepatotoxicity, peripheral neuropathy, photosensitivity, skin discoloration, and ocular deposits (19,28,53,67,68,74,81,96,116,120).

(2) However, many of these side effects appear to be dose related. For example, pulmonary fibrosis appears to be uncommon in patients receiving <300 mg/day, a dose found to be effective for suppression of AF in some studies (53,68). Furthermore, compared with class Ia or Ic agents, cardiac toxicity appears to be less significant with amiodarone (30,73,110,120).

c. Sotalol Compared With Quinidine—Juul-Moller compared sotalol (80 to 160 mg BID) versus quinidine sulfate (600 mg BID) in 183 patients who were in sinus rhythm after reversion from chronic AF. The duration of AF ranged from 2 months to 1 year. Patients with CHF, diabetes mellitus, thyrotoxicosis, recent MI, pulmonary hypertension, or significant conduction system disease were excluded. Except for digoxin, other drugs with antiarrhythmic, negative inotropic, or dromotropic effects were not permitted. The results derived by intention-to-treat analysis are presented in the following sections (85) (see Table 1-18).

(1) There was no significant difference in efficacy between sotalol and quinidine. The recurrence rate of AF was 37% with sotalol and 28% with quinidine. At the end of the 6-month study, 49% of the sotalol-treated patients were in sinus rhythm, compared with 42% of the quinidine-treated patients. However, among the patients who relapsed into AF, the ventricular rate was significantly slower with sotalol.

(2) In addition, sotalol was better tolerated than quinidine, with 28% versus 50% of patients reporting side effects, respectively. In particular, gastrointestinal, skin, and allergic side effects were more common with quinidine. The rate of discontinuation because of side effects was similar in the two groups. One patient in each group experienced a nonfatal ventricular arrhythmia with circulatory collapse.

4. Summary of Maintenance Therapy After Cardioversion—After cardioversion, quinidine can maintain sinus rhythm in about 50% of patients for 1 year. Class Ic and III agents are also effective for this purpose. Class Ia agents may be associated with an increase in the ventricular response because they can decrease the refractoriness of the AV node. Therefore, these drugs should be used in combination with digoxin, calcium channel blockers, or β-blockers to prevent excessive tachycardia. Recent studies have noted an association between use of class Ia or Ic agents and an increase in the risk of sudden cardiac death in susceptible patients. Because of its lower risk of cardiac toxicity, amiodarone has been favored by some authors. In addition, at doses used for treat-

Table 1-18 Soltalol vs. quinidine for maintenance of sinus rhythm (85)

	Sotalol (n=98)	Quinidine (n=85)	*P*
Sinus rhythm at 6 mo	49%	42%	NS
Recurrence of AF	34%	22%	NS
Side effects	28%	50%	<0.01

ment of AF (<300 mg/day), some of its the well-known noncardiac side effects of this drug appear to be less common.

E. Prevention of Thromboembolism—One of the well-known complications of AF is the risk of thromboembolism. To decrease this risk, prophylactic anticoagulation is recommended for most patients with AF. However, anticoagulation should be considered only if the patient's risk of thromboembolism without anticoagulation is greater than the risk of major hemorrhage with anticoagulation. For the purpose of discussion, it is useful to group patients according to their risk of thromboembolism: namely, those with valvular AF, nonvalvular AF, or lone AF.

1. **Valvular AF**—Despite the lack of randomized controlled trials, long-term anticoagulation has become standard therapy in patients with AF and valvular heart disease because of the relatively high risk of thromboembolism (3,128). In a retrospective study, Szekely analyzed the risk of thromboembolism in 754 patients with rheumatic valvular heart disease (151). Overall, 22.3% of the 219 patients in AF had a thromboembolic complication, compared with 3.8% of the 663 patients in sinus rhythm. This translates into an adjusted risk of thromboembolism of 5.2% per patient-year for patients in AF with rheumatic valvular heart disease. In patients with a thromboembolic complication, the risk of recurrence with anticoagulation was 3.4% per patient-year, compared with 9.6% without anticoagulation. Similarly, in patients with AF and no prior history of thromboembolism, two embolic episodes occurred among 30 anticoagulated patients, compared with 34 episodes among 98 non-anticoagulated patients.
2. **Lone AF**—Lone AF usually refers to AF that occurs in patients without clinical heart disease. The risk of thromboembolism in this population appears to be low but it differs depending on the precise definition of lone AF. For example, in the Framingham Heart Study, the age-adjusted risk of stroke was 28.2% among 43 patients with lone AF, compared with 6.8% among age- and sex-matched control patients without AF (26). On the other hand, in a report from the Mayo Clinic, the risk of stroke was only 0.35 events per 100 patient-years among 97 patients with lone AF (95). In the latter study, the definition of lone AF was very strict, excluding all patients with coronary artery disease, hyperthyroidism, valvular heart disease including mitral valve prolapse, CHF, cardiomyopathy, chronic obstructive pulmonary disease, cardiomegaly on chest film, hypertension, diabetes mellitus, or age >60 years. Altogether, >97% of patients with AF were excluded. On the other hand, the Framingham Heart Study excluded only those with coronary artery disease, CHF, rheumatic heart disease, and hypertensive cardiovascular disease. There was no age limit in the Framingham study, and consequently the average age was 70 years. If lone AF is defined as outlined by the Mayo study, prophylactic anticoagulation does not appear to be necessary because the risk of thromboembolism is very low. However, only 2.7% of patients with AF fulfilled this strict definition of lone AF.
3. **Nonvalvular AF**—In modern series, most patients with AF fall into the category of nonvalvular AF. Until recently the value of prophylactic therapy to decrease the risk of stroke in this population was controversial. However, several prospective randomized control trials have clarified this issue (25,38,56,57, 124,145,148).
   - a. **Coumadin**—Six of these studies compared Coumadin versus placebo or Coumadin versus no treatment (25,38,56,57,124,145). One study was a secondary prevention trial (56) and one included patients for both primary and secondary prevention (57); the rest were studies of primary prevention (25,38,124,145). These studies differed somewhat in design, size, exclusion criteria, blinding of treatment assignment, length of follow-up, definition of major bleeding, and specific end points of the study. They also differed in intensity of anticoagulation. The major features of these studies are summarized in Table 1-19.
     - **(1)** Five of the six studies found that warfarin significantly decreased the risk of stroke compared with placebo or no therapy. The average risk reduction ranged from 58% to 86% (25,56,57,124,145). This benefit appeared to extend to both sexes and to patients older than 75 years of

Table 1-19 Prevention of stroke in nonvalvular AF: summary of major trials

Study (Reference)	Year	N	Design	Anticoagulation Target	Reduction in Risk of Stroke With Warfarin
AFASAK (124)	1989	1007	Warfarin vs. placebo vs. aspirin for primary prevention	INR 2.8–4.2	58% (*P* <0.03)
BAATAF (25)	1990	420	Warfarin vs. control for primary prevention	PT ratio 1.2–1.5	86% (*P* <0.002)
SPAF I (145)	1991	1330	Warfarin vs. placebo vs. aspirin for primary prevention	PT ratio 1.3–1.8	67% (*P* <0.01)
CAFA (38)	1991	378	Warfarin vs. placebo for primary prevention	INR 2.0–3.0	37% (NS)
SPINAF (57)	1992	571	Warfarin vs. placebo for primary (n=525) and secondary prevention (n=46)	PT ratio 1.2–1.5	79% (*P* <0.001)
EAFT (56)	1993	1007	Warfarin vs. placebo vs. aspirin in patients eligible for warfarin (n=669) and aspirin vs. placebo in patients not eligible for warfarin (n=338) for secondary prevention	INR 2.5–4.0	69% (*P*=0.04)

age. The sixth study also favored warfarin but the benefit of 37% risk reduction was not statistically significant (38). The risk of hemorrhage leading to death, hospitalization, or transfusion was not significantly different in the Coumadin and control groups (25,57,145). However, the risk of less severe bleeding was substantially higher with warfarin (25,57,124).

(2) A representative study using low-intensity anticoagulation is described for illustration (57). In a double-blind, prospective, randomized controlled trial involving 525 men with chronic nonvalvular AF, Ezekowitz compared warfarin (titrated to maintain a prothrombin time ratio of 1.2 to 1.5) versus placebo. The average follow-up was about 1.75 years. Patients with paroxysmal AF, unstable angina, previous stroke, or recent transient ischemic attack (TIA) were excluded. Those with contraindications to warfarin and those with definite indications for aspirin or warfarin were also excluded. The target prothrombin time ratio was maintained 56% of the time. An intention-to-treat analysis was used (see Table 1-20).

(a) The risk of clinically evident stroke was significantly reduced by anticoagulation. With warfarin, the risk of stroke was 0.9% per year, compared with 4.3% with placebo. The average risk reduction was 79%. Similar benefit was observed for patients older than 70 years of age.

(b) The risk of other vascular events such as MI, TIA, and systemic embolism was also lower with warfarin, but the difference was

Table 1-20 Prevention of stroke in nonvalvular AF: VA cooperative study (57)

	Warfarin (n=260)	Placebo (n=265)	*P*
Risk of stroke per year	0.9%	4.3%	0.001
Risk of other vascular events	2.0%	3.6%	NS
Mortality per year	3.3%	5.0%	NS
Risk of major hemorrhage	1.3%	0.9%	NS
Risk of minor hemorrhage	14.0%	10.5%	0.04

not statistically significant. There was no significant difference in mortality.

(c) The risk of major bleeding leading to an intensive care unit admission, transfusion, surgery, or an intensive medical procedure was similar in the warfarin and placebo groups. The risk of less severe bleeding was greater with warfarin.

b. Aspirin—Four randomized studies have evaluated the role of aspirin in prevention of stroke in AF (56,124,145,148). One was a secondary prevention trial (56), and the others were studies of primary prevention. In the secondary prevention study, 300 mg of aspirin per day was not better than placebo (56). However, warfarin decreased the risk of recurrent stroke by 62% compared with aspirin (4,11). In another study, 75 mg of aspirin per day was also no different than placebo (124); warfarin decreased the risk of stroke by 51% compared with aspirin, but the difference was not statistically significant (4,11). In the Stroke Prevention in Atrial Fibrillation study (SPAF I), 325 mg of aspirin per day reduced the risk of stroke or systemic embolism by 42% compared with placebo (145). Aspirin could not meaningfully be compared with warfarin because there were too few thromboembolic events (11). The second SPAF study (SPAF II) consisted of two parallel trials. One compared aspirin (325 mg/day) versus warfarin (INR 2.0 to 4.5) in 715 patients with AF who were younger than 75 years of age. A similar comparison was made in 385 patients with AF who were >75 years old. All 416 patients from the SPAF I study who had been randomly assigned to receive either warfarin or aspirin were continued on their original assignment, and 265 patients who had been assigned to placebo were randomly reassigned to receive either warfarin or aspirin. In addition, 419 new patients were entered into the trial (148). There was a statistically nonsignificant 32% reduction in the risk of stroke among anticoagulated patients, compared with patients receiving aspirin (4,11). Recently, the investigators of these original studies performed a collaborative analysis of all patients from these trials. When the data from the individual trials were combined into one database, there was a 49% reduction in the risk of stroke with warfarin compared with aspirin (4,11).

c. Predicting the Risk of Stroke for an Individual Patient—The risk of stroke in patients with AF is not uniform. As previously discussed, patients with valvular AF have higher risk of stroke than those with nonvalvular AF. Even among those with nonvalvular AF, there are clinical risk factors that serve as predictors of stroke. These predictors include increasing age (25), previous MI (124), angina (25), prior history of diabetes mellitus (146), thromboembolism (146), hypertension (146), and recent CHF (146). In addition, mitral annular calcification, left ventricular dysfunction, and an enlarged left atrium on echocardiography have also been associated with an increased risk of stroke in patients with AF. (25,147) However, there is little agreement as to which variables are the best predictors of stroke. In a collaborative analysis of the pooled data from five randomized trials (25, 38,57,124,145), the best independent predictors of stroke were increasing age, previous stroke or TIA, hypertension, and diabetes mellitus (11). History of MI, CHF, or angina was also important but none of these factors was independently predictive in multivariate analysis. The incidence of stroke for various combinations of risk factors is summarized in the following sections.

(1) For patients <65 years old with one or more independent predictors of stroke (previous stroke or TIA, hypertension, or diabetes mellitus), the annual incidence of stroke was 4.9%. The annual incidence was 5.7% for similar patients between 65 and 75 years of age and 8.1% for those ≥75 years old. Warfarin reduced the risk of stroke in all of these subgroups.

(2) For patients younger than 65 years of age without any of these independent predictors, the annual incidence of stroke was only 1.0%. The annual incidence was 4.3% for similar patients between 65 and 75 and 3.5% for those ≥75 years old. Warfarin reduced the risk of stroke in the two older subgroups but not in patients <65 years of age.

(3) Patients with lone AF had very low rates of stroke. The annual incidence was 0% among untreated patients <60 years old who were without hypertension, diabetes mellitus, previous stroke, TIA, CHF, angina, or MI. The annual incidence was 1.6%, 2.1%, and 3.0% for patients with lone AF aged 60 to 69, 70 to 79, and 80 or more years, respectively.

(4) Based on these results, anticoagulation is recommended for most patients with nonvalvular AF. However, warfarin does not appear to be necessary for patients with lone AF who are without any clinical risk factors (*i.e.*, previous stroke or TIA, hypertension, or diabetes mellitus). Aspirin may be preferred to warfarin for these low-risk patients.

F. Catheter and Surgical Techniques

1. **Radiofrequency Catheter Ablation**—For patients with AF who remain refractory to medical therapy, radiofrequency catheter ablation of the AV node with pacemaker insertion may provide significant benefit (27,77,90,101, 133,162). For example, in Brignole's randomized study involving 23 patients with chronic, severely symptomatic, and drug-refractory AF or atrial flutter, radiofrequency ablation of the AV node plus rate-responsive VVI pacemaker insertion was significantly better than pacemaker insertion alone for improvement of exercise capacity, left ventricular function, and symptom score (27). More recently, radiofrequency modification rather than ablation of the AV node has been described (162). Because the modification technique slows but does not completely block AV conduction, effective rate control can be achieved without the need for a pacemaker. However, because the atrium remains in fibrillation with either technique, the need for anticoagulation persists and effective atrial contraction is still absent (107).
2. **Atrial Corridor Procedure**—The goal of this operation is to form a corridor that directly connects the sinoatrial (SA) and the AV nodes while electrically isolating the rest of the atria. This procedure preserves the physiologic pacing of the heart by the SA node. Furthermore, because the corridor involves a significant portion of the right atrium, right atrial contraction is preserved in most patients. However, the left atrium continues to fibrillate, so the need for anticoagulation persists and the contribution of the left atrium to left ventricular filling is still lost. Uncontrolled studies have concluded in favor of the corridor operation for patients with symptomatic, drug-refractory AF (48,100,156). The largest of these studies included a series of 36 patients with drug-refractory, symptomatic, paroxysmal AF. Patients with sick sinus syndrome or documented structural heart disease were excluded (156).

   a. After the initial operation, 27 of the 36 patients were free of AF in the corridor without antiarrhythmic therapy. A second surgical exploration allowed 4 more patients to be free of AF, for a total short-term success rate of 86%. After a mean follow-up of 41 months, 69% were free of arrhythmia without any antiarrhythmic therapy.

b. Effective right atrial contraction was observed in 26 of the 31 successfully treated patients. However, effective left atrial contraction was absent in all 31 patients. At the end of follow-up, 81% of the patients had normal chronotropic response to exercise. However, 5 patients required a pacemaker because of abnormal SA-node function after the operation.

c. Two patients had thromboembolic complications perioperatively; both were thought to have been inadequately anticoagulated.

3. **Maze Procedure**—Favorable results have also been reported with the maze operation (23,42,43,111,112). This procedure employs multiple small incisions in the atria to disrupt the potential macro-reentry pathways capable of producing fibrillatory waves. Unlike the corridor procedure or the catheter ablation technique, the maze procedure is designed to completely abolish AF. Therefore, both AV synchrony and the atrial transport function are preserved. In addition, it eliminates the need for chronic anticoagulation or pacemakers. In the largest series reported to date, Cox described the results of the maze operation in 75 patients with symptomatic, drug-refractory AF or atrial flutter (43). Chronic AF, paroxysmal AF, and paroxysmal atrial flutter accounted for 48%, 45%, and 7% of patients, respectively. Sixty-five of the 75 patients were observed for >3 months.

a. As with any other cardiac operation, postoperative AF was common. Within the first 3 months, 47% of patients developed postoperative AF. Fluid retention was also a common problem, but prophylactic diuretic therapy decreased this risk to 6%. One perioperative death and three perioperative neurologic events were reported.

b. Among the 65 patients who were observed for >3 months, 89% were free of arrhythmia without drug therapy. Another 9% remained free of arrhythmia with one antiarrhythmic drug. AV synchrony and effective atrial contraction were preserved in 98% of these patients.

G. Wolff-Parkinson-White Syndrome

1. Management of rapid ventricular response in patients with AF and Wolff-Parkinson-White (WPW) syndrome is complicated by the fact that AF may sometimes degenerate into ventricular fibrillation (93). This risk appears to be increased by the administration of digoxin or verapamil (66,69,70,84,93,114, 115,161). Because they block the AV node and possibly decrease the refractoriness of the bypass tract, these drugs can promote anterograde conduction over the accessory pathway. Enhanced conduction over the bypass tract may paradoxically increase the ventricular rate and precipitate cardiac arrest. Despite this danger, the correct diagnosis is often missed and inappropriate drugs are commonly given. In one study involving 18 patients with rapid AF and WPW syndrome, 56% were inappropriately given verapamil. The correct diagnosis was made in only 17%, although diagnostic electrocardiograms were available for all patients. Sixty percent of patients given verapamil underwent a major clinical deterioration (66).

2. **Catheter Ablation of the Accessory Pathway**—Radiofrequency catheter ablation of the bypass tract is a safe and highly effective treatment for patients with WPW syndrome, including those with AF (32,71,83). In one study involving 166 patients with symptomatic WPW syndrome, successful ablation of the bypass tract was possible in 99% of patients. During an average follow-up of 8 months, 91% of patients remained free of preexcitation or AV nodal reentry tachycardia. The complication rate was only 1.8%; complications included pericarditis, cardiac tamponade, and AV block (83).

3. Various class Ia, Ic, and III antiarrhythmic drugs are also useful for treatment of patients with AF and WPW syndrome (14,16,20,35,37,44,62,64,87,121,132,137). Unlike verapamil or digoxin, these agents maintain patients in sinus rhythm and slow conduction over the accessory pathway. However, most of the data that support the use of these drugs have come from small, uncontrolled studies. Therefore, given the effectiveness and safety record of the radiofrequency catheter ablation technique, these drugs should be reserved for patients who are not candidates for that procedure.

I. Conclusions

1. AF is a common disorder affecting about 2% of unselected adults in the general population. In the Framingham Heart Study, the independent risk factors for development of AF were increasing age, diabetes mellitus, hypertension, valvular heart disease, and CHF. MI was also an independent risk factor, but only for men. Numerous other conditions, including fever, surgery, thyrotoxicosis, alcoholism, pneumonia, pulmonary embolism, and pericarditis, have also been associated with the development of AF. Exceedingly rapid, irregular ventricular response associated with AF may cause palpitations, hemodynamic deterioration, CHF, syncope, or chest pain. The loss of AV synchrony and the lack of atrial contribution to ventricular filling may cause decreased exercise tolerance, CHF, or dyspnea. Formation of intracardiac thrombus increases the risk of systemic embolization.
2. Digoxin is a time-honored therapy for ventricular rate control in patients with chronic AF. Although it is effective for patients at rest, it is generally ineffective during exercise and for paroxysmal AF. IV digoxin slows the ventricular rate in acute AF but only after a mean delay of 5.5 hours. Calcium channel blockers and β-blockers are more effective than digoxin. Unlike digoxin, they decrease the ventricular rate at rest as well as during exercise. Intravenously administered calcium channel blockers and β-blockers work more quickly than digoxin for acute ventricular rate reduction. Although calcium channel blockers and β-blockers are effective, their negative chronotropic and inotropic activity may cause fatigue, heart failure, hypotension, or bradycardia. In addition, β-blockers may induce bronchospasm. Some patients may require insertion of a pacemaker to allow therapy with these drugs. Digoxin or verapamil should be avoided in patients with preexcitation syndrome and AF. Finally, both digoxin and calcium channel blockers have been implicated in prolonging the duration of attack in patients with paroxysmal AF.
3. Restoration of sinus rhythm can be achieved in 80% to 90% of patients with DC cardioversion. However, most of these patients revert to AF unless prophylactic antiarrhythmic therapy is given. Chemical cardioversion can be achieved with class Ia agents (quinidine, disopyramide, or procainamide) with an efficacy rate of 40% to 60%. Patients who have been in AF for longer than 1 year and those with enlarged left atria are less likely to respond to electrical or chemical cardioversion. Class Ic agents (flecainide, encainide, or propafenone) and class III agents (amiodarone, sotalol) are comparable to class Ia agents in efficacy. Digoxin, calcium channel blockers, and β-blockers are no more effective than placebo for conversion of AF to sinus rhythm.
4. Before elective cardioversion, it is now common practice to anticoagulate patients who have been in AF for >2 days in order to decrease the risk of systemic embolism. Generally, anticoagulation therapy is recommended for 2 to 4 weeks before cardioversion and is continued for 4 weeks thereafter. Alternatively, transesophageal echocardiography may be helpful in excluding the presence of atrial thrombi before cardioversion. However, in one study, the rate of embolic complications was still 2.4% despite negative findings on transesophageal echocardiography before cardioversion.
5. After cardioversion, quinidine can maintain sinus rhythm in about 50% of patients for 1 year. Class Ic and class III agents are also effective for this purpose. Class Ia agents may be associated with an increase in the ventricular response because they can decrease the refractoriness of the AV node; these drugs should be used in combination with digoxin, calcium channel blockers, or β-blockers to prevent excessive tachycardia. Recent studies have noted an association between use of class Ia or Ic agents and an increase in the risk of sudden cardiac death in susceptible patients. Amiodarone has a lower risk of cardiac toxicity but noncardiac side effects are common and limit the utility of this drug.
6. The risk of stroke for patients with AF is not uniform. Patients with valvular AF have a higher risk of stroke than those with nonvalvular AF. Among those with nonvalvular AF, the best independent predictors of stroke are increasing age,

previous stroke or TIA, hypertension, and diabetes mellitus. History of MI, CHF, or angina is also important, but in multivariate analysis these factors were not independent predictors for stroke. Recent randomized trials have shown that chronic anticoagulation can decrease the risk of stroke in patients with AF. However, this treatment does not appear to be necessary for patients younger than 65 years of age who do not have a history of diabetes mellitus, hypertension, or previous stroke or TIA. Similarly, patients with lone AF who are <70 years old also may not need anticoagulation. Aspirin may be preferred to warfarin for these low-risk patients. However, the utility of aspirin for prevention of stroke in patients with AF is still controversial. In a pooled analysis of data from major randomized trials, aspirin was more effective than placebo but 50% less effective than warfarin.

7. Nonmedical options for treatment of AF include radiofrequency ablation of the AV node, the atrial corridor procedure, and the maze operation. For patients who remain refractory to drug therapy, radiofrequency catheter ablation of the AV node with pacemaker insertion may improve symptoms and control the ventricular rate. However, because the atrium continues in fibrillation, anticoagulation is still necessary and the atrial contribution to ventricular filling is still absent. The atrial corridor procedure creates a direct connection between the SA and AV nodes while electrically isolating the rest of the atria from this corridor. After a mean follow-up of 41 months in one study, 69% of patients remained free of arrhythmia in the corridor without any antiarrhythmic therapy. However, because the left atrium continues to fibrillate, anticoagulation is still necessary and the atrial contribution to ventricular filling is still absent. The maze procedure uses multiple small incisions in the atria to disrupt the potential macro-reentry pathways capable of producing fibrillatory waves. It is the only procedure that restores sinus rhythm. Anticoagulation is unnecessary, and atrial contribution to ventricular filling is restored. In one study, the maze procedure was effective in 89% of patients who were observed for >3 months.
8. Radiofrequency catheter ablation of the bypass tract can be used for effective treatment of patients with symptomatic WPW, including those with AF. Digoxin or verapamil should be avoided in patients with both preexcitation and AF, because these drugs can increase anterograde conduction over the accessory pathway and precipitate cardiac arrest. Class Ia, Ic or III drugs may be useful in this setting because they help maintain patients in sinus rhythm and slow conduction over the bypass tract. However, given the favorable efficacy and safety record of the radiofrequency catheter ablation technique, these drugs should be reserved for patients who are not candidates for the ablation procedure.

Abbreviations used in Chapter 1

AF = atrial fibrillation
AV = atrioventricular
BID = twice daily
bpm = beats per minute
CHF = congestive heart failure
DC = direct current
INR = international normalized ratio
IV = intravenous
MI = myocardial infarction
n = number of patients in sample
NS = not significant
P = probability value
PO = by mouth, orally
q = every
QID = four times daily

SA = sinoatrial
TIA = transient ischemic attack
TID = three times daily
WPW syndrome = Wolff-Parkinson-White syndrome

References

1. Aberg. Atrial fibrillation: a review or 463 cases from Philadelphia General Hospital from 1955 to 1965. *Acta Medica Scandinavica* 1968;184:425.
2. Aberg. Direct current conversion of atrial fibrillation: long-term results. *Acta Medica Scandinavica* 1968;184:433.
3. Albers. Stroke prevention in nonvalvular atrial fibrillation. *Ann Intern Med* 1991;115:727.
4. Albers. Atrial fibrillation and stroke: three new studies, three remaining questions. *Arch Intern Med* 1994;154:1443.
5. Alboni. Hemodynamic effects of oral sotalol during both sinus rhythm and atrial fibrillation. *J Am Coll Cardiol* 1993;22:1373.
6. Anderson. Prevention of symptomatic recurrences of paroxysmal atrial fibrillation in patients initially tolerating antiarrhythmic therapy: a multicenter, double-blind, crossover study of flecainide and placebo with transtelephonic monitoring. Flecainide Supraventricular Tachycardia Study Group. *Circulation* 1989;80:1557.
7. Anderson. Comparison of the efficacy and safety of esmolol, a short acting beta blocker, with placebo in the treatment of supraventricular tachyarrhythmias. *Am Heart J* 1986;111:42.
8. Ang. Placebo controlled trial of xamoterol versus digoxin in chronic atrial fibrillation. *Br Heart J* 1990;64:256.
9. Antman. Therapy of refractory symptomatic atrial fibrillation and atrial flutter: a staged care approach with new antiarrhythmic drugs. *J Am Coll Cardiol* 1990;15:698. See comments.
10. Arnold. Role of prophylactic anticoagulation for direct current cardioversion in patients with atrial fibrillation or atrial flutter. *J Am Coll Cardiol* 1992;19:851. See comments.
11. Atrial Fibrillation Investigators. Risk factors for stroke and efficacy of antithrombotic therapy in atrial fibrillation: Analysis of pooled data from five randomized controlled trials. Atrial Fibrillation Investigators: Atrial Fibrillation, Aspirin, Anticoagulation Study; Boston Area Anticoagulation Trial for Atrial Fibrillation Study; Canadian Atrial Fibrillation Anticoagulation Study; Stroke Prevention in Atrial Fibrillation Study; Veterans Affairs Stroke Prevention in Nonrheumatic Atrial Fibrillation Study. *Arch Intern Med* 1994;154:1449.
12. Atwood. Diltiazem and exercise performance in patients with chronic atrial fibrillation. *Chest* 1988;93:20.
13. Atwood. Effect of beta-adrenergic blockade on exercise performance in patients with chronic atrial fibrillation. *J Am Coll Cardiol* 1987;10:314.
14. Auricchio. Reversible protective effect of propafenone or flecainide during atrial fibrillation in patients with an accessory atrioventricular connection. *Am Heart J* 1992;124:932.
15. Benjamin. Independent risk factors for atrial fibrillation in a population based cohort: the Framingham Heart Study. *JAMA* 1994;271:840.
16. Bennett. Disopyramide in patients with the Wolff-Parkinson-White syndrome and atrial fibrillation. *Chest* 1978;74:624.
17. Bjerkelund. The efficacy of anticoagulant therapy in preventing embolism related to D.C. electrical conversion of atrial fibrillation. *Am J Cardiol* 1969;23:208.
18. Black. Exclusion of atrial thrombus by transesophageal echocardiography does not preclude embolism after cardioversion of atrial fibrillation: a multicenter study. *Circulation* 1994;89:2509.
19. Blevins. Amiodarone in the management of refractory atrial fibrillation. *Arch Intern Med* 1987;147:1401.

20. Boahene. Termination of acute atrial fibrillation in the Wolff-Parkinson-White syndrome by procainamide and propafenone: importance of atrial fibrillatory cycle length. *J Am Coll Cardiol* 1990;16:1408. See comments.
21. Bohm. Different cardiodepressant potency of various calcium channel antagonists in human myocardium. *Am J Cardiol* 1990;65:1039.
22. Boissel. Controlled trial of a long-acting quinidine for maintenance of sinus rhythm after conversion of sustained atrial fibrillation. *Eur Heart J* 1981;2:49.
23. Bonchek. Cox/maze procedure for atrial septal defect with atrial fibrillation: management strategies. *Ann Thorac Surg* 1993;55:607. See comments.
24. Borgeat. Flecainide versus quinidine for conversion of atrial fibrillation to sinus rhythm. *Am J Cardiol* 1986;58:496.
25. Boston Area Anticoagulation Trial for Atrial Fibrillation Investigators. The effect of low-dose warfarin on the risk of stroke in patients with nonrheumatic atrial fibrillation. *N Engl J Med* 1990;323:1505.
26. Brand. Characteristics and prognosis of lone atrial fibrillation: 30 year follow-up in the Framingham study. *JAMA* 1985;254:3449.
27. Brignole. Influence of atrioventricular junction radiofrequency ablation in patients with chronic atrial fibrillation and flutter on quality of life and cardiac performance. *Am J Cardiol* 1994;74:242.
28. Brodsky. Amiodarone for maintenance of sinus rhythm after conversion of atrial fibrillation in the setting of a dilated left atrium. *Am J Cardiol* 1987;60:572.
29. Brown. Effect of propranolol on exercise tolerance in patients with atrial fibrillation. *Br Med J* 1969;2:279.
30. Burkart. Effect of antiarrhythmic therapy on mortality in survivors of myocardial infarction with asymptomatic complex ventricular arrhythmias: Basel Antiarrhythmic Study of Infarct Survival (BASIS). *J Am Coll Cardiol* 1990;16:1711.
31. Byrne-Quinn. Maintenance of sinus rhythm after DC reversion of atrial fibrillation. *Br Heart J* 1970;32:370.
32. Calkins. Diagnosis and cure of the Wolf-Parkinson-White syndrome or paroxysmal supraventricular tachycardias during a single electrophysiologic test. *N Engl J Med* 1991;324:1612.
33. Campbell. Intravenous sotalol for the treatment of atrial fibrillation and flutter after cardiopulmonary bypass: comparison with disopyramide and digoxin in a randomised trial. *Br Heart J* 1985;54:86.
34. Capucci. Conversion of recent-onset atrial fibrillation by a single oral loading dose of propafenone or flecainide. *Am J Cardiol* 1994;74:503.
35. Chamberlain. Atrial fibrillation complicating Wolff-Parkinson-White syndrome treated with amiodarone. *Br Med J* 1977;2:1519.
36. Chamberlain. Plasma digoxin concentrations in patients with atrial fibrillation. *Br Med J* 1970;3:429.
37. Chimienti. Electrophysiologic and clinical effects of intravenous and oral encainide in patients with Wolf-Parkinson-White syndrome and paroxysmal atrial fibrillation. *Eur Heart J* 1987;8:282.
38. Connolly. Canadian atrial fibrillation anticoagulation study. *J Am Coll Cardiol* 1991;18:349.
39. Connolly. Usefulness of propafenone for recurrent paroxysmal atrial fibrillation. *Am J Cardiol* 1989;63:817.
40. Coplen. Efficacy and safety of quinidine therapy for maintenance of sinus rhythm after cardioversion: a meta-analysis of randomized controlled trials. *Circulation* 1990;82:1106.
41. Coplen. Erratum. *Circulation* 1990;83:714.
42. Cox. Successful surgical treatment of atrial fibrillation. Review and clinical update. *JAMA* 1991;266:1976. Review. See comments.
43. Cox. Five-year experience with the maze procedure for atrial fibrillation. *Ann Thorac Surg* 1993;56:814.
44. Crijns. Successful use of flecainide in atrial fibrillation with rapid ventricular rate in the Wolff-Parkinson-White syndrome. *Am Heart J* 1988;115:1317.
45. Crijns. Serial antiarrhythmic drug treatment to maintain sinus rhythm after elec-

trical cardioversion for chronic atrial fibrillation or atrial flutter. *Am J Cardiol* 1991;68:335.
46. Dalzell. Factors determining success and energy requirements for cardioversion of atrial fibrillation. *Q J Med* 1990;76:903.
47. David. Inefficacy of digitalis in the control of heart rate in patients with chronic atrial fibrillation: beneficial effect of an added beta adrenergic blocking agent. *Am J Cardiol* 1979;44:1378.
48. Defauw. Surgical therapy of paroxysmal atrial fibrillation with the "corridor" operation. *Ann Thorac Surg* 1992;53:564.
49. DiBianco. Effects of nadolol on the spontaneous and exercise-provoked heart rate of patients with chronic atrial fibrillation receiving stable dosages of digoxin. *Am Heart J* 1984;108:1121.
50. Disch. Managing chronic atrial fibrillation: a Markov decision analysis comparing warfarin, quinidine, and low-dose amiodarone. *Ann Intern Med* 1994;120:449. See comments.
51. Dittrich. Echocardiographic and clinical predictors for outcome of elective cardioversion of atrial fibrillation. *Am J Cardiol* 1989;63:193.
52. Donovan. Efficacy of flecainide for the reversion of acute onset atrial fibrillation. *Am J Cardiol* 1992;70:50A.
53. Dusman. Clinical features of amiodarone-induced pulmonary toxicity. *Circulation* 1990;82:51.
54. Echt. Mortality and morbidity in patients receiving encainide, flecainide, or placebo. *N Engl J Med* 1991;324:781.
55. Ellenbogen. A placebo-controlled trial of continuous intravenous diltiazem infusion for 24-hour heart rate control during atrial fibrillation and atrial flutter: a multicenter study. *J Am Coll Cardiol* 1991;18:891.
56. European Atrial Fibrillation Trial Study Group. Secondary prevention in non-rheumatic atrial fibrillation after transient ischaemic attack or minor stroke. *Lancet* 1993;342:1255.
57. Ezekowitz. VA cooperative study of warfarin in the prevention of stroke associated with nonrheumatic atrial fibrillation. *N Engl J Med* 1992;327:1406.
58. Falk. Flecainide-induced ventricular tachycardia and fibrillation in patients treated for atrial fibrillation. *Ann Intern Med* 1989;111:107.
59. Falk. Proarrhythmia in patients treated for atrial fibrillation or flutter. *Ann Intern Med* 1992;117:141.
60. Falk. Digoxin for converting recent-onset atrial fibrillation to sinus rhythm: a randomized, double-blinded trial. *Ann Intern Med* 1987;106:503.
61. Falk. Digoxin for atrial fibrillation: a drug whose time has gone? *Ann Intern Med* 1991;114:573.
62. Feld. Clinical and electrophysiologic effects of amiodarone in patients with atrial fibrillation complicating the Wolff-Parkinson-White syndrome. *Am Heart J* 1988;115:102.
63. Fenster. Conversion of atrial fibrillation to sinus rhythm by acute intravenous procainamide infusion. *Am Heart J* 1983;106:501.
64. Fujimura. Acute effect of disopyramide on atrial fibrillation in the Wolff-Parkinson-White syndrome. *J Am Coll Cardiol* 1989;13:1133.
65. Galun. Failure of long-term digitalization to prevent rapid ventricular response in patients with paroxysmal atrial fibrillation. *Chest* 1991;99:1038.
66. Garratt. Misuse of verapamil in pre-excited atrial fibrillation. *Lancet* 1989;1:367.
67. Gold. Amiodarone for refractory atrial fibrillation. *Am J Cardiol* 1986;57:124.
68. Graboys. Efficacy of amiodarone for refractory supraventricular tachyarrhythmias. *Am Heart J* 1983;106:870.
69. Gulamhusein. Acceleration of the ventricular response during atrial fibrillation in the Wolff-Parkinson-White syndrome after verapamil. *Circulation* 1982;65:348.
70. Gulamhusein. Ventricular fibrillation following verapamil in the Wolf-Parkinson-White syndrome. *Am Heart J* 1983;106:145.
71. Haissaguerre. Frequency of recurrent atrial fibrillation after catheter ablation of overt accessory pathways. *Am J Cardiol* 1992;69:493.

72. Halpern. Efficacy of intravenous procainamide infusion in converting atrial fibrillation to sinus rhythm: relation to left atrial size. *Br Heart J* 1980;44:589.
73. Hamer. Beneficial effects of low dose amiodarone in patients with congestive heart failure: a placebo-controlled trial. *J Am Coll Cardiol* 1989;14:1768.
74. Harris. Side effects of long-term amiodarone therapy. *Circulation* 1983;67:45.
75. Hartel. Disopyramide in the prevention of recurrence of atrial fibrillation after electroconversion. *Clin Pharmacol Ther* 1974;15:551.
76. Hartel. Value of quinidine in maintenance of sinus rhythm after electric conversion of atrial fibrillation. *Br Heart J* 1970;32:57.
77. Heinz. Improvement in left ventricular systolic function after successful radiofrequency His bundle ablation for drug refractory, chronic atrial fibrillation and recurrent atrial flutter. *Am J Cardiol* 1992;69:489.
78. Henry. Relation between echocardiographically determined left atrial size and atrial fibrillation. *Circulation* 1976;53:273.
79. Heywood. Effects of intravenous diltiazem on rapid atrial fibrillation accompanied by congestive heart failure. *Am J Cardiol* 1991;67:1150.
80. Hillestad. Quinidine in maintenance of sinus rhythm after electroconversion of chronic atrial fibrillation: a controlled clinical study. *Br Heart J* 1971;33:518.
81. Horowitz. Use of amiodarone in the treatment of persistent and paroxysmal atrial fibrillation resistant to quinidine therapy. *J Am Coll Cardiol* 1985;6:1402.
82. Hwang. Double-blind crossover randomized trial of intravenously administered verapamil: its use for atrial fibrillation and flutter following open heart surgery. *Arch Intern Med* 1984;144:491.
83. Jackman. Catheter ablation of accessory atrioventricular pathways (Wolf-Parkinson-White syndrome) by radiofrequency current. *N Engl J Med* 1991;324:1605.
84. Jacob. Fatal ventricular fibrillation following verapamil in Wolf-Parkinson-White syndrome with atrial fibrillation. *Ann Emerg Med* 1985;14:159.
85. Juul-Moller. Sotalol versus quinidine for the maintenance of sinus rhythm after direct current conversion of atrial fibrillation. *Circulation* 1990;82:1932. See comments.
86. Kannel. Epidemiologic features of chronic atrial fibrillation: the Framingham Study. *N Engl J Med* 1982;306:1018.
87. Kappenberger. Evaluation of flecainide acetate in rapid atrial fibrillation complicating Wolf-Parkinson-White syndrome. *Clin Cardiol* 1985;8:321.
88. Karlson. Disopyramide in the maintenance of sinus rhythm after electroconversion of atrial fibrillation: a placebo-controlled one-year follow-up study. *Eur Heart J* 1988;9:284.
89. Kastor. The electrical conversion of atrial fibrillation. *Am J Med Sci* 1967;253:511.
90. Kay. Effect of catheter ablation of the atrioventricular junction on quality of life and exercise tolerance in paroxysmal atrial fibrillation. *Am J Cardiol* 1988;62:741.
91. Kerin. The effectiveness and safety of the simultaneous administration of quinidine and amiodarone in the conversion of chronic atrial fibrillation. *Am Heart J* 1993;125:1017.
92. Kingma. Acute pharmacologic conversion of atrial fibrillation and flutter: the role of flecainide, propafenone, and verapamil. *Am J Cardiol* 1992;70:56A.
93. Klein. Ventricular fibrillation in the Wolf-Parkinson-White syndrome. *N Engl J Med* 1979;301:1080.
94. Klein. The beneficial effects of verapamil in chronic atrial fibrillation. *Arch Intern Med* 1979;139:747.
95. Kopecky. The natural history of lone atrial fibrillation: a population-based study over three decades. *N Engl J Med* 1987;317:669.
96. Kowey. Safety and efficacy of amiodarone: the low dose perspective. *Chest* 1988;93:54.
97. Lang. Verapamil improves exercise capacity in chronic atrial fibrillation: double-blind crossover study. *Am Heart J* 1983;105:820.
98. Lang. Superiority of oral verapamil therapy to digoxin in treatment of chronic atrial fibrillation. *Chest* 1983;83:491.

99. Lau. A randomized double-blind crossover study comparing the efficacy and tolerability of flecainide and quinidine in the control of patients with symptomatic paroxysmal atrial fibrillation. *Am Heart J* 1992;124:645.
100. Leitch. Sinus node–atrioventricular node isolation: long-term results with the "corridor" operation for atrial fibrillation. *J Am Coll Cardiol* 1991;17:970. See comments.
101. Lemery. Reversibility of tachycardia-induced left ventricular dysfunction after closed-chest catheter ablation of the atrioventricular junction for intractable atrial fibrillation. *Am J Cardiol* 1987;60:1406.
102. Lloyd. The efficacy of quinidine and disopyramide in the maintenance of sinus rhythm after electroconversion from atrial fibrillation: a double blind study comparing quinidine, disopyramide and placebo. *S Afr Med J* 1984;65:367.
103. Lundstrom. Differential effects of xamoterol and verapamil on ventricular rate regulation in patients with chronic atrial fibrillation. *Am Heart J* 1992;124:917.
104. Lundstrom. Chronic atrial fibrillation: long-term results of direct current conversion. *Acta Medica Scandinavica* 1988;223:53.
105. Lundstrom. Ventricular rate control and exercise performance in chronic atrial fibrillation: effects of diltiazem and verapamil. *J Am Coll Cardiol* 1990;16:86.
106. Manning. Cardioversion from atrial fibrillation without prolonged anticoagulation with use of transesophageal echocardiography to exclude the presence of atrial thrombi. *N Engl J Med* 1993;328:750. See comments.
107. Manolis. Radiofrequency catheter ablation for cardiac tachyarrhythmias. *Ann Intern Med* 1994;121:452.
108. Maragno. Low- and medium-dose diltiazem in chronic atrial fibrillation: comparison with digoxin and correlation with drug plasma levels. *Am Heart J* 1988; 116:385.
109. Martin. Comparison of amiodarone and disopyramide in the control of paroxysmal atrial fibrillation and atrial flutter (interim report). *Br J Clin Pract Symp Suppl* 1986;44:52.
110. Mattioni. Amiodarone in patients with previous drug-mediated torsade de pointes: long-term safety and efficacy. *Ann Intern Med* 1989;111:574.
111. McCarthy. Initial experience with the maze procedure for atrial fibrillation. *J Thorac Cardiovasc Surg* 1993;105:1077.
112. McCarthy. Combined treatment of mitral regurgitation and atrial fibrillation with valvuloplasty and the maze procedure. *Am J Cardiol* 1993;71:483.
113. McEachern. Auricular fibrillation: its etiology, age incidence and production by digitalis therapy. *Am J Med Sci* 1932;183:35.
114. McGovern. Precipitation of cardiac arrest by verapamil in patients with Wolf-Parkinson-White syndrome. *Ann Intern Med* 1986;104:791.
115. Merrill. Magnesium reversal of digoxin-facilitated ventricular rate during atrial fibrillation in the Wolff-Parkinson-White syndrome. *Am J Med* 1994;97:25.
116. Middlekauff. Low-dose amiodarone for atrial fibrillation: time for a prospective study. *Ann Intern Med* 1992;116:1017.
117. Miller. Synchronized precordial electroshock for control of cardiac arrhythmias: initial results of cardiac arrhythmias. *JAMA* 1964;189:549.
118. Molajo. Effect of Corwin (ICI 118587) on resting and exercise heart rate and exercise tolerance in digitalised patients with chronic atrial fibrillation. *Br Heart J* 1984;52:392.
119. Morris. Electric conversion of atrial fibrillation: immediate and long-term results and selection of patients. *Ann Intern Med* 1966;65:216.
120. Naccarelli. Amiodarone: pharmacology and antiarrhythmic and adverse effects. *Pharmacotherapy* 1985;5:298.
121. Neuss. Effects of flecainide on electrophysiological properties of accessory pathways in the Wolf-Parkinson-White syndrome. *Eur Heart J* 1983;4:347.
122. Noc. Intravenous amiodarone versus verapamil for acute conversion of paroxysmal atrial fibrillation to sinus rhythm [see comments]. *Am J Cardiol* 1990;65:679.
123. Perelman. A comparison of bepridil with amiodarone in the treatment of established atrial fibrillation. *Br Heart J* 1987;58:339.

124. Petersen. Placebo-controlled, randomized trial of warfarin and aspirin for prevention of thromboembolic complications in chronic atrial fibrillation: The Copenhagen AFASAK study. *Lancet* 1989;1:175.
125. Pietersen. Usefulness of flecainide for prevention of paroxysmal atrial fibrillation and flutter: Danish-Norwegian Flecainide Multicenter Study Group. *Am J Cardiol* 1991;67:713.
126. Platia. Esmolol versus verapamil in the acute treatment of atrial fibrillation or atrial flutter. *Am J Cardiol* 1989;63:925.
127. Pritchett. Flecainide acetate treatment of paroxysmal supraventricular tachycardia and paroxysmal atrial fibrillation: dose-response studies. The Flecainide Supraventricular Tachycardia Study Group. *J Am Coll Cardiol* 1991;17:297.
128. Pritchett. Management of atrial fibrillation. *N Engl J Med* 1992;326:1264.
129. Pritchett. Propafenone treatment of symptomatic paroxysmal supraventricular arrhythmias: a randomized, placebo-controlled, crossover trial in patients tolerating oral therapy. *Ann Intern Med* 1991;114:539.
130. Rawles. Time of occurrence, duration, and ventricular rate of paroxysmal atrial fibrillation: the effect of digoxin [see comments]. *Br Heart J* 1990;63:225.
131. Reimold. Propafenone versus sotalol for suppression of recurrent symptomatic atrial fibrillation. *Am J Cardiol* 1993;71:558.
132. Rinkenberger. Encainide for atrial fibrillation associated with Wolff-Parkinson-White syndrome. *Am J Cardiol* 1988;62:26L.
133. Rodriguez. Improvement in left ventricular function by ablation of atrioventricular nodal conduction in selected patients with lone atrial fibrillation. *Am J Cardiol* 1993;72:1137.
134. Roth. Efficacy and safety of medium- and high-dose diltiazem alone and in combination with digoxin for control of heart rate at rest and during exercise in patients with chronic atrial fibrillation. *Circulation* 1986;73:316.
135. Salerno. Efficacy and safety of intravenous diltiazem for treatment of atrial fibrillation and atrial flutter: The Diltiazem-Atrial Fibrillation/Flutter Study Group. *Am J Cardiol* 1989;63:1046.
136. Sawyer. Atrial fibrillation: Its etiology, treatment and association with embolization. *South Med J* 1958;51:84.
137. Sellers. Effects of procainamide and quinidine sulfate in the Wolf-Parkinson-White syndrome. *Circulation* 1977;55:15.
138. Shenasa. Effect of intravenous and oral calcium antagonists (diltiazem and verapamil) on sustenance of atrial fibrillation. *Am J Cardiol* 1988;62:403.
139. Shettigar. Combined use of esmolol and digoxin in the acute treatment of atrial fibrillation or flutter. *Am Heart J* 1993;126:368.
140. Singh. Efficacy and safety of sotalol in digitalized patients with chronic atrial fibrillation: The Sotalol Study Group. *Am J Cardiol* 1991;68:1227.
141. Skoularigis. Effectiveness of amiodarone and electrical cardioversion for chronic rheumatic atrial fibrillation after mitral valve surgery. *Am J Cardiol* 1993;72:423.
142. Sodermark. Effect of quinidine on maintaining sinus rhythm after conversion of atrial fibrillation or flutter: a multicentre study from Stockholm. *Br Heart J* 1975;37:486.
143. Steinberg. Efficacy of oral diltiazem to control ventricular response in chronic atrial fibrillation at rest and during exercise. *J Am Coll Cardiol* 1987;9:405.
144. Stern. Clinical use of oral verapamil in chronic and paroxysmal atrial fibrillation. *Chest* 1982;81:308.
145. Stroke Prevention in Atrial Fibrillation Investigators. The stroke prevention in atrial fibrillation study: final results. *Circulation* 1991;84:527.
146. Stroke Prevention in Atrial Fibrillation Investigators. Predictors of thromboembolism in atrial fibrillation, I: clinical features of patients at risk. *Ann Intern Med* 1992;116:1.
147. Stroke Prevention in Atrial Fibrillation Investigators. Predictors of thromboembolism in atrial fibrillation, II: echocardiographic features of patients at risk. *Ann Intern Med* 1992;116:6.

148. Stroke Prevention in Atrial Fibrillation Investigators. Warfarin versus aspirin for prevention of thromboembolism in atrial fibrillation: Stroke Prevention in Atrial Fibrillation II study. *Lancet* 1994;343:687.
149. Suttorp. The value of class IC antiarrhythmic drugs for acute conversion of paroxysmal atrial fibrillation or flutter to sinus rhythm. *J Am Coll Cardiol* 1990;16:1722.
150. Suttorp. Intravenous flecainide versus verapamil for acute conversion of paroxysmal atrial fibrillation or flutter to sinus rhythm. *Am J Cardiol* 1989;63:693.
151. Szekely. Systemic embolism and anticoagulant prophylaxis in rheumatic heart disease. *Br Med J* 1964;1:1209.
152. Szekely. Maintenance of sinus rhythm after atrial defibrillation. *Br Heart J* 1970;32:741.
153. Tommaso. Atrial fibrillation and flutter: immediate control and conversion with intravenously administered verapamil. *Arch Intern Med* 1983;143:877.
154. Van Gelder. Efficacy and safety of flecainide acetate in the maintenance of sinus rhythm after electrical cardioversion of chronic atrial fibrillation or atrial flutter. *Am J Cardiol* 1989;64:1317.
155. Van Gelder. Prediction of uneventful cardioversion and maintenance of sinus rhythm from direct-current electrical cardioversion of chronic atrial fibrillation and flutter. *Am J Cardiol* 1991;68:41.
156. van Hemel. Long-term results of the corridor operation for atrial fibrillation. *Br Heart J* 1994;71:170.
157. Vitolo. Amiodarone versus quinidine in the prophylaxis of atrial fibrillation. *Acta Cardiologia* 1981;36:431.
158. Waxman. Verapamil for control of ventricular rate in paroxysmal supraventricular tachycardia and atrial fibrillation or flutter: a double-blind randomized crossover study. *Ann Intern Med* 1981;94:1.
159. Weiner. Clinical course of acute atrial fibrillation treated with rapid digitalization. *Am Heart J* 1983;105:223.
160. Weiner. Clinical course of recent-onset atrial fibrillation treated with oral propafenone. *Chest* 1994;105:1013.
161. Wellens. Effect of digitalis on atrioventricular conduction and circus-movement tachycardias in patients with Wolff-Parkinson-White syndrome. *Circulation* 1973; 47:1229.
162. Williamson. Radiofrequency catheter modification of atrioventricular conduction to control the ventricular rate during atrial fibrillation. *N Engl J Med* 1994;331: 910. See comments.
163. Wolf. Atrial fibrillation as an independent risk factor for stroke: The Framingham Study. *Stroke* 1991;22:983.
164. Wong. Usefulness of labetalol in chronic atrial fibrillation. *Am J Cardiol* 1990; 66:1212.
165. Yahalom. Beta-adrenergic blockade as adjunctive oral therapy in patients with chronic atrial fibrillation. *Chest* 1977;71:592.
166. Zehender. Effects of amiodarone versus quinidine and verapamil in patients with chronic atrial fibrillation: results of a comparative study and a 2-year follow-up. *J Am Coll Cardiol* 1992;19:1054.

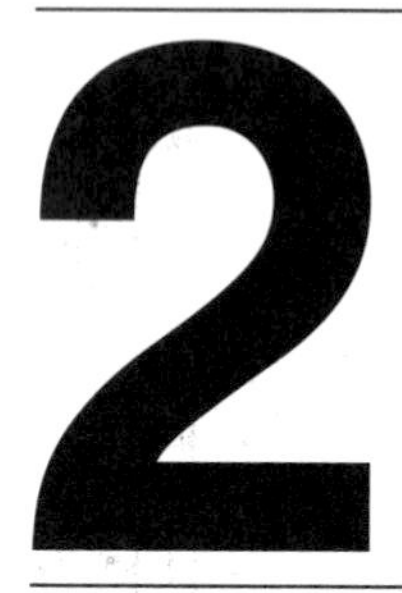

Unstable Angina Pectoris

Donald M. Lloyd-Jones and
Patrick T. O'Gara

A. Introduction

1. Historically, unstable angina pectoris (UA) refers to angina that is recent in onset, increasing in frequency or severity compared with baseline, or occurring with less than the usual amount of provocation or at rest. In contrast, stable angina pectoris is a syndrome in which patients have reliably reproducible symptoms with exertion that do not change in frequency, duration, or severity over time. A variety of other terms have been used to refer to UA, including crescendo angina, preinfarction angina, and intermediate coronary syndrome. The 1994 Agency for Health Care Policy and Research (AHCPR) Clinical Practice Guideline defines UA operationally as a clinical syndrome between stable angina pectoris and acute myocardial infarction (MI); this definition includes all acute presentations of coronary artery disease (CAD) except the so-called reperfusion-eligible acute MI (*i.e.*, acute ST elevation) (11). As discussed later in this chapter, optimal management strategies for UA differ significantly from those for stable angina pectoris or reperfusion-eligible MI.
2. In 1992, UA was the primary diagnosis for approximately 651,000 patients discharged from nonfederal acute care hospitals in the United States. Forty-eight percent of these patients were female, 58% were age 65 years or older, and 36% were between the ages of 45 and 64 years. These admissions represented more than 3.5 million days of inpatient care, with an average of 5.4 days per hospital stay (22).
3. Most practitioners use the Canadian Cardiovascular Society Classification (CCSC) of angina pectoris to describe the severity of limitation caused by angina for a given patient (15).
   a. Class I patients may experience angina only with strenuous, rapid, or prolonged exertion.
   b. Class II patients may experience angina when exerting after meals, in the cold, or when under emotional stress. Symptoms occur at levels of exertion intermediate between those of classes I and III.
   c. Class III patients may experience angina while walking one to two blocks on a level surface or while climbing one flight of stairs at a normal pace.
   d. Class IV patients may have angina with minimal activity or at rest.
4. The three principal presentations of UA are angina occurring at rest within 1 week of presentation; new onset of CCSC III or IV angina within 2 months of presentation; and previously diagnosed angina increasing in severity by at least one CCSC class to CCSC III or IV within 2 months of presentation (11).
5. In 1989, Braunwald (12) proposed a classification scheme for UA taking into account the severity of the symptoms, the clinical circumstances in which they occur, the presence or absence of electrocardiographic (ECG) changes, and the intensity of medical therapy. Under this scheme, UA is categorized as class I (new or accelerated angina without rest pain), class II (subacute rest angina), or class III (acute rest angina within 48 hours). In each of these groups, patient subcategories indicate the clinical circumstances under which UA develops. Class A refers to UA that develops in the setting of noncardiac events that provoke myocardial ischemia (secondary UA); class B refers to UA that develops

in the absence of such provocation (primary UA); and class C refers to UA that develops within 2 weeks after MI (postinfarction UA). Finally, patients are further categorized according to the intensity of medical therapy under which UA develops. Subscript 1 refers to UA that occurs in the setting of no or minimal therapy; subscript 2 refers to UA that occurs in the setting of appropriate oral therapy for stable angina; subscript 3 refers to UA that occurs in the setting of maximally tolerated therapy with calcium channel antagonists, ß-blockers, and IV trinitroglycerin (TNG). For example, a class $IIIB_1$ patient would have acute angina at rest within 48 hours before presentation, have no clear precipitant or recent MI, and be taking no or minimal antiischemic medications. This classification scheme has a pathophysiologic basis (see later discussion) and has been prospectively validated to predict prognosis in patients with UA (14,93).

B. Pathogenesis (27,28,72)

1. **Atherogenesis**—Coronary artery atherosclerosis probably begins as a response to vascular injury in the presence of risk factors or as a result of direct physical injury such as endothelial denudation at sites of nonlaminar blood flow. Cholesterol deposition or physicochemical injury then leads to endothelial dysfunction. However, endothelial dysfunction may be observed even in the absence of clear changes in the vascular wall and may be an important early marker of atherogenesis (56,68). Under normal conditions, the endothelium maintains a baseline vasodilator tone by producing nitric oxide (endothelium-derived relaxing factor), which causes vascular smooth muscle relaxation. The endothelium also produces certain prostaglandins which, along with nitric oxide, have antiplatelet activity and prevent luminal thrombosis. In the presence of endothelial dysfunction, intimal uptake of circulating low-density lipoprotein (LDL) cholesterol is enhanced. Oxidation of LDL in the tissues initiates a complex chain of events, including release of chemoattractants and expression of cell adhesion molecules, recruitment of circulating granulocytes and monocytes into the vessel wall, transformation of monocytes into activated tissue macrophages and foam cells, and secretion of proteases and growth factors, all of which perpetuate the damage to the vessel wall. Proliferation of smooth muscle cells and fibroblasts in response to growth factors and accumulation of lipid and fibrocellular material in the intima and media lead to formation of plaques that can protrude into the vessel lumen.
2. **Plaque Rupture and Thrombosis**—The atherosclerotic plaque is susceptible to rupture because of the shear stress of pulsatile blood flow and the internal degradation of the plaque by products of activated foam cells. Plaque rupture and thrombosis may lead to rapid acceleration of atherogenesis and luminal stenosis, which may cause symptoms if disruption of blood flow causes myocardial ischemia in the territory supplied by that coronary artery. Plaque rupture may expose the extremely thrombogenic substances in the core of the plaque (*e.g.*, lipid, tissue factor) to circulating platelets and coagulation factors, which may lead to further thrombosis and progression of luminal stenosis. In addition, vasoconstriction at the site of the plaque can limit distal blood flow in unstable coronary syndromes (101). If the thrombotic process stabilizes, the plaque may become a site of fixed stenosis and the patient may experience stable clinical symptoms. Alternatively, if the thrombotic process persists, it can lead to acute or subacute occlusion of the vessel and the patient may present with an acute coronary syndrome such as MI or primary UA.
3. Numerous studies have confirmed the important role of thrombosis in UA. Some of these are described for illustration (2,19,23,36,38,40,77,78).
   a. In a study involving 25 cases of sudden death due to acute coronary thrombosis, Falk noted laminated thrombi of differing ages in 81% of infarct-related arteries, with an identical proportion demonstrating underlying plaque rupture. Acute thrombosis was uniformly associated with a platelet- and fibrin-rich occlusive thrombus. Of the 15 patients who had a prodromal syndrome compatible with UA leading up to their fatal MI, 14 had evidence of repetitive episodes of thrombus formation (23).

b. Gurfinkel observed *in vivo* evidence of dynamic thrombus formation and endogenous thrombolysis in 12 patients with UA by measuring the blood levels of tissue-type plasminogen activator (tPA), urokinase, plasminogen activator inhibitor-1 (PAI-1), fibrin degradation products, thrombin/antithrombin complexes, and von Willebrand's factor at baseline and during ischemic episodes (38).

c. Platelet function is also radically altered in patients with UA. In a study involving 47 subjects (13 with ST depression and angina at rest, 14 with progressive angina but not at rest, and 20 healthy controls), Grande measured *ex vivo* platelet aggregation and plasma levels of ß-thromboglobulin, platelet factor 4, and serum thromboxane B_2 (36). Both groups with angina had platelets that exhibited hyperaggregation in response to arachidonic acid, compared with platelets from healthy controls ($P<0.01$). Over the entire 14-day study period, the patients with rest angina had significantly higher levels of thromboxane B_2, ß-thromboglobulin, and platelet factor 4 (putative indicators of platelet activation) than did the subjects in the other two groups ($P<0.01$).

d. Haft histologically compared the atherectomy specimens from 91 patients with coronary lesions that appeared complex on angiography and 20 patients with smooth coronary lesions (40). Thrombus was noted in 81% of the complex and 15% of the smooth lesions ($P<0.001$). Evidence of plaque rupture was noted in 57% of the complex lesions, compared with 10% of the smooth lesions ($P<0.001$). Clinical information was available on 86 patients. Among those with UA, 83% had a thrombus and 63% had evidence of plaque rupture; in contrast, among those with stable angina, 27% had a thrombus and 23% had evidence of plaque rupture ($P<0.001$ for both comparisons). On the other hand, the angiographic appearances of the culprit lesions responsible for UA appeared to be similar to those of lesions associated with non–Q-wave MI (NQWMI) (2).

e. In a study of intraoperative coronary angioscopy involving 27 subjects, all 3 patients with accelerated angina had complex plaques on angioscopy (defined as irregular surface, intimal flap, or intramural hemorrhage); all 7 patients with rest angina had thrombus; and neither of these features was present in any of the 17 patients with stable angina (77). Similarly, in another angioscopic study involving 67 patients undergoing coronary intervention procedures, plaque rupture and thrombosis were present in 68% of the 44 patients with UA versus 17% of the 23 patients with stable angina ($P<0.001$) (19). Ulcerated plaque and thrombi appear to be particularly prevalent among diabetic patients with UA (78). The angioscopic appearance of thrombi in patients with UA appears to be different from the appearance in patients with acute MI associated with ST-segment elevation; the UA lesions appear gray-white and MI lesions appear reddish, which probably reflects the composition or age of the thrombi and perhaps may explain the differential response of these two populations to thrombolytic therapy (see later discussion) (60).

4. Differences in the Pathogenesis of UA and NQWMI

a. In patients with UA, rupture of a relatively small plaque may lead to formation of a nonocclusive thrombus, reduction of the coronary lumen diameter, and exacerbation of anginal symptoms. Vasospasm and transient (typically <20 minutes) occlusion of the vessel by a thrombus may cause rest angina. Approximately two-thirds of UA episodes appear to be caused by decreased coronary perfusion by these mechanisms; the remaining one-third appear to be caused by an increase in myocardial oxygen demand (28).

b. In contrast, NQWMI appears to be associated with severe fissuring of the plaque, a more fibrin-rich thrombus, and prolonged occlusion of the coronary vessel. A transmural MI may develop in this zone unless spontaneous thrombolysis occurs or the zone is supplied by collateral circulation (28).

C. Prognosis—The major potential complications of UA are progression to acute MI and death. The mortality associated with UA appears to be highest at the time of hospitalization and declines over the ensuing 2 months (11). Other potential complications of UA include congestive heart failure (CHF), bradyarrhythmias, tachyarrhythmias, and sudden death. Using clinical, ECG, or other predictors of adverse outcome, numerous investigators have sought to identify the subset of patients with UA who are at high risk for these complications.

1. Gazes published the first case series defining the long-term prognosis of patients with preinfarction angina (30). The study included 140 consecutive patients admitted before 1961 with new onset of progressive rest angina, increasing severity of angina compared with baseline, or >15 minutes of pain at rest without an obvious precipitant. Those with acute MI at presentation, CHF, or cardiomegaly were excluded. Of the 113 patients for whom 10-year follow-up data were available, 80% were male, 17% had normal ECGs, and 83% had abnormalities consistent with acute or chronic ischemia. Twenty-nine patients (21%) had an acute MI within 3 months of the index admission for UA and 41% of these patients died. Seventy-seven patients died over the next 10 years (73 from coronary events). The authors identified a subgroup of 54 patients who had a 35% risk of MI at 3 months and an associated mortality of 63%. The risk factors for this high-risk subgroup were (a) prior history of angina, (b) frequent angina in the hospital, and (c) ischemic ST-segment changes during pain. This initial study led to the understanding that some patients with UA have a significantly elevated risk of death, especially during the first year after diagnosis (30). The cumulative survival rates for all patients and for those in the high-risk group are shown in Table 2-1.
2. Two studies have now prospectively validated the Braunwald classification of UA as an instrument for risk stratification.
   a. In one study, 417 consecutive patients admitted for suspected UA were classified according to the Braunwald criteria and then observed for 6 months; 26 had an acute MI and 109 had noncardiac causes of chest pain, leaving 282 patients with UA (93).
      (1) Classification of these patients according to the Braunwald criteria is summarized in Table 2-2. The numbers in Table 2 refer to the percentage of the patients who met the description for each category. (See introduction to this chapter for a discussion of the Braunwald classification scheme.)
      (2) Recurrent chest pain occurred significantly more often (P=0.0001) among class III patients (64%) than among class I (28%) or class II patients (45%). There was no difference in the rate of recurrent chest pain between classes B (49%) and C (53%).
      (3) The rates of survival and of infarct-free survival at 6 months were not different among the three classes of severity. However, class B patients had better rates (97% and 89%, respectively) than those in class C (89% and 80%, respectively; P=0.01 for both end points).
      (4) Therefore, those in classes III (acute rest angina) and C (UA occurring after recent MI) appear to be particularly high-risk patients who should be treated aggressively. Multivariate analysis revealed the independent predictors of adverse outcome at 6 months seen in Table 2-3.

Table 2-1 Survival after diagnosis of UA in Gazes' cohort (30)

Cumulative Survival	12 Mo	24 Mo	36 Mo	60 Mo	120 Mo
All patients	82%	75%	69%	61%	48%
High-risk subgroup	57%	47%	37%	27%	19%

Table 2-2 Distribution of patients according to Braunwald classification (93)

	Severity of Suspected UA			Clinical Setting			EGG Change	Therapy	
	Class I	Class II	Class III	Class A	Class B	Class C		Minimal	Oral
All patients (n=417)	25%	1%	74%	0%	92%	8%	51%	73%	27%
UA patients (n=282)	28%	1%	71%	0%	88%	12%	61%	67	33%

Table 2-3 Significant predictors of adverse outcome in UA (93)

End Point at 6 Mo	Multivariate Predictors
Death	Age >70, male, hypertension, class C, need for maximal therapy
Death or infarction	Age >70, class C
Death, infarction, or intervention	Male, class III, class C, ECG changes, need for maximal therapy

b. In another study involving 383 patients admitted to a coronary care unit for UA, the independent risk factors for adverse outcome (death, MI, CHF, ventricular tachycardia or fibrillation) were Braunwald class C (OR, 5.72; 95% CI, 1.92 to 16.97); need for maximally intense therapy with IV TNG (OR, 2.33; 95% CI, 1.31 to 4.17); minimal or no therapy before admission (OR, 3.83; 95% CI, 1.55 to 9.42); and baseline ST depression (OR, 2.81; 95% CI, 1.45 to 5.47) (14). Diabetes and age were also significant independent predictors of adverse outcome.

3. In a study involving 1387 consecutive patients with UA, Rizik proposed and prospectively validated an alternative classification scheme based solely on the presenting pattern of angina and ECG changes (69). The combined in-hospital event rates for MI, refractory angina, and death are shown in Table 2-4.

4. Numerous other clinical or laboratory predictors of adverse outcome have been proposed, including classification as definite versus suspected UA at the time of admission by an attending cardiologist (97); history of previous coronary artery bypass graft (CABG) surgery (96); the number of involved leads and the total amount of ST-segment deviation on admission ECG (17,34,64); ST-segment deviation and the duration of silent ischemia on continuous ECG monitoring in the hospital (51,53,70); depression of normal heart rate variability on continuous ECG monitoring in the hospital (45); recurrence of chest pain within 48 hours after admission (9); and lack of preadmission therapy with aspirin (29).

5. One final predictor of adverse outcome deserves mention. Two studies have evaluated the prognostic utility of serum cardiac troponin T levels at the time of admission. In one study involving 131 patients with UA (27 with elevated and 104 with normal troponin T levels), the total event rate for MI, refractory angina, and revascularization was 96% for patients with elevated levels of troponin T versus 44% for those with normal levels (RR, 33; 95% CI, 4.3 to 251; P=0.001) (98). The elevated levels of troponin T were observed equally in all Braunwald severity classes. In another study involving 109 patients with suspected UA (33 with elevated and 76 with normal levels of troponin T), the risk

Table 2-4 Occurrence of death, MI, or refractory angina by clinical class (69)

Class	Description	Event Rate	*P* vs. Next Lower Class
IA	Acceleration of previous angina without ECG changes	2.7%	—
IB	Acceleration of previous angina with ECG changes	9.1%	<0.005
II	New-onset exertional angina	9.7%	NS
III	New-onset rest angina	20.1%	0.0002
IV	Protracted rest angina with ECG changes	42.8%	0.0001

of MI and death was similarly increased for those with elevated troponin T levels ($P<0.05$) (41). In contrast to the first study (98), elevated levels of troponin T were observed only in Braunwald class III (acute rest angina) patients. In both studies, the serum level of troponin T was a significantly better predictor of adverse outcome than the level of the cardiac-specific isoenzyme of creatine kinase (CK-MB).

6. **Risk Classification in the AHCPR Guideline**
   a. **High Risk**—High-risk patients have at least one of the following: >20 minutes of ongoing rest pain; ischemia-related pulmonary edema; angina at rest with dynamic ST changes ≥1 mm; angina with new or worsening mitral regurgitation murmur, third heart sound (S_3), or rales; or angina with hypotension (11).
   b. **Intermediate Risk**—Patients at intermediate risk have no high-risk features but do have any of the following features: prolonged rest angina, now resolved, with moderate or high likelihood of CAD; rest angina lasting >20 minutes; nocturnal angina; dynamic T-wave changes; new-onset CCSC III or IV angina within 2 weeks, with moderate or high likelihood of CAD; pathologic Q waves or resting ST depression in multiple leads; or age >65 years (11).
   c. **Low Risk**—Patients at low risk are defined as those without high or intermediate risk features who have either increased frequency, severity, or duration of angina occurring at a lower threshold or new-onset angina of 2 to 8 weeks' duration and either normal or unchanged ECG (11).

D. **Acute Medical Therapy**—The major categories of drugs that have been evaluated for treatment of UA (with varying degrees of efficacy) are the antiplatelet, antithrombin, thrombolytic, antiischemic, and antiarrhythmic agents.

1. **Antiplatelet Agents**
   a. **Aspirin**—Aspirin prevents platelet activation by irreversibly inhibiting cyclooxygenase. To date, it has been the most widely studied antiplatelet agent, although newer drugs show promise for the future.
      (1) The Veterans Administration Cooperative Study is the largest trial to date that has evaluated the efficacy of aspirin for treatment of UA (55). This multicenter, double-blind, prospective randomized controlled trial (PRCT) enrolled 1338 men with evidence of CAD and symptoms consistent with UA occurring within 1 week of enrollment; those with evidence of acute MI on the entry ECG were excluded. Patients were randomly assigned to receive either aspirin (324 mg of buffered aspirin QD for 12 weeks) or placebo. Thirty-six patients from each group were excluded from analysis because subsequent cardiac enzyme determinations suggested that they had an acute MI at entry.
         (a) Aspirin was significantly better than placebo for reducing the risk of various adverse outcomes at 12 weeks. These findings are summarized in Table 2-5.
         (b) Among those who had an MI during the 12-week study period, the average peak total CK-MB level was lower for aspirin-treated patients than for placebo-treated patients, suggesting that the amount of myocardial damage may be less if MI occurs while a

Table 2-5 Results of the VA Cooperative Study of Aspirin for UA (55)

Outcome	Placebo (n=641)	ASA (n=625)	RRR*	Adjusted *P*
Death or MI	10.1%	5.0%	51%	0.0002
Any MI	7.8%	3.5%	55%	0.0003
Nonfatal MI	6.9%	3.4%	51%	0.002
Death	3.3%	1.6%	51%	0.059

*Relative risk reduction vs. placebo.

patient is receiving aspirin therapy. At 1 year of follow-up (data available for 86% of patients), there was still a persistent mortality benefit with aspirin (5.5% versus 9.6%; RRR, 43%; *P*=0.008).

(c) There was no difference in the risk of adverse reactions between the two arms.

(2) Cairns' Canadian multicenter double-blind PRCT enrolled patients with a clinical diagnosis of UA (crescendo pattern of pain, pain at rest lasting >15 minutes, no evidence of acute MI) within 8 days of admission to a coronary care unit (13). Patients older than 70 years of age, those who had had an MI within the preceding 12 weeks, and those with a history of peptic ulcer disease or gastrointestinal bleeding were excluded. Patients were randomly assigned in a 2×2 factorial design to receive aspirin (325 mg QID), sulfinpyrazone (200 mg QID), both, or neither. The mean age was 57 years, and 73% of the subjects were men. Over a mean follow-up period of 18 months, there was a 30% reduction (*P*=0.072) in the combined risk of death or nonfatal MI and a 56% reduction (*P*=0.009) in the risk of cardiac death for patients treated with aspirin (intention-to-treat analysis). There was no observable benefit of sulfinpyrazone (another antiplatelet agent), either with or without aspirin.

(3) As little as 75 mg of aspirin per day may be beneficial for patients with UA. In the Swedish RISC Trial, a double-blind PRCT involving 796 men with UA (51%) or NQWMI (49%), ingestion of 75 mg of aspirin per day for 1 year significantly reduced the combined risk of death or MI by 48% (21% versus 11%; *p*=0.0001). All subjects in the study were younger than 70 years of age (95).

(4) Metaanalysis

(a) Yusuf (99) pooled the data from three trials (13,55,86) of aspirin in UA and found a 40% reduction in the risk of nonfatal MI and in the risk of death (*P*<0.001).

(b) A recent analysis by the Antiplatelet Trialists Collaboration (5) included 174 published randomized trials of antiplatelet therapy for a variety of vascular conditions. Seven trials looked at the effects of antiplatelet therapy in patients with UA, most of whom received aspirin. The 6-month event rate was 9.1% for treated patients and 14.1% for control patients (see Table 2-6). An event was defined as MI, stroke, or vascular death. This represents a 35% reduction in risk compared with placebo (*P*<0.00001) and approximately 50 fewer events per 1000 patients treated at 6 months.

b. Ticlopidine—Ticlopidine appears to inhibit platelet activation by interfering with the platelet fibrinogen receptor, gp IIb/IIIa. It does not appear to have any significant effect on cyclooxygenase. In an Italian PRCT, Balsano compared ticlopidine plus standard therapy versus standard therapy alone among patients with UA (defined as new-onset, worsened, or rest angina; transient ST depression or T-wave inversion with symptoms; and no elevation of cardiac enzymes) (7). Patients who had taken an antiplatelet agent within 4 days of enrollment were excluded, and other antiplatelet agents (including aspirin) were not allowed during the study. All patients were treated initially with conventional therapy for 48 hours, including β-blockers, calcium channel antagonists, and nitrates; patients were subsequently

Table 2-6 6-m event rate in pooled analysis of antiplatelet therapy for UA (5)

	Control (n=2027)	Antiplatelet Therapy (n=1991)	*P*
MI, stroke, or vascular death	9.1%	14.1%	<0.00001

randomly assigned to receive ticlopidine (250 mg BID) in addition to this therapy or to continue with the conventional therapy alone. At the time of the study, the accepted conventional therapy for UA did not include aspirin. Seventy-two percent of the subjects were men, and 75% had angina at rest. Patients were observed for 6 months.

(1) Ticlopidine plus conventional therapy was significantly better than conventional therapy alone for reducing the risk of various adverse outcomes at 6 months. These findings are summarized in Table 2-7.

(2) In addition, the cumulative risk of adverse events reached a plateau after 3 weeks for those receiving ticlopidine, but for those given conventional therapy alone, this risk continued to rise for the duration of the study.

c. Platelet gp IIb/IIIa Receptor Blockers—The platelet membrane gp IIb/IIIa receptor antagonists are potent inhibitors of platelet aggregation and therefore may play a significant role in future therapy for UA. Although several agents belonging to this class of antiplatelet agents now exist, the best studied is c7E3, a chimeric mouse antigen-binding antibody fragment (Fab) that has a high affinity and specificity for the gp IIb/IIIa receptor. Other agents are being tested for treatment of UA but no large randomized trials have been reported to date. In addition to their antiplatelet effect, many of these drugs also block the integrin and vitronectin receptors, which may potentially limit leukocyte diapedesis and progression of atherosclerosis. The European Cooperative Study Group reported the results of a pilot study involving 60 patients with UA and ECG changes who were found on angiography to have a single culprit lesion amenable to percutaneous transluminal coronary angioplasty (PTCA) (79). Patients were randomly assigned in a double-blind fashion to receive either c7E3 or placebo for 18 to 24 hours. In addition, all patients received IV TNG, adjusted IV heparin, aspirin, and other antiischemic medications as dictated by their clinical course. Patients then underwent repeat angiography and PTCA; the study drugs were continued until 1 hour after the procedure.

(1) Despite randomization, 15 of the 30 placebo patients had multivessel CAD, compared with only 6 of the 30 patients assigned to receive c7E3 ($P<0.05$); this may have biased the outcome against the placebo group.

(2) In the placebo group, 12 major events occurred in 7 patients (23%), including 1 death, 4 MIs, and 7 urgent interventions. In comparison, only one major event (an MI) occurred in the c7E3 group (3%; $P=0.03$).

(3) Five patients required blood transfusions, including three who were receiving c7E3 and two who were receiving placebo (P=NS). For patients assigned to the c7E3 arm, *in vivo* and *in vitro* studies demonstrated >90% blockade of the gp IIb/IIIa receptors. However, the risk of clinically significant bleeding was low in both arms of the study. From these results, addition of c7E3 to heparin and aspirin appears to be safe.

Table 2-7 Effect of adding ticlodipine to conventional therapy for UA (7)

	Conventional Therapy (n=338)	Conventional Therapy Plus Ticlopidine (n=314)	RRR*	*P*
Total events	13.6%	7.3%	46%	0.009
Fatal MI or vascular death	4.7%	2.5%	47%	0.139
Nonfatal MI	8.9%	4.8%	46%	0.039
Any MI	10.9%	5.1%	53%	0.006

*Relative risk reduction vs. conventional therapy.

d. **Summary**—There is compelling evidence that antiplatelet agents (aspirin, ticlopidine, or gp IIb/IIIa antagonists) are beneficial for treatment of patients with UA. Among these agents, aspirin is the best studied to date. In the absence of a significant contraindication, all patients with UA should be given aspirin at the time of presentation and indefinitely thereafter (preferably 160 to 325 mg QD, but at least 75 mg QD). Ticlopidine and gp IIb/IIIa antagonists show promise for the future, but further studies are needed.

2. **Antithrombin Agents**—Because thrombosis appears to be important in the pathogenesis of UA, a significant research effort has been aimed at inhibiting thrombin (*i.e.*, factor II). Heparin is the best studied antithrombotic drug, but many newer agents are being tested. Heparin is an endogenously produced substance made up of proteoglycans of various sizes which combines with antithrombin III to inhibit thrombin. Exogenously administered heparin also increases the levels of plasma tPA antigen in patients with UA, possibly contributing to the pro-fibrinolytic milieu in these patients (46). Heparin also may have direct antiplatelet effects. The major studies that have evaluated the role of heparin for management of patients with UA are described here.

a. Theroux's double-blind PRCT (86) involved 479 patients younger than 75 years of age with accelerating or prolonged angina, ischemic ECG changes, and admission CK less than twice the upper limit of normal. The study excluded patients who were regular aspirin users and those who had undergone PTCA within 6 months or CABG within 12 months. Patients were randomly assigned in a 2×2 factorial design to receive aspirin (325 mg BID) versus placebo and heparin (5000 U IV bolus, then 1000 U/hour) versus placebo and were treated for a mean of 6 days. Heparin was subsequently adjusted by an unblinded pharmacist to keep the activated partial thromboplastin time (aPTT) at 1.5 to 2 times control. Other antianginal medications were given at the discretion of the patients' physicians. Coronary angiography was performed at a mean of 4 days.

(1) The study was discontinued prematurely after the first interim data analysis. As shown in Table 2-8, all three treatment groups were superior to placebo. There were too few deaths in the study to allow meaningful comparison among the groups. There was a trend favoring heparin alone over aspirin alone and heparin alone over the combination of heparin plus aspirin, but the differences were not statistically significant. Although the risk of bleeding was relatively low (6% of all patients), it was slightly higher for patients receiving heparin compared with those not receiving heparin and was highest for those receiving the combination of heparin and aspirin.

(2) Theroux then eliminated the placebo and combination study arms and enrolled an additional 245 patients into the remaining two arms (aspirin alone versus heparin alone) (87). MI occurred in 2 (0.8%) of

Table 2-8 Comparison of ASA, heparin, and their combinations in UA (86)

	Placebo (n=118)	ASA Alone (n=121)	Heparin Alone (n=118)	ASA Plus Heparin (n=122)
Refractory angina	23%	17%	9%	11%
RRR*	—	28%	63%	53%
P vs. placebo	—	0.217	0.002	0.011
Fatal or nonfatal MI	12%	3%	0.8%	1.6%
RRR*	—	72%	93%	86%
P vs. placebo	—	0.012	<0.001	0.001

*Relative risk reduction vs. placebo.

240 patients receiving heparin, compared with 9 (3.7%) of 244 patients receiving aspirin, for a risk reduction of 78% (P=0.035). From these data, 29 additional MIs would be prevented for every 1000 patients treated by the use of heparin rather than aspirin.

(3) In his original study population, Theroux observed an important rebound phenomenon that may occur with discontinuation of heparin. Specifically, 13% of patients treated with heparin alone had reactivation of UA or MI, compared with 5% of all other patients combined (P<0.01). For patients in the heparin group, these reactivation events occurred in a cluster at a mean of 9.5 hours after discontinuation of drug, but events were randomly distributed over 96 hours for the patients in the other three arms. Because patients in the combination arm had a risk of reactivation similar to that seen in the placebo group, aspirin may have significantly blunted the adverse effects of withdrawal from heparin. Therefore, concomitant therapy with aspirin may be important when heparin is being withdrawn (88). A part of the mechanism for this rebound phenomenon may be a transient increase in thrombin activity after heparin is withdrawn abruptly. The increased thrombin activity may lead to symptomatic (88) or silent (37) ischemia in this population.

b. Other studies have added to the debate on the use of heparin, aspirin, or both for management of UA. The Swedish RISC trial (84) used a similar double-blind 2×2 factorial design to randomly assign 796 patients, approximately half with UA and half with NQWMI, to receive aspirin (75 mg QD), heparin (5000 U IV bolus q 6 hours for 24 hours, then 3750 U thereafter for a total treatment period of 5 days), both aspirin and heparin, or neither drug. Patients presenting with ST-segment elevations were included in the study if they did not subsequently develop Q waves.

(1) Aspirin reduced the rate of MI or death by 57% during the 90-day follow-up period. Conversely, heparin did not significantly alter the rates of MI and death at any time point.

(2) However, all of the early benefit of aspirin was observed among those who were also receiving heparin (*i.e.*, combination therapy); there was a 75% reduction in the risk of death or MI in that group during first 5 days, compared with either placebo or heparin alone.

(3) Furthermore, there was a median delay of 33 hours before treatment was actually started. In 81% of patients treatment began after 24 hours, which may have limited the potential benefit that could have been derived with heparin. In addition, the study used a nonstandard method of administering heparin (intermittent boluses without adjustment for aPTT instead of adjusted continuous infusion); this also may have biased the outcome against heparin.

c. The ATACS trial (18) randomly assigned 214 patients with UA or NQWMI who had not previously used aspirin to receive either aspirin alone (162.5 mg QD) or aspirin (162.5 mg QD) plus heparin (100 U/kg bolus, then continuous infusion for 3 to 4 days) plus warfarin (adjusted with an INR goal of 2.0 to 3.0 for 12 weeks). Therapy was begun at a mean of 9.5 hours after admission (median, 6.8 hours). The primary end points were recurrent angina, MI, and death at 12 weeks. By intention-to-treat analysis, the combination therapy was clearly superior to aspirin alone in terms of reducing the risk of adverse events at 14 and 30 days; however, the difference was no longer statistically significant at 12 weeks (see Table 2-9). Major bleeding complications occurred in 3% of the patients in the combination group but in none of the patients in the aspirin group.

d. Conversely, Holdright (43) compared aspirin (150 mg QD) versus the combination of aspirin plus heparin (5000 U IV bolus and adjusted infusion) in a single-blind PRCT. There was no statistically significant difference in the number of ischemic episodes, total duration of ischemia, or in-hospital prognosis between the two groups.

Table 2-9 Occurrence of death, MI, or recurrent angina in the ATACS trial (18)

Any Event by Time Indicated	ASA Alone (n=109)	ASA Plus Heparin/Warfarin (n=105)	RRR*	*P*
14 d	27%	11%	59%	0.004
30 d	27%	14%	48%	0.03
12 wk	28%	19%	32%	0.09

*Relative risk reduction vs. ASA alone.

e. It is difficult to compare these studies of heparin directly, given the different definitions of UA used and the different methods of heparin administration. There is now significant evidence that a therapeutic aPTT is best achieved with continuous IV infusion and use of a weight-based heparin nomogram, so many of these studies may have been biased against heparin by use of a suboptimal dose or mode of administration. Despite this potential bias, Theroux demonstrated a significant benefit of heparin versus aspirin in preventing complications of UA. Therefore, appropriate dosing of IV heparin should be a mainstay of current standard therapy for UA.

f. Subcutaneous unfractionated heparin may also be effective for patients with UA. Serneri administered aspirin, nitrates, nifedipine, and metoprolol to 399 patients who had chest pain occurring at rest or with minimal exertion and either reversible ST-segment changes or a CK value less than twice the upper limit of normal (75). At the end of 24 hours of this therapy, 108 patients who had had either three or more ischemic episodes by Holter monitoring or one symptomatic anginal episode were randomly assigned to receive aspirin (325 mg QD), adjusted IV heparin, or adjusted SQ heparin for 3 days. Both SQ and IV heparin significantly decreased the number and the duration of ischemic episodes by a similar degree compared with baseline. The design of the study has been criticized because UA may remit spontaneously and because aspirin was withdrawn from two thirds of the patients (*i.e.*, those treated with IV or SQ heparin) (see Table 2-10).

g. Gurfinkel (39) conducted a double-blind PRCT comparing the efficacy of aspirin alone or in combination with conventional heparin or nadroparin (a low-molecular-weight heparin) in patients with UA. Two hundred nineteen patients entered the study at a mean of 6 hours after their last episode of rest pain. They were randomly assigned to receive either aspirin (200 mg QD), aspirin plus conventional heparin (5000 U IV bolus followed by infusion at 400 U/kg/day and adjusted for aPTT), or aspirin plus nadroparin (BID SQ without adjustment for aPTT), with appropriate placebos, for 5 to 7 days. The primary end points were recurrent angina, acute MI, requirement for urgent coronary revascularization, major bleeding, and death.

(1) The overall risk of adverse events or recurrent angina was signifi-

Table 2-10 ASA vs. IV heparin vs. SQ heparin for UA (75)

	ASA (n=36)	IV Heparin (n=37)	SQ Heparin (n=35)
Number of ischemic episodes vs. prerandomization	8% decrease	63% decrease	56% decrease
P	NS	<0.001	<0.001
Duration of ischemia vs. prerandomization	6% decrease	66% decrease	61% decrease
P	NS	<0.001	<0.001

cantly lower for those treated with aspirin plus nadroparin than for those in the other two study arms. There were no deaths in any group (see Table 2-11).

(2) In addition, significantly fewer patients receiving aspirin plus nadroparin had silent ischemia documented on continuous ST-segment monitoring during the first 48 hours of the study, compared with those on aspirin plus conventional heparin (25% versus 41%, respectively; P=0.04).

(3) Therefore, low-molecular-weight heparin appears promising for treatment of UA and warrants further study.

h. Direct Antithrombin Agents—Examples of newer antithrombin agents include recombinant hirudin, the anticoagulant produced by leeches; hirulog, a similar synthetic peptide; and argatroban. These drugs all inhibit thrombin directly by binding to the active site of the enzyme. These compounds are still in the early stages of testing, and little efficacy data are available for patients with UA.

(1) Topol conducted a multicenter PRCT comparing hirudin versus conventional heparin among patients with chest pain and ECG changes caused by angiographically documented coronary artery stenosis (>60%) and evidence of a thrombus (92). Patients assigned to receive hirudin tended to have small, but improved, angiographic appearance of the culprit lesion, compared with those receiving heparin. However, there was no statistically significant difference in clinical outcome (*e.g.*, death, MI, recurrent angina, need for a revascularization procedure).

(2) Efficacy results from the Global Use of Strategies to Open Occluded Coronary Arteries (GUSTO-2a) trial, which enrolled patients with any acute coronary syndrome (*e.g.*, UA, MI), are not available because the trial was terminated prematurely after interim analysis revealed an excess of hemorrhagic stroke in all patients receiving recombinant hirudin (1.7%) compared with those receiving heparin (0.8%; P=0.11). Hemorrhage was particularly prevalent among the acute MI patients treated with thrombolysis, but no information is available about the subset of patients with UA who would not have received thrombolysis (83).

(3) Hirulog was studied in the dose-ranging Thrombolysis in Myocardial Ischemia. (TIMI-7) trial without a placebo arm and was associated with a very low risk of major bleeding (0.5%) (26). Other trials are planned to further evaluate the potential role of direct antithrombin agents for treatment of UA.

i. Summary—Blockade of thrombin activity has a sound pathophysiologic basis in the treatment of UA. The best studied drug in this class is heparin, which appears to be very effective in reducing the risk of complications.

Table 2-11 Nadroparin vs. conventional heparin vs. control of UA (39)

	ASA Alone (n=73)	ASA Plus Conventional Heparin (n=70)	ASA Plus Nadroparin (n=68)	*P* for ASA/Nadroparin vs. ASA/Heparin
Total events	59%	63%	22%	0.00001
Recurrent angina	37%	44%	21%	0.002
Acute MI	9.5%	6%	0%	0.1
Urgent revascularization	12%	10%	1.5%	0.07
Major bleeding	0%	3%	0%	0.4

However, it is important that the appropriate dose and mode of administration be used. Other antithrombin drugs, including low-molecular-weight heparin and hirudin, are promising for the future but require further study.

3. Thrombolytic Agents

a. Before the completion of the larger TIMI-3A and -3B trials, numerous small studies had evaluated the role of thrombolytic therapy for patients with UA but had reported mixed results (3,6,8,25,33,54,63,74,94). The TIMI-3A trial (90) analyzed the angiographic effects of tPA when added to conventional therapy for patients with UA or NQWMI. The study enrolled 306 patients with either a known history of CAD or 5 to 360 minutes of chest pain at rest and ischemic ECG changes who presented within 12 hours of onset of symptoms. All patients received standard antiischemic therapy as well as heparin (IV bolus followed by adjusted infusion). Aspirin was not administered until just before the patient was to undergo PTCA or until heparin was to be discontinued. After the probable culprit coronary lesion was identified on angiography, patients were randomly assigned to receive either tPA (0.8 mg/kg IV, maximum 80 mg, one-third as a bolus and the rest over 90 minutes) or placebo. Repeat coronary angiography was performed at 18 to 48 hours. The primary end point was measurable improvement in the culprit lesion at repeat angiography, defined as ≥10% reduction of stenosis or improvement of flow by two TIMI grades; substantial improvement was defined as ≥20% reduction of stenosis or improvement of flow by two TIMI grades. Ninety-seven patients (32%) had NQWMI based on enzyme analysis, and 209 (68%) had UA. Only 107 patients (35%) had angiographically apparent thrombus at the time of initial catheterization (see Table 2-12).

(1) Angiographic improvement was significantly more likely with tPA than with placebo. Nevertheless, only 15% of the patients treated with tPA derived this benefit.

(2) Essentially all of the significant angiographic improvement was observed among patients with a thrombus or NQWMI (or both). Both subgroups were prespecified at the time of study design.

(3) Questions remained as to whether withholding aspirin or performing angiography too early had limited the apparent benefit of tPA.

b. The TIMI-3B trial randomly assigned 1473 patients (similar to those in the TIMI-3A trial but presenting within 24 hours of onset of chest pain at rest) in a 2×2 factorial design to tPA versus placebo plus early invasive therapy (angiography with revascularization if necessary) versus early conservative therapy (invasive therapy only after failure of medical therapy) (91). All patients received antiischemic medications, aspirin, and adjusted IV heparin. Again, 32% met the criteria for the diagnosis of NQWMI. The comparison between tPA and placebo is presented here; comparison of conservative versus invasive strategies is discussed in section E of this chapter. The primary end point was combined risk of death, nonfatal MI, or failure of initial therapy at 6 weeks (see Table 2-13).

Table 2-12 Results of the TIMI-3A angiographic trial (90)

	Placebo (n=156)	tPA (n=150)	*P*
Measurable improvement	19%	25%	0.25
Substantial improvement			
All patients	5%	15%	0.003
Patients with thrombus	15%	36%	0.01
Patients with NQWMI	8%	33%	0.003
Patients with UA	4%	7%	NS

Table 2-13 Results of the TIMI-3B trial for thrombolytic therapy (91)

Outcome	Placebo (n=744)	tPA (n=729)	*P*
Primary end point	55.5%	54.2%	0.61
Intracranial hemorrhage	0%	0.55%	0.06
Death	2.0%	2.3%	0.67
MI	4.9%	7.4%	0.04
Death or MI	6.2%	8.8%	0.05

(1) There was no difference in the likelihood of reaching a primary end point between the two groups.

(2) However, there was a trend toward increased risk of intracranial hemorrhage with tPA (0.55% versus 0% with placebo; *P*=0.06). In addition, the risk of death or MI was marginally higher with tPA (8.8% versus 6.2% with placebo; *P*=0.05). The authors concluded that routine thrombolytic therapy for UA is not beneficial and may even be detrimental.

c. In the TIMI-3B trial, tPA was administered over a short time period and in doses approaching those used for acute MI. Romeo (71) conducted a double-blind PRCT comparing prolonged low-dose tPA (20-mg bolus plus infusion at 0.03 mg/kg/hour) versus placebo in 67 patients with refractory UA (rest or increasing angina and reversible ECG changes with ongoing symptoms despite antianginal and aspirin therapy). All patients received IV heparin continuously for 3 days, and the activated clotting time was maintained between 250 and 400 seconds (see Table 2-14).

(1) During the index hospitalization, patients with UA who were treated with a prolonged low-dose infusion of tPA were significantly less likely to have recurrent angina, to need emergency CABG or PTCA, or to experience any adverse event than were patients who received placebo. They were also more likely to be free of angina and less likely to require another admission for MI or UA at 14 months.

(2) There were no episodes of major bleeding in either group.

(3) Based on the results of this small study, a prolonged low-dose infusion of tPA may be safer and more effective than the standard regimen of tPA for patients with UA. However, more studies are needed.

d. Summary—At the present time, thrombolytic therapy for UA is not recommended.

4. Antiischemic and Antianginal Agents

a. Nitrates—Nitrates may improve myocardial ischemia by several mechanisms. First, they decrease myocardial oxygen consumption in some pa-

Table 2-14 Efficacy of prolonged low-dose tPA infusion in UA (71)

	Placebo (n=31)	tPA (n=36)	*P*
In-hospital Risk (no. patients)			
Recurrent angina	13	5	<0.03
Acute MI	4	1	NS
Needing emergency CABG/PTCA	8	0	<0.01
Any adverse event	21	7	<0.01
Risk at 14 Mo (no. patients)			
Death	4	3	NS
Admission for MI or UA	11	7	<0.05
CABG/PTCA	18	20	NS
Being angina-free	1	8	<0.01

tients by decreasing preload and afterload (21). Second, they can directly vasodilate the coronary arteries and thereby improve coronary blood flow (21). Finally, nitrates, including IV TNG, can inhibit the cyclic guanosine monophosphate–dependent steps of platelet activation and aggregation (52). Among the available routes for delivery of nitrates, IV TNG is the best studied mode for UA.

(1) In an uncontrolled study, Kaplan (49) administered IV TNG to 35 patients who had rest angina that was refractory to oral or topical nitrates and either transient ECG changes or thallium defects during pain. Seventeen of the 35 patients were also receiving propranolol. Compared with baseline (*i.e.*, with oral or topical nitrates), IV TNG markedly reduced the number of anginal episodes (3.5 versus 0.3 per day) as well as the requirement for sublingual TNG or morphine. Twenty-five patients responded completely to IV TNG (*i.e.*, no angina), 8 responded partially, and 2 did not respond significantly. The results of this and other studies suggest that IV TNG is effective in relieving angina in patients with UA. However, other than pain relief, no study has demonstrated a significant mortality or morbidity benefit in this population.

(2) In Yusuf's metaanalysis of 10 randomized trials evaluating the benefit of IV nitrates in patients with acute MI, IV TNG reduced mortality by approximately 35% (95% CI, 16% to 50%; $P<0.001$) compared with control (100). No such data exist for UA, and it is unclear whether the data from patients with an MI can be extrapolated to those with UA.

(3) Just as abrupt withdrawal of heparin can cause rebound ischemia, abrupt cessation of IV TNG can precipitate coronary ischemia. Figueras found that 55% of 46 patient with UA developed ischemic ECG changes within 10 minutes after abrupt cessation of IV TNG. This result was highly reproducible for a given patient. Rebound coronary vasoconstriction may be the underlying pathophysiologic mechanism for this phenomenon (24). Therefore, tapering of IV TNG, with or without substitution of oral nitrates, may be prudent for some patients.

b. β-Adrenergic Receptor Antagonists and Calcium Channel Blockers (66)—β-Adrenergic receptor antagonists (β-blockers) can improve myocardial ischemia by decreasing heart rate, blood pressure, and myocardial contractility, all of which are major determinants of myocardial oxygen demand. In addition, they may improve coronary blood flow by prolonging the diastolic perfusion time, allowing more blood to flow across stenotic lesions. Calcium channel blockers appear to improve coronary blood flow by direct smooth muscle relaxation and vasodilation. They may also block coronary vasoconstriction, which can precipitate or accompany myocardial ischemia. Furthermore, they may dilate collateral vessels that could be supplying an area of ischemic myocardium, thereby reducing myocyte damage or necrosis. These agents also may promote ventricular relaxation, enhancing subendocardial blood flow and improving ischemia. The major trials that have evaluated the benefit of these agents for patients with UA are discussed here.

(1) In the Telford study, which compared IV heparin, atenolol, both, or neither in patients with UA, atenolol (100 mg QD) did not significantly improve the risk of death or transmural MI (81).

(2) The Holland Interuniversity Nifedipine/Metoprolol Trial (HINT) has had the greatest impact in confirming the role of β-blockers for patients with UA (57). This was a double-blind PRCT with two major arms. In the larger arm of the trial, 338 patients with chest pain and either reversible ECG changes or known history of CAD were randomly assigned in a 2×2 factorial design to receive nifedipine (10 mg q 4 hours), metoprolol (100 mg BID), both nifedipine and metoprolol, or double placebo. Only those who had not been taking β-blockers before the study were enrolled in this arm. Most were younger than 65 years of age, 75% were male, and up to 20% had transient ST-segment elevation on ECG with pain. The 177 patients in the second arm of the trial had presentations similar to those in the first arm but were receiving chronic β-blocker therapy before admission. These patients were either maintained on their usual dose or switched to metoprolol 100 mg BID. In addition to the β-blockers, they were also randomly assigned to receive nifedipine (10 mg q 4 hours) or placebo.

(a) In the first arm of the study (previous nonusers of β-blockers), there was a trend toward a lower risk of recurrent ischemia or MI at 48 hours with metoprolol, compared with placebo (OR, 0.76; 95% CI, 0.49 to 1.16). The risk of recurrent ischemia or MI at 48 hours was significantly lower with metoprolol than with nifedipine (OR, 0.66; 95% CI, 0.43 to 0.98). For the same end point, combination therapy was significantly better than nifedipine alone (OR, 0.68; 95% CI, 0.47 to 0.97) but not better than metoprolol alone (OR, 1.06; 95% CI, 0.67 to 1.70) (see Table 2-15). Therefore, for patients not receiving chronic β-blocker therapy who develop UA, addition of metoprolol is beneficial. However, addition of nifedipine did not offer any significant benefit over placebo, and combination therapy (nifedipine plus metoprolol) provided no additional benefit over metoprolol alone.

(b) In the second arm of the trial (previous users of β-blockers), the risk of recurrent ischemia or MI at 48 hours was significantly lower with nifedipine than with placebo (OR, 0.68; 95% CI, 0.47 to 0.97). Therefore, for patients who develop UA while receiving chronic β-blocker therapy, the addition of nifedipine appears to be beneficial (see Table 2-16).

(3) In another double-blind PRCT, Muller also found the addition of nifedipine to be beneficial for UA patients receiving chronic β-blocker therapy. However, for those not previously receiving β-block-

Table 2-15 Results of the HINT trial in previous nonusers of β-blockers (57)

	Placebo (n=84)	Nifedipine (n=89)	Metoprolol (n=79)	Combination (n=86)
Recurrent ischemia or MI at 48 h	37%	47%	28%	30%
Adjusted OR vs. placebo (95% CI)	—	1.15 (0.83–1.64)	0.76 (0.49–1.16)	0.80 (0.53–1.19)
MI at 48 h	15%	28%	16%	14%
Adjusted OR vs. placebo (95% CI)	—	1.51 (0.87–2.74)	1.07 (0.54–2.09)	0.88 (0.44–1.74)

Table 2-16 Results of the HINT trial in previous users of β-blockers (57)

	Continued β-Blocker Only (n=81)	Nifedipine Added (n=96)
Recurrent ischemia or MI at 48 h	51%	30%
Adjusted OR (95% CI)	—	0.68 (0.47–0.97)
MI at 48 h	20%	14%
Adjusted OR (95% CI)	—	0.86 (0.45–1.61)

ers, addition of propranolol produced more rapid symptom relief than addition of nifedipine, which tended to increase the heart rate (62).

(4) Gerstenblith's double-blind PRCT examined the benefit of adding nifedipine (10 to 20 mg q 6 hours) for UA patients receiving chronic nitrate and β-blocker therapy. (31) Patients were included if they had rest pain with ECG changes but had no evidence of an MI. The average duration of angina was remarkably long, at 1200 days. The primary end point of the study was failure of medical therapy at 3 months, defined as sudden death, MI, or need for surgery. Prespecified subgroups included patients with and patients without ST-segment elevations (see Table 2-17).

(a) Overall, patients treated with nifedipine were significantly less likely to fail therapy.

(b) Thirty-eight percent of the 138 patients had ST-segment elevation on the enrollment ECG. Many of these patients may have had variant (vasospastic) angina, which would have biased the study in favor of nifedipine. In fact, most of the benefit was observed among those with ST-segment elevations.

(5) As a variation on the theme, Gottlieb examined the benefit of adding β-blocker therapy for patients who develop UA while receiving chronic nifedipine therapy (35). Over a 4-day treatment period, propranolol (at least 160 mg total daily dose), when added to nifedipine and nitrates, significantly reduced the risk of recurrent angina, the duration of angina, the need for TNG, and the number of ischemic episodes on continuous ECG monitoring, compared with placebo.

(6) Theroux and colleagues randomly compared diltiazem (120 mg TID) versus propranolol (80 mg TID) in 100 patients with UA in a single-blind fashion. Patients with ST elevations were specifically not included in order to exclude those with vasospastic (Prinzmetal) angina. Patients were observed for a mean of 5.1 months (89).

(a) Both drugs decreased the heart rate and the systolic blood pressure to similar degrees compared with baseline. The two therapies were also similar in their ability to reduce symptoms and maintain patients free of symptoms. There were no differences in the risk of death or the need for surgery.

(b) The authors concluded that diltiazem could be a useful alternative to β-blockers for treatment of UA.

(7) A more recent double-blind study randomly compared IV TNG versus IV diltiazem in 121 patients with UA (32). The risk of refractory angina and MI was significantly lower in patients who were receiving diltiazem (20%) than in patients receiving IV TNG (41%, P=0.02). Conduction disturbances occurred in 8% of the diltiazem-treated patients, all of which resolved with reduction of the dose. None of the patients in the IV TNG group had this complication. Although fewer patients in

Table 2-17 Efficacy of nifedipine in previous users of β-blockers with UA (31)

	Placebo (n=70)	Nifedipine (n=68)	RRR*	*P*
Failure of therapy—all patients	61%	44%	28%	0.03
Failure of therapy—with ST elevation	67%	36%	46%	0.02
Failure of therapy—without ST elevation	58%	49%	—	NS
Surgery	41%	26%	37%	0.04

*Relative risk reduction vs. placebo.

the IV TNG group received β-blockers (23% versus 37%), this did not appear to affect the statistical benefit of diltiazem on multivariate analysis.

c. **Summary**—IV TNG appears to be helpful for relieving symptoms in patients with UA, but no study has demonstrated a reduction in the risk of death or MI in this population. In the absence of contraindications, β-blockers should be administered to almost all patients with UA. Nifedipine probably should not be used as monotherapy, but it may be beneficial for patients with vasospastic angina and for those with refractory symptoms despite treatment with β-blockers and other conventional drugs. Diltiazem may be an effective alternative for patients in whom β-blockers are contraindicated or for whom vasospasm is suspected. Although a combination of β-blockers and calcium channel blockers may be helpful for patients with refractory UA, the routine use of combined therapy is not recommended. It should be noted that patients with significant left ventricular (LV) dysfunction, CHF, or preexisting conduction system disease were routinely excluded from the trials that evaluated these therapies; for this reason, β-blockers and calcium channel blockers should be used with caution in these settings.

5. **Antiarrhythmic Agents**—In a non-blinded prospective randomized study without placebo control, the role of prophylactic lidocaine was evaluated in patients with chest pain of suspected cardiac origin (42). Of 1427 patients, 31% proved to have an acute MI and 33% to have UA. Patients with warning ventricular ectopy, second- or third-degree heart block, or hypotension were excluded. Cardiac arrest and death occurred in 1.5% and 7.4% of patients, respectively; most of the patients with these complications had an acute MI. There was no significant benefit of lidocaine even when the analysis was restricted to patients with an MI. Although a specific analysis for patients with UA was not done, prophylactic lidocaine does not appear to be warranted for electrically stable patients with UA.

E. Further Management of Unstable Angina

1. Patients with UA who are thought to be at high risk for death or complications during the acute phase of their illness should be referred for emergent or urgent cardiac catheterization and considered for a revascularization procedure. The features defining a high-risk patient in the AHCPR Guideline for UA were described in section C of this chapter (11). Other predictors of poor prognosis include Braunwald class III (acute rest angina within 48 hours), Braunwald class C (postinfarction UA), angina refractory to maximal medical therapy, recurrence of angina after stabilization, diabetes mellitus, and older age (9,12, 14,69,93).

2. The TIMI-3B study was specifically designed to address whether cardiac catheterization and revascularization should be performed routinely in all patients who present with UA. In this trial, 740 patients were randomly assigned to undergo cardiac catheterization at 18 to 48 hours after presentation (the early invasive group). If feasible, angioplasty was performed on the culprit lesion and on any other vessel with >60% stenosis. Patients were referred for CABG if they had ≥50% left main CAD, three-vessel disease with ejection fraction (EF) <40%, or recurrent angina after PTCA. Patients were also referred for CABG if the lesion was not amenable to PTCA. In the other arm of the trial, 733 patients who were randomly assigned to the early conservative group were treated medically and underwent cardiac catheterization only for one of the following indications: recurrent symptomatic or silent ischemia; unsatisfactory result on predischarge low-level exercise tolerance testing (ETT) with thallium; or CCSC III or IV angina with a positive stress test (91).

   a. The risk of rehospitalization at 6 weeks was lower with the invasive strategy. However, as summarized in Table 2-18, there were no significant differences in other outcome measures.

   b. At 1-year follow-up, the severity of angina was not different between the two

Table 2-18 6-Week results of the TIMI-3B trial (91)

6-Wk End Point	Invasive (n=740)	Conservative (n=733)	*P*
Death, MI, failed ETT	16.2%	18.1%	NS
Rehospitalization	7.8%	14.1%	<0.001
CCSC class I/II	16.4%	17.1%	NS
CCSC class III/IV	7.6%	9.5%	NS

Table 2-19 1-Year results of the TIMI-3B trial (91)

One-Yr End Point	Invasive	Conservative	*P*
Death or nonfatal MI	10.8%	12.2%	NS
Revascularization	64%	58%	<0.001
PTCA	39%	32%	<0.001
CABG	30%	30%	NS
Rehospitalization	26%	33%	<0.005

groups. Patients who received the early invasive strategy did undergo more revascularization procedures, as shown in Table 2-19, but there was no clear precipitant. The authors concluded that either strategy was acceptable for appropriately selected patients whose condition stabilizes after UA (4).

3. For patients with UA whose condition stabilizes with medical therapy, four factors are consistently related to short-term and long-term prognosis: LV systolic function, the extent and severity of CAD, age, and comorbid conditions (11). One of the major goals in the postacute setting should be to stratify patients according to their risk of subsequent morbidity and mortality, so that high-risk patients can undergo a revascularization procedure if appropriate and low-risk patients can be monitored closely under medical therapy. For example, CABG studies have demonstrated that patients with significant left main CAD or depressed LV function have a high mortality rate when treated medically and that CABG can improve survival in these patients (1,16). Risk stratification should attempt to identify patients who may have these conditions. (See Chap. 8).

a. Determination of LV Function—Except for patients whose LV function is clearly preserved based on clinical assessment, it is often helpful to objectively measure the global LV function with echocardiography, radionuclide ventriculography, or left ventriculography.

b. Stress Testing—Patients whose condition stabilizes clinically and who experience no further angina with therapy require risk stratification to rule out life-limiting or activity-limiting CAD. This should be accomplished with the use of treadmill ETT only after the patient has been asymptomatic and without objective signs of ischemia for approximately 48 hours (11).

(1) Moss, writing for the Multicenter Myocardial Ischemia Research Group, reported the results of noninvasive testing on 936 patients who had been stable for 1 to 6 months after an admission for Q-wave MI (44%), NQWMI (26%), or UA (30%). None had undergone CABG and all had interpretable ECGs. Patients underwent ECG monitoring with thallium scintigraphy under rest, ambulatory, and stress conditions. On multivariate analysis, ST depression on the resting ECG was a significant predictor of a combined end point of death, nonfatal MI, or UA (OR, 1.50, 95% CI, 1.00 to 2.25; P=0.05). In addition, exercise-induced ischemic ST depression with poor exercise tolerance (<6 to 9 minutes on a modified Bruce protocol) and increased thallium lung uptake with reversible thallium defects were predictors of increased risk, but these findings accounted for only 6% of the patients who developed adverse outcome (61).

(2) Conversely, in a study of 400 men hospitalized for suspected unstable CAD, the independent predictors of death, MI, or need for CABG were (a) exercise-induced ST depression, (b) exercise-limiting chest pain, and (c) low exercise capacity on a predischarge stress test (80). Similar findings were reported in a study of 740 men with UA (51%) or NQWMI (49%). Again, the independent predictors of MI at 1 year were (a) the number of involved leads with exercise-induced ST depression and (b) poor exercise tolerance (65).

(3) Whether or not a nuclear perfusion imaging agent (*e.g.*, thallium, sestamibi) should be added to the ETT depends on the patient's baseline ECG, the importance of assessing perfusion to multiple coronary territories, and local expertise with the procedure. The results of numerous small studies that included patients with UA indicate that the diagnostic accuracy for discriminating between patients at high versus low risk of subsequent morbidity and mortality is approximately the same for ETT alone, ETT with thallium, and testing with dipyridamole (Persantine)–thallium (11). Patients who are not candidates for catheterization or revascularization on clinical grounds may not require any functional testing, in which case palliation of symptoms should be the goal.

4. Patients who present with UA should receive appropriate counseling about their illness, including relevant information about modification of risk factors for CAD (*e.g.*, smoking cessation, dietary changes, weight loss, exercise, control of diabetes and hypertension). In addition, patients with elevated cholesterol should be treated to reduce subsequent morbidity and mortality. In a secondary prevention study, the Scandinavian Simvastatin Survival Study (4S Study), 4444 patients with known CAD (angina or history of MI >6 months prior to enrollment) were randomly assigned to receive either simvastatin or placebo. The total cholesterol levels ranged from 213 to 310 mg/dl. After a mean follow-up of 5.4 years, the total mortality rate was lower with simvastatin than with placebo (8.2% versus 11.5%; RRR 30%; $P=0.0003$). There was also a 34% reduction in risk of major coronary events ($P<0.00001$) and a 37% reduction in need for a revascularization procedure ($P<0.00001$) with simvastatin (73).

F. Revascularization for UA

1. PTCA—Several large series have demonstrated the effectiveness of PTCA for relieving symptoms in UA. In one series of 840 consecutive patients undergoing PTCA for either stable (n=506) or unstable (n=334) angina, the event-free survival rates were similar between the two groups at 2 years (68% versus 62%; *P*=NS) (48). However, compared with stable angina patients, those with UA who underwent PTCA had a higher event rate (death, nonfatal MI, recurrent angina requiring PTCA or CABG) within 24 hours of the procedure (15.8% versus 6.3%; *P*,0.01). De Feyter reported similar outcomes after 2 years in 200 consecutive patients undergoing PTCA for UA. In this series, 3% of the patients died, 12% had nonfatal MI, 13% were still symptomatic but had improved to a better functional class, and 32% had restenosis on repeat angiography (20).

2. CABG

a. The Veterans Administration Cooperative Study for UA was a multicenter PRCT comparing CABG plus medical therapy versus medical therapy alone in 468 selected men with UA. Patients with a history of MI within 3 months, LV EF <30%, or significant left main CAD were excluded (see Table 2-20).

(1) By intention-to-treat analysis, the overall 2-year survival rates were not different between the two arms (approximately 93%). However, 34% of the patients assigned to medical therapy had crossed over to CABG during this period. At 5 and 8 years, there was still no significant difference in overall survival between the two groups (58,67,76).

Table 2-20 Results of the VA Cooperative Study of CABG after UA (58,67,76)

Follow-Up (Reference)	Medical (n=237)	CABG + Medical (n=231)	*P*
5 Y (67)			
Survival—all patients	81%	84%	NS
Survival—three-vessel CAD	755	89%	<0.02
Nonfatal MI	18%	16%	NS
8 Y (76)			
Survival—all patients	71%	72%	NS
Survival—depressed LV EF	54%	87%	0.04
Nonfatal MI	19%	17%	NS

(2) However, CABG did improve survival in a subset of patients with three-vessel CAD at 5 years (75% versus 89%; *P*<0.02) and in those with LV EFs between 30% and 59% at 8 years (54% versus 87%; *P*=0.04) (58,67,76).

(3) In addition, compared with patients treated medically, CABG patients reported significant improvement in symptoms and quality of life during the first 5 years of the study (10).

b. A review by Kaiser summarized the results of 14 reports of CABG (performed in the 1970s and early 1980s) in patients with UA; the review included a total of 6136 patients from these studies (47).

(1) The mean operative mortality rate was 3.7%, the perioperative MI rate was 9.9%, and the incidence of need for prolonged inotropic or intraaortic balloon pump support because of low cardiac output was 16%. Overall, these data appear to be quite similar to the results of CABG in stable angina patients.

(2) At 7 to 10 years, approximately 80% of the patients who had undergone CABG had minimal or no angina symptoms. Late nonfatal MI occurred at a rate of 3% to 4% per year. The 5-year survival rate was approximately 90%, and the 10-year survival rate was higher than 80%. These are somewhat better than the survival rates for comparable patients in natural history studies or randomized trials.

3. PTCA versus CABG—Several large trials have compared PTCA versus CABG in patients with CAD (50,82,85). All of the reported findings were similar, with no major differences in survival between the two procedures, but patients treated with PTCA were two to three times more likely to require another revascularization procedure (PTCA or CABG) than those treated with CABG. For illustration, the results of the Bypass Angioplasty Revascularization Investigation (BARI) trial are discussed here (82). To date, the BARI trial is the largest reported randomized study (N=1829) to compare PTCA versus CABG. Selected patients with clinically severe angina or objective evidence of ischemia and multivessel CAD were randomly assigned to undergo either PTCA or CABG; 64% of the patients had symptoms of UA at the time of randomization. To be included, the patients had to have lesions amenable to treatment by either procedure. The mean age was 61 years, and 55% had a history of MI; patients were observed for a mean of 5.4 years (see Table 2-21).

a. There was no significant difference in overall survival between the two groups. However, for diabetic patients requiring insulin or oral hypoglycemic therapy (not a prespecified subgroup), the 5-year survival rate was significantly better with CABG than with PTCA (81% versus 65%, *P*=0.003).

b. The need for a subsequent revascularization procedure was substantially higher with PTCA than with CABG (54% versus 8%; *P*<0.001). Further-

Table 2-21 Results of the BARI trial (82)

	CABG (n=892)	PTCA (n=904)	*P*
Survival	89%	86%	NS
Survival without Q-wave MI	80%	79%	NS
Subsequent revascularization	8%	54%	<0.001
Average hospitalizations	1.9	2.5	<0.001

more, CABG patients were somewhat less likely to require subsequent hospitalization.

G. Conclusions

1. The Braunwald classification for UA has been prospectively validated to predict prognosis in patients with UA. This scheme takes into account the severity of symptoms, the clinical circumstances in which they occur, the presence or absence of ECG changes, and the intensity of medical therapy. There are three levels of classification: class I (new or accelerated angina without rest pain), II (subacute rest angina), or III (acute rest angina within 48 hours); class A (secondary UA), B (primary UA), or C (postinfarction UA); and subscript 1 (occurs in the setting of no or minimal therapy), 2 (occurs in the setting of appropriate oral therapy for stable angina), or 3 (occurs in the setting of maximally tolerated therapy with calcium channel blockers, β-blockers, and IV TNG).
2. Coronary artery atherosclerosis probably begins as a response to vascular injury. A complex set of events ultimately leads to proliferation of smooth muscle cells and fibroblasts and accumulation of lipid and fibrocellular material in the intima and media of the coronary vessels. These atherosclerotic plaques are susceptible to rupture. Plaque rupture and associated thrombosis may lead to rapid acceleration of atherogenesis and luminal stenosis. If this process stabilizes, the plaque may become a site of fixed stenosis and the patient may experience stable clinical symptoms. Alternatively, if the thrombotic process persists, it can lead to acute or subacute occlusion of the vessel and the patient may present with an acute coronary syndrome such as an acute MI or primary UA. Vasoconstriction at the site of the plaque also can contribute to coronary ischemia. For some patients, the major cause for the UA is a sudden increase in myocardial oxygen demand (*e.g.*, because of stress due to another illness) rather than plaque rupture or thrombosis.
3. Prognosis in UA is related to a number of clinical features. The AHCPR Guideline for UA defines a high-risk patient as a patient having at least one of the following: >20 minutes of ongoing rest pain; ischemia-related pulmonary edema; angina at rest with dynamic ST changes ≥1 mm; angina with new or worsening mitral regurgitation murmur, S_3, or rales; or angina with hypotension. Other predictors of poor prognosis include Braunwald class III (acute rest angina within 48 hours), Braunwald class C (postinfarction UA), angina refractory to maximal medical therapy, recurrence of angina after stabilization, diabetes mellitus, and older age.
4. The AHCPR Guideline has numerous recommendations for management of patients with UA. These recommendations were formulated by an expert panel and were based on much of the data presented in this chapter. Each recommendation is graded according to the strength of evidence available in the literature. Grade A recommendations are supported by at least one well-designed randomized controlled study; grade B recommendations are supported by well-designed clinical studies but no randomized trials; and grade C recommendations are reached by consensus of the panel in the absence of directly applicable clinical studies of adequate quality. Table 2-22 lists selected recommendations from the AHCPR Guideline (11). All of the grade A recommendations are presented, along with some of the grade B and grade C recommendations.

Table 2-22 Selected recommendations from the AHCPR Guideline (11)

Recommendation	Strength-of-Evidence Grade
Initial Evaluation and Treatment	
Patients with symptoms suggestive of UA should be evaluated by a medical practitioner in a facility equipped to perform an ECG.	B
Physicians should rapidly assess the risk of immediate adverse outcomes and the need for emergency diagnostic and therapeutic interventions.	B
Patients should be placed on continuous ECG monitoring.	C
IV thrombolytic therapy is not indicated if there is no acute ST segment elevation or left bundle branch block on the ECG.	A
In the absence of a definite contraindication, ASA (160–324 mg) should be given to all patients with suspected UA as soon as possible.	A
IV heparin should be started as soon as a diagnosis of intermediate- or high-risk angina is made.	A
Antiischemic medication should be used to relieve symptoms.	C
High-risk patients should be admitted to an ICU.	B
Intensive Medical Management	
IV or oral β-blockers should be started in the absence of contraindications.	B
IV TNG should be added if the patients remain symptomatic.	B
Nifedipine should not be used without concurrent administration of β-blockers.	A
ASA (80–324 mg/d) should be continued indefinitely.	A
Heparin infusion should be continued for 2–5 d or until revascularization.	C
Serum lipids may be measured within 24 h of presentation.	C
After patients have been stabilized on a medical regimen, consideration should be given to early invasive management.	A
Recurrent symptoms after initial stabilization may be regarded as a failure of therapy and should prompt consideration of urgent cardiac catheterization.	C
If ischemia persists ≥1 h on aggressive therapy, emergent catheterization should be considered.	B
Noninvasive Testing	
Unless catheterization is indicated, stress testing should be performed in low- and intermediate-risk patients who are free of angina and CHF for ≥48 h.	B
Patients with low-risk stress test results can be managed medically; those with intermediate-risk results should be referred for catheterization or additional functional testing with imaging; those with high-risk results should undergo cardiac catheterization.	B/C
Catheterization and Revascularization	
If an early invasive strategy is chosen, catheterization should be performed within 48 h.	A
Routine catheterization should be performed in all patients with UA who are candidates for revascularization and have one or more of the following: prior PTCA or CABG; associated CHF or depressed LV function; malignant ventricular arrhythmia; persistent or recurrent ischemia; high-risk functional study.	A
Patients with significant left main stenosis (≥50%) or significant three-vessel CAD with depressed LV function (ejection fraction <0.50) should be referred for CABG.	A
Patients with two-vessel disease including ≥95% stenosis of the LAD and decreased LV ejection fraction should be revascularized with either CABG (B) or PTCA (C).	B/C

Table 2-22 (continued)

Recommendation	Strength-of-Evidence Grade
Patients with other significant CAD may be managed with early revascularization or early conservative therapy (with revascularization performed only for those who fail medical therapy).	A
Patients should be counseled about the nature of UA and the need for lifestyle changes including smoking cessation, appropriate levels of daily exercise, and diet.	B/C

Abbreviations used in Chapter 2

AHCPR = Agency for Health Care Policy and Research of the US Department of Health and Human Services
aPTT = activated partial thromboplastin time
BID = twice daily
CABG = coronary artery bypass graft surgery
CAD = coronary artery disease
CCSC = Canadian Cardiovascular Society Classification of angina pectoris
CHF = congestive heart failure
CI = confidence interval
CK = creatine kinase
CK-MB = creatine kinase, cardiac-specific isoform
ECG = electrocardiogram
EF = ejection fraction
ETT = exercise tolerance testing
Fab = antigen-binding fragment (of immunoglobulins)
gp IIb/IIIa = platelet membrane glycoprotein IIb-IIIa, the platelet fibrinogen receptor
INR = international normalized ratio
IV = intravenous
LDL = low-density lipoprotein
LV = left ventricle, left ventricular
LV EF = left ventricular ejection fraction
MI = myocardial infarction
N = number of patients in population
n = number of patients in sample
NQWMI = non–Q-wave myocardial infarction
NS = not significant
OR = odds ratio
P = probability value
PAI-1 = plasminogen activator inhibitor-1
PRCT = prospective randomized controlled trial
PTCA = percutaneous transluminal coronary angioplasty
q = every
QD = daily
QID = four times daily
OR = odds ratio
RR = relative risk
RRR = Relative risk reduction
S_3 = third heart sound
SQ = subcutaneous

TID = three times daily
TNG = trinitroglycerin
tPA = tissue-type plasminogen activator
UA = unstable angina pectoris

References

1. Alderman. Ten-year follow-up of survival and myocardial infarction in the randomized coronary artery surgery study. *Circulation* 1990;82:1629.
2. Ambrose. Angiographic demonstration of a common link between unstable angina pectoris and non–Q wave acute myocardial infarction. *Am J Cardiol* 1988;61:244.
3. Ambrose. Quantitative and qualitative effects of intracoronary streptokinase in unstable angina and non–Q wave infarction. *J Am Coll Cardiol* 1987;9:1156.
4. Anderson. One year results of the TIMI-IIIB clinical trial. *J Am Coll Cardiol* 1995;26:1643.
5. Antiplatelet Trialists Collaboration. Collaborative overview of randomised trials of antiplatelet therapy: I. Prevention of death, myocardial infarction, and stroke by prolonged antiplatelet therapy in various categories of patients. *Br Med J* 1994;308:81. Review.
6. Ardissino. Recombinant tissue-type plasminogen activator followed by heparin compared with heparin alone for refractory unstable angina pectoris. *Am J Cardiol* 1990;66:910.
7. Balsano. Antiplatelet treatment with ticlopidine in unstable angina. *Circulation* 1990;82:17.
8. Bar. Thrombolysis in patients with unstable angina improves the angiographic but not the clinical outcome. *Circulation* 1992;86:131.
9. Betriu. Unstable angina: outcome according to clinical presentation. *J Am Coll Cardiol* 1992;19:1659.
10. Booth. Quality of life after bypass surgery for unstable angina. *Circulation* 1991; 83:87.
11. Braunwald. *Unstable Angina: Diagnosis and Management. Clinical Practice Guidelines*, vol 10. Washington: Agency for Health Care Policy and Research, 1994. Review.
12. Braunwald. Unstable angina: a classification. *Circulation* 1989;80:410.
13. Cairns. Aspirin, sulfinpyrazone, or both in unstable angina. *N Engl J Med* 1985;313:1369.
14. Calvin. Risk stratification in unstable angina. *JAMA* 1995;273:136.
15. Campeau. Grading of angina pectoris. *Circulation* 1976;54:522. Letter.
16. Chaitman. Effect of coronary bypass surgery on survival patterns in subsets of patients with left main coronary artery disease. *Am J Cardiol* 1981;48:765.
17. Cohen. Usefulness of ST-segment changes in ≥2 leads on the emergency room electrocardiogram in either unstable angina pectoris or non–Q wave myocardial infarction in predicting outcome. *Am J Cardiol* 1991;67:1368.
18. Cohen. Combination antithrombotic therapy in unstable rest angina and non–Q-wave infarction in nonprior aspirin users: primary endpoints analysis from the ATACS Trial. *Circulation* 1994;89:81.
19. de Feyter. Ischemia-related lesion characteristics in patients with stable or unstable angina. *Circulation* 1995;92:1408.
20. de Feyter. Coronary angioplasty for unstable angina: immediate and late results in 200 consecutive patients with identification of risk factors for unfavorable early and late outcome. *J Am Coll Cardiol* 1988;12:324.
21. DePace. Intravenous nitroglycerin for rest angina. *Arch Intern Med* 1982; 142:1806.
22. Detailed diagnoses and procedures: National Hospital Discharge Survey, 1992, Series 13, Number 118. Hyattsville, MD: US Department of Health and Human Services, 1994.

23. Falk. Unstable angina with fatal outcome: dynamic coronary thrombosis leading to infarction and/or sudden death. *Circulation* 1985;71:699.
24. Figueras. Rebound myocardial ischaemia following abrupt interruption of intravenous nitroglycerin infusion in patients with unstable angina at rest. *Eur Heart J* 1991;12:405.
25. Freeman. Thrombolysis in unstable angina. *Circulation* 1992;85:150.
26. Fuchs. Hirulog in the treatment of unstable angina. *Circulation* 1995;92:727.
27. Fuster. The pathogenesis of coronary artery disease and the acute coronary syndromes. *N Engl J Med* 1992;326:242,310. Review.
28. Fuster. Mechanisms leading to myocardial infarction: insights from studies of vascular biology. *Circulation* 1994;90:2126. Review.
29. Garcia-Dorado. Previous aspirin use may attenuate the severity of the manifestation of acute ischemic syndromes. *Circulation* 1995;92:1743.
30. Gazes. Preinfarctional (unstable) angina: a prospective study. Ten-year follow-up. *Circulation* 1973;68:331.
31. Gerstenblith. Nifedipine in unstable angina. *N Engl J Med* 1982;306:885.
32. Gobel. Randomised, double-blind trial of intravenous diltiazem versus glyceryl trinitrate for unstable angina pectoris. *Lancet* 1995;346:1653.
33. Gold. A randomized, blinded, placebo-controlled trial of recombinant human tissue-type plasminogen activator in patients with unstable angina pectoris. *Circulation* 1987;75:1192.
34. Gorgels. Value of the electrocardiogram in diagnosing the number of severely narrowed coronary arteries in rest angina pectoris. *Am J Cardiol* 1993;72:999.
35. Gottlieb. Effect of the addition of propranolol to therapy with nifedipine for unstable angina pectoris: a randomized, double-blind, placebo-controlled trial. *Circulation* 1986;73:331.
36. Grande. Unstable angina pectoris: platelet behavior and prognosis in progressive angina and intermediate coronary syndrome. *Circulation* 1990;81:I-16.
37. Granger. Rebound increase in thrombin generation and activity after cessation of intravenous heparin in patients with acute coronary syndromes. *Circulation* 1995;91:1929.
38. Gurfinkel. Importance of thrombosis and thrombolysis in silent ischaemia: comparison of patients with acute myocardial infarction and unstable angina. *Br Heart J* 1994;71:151.
39. Gurfinkel. Low molecular weight heparin versus regular heparin or aspirin in the treatment of unstable angina and silent ischemia. *J Am Coll Cardiol* 1995;26:313.
40. Haft. Correlation of atherectomy specimen histology with coronary arteriographic lesion morphologic appearance in patients with stable and unstable angina. *Am Heart J* 1995;130:420.
41. Hamm. The prognostic value of serum troponin T in unstable angina. *N Engl J Med* 1992;327:146.
42. Hargarten. Prehospital prophylactic lidocaine does not favorably affect outcome in patients with chest pain. *Ann Emerg Med* 1990;19:1274.
43. Holdright. Comparison of the effect of heparin and aspirin versus aspirin alone on transient myocardial ischemia and in-hospital prognosis in patients with unstable angina. *J Am Coll Cardiol* 1994;24:39.
44. Horowitz. Combined use of nitroglycerin and *N*-acetylcysteine in the management of unstable angina pectoris. *Circulation* 1988;77:787.
45. Huang. Heart rate variability depression in patients with unstable angina. *Am Heart J* 1995;130:772.
46. Huber. Heparin induced increase of tPA antigen plasma levels in patients with unstable angina. *Thromb Res* 1989;55:779.
47. Kaiser. Myocardial revascularization for unstable angina pectoris. *Circulation* 1989;79:I-60. Review.
48. Kamp. Short-, medium-, and long-term follow-up after percutaneous transluminal coronary angioplasty for stable and unstable angina pectoris. *Am Heart J* 1989; 117:991.
49. Kaplan. Intravenous nitroglycerin for the treatment of angina at rest unresponsive to standard nitrate therapy. *Am J Cardiol* 1983;51:694.

50. King. A randomized trial comparing coronary angioplasty with coronary bypass surgery. *N Engl J Med* 1994;331:1044.
51. Langer. ST segment shift in unstable angina: pathophysiology and association with coronary anatomy and hospital outcome. *J Am Coll Cardiol* 1989;13:1495.
52. Langford. Platelet activation in acute myocardial infarction and unstable angina is inhibited by nitric oxide donors. *Arterioscler Thromb Vasc Biol* 1996;16:51.
53. Larsson. Diagnostic and prognostic importance of ST recording after an episode of unstable angina or non–Q-wave myocardial infarction. *Eur Heart J* 1992;13: 207.
54. Lawrence. Fibrinolytic therapy in unstable angina pectoris: a controlled clinical trial. *Thromb Res* 1980;17:767.
55. Lewis. Protective effects of aspirin against acute myocardial infarction and death in men with unstable angina. *N Engl J Med* 1983;309:396.
56. Lloyd-Jones. The vascular biology of nitric oxide and its role in atherogenesis. *Annu Rev Med* 1996;47:365. Review.
57. Lubsen. Early treatment of unstable angina in the coronary care unit: a randomised, double-blind, placebo-controlled comparison of recurrent ischemia in patients with nifedipine or metoprolol or both. *Br Heart J* 1986;56:400.
58. Luchi. Comparison of medical and surgical treatment for unstable angina pectoris. *N Engl J Med* 1987;316:977.
59. Mark. Clinical characteristics and long-term survival of patients with variant angina. *Circulation* 1984;69:880.
60. Mizuno. Angioscopic evaluation of coronary artery thrombi in acute coronary syndromes. *N Engl J Med* 1992;326:287.
61. Moss. Detection and significance of myocardial ischemia in stable patients after recovery from an acute coronary event. *JAMA* 1993;269:2379.
62. Muller. Nifedipine and conventional therapy for unstable angina pectoris: a randomized, double-blind comparison. *Circulation* 1984;69:728.
63. Nicklas. Randomized, double-blind, placebo-controlled trial of tissue plasminogen activator in unstable angina. *J Am Coll Cardiol* 1989;13:434.
64. Nyman. Very early risk stratification by electrocardiogram at rest in men with suspected unstable coronary heart disease. *J Intern Med* 1993;234:293.
65. Nyman. The predictive value of silent ischemia at an exercise test before discharge after an episode of unstable coronary artery disease. *Am Heart J* 1992; 123:324.
66. Packer. Combined beta-adrenergic and calcium-entry blockade in angina pectoris. *N Engl J Med* 1989;320:709. Review.
67. Parisi. Medical compared with surgical management of unstable angina: 5-year mortality and morbidity in the Veterans Administration Study. *Circulation* 1989;80:1176.
68. Reddy. Evidence that selective endothelial dysfunction may occur in the absence of angiographic or ultrasound atherosclerosis in patients with risk factors for atherosclerosis. *J Am Coll Cardiol* 1994;23:833.
69. Rizik. A new clinical classification for hospital prognosis of unstable angina pectoris. *Am J Cardiol* 1995;75:993.
70. Romeo. Unstable angina: role of silent ischemia and total ischemic time (silent plus painful ischemia): a 6-year follow-up. *J Am Coll Cardiol* 1992;19:1173.
71. Romeo. Effectiveness of prolonged low dose recombinant tissue-type plasminogen activator for refractory unstable angina. *J Am Coll Cardiol* 1995;25: 1295.
72. Ross. The pathogenesis of atherosclerosis: a perspective for the 1990s. *Nature* 1993;362:801. Review.
73. Scandinavian Simvastatin Survival Study Group. Randomised trial of cholesterol lowering in 4444 patients with coronary heart disease: the Scandinavian Simvastatin Survival Study (4S). *Lancet* 1994;344:1383.
74. Schreiber. Randomized trial of thrombolysis versus heparin in unstable angina. *Circulation* 1992;86:1407.
75. Serneri. Randomised comparison of subcutaneous heparin, intravenous heparin, and aspirin in unstable angina. *Lancet* 1995;345:1201.

76. Sharma. Coronary bypass surgery improves survival in high-risk unstable angina. *Circulation* 1991;83:III-260.
77. Sherman. Coronary angioscopy in patients with unstable angina pectoris. *N Engl J Med* 1986;315:913.
78. Silva. Unstable angina: a comparison of angioscopic findings between diabetic and nondiabetic patients. *Circulation* 1995;92:1731.
79. Simoons. Randomized trial of a GPIIb/IIIa platelet receptor blocker in refractory unstable angina. *Circulation* 1994;89:596.
80. Swahn. Predictive importance of clinical findings and a predischarge exercise test in patients with suspected unstable coronary artery disease. *Am J Cardiol* 1987;59:208.
81. Telford. Trial of heparin versus atenolol in prevention of myocardial infarction in intermediate coronary syndrome. *Lancet* 1981;1:1225.
82. The BARI Investigators. Comparison of coronary bypass surgery with angioplasty in patients with multivessel disease. *N Engl J Med* 1996;335:217.
83. The GUSTO IIa Investigators. Randomized trial of intravenous heparin versus recombinant hirudin for acute coronary syndromes. *Circulation* 1994;90:1631.
84. The RISC Group. Risk of myocardial infarction and death during treatment with low dose aspirin and intravenous heparin in men with unstable coronary artery disease. *Lancet* 1990;336:827.
85. The RITA Investigators. Coronary angioplasty versus coronary artery bypass surgery: the Randomized Intervention Treatment of Angina (RITA) trial. *Lancet* 1993;341:573.
86. Theroux. Aspirin, heparin, or both to treat acute unstable angina. *N Engl J Med* 1988;319:1105.
87. Theroux. Aspirin versus heparin to prevent myocardial infarction during the acute phase of unstable angina. *Circulation* 1993;88:2045.
88. Theroux. Reactivation of unstable angina after the discontinuation of heparin. *N Engl J Med* 1992;327:141.
89. Theroux. A randomized study comparing propranolol and diltiazem in the treatment of unstable angina. *J Am Coll Cardiol* 1985;5:717.
90. The TIMI-IIIA Investigators. Early effects of tissue-type plasminogen activator added to conventional therapy on the culprit coronary lesion in patients presenting with ischemic cardiac pain at rest. *Circulation* 1993;87:38.
91. The TIMI-IIIB Investigators. Effects of tissue plasminogen activator and a comparison of early invasive and conservative strategies in unstable angina and non–Q-wave myocardial infarction. *Circulation* 1994;89:1545.
92. Topol. Recombinant hirudin for unstable angina pectoris. *Circulation* 1994;89:1557.
93. van Miltenburg-van Zijl. Incidence and follow-up of Braunwald subgroups in unstable angina pectoris. J Am Coll Cardiol 1995;25:1286.
94. Vetrovec. Intracoronary thrombolysis in syndromes of unstable ischemia: angiographic and clinical results. *Am Heart J* 1982;104:946.
95. Wallentin. Aspirin (75 mg/day) after an episode of unstable coronary artery disease: long-term effects on the risk for myocardial infarction, occurrence of severe angina and the need for revascularization. *J Am Coll Cardiol* 1991;18:1587.
96. Waters. Previous coronary artery bypass grafting as an adverse prognostic factor in unstable angina pectoris. *Am J Cardiol* 1986;58:465.
97. Wilcox. Risk of adverse outcome in patients admitted to the coronary care unit with suspected unstable angina pectoris. *Am J Cardiol* 1989;64:845.
98. Wu. Prognostic value of cardiac troponin T in unstable angina pectoris. *Am J Cardiol* 1995;76:970.
99. Yusuf. Overview of results of randomised clinical trials in heart disease. *JAMA* 1988;260:2259. Review.
100. Yusuf. Effect of intravenous nitrates on mortality in acute myocardial infarction: an overview of the randomised trials. *Lancet* 1988;1:1082. Review.
101. Zeiher. Tissue endothelin-1 immunoreactivity in the active coronary atherosclerotic plaque. *Circulation* 1995;91:941.

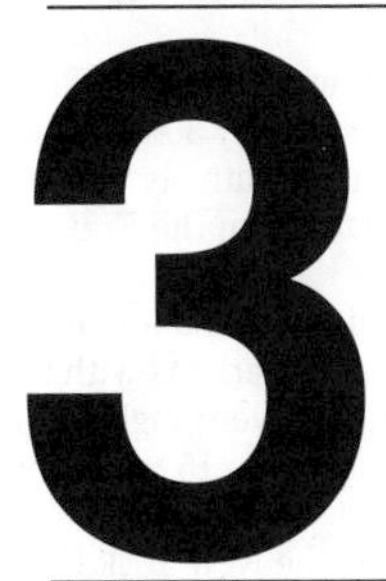

Congestive Heart Failure: Systolic Failure

Stephen I. Hsu and
Patrick T. O'Gara

A. Introduction

1. Congestive heart failure (CHF) is a common and highly lethal condition in the United States. About 400,000 patients with CHF entered the health care system in 1980, generating more than 900,000 hospitalizations at an estimated annual cost of almost $9 billion (177). In the population-based Framingham Heart Study, in which 5192 persons initially free of cardiac disease were observed over a 34-year period (1949 through 1983), the overall annual incidence of CHF was 1.3% in men and 1.0% in women (98,119).
   a. At all ages, men had a higher incidence of CHF than women. This gender difference most likely reflected the higher rate of coronary artery disease (CAD) among men, which conferred a fourfold increased risk of CHF (98).
   b. Advanced age was a major risk factor for the development of CHF; the incidence of CHF was 0.2% for 45- to 55-year-old subjects but roughly doubled with each decade of age increment (98).
   c. Hypertension, with or without CAD, preceded the onset of CHF in 76% of men and 79% of women at 32-year follow-up. CAD was present in 46% of men and 27% of women (98).
2. Isolated systolic failure arises from a defect in the ability of myofibrils to shorten against a load, which results in a depressed ejection fraction (EF), pulmonary or systemic venous congestion (or both), and low cardiac output. Clinical manifestation of isolated systolic failure can include exercise intolerance, dyspnea, fatigue, prerenal azotemia, cool skin, and mental obtundation. In contrast, isolated diastolic failure arises from an increased resistance to ventricular filling, which results primarily in pulmonary or systemic venous congestion (or both). Clinical manifestation of isolated diastolic failure include exercise intolerance, dyspnea, and fatigue (72). Although most patients with CHF have components of both systolic and diastolic dysfunction, recognition of the predominant abnormality has important therapeutic and prognostic implications. The focus of this chapter is on systolic heart failure; diastolic heart failure is discussed in Chapter 4.
   a. A consideration of the patient's history, physical findings, electrocardiogram, and chest film may sometimes offer clues that help distinguish systolic from diastolic CHF. A history of multiple myocardial infarctions (MIs), Q waves on the electrocardiogram, third heart sound (S_3 gallop), and cardiomegaly favor the diagnosis of systolic CHF (78).
   b. However, clinical criteria alone lack sufficient sensitivity and specificity to accurately differentiate systolic from diastolic CHF. In a study of 407 patients referred for resting radionuclide ventriculography to assess left ventricular (LV) EF, 20% of the 153 patients with LV EF ≤40% met none of the clinical criteria for systolic CHF, whereas 51% of the 204 patients with LV EF ≥50% met at least one criterion (115). A combination of clinical features and an objective assessment of LV function (*e.g.*, echocardiography, radionuclide scanning) is usually necessary for appropriate management of systolic CHF.

3. **Prognosis**—The morbidity and mortality associated with overt CHF is extraordinarily high and rivals that of cancer (119). Approximately 30% to 50% of all cardiac deaths in patients with CHF are sudden and relatively unexpected (118). For illustration, the mortality and morbidity data from the Framingham Heart Study are summarized in Table 3-1 (98).
   a. **Age and Gender**—In the NHANES-I Epidemiologic Follow-up Study (1982 to 1986), the 10- and 15-year mortality rates for persons with CHF increased in a graded fashion with advancing age and were higher for men than for women at all ages. For patients ≥55 years old, the 15-year mortality rate was 71.8% for men and 39.1% for women (153).
   b. **Functional Class**—The severity of CHF based on the New York Heart Association (NYHA) functional classification of heart disease also correlates with mortality (32,38,175). For example, in one study, the 1-year mortality rate for patients in NYHA class IV was 66%, compared with 22% for those in classes I through III (19).
   c. **Ejection Fraction**—The severity of CHF based on LV EF was the strongest predictor of survival in several major prospective studies (19,33,82). These findings are summarized in Table 3-2. Cohn also emphasized the importance of low exercise capacity and high serum catecholamine concentrations as independent predictors of survival (33).
   d. **Presence of CAD**—As shown in Table 3-3, the mortality rate for heart failure patients with CAD is significantly higher than for those with idiopathic dilated cardiomyopathy (IDCM) (32,66). In one study, the excess mortality in the CAD group occurred mostly in the initial 6 months after an MI (66). In contrast, Wilson found no difference in mortality between these two groups, but Wilson's study excluded patients who had had an acute MI during the previous 6 months (175).
   e. **Systolic Versus Diastolic CHF**—As is discussed in Chapter 4, the mortality rate for patients with primary systolic failure and low LV EF is signifi-

Table 3-1 Mortality and morbidity associated with CHF (98)

Outcome	Men	Women
Mortality at 2y	37%	38%
Mortality at 6y	82%	67%
Sudden Death*	28%	14%
Recurrent CHF at 6y	70%	63%
Risk of stroke	Fourfold increase	

*Expressed as percentage of cardiovascular deaths.

Table 3-2 Survival as a function of LV EF in major prospective studies of CHF

Study (Reference)	Length of Follow-Up	LV EF (%)	Probability of Survival (%)
Califf (19)	3y	10	21
		20	32
		30	47
		40	69
Cohn (33)	1y	13±2	47±11
		20±3	91±6
		25±2	77±8
		40±8	85±7
Gradman (82)	16 mo	≤20	73
		≥30	93

Table 3-3 Comparison of mortality in patients with CHF due to CAD vs. IDCM

	Cumulative Mortality (%)						
	CAD			IDCM			
Study (Reference)	1 Y	2 Y	3 Y	1 Y	2 Y	3 Y	*P*
Franciosa (66)	34	59	76	23	48	—	<0.01
Cohn (32)	23	40	60	17	29	40	<0.02

cantly higher than for those with primary diastolic failure and preserved LV EF (34).

B. Pathophysiology of Systolic Heart Failure

1. Circulatory Pathophysiology of Systolic Failure

a. Impaired Cardiac Performance—The primary abnormality in systolic failure is impaired myocardial contractility. This may be expressed as a downward shift in the Frank–Starling curve, which relates stroke volume (cardiac performance) to preload (or end-diastolic fiber length) for a given afterload and inotropic state. Fatigue, dyspnea, and exercise intolerance result from limited ability to increase the stroke volume during exercise and from the high LV filling pressures required to maintain adequate cardiac output (72,78).

b. Ventricular Remodeling

(1) Hypertrophic Response to Chronic Overload—Heart failure can result from various causes of ventricular overload such as chronic hypertension or valvular heart disease (160). The myocardial response to sustained pressure or volume overload is hypertrophy, which tends to normalize wall tension by distributing excess load among an increased number of sarcomeres. This response is predicted by Laplace's Law: $T=Pr/2h$, where T is wall tension, P is the chamber pressure, r is the radius of the chamber, and h is the thickness of the wall. The addition of new sarcomeres has an energy-sparing effect because it decreases the rate of expenditure of mechanical energy by the overloaded sarcomeres (102).

(2) Hypertrophic Response to Acute Myocardial Injury—In the setting of loss of cardiac myocytes, as may occur with an MI, the end-diastolic volume may increase as a result of infarct expansion or a rise in filling pressure, or both. To compensate for the depressed EF in the acute setting, ventricular dilation takes advantage of the Frank–Starling mechanism to maintain stroke volume (138). As the ventricle dilates, the ventricular wall becomes thinner. As predicted by Laplace's law, the dilation of the chamber (higher r) and thinning of the wall (lower h) increase the wall stress and thereby augment the degree of hypertrophy required to normalize wall tension (160). With a large transmural infarct, the hypertrophic response may prove inadequate, and a vicious cycle of progressive LV enlargement and reduced EF may ensue (138).

c. Compensatory Neurohormonal Activation in Response to Low Output State—As cardiac output drops, a series of neurohormonal compensatory mechanisms is activated in an attempt to maintain adequate tissue perfusion. Reflex activation of the sympathetic nervous system (SNS) and the renin-angiotensin-aldosterone system (RAAS) causes arteriolar vasoconstriction. Furthermore, activation of RAAS and secretion of antidiuretic hormone (vasopressin) cause salt and water retention. The degree to which these systems are activated is proportional to the severity of heart failure (30,53,78). Although vasoconstriction and volume retention typically help in the short term, they can be detrimental in the long term and largely account for the clinical syndrome of heart failure (102). The impedance to ejection of blood during systole is often increased beyond the level necessary to maintain effective perfusion pressure (29). Under these circumstances, the impaired left ventricle may not be able to compensate for the increased afterload. As a result, the EF and stroke volume fall even further, creating a vicious cycle of progressive reduction in cardiac output and progressive rise in afterload (30).

d. Role of Counterregulatory Hormones

(1) **Atrial Natriuretic Peptide (ANP)**—This peptide hormone is released from the atria in response to increased central cardiac pressures. ANP levels are increased in CHF. In early stages of CHF, ANP antagonizes the effects of angiotensin II (AT II), promoting vasodilation and renal salt excretion. It may also counter SNS activation by modulating the baroreceptor reflexes. In later stages of CHF, there is a diminished responsiveness to ANP which may be related to receptor downregulation (28). The circulating levels of ANP correlate with the levels of norepinephrine (NE) and the plasma renin activity (PRA). In a study from the Studies of Left Ventricular Dysfunction (SOLVD) registry, the level of ANP correlated better with LV EF than did NE, PRA, or arginine vasopressin (AVP) (8). High levels of ANP predict poor survival in patients with chronic CHF (81,162). The ANP level likely reflects the severity of CHF and the degree of neurohormonal response, which may contribute to mortality in this disease (see later discussion).

(2) **Prostaglandins**—During states of hypoperfusion, vasodilatory prostaglandins are released locally and act to preserve renal and coronary blood flow in the setting of high circulating levels of AT II and NE (48). The importance of prostaglandins in modulating the effects of the activated SNS and RAAS is emphasized by the observation that acute cardiac decompensation has been associated with indomethacin use in hyponatremic patients with CHF (48).

(3) **Endothelium-Derived Relaxing Factor**—Endothelial cells produce a number of substances (including nitric oxide) that are collectively termed endothelium-derived relaxing factor (EDRF) and that cause relaxation of local vascular smooth muscle cells. Endothelium-dependent vasodilation is impaired in patients with CHF, as documented by a decrease in vasodilatory response to methacholine, a known stimulus of EDRF release (107).

e. Prognostic Significance of Neurohormonal Activation—Neuroendocrine activation occurs in the very early stages of ventricular dysfunction and typically before the onset of symptoms. The degree of activation increases in proportion to the extent of ventricular dysfunction and correlates with poor survival (31,68,69,139,162).

(1) Cohn reported that an increased level of NE was an independent predictor of poor survival by multivariate analysis (P=0.002) in patients with CHF. In fact, a single resting value of NE was a better prognostic indicator than the commonly measured indices of cardiac performance (31). These findings were also confirmed in the Vasodilators in Heart Failure Trial II (V-HeFT II) (69).

(2) In a substudy from the SOLVD registry, the median values for plasma NE (P=0.0001), ANP (P<0.0001), AVP (P=0.006), and PRA (P=0.03) were significantly higher in patients with impaired LV function (EF <35%) than in control subjects. Furthermore, independent of functional class or concomitant drug therapy, the degree of neurohormonal activation correlated inversely with the LV EF (68).

(3) In the Survival and Ventricular Enlargement (SAVE) trial, Rouleau reported increased levels of PRA, NE, AVP, and ANP immediately after an acute MI in a large number of patients who had asymptomatic LV dysfunction (LV EF ≤40%). Therefore, it appears that a subgroup of patients undergo neurohormonal activation after an acute MI even in

the absence of overt CHF. It is likely that the improved survival with captopril in these patients (see later discussion) is a result of attenuation of the neurohormonal activation in the post-MI period (150).

(4) Finally, the placebo arm of the Cooperative North Scandinavian Enalapril Survival (CONSENSUS) study demonstrated a significant positive correlation between mortality and the levels of AT II ($P<0.05$), aldosterone ($P=0.003$), NE ($P<0.001$), epinephrine ($P=0.001$), and ANP ($P=0.003$). Treatment with enalapril was associated with a significant reduction in the levels of these hormones and improved survival. The survival benefit was observed mainly among those patients with the highest hormone levels at baseline (162).

2. Consequences of Chronic Activation of the β-Adrenergic System

a. Myocardial contractility is regulated principally by the SNS (53). In normal hearts, the ratio of β_1- to β_2-adrenergic receptors is approximately 80:20 (14). The binding of a β-agonist (*e.g.*, NE) to the β_1 receptor causes the G_s protein (the stimulatory component of the G protein–adenylate cyclase complex) to activate adenylate cyclase. Adenylate cyclase converts adenosine triphosphate to cyclic adenosine monophosphate (cAMP), which in turn phosphorylates sarcolemmal and sarcoplasmic reticulum proteins. Phosphorylation of these proteins increases the intracellular calcium ion (Ca^{2+}) flux and promotes cardiac excitation-contraction coupling. The G_s protein also directly stimulates the sarcolemmal Ca^{2+} channels and inhibits the sarcolemmal sodium (Na^+) channels, further increasing the intracellular Ca^{2+} ion concentration and augmenting myocardial contractility.

b. In the setting of CHF, aortic and cardiac baroreceptors are reset, and therefore their chronic inhibitory effect on SNS traffic is attenuated. (53,110) This leads to chronic sympathetic activation and vasoconstriction (31).

c. Furthermore, a deficiency in cAMP production appears to be a fundamental defect in end-stage failing hearts (58). One mechanism for this deficiency may be a progressive downregulation of the myocardial β_1-adrenergic receptors in response to high synaptic levels of NE. Another mechanism may be an uncoupling of the β_2-adrenergic receptor from adenylate cyclase, mediated by the G_i protein (the inhibitory component of the G protein–adenylate cyclase complex) (15,59). In addition, the ratio of β_1- to β_2-receptors is reduced (to approximately 60:40) in comparison with the normal heart, so that the failing ventricle becomes less inotropically responsive to a given level of β-adrenergic stimulation (14).

d. High catecholamine levels may be directly toxic to the myocardium. For example, NE activation of the α-adrenergic system has been shown to cause a cardiomyopathy in rabbits that is characterized by focal or diffuse interstitial myonecrosis (47,73). Similar lesions have been described in patients with pheochromocytoma who died of cardiac causes (171). β-Blocker therapy has been reported to reverse the ventricular dysfunction in patients with presumed catecholamine-induced dilated cardiomyopathy (85,92).

e. Myocardial energy expenditure is increased by the inotropic and chronotropic effects of sympathetic-adrenergic stimulation. In the chronically overloaded heart, this response may exaggerate the existing imbalance between energy supply and energy demand (101). Because ventricular relaxation is an energy-dependent process, depletion of high-energy phosphates may lead to worsening diastolic dysfunction (see Chapter 4). Furthermore, a sustained energy deficit may accelerate the rate of myocardial cell death (102). Finally, chronic inotropic stimulation may increase the risk of arrhythmias (100).

3. Consequences of Chronic Activation of the RAAS

a. Normal Heart

(1) Circulatory RAAS—The hormone renin is released by the macula densa in response to β_1-adrenergic stimulation or hyponatremia. It is also released in response to decreased volume and perfusion pressure as sensed by the juxtaglomerular apparatus. Renin acts on angiotensinogen to form angiotensin I (AT I), which is then converted into AT II by angiotensin-converting enzyme (ACE). AT II is a potent arteriolar vasoconstrictor and also promotes Na^+ and water retention in the renal proximal tubule. In addition, AT II induces aldosterone release from the adrenal cortex, resulting in enhanced Na^+ reabsorption in the renal distal tubule (51).

(2) **Tissue RAAS**—Studies have documented that 90% to 99% of ACE in the body is expressed on the endothelium of vascular tissue (tissue RAAS), and that only 1% to 10% is found in the circulation (circulatory RAAS) (51). Indeed, all components of the RAAS are found at various tissue sites and act locally (most notably in the heart and kidney). Cardiac tissue RAAS appears to exert long-term effects on the structure and the function of the heart and likely plays a key role in the pathophysiology of CHF (49).

b. The Failing Heart

(1) **Circulatory RAAS**—Aldosterone and AT II promote vasoconstriction and retention of Na^+ and water and thereby maintain blood pressure in the setting of acute cardiovascular decompensation. Circulating AT II has a short half-life, and circulating RAAS is turned off after cardiovascular stability is achieved (90).

(2) **Cardiac RAAS**—Several pathophysiologic roles of the cardiac tissue RAAS have been proposed by Hirsch and are shown in Table 3-4 (90). In contrast to the circulatory RAAS, cardiac tissue RAAS is activated in the setting of chronic compensated CHF, at a time when the circulatory RAAS activity is normal or only mildly increased. The cardiac tissue RAAS may be activated in response to increased wall tension and likely plays a key role in cardiac remodeling (see Chapter 4). (90) Inhibition of tissue RAAS (rather than circulatory RAAS) may be the basis for the well-documented benefit of ACE inhibitors on ventricular remodeling after MI (51). In addition, AT II has been shown to have direct cardiotoxic effects independent of its hypertensive effect. The cardiotoxic effect of AT II was not attenuated by β-blockade but was prevented by ACE inhibition (164).

(3) **Vascular RAAS**—A complete tissue RAAS has been localized to the vascular endothelium in arteries and veins (50). AT II that is formed within large vessels can increase afterload and augment preload (49). Furthermore, AT II induces protooncogene and autocrine growth factor expression in vascular smooth muscle cells. It may therefore be important in the pathogenesis of hypertensive vascular hypertrophy, neointimal hyperplasia, and atherosclerosis (128).

(4) **Renal RAAS**—Angiotensin is produced locally at the proximal tubule, glomerulus, and renal blood vessels (including vasa recta).

Table 3-4 Proposed role of the cardiac tissue RAAS in chronic compensated CHF

Potential Tissue Effects	Pathophysiological Consequences
Direct cellular AT II effects on cardiac myocytes	Positive inotropic effect, diastolic dysfunction
AT II–mediated stimulation of NE release from sympathetic nerve endings	Positive inotropic effect, dysrhythmia induction
Coronary artery vasoconstriction	Subendocardial ischemia
Protooncogene expression	Cardiac hypertrophy and remodeling

Adapted from Hirsch (90).

Along with the cardiac tissue RAAS, renal tissue RAAS is preferentially activated in the setting of chronic compensated CHF. It may regulate glomerular and intrarenal hemodynamics and stimulate proximal tubular AT II receptors, which are important in Na^+ reabsorption and pH regulation. Chronic activation may lead to glomerular hypertension (50).

4. **Role of Arginine Vasopressin**—The antidiuretic hormone AVP is a powerful endogenous vasoconstrictor that can potentiate the effects of AT II and NE (67). The stimuli for the increase in AVP levels are not well defined for patients with CHF but probably involve nonosmotic factors such as an impairment in baroreceptor-mediated inhibition of brainstem centers and direct stimulation of hypophyseal production of AVP by AT II (67,77).
5. **Role of Endothelins**—This family of endothelium-derived peptides is the most potent class of vasoconstrictors known for arterial and venous smooth muscle cells. These peptides cause coronary, renal, and systemic vasoconstriction at physiologic doses (121). The level of endothelins may be increased twofold in patients with severe CHF and is inversely correlated with the LV EF ($r=-0.279$; $P=0.037$) (148). Therefore, endothelins may also contribute to the high systemic vascular tone that characterizes chronic CHF. In vitro studies suggest that endothelins may enhance smooth muscle and cardiac cell growth, which lends support for their potential role in ventricular hypertrophy and remodeling (96,129).
6. **Cardiomyopathy of Overload**—Katz coined the phrase "cardiomyopathy of overload" to describe the deleterious effects of sustained overload and the cellular abnormalities that characterize the hypertrophic response (102). The latter include (a) expression of new isoforms of actin and myosin, which may represent an adaptive response to the changes in cardiac loading conditions; (b) reduced concentrations of calcium-pump adenosine triphosphatase (Ca^{2+}-ATPase) molecules in the sarcoplasmic reticulum, which may slow Ca^{2+} uptake during myocardial relaxation and lead to diastolic dysfunction; and (c) expression of abnormal isoforms of various ion channels, which may play a role in the development of arrhythmias in the failing heart.

C. **Drug Therapy for Systolic Failure**—The physiologic goals of drug therapy are to decrease the ventricular filling pressure and to improve the systolic performance of the failing heart. The former can be accomplished by reducing preload. The latter can be achieved by directly increasing stroke volume, treating ischemia, preserving atrial contraction by maintenance of sinus rhythm, preventing tachycardia, and reducing afterload. Additional physiologic goals are to limit ventricular enlargement and to reverse the compensatory vascular and neurohormonal changes that contribute to the pathogenesis of chronic CHF. The clinical goals of drug therapy (see Table 3-5) include symptom relief, enhanced exercise tolerance, prevention of complications (*e.g.*, stroke), and improved survival (78). With these goals in mind, each class of medications used for treatment of systolic CHF is discussed in further detail in the sections that follow.

1. **Vasodilators**—LV systolic function is exquisitely sensitive to changes in afterload, so that even a small reduction in afterload can significantly increase the stroke volume, provide long-term symptom relief, and enhance exercise tolerance (30,78). Furthermore, in several large multicenter trials (discussed later), vasodilator therapy has significantly improved survival in patients with LV dysfunction.

a. **Direct-Acting Vasodilators: Nitrates, Hydralazine, and α-Antagonists**

(1) A metaanalysis of 28 prospective randomized controlled trials (PRCTs) of vasodilator therapy in chronic CHF showed that all classes of vasodilators except hydralazine were associated with a statistically significant improvement in functional status. α-Antagonists such as prazosin and trimazosin were consistently associated with the greatest functional improvement (OR, 10.17; 95% CI, 5.25 to 19.7). No survival benefit was observed for nitrates, hydralazine, or α-antagonists. In fact, nitrates were associated with a statistically nonsignifi-

Table 3-5 Goals of therapy for systolic dysfunction

Goal	Pharmacologic Approach
Promote myocardial contractility	
Increase stroke volume	Inotropic agents Digoxin β-Adrenergic Agonists Dopaminergic Agonists Phosphodiesterase Inhibitors Calcium-sensitizing Agents
Prevent/treat ischemia	Antiischemic drugs β-Adrenergic blockers Ca^{2+} channel blockers Nitrates
Maintain atrial contraction	Cardioversion for AF Sequential AV Pacemaker Antiarrhythmic Drugs
Reduce heart rate	β-adrenergic blockers Ca^{2+} Channel blockers
Reduce afterload	Vasodilators ACE inhibitors Hydralazine Nitrates α-Antagonists
Reduce preload	Diuretics Salt restriction Nitrates
Prevent/reduce ventricular enlargement	Remodeling drugs: ACE inhibitors Surgery: valve reconstruction or replacement
Prevent clot formation	Anticoagulant drugs

cant trend toward increased mortality (OR, 2.26; 95% CI, 0.58 to 8.84). Only ACE inhibitors improved both survival and functional status (see later discussion) (125).

(2) The V-HeFT I Study—This landmark study included 642 men with mild to moderate symptoms of chronic CHF and LV EF <45% (mean, 30%) who were receiving optimal doses of digoxin and diuretics (32). Patients were randomly assigned to receive prazosin (5 mg PO QID), a combination of isosorbide dinitrate (20 to 40 mg PO QID) and hydralazine (37.5 to 75 mg PO QID), or placebo. The average length of follow-up was 2.3 years. Treatment with the isosorbide-hydralazine combination was associated with reductions in mortality of 38% and 23% at 1 and 3 years, respectively (see Table 3-6). A small increase in LV EF was also observed in this group. Prazosin showed no advantage over placebo. However, side effects were more common with the

Table 3-6 V-HeFT I: Isosorbide-hydralazine combination for chronic CHF (32)

	Isosorbide Dinitrate–Hydralazine (n=186)	Placebo (n=273)	*P*
2-Y mortality EF	25.6%	34.3%	<0.028
Change in LV EF at 1 y	+1.4%	−0.1%	<0.001

isosorbide-hydralazine combination; only 55% of the patients were taking full doses of both drugs at 6 months. In a follow-up report of V-HeFT I, the absolute change in LV EF at 8 weeks was highly correlated with subsequent survival after adjusting for all other significant prognostic variables, including the treatment assignment ($P<0.0004$) (4).

(3) Based on another PRCT of 49 patients randomly assigned to receive hydralazine (225 mg PO QD), isosorbide dinitrate (160 mg PO QD), hydralazine-isosorbide combination, or placebo, Packer argued that the beneficial effect of the isosorbide-hydralazine combination was most likely related to hydralazine than to isosorbide. After 3 months of therapy, LV systolic function was significantly improved in patients taking either hydralazine alone or the isosorbide-hydralazine combination, but not in those taking isosorbide dinitrate alone (133,165). Similarly, in the Gruppo Italiano per lo Studio della Sopravvivena nell Infarto Miocardico (GISSI-3) trial, nitrates were no better than placebo in terms of survival benefit (see later discussion) (122).

b. Angiotensin-Converting Enzyme Inhibitors—ACE inhibitors improve symptoms and prolong survival in patients with LV systolic failure. ACE inhibitors increase coronary blood flow, decrease afterload, and attenuate the maladaptive compensatory neurohormonal activation that is characteristic of compensated CHF. In addition, they may improve LV function through their beneficial effects on ventricular remodeling and wall stress (62,140).

(1) Role of ACE Inhibitors for Patients with Symptomatic LV Dysfunction—Several PRCTs have demonstrated that ACE inhibitors significantly improve mortality and morbidity in patients with symptomatic LV dysfunction (35,38,106,158). Three of these trials are described for illustration (35,38,158).

(a) The V-HeFT II Study—This PRCT included 804 men with chronic stable CHF (NYHA classes II or III) and LV EF <45% (mean 29%) who were receiving optimal conventional therapy for CHF (vasodilators in 60%). Patients were randomly assigned to receive either enalapril (5 to 10 mg PO BID) or a combination of hydralazine (37.5 to 75 mg PO QID) plus isosorbide dinitrate (20 to 40 mg PO QID). The average length of follow-up was 2.5 years. Treatment with enalapril was associated with a 28% reduction in mortality, which was attributable to a reduction in the incidence of sudden death but not death due to pump failure (see Table 3-7). The benefit of enalapril was observed only for those with less severe symptoms at the time of randomization (NYHA classes I or II). Only those patients treated with the hydralazine-isosorbide combination had an improved exercise tolerance as measured by the level of systemic oxygen consumption at peak exercise ($P<0.0001$). Both treatments significantly improved the LV EF at 3 years ($P<0.0001$), but the hydralazine-isosorbide combination was superior to enalapril in this respect at 13 weeks ($P=0.026$) (35).

Table 3-7 V-HeFT II: Enalapril vs. isosorbide-hydralazine for CS-CHF* (35)

	Enalapril (n=403)	Isosorbide-Hydralazine (n=401)	*P*
Mortality	18%	25%	0.016
Sudden death without warning	16%	25%	0.015
Death from CHF	23%	19%	NS

*Chronic Symptomatic CHF

(b) **Treatment Arm of the SOLVD Trial**—This large PRCT included 2569 patients with LV EF ≤35% (mean, 25%) and mild to moderate symptoms of CHF (90% NYHA class II or III) who were receiving conventional therapy for CHF including other vasodilators (nitrates in 40%). Patients were randomly assigned to receive either enalapril (2.5 to 10 mg PO BID) or placebo. The average length of follow-up was 41.4 months. Enalapril significantly reduced the overall mortality as well as the risk for development of CHF leading to death or hospitalization (see Table 3-8). Most of this survival benefit was attributable to a 22% reduction in the risk of death from worsening CHF; the risk of sudden death was similar between the two groups. Patients with LV EF >30% did not benefit from enalapril in subgroup analysis. (158).

(c) **The CONSENSUS I Study**—This PRCT included 253 patients with severe symptomatic CHF (NYHA class IV) who were receiving optimal conventional therapy for CHF including other vasodilators (nitrates in 50%). Patients were randomly assigned to receive either enalapril (2.5 mg PO QD to 20 mg PO BID) or placebo. The average length of follow-up was 188 days. The study was terminated early after a 40% reduction in crude mortality was observed with enalapril at 6 months (see Table 3-9). The entire survival benefit was attributable to enalapril's effect on death from worsening CHF (50% reduction); the risk of sudden death was similar between the two groups. In addition to this dramatic survival benefit, treatment with enalapril was associated with reduction in heart size, improvement of NYHA classification, and fewer days of hospitalization. Furthermore, patients assigned to enalapril were less likely to require other medications for CHF (38).

(2) **Role of ACE Inhibitors in Asymptomatic LV Dysfunction**—In the prevention arm of the SOLVD trial, 4228 patients with asymptomatic LV dysfunction (LV EF ≤35%) were randomly assigned to receive either enalapril (2.5 mg PO QD to 10 mg PO BID) or placebo. The average length of follow-up was 37.4 months. There was no statistically significant difference in mortality between the two groups (see Table 3-10). However, patients assigned to enalapril were significantly less

Table 3-8 SOLVD: Enalapril for chronic symptomatic CHF (158)

	Enalapril (n=1285)	Placebo (n=1284)	*P*
Mortality	35.2%	39.7%	0.0036
CHF leading to death	16.3%	19.5%	<0.0045
CHF leading to death or hospitalization	47.7%	57.3%	<0.001

Table 3-9 CONSENSUS I: Enalapril for chronic symptomatic CHF (38)

	Enalapril (n=127)	Placebo (n=126)	*P*
Mortality			
6 mo	26%	44%	0.002
12 mo	36%	52%	0.001
Total	39%	54%	0.003
Sudden cardiac death	11%	11%	NS
Death from CHF	17%	35%	0.001

Table 3-10 SOLVD: Enalapril for asymptomatic LV dysfunction (159)

	Enalapril (n=2111)	Placebo (n=2117)	*P*
Mortality	14.8%	15.8%	NS
Onset of symptomatic CHF	20.7%	30.2%	<0.001
CHF leading to death or hospitalization	20.6%	24.5%	<0.001

likely to develop symptomatic CHF or CHF leading to death or hospitalization. In subgroup analysis, this benefit was primarily conferred on those with LV EF ≤28% (159).

(3) Role of ACE Inhibitors After Acute MI

(a) The SAVE Trial—This large PRCT included 2231 patients with asymptomatic LV dysfunction (mean LV EF, 31%) who were receiving conventional therapy for acute MI (nitrates in 50%). Patients were randomly assigned to receive either captopril (12.5 to 50 mg PO TID) or placebo, and therapy was begun 3 to 16 days after the onset of acute MI. Fifty-five percent of the patients had had anterolateral Q-wave infarctions; 50% had undergone thrombolysis or angioplasty. The average length of follow-up was 42 months. There was a statistically significant reduction in mortality with captopril (20.4% versus 24.6%; *P*=0.019) (see Table 3-11). Patients assigned to captopril were less likely to develop CHF, to die from progressive CHF, to be hospitalized for CHF, or to experience reinfarction. Most of the survival benefit was attributable to captopril's salutary effect on the risk of death from progressive CHF (22%); the risks of sudden death and of death from acute MI were similar between the two groups. In subgroup analysis, captopril was particularly beneficial for elderly patients (age >65 years), those with LV EF ≤32%, and those in Killip class I (*i.e.*, no evidence of pulmonary congestion) at the time of acute MI. (139).

(b) The CONSENSUS II Study—This large multicenter PRCT included 6090 patients without overt CHF who were receiving conventional therapy for acute MI including vasodilators (nitrates in 50%). Patients were randomly assigned to receive either enalaprilat (1 mg IV) followed 6 hours later by enalapril (5 to 10 mg PO QD) or placebo. Therapy was begun within 24 hours after the onset of chest pain; 41% had suffered anterior infarcts and 56% had received thrombolysis. The length of follow-up was 6 months. The study was stopped early because of a trend toward increased mortality in the treatment arm (see Table 3-12). Enalapril was associated with an increased risk of death from progressive CHF and early hypotension (163). The results of this study are in sharp

Table 3-11 SAVE: Captopril for asymptomatic LV dysfunction after acute MI (139)

	Captopril (n=1115)	Placebo (n=1116)	*P*
Total mortality	20.4%	24.6%	0.019
Death from CHF	3%	5%	0.032
Sudden death	9%	11%	NS
Hospitalizations for CHF	14%	17%	0.019
Recurrent MI	12%	15%	0.015
Decrease in LV EF of >9%	13%	16%	0.168

Table 3-12 CONSENSUS II: Enalapril for asymptomatic LV dysfunction (163)

	Enalapril (n=3044)	Placebo (n=3046)	*P*
Total mortality	11.0%	10.2%	NS
Death from CHF	4.3%	3.4%	0.06
Sudden death	2.8%	2.8%	NS
Early hypotension	12%	3%	<0.001
Change in therapy due to CHF	27%	30%	<0.006
Reinfarction	9%	9%	NS

contrast to those of the SAVE trial, which reported a higher mortality rate with placebo than with ACE inhibition (24.6% versus 20.4%) (139). It has been proposed that AT II is important in the healing process during the immediate post-MI period, so the timing of initiation of drug therapy (*i.e.*, within 24 hours versus 3 to 16 days) may influence whether a patient benefits from ACE inhibition. Alternatively, hypotension caused by enalaprilat infusion may have caused infarct expansion in areas of hibernating myocardium.

(c) **The Acute Infarction Ramipril Efficacy Study (AIRE)**—This large PRCT included 1986 patients with mild to moderate CHF symptoms (NYHA classes I through III) who were receiving conventional therapy for acute MI (nitrates in 55%). Patients were randomly assigned to receive either ramipril (2.5 to 5.0 mg PO BID) or placebo. Therapy was begun at a mean of 5.4 days after acute MI (range, 3 to 10 days). Sixty percent of patients had suffered anterior infarcts and 58% had received thrombolysis. The average length of follow-up was 15 months. On an intention-to-treat analysis, ramipril treatment was associated with a 27% reduction in all-cause mortality and a 19% reduction in the combined secondary end points of death, severe CHF, reinfarction, or stroke (see Table 3-13). The benefit of ramipril was consistent over a wide range of subgroups and was particularly strong for for elderly patients (age >65 years). The incidence of sudden death and the risk of death from reinfarction were not reported (1).

(d) **The GISSI-3 Study**—This very large multicenter PRCT was designed to reexplore two issues. The first was the unexpected and disappointing results of the CONSENSUS II trial, which had found no mortality benefit when ACE inhibition was started within 24 hours of acute MI (see previous discussion). The second was a controversial metaanalysis which found a strong survival benefit for nitrates when used to treat acute MI (163,179). In the GISSI-3 trial, 19,394 patients with acute MI were randomly assigned in a 2×2 factorial design to receive lisinopril (5 to 10 mg PO QD) versus placebo and nitrates (IV trinitroglycerin [TNG] for the first 24

Table 3-13 AIRE: Ramipril for symptomatic CHF after acute MI (1)

	Ramipril (n=1004)	Placebo (n=982)	*P*
Total mortality	17%	23%	0.002
Death, severe CHF, reinfarction, or stroke	28%	34%	0.008

hours followed by transdermal TNG 10 mg QD) versus placebo. Therapy was begun within 24 hours of symptom onset; 27% of patients had suffered anterior infarcts, 72% had undergone thrombolysis, and 85% were in Killip class I. Patients with severe CHF, cardiogenic shock, or systolic blood pressure ≤100 mm Hg were excluded. The length of follow-up was 6 weeks. Lisinopril (with or without nitrates) was associated with a modest reduction in both mortality and the combined end point of mortality or severe LV dysfunction (see Table 3-14). Severe LV dysfunction was defined as clinically overt CHF with LV EF ≤35%. Nitrates were no better than placebo. The combination of lisinopril plus nitrates was even more effective in reducing mortality than lisinopril alone (P=0.021). In subgroup analysis, lisinopril was beneficial in all subgroups including women and the elderly (122).

(e) **The Survival of Myocardial Infarction Long-Term Evaluation Study (SMILE)**—This large PRCT included 1556 patients with acute anterior MI who were receiving conventional therapy. Patients were randomly assigned to receive either zofenopril (7.5 to 30 mg PO BID) or placebo. Therapy was begun within 24 hours of symptom onset; 85% of the patients were in Killip class I at the time of randomization; LV EF was not assessed. Patients with cardiogenic shock, history of CHF, systolic blood pressure ≤100 mm Hg, or history of outpatient use of ACE inhibitors were excluded. Patients were treated with study medications for 6 weeks and then continued on standard therapy (ACE inhibitors excluded) for 1 year. Zofenopril significantly improved survival at 1 year and also reduced the incidence of CHF at 6 weeks (see Table 3-15). These findings support the early use of ACE inhibition after acute MI and suggest that the lack of mortality benefit in CONSENSUS II may have resulted from the relatively short follow-up time of 6 months (2).

(f) **Fourth International Study of Infarct Survival (ISIS-4)**—This extremely large PRCT included 58,050 patients with suspected acute MI that was not complicated by cardiogenic shock or severe CHF. Patients were randomly assigned in a multifactorial design to receive captopril (6.25 to 50 mg PO BID) versus placebo and controlled-release mononitrate (30 to 60 mg PO QD) versus placebo. Magnesium was compared with placebo in a third factorial, but this comparison is not discussed in this chap-

Table 3-14 GISSI-3: Lisinopril, nitrates, both, or neither for acute MI (122)

	Lisinopril (n=9435)	Placebo (n=9450)	P	Nitrates (n=9453)	Placebo (n=9442)	P
Mortality	6.3%	7.1%	0.03	6.5%	6.9%	NS
Death or severe LV dysfunction	15.6%	17.0%	0.009	15.9%	16.7%	NS

Table 3-15 SMILE: Zofenopril for acute anterior MI (2)

	Zofenopril (n=772)	Placebo (n=784)	P
Total mortality—6 wk	4.9%	6.5%	NS
Severe CHF—6 wk	2.2%	4.1%	0.018
Total mortality—1 y	10%	14.1%	0.011

ter. Therapy was begun within 24 hours of symptom onset (median, 8 hours); 92% of patients had a confirmed MI; 70% had received thrombolysis. The length of follow-up was 12 months. Treatment with captopril was associated with 4.9±2 fewer deaths per 1000 patients at 1 month and 5.4±2.8 fewer deaths per 1000 patients at 12 months (see Table 3-16). The absolute benefit was even larger for higher-risk patients such as those presenting with a history of previous MI or with CHF (about 10 fewer deaths per 1000). Although patients on captopril were more likely to experience treatment-limiting hypotension (10.0% versus 4.8%; $P<0.0001$), there was no difference in mortality on day 0 or day 1. Mononitrate therapy was no better than placebo in terms of short- or long-term mortality (94).

(g) **The Chinese Cardiac Study (CCS-1)**—This PRCT included 13,634 patients with suspected acute MI not complicated by persistent hypotension. Patients were randomly assigned to receive either captopril (12.5 mg PO TID) or placebo for 1 month. Therapy was begun within 36 hours after the onset of symptoms; 39% of patients had received IV nitrates and 27% had undergone thrombolysis. At 1 month, there was a nonsignificant trend toward reduced mortality with captopril (9.05% versus 9.59%; $P=0.3$). Captopril also increased the risk of persistent hypotension (16.3% versus 10.8%; $P=0.0001$), particularly with initiation of therapy, but did not cause excess deaths (2.8% versus 3.2% on day 0 and day 1; $P=$NS) (27). The long-term follow-up of this cohort is to be reported in the near future.

c. Summary of the Role of Vasodilators for Treatment of Systolic CHF

(1) **Patients With Chronic Symptomatic CHF**—Nitrates, hydralazine, α-antagonists, and ACE inhibitors all appear to improve the functional status in patients with chronic symptomatic CHF. However, only ACE inhibitors and the combination of nitrates plus hydralazine have been shown to improve survival. The mortality benefit of ACE inhibition was primarily attributable to a reduction in the number of deaths from progressive CHF in the SOLVD and CONSENSUS trials and to a reduction in the risk of sudden death in the V-HeFT II study. In the SOLVD trial, the mortality benefit of enalapril was evident only in those with LV EF <30%.

(2) **Patients With Chronic Asymptomatic CHF**—ACE inhibitors reduce the incidence of overt CHF and the risk of death or hospitalization from progressive pump failure in patients with asymptomatic LV dysfunction. This benefit is observed primarily among those with LV EF ≤28%.

(3) **Patients With Acute MI**—In patients with acute MI, the addition of captopril (SAVE, ISIS-4), ramipril (AIRE), lisinopril (GISSI-3), or zofenopril (SMILE) to a conventional drug regimen significantly improves short- and long-term survival and also reduces the incidence of progressive pump failure. In the SMILE study, the mortality benefit was apparent at 1 year even though therapy was given for only 6 weeks after acute MI. The morbidity and mortality benefits observed with ACE inhibition were consistent among various subgroups and were particularly beneficial for the elderly and for those with severe

Table 3-16 ISIS-4: Captopril for suspected acute MI (94)

	Captopril (n=29,028)	Placebo (n=29,022)	*P*
Mortality—1 mo	7.19%	7.69%	0.02

LV dysfunction. In contrast, the CONSENSUS II trial failed to find a significant mortality benefit with early administration of IV enalaprilat in MI patients (*i.e.*, within 24 hours). However, other studies (GISSI-3, ISIS-4, SMILE) have shown that ACE inhibitors may safely be given within 24 hours of onset of acute MI with reduction in mortality. Patients were more likely to experience treatment-limiting hypotension with ACE inhibition but this did not lead to increased mortality (ISIS-4, CCS-1).

(4) **Alternatives to ACE Inhibitors**—For patients with chronic CHF, a hydralazine-isosorbide combination is a reasonable alternative to ACE inhibitors if the latter are contraindicated. However, the risk of treatment-limiting side effects may be significant. In the V-HeFT II study, the hydralazine-isosorbide combination had a greater beneficial effect on exercise tolerance and LV EF than did enalapril. Cohn has suggested that a combination of enalapril and hydralazine-nitrates may confer even greater benefit than either regimen alone, but this hypothesis has not been studied rigorously (35).

2. **Calcium Channel Blockers**-For patients with CHF, the antihypertensive and antiischemic properties of calcium channel blockers predict a beneficial effect, although resultant neurohormonal activation and negative inotropic properties predict detrimental effects on LV function (39,56). The negative inotropic effects are particularly important for the first-generation calcium channel blockers (nifedipine, diltiazem, and verapamil). In theory, they may be less of a problem for the second-generation dihydropyridines (amlodipine, nitrendipine, nisoldipine, nicardipine, isradipine, and felodipine), which appear to have less negative inotropy and to be more selective in terms of their vasodilatory properties (36,70).

a. **Role in Post-MI Patients**—Numerous PRCTs have evaluated the role of calcium channel blockers in management of post-MI patients. Most evaluated the role of nifedipine (80,95,124,156,174), but others evaluated the role of diltiazem (79,126) or verapamil (43,44). In most of these studies, treatment was started within 24 hours of an acute MI (early intervention) (44,80,124,156,174). In a few studies, treatment was started 3 to 21 days after MI (delayed intervention) (44,95,126). None of the early intervention studies was able to demonstrate a significant survival benefit in patients with acute MI. Similarly, except for metaanalyses (44) and subgroup analyses (126), none of the delayed intervention studies was able to demonstrate a significant survival benefit in the original study population of post-MI patients (44,95,126). The studies that are particularly relevant to patients with CHF are discussed in the following sections (44,126).

(1) **The Danish Study Group on Verapamil in Myocardial Infarction (DAVIT II)**—This study randomly assigned 1775 post-MI patients to receive either verapamil (120 mg PO TID) or placebo for 12 to 18 months. Therapy was not started until 7 to 15 days after MI (mean, 9±2.7 days). Patients with CHF were included in the study if they could be managed with ≤160 mg per day of furosemide. Based on an intention-to-treat analysis at 18 months, there was a nonsignificant trend toward a reduction in mortality with verapamil (see Table 3-17). However, there was a significant reduction in the risk of first reinfarction and in the combined risk of first major event (first reinfarction or

Table 3-17 DAVIT II: Verapamil for acute MI (44)

	Verapamil (n=878)	Placebo (n=897)	*P*
Mortality	11.1%	13.8%	NS
First reinfarction	11.0%	13.2%	0.044
First major event	18.0%	21.6%	0.027

death). No difference was observed in the rate of sudden death. Subgroup analysis showed that the benefit of verapamil was limited to men (*P*=0.035) and to patients without CHF (*P*=0.024). In part, the gender difference may have resulted from the higher prevalence of CHF among women in the study (39.2% versus 33.4%; *P*=0.04) (44).

(2) The Multicenter Diltiazem Postinfarction Trial (MDPIT)—In this large PRCT, 2466 patients with acute MI who were receiving conventional therapy including vasodilators were randomly assigned to receive either diltiazem (60 mg PO QID) or placebo. Therapy was begun 3 to 15 days after MI; about 70% of patients had LV EF ≥40% at the time of randomization; those in cardiogenic shock were excluded. The mean length of follow-up was 25 months. The total mortality rate was almost identical in the two groups (126) (see Table 3-18). Subgroup analysis suggested that the lack of survival benefit with diltiazem treatment may have resulted because the lower mortality among those without CHF was negated by higher mortality among those with CHF. For example, the Cox hazard ratio of first recurrent cardiac event was 1.41 (95% CI, 1.41 to 1.96) for those with CHF, compared with 0.77 (95% CI, 0.61 to 0.98) for those without CHF. This type of bidirectional interaction between diltiazem and CHF was also observed between diltiazem and LV EF (dichotomized at 40%) and between diltiazem and the presence or absence of anterior Q-wave MI (79).

b. Role of Calcium Channel Blockers for Management of Chronic CHF

(1) First-Generation Agents—In a small PRCT with crossover design, nifedipine, isosorbide dinitrate, and their combination were compared among 28 patients with chronic systolic CHF (NYHA class II or III and LV EF <40%). After 8 weeks of treatment with the randomly assigned drugs, patients were crossed over to another treatment arm for

Table 3-18 MDPIT: Diltiazem for acute MI (79)

	Diltiazem (n=1232)	Placebo (n=1234)	Hazard Ratio (95% CI)
Overall mortality	13.5%	13.5%	NS
First recurrent cardiac event (CHF)	26%	18%	1.41 (1.01–1.96)
First recurrent cardiac event (No CHF)	8%	11%	0.77 (0.61–0.98)
First recurrent cardiac event (LV EF <40%)	26%	20%	1.31 (0.87–1.98)
First recurrent cardiac event (LV EF ≥40%)	6%	10%	0.73 (0.48–1.11)
First recurrent cardiac event (AQWMI)	15%	15%	NS
First recurrent cardiac event (No AQWMI)	9%	12%	0.74 (0.57–0.96)
Late CHF (LV EF <40%)	21%	12%	*P*=0.004
Late CHF (LV EF ≥40%)	4.0%	4.2%	NS

Table 3-19 Nitrates, nifedipine, or both for chronic CHF (55)

	Nitrates Alone	Nifedipine Alone	Combination	*P* (Nifedipine vs. Nitrates)	*P* (Combination vs. Nitrates)
Hospitalization due to worsening CHF	0%	24%	26%	<0.05	<0.05
Number of episodes of worsening CHF	3	9	21	NS	<0.0001

additional 8 weeks. This process was repeated until all patients had received all three treatments. The risk of worsening CHF was significantly higher while patients were receiving nifedipine (alone or in combination with nitrates) than while they were taking nitrates alone (55) (see Table 3-19).

(2) **Second-Generation Agents**—In one PRCT, 118 patients with mild to moderate LV dysfunction (NYHA class II or III and LV EF <40%) who were receiving conventional therapy for CHF (ACE inhibitors in 68%) were randomly assigned to receive either amlodipine (10 mg PO QD) or placebo. The length of follow-up was 2 months. Treatment with amlodipine was associated with improvement of symptoms, increase in exercise tolerance, and reduction of serum NE level (see Table 3-20) (135). The study did not address the effect of amlodipine on survival.

c. **Summary of the Role of Calcium Channel Blockers in Management of Systolic CHF**

(1) The current data do not support the use of calcium channel blockers for routine management of patients with acute MI, and there is some evidence that these agents may actually be harmful for the subgroup with poor LV function.

(2) Similarly, for patients with chronic CHF, nifedipine (a first-generation agent) appears to increase the risk of worsening CHF. In theory, second-generation dihydropyridines may be more useful because they appear to have less negative inotropy and to be more selective in terms of their vasodilatory properties than first-generation agents. The only study involving a second-generation agent in patients with mild to moderate CHF showed that amlodipine therapy was associated with a significant improvement in CHF symptoms and exercise tolerance; this study did not examine the effect of amlodipine on survival.

(3) Several ongoing trials should clarify the safety and efficacy of the second-generation calcium channel blockers in chronic CHF when used in combination with ACE inhibitors. The V-HeFT III trial is evaluating the effect of felodipine versus placebo on morbidity and mortality in patients with mild to moderate CHF treated with diuretics and ACE inhibitors, with and without digoxin. The Prospective Randomized Amlodipine Survival Evaluation (PRAISE) is studying the effects of amlodipine versus placebo on survival in patients with NYHA class III or IV chronic CHF treated concomitantly with ACE inhibitors.

3. **β-Adrenergic Receptor Blockers**

a. **β-Blockers in Chronic CHF**—In addition to their antiischemic and antiarrhythmic properties, β-blockers may improve contractile function in patients with LV dysfunction by attenuating the potentially toxic effects of catecholamines on myocytes and upregulating the myocardial β-adrenergic receptors (45,62,65,75,88,92,149). Several PRCTs have found that β-blocker therapy can relieve symptoms and improve exercise tolerance in patients with chronic CHF, regardless of whether the LV dysfunction is caused by IDCM or by CAD (3,172,176). However, none of these studies was able to demonstrate a statistically significant survival benefit. The two largest studies are described in the following sections. (45,75).

(1) **The Metoprolol in Idiopathic Dilated Cardiomyopathy Study**

Table 3-20 Amlodipine for chronic CHF (135)

	Amlodipine (n=58)	Placebo (n=60)	*P*
Percent with improved symptoms	55	29	<0.05
Increase in exercise duration	62±17 s	22±13 s	<0.05
Change in norepinephrine level	−95 pg/ml	+30 pg/ml	<0.05

(MDC Study)—This PRCT included 383 patients with mild to moderate chronic stable CHF (NYHA class II or III; mean LV EF, 22%) who were receiving conventional therapy (ACE inhibitors in 80%). Patients were randomly assigned to receive either metoprolol (50 to 75 mg PO BID) or placebo. Patients requiring inotropic agents (other than digoxin) and those who had received β-blockers or calcium channel blockers were excluded. The length of follow-up was 12 months. Metoprolol was associated with a reduction in the number of patients who had progressive LV dysfunction to the point of requiring transplantation. It also improved symptoms and LV EF but had no significant effect on survival (172) (see Table 3-21).

(2) **The Xamoterol in Severe Heart Failure Study**—This PRCT included 516 patients who had moderate to severe chronic CHF (NYHA class III or IV; mean LV EF, 25%) despite stable therapy with diuretics and ACE inhibitors. Patients were randomly assigned to receive either placebo or xamoterol (200 mg PO BID), which functions as a β_1-selective partial agonist at rest or with mild exercise but a β_1-selective antagonist at high levels of sympathetic tone or during heavy exercise. Approximately 30% of patients had IDCM and 60% had CAD. The length of follow-up was 13 weeks. On an intention-to-treat analysis, xamoterol was associated with a significant increase in mortality (9.1% versus 3.7% at 100 days; P=0.02). The investigators suggested that its partial β_1-agonist activity may have contributed to the increased risk of death (176).

b. **β-Blockers in Post-MI Patients With Poor LV Function**—There is now convincing evidence that β-blockers confer a significant survival benefit in patients with acute MI. Not only are β-blockers safe in post-MI patients with CHF, but those with the most severe LV dysfunction have the greatest survival benefit from β-blockade. Representative studies are described here.

(1) **The Beta-Blocker Heart Attack Trial (BHAT Trial)**—In this large PRCT, 3837 patients with acute MI were randomly assigned to receive either propranolol (60 to 80 mg PO TID) or placebo; therapy was begun 5 to 21 days after infarction; (26% of patients had anterior infarcts). Post-MI patients with mild or compensated CHF were included in the study. The length of follow-up averaged 25 months.

(a) Propranolol significantly reduced not only the total mortality rate but also the risk of cardiovascular death and the risk of sudden cardiac death (10) (see Table 3-22).

Table 3-21 MDC: Metoprolol for chronic CHF (172)

	Metoprolol (n=194)	Placebo (n=189)	*P*
Total mortality (%)	11.9	10.1	NS
Need for transplantation (%)	1.0	10.1	0.0001
Change in LV EF (%)	13	6	<0.0001
Change in PCWP (mm HG)	−5	−2	0.06

Table 3-22 BHAT: Propranolol for acute MI (10)

	Propranolol (n=1916)	Placebo (n=1921)	*P*
Total mortality	7.2%	9.8%	<0.005
Cardiac mortality	6.6%	8.9%	<0.01
Sudden cardiac death	3.3%	4.6%	<0.05
Nonsudden cardiac death	2.9%	3.9%	NS

(b) Two subgroup analyses have been reported from the BHAT data. In the analysis by Chadda, patients with a history of CHF were more likely than those without CHF to derive benefit from propranolol in terms of the percentage of reduction in the relative risk of total cardiac death, sudden death, or nonfatal reinfarction. Probability values were not provided (see Table 3-23) (26).

(c) In the analysis by Viscoli, patients were stratified according to their clinical course during the first year after MI. Only the high-risk patients (recurrent ischemic events, arrhythmias, CHF, or severe comorbidity) derived a significant survival benefit from propranolol during subsequent follow-up; they had a 43% decline in the risk of death (P=0.01). (170) Analysis of the Norwegian Timolol Trial yielded similar findings (131).

(2) The Beta-Blocker Pooling Project—In this metaanalysis, 1-year all-cause mortality data from nine β-blocker postinfarction trials (13,679 patients) were analyzed. Use of β-Blockers was associated with a 24% reduction in overall mortality (P<0.0001). In subgroup analysis, β-blockers significantly reduced the mortality rate in patients who developed pump or mechanical failure between the onset of the qualifying MI and the time of randomization (9.6% versus 12.8%; P=0.004) (11).

(3) The MDPIT Study (Placebo Arm)—This PRCT examined the effect of diltiazem on mortality in the postinfarction period (see previous discussion). In a retrospective Kaplan–Meier analysis of patients in the placebo arm whose LV EF was known (n=1084), β-blockers were associated with a significant reduction in the 2.5-year relative risk of death; this result included patients with poor LV function (LV EF >30% or CHF on chest film) (112) (see Table 3-24).

(4) A similar multivariate analysis of the Cardiac Arrhythmia Suppression Trial (CAST) study showed that β-blocker therapy was associated with significant reductions in the risk of arrhythmic death or cardiac arrest (P=0.036) and in the occurrence of new or worsened CHF (P=0.015) at 30 days and at 1 and 2 years (105).

c. Summary of the Role of β-Blocker Therapy on Systolic Dysfunction

(1) Although β-blockers appear to improve morbidity in patients with chronic CHF, no survival benefit has yet been demonstrated in a PRCT. Two large PRCTs are underway to clarify the role of β-blocker

Table 3-23 BHAT subgroup analysis: outcome in patients with or without CHF (26)

Relative Reduction in Outcome Indicated	History of CHF	No History of CHF
Total mortality	27%	25%
Total cardiac death	32%	21%
Sudden death	47%	13%
Nonfatal infarction	42%	6%

Table 3-24 MDPIT (Placebo Arm): Effect of β-blockers on survival (112)

	2.5-Y Mortality Risk on β-Blockers	2.5-Y Mortality Risk not on β-Blockers	Relative Risk	95% CI
LV EF <30%	23.5%	44.6%	0.53	?
LV EF 30%–39%	8.5%	19.0%	0.45	0.18–1.10
LV EF ≥40%	7.7%	12.6%	0.61	0.38–0.99
CHF on chest film	13.4%	30.3%	0.44	0.22–0.90

therapy in chronic CHF. The Cardiac Insufficiency Bisoprolol Study involves 630 patients with NYHA class II or III symptoms. A trial of carvedilol by the Australia and New Zealand Heart Failure Research Collaborative Group will eventually include 3000 subjects.

(2) There is convincing evidence from numerous sources that β-blockers confer significant mortality benefit in post-MI patients. β-Blockers are not only safe in patients with CHF but appear to provide the greatest survival benefit in this group. This benefit is attributable primarily to a reduction in the rates of sudden death and reinfarction.

4. Positive Inotropic Agents

a. Digoxin—The positive inotropic effect of digoxin results from inhibition of the sodium-potassium ATPase pump in the sarcolemmal membrane of the cardiac myocyte. This leads ultimately to increased calcium influx and enhanced myocardial contraction (157). Digoxin also enhances vagal tone, augments baroreceptor sensitization, and reduces sympathetic outflow, all of which may be clinically more important that its modest inotropic effects (63,64,113).

(1) Morbidity Studies

(a) In a metaanalysis of seven trials that evaluated the role of digoxin for management of patients in sinus rhythm with CHF, the pooled odds ratio of worsening CHF was 0.28 (95% CI, 0.16 to 0.49), favoring digoxin over control. On average, 12% of patients derived a clinically important benefit such as improved symptoms, fewer hospitalizations, or lower risk of progressive pump failure (97). In two of the trials examined, the presence of an S_3 gallop and more severe CHF (greater LV dilation and depressed LV EF) predicted a clinically beneficial response to digoxin (83,109).

(b) Prospective Randomized Study of Ventricular Failure and the Efficacy of Digoxin (PROVED) Study—This small PRCT included 88 patients with mild to moderate chronic stable CHF (NYHA class II or III; mean LV EF, 28%) who were receiving long-term therapy with diuretics and digoxin. Patients were randomly assigned to either withdrawal or continuation of digoxin. CHF was caused by CAD in 64% of the patients; the length of follow-up was 3 months. Withdrawal of digoxin was associated with a significant worsening of maximal exercise capacity and an increased rate of treatment failure (see Table 3-25). Patients who continued to receive digoxin had a significantly higher LV EF. (167).

(c) Randomized Assessment of (the Effect of) Digoxin on Inhibitors of the Angiotensin-Converting Enzyme (RADIANCE) Study—This PRCT included 178 patients with mild to moderate chronic stable CHF (NYHA class II or III; LV EF, ≤35%) who were receiving long-term therapy with diuretics, digoxin, and ACE inhibitors. Patients were randomly assigned to withdrawal or continuation of digoxin. CHF was caused by CAD in 54% of the patients; the length of follow-up was 3 months. Dis-

Table 3-25 PROVED: Effect of withdrawal of digoxin in chronic CHF (167)

	Digoxin Continued (n=42)	Digoxin Withdrawn (n=46)	*P*
Change in median exercise time	+4.5 s	−96 s	0.003
Treatment failure	19%	39%	0.039
Change in LV EF	+2±2%	−3±2%	0.016

continuation of digoxin significantly increased the rate of worsening CHF sufficient to require withdrawal from the study. In addition, various measures of functional capacity or cardiac function (NYHA class, LV EF, weight change) worsened with withdrawal of digoxin (137) (see Table 3-26).

(2) Mortality Studies

(a) In one prospective cohort study of 134 patients, those with a digoxin level >1 ng/ml had a higher 1-year mortality rate than those with a digoxin level ≤1 ng/ml (47% versus 32%; P=0.02). However, when the indices of CHF severity were included in a Cox regression model, digoxin level had no independent prognostic value (151).

(b) In a retrospective subgroup analysis of the PROMISE (Prospective Randomized Milrinone Survival Evaluation) study (see Chapter 4), a digoxin level of >1.1 ng/ml was associated with a 34% increased risk of death, independent of LV EF and renal function (114).

(c) A review of eight retrospective analyses of digoxin therapy in post-MI patients was previously reported (181). Several of these studies suggested that digoxin may increase the risk of sudden death or overall mortality in a subgroup of patients with frequent ventricular ectopy. However, most of the studies concluded that the higher mortality rate observed among digoxin-treated patients more likely reflected the higher incidence of poor prognostic factors in these patients rather than an independent deleterious effect on survival.

(d) A large multicenter PRCT designed to evaluate the effect of digoxin on mortality in patients with moderate to severe chronic CHF and sinus rhythm has recently been completed. Preliminary analysis reportedly suggests that digoxin does not alter mortality but does reduce the incidence of worsening CHF. Peer review and publication of this study are awaited (44a).

b. β-Adrenergic Agonists and Phosphodiesterase Inhibitors—Both β-agonists and phosphodiesterase inhibitors have well-known inotropic effects that are mediated by cAMP-dependent protein kinase activity (99). Although these agents can provide short-term symptomatic and hemodynamic improvements, long-term use may be associated with an increased risk of arrhythmia and sudden death. Representative studies are discussed here.

(1) Oral β-Agonists—In general, oral β-agonists such as salbutamol, pirbuterol, and terbutaline offer only short-term hemodynamic and symptomatic improvements (147). These agents are rarely used, because a pooled analysis revealed a twofold higher mortality rate for patients treated with oral β-agonists compared with control patients (P<0.001) (180).

(2) Dobutamine—This parenteral β_1-agonist is commonly used for acute management of severe LV dysfunction in a coronary care unit setting. One small PRCT comparing a 72-hour continuous infusion of dobuta-

Table 3-26 RADIANCE: Effect of withdrawal of digoxin in chronic CHF (137)

	Digoxin Continued (n=85)	Digoxin Withdrawn (n=93)	P
Worsening CHF	4%	23%	<0.001
Decreased NYHA class	10%	27%	0.019
Change in LV EF	−1±1%	−4±1%	0.001
Change in body weight	−1±2 kg	+1±3 kg	<0.001

mine versus placebo in 15 patients with IDCM (NYHA class III or IV) reported sustained improvements in resting hemodynamics, exercise tolerance, LV EF, and symptoms that persisted for 2 to 4 weeks ($P<0.05$) (111). However, another PRCT involving patients with CHF was stopped early after a twofold higher mortality rate was observed with dobutamine, compared with placebo (39% versus 17%; $P=0.08$).

(3) Ibopamine—This oral dopaminergic agonist with selective dopamine$_2$-receptor specificity was developed because of a desire to extend the favorable hemodynamic effects of IV dopamine to the outpatient setting (23,147). A number of small PRCTs have reported conflicting results in regard to the relative predominance of vasodilatory versus inotropic effects and whether these effects are sustained with long-term therapy (6,21,37,104,144). However, ibopamine appears to consistently attenuate the extent of neurohormonal activation. Furthermore, it does not appear to have significant proarrhythmic effects (22,76,123,143,168,169).

(4) Phosphodiesterase Inhibitors

(a) An early uncontrolled study involving eight patients with CHF (NYHA class III or IV) demonstrated a significant immediate hemodynamic benefit with IV infusion of amrinone (9). However, in a PRCT involving 99 patients with severely depressed LV EF, 3 months of oral amrinone therapy was no better than placebo in terms of symptom relief, NYHA class, LV EF, or survival. On the other hand, nonarrhythmogenic adverse reactions necessitating withdrawal of treatment occurred more frequently with amrinone (34% versus 3%; $P<0.01$) (116).

(b) A multicenter PRCT involving patients with severely depressed LV EF failed to demonstrate improvements in exercise capacity or symptoms after 4 months of therapy with enoximone (12,166). In fact, enoximone was associated with poorer survival.

(c) Finally, in the PROMISE trial, long-term oral therapy with milrinone was associated with a 34% increase in cardiovascular mortality in patients with severely depressed LV EF (see Chapter 4) (134).

c. Vesnarinone (OPC-8212)—This quinolinone derivative is an oral inotropic agent that augments myocardial contractility by modulating cardiac potassium and sodium channels. It does not cause tachycardia or increase myocardial oxygen consumption. Vesnarinone also has mild phosphodiesterase inhibitor activity and class III antiarrhythmic properties but no important vasodilatory or neurohormonal modifying effects at standard doses. All three PRCTs that have examined the effect of vesnarinone therapy on morbidity and mortality in patients with chronic CHF have reported encouraging results (60,61,132). The largest PRCT included 474 patients with symptomatic LV dysfunction and LV EF ≤30% (69% NYHA class III; mean LV EF, 20%) despite conventional therapy for CHF (including ACE inhibitors in 89%). Patients were randomly assigned to receive vesnarinone (either 60 mg PO QD or 120 mg PO QD) or placebo. CHF was caused by CAD in 52%; the length of follow-up was 6 months. Randomization to the higher-dose vesnarinone arm was stopped after an excess early mortality was observed in this group. However, use of 60 mg of vesnarinone was associated with a significant reduction in overall mortality, risk of sudden death, and risk of progressive pump failure leading to death (see Table 3-27). The overall quality of life also improved significantly with vesnarinone, although length of life was an important variable in the quality of life index. More patients in the placebo group were treated with conventional antiarrhythmic therapy than in the treatment group; it is unclear whether this difference had any influence on outcome. The main side effect of vesnarinone was reversible neutropenia, which affected 2.5% of patients (61).

Table 3-27 Vesnarinone for refractory CHF (61)

	Vesnarinone (n=239)	Placebo (n=238)	*P*
Total mortality	5.4%	13.9%	0.002
Sudden death	2.1	6.3%	Not reported
Worsening CHF	2.9%	7.6%	Not reported

d. Flosequinan—This oral agent belongs to a new class of fluoroquinolones which modulate all three of the second-messenger systems that regulate the intracellular calcium concentration: cAMP, cyclic guanine monophosphate (cGMP), and inositol 1,4,5-triphosphate (IP_3) (7). Clinically, flosequinan has potent arterial and venous vasodilatory properties (178). In the failing human heart, flosequinan also appears to have cAMP-independent inotropic effects (17,40,120,173). It also has direct positive chronotropic properties and can cause tachycardia (13,74). In eight PRCTs ranging in size from 16 to 322 patients (1 to 12 months of follow-up), flosequinan significantly improved the indices of functional status and exercise capacity. The magnitude of these benefits was comparable to that observed with ACE inhibitors (41,42,54,84,117,136,142,154). However, despite convincing symptomatic benefits, its use cannot be advised because it appears to increase the risk of death (93). Representative studies are described here.

(1) Randomized Evaluation of Flosequinan on Exercise Tolerance (REFLECT)—This PRCT included 193 patients with mild to moderate CHF (NYHA class II or III) who were receiving digoxin and diuretics. Patients were randomly assigned to receive either flosequinan or placebo. Flosequinan (for 12 weeks) improved symptoms and increased both exercise duration and peak oxygen consumption (see Table 3-28). It also significantly increased the heart rate compared with baseline ($P<0.001$), but indices of neurohormonal activation remained unchanged (136).

(2) Flosequinan–Angiotensin Converting Enzyme Inhibitor Trial (FACET)—This PRCT included 322 patients with mild to moderate CHF (NYHA class II or III) who remained symptomatic despite conventional therapy with diuretics, digoxin, and ACE inhibitors. These patients were randomly assigned to receive flosequinan (either 100 mg PO QD or 75 mg PO BID) or placebo, in addition to their conventional therapy. Add-on therapy with 100 mg of flosequinan daily for 4 months was associated with improvements in maximal exercise capacity and symptom scores ($P<0.05$) (117).

(3) However, the Prospective Randomized Flosequinan Longevity Evaluation (PROFILE) was terminated early because of excess mortality in the flosequinan group (93). This PRCT had included about 3500 patients with severe CHF and was designed to assess mortality differences between patients randomly assigned to receive flosequinan (100 mg PO QD) or placebo.

e. Pimobendan—This oral agent has partial phosphodiesterase-inhibiting

Table 3-28 REFLECT: Flosequinan for chronic CHF (136)

	Flosequinan	Placebo	*P*
Change in exercise duration	+96 s	+47 s	0.022
Change in peak oxygen uptake	+1.7 ml/kg/min	+0.6 ml/kg/min	0.05
Improved symptoms	55%	36%	0.018

and significant calcium-sensitizing properties and offers a combination of positive inotropic and arterial vasodilatory effects. Its inotropic effect is largely mediated by an increase in calcium occupancy of the low-affinity calcium-specific regulatory site of troponin C. Its vasodilatory effect results from increased levels of intracellular cAMP (87). Pimobendan decreases preload and afterload but does not cause neurohormonal activation (145). In six studies (five PRCTs) that ranged in size from 21 to 242 patients (with 1 to 6 months of follow-up), pimobendan significantly improved the indices of functional status and exercise capacity. The magnitude of these benefits was comparable to that observed with enalapril in parallel-design studies (57,86,103,108,146,152). Clinically significant proarrhythmic effects have not been observed with pimobendan. Representative studies are described here.

(1) One PRCT included 198 patients with moderate CHF symptoms (NYHA class III; mean LV EF, 22%) despite conventional therapy (including ACE inhibitors in 80%). Patients were randomly assigned to receive either pimobendan (2.5 to 10 g PO QD) or placebo. Therapy with 5 mg of pimobendan for 12 weeks was associated with a significant increase in exercise duration, peak oxygen uptake, and quality of life measures (see Table 3-29). There were no significant differences in LV EF, levels of plasma NE, or frequency of arrhythmia (108).

(2) A similar PRCT found that pimobendan can reduce morbidity in patients who have severe refractory CHF symptoms despite optimal therapy with diuretics, digoxin, and ACE inhibitors (103).

(3) In a double-blind parallel-design study, 242 patients with mild to moderate CHF symptoms (NYHA class II or III) despite therapy with diuretics and digoxin were randomly assigned to receive either pimobendan (average dose, 10.3 mg PO QD) or enalapril (average dose, 10.7 mg PO QD). After 6 months of therapy, the two drugs had produced similar degrees of improvement in exercise duration (the primary end point), NYHA class, and hemodynamic indices at rest compared with baseline ($P<0.05$). However, only enalapril improved the hemodynamic indices during exercise ($P<0.05$) (146).

f. Summary of the Role of Positive Inotropic Agents in Systolic Failure

(1) A metaanalysis of morbidity studies supports the safety and efficacy of digoxin therapy in patients with chronic CHF and sinus rhythm. The benefit of digoxin may derive more from an autonomic sympathoinhibitory effect than from a modest inotropic effect. In several well-designed studies that withdrew digoxin from patients with CHF, it was concluded that digoxin offers significant symptomatic benefits, even for those already being treated with ACE inhibitors. A large multicenter PRCT designed to evaluate the effect of digoxin on mortality in patients with moderate to severe chronic CHF and sinus rhythm has recently been completed. Preliminary analysis reportedly suggests that digoxin does not alter mortality but does reduce the incidence of worsening CHF.

(2) Although β-agonists and phosphodiesterase inhibitors can be helpful for short-term management of patients with severe LV dysfunction in the coronary care unit setting, the absence of sustained benefit and the potential for increased mortality preclude their routine use for

Table 3-29 Pimobendam for refractory CHF (108)

	Pimobendan (n=51)	Placebo (n=49)	*P*
Change in exercise duration	+121.6 s	+29.6 s	<0.001
Change in peak oxygen uptake	+2.23 ml/kg/min	Fell slightly	<0.01

long-term management of systolic dysfunction. For the future, the oral dopaminergic agonist, ibopamine, shows some promise as a modulator of sympathetic tone and aldosterone secretion. Along with digoxin, ibopamine may help define a new class of agents that act primarily as neurohormonal antagonists.

(3) In patients with moderate to severe chronic CHF, vesnarinone (60 mg PO QD) decreased mortality by 62% at 6 months. This dose was not associated with any significant hemodynamic or inotropic effects. The mechanism for the clinical benefit remains unclear. Vesnarinone may be a useful option for patients with refractory symptoms despite optimal conventional therapy.

(4) Although flosequinan has consistently been shown to improve symptoms, its routine use is not recommended because it was associated with excess mortality in the PROFILE study.

(5) Preliminary morbidity studies have demonstrated that pimobendan is safe and efficacious when administered for up to 6 months. Its beneficial effects on functional capacity, exercise tolerance, and hemodynamics are comparable to those of enalapril. It may prove useful as an alternative or adjunct therapy to ACE inhibitors. However, given the excess mortality observed with many other positive inotropic agents, further studies are needed before its routine use can be recommended.

5. Antiarrhythmic Agents—In patients with chronic CHF, up to 50% of cardiac deaths are sudden and presumably caused by an arrhythmia (118). In addition, post-MI patients with premature ventricular contractions (PVCs) have a higher risk of death (89). Various antiarrhythmic drugs have been tried in an attempt to suppress PVCs (symptomatic and asymptomatic) in patients with chronic CHF and in post-MI patients.

a. Class I Antiarrhythmic Agents—The CAST I and II studies found that therapy with encainide, flecainide, or moricizine effectively suppressed PVCs in post-MI patients but also increased their risk of death (see Chapter 5) (20,52). These findings were confirmed in a metaanalysis of 11 studies involving 4122 patients. (89).

b. Amiodarone—Amiodarone is a class III antiarrhythmic agent that lengthens the refractory period and the duration of the action potential. It also has coronary and peripheral vasodilatory effects as well as bradycardic effects (127). Amiodarone has been studied in patients with chronic CHF and in post-MI patients.

(1) Amiodarone in Chronic CHF—Five PRCTs, ranging in size from 34 to 674 patients, have examined the effect of amiodarone in patients with chronic CHF (1 to 6 years of follow-up). These studies have reported mixed results (24,46,130,155,161). Representative studies are described here.

(a) Grupo de Estudio de la Sobrevida en la Insuficiencia Cardiaca en Argentina (GESICA Study)—This randomized but not double-blind study included 516 patients with severe chronic CHF (80% NYHA class III or IV; mean LV EF, 20%) who were receiving conventional therapy for CHF (including ACE inhibitors in 90%). Patients were randomly assigned to receive either low-dose amiodarone (300 mg PO QD) or placebo. CHF was caused by CAD in 40%; the length of follow-up was 2 years. In an intention-to-treat analysis, amiodarone significantly reduced the risk of overall mortality and the risk of death or hospitalization from to progressive pump failure (see Table 3-30). There was also a trend toward lower risk of sudden death. The benefits were consistent for all subgroups examined and were independent of the presence or absence of nonsustained ventricular tachycardia. Side effects were reported in 6.1% of those assigned to amiodarone. (46).

Table 3-30 GESICA: Amiodarone for chronic CHF (46)

	Amiodarone (n=260)	Placebo (n=256)	*P*
Total mortality	33.5%	41.4%	0.024
Death or hospitalization due to progressive pump failure	45.8%	58.2%	0.0024
Sudden death	12.3%	15.2%	0.16

(b) The CASCADE Study—This PRCT randomly assigned 228 survivors of out-of-hospital ventricular fibrillation to receive either empiric therapy with amiodarone or conventional antiarrhythmic therapy guided by electrophysiologic testing. The mean LV EF was 35%; 82% had CAD, 45% had CHF, and 46% had an automatic implanted defibrillator. Amiodarone significantly improved the rate of event-free survival at 6 years (defined as survival free of resuscitation for ventricular fibrillation or syncope despite defibrillator shock). However, patients in the amiodarone group had to discontinue the drug or be switched to an alternative therapy more often than those in the conventional therapy group (24) (see Table 3-31).

(c) The Survival Trial of Antiarrhythmic Therapy in Congestive Heart Failure (The STAT-CHF Trial)—This PRCT included 674 patients with chronic CHF (43% NYHA class III or IV) and asymptomatic ventricular arrhythmia (≥10 PVCs/hour by Holter monitoring). Patients were receiving conventional therapy, including ACE inhibitors in >90%. Patients were randomly assigned to receive either amiodarone (800 mg PO QD for 14 days, then 400 mg PO QD for 50 weeks, then 300 mg PO QD) or placebo. CHF was caused by CAD in 71%; the median length of follow-up was 45 months. Although amiodarone was more effective at suppressing ventricular arrhythmias ($P<0.001$), there was no difference in the 2-year overall mortality rate between the two groups (155).

(d) A smaller study using similar design also failed to demonstrate a mortality benefit with amiodarone in patients with either ischemic or nonischemic cardiomyopathy (130).

(2) Amiodarone in Post-MI Patients—Four PRCTs, ranging in size from 77 to 613 patients (6 to 20 months of follow-up), have evaluated the role of amiodarone in post-MI patients (16,18,25,91,141). Representative studies are described here.

(a) In the largest PRCT, 613 patients with acute MI and contraindications to β-blockade (*e.g.*, CHF, diabetes, asthma) were randomly assigned to receive either amiodarone (800 mg PO QD for 7 days, then 100 to 400 mg PO for 6 days each week) or placebo. Therapy was begun 5 to 7 days after hospital admission; 51% of the patients had anterior infarcts. The length of follow-up was 1 year.

Table 3-31 CASCADE: Amiodarone in survivors of ventricular fibrillation (24)

	Amiodarone (n=113)	Conventional Therapy (n=115)	*P*
Survival free of combined end points	53%	40%	0.007
Survival free of cardiac death and sustained arrhythmias	41%	20%	<0.001
Discontinuation of assigned therapy or crossing over to alternative therapy	41%	21%	0.13

Amiodarone was associated with a marginally significant reduction in cardiac deaths (19% versus 33%; *P*=0.048) (25).

(b) Basel Antiarrhythmia Study of Infarct Survival (BASIS)—In this PRCT, 312 infarct survivors with asymptomatic complex ventricular arrhythmias were randomly assigned to receive low-dose amiodarone (200 mg PO QD), individualized therapy with other conventional antiarrhythmic agents, or placebo. The mean LV EF was 43%; 40% of patients had anterior infarcts; and the length of follow-up was 1 year. Amiodarone significantly improved survival but individualized therapy was no better than placebo (16). In subgroup analysis, the survival benefit was limited to patients with LV EF ≥40% (141) (see Table 3-32).

(c) Canadian Amiodarone Myocardial Infarction Arrhythmia Trial (CAMIAT)—This pilot study involving 77 post-MI patients (about 30% with CHF) found that moderate-dose amiodarone therapy was associated with a reduction in all-cause mortality at a mean follow-up of 20 months (10% versus 21%; no probability values reported) (18).

(d) A multicenter trial of amiodarone for post-MI patients with high-grade ventricular ectopic activity (irrespective of LV EF) is in progress.

c. Summary of the Role of Antiarrhythmic Agents in Systolic Dysfunction

(1) Because class I agents appear to increase mortality in post-MI patients, much of the recent research on antiarrhythmic therapy has centered on evaluation of amiodarone. Studies of amiodarone in patients with chronic CHF (with or without documented ventricular arrhythmia) have yielded mixed results. A large Veterans Administration trial is in progress to better assess the benefit of amiodarone in patients with NYHA class III or IV CHF and PVCs.

(2) Studies of amiodarone in patients with acute MI have also been inconclusive. The European Myocardial Infarction Arrhythmia Trial will evaluate the effect of amiodarone in a large group of early post-MI patients who have low LV EF.

6. Diuretics—Diuretics have been used for more than 50 years to treat CHF. They are clearly effective for symptom relief and are assumed to be safe. An ideal diuretic should achieve natriuresis without promoting further neurohormonal activation. However, diuretics have not been subjected to rigorous study.

7. Anticoagulation—A retrospective analysis of 104 patients with IDCM found that anticoagulation was associated with a highly significant reduction in the number of embolic events; the benefit was greatest for patients with atrial fibrillation and LV EF <30% (see Chapter 32) (71). However, no controlled trial has evaluated the benefits or risks of anticoagulation for patients with CHF and sinus rhythm; a low frequency of embolic events has hampered the efforts to prospectively evaluate this issue. The precise role of anticoagulation for prevention of embolic stroke in patients with systolic CHF and sinus rhythm remains unknown (5). (See Chapter 32 for further discussion.)

D. Summary

1. Numerous large PRCTs have shown that ACE inhibition significantly reduces

Table 3-32 BASIS: Amiodarone in infarct survivors with complex arrhythmias (16)

	Amiodarone (n=98)	Placebo (n=114)	*P*
Total mortality	5%	13%	<0.05
Cardiac death (LV EF ≥40%)	1.5%	8.9%	<0.03
Cardiac death (LV EF <40%)	13.3%	13.8%	NS

morbidity and mortality for patients with chronic CHF and after an acute MI. For patients with asymptomatic LV dysfunction, ACE inhibitors also prevent progression to overt CHF and worsening pump failure. In all of these clinical settings, ACE inhibition was especially beneficial for the elderly and for those with severe LV dysfunction. Hydralazine-isosorbide combination is a reasonable alternative to ACE inhibition if the latter is contraindicated.

2. The first-generation calcium channel blockers are not recommended for routine management of patients with chronic CHF or acute MI. The role of second-generation calcium channel blockers such as amlodipine and felodipine is currently being evaluated.
3. The mortality benefit of β-blockers in patients with chronic CHF is unknown and is presently under study. However, numerous studies have consistently shown that β-blockers significantly reduce the rates of sudden death and reinfarction in post-MI patients. Those patients with overt CHF in this setting appeared to benefit the most.
4. Several well-designed studies have demonstrated that digoxin offers significant symptom relief even for patients already receiving long-term ACE inhibition. A large multicenter PRCT designed to evaluate the effect of digoxin on mortality in patients with moderate to severe chronic CHF and sinus rhythm has recently been completed. Preliminary analysis reportedly suggests that digoxin does not alter mortality but does reduce the incidence of worsening CHF. Peer review and publication of this study are awaited.
5. Vesnarinone (60 mg PO QD) is the only positive inotropic agent that has been shown to improve survival in patients with chronic CHF. However, at higher doses (120 mg) it appears to increase mortality. Although β-adrenergic agonists, dopaminergic agonists, and phosphodiesterase inhibitors can be helpful for short-term management of patients with severe LV dysfunction, long-term therapy with these agents has been associated with increased mortality. Similarly, flosequinan significantly improves symptoms but appears to increase mortality. Therefore, its use should be limited to patients whose desire for short-term improvement in quality of life significantly outweighs the potential reduction in the duration of life. Newer drugs such as ibopamine and pimobendan show promise, but further studies are needed.
6. Large PRCTs are in progress to examine the role of amiodarone in patients with severe chronic CHF and PVCs. Other studies are underway to evaluate the role of amiodarone in patients with low LV EF in the early post-MI period. Class I agents should be avoided because they can increase mortality, especially in those with ischemic heart disease.
7. Diuretics are clearly effective for symptom relief and are generally assumed to be safe. The precise role of anticoagulation for prevention of embolic stroke in patients with systolic CHF and sinus rhythm is unknown at this time.

Abbreviations used in Chapter 3

ACE = angiotensin-converting enzyme
ANP = atrial natriuretic peptide
AT I = angiotensin I
AT II = angiotensin II
ATPase = adenosine triphosphatase
AVP = arginine vasopressin
BID = twice daily
Ca^{2+} = calcium
CAD = coronary artery disease
cAMP = cyclic adenosine monophosphate
cGMP = cyclic guanine monophosphate

CHF = congestive heart failure
CI = confidence interval
EDRF = endothelium-derived relaxing factor
EF = ejection fraction
IDCM = idiopathic dilated cardiomyopathy
IP_3 = inositol 1,4,5-triphosphate
IV = intravenous
LV = left ventricular
LVEDP = left ventricular end-diastolic pressure
LVEDVI = left ventricular end-diastolic volume index
LV EF = left ventricular ejection fraction
MI = myocardial infarction
N = number of patients in population
n = number of patients in sample
Na^+ = sodium
NE = norepinephrine
NS = not significant
NYHA = New York Heart Association
OR = odds ratio
P = probability value
PCWP = pulmonary capillary wedge pressure
PO = per os
PRA = plasma renin activity
PRCT = prospective randomized controlled trial
PVC = premature ventricular contraction
QD = every day
QID = four times daily
r = correlation coefficient
RAAS = renin-angiotensin-aldosterone system
S_3 = third heart sound
SNS = sympathetic nervous system
TID = three times daily
vs. = versus

References

1. Acute Infarction Ramipril Efficacy (AIRE) Study Investigators. Effect of ramipril on mortality and morbidity of survivors of acute myocardial infarction with clinical evidence of heart failure. *Lancet* 1993;342:821.
2. Ambrosioni. The effect of the angiotension-converting-enzyme inhibitor zofenopril on mortality and morbidity after anterior myocardial infarction. *N Engl J Med* 1995;332:80.
3. Anderson. A randomized trial of low-dose beta-blockade therapy for idiopathic dilated cardiomyopathy. *Am J Cardiol* 1985;55:471.
4. Archibald. A treatment-associated increase in ejection fraction predicts long-term survival in congestive heart failure: the V-HeFT study. *Circulation* 1986;74 (Suppl II): II-309.
5. Baker. Management of heart failure: IV. Anticoagulation for patients with heart failure due to left ventricular systolic dysfunction. *JAMA* 1994;272:1614.
6. arabino. Comparative effects of long-term therapy with captopril and ibopamine in chronic congestive heart failure in old patients. *Cardiology* 1991;78:243.
7. Barnett. Flosequinan. *Lancet* 1993;341:733.
8. Benedict. Relation of neurohumoral activation to clinical variables and degree of ventricular dysfunction: a report from the Registry of Studies of Left Ventricular Dysfunction. *J Am Coll Cardiol* 1994;23:1410.
9. Benotti. Hemodynamic assessment of amrinone: a new inotropic agent. *N Engl J Med* 1978;299:1373.

10. Beta-Blocker Heart Attack Trial Research Group. A randomized trial of propranolol in patients with acute myocardial infarction: I. Mortality results. *JAMA* 1982;247:1707.
11. Beta-Blocker Pooling Project Research Group. The Beta-Blocker Pooling Project (BBPP): subgroup findings from randomized trials in post infarction patients. *Eur Heart J* 1988;9:8.
12. Binkley. Augmentation of diastolic function with phosphodiesterase inhibition in congestive heart failure. *J Lab Clin Med* 1989;114:266.
13. Binkley. Influence of flosequinan on autonomic tone in congestive heart failure: implications for the mechanism of the positive chronotropic effect and survival influence of long-term vasodilator administration. *Am Heart J* 1994;1994:128.
14. Bristow. β_1- and β_2-adrenergic-receptor subpopulations in nonfailing human –ventricular myocardium: coupling of both receptor subtypes to muscle contraction and selective β_1-receptor down-regulation in heart failure. *Circ Res* 1986;59: 297.
15. Bristow. Beta-adrenergic pathways in nonfailing and failing human ventricular myocardium. *Circulation* 1990;82(Suppl I):12.
16. Burkart. Effect of antiarrhythmic therapy on mortality in survivors of myocardial infarction with asymptomatic complex ventricular arrhythmias: Basel Antiarrhythmic Study of Infarct Survival (BASIS). *J Am Coll Cardiol* 1990;16:1711.
17. Burstein. Positive inotropic and lusitropic effects of intravenous flosequinan in patients with heart failure. *J Am Coll Cardiol* 1992;20:822.
18. Cairns. Post-myocardial infarction mortality in patients with ventricular premature depolarizations: Canadian Amiodarone Myocardial Infarction Arrhythmia Trial Pilot Study. *Circulation* 1991;84:550.
19. Califf. The prognosis in the presence of coronary artery disease. In: Braunwald, ed. *Congestive Heart Failure: Current Research and Clinical Applications.* New York: Grune & Stratton, 1992:31.
20. Cardiac Arrhythmia Suppression Trial II Investigators. Effect of the antiarrhythmic agent moricizine on survival after myocardial infarction. *N Engl J Med* 1992; 327:227.
21. Cas. Multicenter study on the clinical efficacy of chronic ibopamine administration. *Arzneimittelforschung* 1986;36:383.
22. Cas. Effects of acute and chronic ibopamine administration on resting and exercise hemodynamics, plasma catecholamines and functional capacity of patients with chronic congestive heart failure. *Am J Cardiol* 1992;70:629.
23. Cas. Clinical pharmacology of inodilators. *J Cardiovasc Pharmacol* 1989;14 (Suppl8):S60.
24. CASCADE Investigators. Randomized antiarrhythmic drug therapy in survivors of cardiac arrest (the CASCADE Study). *Am J Cardiol* 1993;72:280.
25. Ceremuzynski. Effect of amiodarone on mortality after myocardial infarction: a double-blind, placebo-controlled, pilot study. *J Am Coll Cardiol* 1992;20:1056.
26. Chadda. Effect of propranolol after acute myocardial infarction in patients with congestive heart failure. *Circulation* 1986;73:503.
27. Chinese Cardiac Study Collaborative Group. Oral captopril versus placebo among 13,634 patients with suspected acute myocardial infarction: interim report from the Chinese Cardiac Study (CCS-1). *Lancet* 1995;345:686.
28. Cody. Atrial natriuretic factor in normal subjects and heart failure patients: plasma levels and renal, hormonal, and hemodynamic responses to peptide infusion. *J Clin Invest* 1986;78:1362.
29. Cohn. Paroxysmal hypertension and hypovolemia. *N Engl J Med* 1966;275:643.
30. Cohn. Vasodilator therapy for heart failure: the influence of impedance on left ventricular performance. *Circulation* 1973;48:5.
31. Cohn. Plasma norepinephrine as a guide to prognosis in patients with chronic congestive heart failure. *N Engl J Med* 1984;311:819.
32. Cohn. Effect of vasodilator therapy on mortality in chronic congestive heart failure. *N Engl J Med* 1986;314:1547.
33. Cohn. Prognosis of congestive heart failure and predictors of mortality. *Am J Cardiol* 1988;62:25A.

34. Cohn. Heart failure with normal ejection fraction: the V-HeFT study. *Circulation* 1990;81:48.
35. Cohn. A comparison of enalapril with hydralazine-isosorbide dinitrate in the treatment of chronic congestive heart failure. *N Engl J Med* 1991;325:303.
36. Cohn. Vasodilators in heart failure: conclusions from V-HeFT II and rationale for V-HeFT III. *Drugs* 1994;47(Suppl 4):47.
37. Condorelli. The long-term efficacy of ibopamine in treating patients with severe heart failure: a multicenter investigation. *J Cardiovasc Pharmacol* 1989;14(Suppl 8):S83.
38. CONSENSUS Trial Study Group. Effects of enalapril on mortality in severe congestive heart failure. *N Engl J Med* 1987;316:1429.
39. Conti. Use of calcium antagonists to treat heart failure. *Clin Cardiol* 1994;17:101.
40. Corin. Flosequinan: a vasodilator with positive inotropic activity. *Am Heart J* 1991;121:537.
41. Cowley. Flosequinan in heart failure: acute haemodynamic and longer term symptomatic effects. *Br Med J* 1988;297:169.
42. Cowley. Long-term evaluation of treatment for chronic heart failure: a 1 year comparative trial of flosequinan and captopril. *Cardiovasc Drugs Ther* 1994;8:829.
43. Danish Study Group on Verapamil in Myocardial Infarction. Verapamil in acute myocardial infarction. *Eur Heart J* 1984;5:516.
44. Danish Study Group on Verapamil in Myocardial Infarction. Secondary prevention with verapamil after myocardial infarction. *Am J Cardiol* 1990;66:33I.
44a. The Digitalis Investigation Group. The effect of digoxin on mortality and morbidity in patients with heart failure. *N Engl J Med* 1997;336:525.
45. Doughty. Beta-blockers in heart failure: promising or proved. *J Am Coll Cardiol* 1994;23:814.
46. Doval. Randomised trial of low-dose amiodarone in severe congestive heart failure. *Lancet* 1994;344:493.
47. Downing. Contribution α-adrenoceptor activation to the pathogenesis of norepinephrine cardiomyopathy. *Circ Res* 1983;52:471.
48. Dzau. Prostaglandins in severe congestive heart failure: relation to activation of the renin-angiotensin system and hyponatremia. *N Engl J Med* 1984;310: 347.
49. Dzau. Circulating versus local renin-angiotensin system in cardiovascular homeostasis. *Circulation* 1988;7(Suppl I):I.
50. Dzau. Evolving concepts of the renin-angiotensin system: focus on renal and vascular mechanisms. *Am J Hypertens* 1988;1:334.
51. Dzau. Tissue renin-angiotensin system in myocardial hypertrophy and failure. *Arch Intern Med* 1993;153:937.
52. Echt. Mortality and morbidity in patients receiving encainide, flecainide, or placebo: the Cardiac Arrhythmia Suppression Trial. *N Engl J Med* 1991;324:781.
53. Eichhorn. The paradox of β-adrenergic blockade for the management of congestive heart failure. *Am J Med* 1992;92:527.
54. Elborn. Effect of flosequinan on exercise capacity and symptoms in severe heart failure. *Br Heart J* 1989;61:331.
55. Elkayam. A prospective, randomized double-blind, crossover study to compare the efficacy and safety of chronic nifedipine therapy with that of isosorbide dinitrate and their combination in the treatment of chronic congestive heart failure. *Circulation* 1990;82:1954.
56. Elkayam. Calcium channel blockers in heart failure. *J Am Coll Cardiol* 1993;22(Suppl A):139A.
57. Erlemeier. Comparison of hormonal and haemodynamic changes after long-term oral therapy with pimobendan or enalapril: a double-blind randomized study. *Eur Heart J* 1991;12:889.
58. Feldman. Deficient production of cyclic AMP: pharmacologic evidence of an important cause of contractile dysfunction in patients with end-stage heart failure. *Circulation* 1987;75:331.
59. Feldman. Increase of the 40,000-mol wt pertussis toxin substrate (G protein) in the failing human heart. *J Clin Invest* 1988;82:189.

60. Feldman. Usefulness of OPC-8212, a quinolinone derivative, for chronic congestive heart failure in patients with ischemic heart disease or idiopathic dilated cardiomyopathy. *Am J Cardiol* 1991;68:1203.
61. Feldman. Effects of vesnarinone on morbidity and mortality in patients with heart failure. *N Engl J Med* 1993;329:149.
62. Feldman. Can we alter survival in patients with congestive heart failure. *JAMA* 1992;267:1956.
63. Ferguson. Sympathoinhibitory responses to digitalis glycosides in heart failure patients: direct evidence from sympathetic neural recordings. *Circulation* 1989;80:65.
64. Ferguson. Digitalis and neurohormonal abnormalities in heart failure and implications for therapy. *Am J Cardiol* 1992;69:24G.
65. Fowler. Rationale for β-adrenergic blocking drugs in cardiomyopathy. *Am J Cardiol* 1985;55:D120.
66. Franciosa. Survival in men with severe chronic left ventricular failure due to either coronary heart disease or idiopathic dilated cardiomyopathy. *Am J Cardiol* 1983;51:831.
67. Francis. Neuroendocrine manifestations of congestive heart failure. *Am J Cardiol* 1988;62:9A.
68. Francis. Comparison of neuroendocrine activation in patients with left ventricular dysfunction with and without congestive heart failure: a substudy of the Studies of Left Ventricular Dysfunction (SOLVD). *Circulation* 1990;82:1724.
69. Francis. Plasma norepinephrine, plasma renin activity, and congestive heart failure. *Circulation* 1993;87(Suppl VI):VI.
70. Francis. Calcium channel blockers and congestive heart failure. *Circulation* 1991;83:336.
71. Fuster. The natural history of idiopathic dilated cardiomyopathy. *Am J Cardiol* 1981;47:525.
72. Gaasch. Diagnosis and treatment of heart failure based on left ventricular systolic or diastolic dysfunction. *JAMA* 1994;271:1276.
73. Gavras. Angiotensin- and norepinephrine-induced myocardial lesions: experimental and clinical studies in rabbits and man. *Am Heart J* 1975;89:321.
74. Gilbert. Flosequinan selectively lowers cardiac adrenergic drive in the failing human heart. *Circulation* 1992;86(Suppl I):I.
75. Gilbert. Therapy of idiopathic dilated cardiomyopathy with chronic β-adrenergic blockade. *Heart Vessels* 1991;6(Suppl):29.
76. Girbes. Effects of ibopamine on exercise-induced increase in norepinephrine in normal men. *J Cardiovasc Pharmacol* 1992;19:371.
77. Goldsmith. Increased plasma arginine vasopressin levels in patients with congestive failure. *J Am Coll Cardiol* 1983;1:1385.
78. Goldsmith. Differentiating systolic from diastolic heart failure: pathophysiologic and therapeutic considerations. *Am J Med* 1993;95:645.
79. Goldstein. Diltiazem increases late-onset congestive heart failure in postinfarction patients with early reduction in ejection fraction. *Circulation* 1991;83:52.
80. Gottlieb. Nifedipine in acute myocardial infarction: an assessment of left ventricular function, infarct size and infarct expansion: a double blind, randomised, placebo controlled trial. *Br Heart J* 1988;59:411.
81. Gottlieb. Prognostic importance of atrial natriuretic peptide in patients with chronic heart failure. *J Am Coll Cardiol* 1989;13:1534.
82. Gradman. Predictors of total mortality and sudden death in mild to moderate heart failure. *J Am Coll Cardiol* 1989;14:564.
83. Guyatt. A controlled trial of digoxin in congestive heart failure. *Am J Cardiol* 1988;61:371.
84. Haas. Chronic vasodilator therapy with flosequinan in congestive heart failure. *Clin Cardiol* 1990;13:414.
85. Haft. Cardiovascular injury induced by sympathetic catecholamines. *Prog Cardiovasc Dis* 1974;17:73.
86. Hagemeijer. Intractable heart failure despite angiotensin-converting enzyme inhibitors, digoxin, and diuretics: long-term effectiveness of add-on therapy with pimobendan. *Am Heart J* 1991;122:517.

87. Hagemeijer. Calcium sensitization with pimobendan: pharmacology, haemodynamic improvement, and sudden death in patients with chronic congestive heart failure. *Eur Heart J* 1993;14:551.
88. Heilbrunn. Increased β-receptor density and improved hemodynamic response to catecholamine stimulation during long-term metoprolol therapy in heart failure from dilated cardiomyopathy. *Circulation* 1989;79:483.
89. Hine. Meta-analysis of empirical long-term antiarrhythmic therapy after myocardial infarction. *JAMA* 1989;262:3037.
90. Hirsch. Potential role of the tissue renin-angiotensin system in the pathophysiology of congestive heart failure. *Am J Cardiol* 1990;66:22D.
91. Hockings. Effectiveness of amiodarone on ventricular arrhythmias during and after acute myocardial infarction. *Am J Cardiol* 1987;60:967.
92. Imperato-McGinley. Reversibility of catecholamine-induced dilated cardiomyopathy in a child with pheochromocytoma. *N Engl J Med* 1987;316:793.
93. *Informational Letter to Physicians: Flosequinan.* Boots Pharmaceutical, 1993.
94. ISIS-4 (Fourth International Study of Infarct Survival) Collaborative Group. ISIS-4: a randomised factorial trial assessing early oral captopril, oral mononitrate, and intravenous magnesium sulphate in 58,050 patients with suspected acute myocardial infarction. *Lancet* 1995;345:669.
95. Israeli SPRINT Study Group. Secondary Prevention Reinfarction Israeli Nifedipine Trial (SPRINT): a randomized intervention trial of nifedipine in patients with acute myocardial infarction. *Eur Heart J* 1988;9:354.
96. Ito. Endothelin-1 induces hypertrophy with enhanced expression of muscle-specific genes in cultured neonatal rat cardiomyocytes. *Circ Res* 1991;69:209.
97. Jaeschke. To what extent do congestive heart failure patients in sinus rhythm benefit from digoxin therapy? A systematic overview and meta-analysis. *Am J Med* 1990;88:279.
98. Kannel. Epidemiology in heart failure. *Am Heart J* 1991;121:951.
99. Katz. Cyclic adenosine monophosphate effects on the myocardium: a man who blows hot and cold with one breath. *J Am Coll Cardiol* 1983;2:143.
100. Katz. Potential deleterious effects of inotropic agents in the the therapy of chronic heart failure. *Circulation* 1986;73(Suppl III):III.
101. Katz. Cellular mechanisms in congestive heart failure. *Am J Cardiol* 1988;62:3A.
102. Katz. Cardiomyopathy of overload: a major determinant of prognosis in congestive heart failure. *N Engl J Med* 1990;322:100.
103. Katz. A multicenter, randomized, double-blind, placebo-controlled trial of pimobendan, a new cardiotonic and vasodilator agent, in patients with severe congestive heart failure. *Am Heart J* 1992;123:95.
104. Kayanakis. Comparison of ibopamine and placebo in the treatment of chronic congestive heart failure NYHA class II-III. *Cardiovascular Drugs Ther* 1987;1:255.
105. Kennedy. Beta-blocker therapy in the cardiac arrhythmia suppression trial. *Am J Cardiol* 1994;74:674.
106. Kleber. Impact of converting enzyme inhibition on progression of chronic heart failure: results of the Munich Mild Heart Failure Trial. *Br Heart J* 1992;67:289.
107. Kubo. Endothelium-dependent vasodilation is attenuated in patients with heart failure. *Circulation* 1991;84:1589.
108. Kubo. Beneficial effects of pimobendan on exercise tolerance and quality of life in patients with heart failure: results of a multicenter trial. *Circulation* 1992;85:942.
109. Lee. Heart failure in outpatients: a randomized trial of digoxin versus placebo. *N Engl J Med* 1982;306:699.
110. Leimbach. Direct evidence from intraneural recordings for increased central sympathetic outflow in patients with heart failure. *Circulation* 1986;5:913.
111. Liang. Sustained improvement of cardiac function in patients with congestive heart failure after short-term infusion of dobutamine. *Circulation* 1984;69:113.
112. Lichstein. Relation between beta-adrenergic blocker use, various correlates of left ventricular function and the chance of developing congestive heart failure. *J Am Coll Cardiol* 1990;16:1327.
113. Mancia. Reflex cardiovascular control in congestive heart failure. *Am J Cardiol* 1992;69:17G.

114. Mancini. Antiarrhythmic drug use and high serum levels of digoxin are independent adverse prognostic factors in patients with chronic heart failure. *Circulation* 1991;84(Suppl II):243.
115. Marantz. The relationship between left ventricular systolic function and congestive heart failure diagnosed by clinical criteria. *Circulation* 1988;77:607.
116. Massie. Long-term oral administration of amrinone for congestive heart failure: lack of efficacy in a multicenter controlled trial. *Circulation* 1985;71:963.
117. Massie. Can further benefit be achieved by adding flosequinan to patients with congestive heart failure who remain symptomatic on diuretic, digoxin, and an angiotensin converting enzyme inhibitor? *Circulation* 1993;88:492.
118. Massie. Survival of patients with congestive heart failure: past, present, and future prospects. *Circulation* 1987;75(Suppl IV):IV.
119. McKee. The natural history of congestive heart failure: The Framingham study. *N Engl J Med* 1971;285:1441.
120. Miao. Cyclic AMP–independent inotropic action of flosequinan. *Circulation* 1992;86(Suppl I):I.
121. Miller. Integrated cardiac, renal, and endocrine actions of endothelin. *J Clin Invest* 1989;83:317.
122. Miocardico. GISSI-3: effects of lisinopril and transdermal glyceryl trinitrate singly and together on 6-week mortality and ventricular function after acute myocardial infarction. *Lancet* 1994;343:1115.
123. Missale. Inhibition of aldosterone secretion by dopamine, ibopamine, and dihydroergotoxine in patients with congestive heart disease. *J Cardiovasc Pharmacol* 1989;14(Suppl 8):S72.
124. Muller. Nifedipine therapy for patients with threatened and acute myocardial infarction: a randomized, double-blind, placebo-controlled comparison. *Circulation* 1984;69:740.
125. Mulrow. Relative efficacy of vasodilator therapy in chronic congestive heart failure: implications of randomized trials. *JAMA* 1988;259:3422.
126. Multicenter Diltiazem Postinfarction Trial Research Group. The effect of diltiazem on mortality and reinfarction after myocardial infarction. *N Engl J Med* 1988;319:385.
127. Nademanee. Amiodarone and post-MI patients. *Circulation* 1993;88:764.
128. Naftilan. Induction of platelet-growth factor A-chain and *c-myc* gene expressions by angiotensin II in cultured rat vascular smooth muscle cells. *J Clin Invest* 1989;83:1419.
129. Neuser. Mitogenic activity of endothelin-1 and -3 on vascular smooth muscle cells is inhibited by atrial natriuretic peptides. *Artery* 1990;17:311.
130. Nicklas. Prospective, double-blind, placebo-controlled trial of low-dose amiodarone in patients with severe heart failure and asymptomatic frequent ventricular ectopy. *Am Heart J* 1991;122:1016.
131. Norwegian Multicenter Study Group. Timolol-induced reduction in mortality and reinfarction in patients surviving acute myocardial infarction. *N Engl J Med* 1981;304:801.
132. OPC-8212 Multicenter Research Group. A placebo-controlled, randomized, double-blind study of OPC-8212 in patients with mild chronic heart failure. *Cardiovasc Drugs Ther* 1990;4:419.
133. Packer. Are nitrates effective in the treatment of chronic heart failure? Antagonist's viewpoint. *Am J Cardiol* 1990;66:458.
134. Packer. Effect of oral milrinone on mortality in severe chronic heart failure. *N Engl J Med* 1991;325:1468.
135. Packer. Randomized, multicenter, double-blind, placebo-controlled evaluation of amlodipine in patients with mild-to-moderate heart failure. *J Am Coll Cardiol* 1991;17:274A.
136. Packer. Double-blind, placebo-controlled study of the efficacy of flosequinan in patients with chronic heart failure. *J Am Coll Cardiol* 1993;22:65.
137. Packer. Withdrawal of digoxin from patients with chronic heart failure treated with angiotensin-converting-enzyme inhibitors. *N Engl J Med* 1993;329:1.

138. Pfeffer. Ventricular remodeling after myocardial infarction: experimental observations and clinical implications. *Circulation* 1990;81:1161.
139. Pfeffer. Effect of captopril on mortality and morbidity in patients with left ventricular dysfunction after myocardial infarction: results of the survival and ventricular enlargement trial. *N Engl J Med* 1992;327:669.
140. Pfeffer. Development and prevention of congestive heart failure following myocardial infarction. *Circulation* 1993;87(Suppl IV):IV.
141. Pfisterer. Beneficial effect of amiodarone on cardiac mortality in patients with asymptomatic complex ventricular arrhythmias after acute myocardial infarction and preserved but not impaired left ventricular function. *Am J Cardiol* 1992;69:1399.
142. Pitt. A randomized, multicenter, double-blind placebo controlled study of the efficacy of flosequinan in patients with chronic heart failure. *Circulation* 1991;84(Suppl II):II.
143. Rafjer. Effects of long-term therapy with oral ibopamine on resting hemodynamics and exercise capacity in patients with heart failure: relationship to the generation of *N*-methyldopamine and to plasma norepinephrine levels. *Circulation* 1986;73:740.
144. Reffo. Double-blind acute hemodynamic invasive evaluation in congestive heart failure before and after open sustained treatment with ibopamine. *Current Therapeutic Research* 1988;44:723.
145. Remme. Hemodynamic, neurohumoral, and myocardial energetic effects of pimobendan, a novel calcium-sensitizing compound, in patients with mild to moderate heart failure. *J Cardiovasc Pharmacol* 1994;24:730.
146. Remme. Long-term efficacy and safety of pimobendan in moderate heart failure: a double-blind parallel 6-month comparison with enalapril. *Eur Heart J* 1994;15:947.
147. Remme. Inodilator therapy for heart failure: early, late, or not at all? *Circulation* 1993;87(Suppl IV):IV.
148. Rodeheffer. Increased plasma concentrations of endothelin in congestive heart failure in humans. *Mayo Clin Proc* 1992;67:719.
149. Rosenbaum. Effects of adrenergic receptor antagonists on cardiac morphological and functional alterations in rats harboring pheochromocytoma. *J Pharmacol Exp Ther* 1987;241:354.
150. Rouleau. Activation of neurohormonal systems following acute myocardial infarction. *Am J Cardiol* 1991;68:80D.
151. Sackner-Bernstein. Does digoxin exert an adverse effect on survival? Prognostic importance of serum digoxin levels in patients with chronic heart failure. *Circulation* 1991;84(Suppl II):244.
152. Sasayama. Clinical effects of long-term administration of pimobendan in patients with moderate congestive heart failure. *Heart Vessels* 1994;9:113.
153. Schocken. Prevalence and mortality rate of congestive heart failure in the United States. *J Am Coll Cardiol* 1992;20:301.
154. Silke. A double-blind, parallel-group comparison of flosequinan and enalapril in the treatment of chronic heart failure. *Eur Heart J* 1992;13:1092.
155. Singh. Amiodarone in patients with congestive heart failure and asymptomatic ventricular arrhythmia. *N Engl J Med* 1995;333:77.
156. Sirnes. Evolution of infarct size during the early use of nifedipine in patients with acute myocardial infarction: the Norwegian nifedipine multicenter trial. *Circulation* 1984;70:638.
157. Smith. Digitalis: mechanisms of action and clinical use. *N Engl J Med* 1988;318:358.
158. SOLVD Investigators. Effect of enalapril on survival in patients with reduced left ventricular ejection fractions and congestive heart failure. *N Engl J Med* 1991;325:293.
159. SOLVD Investigators. Effect of enalapril on mortality and the development of heart failure in asymptomatic patients with reduced left ventricular ejection fractions. *N Engl J Med* 1992;327:685.
160. Sonnenblick. Heart failure: its progression and its therapy. *Hosp Prac* 1993;28:75.

161. Stewart. Prospective, randomised, double-blind, placebo-controlled trial of low dose amiodarone in patients with severe heart failure and frequent ventricular ectopy. *Eur Heart J* 1989;10:229. Abstract.
162. Swedberg. Hormones regulating cardiovascular function in patients with severe congestive heart failure and their relation to mortality. *Circulation* 1990;82:1730.
163. Swedberg. Effects of the early administration of enalapril on mortality in patients with acute myocardial infarction. *N Engl J Med* 1992;327:678.
164. Tan. Cardiotoxic effects of angiotensin II. *J Am Coll Cardiol* 1989;13:2A.
165. Unverferth. Regression of myocardial cellular hypertrophy with vasodilator therapy in chronic congestive heart failure associated with idiopathic dilated cardiomyopathy. *Am J Cardiol* 1983;51:1392.
166. Uretsky. Multicenter trial of oral enoximone in patients with moderate to moderately severe congestive heart failure: lack of benefit compared with placebo. *Circulation* 1990;82:774.
167. Uretsky. Randomized study assessing the effect of digoxin withdrawal in patients with mild to moderate chronic congestive heart failure: results of the PROVED trial. *J Am Coll Cardiol* 1993;22:955.
168. Veldhuisen. Double-blind placebo-controlled study of ibopamine and digoxin in patients with mild to moderate heart failure: results of the Dutch Ipopamine Multicenter Trial (DIMT). *J Am Coll Cardiol* 1993;22:1564.
169. Veldhuisen. Effects of ibopamine on the increase in plasma norepinephrine levels during exercise in congestive heart failure. *Am J Cardiol* 1993;71:992.
170. Viscoli. Beta-blockers after myocardial infarction: influence of first-year clinical course on long-term effectiveness. *Ann Intern Med* 1993;118:99.
171. Vliet. Focal myocarditis associated with pheochromocytoma. *N Engl J Med* 1966;274:1102.
172. Waagstein. Beneficial effects of metoprolol in idiopathic dilated cardiomyopathy. *Lancet* 1993;342:1441.
173. Weishaar. Direct effect of flosequinan on the contractility of cardiac muscle fibers from patients with and without heart failure. *Circulation* 1991;84(Suppl II):II.
174. Wilcox. Trial of early nifedipine in acute myocardial infarction: the TRENT study. *Br Med J* 1986;293:1204.
175. Wilson. Prognosis in severe heart failure: relation to hemodynamic measurements and ventricular ectopic activity. *J Am Coll Cardiol* 1983;2:403.
176. Xamoterol in Severe Heart Failure Study Group. Xamoterol in severe heart failure. *Lancet* 1990;336:1.
177. Yancy. Congestive heart failure. *Dis Mon* 1988;34:465.
178. Yates. Pharmacology of flosequinan. *Am Heart J* 1991;121:974.
179. Yusuf. Effect of intravenous nitrates on mortality in acute myocardial infarction: an overview of the randomised trials. *Lancet* 1988;1:1088.
180. Yusuf. Inotropic agents increase mortality in patients with congestive heart failure. *Circulation* 1990;82(Suppl III):III.
181. Yusuf. Need for a large randomized trial to evaluate the effects of digitalis on morbidity and mortality in congestive heart failure. *Am J Cardiol* 1992;69:64G.

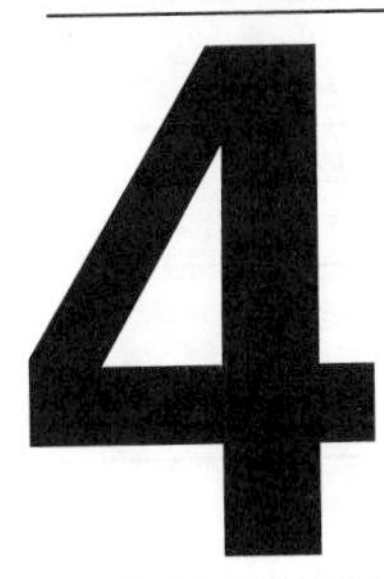

Congestive Heart Failure: Diastolic Failure

Stephen I. Hsu and
Patrick T. O'Gara

A. Introduction

1. Primary diastolic failure has been defined as "a condition with classic findings of congestive failure with abnormal diastolic but normal systolic function at rest" (16). Although most patients with congestive heart failure (CHF) have both systolic and diastolic dysfunction to varying degrees, distinguishing between them is important because the therapeutic implications vary depending on which process is predominant (61).
2. Among patients with clinically evident CHF, 34% to 42% have preserved left ventricular (LV) systolic function (1,25,26,81). Although by implication these patients are presumed to have diastolic dysfunction, actual diastolic abnormalities are documented in only about 40% of these cases. This discrepancy may be caused by the relatively poor accuracy of the noninvasive diagnostic modalities currently used for demonstration of abnormal diastolic filling (see section C of this chapter) and by the role of intermittent ischemia in producing transient diastolic dysfunction and CHF.
   a. In one study involving 151 patients at a referral center who had classic signs and symptoms compatible with CHF, 34% had an LV ejection fraction (LV EF) ≥55% by echocardiography (1).
   b. In Soufer's study of 58 patients with New York Heart Association (NYHA) class III or IV CHF and preserved LV EF (≥45%), the majority had significant (38%) or probable (24%) diastolic dysfunction as inferred from decreased peak filling rates by radionuclide study (see section C2). During a subsequent prospective 3-month sampling period in the same study, 42% of the 74 patients with CHF had preserved LV EF (81).
   c. Because the indices of LV diastolic function worsen during the normal aging process, diastolic dysfunction may be especially important among the elderly (84). In a study of 47 elderly nursing home residents receiving long-term digoxin therapy, 75% of the patients had LV EF ≥50% (29).
3. Although CHF caused by isolated diastolic dysfunction is associated with significant morbidity, it is associated with relatively low cardiac mortality (15,19). However, in the presence of coronary artery disease (CAD), the mortality and morbidity in these patients approach those in patients with CHF caused by systolic dysfunction (46,78).
   a. For example, the annual mortality rate was only 1.3% in Brogan's follow-up study of 51 patients who had isolated diastolic dysfunction (LV EF >50%), few symptoms at presentation, and no CAD by cardiac catheterization. The morbidity was more significant: new-onset CHF developed at an annual rate of 6.9% (15).
   b. In the Vasodilators in Heart Failure Trial (V-HeFT), in which patients with chronic CHF were observed for an average of 2.3 years, the annual mortality rate was significantly lower in patients with normal LV EF (≥45%) than in those with depressed LV EF (<45%). Compared with those with depressed LV EF, patients with normal LV EF were less likely to have CAD and more likely to have a history of hypertension (HTN) (19) (see Table 4-1).

Table 4-1 Mortality as a function of LV EF in chronic CHF (19)

	Normal LV EF (≥45) (n=83)	Low LV EF (<45) (n=540)	*P*
CAD	26.5%	47.2%	<0.01
History of hypertension	53.0%	39.4%	<0.02
Mortality rate	8%	19%	0.0001

c. In a 7-year follow-up of the cohort originally reported by Soufer (see section A2b), the rates of cardiovascular mortality and morbidity (*i.e.*, recurrent CHF, myocardial infarction, unstable angina) were 46% and 29%, respectively (78). In part, the higher mortality rate may have resulted from the fact that 52% of the patients had evidence of CAD by clinical assessment. In addition, Soufer's cohort was older and more critically ill at the time of entry than those in either the V-HeFT or Brogan's study.

d. In a 6-year case-control study of 284 patients from the Coronary Artery Surgery Study (CASS) registry with moderate to severe CHF and preserved LV EF, the mortality rate was significantly higher in the study group than in the control group without CHF (18% versus 9%, respectively, $P<0.0001$) (46). As shown in Table 4-2, the severity of CAD correlated with the risk of death in the study group.

B. Pathophysiology

1. Diastole is most frequently described as a biphasic process. It begins with rapid ventricular filling, during which the left arterial pressure exceeds the LV pressure and the ventricle begins to relax. This phase is followed by a period of relatively slow passive filling (diastasis), which terminates with atrial contraction (61). However, physiologic consideration of the heart as an integrated muscular pump dictates that ventricular contraction (isovolumetric contraction and ejection) and relaxation (isovolumetric relaxation and rapid filling) be considered as parts of one contraction-relaxation cycle or "systole" (16). Both phases of systole are energy-dependent, and they are closely related processes (see section B3b). Diastole may then be defined as the phase during the cardiac cycle that separates two consecutive contraction-relaxation cycles (see Figure 1). It consists of diastasis, during which there is no measurable change in the ventricular volume, and atrial contraction, which contributes the last 5% to 15% of volume change during ventricular filling (16).

a. Diastolic failure results from an increased resistance to filling of one or both ventricles. Symptoms of pulmonary or systemic venous congestion (or both) occur as a result of elevated atrial pressure generated by an inappropriate upward shift of the diastolic pressure-volume curve during the terminal phase of the cardiac cycle (see Figure 4-1) (16).

b. Exercise intolerance, manifesting as dyspnea and fatigue, is considered to be an early sign of diastolic failure (70). This has been attributed to a limited ability of the abnormal ventricle to utilize the Frank–Starling mechanism. Abnormal stiffness of the ventricle causes a rapid increase in the ventricular filling pressures and limits the physiologic increase in end-diastolic and stroke volumes in response to exercise (85).

2. Causes of Diastolic Failure—In the largest series reported to date, CHF and intact systolic function were most frequently associated with CAD, HTN, and

Table 4-2 Mortality as a function of the severity of CAD in chronic CHF (46)

	No CAD	1- or 2-Vessel CAD	3-Vessel CAD	*P*
Mortality rate	8%	17%	32%	0.0001

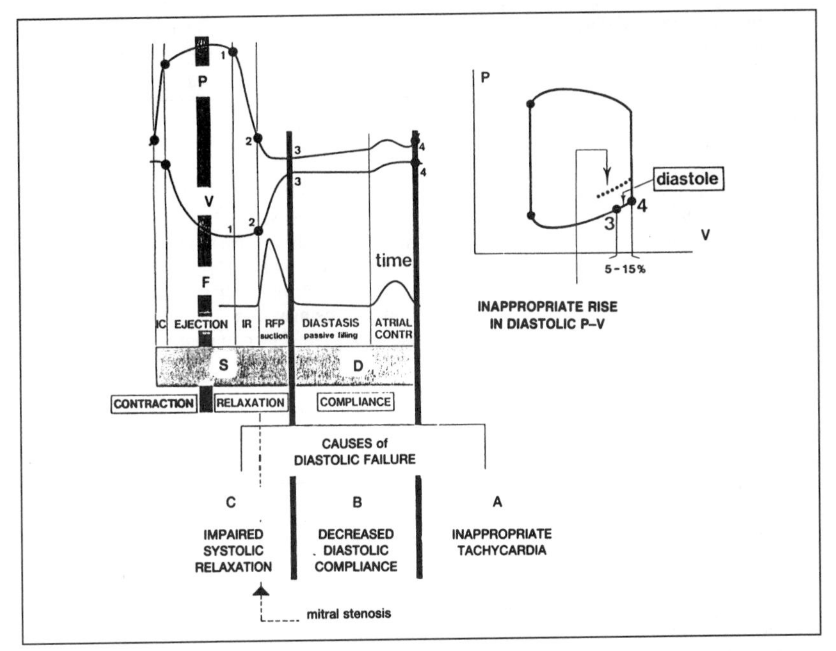

Fig. 4-1 Subdivision of the cardiac cycle into systole (S) and diastole (D), illustrating the causes of diastolic failure: CONTR = contraction; F = flow; IC = isovolumetric contraction; IR = isovolumetric relaxation; P = pressure; RFP = rapid filling phase; V = volume. 1 = aortic valve closure; 2 = mitral valve opening; 3 = end of early rapid filling; 4 = end-diastole. Reproduced with permission from Brutsaert et al, "Diastolic Failure." *JACC*, Vol. 22, No. 1; 1993.

restrictive cardiomyopathy. Among the 58 patients in this study, 28% had CAD without HTN, 10% had HTN without CAD, 22% had both CAD and HTN, and 10% had restrictive cardiomyopathy. In all, 70% of the patients had one or more of these three conditions (81). In physiologic terms, there are three primary causes of diastolic failure (see Figure 4-1): inappropriate tachycardia, decreased diastolic compliance, and impaired systolic relaxation. Whereas systolic relaxation is an active and energy-dependent process, diastolic compliance is determined principally by the passive viscoelastic properties of the heart (49). For many patients with diastolic failure, more than one factor may be present. For example, in patients with hypertrophic cardiomyopathy, the increased resistance to ventricular filling results from decreased diastolic compliance (increased wall thickness and fibrosis) and from impaired systolic relaxation (abnormal calcium handling).

a. **Inappropriate Tachycardia**—Tachycardia shortens the diastolic filling time and limits the end-diastolic volume. Tachycardia may also increase the rate of calcium influx, which causes a net intracellular accumulation of the ion and an increase in diastolic wall tension (see section B3b) (36).
b. **Decreased Diastolic Compliance**
   (1) The major conditions associated with decreased diastolic compliance are listed in Tables 4-3 and 4-4 (16,34,55,81).
   (2) **Hypertrophy and Diastolic Dysfunction**—Hypertrophy is a response of the myocardium to sustained pressure or volume overload. Sustained pressure overload, as occurs in chronic HTN and aortic

Table 4-3 Decreased diastolic compliance due to ventricle structural changes

Condition	Mechanism of Diastolic Dysfunction
Restrictive cardiomyopathy Amyloidosis Hemochromatosis Interstitial fibrosis (scleroderma) Hypothyroidism	Increased resistance to ventricular inflow
Ventricular hypertrophy Hypertrophic cardiomyopathy Chronic hypertension Aortic stenosis	Increased resistance to ventricular inflow due to thick chamber walls and altered collagen matrix; activation of renin-angiotensin system
Ischemic heart disease Postinfarction scarring and aneurysm Dilated cardiomyopathy	Increased resistance to ventricular inflow due to myocardial fibrosis or scar
Obliterative cardiomyopathy Endomyocardial fibroelastosis Loeffler syndrome	Increased resistance to ventricular inflow

Table 4-4 Other causes of decreased diastolic compliance

Condition	Mechanism of Diastolic Dysfunction
Pericardial constraint Effusive/constrictive pericarditis Tamponade Ventricular enlargement	Direct compression of ventricle by diseased pericardium during diastole; or mechanical constraint by normal pericardium during diastole if cardiac dilation or tamponade is present
Cor pulmonale Pulmonary diseases Pulmonary embolism Pulmonary venocclusive disease Primary pulmonary hypertension Other causes of pulmonary hypertension	RV and LV cross-talk: unilateral RV overload, especially in conditions of pericardial constraint, is transmitted to the LV, where it may decrease diastolic compliance Increased RA pressure may lead to engorgement of coronary veins, increased myocardial blood volume, and reduced LV diastolic compliance

stenosis, leads to concentric LV hypertrophy (LVH) and medial wall thickening of the intramyocardial coronary arteries, which results in decreased vasodilator reserve (34). However, LVH alone does not appear to be responsible for the abnormal stiffness of the ventricle. Rather, qualitative and quantitative changes in myocardial collagen lead to increased interstitial and perivascular fibrosis, which correlates with increased myocardial stiffness (13). This process appears to be hormonally regulated and may underlie the transition from compensated LVH to decompensated heart failure. Both circulating and local trophic factors have been implicated in the physiologic adaptation of the heart to pressure overload.

(a) **Role of the Activated Renin-Angiotensin-Aldosterone System (RAAS)**—In a comparison of experimental rat models of HTN, myocardial fibrosis was observed only in those models in which the RAAS was activated (94,95). These animal studies suggest that (a) interstitial and perivascular fibrosis is not a uniform accompaniment to myocyte hypertrophy but is associated with the presence of elevated circulating levels of angiotensin II or aldosterone, or both; (b) increased local angiotensin II production, caused by enhanced expression and activity of a cardiac angiotensin-converting enzyme (ACE), is associated with marked diastolic dysfunction; (c) the reactive and reparative fibrotic process associated with activation of the RAAS can be reversed with administration of an ACE inhibitor (76,94,95).

(b) **Role of Endothelins**—In vitro studies have implicated endothelins, a family of peptide hormones released locally by myocardial vascular endothelial cells, in the stimulation of myocyte hypertrophy and myocardial fibrosis by a paracrine mechanism (35,56,80).

c. **Impaired Systolic Relaxation**

(1) Impaired systolic relaxation may cause an upward shift of the pressure-volume curve if the abnormal systolic relaxation phase (decreased rate or extent of relaxation) extends into true diastole. The major conditions associated with impaired systolic relaxation are listed in Table 4-5 (16,34).

(2) **Clinical and Physiologic Consequences**—Slowing of the relaxation process leads to increased dependence on late diastolic filling and atrial contraction to achieve adequate stretch of the sarcomeres at end-diastole. It also interferes with coronary perfusion by allowing myocardial contraction to persist into early diastole, thereby compressing intramyocardial coronary vessels and reducing the coronary pressure gradient for subendocardial perfusion. Transient subendocardial ischemia may occur in the hypertrophied heart even in the absence of epicardial coronary artery stenoses (34).

(3) Myocardial relaxation is influenced primarily by the intracellular level of calcium (Ca^{2+}). After myocardial contraction, a powerful calcium-transporting adenosine triphosphatase (ATPase) pumps Ca^{2+} back into storage sites in the sarcoplasmic reticulum. Ca^{2+} is also transported out of the cell by sodium-calcium exchange and by calcium pumps located in the myocardial cell membrane (the sarcolemma). Impaired relaxation may result from high levels of intracellular Ca^{2+} that occur because of abnormalities in the key components of this process, which are described in the following sections.

(a) **Depletion of Adenosine Triphosphate (ATP)**—Myocardial relaxation may be impaired during conditions such as ischemia or hypoxia because of a decrease in the availability of high-energy phosphates (67).

(b) **Abnormal Handling of Ca^{2+}**—A diminished capacity to restore low resting levels of intracellular Ca^{2+} during the relaxation phase has been demonstrated in myocardial preparations from patients with end-stage dilated and hypertrophic cardiomyopa-

Table 4-5 Causes of impaired systolic relaxation

Condition	Mechanism of Diastolic Dysfunction
Ischemic heart disease Acute pulmonary edema Dyspnea during angina Acute MI	Impaired myocardial relaxation; calcium overload during diastole
Hypertrophic cardiomyopathy	Impaired myocardial relaxation; calcium overload during diastole; increased susceptibility to ischemia during tachycardia or exercise
Dilated cardiomyopathy	Impaired myocardial relaxation; calcium overload during diastole

thy. (36) This abnormality was more marked with rapid stimulation and in tissue preparations from hypertrophic hearts. Abnormalities in Ca^{2+} handling by both the sarcolemma (increased calcium entry) and the sarcoplasmic reticulum (decreased rate of calcium resequestration) were present in myopathic muscles. Abnormal Ca^{2+} handling may also underlie the impaired diastolic relaxation observed during demand ischemia or hypoxia in the hypertrophic heart, such as that resulting from exercise-induced tachycardia (34,51).

(c) Deficient Production of Cyclic Adenosine Monophosphate (cAMP)—This second messenger enhances diastolic relaxation by causing the phosphorylation of troponin I and phospholamban, thereby promoting the resequestration of Ca^{2+} during myocardial relaxation. Deficient production of cAMP appears to be a fundamental defect in end-stage failing hearts. (27) This deficiency could be a result of decreased β-adrenergic receptor stimulation caused by downregulation of β_1-adrenergic receptors or of uncoupling of the β_2-adrenergic receptor from adenylate cyclase because of increased levels of G_i (the inhibitory component of the G protein–adenylate cyclase complex), both of which have been demonstrated in the failing heart (14,28).

C. Diagnosis of Diastolic Dysfunction

1. Clinical Assessment

a. A consideration of the patient's history, physical findings, and chest radiograph may occasionally offer clues that help distinguish CHF caused by diastolic dysfunction from that caused by systolic dysfunction. The absence of cardiomegaly and the presence of a fourth heart sound (S_4) gallop and LV hypertrophy in an obese, hypertensive female favors the diagnosis of diastolic dysfunction (33). In a study of 82 consecutive patients hospitalized for decompensated CHF, the combination of diastolic blood pressure ≥105 mm Hg plus absence of jugular venous distention was highly predictive of preserved systolic function; if both criteria were met, the specificity and the positive predictive value were 100% (32).

b. However, in the same study, this combination had a sensitivity of only 30% for identification of preserved systolic function (32). Therefore, objective measurement of LV EF and functional assessment of LV diastolic properties by echocardiography, radionuclide scanning, or cardiac catheterization are usually necessary for accurate diagnosis and appropriate therapy. In one study of 20 patients with CHF, the echocardiographic finding of preserved systolic function was unexpected in 90% and led to a change of therapeutic strategy in each case (26). In another study, 51% of 51 patients with preserved LV EF were being treated with digoxin in the absence of atrial arrhythmia (1).

2. Echocardiography

a. In a patient with heart failure, the finding of normal or near-normal LV EF (*i.e.*, ≥45%) on echocardiography suggests diastolic dysfunction as the cause of CHF (85). Echocardiography may also identify other important conditions such as LVH, pericardial effusion, myocardial infiltration, or valvular heart disease.

b. In addition, a pulsed Doppler echocardiographic evaluation of the transmitral velocity patterns is a noninvasive and readily available technique that provides reproducible measurements of LV diastolic function. It compares favorably with radionuclide and angiographically derived hemodynamic indices (3,83). The complexity of diastolic function, however, cannot adequately be reflected in any single parameter of LV filling. Instead, a simultaneous assessment of the ratio of peak early to peak late transmitral velocity (E:A ratio), isovolumic relaxation time (IVRT), and deceleration time (DT) is necessary (89).

(1) **E:A Ratio**—In a normal transmitral filling pattern, the peak E velocity (rapid filling phase) is greater than the peak A velocity (atrial contraction phase). An E:A ratio ≤1.0 has been used by some investigators as an indicator of impaired LV relaxation. However, the E:A ratio may be difficult to interpret in isolation because it decreases with age and is influenced by a variety of factors, including preload, afterload, heart rate, and atrial systole.

(2) **Isovolumic Relaxation Time**—IVRT is measured from the closing of the aortic valve until the opening of the mitral valve. Prolonged IVRT is probably the most sensitive Doppler index of impaired relaxation because it is the first parameter to become abnormal in patients with diastolic dysfunction. It is influenced by the heart rate but appears to be relatively independent of LV loading conditions.

(3) **Deceleration Time**—DT is the measured interval from the peak of the early flow velocity (E) to the return of the flow velocity to baseline. Prolonged DT may be a more sensitive index of impaired relaxation than the E:A ratio. It is altered by changes in LV loading conditions but appears to be independent of the heart rate and the peak E velocity.

c. Table 4-6 shows the characteristic transmitral Doppler inflow velocity (DIV) patterns in patients with diastolic dysfunction caused by impaired relaxation versus decreased compliance.

d. Because the transmitral velocity patterns are influenced by the heart rate and loading conditions of the heart, they cannot be relied on exclusively to establish a diagnosis of diastolic dysfunction (33). Similarly, when used in clinical studies to demonstrate an effect of drug therapy on diastolic function, alterations in transmitral velocity patterns may reflect drug-induced changes in heart rate or loading conditions rather than a true effect on the inherent diastolic properties.

3. **Radionuclide Angiography**—This technique uses radioactively labeled red blood cells to image the heart throughout the cardiac cycle. It can provide an estimate of the LV EF as well as an indirect assessment of ventricular relaxation. Abnormal relaxation is associated with a decreased peak filling rate (PFR), a prolonged time to peak filling (TPFR), and a decreased fraction of filling during the first third of diastole (FF-1/3) (11). Because these measurements are influenced by the heart rate and loading conditions, they cannot independently establish a diagnosis of diastolic heart failure (33).

4. **Invasive Hemodynamic Studies**—Left and right cardiac catheterization remains the gold standard for evaluation of LV diastolic properties, because the ventricular pressures can be measured directly. The rate of LV relaxation has been quantitated by measuring the maximal rate of fall of the LV pressure (peak −dP/dt) and the time constant (T) of an assumed exponential decline in LV pressure during isovolumic relaxation (3). In addition, LV diastolic compliance can be determined from the pressure-volume loops generated during mechanical obstruction of inferior vena caval inflow (49). Despite its superiority to other diagnostic techniques, the routine use of cardiac catheterization for assessment of diastolic function is often not practical given its invasive nature,

Table 4-6 Transmitral DIV patterns in diastolic dysfunction

Pattern	Peak E	Peak A	E:A ratio	IVRT	DT
Impaired relaxation	Decreased	Normal or increased	Decreased	Increased	Increased
Decreased compliance	Normal or increased	Normal or decreased	Increased	Decreased	Decreased

high cost, and risk of complications (55). A reasonable approach may be to reserve cardiac catheterization for cases in which the diagnosis remains unclear after noninvasive assessments and those in which another indication for cardiac catheterization exists.

D. Drug Therapy for Diastolic Dysfunction

1. Goals of Therapy

a. Because HTN, LVH, and CAD are known to be independent risk factors for cardiac death, treatment aimed at these processes may be expected to provide mortality benefit for patients with one of these conditions and diastolic dysfunction (20,46,54,78). Nevertheless, no clinical trial has been conducted specifically to examine the mortality benefit of drug therapy in patients with heart failure and preserved LV EF.

b. As illustrated in Table 4-7, a reasonable therapeutic strategy is to target the three physiologic causes of diastolic dysfunction (inappropriate tachycardia, decreased diastolic compliance, and impaired systolic relaxation) and decrease the pulmonary and systemic venous pressures to relieve the congestive symptoms (16, 85). In addition, restoration of sinus rhythm may be important for patients with atrial fibrillation to provide the needed atrial contribution for adequate ventricular filling.

c. As described previously, radionuclide- and Doppler-derived indices of diastolic function may be influenced by the heart rate and the loading conditions of the heart. Thus, when used in clinical studies to demonstrate an effect of drug therapy on diastolic function, alterations in transmittal velocity patterns may reflect drug-induced changes in the heart rate or the loading conditions rather than a true effect on the inherent diastolic properties. With these limitations in mind, the major drugs used for treatment of diastolic dysfunction are described in greater detail in the following sections.

2. Diuretics and Nitrates—A judicious use of diuretics and nitrates reduces preload and may relieve the symptoms of venous congestion, especially in the setting of acute CHF. Salt restriction is also helpful for this purpose. In addition, nitrates may control ischemia, which can also be an important contributor to diastolic dysfunction. However, the use of these agents may be limited by a relatively steep diastolic pressure-volume curve in some patients with diastolic dysfunction; in such patients, even a modest decrease in LV volume can produce a large drop in LV pressure, leading to hypotension, syncope, or sudden death (33).

Table 4-7 Goals of therapy for diastolic dysfunction

Reduce Preload	Reduce Heart Rate	Promote Myocardial Relaxation	Increase Diastolic Compliance	Maintain Atrial Contraction
Diuretics Salt restriction Nitrates	β-Adrenergic blockers Ca^{2+} channel blockers	*Enhance Ca^{2+} Handling* Ca^{2+} channel blockers PDE inhibitors β-Adrenergic agonists *Prevent/treat ischemia* β-Adrenergic blockers Ca^{2+} channel blockers Nitrates	*Antihypertensive drugs* β-Adrenergic blockers Ca^{2+} channel blockers ACE inhibitors Diuretics *Remodeling drugs* ACE inhibitors Endothelin antagonist? *Surgery* AVR for AS Myomectomy for IHSS	Cardioversion for AF Sequential AV pacing

a. **Diuretics**—In a metaanalysis of 12 studies (mostly uncontrolled) that examined the effect of diuretic monotherapy on LV structure in patients with essential HTN, the average LV mass was reduced by 11% (95% CI, 5.6% to 17%). This improvement resulted mainly from a reduction of the LV volume rather than from reversal of LVH (21).

b. **Nitrates**—In one prospective randomized controlled trial (PRCT), 21 patients with CHF and mildly depressed LV EF (>40%) were randomly assigned to receive either isosorbide dinitrate (40 to 80 mg PO QD) or placebo for 3 months. Nitrate therapy failed to improve the radionuclide indices of diastolic function, and there was no difference in functional status or level of exercise tolerance between the two groups. The mean arterial pressure (MAP) was decreased by nitrate therapy ($P<0.0001$); the effect on the heart rate was not reported (98). In an uncontrolled study of patients with essential HTN, nitrate therapy was associated with a statistically significant impairment of the radionuclide indices of LV relaxation. This impairment was probably caused by a reduction in the preload rather than a genuine alteration in the inherent diastolic properties of the heart (66). In another uncontrolled study of patients with nonobstructive hypertrophic cardiomyopathy, 3 of the 6 patients treated with nitrates experienced severe hypotensive reactions, including one death (91).

c. **Summary of the Role of Diuretics and Nitrates**

(1) Diuretics and nitrates reduce preload and may relieve the symptoms caused by venous congestion.

(2) A metaanalysis of diuretic therapy in patients with essential HTN failed to show statistically significant regression of LVH.

(3) One PRCT and one uncontrolled study of nitrate therapy failed to show any effect on diastolic function beyond preload reduction.

(4) Another uncontrolled study suggests that nitrates should be used with caution in patients with diastolic dysfunction, especially in the setting of idiopathic hypertrophic cardiomyopathy.

3. **Calcium Channel Blockers**—The antihypertensive, antiischemic, and negative chronotropic properties of some calcium channel blockers predict a favorable effect on diastolic function. Amelioration of intracellular Ca^{2+} overload may be an additional benefit for patients with hypertrophic cardiomyopathy. However, firm conclusions regarding the efficacy of calcium channel blockers for treatment of diastolic dysfunction cannot be made, because most of the clinical studies to date have been poorly controlled, very small, and of questionable study design. In addition, only a few studies have used cardiac catheterization to assess diastolic function. A sampling of the available literature is described here for illustration.

a. **Improvement of Diastolic Properties in Patients With Essential Hypertension**

(1) In patients with HTN, there is some evidence that calcium channel blockers may reverse LVH. In a metaanalysis of 30 studies (mostly uncontrolled) that examined the benefit of monotherapy with calcium channel blockers on LV structure in patients with essential HTN, LV mass was reduced by 8.5% (95% CI, 5.1% to 11.8%) due to significant reversal of LVH (21).

(2) Furthermore, in several studies (three PRCTs) ranging in size from 10 to 28 patients, calcium channel blockers significantly improved some of the indices of diastolic function. The length of follow-up ranged from immediately after IV drug administration to after 6 weeks of oral therapy (17,24,77,102). Representative studies are described here.

(a) The least flawed of these trials was a 1-month multiphasic study of nifedipine (20 to 80 mg PO BID) in 22 hypertensive patients (diastolic pressure, 95 to 115 mm Hg). All patients were treated with a diuretic and a placebo initially. After assessment of the diastolic function with a radionuclide study, patients were randomly assigned to a predetermined dose of nifedipine or propranolol that lowered the diastolic pressure to <90 mm Hg. Diuretic therapy was continued. Nifedipine and propranolol were sequentially compared with placebo in such a way that the patients served as their own controls. Compared with placebo, propranolol lowered the blood pressure and the heart rate but did not improve any measure of diastolic function. Nifedipine significantly increased the PFR at rest and during peak exercise, but the TPFR and the filling fraction at midpoint of diastole (DF_{50}) were improved only at rest. The blood pressure was decreased ($P<0.01$) but the heart rate remained unchanged with nifedipine (102) (see Table 4-8).

(b) The only cardiac catheterization study (uncontrolled) examined the effect of IV verapamil on diastolic function in 10 hypertensive patients. Verapamil was titrated to achieve a 20% reduction in the MAP. Patients were then atrially paced to normalize the heart rate. Verapamil increased the LV end-diastolic volume index (LVEDVI) without affecting the LV end-diastolic pressure (LVEDP), consistent with an increase in the LV compliance. However, the indices of isovolumic relaxation were unchanged. The MAP was decreased ($P<0.05$) but the pulmonary capillary wedge pressure (PCWP) was unchanged (46).

(3) Other studies found no statistically significant improvement in the indices of diastolic function during therapy with diltiazem or nifedipine (44,58). For example, in one study of 6 hypertensive patients treated with a diuretic and a β-blocker, addition of nifedipine (20 to 40 mg PO BID) failed to improve the radionuclide indices of diastolic function (PFR, TPFR) at 9 weeks (58). Similarly, in a study of 12 hypertensive patients without CAD, diltiazem (60 to 120 mg TID) did not improve the PFR, TPFR, or FF-1/3 (44).

b. Improvement of Diastolic Properties in Patients With Idiopathic Hypertrophic Cardiomyopathy

(1) Calcium channel blockers were found in 13 studies (one PRCT) to significantly improve the indices of diastolic function or exercise capacity (or both) in patients with idiopathic hypertrophic cardiomyopathy. Study size ranged from 6 to 42 patients, and the length of follow-up ranged from 5 minutes after IV drug administration to after 2 years of oral therapy (8,9,31,40,41,45,47,49,59,62,72,73,87). Representative studies are described here.

(a) The only PRCT compared verapamil (240 to 640 mg PO total per day) versus placebo in 28 patients with idiopathic hypertrophic cardiomyopathy. After 1 to 4 weeks of therapy, radionuclide angiography and graded treadmill exercise tests were performed. Compared with placebo, verapamil significantly improved the PFR (3.1 versus 3.8 end-diastolic volumes per second, respectively; $P<0.005$) and the exercise capacity (5.3 versus 8.5 min-

Table 4-8 Nifedipine for diastolic dysfunction due to hypertension (102)

	At Rest			Peak Exercise		
	Placebo (n=22)	Nifedipine (n=11)	*P*	Placebo (n=22)	Nifedipine (n=11)	*P*
PFR	327±26 ml/s	386±39 ml/s	<0.01	730±53 ml/s	896±94 ml/s	<0.01
TPFR	221±9 ms	203±13 ms	<0.05	113±6 ms	109±7 ms	NS
DF_{50}	0.46±0.03	0.54±0.03	<0.01	0.38±0.01	0.39±0.02	NS

utes, respectively; $P<0.01$). Verapamil also decreased the heart rate and the blood pressure ($P<.001$). A linear regression analysis suggested a weak but significant correlation between change in PFR and change in exercise tolerance ($r=0.38$; $P<0.05$) (50) (see Table 4-9).

(b) In three studies that used cardiac catheterization to measure diastolic function, IV verapamil significantly improved the indices of LV relaxation but compliance was unchanged. Verapamil did not change the heart rate or the loading conditions in any of these studies (40,41,49).

(c) In two other studies that used cardiac catheterization, verapamil significantly decreased the gradient across the LV outflow tract (LVOT) (47,73). Furthermore, verapamil was associated with improved symptoms and increased exercise tolerance during 1 to 2 years of therapy (47).

(d) In two cardiac catheterization studies by the same investigator, sublingual nifedipine appeared to improve LV relaxation and compliance. The heart rate increased slightly ($P<0.05$), whereas the indices of preload and afterload decreased ($P<0.01$) (62,72).

(e) In two studies that used Doppler ultrasonography to assess diastolic function, diltiazem significantly improved the indices of LV relaxation. The heart rate was either decreased slightly ($P<0.05$) or unchanged (45,87).

(2) In contrast, two uncontrolled studies using cardiac catheterization found no statistically significant improvement in diastolic function with calcium channel blockade (4,90). In one small study, IV verapamil given during atrial pacing to normalize the heart rate did not improve the LVEDP or T, whereas peak −dP/dt was significantly decreased in proportion to the decrease in LV systolic pressure (90). In another small study that normalized the heart rate by atrial pacing, sublingual nifedipine markedly reduced the afterload without decreasing the degree of LVOT obstruction or improving diastolic function. Moreover, nifedipine appeared to worsen the degree of LVOT obstruction and to increase the PCWP in patients in whom the systemic vascular resistance fell by ≥25% (4).

c. Improvement of Diastolic Properties in Patients With Ischemic Heart Disease

(1) Calcium channel blockers were found in six PRCTs to significantly improve the indices of diastolic function in patients with CAD. Study size ranged from 12 to 135 patients. The length of follow-up ranged from immediately after IV drug administration to after 6 months of oral therapy (7,22,59,68,99,101). Representative studies are described here.

(a) The largest PRCT compared nisoldipine (20 mg PO QD) versus placebo in 135 postinfarction patients with LV EF <50% (mean LV EF, 42±7%). This study excluded patients with overt heart failure, dilated or hypertrophic cardiomyopathy, ore significant valvular heart disease. Treatment was started 7 to 35 days after the infarction and continued for 4 weeks. Compared with base-

Table 4-9 Verapamil for idiopathic hypertrophic cardiomyopathy (50)

	Placebo (n=28)	Verapamil (n=28)	*P*
PFR (EDV/s)	3.1±1.2	3.8±1.3	<0.005
Exercise capacity	5.3±3.1 min	8.5±4.3 min	<0.01

EDV = End disastolic volume.

line, there was no significant benefit of nisoldipine therapy on IVRT, DT, or E:A ratio at 4 weeks. There was also no significant difference in the indices of diastolic function with nisoldipine therapy compared with placebo. The heart rate, blood pressure, and LV EF remained unchanged. However, through data manipulation, the authors did report a statistically significant improvement of IVRT by 14.7 msec (95% CI, 6.9 to 22.5 msec) with nisoldipine (see Table 4-10). This was achieved by calculating the observed difference in the indices between nisoldipine and placebo as follows: first, the effect of placebo or nisoldipine was calculated by examining the difference in the value of an index at 4 weeks compared with baseline (ΔPlacebo and ΔNisoldipine, respectively); then, the observed difference between the effect of nisoldipine and placebo was calculated by subtracting ΔPlacebo from ΔNisoldipine for a given index. There was also a statistically significant improvement in exercise capacity as measured by peak workload. In addition, ischemic events (angina pectoris or 1 mm ST depression) occurred less frequently during exercise with nisoldipine than with placebo (59).

(b) In a multiphasic crossover study of verapamil (480 mg PO total per day), propranolol (160 to 320 mg PO total per day), and placebo in 16 patients with normal resting LV EF and angina refractory to propranolol and nitrates, verapamil significantly improved the indices of diastolic function (PFR and TPFR) as measured by radionuclide angiography. Verapamil also decreased the heart rate and the blood pressure ($P<0.005$). Propranolol improved neither of the measured indices of diastolic function (see Table 4-11).

(c) In the only calcium channel blocker study that used cardiac catheterization to assess diastolic function in patients with CAD, 20 patients with stable angina and LV EF <40% were randomly assigned to receive IV isradipine or IV nifedipine. The effects of these drugs were assessed at rest and during ischemia (induced

Table 4-10 Nisoldipine for diastolic dysfunction associated with CAD (59)

	Placebo (n=67)			Nisoldipine (n=68)			ΔNisoldipine minus ΔPlacebo (95% CI)
	Baseline	4 Wk	Δ	Baseline	4 Wk	Δ	
E:A ratio	1.11	1.06	−0.04	1.08	1.08	0.00	+0.04 (−0.13–0.20)
IVRT	87.7 ms	94.4 ms	+6.7 ms	85.8 ms	77.8 ms	−8.0 ms	−14.7 (−22.5–6.9)
DT	162.9 ms	171.4 ms	+8.5 ms	160.6 ms	165.2 ms	+4.6 ms	−4.0 (−16.1–8.2)
Peak workload	—	97 W	—	—	109 W	—	12 (0.8–23.3)

Δ, Difference between 4-wk and baseline values.

Table 4-11 Verapamil for diastolic dysfunction associated with CAD (7)

	At Rest			Peak Exercise		
	Placebo (n=16)	Verapamil (n=16)	*P*	Placebo (n=16)	Verapamil (n=16)	*P*
PFR (EDV/s)	1.9±0.6	2.3±0.9	<0.005	3.1±0.9	3.6±1.1	<0.05
TPFR	185±38 ms	161±27 ms	<0.05	108±30 ms	91±17 ms	<0.05

by atrial pacing 20 bpm above the resting rate). Compared with baseline, both drugs improved the indices of LV relaxation and compliance during pacing but neither did so during rest, suggesting that the observed improvement in diastolic properties may have resulted from the antiischemic effects of the drugs. There were no important differences in the effects of the two drugs. Both drugs decreased the blood pressure ($P<0.01$) and the LVEDP ($P<0.05$), but neither changed the heart rate significantly (99). Only the data for nifedipine are shown in Table 4-12.

(2) In contrast, two PRCTs found no statistically significant improvement in the indices of diastolic function with nifedipine or nicardipine. Both studies failed to report drug-induced changes in the heart rate. However, nifedipine significantly improved exercise tolerance and lowered the indices of preload and afterload, especially in patients with increased LVEDV and LVEDP (64,71).

d. Summary of the Role of Calcium Channel Blockers

(1) In patients with essential HTN, a metaanalysis supports the use of calcium channel blockers for regression of LVH. Many studies suggest that calcium channel blockers effectively reduce the afterload in these patients, but the role of these agents in improving the inherent LV diastolic properties has been less convincingly demonstrated. An improvement in the indices of diastolic function (*i.e.*, PFR, TPFR, DF_{50}, or compliance) has been demonstrated with the use of calcium channel blockers in some but not other studies.

(2) In patients with idiopathic hypertrophic cardiomyopathy, one PRCT and most of the well-conducted but uncontrolled catheterization studies found that verapamil significantly improved LV relaxation but not compliance. These favorable changes were associated with an improvement in symptoms, in exercise capacity, and in the degree of LVOT obstruction. A similar benefit was reported with diltiazem in some studies, but the data are more limited. Nifedipine consistently reduced the afterload, but any additional effect on the inherent LV diastolic properties was less convincingly demonstrated. Furthermore, nifedipine may increase the degree of LVOT obstruction in some patients with idiopathic hypertrophic cardiomyopathy.

(3) In patients with ischemic heart disease, many studies have found that calcium channel blockade significantly improves symptoms, exercise capacity, and the indices of diastolic function. In a study that used cardiac catheterization to measure diastolic function, an improvement in LV relaxation and compliance was found only during atrial pacing, suggesting that this result may have been caused by the antiischemic properties of the drugs.

Table 4-12 Nifedipine for diastolic dysfunction associated with CAD (99)

	Rest			Atrial Pacing		
	Baseline (n=10)	Nifedipine (n=10)	*P*	Baseline (n=10)	Nifedipine (n=10)	*P*
Heart rate	72 bpm	81 bpm	NS	126 bpm	126 bpm	NS
Diastolic blood pressure	67 mm Hg	58 mm Hg	<0.01	84 mm Hg	66 mm Hg	<0.01
LVEDP	12 mm Hg	10 mm Hg	<0.05	15 mm Hg	9 mm Hg	<0.01
T	43 ms	42 ms	NS	52 ms	43 ms	<0.02
Stiffness constant	2.6	2.1	NS	7.3	3.8	<0.01

4. β-Blockers—The antihypertensive, antiischemic, and negative chronotropic properties of β-blockers predict a favorable effect on diastolic function in patients with HTN, hypertrophic cardiomyopathy, or ischemic heart disease.

a. Improvement of Diastolic Properties in Patients With Essential Hypertension

(1) In a metaanalysis of 31 studies (mostly uncontrolled) that examined the benefit of monotherapy with β-blockers on the LV structure in patients with essential HTN, the LV mass was reduced by 8.0% (95% CI, 4.8% to 11.2%) due to a significant reversal of LVH (21).

(2) Furthermore, in several uncontrolled studies ranging in size from 9 to 21 patients, a wide variety of β-blockers significantly improved the noninvasive indices of diastolic function in patients with essential HTN (2,30,43,57,92,96,97). The length of follow-up ranged from 1 to 6 months. In two studies, β-blockers improved the rate of rapid LV filling because of regression of LVH (96,97). β-Blockers also improved the rate of rapid LV filling in two other studies, but without a clear relation to regression of LVH. (43,92) Finally, two studies found that β-blockers improved the rate of rapid LV filling only in those patients who exhibited a decrease in arterial blood pressure, suggesting that afterload reduction rather than a direct cardiac effect was responsible for improved transmitral velocity (30,57). β-Blockade caused a statistically significant reduction in heart rate and blood pressure in all but one study (97).

(3) In contrast, three noninvasive studies (two PRCTs) found no statistically significant improvement in the indices of LV relaxation during β-blocker therapy. Study size ranged from 12 to 22 patients, and the length of follow-up ranged from 1 to 3 months (44,100,102). β-Blockade caused a statistically significantly reduction in heart rate and blood pressure in all studies.

b. Improvement of Diastolic Properties in Patients With Idiopathic Hypertrophic Cardiomyopathy

(1) Four studies (one PRCT), ranging in size from 8 to 20 patients, found that β-blockers significantly improved some of the indices of diastolic function in patients with hypertrophic cardiomyopathy. The length of follow-up ranged from 30 minutes after IV drug administration to after 6 months of oral therapy (12,42,75,88). Representative studies are described here.

(a) One PRCT compared propranolol (320 mg PO QD) versus placebo in 16 patients with hypertrophic cardiomyopathy. After 1 month of therapy, propranolol had improved the indices of LV relaxation, as measured by Doppler echocardiography, as well as the symptoms of dyspnea, angina, and palpitation (see Table 4-13). The heart rate was decreased ($P<0.01$) but the blood pressure was unchanged (42).

(b) One uncontrolled study found a dose-dependent effect of oral propranolol on shortening of the IVRT, despite a significant decrease in the heart rate ($P<0.001$) (12).

(c) In an uncontrolled study that used cardiac catheterization to assess diastolic function, acute administration of IV propranolol

Table 4-13 Propranolol for idiopathic hypertrophic cardiomyopathy (42)

	Placebo (n=16)	Propranolol (n=16)	*P*
IVRT	145.6±9.5 ms	122.2±10.3 ms	<0.01
Atrial contribution to diastolic filling	28.7±5.1%	18.0±3.2%	<0.01

increased diastolic compliance. Both the heart rate and the LVEDP were decreased by propranolol ($P<0.02$), but the LV peak systolic pressure (LVSP), a better measure of afterload than blood pressure in the presence of LVOT obstruction, was unchanged (88).

(2) Five uncontrolled studies, ranging in size from 9 to 16 patients, found no statistically significant benefit of propranolol therapy on the indices of LV relaxation or on diastolic compliance in patients with hypertrophic cardiomyopathy. The length of follow-up ranged from 10 minutes after IV drug administration to after 2 weeks of oral therapy (6,40,82,87,90).

(a) Three studies used catheter-derived hemodynamic measurements to assess diastolic function (40,82,90). One study showed further impairment of the indices of LV relaxation with β-blockade (40). In two of the studies, propranolol decreased the heart rate ($P<0.05$) but the preload and the afterload were unchanged (40, 82). In one study, the heart rate was unchanged but the preload and the afterload were decreased ($P<0.02$) (90).

(b) Two studies assessed diastolic function by Doppler echocardiography. Propranolol decreased the heart rate ($P<0.05$), but the blood pressure was unchanged in both studies (6,87).

c. Improvement of Diastolic Properties in Patients With Ischemic Heart Disease—Three studies (two PRCTs) found no statistically significant improvement in the indices of LV relaxation with β-blocker therapy in patients with CAD and diastolic dysfunction (7,37,71).

(1) The larger of the two PRCTs compared atenolol (50 to 100 mg PO QD) versus placebo in 30 patients with chronic stable angina. Radionuclide angiography was used to assess diastolic function after 6 weeks of therapy. No significant improvement in the indices of LV relaxation was noted. The heart rate and the blood pressure were not reported (71).

(2) In the only study that used cardiac catheterization to assess diastolic function, IV propranolol and IV metoprolol decreased the heart rate and the LVSP ($P<0.05$) but the PCWP was unchanged (37).

d. Summary of the Role of β-Blockers

(1) In patients with essential HTN, a metaanalysis supports the use of β-blockers for regression of LVH, but the role of these agents in improving the inherent LV diastolic properties has been less convincingly demonstrated. Several uncontrolled studies found that β-blockade improved the indices of LV relaxation in patients with essential HTN. However, the two PRCTs reported to date failed to confirm these benefits.

(2) In patients with hypertrophic cardiomyopathy, several noninvasive studies (one PRCT) demonstrated that propranolol significantly improved the indices of LV relaxation with a concomitant decrease in the heart rate and no apparent change in the loading conditions. Although most of the studies using cardiac catheterization found no statistically significant improvement in diastolic function with IV propranolol, a drug-induced decrease in heart rate without an alteration in the loading conditions may have masked improvement in diastolic function.

(3) In patients with ischemic heart disease, three studies (two PRCTs) found that β-blockade therapy did not significantly improve the indices of diastolic function.

5. ACE Inhibitors—The strong preload- and afterload-reducing properties of ACE inhibitors predict a favorable effect on congestive symptoms and LVH. In addition, as discussed previously, animal studies suggest that ACE inhibitors may promote regression of interstitial fibrosis (see section B2).

a. In a metaanalysis of 31 studies (mostly uncontrolled) that examined the benefit of monotherapy with ACE inhibitors on the LV structure in patients with essential HTN, the LV mass was reduced by 15% (95% CI, 9.9% to

20.1%) due to a significant reversal of LVH. ACE inhibitors were more effective in this respect than β-blockers (8%) or calcium channel blockers (8.5%) (21).

b. Furthermore, in several studies (two PRCTs) ranging in size from 8 to 43 patients, ACE inhibitors significantly improved the indices of diastolic function, both in patients with essential HTN and preserved LV EF and in those with CAD and depressed LV EF (23,48,52,53,65,74). The length of follow-up ranged from 20 minutes after IV drug administration to after 1 year of oral therapy. Representative studies are described here.

(1) In one PRCT, 10 patients with essential HTN were randomly assigned to receive either quinapril (20 mg PO QD) or placebo. After 4 weeks of therapy, quinapril had improved one of the indices of diastolic function (E:A ratio), as assessed by Doppler echocardiography (see Table 4-14). Quinapril also decreased the blood pressure ($P<0.001$) but not the heart rate (52). However, the design of the study did not allow the benefit derived from afterload reduction to be differentiated from genuine improvement in inherent LV diastolic properties.

(2) In another PRCT, 8 patients with essential HTN were randomly assigned to receive either a single dose of cilazapril (5 mg PO) or placebo (65). Cilazapril decreased the heart rate ($P=0.05$) and the blood pressure ($P=0.02$) slightly. The TPFR expressed as a percentage of diastole (%TPFR) was reduced slightly ($P=0.05$), but the PFR and the absolute TPFR were unchanged with cilazapril. The authors suggest that %TPFR may be a more sensitive index of diastolic function.

(3) In the only study that used cardiac catheterization to assess diastolic function, IV benazeprilat improved the indices of LV compliance but not those of relaxation in patients with mildly depressed LV EF (74). The heart rate and the blood pressure were reduced ($P<0.0003$) but the LVEDP did not change.

(4) The most convincing uncontrolled study was a 1-year Doppler study of monotherapy with trandolapril in 15 patients with untreated essential HTN and LVH (23). Significant blood pressure reduction was associated with an increased E:A ratio and normalization of the LV mass index after 6 and 12 months of therapy. These functional and structural changes were still evident after a 1-month drug washout period, despite return of the blood pressure to baseline values. Therefore, ACE inhibition may have effects on cardiac structure and function that are distinct from its antihypertensive properties.

(5) The Studies Of Left Ventricular Dysfunction (SOLVD) investigators found that IV enalapril improved radionuclide indices of LV relaxation only in the subset of patients with right ventricular dilatation, suggesting a favorable drug effect on pericardial constraint and ventricular interdependence in these patients. The heart rate and the blood pressure were unchanged (53).

c. In contrast, three studies (two PRCTs) found no statistically significant improvement in the indices of diastolic function with ACE inhibitor therapy (79,98,100). One PRCT was a 3-month radionuclide study of lisinopril (20 to 80 mg PO QD) versus placebo in 21 patients with essential HTN (100). Lisinopril decreased the blood pressure ($P<0.01$), but the indices of diastolic function and the heart rate remained unchanged. Similar results were reported in an uncontrolled study of captopril in patients with essential

Table 4-14 Quinapril for diastolic dysfunction due to hypertension (52)

	Placebo (n=10)	Quinapril (n=10)	*P*
E:A ratio	1.12	1.31	<0.02

HTN (79). The other PRCT was a 3-month radionuclide study of captopril versus placebo in 21 patients with moderately depressed LV EF (98). Captopril decreased the MAP ($P<0.0001$), but the indices of diastolic function remained unchanged. The effect on the heart rate was not reported.

d. Summary of the Role of ACE Inhibitors

(1) In patients with essential HTN, a metaanalysis suggests that ACE inhibitors may be superior to β-blockers or calcium channel blockers for reversal of LVH. Most of the studies examining the effect of ACE inhibition on diastolic function were of short duration and yielded mixed results. Large PRCTs of longer duration are needed to confirm the observation that chronic ACE inhibition can lead to regression of LVH and improvement of diastolic function.

(2) In two small PRCTs, ACE inhibitors significantly improved the indices of diastolic function in patients with essential HTN. However, one study may be criticized because its design did not allow the benefit derived from afterload reduction to be differentiated from genuine improvement in the inherent LV diastolic properties. The %TPFR was improved with ACE inhibition in the second study, but the study was unable to demonstrate an improvement in the usual radionuclide indices of diastolic function (*i.e.*, PFR, TPFR, FF-1/3).

6. Agents That Raise cAMP Levels—Both β-adrenergic agonists and phosphodiesterase inhibitors have lusitropic properties that appear to be mediated by their ability to raise cAMP levels in myocytes and to promote Ca^{2+} resequestration by the sarcoplasmic reticulum. In addition to their lusitropic effects, these agents also have well-known inotropic effects that are mediated by cAMP-dependent protein kinase activity and by Ca^{2+} entry across the sarcolemma in response to β-adrenergic stimulation (50). Therefore, sustained elevation of cAMP may eventually lead to cellular calcium overload, tachycardia, arrhythmia, and cell death (60,61,63).

a. β-Adrenergic Agonists

(1) In two small, uncontrolled studies, the administration of a β-agonist (dopamine, dobutamine, or ibopamine) to patients with CHF and severely depressed LV EF was associated with an improvement in the indices of LV relaxation without a change in heart rate, MAP, or LVEDP (18,86).

(2) In another small, uncontrolled study, isoproterenol improved the indices of LV relaxation and compliance in patients with hypertrophic cardiomyopathy. However, it also provoked ischemia and increased the gradient across the LVOT. The heart rate and the LVSP increased ($P<0.001$) but the LVEDP was unchanged (93).

b. Phosphodiesterase Inhibitors

(1) In one small PRCT, oral enoximone was compared with placebo in 13 patients with CHF and severely depressed LV EF. After 3 months of therapy, enoximone significantly improved the radionuclide indices of systolic and diastolic function compared to baseline (see Table 4-15). The heart rate and the blood pressure were unchanged (5).

(2) In one small, uncontrolled study that used cardiac catheterization to assess diastolic function in patients with CHF and severely depressed LV EF, enoximone improved some but not all indices of diastolic func-

Table 4-15 Enoximone for treatment of chronic CHF (5)

	Placebo (n=6)	Enoximone (n=7)	*P*
Change in LV EF (EF units)*	0.2	11±14	<0.05
Change in PFR (EDV/s)*	0.2	0.5	<0.05

*Change at 3 mo compared to baseline.

tion (39). Enoximone increased the heart rate slightly ($P<0.01$), but the LVEDP decreased ($P<0.01$) and the MAP remained unchanged.

(3) However, in the PROMISE (Prospective Randomized Milrinone Survival Evaluation) trial, long-term oral therapy with milrinone significantly increased the mortality rate in patients with severely depressed LV EF (69) (see Table 4-16).

c. Summary of the Role of Agents that Raise cAMP Levels

(1) In patients with dilated or hypertrophic cardiomyopathy, a few small, uncontrolled studies of short-term β-agonist therapy demonstrated a favorable effect on diastolic function. However, these agents may precipitate ischemia in patients with CAD and may increase the degree of LVOT obstruction in patients with hypertrophic cardiomyopathy.

(2) Similarly, in one small PRCT, therapy with a phosphodiesterase inhibitor for 3 months improved the indices of systolic and diastolic function in patients with severely depressed LV EF. However, one large PRCT found that long-term therapy with a phosphodiesterase inhibitor increased the mortality and morbidity in patients with low LV EF (69). Therefore, although β-agonists and phosphodiesterase inhibitors may have some favorable effects on diastolic function, their potential for causing adverse effects precludes their routine use for treatment of diastolic dysfunction.

E. Summary

1. Diuretics and nitrates are effective in reducing preload and are indicated to relieve the symptoms of pulmonary congestion in patients with CHF. However, they should be used with caution, especially in patients with diastolic heart failure caused by idiopathic hypertrophic cardiomyopathy.
2. In patients with isolated diastolic dysfunction secondary to essential HTN, afterload reduction and regression of LVH may be achieved by monotherapy with β-blockers, calcium channel blockers, or ACE inhibitors. ACE inhibitors may be superior for reversal of LVH. However, the role of any of these agents in improving the inherent LV diastolic properties has been less convincingly demonstrated. In general, the clinical studies in this area have been small in size, poorly controlled, and of questionable design; not surprisingly, they have yielded mixed results.
3. In patients with diastolic dysfunction caused by idiopathic hypertrophic cardiomyopathy, verapamil significantly improves LV relaxation but not compliance. These favorable changes are also associated with improved symptoms and exercise capacity and a reduction in the degree of LVOT obstruction. A similar benefit has been reported with diltiazem in some studies, but the data are more limited. Nifedipine should be avoided because it may increase the degree of LVOT obstruction in some patients with idiopathic hypertrophic cardiomyopathy. β-Blockade also appears to improve the indices of LV relaxation and to decrease the severity of symptoms in patients with idiopathic hypertrophic cardiomyopathy.
4. In patients with diastolic dysfunction caused by ischemic heart disease, calcium channel blockade lessens the severity of symptoms, increases the exercise capacity, and improves the indices of diastolic function. In the few small studies that have been reported, β-blockade therapy did not significantly improve the indices of diastolic function in patients with ischemic heart disease.

Table 4-16 Milrinone for treatment of chronic CHF (69)

	Placebo (n=527)	Milrinone (n=561)	P
All-cause mortality	24%	30%	0.060
Cardiac mortality	23%	29%	0.016

Abbreviations used in Chapter 4

ACE = angiotensin-converting enzyme
AS = aortic stenosis
BID = twice daily
bpm = beats per minute
Ca^{2+} = calcium
CAD = coronary artery disease
CHF = congestive heart failure
CI = confidence interval
DF_{50} = fraction of total diastolic filling at midpoint of diastole
DT = deceleration time during isovolumic relaxation
E:A ratio = ratio of peak early (E) to peak late (A) transmitral velocity
EF = ejection fraction
FF-1/3 = filling fraction during the first third of diastole
HTN = hypertension
IHSS = idiopathic hypertrophic subaortic stenosis
IV = intravenous
IVRT = isovolumic relaxation time
LV = left ventricular
LV EF = left ventricular ejection fraction
LVEDP = left ventricular end-diastolic pressure
LVEDVI = left ventricular end-diastolic volume index
LVH = left ventricular hypertrophy
LVOT = left ventricular outflow tract
LVSP = left ventricular peak systolic pressure
MAP = mean arterial pressure
MI = myocardial infarction
N = number of patients in population
n = number of patients in sample
NS = not statistically significant
NYHA = New York Heart Association
P = probability value
PCWP = pulmonary capillary wedge pressure
peak A = late diastolic flow velocity peak (rapid filling phase)
peak E = early diastolic flow velocity peak (atrial contraction phase)
peak −dP/dt = peak negative pressure decline during isovolumic relaxation
PFR = peak filling rate
PO = per os
PRCT = prospective randomized controlled trial
QD = every day
r = correlation coefficient
RAAS = renin-angiotensin-aldosterone system
T = time constant of pressure decline during isovolumic relaxation
TID = three times daily
TPFR = time to peak filling rate
%TPFR = time to peak filling rate expressed as a percentage of diastole
vs. = versus

References

1. Aguirre. Usefulness of Doppler echocardiography in the diagnosis of congestive heart failure. *Am J Cardiol* 1989;63:1098.
2. Allen. Effects of atenolol on left ventricular hypertrophy and early left ventricular function in essential hypertension. *Am J Cardiol* 1989;64:1157.

3. Appleton. Relation of transmitral flow velocity patterns to left ventricular diastolic function: new insights from a combined hemodynamic and Doppler echocardiographic study. *J Am Coll Cardiol* 1988;12:426.
4. Betocchi. Effects of sublingual nifedipine on hemodynamics and systolic and diastolic function in patients with hypertrophic cardiomyopathy. *Circulation* 1985;72:1001.
5. Binkley. Augmentation of diastolic function with phosphodiesterase inhibition in congestive heart failure. *J Lab Clin Med* 1989;114:266.
6. Bonow. Effects of verapamil on left ventricular systolic function and diastolic filling in patients with hypertrophic cardiomyopathy. *Circulation* 1981;64:787.
7. Bonow. Effects of verapamil and propranolol on left ventricular systolic function and diastolic filling in patients with coronary artery disease: radionuclide angiographic studies at rest and during exercise. *Circulation* 1981;65:1337.
8. Bonow. Atrial systole and left ventricular filling in hypertrophic cardiomyopathy: effect of verapamil. *Am J Cardiol* 1983;51:1386.
9. Bonow. Verapamil-induced improvement in left ventricular diastolic filling and increased exercise tolerance in patients with hypertrophic cardiomyopathy: short and long-term effects. *Circulation* 1985;75:853.
10. Bonow. Left ventricular diastolic dysfunction as a cause of congestive heart failure: mechanisms and management. *Ann Intern Med* 1992;117:502
11. Bonow. Radionuclide angiographic evaluation of left ventricular diastolic function. *Circulation* 1991;84(Suppl I):208.
12. Bourmayan. Effect of propranolol on left ventricular relaxation in hypertrophic cardiomyopathy: an echographic study. *Am Heart J* 1985;109:1311.
13. Brilla. Impaired diastolic function and coronary reserve in genetic hypertension: role of interstitial fibrosis and medial thickening of intramyocardial coronary arteries. *Circ Res* 1991;67:107.
14. Bristow. Beta-adrenergic pathways in nonfailing and failing human ventricular myocardium. *Circulation* 1990;82(Suppl I):12.
15. Brogan. The natural history of isolated left ventricular diastolic dysfunction. *Am J Med* 1992;92:627.
16. Brutsaert. Diastolic failure: pathophysiology and therapeutic implications. *J Am Coll Cardiol* 1993;22:318.
17. Brush. Comparative effects of verapamil and nitroprusside on left ventricular function in patients with hypertension. *J Am Coll Cardiol* 1989;14:515.
18. Carroll. The differential effects of positive inotropic and vasodilator therapy on diastolic properties in patients with congestive cardiomyopathy. *Circulation* 1986;74:815.
19. Cohn. Heart failure with normal ejection fraction: the V-HeFT study. *Circulation* 1990;81:48.
20. Cooper. Left ventricular hypertrophy is associated with worse survival independent of ventricular function and number of coronary arteries severely narrowed. *Am J Cardiol* 1990;65:441.
21. Dahlof. Reversal of left ventricular hypertrophy in hypertensive patients: a meta-analysis of 109 treatment studies. *Am J Hypertens* 1992;5:95.
22. De Cock. Effects of nisoldipine on systolic and diastolic function in postinfarction patients with reduced left ventricular function: a randomized, double-blind, placebo controlled study. *Eur Heart J* 1991;12:1012.
23. De Luca. Reversal of cardiac and large artery structural abnormalities induced by long-term antihypertensive treatment with trandolapril. *Am J Cardiol* 1992;70:52D.
24. De Luca. Effects of the single and repeated administration of benazepril on systemic and forearm circulation and cardiac function in hypertensive patients. *Cardiovasc Drugs Ther* 1993;7:211.
25. Dougherty. Congestive heart failure with normal systolic function. *Am J Cardiol* 1984;54:778.
26. Echeverria. Congestive heart failure: echocardiographic insights. *Am J Med* 1983;75:750.

27. Feldman. Deficient production of cyclic AMP: pharmacologic evidence of an important cause of contractile dysfunction in patients with end-stage heart failure. *Circulation* 1987;75:331.
28. Feldman. Increase of the 40,000-mol wt pertussis toxin substrate (G protein) in the failing human heart. *J Clin Invest* 1988;82:189.
29. Forman. Clinical issues related to discontinuing digoxin therapy in elderly nursing home patients. *Arch Intern Med* 1991;151:2194.
30. Fouad. Alterations in left ventricular filling with beta-adrenergic blockade. *Am J Cardiol* 1983;51:161.
31. Friart. Doppler evaluation of left ventricular filling: effect of verapamil on nonobstructive hypertrophic cardiomyopathy. *Eur Heart J* 1990;11:839.
32. Ghali. Bedside diagnosis of preserved versus impaired left ventricular systolic function in heart failure. *Am J Cardiol* 1991;67:1002.
33. Goldsmith. Differentiating systolic from diastolic heart failure: pathophysiologic and therapeutic considerations. *Am J Med* 1993;95:645.
34. Grossman. Diastolic dysfunction in congestive heart failure. *N Engl J Med* 1991;325:1557.
35. Guarda. Effects of endothelins on collagen turnover in cardiac fibroblasts. *Cardiovasc Res* 1993;27:2130.
36. Gwathmey. Abnormal intracellular calcium handling in myocardium from patients with end-stage heart failure. *Circ Res* 1987;61:70.
37. Haber. Why do patients with congestive heart failure tolerate the initiation of β-blocker therapy? *Circulation* 1993;88:1610.
38. Hanrath. Effect of verapamil on left ventricular isovolumic relaxation time and regional left ventricular filling in hypertrophic cardiomyopathy. *Am J Cardiol* 1980;45:1258.
39. Herrmann. Diastolic function in patients with severe heart failure: comparison of the effects of enoximone and nitroprusside. *Circulation* 1987;75:1214.
40. Hess. Diastolic function in hypertrophic cardiomyopathy: effects of propranolol and verapamil on diastolic stiffness. *Eur Heart J* 1983;4:47.
41. Hess. Does verapamil improve left ventricular relaxation in patients with myocardial hypertrophy? *Circulation* 1986;74:530.
42. Hubner. Double-blind trial of propranolol and practolol in hypertrophic cardiomyopathy. *Br Heart J* 1973, 35:1116.
43. Ibrahim. Effect of regression of left ventricular hypertrophy following sotalol therapy on diastolic function in hypertensive patients. *J Hypertens* 1987;5(Suppl 5):S411.
44. Inouye. Failure of antihypertensive therapy with diuretic, beta-blocking and calcium channel-blocking drugs to consistently reverse left ventricular diastolic filling abnormalities. *Am J Cardiol* 1984;53:1583.
45. Iwase. Effects of diltiazem on left ventricular diastolic behavior in patients with hypertrophic cardiomyopathy: evaluation with exercise pulsed Doppler echocardiography. *J Am Coll Cardiol* 1987;9:1099.
46. Judge. Congestive heart failure in patients with preserved left ventricular systolic function: analysis of the CASS registry. *J Am Coll Cardiol* 1991;18:377.
47. Kaltenbach. Treatment of hypertrophic obstructive cardiomyopathy with verapamil. *Circulation* 1979, 59/60(Suppl II):76.
48. Kapuku. Reversal of diastolic dysfunction in borderline hypertension by long-term medical treatment: longitudinal evaluation by pulsed Doppler echocardiography. *Am J Hypertens* 1993;6:547.
49. Kass. Diastolic compliance of hypertrophied ventricle is not acutely altered by pharmacologic agents influencing active processes. *Ann Intern Med* 1993;119:466.
50. Katz. Cyclic adenosine monophosphate effects on the myocardium: a man who blows hot and cold with one breath. *J Am Coll Cardiol* 1983;2:143.
51. Kihara. Direct measurement of changes in intracellular calcium transients during hypoxia, ischemia, and reperfusion of the intact mammalian heart. *Circ Res* 1989;65:1029.

52. Kjeldsen. Does blood pressure reduction necessarily compromise cardiac function or renal hemodynamics? Effects of the angiotensin-converting enzyme inhibitor quinapril. *Am Heart J* 1992;123:1433.
53. Konstam. Effect of acute angiotensin converting enzyme inhibition on left ventricular filling in patients with congestive heart failure. *Circulation* 1990;81 (Suppl III):115.
54. Koren. Relation of left ventricular mass and geometry to morbidity and mortality in uncomplicated essential hypertension. *Ann Intern Med* 1991;114:345.
55. Labovitz. Evaluation of left ventricular diastolic function: clinical relevance and recent Doppler echocardiographic insights. *Am Heart J* 1987;114:836.
56. Laxmansa. Endothelin receptors in cultured adult rat cardiac fibroblasts. *Cardiovasc Res* 1993;27:2125.
57. Lee. Behavioral vs beta-blocker therapy in patients with primary hypertension: effects on blood pressure, left ventricular function and mass, and the pressor surge of social stress anger. *Am Heart J* 1988;116:637.
58. Leenen. Effects of nifedipine versus hydralazine on sympathetic activity and cardiac function in patients with hypertension persisting on diuretic plus beta-blocker therapy. *Cardiovasc Drugs Ther* 1990;4:499.
59. Lewis. The DEFIANT study of left ventricular function and exercise performance after acute myocardial infarction. *Cardiovasc Drugs Ther* 1994;8:407.
60. Litwin. Captopril enhances intracellular calcium handling and beta-adrenergic responsiveness of myocardium from rats with postinfarction failure. *Circ Res* 1992;71:797.
61. Litwin. Diastolic dysfunction as a cause of heart failure. *J Am Coll Cardiol* 1993;22(Suppl A):49A.
62. Lorell. Modification of abnormal left ventricular diastolic properties by nifedipine in patients with hypertrophic cardiomyopathy. *Circulation* 1982;65:499.
63. Lubbe. Potential arrhythmogenic role of cyclic adenosine monophosphate and cytosolic calcium overload: implications for prophylactic effects of beta-blockers in myocardial infarction and proarrhythmic effects of phosphodiesterase inhibitors. *J Am Coll Cardiol* 1992;19:1622.
64. Ludbrook. Influence of nifedipine on left ventricular systolic and diastolic function: relationships to manifestations of ischemia and congestive heart failure. *Am J Med* 1981;71:683.
65. Marmor. A single dose of cilazapril improves diastolic function in hypertensive patients. *Am J Med* 1989;87(Suppl 6B):61.
66. Marmor. Effects of a single dose of isosorbide-5-mononitrate on the left ventricular diastolic function in systemic hypertension. *Am J Cardiol* 1989;63:1235.
67. Morgan. Abnormal intracellular modulation of calcium as a major cause of cardiac contractile dysfunction. *N Engl J Med* 1991;325:625.
68. Otto. The effects of nisoldipine on left ventricular filling rate in patients with ischemic heart disease measured with radionuclide gated blood pool scintigraphy. *Eur J Nucl Med* 1988;14:542.
69. Packer. Effect of oral milrinone on mortality in severe chronic heart failure. *N Engl J Med* 1991;325:1468.
70. Packer. Abnormalities of diastolic function as a potential cause of exercise intolerance in chronic heart failure. *Circulation* 1990;81(Suppl III):III.
71. Parameshwar. Atenolol or nicardipine alone is as efficacious in stable angina as their combination: a double blind randomised trial. *Int J Cardiol* 1993;40:135.
72. Paulus. Comparison of the effects of nitroprusside and nifedipine on diastolic properties in patients with hypertrophic cardiomyopathy: altered left ventricular loading or improved muscle inactivation. *J Am Coll Cardiol* 1983;2:879.
73. Rossing. Verapamil therapy: a new approach to the pharmacologic treatment of hypertrophic cardiomyopathy. I: Hemodynamic effects. *Circulation* 1979, 60: 1201.
74. Rousseau. Effects of benazeprilat on left ventricular systolic and diastolic function and neurohumoral status in patients with ischemic heart disease. *Circulation* 1990;81(Suppl III):123.

75. Saenz de la Calzada. Effect of acute administration of propranolol on ventricular function in hypertrophic obstructive cardiomyopathy measured by non-invasive techniques. *Br Heart J* 1976;38:798.
76. Schunkert. Increased rat cardiac angiotensin converting enzyme activity and mRNA expression in pressure overload left ventricular hypertrophy: effects on coronary resistance, contractility, and relaxation. *J Clin Invest* 1990;86:1913.
77. Setaro. Usefulness of verapamil for congestive heart failure associated with abnormal left ventricular diastolic filling and normal left ventricular systolic performance. *Am J Cardiol* 1990;66:981.
78. Setaro. Long-term outcome in patients with congestive heart failure and intact systolic left ventricular performance. *Am J Cardiol* 1992;69:1212.
79. Shani. Regression of hypertensive left ventricular hypertrophy and left ventricular diastolic function. *Lancet* 1990;336:458.
80. Shubeita. Endothelin induction of inositol phospholipid hydrolysis, sarcomere assembly, and cardiac gene expression in ventricular myocytes. *J Biol Chem* 1990;265:20555.
81. Soufer. Intact systolic left ventricular function in clinical congestive heart failure. *Am J Cardiol* 1985;55:1032.
82. Speiser. Reappraisal of the effect of acute betablockade on left ventricular filling dynamics in hypertrophic obstructive cardiomyopathy. *Eur Heart J* 1981;2:21.
83. Spirito. Noninvasive assessment of left ventricular diastolic function: comparative analysis of Doppler echocardiographic and radionuclide angiographic techniques. *J Am Coll Cardiol* 1986;7:518.
84. Spirito. Influence of aging on Doppler echocardiographic indices of left ventricular diastolic function. *Br Heart J* 1988;59:672.
85. Stauffer. Recognition and treatment of left ventricular diastolic dysfunction. *Prog Cardiovasc Dis* 1990;32:319.
86. Stoddard. Noninvasive assessment of diastolic and systolic properties of ibopamine in patients with congestive heart failure. *Am Heart J* 1989;117:395.
87. Suwa. Improvement in left ventricular diastolic function during intravenous and oral diltiazem therapy in patients with hypertrophic cardiomyopathy: an echocardiographic study. *Am J Cardiol* 1984;54:1047.
88. Swanton. Hemodynamic studies of β-blockade in hypertrophic obstructive cardiomyopathy. *Eur J Cardiol* 1977;5/4:327.
89. Taylor. Doppler assessment of left ventricular diastolic function: a review. *J Am Soc Echocardiogr* 1992;5:603.
90. Thompson. Pressure-derived indices of left ventricular isovolumic relaxation in patients with hypertrophic cardiomyopathy. *Br Heart J* 1983;49:259.
91. Topol. Hypertensive hypertrophic cardiomyopathy of the elderly. *N Engl J Med* 1985;312:277.
92. Trimarco. Improvement of diastolic function after reversal of left ventricular hypertrophy induced by long-term antihypertensive treatment with tertatolol. *Am J Cardiol* 1989;64:745.
93. Udelson. β-Adrenergic stimulation with isoproterenol enhances left ventricular diastolic performance in hypertrophic cardiomyopathy despite potentiation of myocardial ischemia: comparison to rapid atrial pacing. *Circulation* 1989;79:371.
94. Weber. Structural remodeling in hypertensive heart disease and the role of hormones. *Hypertension* 1994;23:869.
95. Weber. Pathological hypertrophy and cardiac interstitium: fibrosis and renin-angiotensin-aldosterone system. *Circulation* 1991;83:1849.
96. White. Regression of left ventricular mass is accompanied by improvement in rapid left ventricular filling following antihypertensive therapy with metoprolol. *Am Heart J* 1989;117:145.
97. Why. Effect of carvedilol on left ventricular function and mass in hypertension. *J Cardiovasc Pharmacol* 1992;19(Suppl 1):S50.
98. Wilkes. Comparison of the immediate and long-term effects of captopril and isosorbide dinitrate as adjunctive treatment in mild heart failure. *Br J Clin Pharmacol* 1989;28:427.

99. Wout van den Toren. Effect of isradipine and nifedipine on diastolic function in patients with left ventricular dysfunction due to coronary artery disease: a randomized, double-blind, nuclear, stethoscope study. *J Cardiovasc Pharmacol* 1994;23:952.
100. Zusman. Comparison of the cardiac and hemodynamic effects of lisinopril and atenolol in patients with hypertension: therapeutic implications. *J Cardiovasc Pharmacol* 1992;20:216.
101. Zusman. Bepridil improves left ventricular performance in patients with angina pectoris. *J Cardiovasc Pharmacol* 1993;22:474.
102. Zusman. Nifedipine, but not propranolol, improves left ventricular systolic and diastolic function in patients with hypertension. *Am J Cardiol* 1989;64:51F.

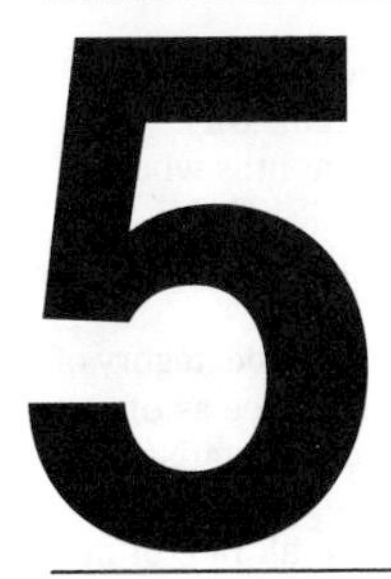

Myocardial Infarction: Standard Drug Therapy

Stephanie A. Coulter,
Gordon S. Huggins, and
Patrick T. O'Gara

A. Introduction

1. In recent years, reperfusion therapy has been the principal therapy for patients with acute myocardial infarction (AMI). In numerous, well-designed trials it has been shown to improve both survival and left ventricular (LV) function (see Chapter 6). However, most patients with AMI are not candidates for this therapy. For example, 20% of patients with AMI die before reaching a hospital, and another 25% have silent infarctions. Among those who do present to a hospital with AMI, reperfusion therapy is instituted less often in the elderly, in women (who tend to be older than their male counterparts), and in patients presenting longer than 6 to 12 hours after symptom onset (38). Furthermore, patients with an AMI associated with ST-segment depression (rather than ST elevation) do not appear to benefit from thrombolytic therapy (16).
2. The indications, benefits, and risks of thrombolytic therapy for acute MI are discussed in Chapter 6. This chapter focuses on other medications that have proved useful for primary prevention, secondary prevention, or acute management of myocardial infarction (MI). These include antiplatelet agents, antithrombin agents, β-adrenergic antagonists (β-blockers), nitrates, angiotensin-converting enzyme (ACE) inhibitors, lipid-lowering agents, and estrogen replacement therapy. More controversial drugs such as magnesium, calcium channel blockers, and antiarrhythmic agents are also discussed.

B. Antiplatelet Therapy—Because platelet aggregation and thrombus formation are the proximate causes of acute coronary syndromes, both antiplatelet and antithrombotic agents have been extensively investigated for treatment and prevention of these syndromes (17). Acetylsalicylic acid (aspirin), the best studied antiplatelet agent, irreversibly acetylates cyclooxygenase and thereby inhibits the production of platelet-derived thromboxane A_2, a potent vasoconstrictor and stimulator of platelet aggregation. Aspirin also inhibits the production by endothelial cells of prostacyclin, a potent vasodilator. The effect of aspirin on platelets is irreversible, but the effect on endothelial cells is transient because of the cells' ability to resynthesize cyclooxygenase. Doses ranging from 75 mg to 1500 mg daily have been used, but high doses of aspirin are associated with a higher risk of adverse effects and are more likely to inhibit the production of endothelial prostacyclin. For acute coronary syndromes, a loading dose of 160 to 325 mg, chewed, produces rapid platelet inhibition (18).

1. Role of Aspirin for Primary Prevention of AMI

a. The United States Physicians Health Study was a double-blind prospective randomized controlled trial (PRCT) in which 22,071 apparently healthy male physicians without a prior diagnosis of cardiovascular disease were randomly assigned to one of four groups using a 2×2 factorial design: aspirin (325 mg every other day) plus β-carotene, aspirin plus placebo, β-carotene plus placebo, or double placebo. The average length of follow-up was 60.2 months. The percentages of subjects with diastolic blood pressures greater than 90 mm Hg, systolic blood pressures greater than 150 mm Hg, and serum cholesterol levels greater than 210 mg/dl were 9.1%, 3.9%, and 18.3%, respectively. About half of the subjects were past or current smokers and 2.4% had diabetes mellitus (44) (see Table 5-1).

(1) The study was stopped prematurely after 57 months when an interim analysis revealed a 44% reduction in the risk of AMI with aspirin ($P<0.00001$). Subgroup analysis suggested that only subjects older than 50 years of age benefited from aspirin.

(2) Aspirin did not reduce the risk of stroke or any subcategory of stroke. In fact, hemorrhagic strokes occurred almost twice as often with aspirin as with placebo, but the difference was not statistically significant ($P=0.06$).

(3) There was no significant difference in the overall rate of death or in the rate of cardiovascular death between the two groups. However, the combined risk of MI, stroke, or cardiovascular death was significantly lower with aspirin than with placebo ($P=0.01$).

(4) Bleeding episodes severe enough to require blood transfusions were uncommon in both groups but did occur more frequently with aspirin than with placebo (48 versus 28 events; $P=0.02$).

b. The British Doctors' Trial was an unblinded PRCT in which 5139 apparently healthy male physicians were randomly assigned to receive aspirin (500 mg PO QD) or to "avoid aspirin" for primary prevention of AMI (35). The control group did not receive placebo. In contrast to the United States Physicians Health Study, there was no difference in the rate of AMI between the two groups (see Table 5-2). In addition, the risk of disabling stroke was higher in the aspirin group ($P<0.05$) than in the control group. The lack of benefit observed in this study may have been caused in part by the relatively smaller study population (*i.e.*, β error). Furthermore, 24.8% of patients assigned to aspirin stopped taking the drug, and 9.2% of patients assigned to control took aspirin; these crossover patients may have further obscured any benefit of aspirin. Finally, the relatively high doses of aspirin used in this study may have contributed to the higher rate of disabling strokes among aspirin users.

c. The ongoing Nurses' Health Study was a retrospective study of the effect of chronic aspirin use on the incidence of AMI. Data were ascertained from

Table 5-1 Physicians' Health Study: aspirin for primary prevention of AMI (44)

	Aspirin (54,560 Patient-Years)	Control (54,356 Patient-Years)	*P*
Fatal and Nonfatal AMI	139	239	<0.00001
Fatal and Nonfatal stroke	119	98	NS
Hemorrhagic stroke	23	12	NS, 0.06
Cardiovascular deaths	81	83	NS
All deaths	217	227	NS

Table 5-2 British Doctors' Trial: aspirin for primary prevention of AMI (35)

	Aspirin* (18,820 Patient-Years)	Control* (9,470 Patient-Years)	*P*
Confirmed nonfatal AMI	42.5	43.3	NS
Confirmed stroke	32.4	28.5	NS
Disabling stroke	19.1	7.4	<0.05
All-cause mortality	143.5	159.5	NS

*No. events per 10,000 patient-years.

87,678 apparently healthy women older than 45 years of age (31). Women who took 1 to 6 aspirins per week (325 mg tablets) had a 32% reduction in the age-adjusted risk of AMI (RR=0.68; 95% CI, 0.52 to 0.89; *P*=0.005). However, women who used 7 to 14 aspirins per week had no reduction in the risk of AMI. Aspirin use did not increase the risk of hemorrhagic or nonhemorrhagic stroke.

2. **Role of Aspirin for Management of AMI**—The Second International Study of Infarct Survival (ISIS-2) was a PRCT in which 17,187 patients presenting within 24 hours of suspected AMI were randomly assigned to receive aspirin alone (160 mg PO QD), streptokinase alone, both agents, or neither agent (27) (see Table 5-3).
   a. Aspirin was associated with a 23% reduction in cardiovascular mortality at 5 weeks, compared with placebo (2*P*<0.00001), a benefit comparable to that of streptokinase. In addition, the combination of aspirin plus streptokinase was significantly better than either agent alone (2*P*<0.00001).
   b. Aspirin also reduced the rates of nonfatal reinfarction and nonfatal stroke. There was no significant increase in the risk of major bleeding events with aspirin.
3. **Role of Aspirin for Secondary Prevention of AMI**
   a. No single study has shown a statistically significant survival benefit of aspirin when used for secondary prevention of AMI. The published studies were relatively small and probably lacked the statistical power to find modest but clinically significant differences in outcome (5).
   b. However, a metaanalysis of these randomized trials revealed that aspirin reduced the vascular mortality rate by 13% (*P*=0.005), the rate of nonfatal reinfarction by 31% (*P*<0.0001), and the risk of nonfatal stroke by 42% (*P*<0.0001) (4).
4. **Conclusions Regarding the Role of Aspirin**
   a. **Primary Prevention of AMI**—For asymptomatic men older than 50 years of age, aspirin (325 mg PO every other day) is effective for primary prophylaxis against development of AMI. However, aspirin use may increase the risk of hemorrhagic stroke (*P*=NS in the Physicians Health Study). Preliminary results from the Nurses Health Study suggest that the benefit of aspirin use also extends to women.
   b. **Management of AMI**—Aspirin should be an integral component of standard medical therapy for patients presenting with AMI, regardless of whether thrombolytic therapy is administered. Aspirin reduces the risk of cardiovascular death as well as the risks of nonfatal stroke or reinfarction.
   c. **Secondary Prevention of AMI**—Aspirin should be an integral component of standard medical therapy for prevention of recurrent AMI. Aspirin reduces the risk of cardiovascular death as well as the risks of nonfatal stroke or reinfarction.

C. **Antithrombin Therapy**

1. **Role of Heparin for Management of AMI**—The antithrombotic effect of heparin is mediated through antithrombin III; the heparin–antithrombin III complex inhibits thrombin-mediated polymerization of fibrin (factor Ia). It also inhibits procoagulant factors IXa, Xa, XIa, and XIIa. High-molecular-weight

Table 5-3 ISIS-2: Role of aspirin for management of AMI (27)

	Aspirin (n=8587)	Control (n=8600)	*P*
Cardiovascular deaths	9.4%	11.8%	<0.00001
Nonfatal reinfarction	1.0%	2.0%	<0.00001
Nonfatal stroke	0.3%	0.6%	<0.01

fractions of heparin have a low affinity for antithrombin III but can prolong bleeding time through an antiplatelet effect. Low-molecular-weight fractions exert a strong anticoagulant effect through preferential inhibition of factor Xa. For patients with AMI, systemic anticoagulant therapy with heparin is used to improve the patency of infarct-related arteries and to limit infarct size. It also provides prophylaxis against formation of LV mural thromi (22, 23).

a. **Prevention of Left Ventricular Mural Thrombi**—Mural thrombi can be detected in as many as 30% of patients with anterior transmural AMI; they are relatively uncommon with isolated inferior AMI. Apical akinesis-dyskinesis, depressed LV systolic function (LV ejection fraction [EF] <35%), and abnormal cavitary blood flow are the principal risk factors for mural thrombus formation. Mural thrombi typically form early after transmural AMI, and the subsequent risk of systemic thromboembolism is highest in the weeks to months after infarction (25).

   (1) In one small PRCT, 221 patients presenting with acute anterior wall MI were randomly assigned to receive either low-dose heparin (5000 IU SQ BID) or high-dose heparin (12,500 IU SQ BID) (47). The activated partial thromboplastin times were 34.8 and 47.8 seconds, respectively. After 10 days, 32% of the patients in the low-dose group had an LV thrombus detectable by two-dimensional echocardiography, compared with only 11% of those in the high-dose group (P=0.0004). However, there was no significant difference in the rate of clinically evident thromboembolic events between the two groups.

   (2) According to the second report of the Cerebral Embolism Task Force, an aggregate of all randomized trials of heparin versus control in patients with AMI suggests that anticoagulation decreases the risk of LV thrombus formation from 19.8% to 8.0% (a reduction of about 60%) and the risk of stroke from 2.8% to 1.1% (11). Therefore, for the purpose of preventing strokes, it is reasonable to anticoagulate patients with anterior transmural infarctions who do not have contraindications to heparin therapy (see Chapter 32).

b. Heparin is also used, with or without thrombolysis, to improve the patency of infarct-related arteries and to limit infarct size. Heparin as an adjunct to thrombolytic therapy is described in detail in Chapter 6. Only a few studies have investigated the role of heparin apart from thrombolysis, and they reported conflicting results.

   (1) In one study, heparin therapy alone for AMI was associated with a 10% to 30% mortality reduction and a reduced incidence of reinfarction, stroke, and pulmonary embolism (34).

   (2) The Late Assessment of Thrombolytic Efficacy (LATE) Trial was a brief observational study that included a comparison of aspirin plus heparin versus aspirin alone for the management of AMI (29). After 35 days, 8.7% of patients treated with heparin plus aspirin had died, compared with 12.9% of patients treated with aspirin alone (P<0.001).

   (3) In contrast, patients treated with heparin in the aspirin arm of the ISIS-2 study derived no survival advantage at 35 days, compared with patients treated with aspirin alone (27). Anticoagulant therapy was not randomized in either of these studies. Furthermore, the benefit of heparin may have been lost between the time of discharge and the follow-up evaluation at 35 days.

2. **Role of Warfarin for Secondary Prevention of AMI**—Warfarin produces its anticoagulant effect by interfering with the vitamin K–dependent carboxylation of coagulation factors II (prothrombin), VII, IX, and X and the regulatory proteins C and S (22). Warfarin is commonly dosed according to the international normalized ratio (normal INR=1.0), which standardizes prothrombin time measurements, making interlaboratory comparisons possible.

   a. The Warfarin Reinfarction Study (WARIS) was a double-blind PRCT in which 1214 patients were randomly assigned to receive either warfarin (target INR, 2.8 to 4.8) or placebo starting 27 days after AMI (42). Patients taking antiplatelet medications such as aspirin were excluded. The mean length of follow-up was 37 months (see Table 5-4).

(1) Warfarin therapy was associated with a 24% reduction in mortality (*P*=0.0267).

(2) Warfarin also reduced the incidence of reinfarction by 34% (*P*=0.0007) and the rate of stroke by 55% (*P*=0.0015). All of the fatal strokes in the warfarin arm were hemorrhagic (4 patients), whereas all of the fatal strokes in the placebo arm were nonhemorrhagic (10 patients).

(3) Five intracranial and eight nonintracranial major bleeding episodes were associated with warfarin, for an overall risk for major bleeding of 0.6% per year.

b. The Anticoagulants in the Secondary Prevention of Events in Coronary Thrombosis (ASPECT) trial compared nicoumalone or phenprocoumon (started within 6 weeks of discharge with INR goal of 2.8 to 4.8) versus placebo among 3404 survivors of MI. The use of antiplatelet drugs was discouraged. An intention-to-treat analysis was used (3).

(1) The rate of recurrent AMI was reduced from 14.2% to 6.7% with anticoagulation. In addition, the rate of all cerebrovascular events (cerebral infarctions, intracranial hemorrhages, transient ischemic attacks, and unspecified strokes) was reduced from 3.6% to 2.2%.

(2) However, there was no significant difference in survival, and there was an increase in the rate of intracranial bleeding from 0.1% to 1.0% with anticoagulation (see Table 5-5).

c. Conclusions Regarding the Role of Warfarin for Secondary Prevention of AMI

(1) For survivors of AMI, long-term therapy with warfarin (to an INR of 2.8 to 4.8) significantly reduces the risk of cardiovascular morbidity and/or mortality. The incidence of major bleeding episodes appears to be low.

(2) However, because the patients in these trials were not receiving antiplatelet therapy, it is unknown whether the benefit of anticoagulation persists for those who are concomitantly treated with aspirin. Ongoing studies are investigating the role of combined aspirin and warfarin therapy for secondary prevention of AMI.

Table 5-4 WARIS: Role of warfarin for secondary prevention of AMI (42)

	Placebo (n=607)	Warfarin (n=607)	*P*
Cerebrovascular events	7.2%	3.3%	0.0015
Recurrent MI	20.4%	13.5%	0.0007
Overall mortality	20.3%	15.5%	0.027
Intracranial hemorrhagic	0%	1.0%	NS
Major bleeding	0%	2.1%	<0.05

Table 5-5 ASPECT: Role of anticoagulation for secondary prevention of AMI (3)

	Placebo (n=1704)	Anticoagulant (n=1700)	*P*
Cerebrovascular events	3.6%	2.2%	<0.05
Recurrent MRI	14.2%	6.7%	<0.05
Overall mortality	11.1%	10.0%	NS
Intracranial hemorrhage	0.1%	1.0%	?
Major bleeding	1.1%	4.3%	<0.05

D. β-Adrenergic Receptor Blocker Therapy—The negative inotropic effects of β_1-adrenergic receptor blockade may reduce myocardial wall stress and myocardial oxygen demand. The associated negative chronotropic effects may prolong the time for diastolic coronary artery perfusion, thereby improving blood flow to myocardial zones subserved by severely diseased coronary arteries. Inhibition of the sympathetic nervous system may also serve to suppress the renin-angiotensin-aldosterone system, which is activated in the setting of AMI and which plays an important role in the development of LV dilatation and progression to dilated cardiomyopathy (see Chapter 3 for detailed discussion). Finally, β-adrenergic blockers may favorably effect the balance of the sympathetic and parasympathetic nervous systems, thereby reducing the tendency toward life-threatening arrhythmias in patients with ischemic heart disease.

1. **Delayed β-Blocker Therapy in Post-MI Patients**—In the era before thrombolytic agents were available, the benefit of β-blocker therapy was first studied in patients who had survived at least a few days after an AMI. The details of the β-Blocker Heart Attack Trial (BHAT), the Norwegian Timolol Trial, and other studies were described in Chapter 3 (7,12,33,48). Only the conclusions from these studies are summarized here.
   - **a.** Overall, β-blocker therapy was associated with significant reductions in the risks of all-cause death, cardiovascular death, and reinfarction.
   - **b.** Subgroup analysis, metaanalysis, and retrospective analysis of a number of large postinfarction trials consistently found that β-blocker therapy was associated with a significant survival benefit after AMI. β-Blockers were not only safe in patients with congestive heart failure (CHF) but appeared to have the greatest mortality benefit in this group. The mechanism of this survival benefit was primarily through a reduction in the rates of sudden death and reinfarction.
2. **Early β-Blocker Therapy for AMI**—Following the favorable results obtained with delayed β-blocker therapy (*i.e.*, days to weeks after infarction) in post-MI patients, a number of large PRCTs evaluated the role of β-blocker therapy given within hours of infarction.
   - **a.** ISIS-1 was an open-labeled PRCT in which 16,027 patients who presented with suspected AMI were randomly assigned to receive immediate atenolol (5 to 10 mg IV, followed by 100 mg PO daily for 7 days) or standard therapy without a β-blocker (26).
     - **(1)** After 7 days of therapy, the vascular mortality was 15% lower in the atenolol arm than in the control arm (95% CI, 1% to 27%). There was also a trend toward a lower in-hospital risk of reinfarction and cardiac arrest. These benefits were achieved largely during the first day of hospitalization.
     - **(2)** Subgroup analysis found that patients older than 65 years of age and those with extensive infarctions were most likely to benefit from immediate atenolol therapy. The latter result may reflect a lower incidence of free-wall rupture.
   - **b.** Hjalmarson also conducted a PRCT of metoprolol (15 mg IV, followed by 100 mg PO BID) versus placebo in 1395 patients with suspected AMI (24). The length of follow-up was 3 months.
     - **(1)** Metoprolol therapy was associated with a 36% reduction in the relative risk of death ($P<0.03$).
     - **(2)** Subgroup analysis found that the survival benefit was greatest in elderly persons.
3. **β-Blocker Therapy and Thrombolysis**—The Thrombolysis in Myocardial Infarction 2B Study (TIMI-2B) was a PRCT in which 1434 patients undergoing thrombolysis with recombinant tissue plasminogen activator were randomly assigned to receive either early metoprolol therapy (15 mg IV over 6 minutes, 50 mg PO BID on day 1, then 100 mg PO BID thereafter) or delayed metoprolol therapy (50 mg PO BID on day 6, then 100 mg PO BID thereafter) (37).
   - **a.** There were no differences in mortality or LV EF between the two treatment groups at 6 days, 6 weeks, or 1 year. Because thrombolytic therapy can re-

duce infarction-related mortality by as much as 27%, the additional survival benefit of immediate β-blocker therapy may have been difficult to demonstrate in this population.

b. However, there was a lower risk of reinfarction (2.7% versus 5.1%; $P=0.02$) or recurrent chest pain (18.8% versus 24.1%; $P<0.02$) at 6 days in the immediate therapy group.

4. Conclusions Regarding the Role of β-Blocker Therapy in the Management of AMI

a. β-Blockers should be an integral component of standard medical therapy for management of AMI. β-Blocker therapy initiated early in the course of AMI is associated with significant reductions in morbidity and mortality. These benefits persist in patients maintained chronically on β-blocker therapy. In patients undergoing thrombolysis, the addition of β-blocker therapy may reduce the incidence of reinfarction.

b. Despite concern for the potential adverse effects of β-blocker therapy in certain subgroups of patients with AMI (*i.e.*, those with advanced age, overt CHF, transient hypotension, large MI, or arrhythmic complications), the data have consistently shown that it is precisely these patients who derive the greatest benefit from β-blocker therapy.

E. Angiotensin Converting Enzyme Inhibitors—A detailed discussion of the pathophysiology of CHF and the role of the renin-angiotensin-aldosterone system in the maladaptive response to loss of LV systolic function after MI is presented in Chapter 3, Section B. The results of seven large PRCTs of ACE inhibitor therapy in post-MI patients, including the Survival and Ventricular Enlargement (SAVE) trial, the Cooperative North Scandinavian Enalapril Survival Study II (CONSENSUS II), the Gruppo Italiano per lo Studio della Sopravvivena nell Infarto Miocardico Trial (GISSI-3), and the ISIS-4 trial, are presented in Chapter 3, Section C (1,2,20,28, 36,46). Only the conclusions from these studies are summarized here.

1. For patients presenting with AMI, the addition of an oral ACE inhibitor to a conventional drug regimen was associated with a modest but significant reduction in both short-term and long-term mortality as well as a reduction in the incidence of progressive pump failure.

2. The morbidity and mortality benefits observed with ACE inhibitor therapy were consistent among all subgroups analyzed and were particularly impressive in elderly patients and those with severe LV dysfunction.

3. In general, ACE inhibitors may be given safely within 24 hours of onset of acute MI. Although patients were more likely to experience treatment-limiting hypotension with ACE inhibition, this effect was not associated with increased mortality.

F. Nitrate Therapy—Nitroglycerin (TNG) is predominantly a venodilator, whereas sodium nitroprusside has both arterial and venous vasodilatory activity. Although both agents can reduce LV preload, TNG has the theoretical advantage of improving regional myocardial blood flow to ischemic tissue. Nitroprusside may actually "steal" coronary blood flow away from infarct-related arteries through its arterial vasodilatory effects.

1. Yusuf conducted a metaanalysis of 10 controlled trials of TNG or nitroprusside therapy for the management of AMI. The analysis included approximately 2000 patients (51). IV TNG therapy was associated with a 49% reduction in mortality ($P<0.05$). The survival benefit was largely achieved during the acute hospitalization, and there was little long-term benefit. In contrast, IV nitroprusside therapy was not associated with a statistically significant mortality benefit.

2. GISSI-3 was a large PRCT in which 17,817 patients with AMI were randomly assigned in a 2×2 factorial design to one of four groups: lisinopril alone (5 to 10 mg PO QD) versus nitrates alone (IV TNG for the first 24 hours, followed by transdermal TNG 10 mg QD) versus nitrates plus lisinopril versus double placebo. Therapy was begun within 24 hours of symptom onset (20). The length of follow-up was 6 weeks. Further details of this study are presented in Chapter 3.

a. Lisinopril (with or without concomitant nitrates) was associated with a modest reduction in both mortality ($P=0.03$) and the combined end point of mortality or severe LV dysfunction ($P=0.009$). The combination of lisinopril and nitrates was even more effective in reducing mortality than lisinopril alone ($P=0.021$).

b. Nitrates alone were no better than placebo in terms of survival benefit. However, nitrate therapy was associated with a lower incidence of cardiogenic shock and postinfarction angina ($P<0.05$).

3. ISIS-4 was a large PRCT in which 58,050 patients with suspected acute MI (not complicated by cardiogenic shock or severe CHF) were randomly assigned in a multifactorial design to receive captopril (6.25 to 50 mg PO BID) versus placebo, oral controlled-release mononitrate (30 to 60 mg PO QD) versus placebo, or magnesium versus placebo. The length of follow-up was 12 months (28). Nitrate therapy was no better than placebo in terms of short- or long-term mortality. The details of this study are presented in Chapter 3.

4. Conclusions Regarding the Role of Nitrate Therapy in the Management of AMI

a. In Yusuf's controversial metaanalysis, IV nitrates were found to significantly improve survival in patients with AMI. However, no single PRCT has been able to confirm this finding. Nevertheless, GISSI-3 does support a role for IV nitrates as an adjunct to ACE inhibition for reducing postinfarction mortality.

b. There are no data to support the long-term use of nitrates in patients without active ischemia in the postinfarction period.

G. Calcium Channel Blocker Therapy—Calcium channel blockers are a diverse class of drugs with varying effects on vasomotor tone, LV contractility, and pacemaker cell automaticity. Verapamil's principal effects are negative inotropy and negative chronotropy without significant vasodilator properties. Diltiazem has an additional peripheral arteriolar vasodilatory effect. Nifedipine produces a prominent relaxation of vasomotor tone and reflex tachycardia. Despite numerous theoretical reasons why these agents should be able to limit infarction size, improve symptoms, and reduce mortality after AMI, results from studies of the first-generation agents (nifedipine, diltiazem, and verapamil) have been disappointing. However, second-generation dihydropyridine agents such as amlodipine, which exhibit less negative inotropy and which are more potent and selective in terms of vasodilatory properties, may yet prove to have beneficial effects on symptoms and survival after AMI. The results of all major PRCTs of calcium channel blocker therapy after AMI, including the Danish Study Group on Verapamil in Myocardial Infarction (DAVIT) and the Multicenter Diltiazem Postinfarction Trial (MDPIT), are presented in detail in Chapter 3 (13,14,32). Only the conclusions from these studies are summarized here.

1. The only evidence of a survival benefit associated with calcium channel blocker therapy after acute MI was derived from the DAVIT studies. However, the benefit of verapamil was limited to patients without overt CHF. In addition, early treatment with verapamil was associated with a significantly increased incidence of death due to cardiogenic shock.

2. In the MDPIT study, diltiazem was found to be harmful in patients with reduced LV EF after acute MI.

3. In summary, the results of PRCTs reported to date do not support a role for calcium channel blocker therapy in the routine management of AMI. Caution must be exercised if they are used as alternative antihypertensive or antiischemic therapy in patients who are intolerant of β-blockers.

H. Magnesium—Magnesium is considered a physiologic calcium channel blocker that produces coronary and systemic vasodilatation, inhibits platelet aggregation, and suppresses ventricular ectopy.

1. The Leicester Intravenous Magnesium Intervention Trial (LIMIT-2) was a PRCT in which 2316 patients with suspected AMI were randomly assigned to receive either high-dose IV magnesium sulfate or placebo (49). Only 65% of this cohort proved to have had a true AMI; 35% had received thrombolysis. Magnesium therapy was associated with a 24% reduction in the risk of death (95% CI, 1% to 43%) and a 25% reduction in the risk of LV systolic failure (95% CI, 7% to 39%).

2. ISIS-4 was an open-label PRCT that compared IV magnesium sulfate versus placebo in patients presenting with AMI (28). More than 23,000 patients were randomly assigned within 6 hours of symptom onset. A double-blind design was not attempted because the investigators reasoned that the systemic effects of IV magnesium (flushing and bradycardia) would effectively unblind the treatment. The length of follow-up was 5 weeks.
   a. Overall, high-dose magnesium therapy was not associated with a significant survival benefit. In fact, there was an increase in the risk of CHF and death attributed to cardiogenic shock during the infusion period (1.62% versus 1.26%; $P<0.001$).
   b. Subgroup analysis found that magnesium therapy was associated with a marginally increased risk of death in patients presenting with bradycardia and hypotension.
3. **Conclusions Regarding the Role of High-Dose Intravenous Magnesium Therapy in the Management of AMI**—High-dose IV magnesium therapy in the setting of AMI may be associated with an increased risk of death in hemodynamically unstable patients. Therefore, this therapy is not recommended for the routine management of patients with AMI.

I. Role of Empiric Antiarrhythmic Therapy for AMI—The presence of premature ventricular contractions (PVCs) after acute MI has been shown to be a risk factor for increased mortality (21). For this reason, there has been much enthusiasm for the use of antiarrhythmic drugs to suppress symptomatic and asymptomatic PVCs, with the goal of decreasing the risk of sudden cardiac death. However, as discussed later, the results of such attempts have been largely disappointing. For purposes of discussion, studies that evaluated the role of empiric antiarrhythmic therapy for suppression of PVCs in the acute setting (*i.e.*, with IV lidocaine) are separated from studies that evaluated the role of these drugs for long-term suppression of PVCs in the nonacute setting (*i.e.*, with oral agents such as encainide, flecainide, and amiodarone).

1. **Empiric Therapy in the Acute Setting**
   a. Fourteen PRCTs, involving a total of about 8000 patients, have compared the routine use of prophylactic lidocaine versus placebo in patients with suspected AMI. These studies were reviewed by McMahon in 1988 (30). Eight studies used IV lidocaine, and clinical outcomes were measured mostly at 48 hours. The other six studies used a single dose of intramuscular lidocaine, and clinical outcomes were measured mostly at 1 hour. Only one study showed a significant decrease in the subsequent risk of ventricular fibrillation (VF), and none showed a mortality benefit.
      (1) If the data from the 14 studies are pooled, lidocaine lowered the risk of VF arrest but not the mortality rate. In fact, there was a nonsignificant trend toward higher mortality with lidocaine (see Table 5-6).
      (2) If the pooled data are limited only to the eight studies that used IV lidocaine, lidocaine had no effect on the risk of VF but increased the risk of death (see Table 5-7).
   b. An alternative to routine prophylactic use of lidocaine is to target only those who actually experience PVCs in the post-MI period. One problem with this strategy is that about 50% of primary VF arrests occur without

Table 5-6 Role of prophylactic use of IV or IM lidocaine for AMI (30)

	Lidocaine (n=4616)	Placebo (n=4539)	*P*
In-hospital risk of VF	1.0%	1.3%	0.04
In-hospital mortality rate	1.8%	1.2%	NS

Table 5-7 Role of prophylactic use of IV lidocaine for AMI (30)

	Lidocaine (n=1157)	Placebo (n=1037)	*P*
In-hospital risk of VF	2.7%	3.3%	NS
In-hospital mortality rate	5.2%	3.2%	<0.05

warning (*i.e.*, prior PVCs). Nevertheless, selective use of lidocaine does not appear to be associated with poorer outcome when compared with prophylactic lidocaine use. For example, in one study, there were no significant differences in mortality or in the risk of ventricular tachycardia or VF between the two strategies (50) (see Table 5-8). In fact, there was a trend toward higher risk of drug toxicity with the routine prophylactic strategy, especially for elderly patients.

2. **Empiric Therapy for Long-Term Suppression**—As noted previously, post-MI patients with PVCs have a higher risk of death. Therefore, various antiarrhythmic drugs have been used in an attempt to suppress symptomatic and asymptomatic PVCs in these patients. The results of all major PRCTs of antiarrhythmic therapy in patients with AMI, including the Cardiac Arrhythmia Suppression Trials I and II (CAST), the Basel Antiarrhythmia Study of Infarct Survival (BASIS), the Canadian Amiodarone Myocardial Infarction Arrhythmia Trial (CAMIAT Pilot Study), and others, are provided in Chapter 3 (8–10, 15). Only the conclusions from these studies are summarized here.
   a. The class I agents (encainide, flecainide, and moricizine) do effectively suppress PVCs but are associated with increased mortality when used for suppression of asymptomatic complex ventricular arrhythmias in the postinfarction period.
   b. Studies of amiodarone therapy in patients with acute MI have reported mixed results. Three of four PRCTs reported a survival benefit with amiodarone when given empirically or when used for suppression of asymptomatic complex ventricular arrhythmias in the postinfarction period. However, the beneficial effect on survival barely reached statistical significance in one study; the survival benefit reported in another study (BASIS) was limited to patients with LV EF ≥40%; and two of the four studies were pilot studies.
3. In summary, available data do not support the routine use of prophylactic lidocaine for suppression of asymptomatic ventricular arrhythmias in patients with MI in the acute setting. For post-MI patients in the nonacute setting, class I agents appear to increase mortality and therefore should be avoided. Preliminary studies of amiodarone in this setting are more promising but are still inconclusive. The European Myocardial Infarction Arrhythmia Trial will evaluate the effect of amiodarone in a large group of early postinfarction patients who have low LV EF.

J. Lipid-Lowering Therapy

1. **Angiographic Regression Trials**—Atherosclerosis was previously been considered to be a progressive and irreversible process amenable only to revascu-

Table 5-8 Role of prophylactic vs. selective use of lidocaine for AMI (50)

	Prophylactic Lidocaine (n=168)	Selective Lidocaine (n=165)	*P*
Lidocaine toxicity	2.4%	0.0%	NS
In-hospital VT or VF	0.0%	1.2%	NS
In-hospital mortality rate	5.0%	3.0%	NS

larization therapy. More recent studies have demonstrated that medical therapy with lipid-lowering agents can slow progression and actually promote regression of atherosclerotic disease. A metaanalysis of 10 randomized controlled trials involving a total of 2095 patients examined the effect of lipid-lowering therapy on the natural history of atherosclerotic lesions as assessed by angiography (45). Aggressive lipid-lowering therapy (mean reduction of low-density lipoprotein [LDL] cholesterol, 28%) was associated with a 21.2% reduction in the extent of progression and a 10.1% increase in the extent of regression of atherosclerotic lesions, compared with control. Of note, smaller and hemodynamically less significant lipid-rich plaques were more likely to regress than severe stenotic lesions, which tended to be more fibrotic. Smaller plaques are more often responsible for acute infarctions than stenotic plaques.

2. **Lipid-Lowering Therapy for the Primary Prevention of AMI**—The West of Scotland Coronary Prevention Study Group was a PRCT in which 6595 men aged 45 to 64 years were randomly assigned to receive either pravastatin or placebo for the prevention of coronary artery disease (CAD)–related morbidity and mortality (41). At the start of the study, only 5% of the patients had angina and 3% had claudications. The average baseline LDL cholesterol level was 192 mg/dl; this level had decreased by 26% at mean follow-up of 4.9 years.
   a. Therapy with pravastatin was associated with a 32% reduction in the risk of cardiac death (P=0.033) and a 22% reduction in all-cause mortality (95% CI, 0% to 40%; P=0.051), compared with placebo.
   b. The treatment group also had a 33% lower risk of nonfatal MI and a 37% lower risk of need for angioplasty or coronary artery bypass surgery.
3. **Lipid-Lowering Therapy for the Secondary Prevention of AMI**—The Scandinavian Simvastatin Survival Study (4S Study) randomly assigned 4444 patients with a history of angina or MI to receive either simvastatin or placebo. (40) At mean follow-up of 5.4 years, the treatment group had a 35% reduction of LDL cholesterol and an 8% increase in high-density lipoprotein cholesterol; the control group had little change in lipid parameters.
   a. Therapy with simvastatin was associated with a relative risk of death of 0.70 (95% CI, 0.58 to 0.85; P=0.0003) and a relative risk of cardiovascular death of 0.58 (95% CI, 0.46 to 0.73).
   b. The treatment group also had reduction of >30% in the risk of major coronary events and need for revascularization.
   c. Subgroup analysis showed that the benefits of simvastatin were independent of age or sex.
4. **Conclusions Regarding the Role of Lipid-Lowering Therapy for Management of Atherosclerotic Heart Disease**
   a. Lipid-lowering therapy should be an integral component of standard therapy for primary and secondary prevention of cardiovascular morbidity and mortality in patients with elevated cholesterol levels. Lipid-lowering therapy may slow progression and promote regression of established atherosclerotic disease.
   b. Patients with AMI should have a complete lipid panel analysis soon after admission. If the fasting LDL cholesterol level is >160 mg/dl, the patient should be discharged on a lipid-lowering medication, because dietary therapy alone is usually insufficient to achieve the desired level of <100 mg/dl or 25% to 35% reduction in the level of LDL cholesterol. For patients with an LDL cholesterol level <130 mg/dl, modifications of diet and exercise may be adequate. A repeat lipid panel should be obtained weeks to months after discharge, because in-hospital lipid values may be spuriously low.

K. **Smoking Cessation**—Tobacco exposure produces diffuse arterial injury and increases the risk of AMI by promoting vasoconstriction, enhancing platelet aggregation, and increasing lipoprotein oxidation. In one representative study, among men younger than 55 years of age, the relative risk of AMI was 2.9 (95% CI, 2.4 to 3.4) for current smokers, compared with those who had never smoked (39). After 2 years of abstinence, the risk of AMI fell to the same level as in control patients. Therefore, all active smokers should be encouraged to abstain from tobacco use.

L. Estrogen Replacement Therapy for Prevention of CAD Among Women—The risk of AMI increases significantly in women after menopause, quickly reaching a level comparable to that of age-matched men. Estrogen has numerous biologic effects that may lower the risk of coronary atherosclerosis. These include increasing high-density lipoprotein levels, decreasing fibrinogen levels, reducing blood pressure, and enhancing peripheral vasodilation. Estrogen also may favorably affect carbohydrate metabolism by enhancing insulin sensitivity (6).

1. The 10-year follow-up report of the Nurses Health Study found that the relative risk of cardiovascular mortality, adjusted for age and other risk factors, was 0.72 (95% CI, 0.55 to 0.95) for women who had used estrogen replacement therapy at any time (43). Compared with nonusers, current users of estrogen had a lower risk of major CAD (RR 0.51; 95% CI, 0.37 to 0.70). However, former users had a risk similar to that of the nonusers (RR 0.91; 95% CI, 0.73 to 1.14).
2. In the 16-year follow-up report of the Nurses Health Study, the relative risk of major CAD was 0.60 (95% CI, 0.43 to 0.83) for women who had used estrogen replacement therapy at any time, compared with those who had never received hormone replacement therapy. The relative risk of CAD was 0.39 (95% CI, 0.19 to 0.78) for women who had used the combination of estrogen and progestin. There was no significant reduction in the risk of stroke (19).
3. A metaanalysis of 18 controlled observational studies showed that estrogen replacement therapy was associated with significant reductions in the risk of fatal and nonfatal cardiovascular disease (range, 46% to 84%), independent of other known coronary risk factors (6).
4. **Conclusions Regarding the Role of Estrogen Therapy for Prevention of CAD**
   a. Estrogen replacement therapy should be considered for all women who are postmenopausal, who have premature ovarian failure, or who have undergone bilateral oophorectomy, especially if they have known risk factors for CAD or a prior history of AMI.
   b. The addition of a progestin is appropriate in women who still have a uterus to reduce the risks of unopposed estrogen therapy.

M. Recommendations

1. Aspirin is effective for primary prevention, secondary prevention, and acute treatment of AMI. For asymptomatic men older than 50 years of age, aspirin (325 mg PO every other day) is effective for primary prophylaxis against development of AMI. However, there may be a statistically nonsignificant trend toward a higher rate of hemorrhagic stroke with aspirin. Preliminary results from the Nurses Health Study suggest that the benefit of aspirin also extends to women. When used for acute treatment of AMI, aspirin reduces the risk of cardiovascular death as well as the risks of nonfatal stroke or reinfarction; patients should immediately receive 325 mg of aspirin (chewed). The benefits of aspirin apply regardless of age, gender, time of presentation, or use of thrombolytic therapy. Aspirin in moderate doses should be continued indefinitely after AMI to reduce the rates of reinfarction, stroke, and death.
2. Heparin is frequently used, with or without thrombolysis, to improve the patency of infarct-related arteries and to limit the infarct size. Heparin as an adjunct to thrombolytic therapy is detailed in Chapter 6. Only a few have investigated the role of heparin apart from thrombolysis, and they have reported conflicting results. Nevertheless, heparin does appear to reduce the incidence of LV mural thrombus formation after AMI.
3. Although long-term therapy with warfarin significantly reduced the risk of cardiovascular morbidity and/or mortality in post-MI patients, the patients in these trials were not receiving antiplatelet therapy. Therefore, it is unknown whether the benefit of anticoagulation persists for those who are concomitantly treated with aspirin.
4. β-Blocker therapy initiated early in the course of AMI is associated with significant reductions in morbidity and mortality. These benefits persist when patients are maintained chronically on β-blocker therapy. In patients undergoing thrombolysis, the addition of β-blockers may reduce the incidence of reinfarc-

tion. Despite concerns of potential adverse effects of β-blocker therapy in certain subgroups of patients with AMI (advanced age, overt CHF, transient hypotension, large MI, arrhythmia), the data have consistently shown that it is precisely these patients who derive the greatest benefit from β-blocker therapy.

5. For patients presenting with AMI, the addition of an oral ACE inhibitor to a conventional drug regimen was associated with reductions in short-term and long-term mortality and in the incidence of progressive pump failure. The benefits of ACE inhibitor therapy were consistent among all subgroups analyzed and were particularly impressive for the elderly and for those with severe LV dysfunction. In general, ACE inhibitors may be given safely within 24 hours of onset of acute MI. Although patients were more likely to experience treatment-limiting hypotension with ACE inhibition, this effect was not associated with increased mortality.
6. In Yusuf's controversial metaanalysis, IV nitrates significantly improved survival in patients with AMI. However, no single PRCT has confirmed this finding. Nevertheless, GISSI-3 did support a role of IV nitrates as an adjunct to ACE inhibition for reduction of early postinfarction mortality. There are no data to support the long-term use of nitrates in patients without active ischemia in the postinfarction period.
7. The current data do not support a role for calcium channel blockers or high-dose IV magnesium for routine management of AMI.
8. There are insufficient data to support the routine use of prophylactic lidocaine for suppression of asymptomatic ventricular arrhythmias in patients with MI in the acute setting. For post-MI patients in the nonacute setting, class I agents appear to increase the mortality and should be avoided. Preliminary studies of amiodarone in this setting are more promising but are still inconclusive.
9. Lipid-lowering therapy should be an integral component of standard therapy for primary and secondary prevention of cardiovascular morbidity and mortality in patients with elevated cholesterol levels. Lipid-lowering therapy may slow progression and promote regression of established atherosclerotic disease. Although lipid-lowering agents may increase the minimal luminal diameter of coronary vessels to only a small extent, the use of these drugs has been associated with marked reductions in the risk of death, the risk of nonfatal MI, and the need for angioplasty or coronary artery bypass surgery.
10. Estrogen replacement therapy should be considered for all postmenopausal women, especially if they have known risk factors for CAD or a prior history of AMI. The addition of a progestin is appropriate for women with an intact uterus.

Abbreviations used in Chapter 5

ACE = angiotensin-converting enzyme
AMI = acute myocardial infarction
BID = twice daily
CAD = coronary artery disease
CHF = congestive heart failure
CI = confidence interval
EF = ejection fraction
INR = international normalized ratio
IV = intravenous
LDL = low-density lipoprotein
LV = left ventricular
LV EF = left ventricular ejection fraction
MI = myocardial infarction

N = number of patients in population
n = number of patients in sample
NS = not significant
P = probability value
PO = per os
PRCT = prospective randomized controlled trial
PVC = premature ventricular contraction
QD = daily
RR = relative risk
SQ = subcutaneous
VF = ventricular fibrillation

References

1. Acute Infarction Ramipril Efficacy (AIRE) Study Investigators. Effect of ramipril on mortality and morbidity of survivors of acute myocardial infarction with clinical evidence of heart failure. *Lancet* 1993;342:821.
2. Ambrosioni. The effect of the angiotension-converting-enzyme inhibitor zofenopril on mortality and morbidity after anterior myocardial infarction. *N Engl J Med* 1995;332:80.
3. Anticoagulants in the Secondary Prevention of Events in Coronary Thrombosis (ASPECT) Research Group. Effect of long-term oral anticoagulant treatment on mortality and cardiovascular morbidity after myocardial infarction. *Lancet* 1994; 343:499.
4. Antiplatelet Trialists Collaboration. Secondary prevention of vascular disease by prolonged antiplatelet treatment. *Br Med J* 1988;296:320.
5. Aspirin Myocardial Infarction Study Research Group. A randomized, controlled trial of aspirin in persons recovered from myocardial infarction. *JAMA* 1980;243: 661.
6. Barrett-Conner. Estrogen and coronary heart disease in women. *Journal of the American Heart Association* 1991;265:1861.
7. Beta-Blocker Heart Attack Trial Research Group. A randomized trial of propranolol in patients with acute myocardial infarction: I. Mortality results. *JAMA* 1982;247:1707.
8. Burkart. Effect of antiarrhythmic therapy on mortality in survivors of myocardial infarction with asymptomatic complex ventricular arrhythmias: Basel Antiarrhythmic Study of Infarct Survival (BASIS). *J Am Coll Cardiol* 1990;16:1711.
9. Cairns. Post-myocardial infarction mortality in patients with ventricular premature depolarizations: Canadian Amiodarone Myocardial Infarction Arrhythmia Trial Pilot Study. *Circulation* 1991;84:550.
10. Cardiac Arrhythmia Suppression Trial II Investigators. Effect of the antiarrhythmic agent moricizine on survival after myocardial infarction. *N Engl J Med* 1992;327:227.
11. Cerebral Embolism Task Force. Cardiogenic brain embolism: the second report of the cerebral embolism task force. *Arch Neurol* 1989;46:727.
12. Chadda. Effect of propranolol after acute myocardial infarction in patients with congestive heart failure. *Circulation* 1986;73:503.
13. Danish Study Group on Verapamil in Myocardial Infarction. Verapamil in acute myocardial infarction. *Eur Heart J* 1984;5:516.
14. Danish Study Group on Verapamil in Myocardial Infarction. Secondary prevention with verapamil after myocardial infarction. *Am J Cardiol* 1990;66:33I.
15. Echt. Mortality and morbidity in patients receiving encainide, flecainide, or placebo: The Cardiac Arrhythmia Suppression Trial. *N Engl J Med* 1991;324:781.
16. Fibrinolytic Therapy Trialists (FTT) Collaborative Group. Indications for fibrinolytic therapy in suspected acute myocardial infarction: collaborative overview

of early mortality and major morbidity results from all randomized trials of more than 1000 patients. *Lancet* 1994;343:311.

17. Fuster. The pathogenesis of coronary artery disease and the acute coronary syndromes. *N Engl J Med* 1992;326:242.
18. Fuster. Aspirin as a therapeutic agent in cardiovascular disease. *Circulation* 1993;87:659.
19. Grodstein. Postmenopausal estrogen and progestin use and the risk of cardiovascular disease. *N Engl J Med* 1996;335:453.
20. Gruppo Italiano per lo Studio della Sopravvivena nell Infarto Miocardico. GISSI-3: effects of lisinopril and transdermal glyceryl trinitrate singly and together on 6-week mortality and ventricular function after acute myocardial infarction. *Lancet* 1994;343:1115.
21. Hine. Meta-analysis of empirical long-term antiarrhythmic therapy after myocardial infarction. *JAMA* 1989;262:3037.
22. Hirsh. Guide to anticoagulant therapy: Part 2. Oral anticoagulants. *Circulation* 1994;89:1469.
23. Hirsh. Guide to anticoagulant therapy: Part 1. Heparin. *Circulation* 1994;89:1449.
24. Hjalmarson. Effect on mortality of metoprolol in acute myocardial infarction: a double blind randomized trial. *Lancet* 1981;ii:823.
25. Huggins. Left ventricular thromboembolism after myocardial infarction. *Heart Disease and Stroke* 1994:355.
26. ISIS-1 Collaborative Group. Randomized trial of intravenous atenolol among 16,027 cases of suspected acute myocardial infarction: ISIS-1. *Lancet* 1986;ii:57.
27. ISIS-2 (Second International Study of Infarct Survival) Collaborative Group. Randomized trial of intravenous streptokinase, oral aspirin, both, or neither among 17,187 cases of suspected acute myocardial infarction: ISIS-2. *Lancet* 1988;ii:349.
28. ISIS-4. ISIS-4: a randomized factorial trial assessing early oral captopril, oral mononitrate, and intravenous magnesium sulphate in 58,050 patients with suspected acute myocardial infarction. *Lancet* 1995;345:669.
29. LATE Study Group. Late assessment of thrombolytic efficacy (LATE) study with alteplase 6–24 hours after acute myocardial infarction. *Lancet* 1993;342:759.
30. MacMahon. Effects of prophylactic lidocaine in suspected acute myocardial infarction. *JAMA* 1988;260:1910.
31. Manson. A prospective study of aspirin use and primary prevention of cardiovascular disease in women. *JAMA* 1991;266:521.
32. Multicenter Diltiazem Postinfarction Trial Research Group. The effect of diltiazem on mortality and reinfarction after myocardial infarction. *N Engl J Med* 1988;319:385.
33. Norwegian Multicenter Study Group. Timolol-induced reduction in mortality and reinfarction in patients surviving acute myocardial infarction. *N Engl J Med* 1981;304:801.
34. O'Donnell. Antithrombotic therapy for acute myocardial infarction. *J Am Coll Cardiol* 1995;25(Suppl):23S.
35. Peto. Randomized trial of prophylactic daily aspirin in British male doctors. *Br Med J* 1988;296:313.
36. Pfeffer. Effect of captopril on mortality and morbidity in patients with left ventricular dysfunction after myocardial infarction: results of the Survival and Ventricular Enlargement trial. *N Engl J Med* 1992;327:669.
37. Roberts and the TIMI investigators. Immediate versus deferred β-blockade following thrombolytic therapy in patients with acute myocardial infarction. *Circulation* 1991;83:422.
38. Rogers and the Participants in the National Registry of Myocardial Infarction. Treatment of myocardial infarction in the United States (1990–1993). *Circulation* 1994;90:2103.
39. Rosenberg. The risk of myocardial infarction after quitting smoking in men under 55 years of age. *N Engl J Med* 1985;313:1511.

40. Scandinavian Simvastatin Study Group. Randomized trial of cholesterol lowering in 4444 patients with coronary heart disease: the Scandinavian Simvastatin Survival Study (4S). *Lancet* 1994;344:1383.
41. Shepherd. Prevention of coronary heart disease with pravastatin in men with hypercholesterolemia. *N Engl J Med* 1995;333:1301.
42. Smith. The effect of warfarin on mortality and reinfarction after myocardial infarction. *N Engl J Med* 1990;323:147.
43. Stampfer. Postmenopausal estrogen therapy and cardiovascular disease: Ten year follow-up from the Nurses Health Study. *N Engl J Med* 1991;325:756.
44. Steering Committee of the Physicians Health Study Research Group. Final report of the aspirin component of the ongoing Physicians Health Study. *N Engl J Med* 1989;321:129.
45. Superko. Coronary artery disease regression. Convincing evidence for the benefit of aggressive lipoprotein management. *Circulation* 1994;90:1056.
46. Swedberg. Effects of the early administration of enalapril on mortality in patients with acute myocardial infarction. *N Engl J Med* 1992;327:678.
47. Turpie. Comparison of high-dose with low-dose subcutaneous heparin to prevent left ventricular mural thrombosis in patients with acute transmural anterior myocardial infarction. *N Engl J Med* 1989;320:352.
48. Viscoli. Beta-blockers after myocardial infarction: influence of first-year clinical course on long-term effectiveness. *Ann Intern Med* 1993;118:99.
49. Woods. Intravenous magnesium sulphate in suspected acute myocardial infarction: results of the second Leicester Intravenous Magnesium Intervention Trial (LIMIT-2). *Lancet* 1992;339:1553.
50. Wyse. Prophylactic vs. selective lidocaine for early ventricular arrhythmias of MI. *J Am Coll Cardiol* 1988;12:507.
51. Yusuf. Effect of intravenous nitrates on mortality in acute myocardial infarction: an overview of the randomized trials. *Lancet* 1988;i:1088.

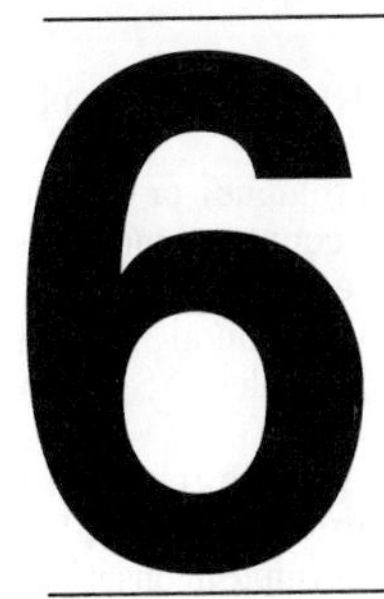

Myocardial Infarction: Thrombolytic Therapy

Gordon S. Huggins and
Patrick T. O'Gara

A. Introduction

1. For patients presenting with acute myocardial infarction (AMI), large randomized clinical trials have convincingly demonstrated that prompt restoration and maintenance of brisk antegrade flow in the infarct-related artery (IRA) can limit infarct size, preserve left ventricular (LV) function, attenuate LV remodeling, and improve survival. In general, thrombolytic therapy administered within 6 hours of symptom onset is associated with a 25% reduction in mortality. However, the benefit of prompt restoration of blood flow in the IRA must be weighed against the risk of serious bleeding, particularly intracerebral hemorrhage.
2. Although the efficacy of reperfusion therapy is widely accepted, more recent studies have addressed the relative merits of pharmacologic versus mechanical intervention for patients with AMI. Encouraging results from several trials of primary percutaneous transluminal coronary angioplasty (PTCA) for AMI have heightened the interest in this modality. However, the requirement for a dedicated cardiac catheterization facility may limit the availability of primary PTCA to tertiary care centers (see Chapter 7). In contrast, thrombolytic therapy is widely available, and it remains the principal therapeutic modality for most presenting with AMI. Future studies will probably focus on the effect of earlier administration of thrombolytic therapy, the role of adjunctive antithrombotic therapies, and simplified dosing with the use of genetically altered thrombolytic agents (10).
3. Recent statistics suggest that thrombolytic therapy is still being underutilized.
   a. Investigators of the National Registry of Myocardial Infarction (NRMI) found that only one-third of the 240,989 patients with AMI had been treated with thrombolytic therapy (34). Elderly patients and those who presented more than 12 hours after symptom onset were less likely to have received thrombolytic therapy.
   b. The current in-hospital mortality rate for AMI is approximately 10%, and another 10% of hospital survivors die within the first year (2). However, up to 20% of patients with AMI die at home. Despite public awareness campaigns, two-thirds of the delay from symptom onset to therapeutic intervention is attributable to patient-related procrastination (39). Forty percent of patients delay more than 4 hours after the onset of symptoms, and 10% to 15% present after a 12-hour delay. The "door-to-drug" time may be reduced to less than 30 minutes through the use of prehospital electrocardiography (ECG) and dedicated thrombolytic protocols, which serve to stream-line decision making and facilitate patient care (39).

B. Pathophysiology of Acute Myocardial Infarction

1. **The Acute Coronary Syndrome** (See Chapter 2 for further discussion.)
   a. The most common precipitant of AMI is acute coronary artery occlusion caused by thrombosis at a site of atherosclerotic plaque rupture. Alternatively, infarction may be caused by sustained increase in myocardial oxygen demand (*e.g.*, exercise, sepsis, anemia, β-blocker withdrawal, thyrotoxicosis) in the setting of restricted coronary flow reserve (*e.g.*, fixed

atherosclerotic coronary artery disease, aortic stenosis, hypertrophic cardiomyopathy).

b. The thrombus may be either fibrin-rich (red thrombus) or platelet-rich (white thrombus). Fibrin-rich thrombi, which account for most cases of AMI associated with ST elevation, are susceptible to fibrinolysis; platelet-rich thrombi are relatively resistant. Nonocclusive mural thrombi may cause unstable or progressive angina, whereas complete occlusion typically results in AMI (14).

c. An acute thrombotic occlusion is a dynamic event, with recurrent vessel opening and closing (20). Before the era of reperfusion therapy, DeWood studied 332 patients within the first 24 hours after symptom onset with serial coronary angiography to determine the natural history of thrombotic coronary occlusion (12). The prevalence of vessel occlusion was 87% at 4 hours from symptom onset but fell progressively to 65% at 12 to 24 hours. Stable recanalization requires tipping the balance of local fibrinolytic, thrombotic, and vasoactive influences at the site of endothelial injury toward vessel patency.

2. The Open Artery Theory

a. Early Benefit—Acute occlusion of a coronary artery produces an advancing wave of myocyte necrosis from the subendocardium to the subepicardium. The infarct zone is bordered by a rim of ischemic myocardium which may be salvaged by restoration of blood flow. According to the open artery theory, early recanalization of the IRA may limit the infarction to the subendocardium, reduce the extent of infarction, and restore coronary blood flow to viable myocardium. Larger infarctions result in a greater impairment of LV systolic function and an increased risk of cardiac complications. Consequently, reestablishment of antegrade IRA blood flow should be the primary goal during the acute phase of AMI.

(1) The Global Use of Strategies to Open Occluded Coronary Arteries (GUSTO) Angiographic Investigators reported a large angiographic study of 2431 patients treated with thrombolytic therapy within 6 hours of AMI to determine the relation between IRA patency, infarction size, and 30-day mortality (18).

(a) Patients with normal coronary flow (TIMI grade 3, on a scale of 0 to 3) at 90 minutes after the initiation of thrombolytic therapy had the greatest preservation of left ventricular ejection fraction (LV EF) and regional wall motion, compared with patients who had persistently occluded or almost occluded arteries (TIMI grade 0 or 1 flow, respectively). In addition, the left ventricular end-systolic volume index (LVESVI), a reflection of infarct size and LV remodeling, was significantly lower in patients with TIMI grade 3 flow at 90 minutes, compared with those with flows of grade 0, 1, or 2 (see Table 6-1).

(b) The presence of brisk antegrade flow (TIMI grade 3) at 90 minutes was associated with a significantly lower 30-day mortality rate, compared with persistently occluded arteries, regardless of the thrombolytic agent used.

b. Late Benefit—Extensive myocyte necrosis produces LV systolic dysfunction, reduces cardiac output, and increases LV filling pressures. During the

Table 6-1 IRA patency, infarct size, and mortality after thrombolysis (18)

	TIMI 0	TIMI 1	TIMI 2	TIMI 3
30-Day mortality	Combined 8.9%		7.4%	4.4%
5–7 Day LV EF	56±14%	54±12%	56±14%	61±14%
5–7 Day LVESVI	32±16 ml/m^2	34±13 ml/m^2	30±13 ml/m^2	26±14 ml/m^2

weeks following AMI, compensatory dilatation of infarcted areas and hypertrophy of noninfarcted areas serve to restore cardiac output and reduce filling pressures (28). Although cavitary dilation provides short-term hemodynamic benefit, the long-term consequences of infarct remodeling include heart failure, ventricular arrhythmia, LV thromboembolism, and death (see Chapter 3). Restoration of antegrade IRA blood flow may improve infarct healing by preserving viable myocardial tissue within and around the infarct zone.

(1) Pfeffer found that among patients not treated with thrombolysis, those with a patent left anterior descending artery after transmural anterior AMI had significantly less postinfarction cavitary dilation than patients with a persistently occluded artery (32).

(2) The Thrombolysis and Angioplasty in Myocardial Infarction-6 (TAMI-6) Study Group found that patients treated with recombinant tissue plasminogen activator (rtPA) more than 6 hours after the onset of symptoms had stable LV size 6 months after AMI, whereas placebo-treated patients had a 25% increase in left ventricular end-diastolic volume (LVEDV) (37).

C. Criteria for Thrombolytic Therapy

1. Indications for Thrombolysis—The Fibrinolytic Therapy Trialists (FTT) Collaborative Group combined data from nine large prospective randomized controlled trials (PRCTs) of thrombolytic therapy. The analysis included a total of 58,000 patients and attempted to determine which patient characteristics were associated with improved survival at 35 days (13). Despite the wide range of thrombolytic agents and adjuvant therapies employed in these studies, several generalizations regarding the indication for fibrinolytic therapy can be made.

a. Duration of Chest Pain—Survival was inversely related to the number of hours from symptom onset to initiation of fibrinolytic therapy. The confidence interval of this relation crossed the point of no added survival benefit after 12 hours. One concern regarding late thrombolytic therapy in the setting of a fresh transmural infarction is the risk of subsequent free wall rupture. A metaanalysis from trials using streptokinase (SK) found that early thrombolytic therapy reduced the relative risk of free wall rupture in treated patients, compared with control patients, whereas thrombolytic therapy after 17 to 21 hours of symptoms was associated with an increased risk (21). In contrast, the Late Assessment of Thrombolytic Efficacy (LATE) investigators found that therapy with rtPA initiated 12 hours after onset of symptoms was not associated with an increased risk of rupture, compared earlier thrombolytic therapy. The small percentage of patients treated with rtPA who did suffer free wall rupture were more likely to have their event on the first day after AMI, whereas placebo-treated patients were more likely to rupture in the first week after AMI (7).

b. Electrocardiographic Findings—The ECG findings for which thrombolytic therapy has been shown to confer a survival benefit are listed in Table 6-2. Although some clinical trials have found a survival benefit only in patients with anterior AMI, the FTT Collaborative Group reported a survival benefit in patients with either anterior or inferior infarcts (13). An ECG injury current may be confused with ST-segment elevation resulting from pericarditis, LV aneurysm, or normal early repolarization; comparison with prior studies may help distinguish acute from chronic abnormalities.

2. Relative and Absolute Contraindications for Thrombolysis—Increased risk of bleeding is the major adverse effect associated with thrombolytic therapy. Some bleeding risks have been termed relative contraindications, reflecting the need to weigh modest risks against substantial benefits. In contrast, absolute contraindications to thrombolysis denote conditions associated with a high risk of morbidity or mortality from bleeding (3). If mechanical revascularization is an option, then the presence of numerous relative contraindications may make primary angioplasty more attractive. Alternatively, thrombolytic therapy in the setting of relative contraindications is acceptable if valuable

Table 6-2 ECG findings and survival benefit with thrombolysis for AMI

Electrocardiographic Finding	Survival Benefit With Thrombolytic Therapy
≥1 mm ST elevation in two contiguous leads	Yes
New left bundle branch block	Yes
ST depression in leads V_2–V_4 (posterior infarction)	Yes
ST depression in other leads (unstable angina)	No

time may be lost during patient transfer. The presence of absolute contraindications in an otherwise suitable patient mandates mechanical revascularization, because the risk of bleeding with PTCA is lower and more easily controlled.

a. **Blunt or Sharp Trauma**—Major surgery, trauma, or organ biopsy within 6 weeks of presentation should be considered an absolute contraindication to thrombolytic therapy. Standard chest compressions lasting <10 minutes typically do not cause significant myocardial or pericardial trauma; in these cases, thrombolytic therapy may be given with only a minor risk of bleeding. More prolonged duration of chest compressions may carry a greater risk of major bleeding. Arterial punctures and venous punctures of noncompressible sites should be strictly avoided (29).

b. **Age**—Irrespective of whether a patient receives thrombolytic therapy, advanced age is associated with increased in-hospital mortality after AMI. Few individual studies have had sufficient power to study the utility of thrombolytic therapy in patients older than 75 years of age.

   (1) Subgroup analysis in the FTT Collaborative Group Study found a significant survival benefit associated with thrombolysis in patients <75 years old. Patients ≥75 years old had an increased mortality during the first 24 hours after thrombolysis (26 per 1000 excess deaths) but had a significant improvement in survival from day 2 through day 35 (35 per 1000 fewer deaths); overall, a nonsignificant trend toward improved 35-day survival was observed in this age group (13). The poorer early outcome in elderly patients may reflect the increased time from symptom onset to initiation of therapy for this group of patients as well as the increased incidence of early strokes. This paradox of an early hazard in elderly patients and substantial gains during subsequent days should not exclude such patients from acute reperfusion therapy.

   (2) Randomized studies using SK, such as the Gruppo Italiano per lo Studio della Sopravvivenza nell Infarto Miocardico (GISSI-1) Trial and the Second International Study of Infarct Survival (ISIS-2), found a substantial and significant survival benefit of thrombolysis in elderly patients, at least rivaling that in younger patients (25).

   (3) The risk of hemorrhagic stroke may be decreased in elderly patients by use of less intensive thrombolytic and antithrombotic regimens; rtPA should be administered in a weight-adjusted manner. The present challenge is to formulate reperfusion regimens that safely extend the survival advantage of thrombolytic therapy to a greater portion of the elderly population (38).

c. **Hypertension**—Patients who present with transient severe hypertension (systolic blood pressure [SBP], >180 mm Hg; diastolic blood pressure [DBP], >110 mm Hg) in the setting of AMI have a relative contraindication to thrombolytic therapy. Subgroup analysis of the FTT Collaborative Group found no statistically significant difference in survival at 35 days between patients in the thrombolysis and placebo groups who presented with an SBP >175 mm Hg. Although an absolute excess of early deaths (*i.e.*, in the first 24 hours) was observed with increasing blood pressure, a substantial survival benefit was evident during day 2 through day 35 (13).

d. **Cardiogenic Shock**—Hypotension due to pump failure at the time of presentation is associated with a very high risk of death. Subgroup analysis of the FTT Collaborative Group revealed that thrombolytic therapy was associated with a substantial survival benefit at 35 days in each category of blood pressure. However, an early survival benefit (first 24 hours) was observed only in patients presenting with an SBP <100 mm Hg (33 per 1000 fewer deaths). This group also benefited the most during the entire period of follow-up (60 per 1000 fewer deaths) (13). However, there is convincing evidence that patients presenting with cardiogenic shock in the setting of AMI may benefit more from angioplasty than from thrombolytic therapy with respect to survival. Initiation of thrombolytic therapy may only delay an inevitable catheterization and increase the procedural risk of bleeding (6). Nevertheless, if coronary angiography and intraaortic balloon counterpulsation are not immediately available, then early initiation of thrombolytic therapy may speed the time to vessel patency.

e. **Risk of Stroke**—Without thrombolytic therapy, there is a 0.5% to 1.0% risk of either hemorrhagic or thromboembolic stroke within the first 35 days of AMI.

   (1) Thrombolytic therapy was associated with a small but significantly increased incidence of stroke within the first 24 hours (4.3 per 1000 excess strokes) and a lower incidence between day 2 and day 35 (0.4 per 1000 fewer strokes). The increase in early events (mostly hemorrhagic) and the decrease in later events (mostly thromboembolic) resulted in an overall incidence of stroke associated with thrombolytic therapy that was not significantly higher than that seen in control patients (13).

   (2) GISSI-2 found that patients treated with rtPA had a small but significantly higher risk of stroke than patients treated with SK (adjusted OR, 1.42; 95% CI, 1.09 to 1.84) (27). Subgroup analysis also found that female gender was associated with hemorrhagic stroke (adjusted OR, 1.72, 95% CI, 1.04 to 2.85), whereas advanced age was associated with thromboembolic stroke (adjusted OR, 3.44; 95% CI, 1.84 to 5.98) without an increased risk of hemorrhagic stroke.

   (3) In general, in patients without a known risk for intracranial bleeding, the benefits of myocardial salvage and reduction in cardiovascular mortality greatly outweigh the risk of hemorrhagic stroke associated with thrombolytic therapy. A remote history of thromboembolic stroke or a recent transient ischemic attack should be considered a relative contraindication to thrombolytic therapy. A history of a hemorrhagic or undefined stroke, an intracranial tumor, prior neurosurgery, and recent head trauma are absolute contraindications to thrombolytic therapy.

f. **Major Bleeding**—Major bleeding, as defined by the requirement for blood transfusion or the occurrence of life-threatening bleeding, occurs in about 1% of patients treated with thrombolytic therapy.

   (1) Patients with melena, marked hematuria, or recent major surgery have an absolute contraindication to thrombolysis, whereas patients with occult fecal blood have a relative contraindication to thrombolysis.

   (2) Warfarin therapy depletes the vitamin K–dependent coagulation factors (thrombin, VII, IX, and X), whereas thrombolytic therapy degrades fibrinogen and factors V and VIII. The potential for a severe combined coagulopathic state makes thrombolytic therapy relatively contraindicated in the setting of warfarin therapy, depending on the extent of prolongation of the prothrombin time.

   (3) Thrombolytic therapy should be considered contraindicated in patients with a defined bleeding diathesis such as hemophilia (3).

g. **Summary Table of Relative and Absolute Contraindications for Thrombolysis** (see Table 6-3)

D. **Clinical Trials of Thrombolytic Therapy for AMI**

1. **Streptokinase**—SK is a product of group C b-hemolytic streptococci; it forms a heterodimer with plasminogen that is capable of degrading fibrin, fibrinogen, and factors V and VIII. The systemic hypofibrinogenemia that follows SK administration results in a residual lytic state lasting for 24 hours. Hypotension and bradycardia may develop in as many as 10% of patients during the administration of SK. Volume resuscitation and brief cessation of the SK infusion are usually required for hemodynamic stabilization. SK may be resumed at a slower rate, or rtPA may be substituted. Prior pharmacologic exposure to SK may stimulate the formation of anti-SK antibodies, which may inhibit the enzymatic activity of SK. In addition, cutaneous or anaphylactic allergic reactions may follow SK administration in presensitized patients. Therefore, rtPA should be used for subsequent thrombolytic interventions in patients who previously been treated with SK.

a. **The Gruppo Italiano per lo Studio Della Sopravvivenza nell' Infarto Miocardico (GISSI-1) Trial**—This early study was an unblinded comparison of SK (1.5 million U IV over 60 minutes) versus no thrombolytic therapy in 11,806 patients who presented within 12 hours after the onset of symptoms of AMI (15). Unlike subsequent large-scale thrombolysis studies, routine adjunctive therapy was not administered in this trial.

(1) SK therapy was associated with a significant reduction in mortality at 21 days (see Table 6-4).

(2) The survival benefit was restricted to patients presenting with anterior AMI who received therapy within 6 hours of symptom onset, and it persisted beyond 1 year after initial therapy (16).

(3) The relative risk of reinfarction in patients who received SK was 1.42 (95% CI, 1.11 to 1.81), compared with the control group, reflecting reocclusion of the IRA after initially successful recanalization (16).

(4) Subgroup analysis suggested that the survival benefit was restricted to patients ≤65 years of age, those with AMI involving the anterior wall or occurring in multiple locations (but not isolated inferior or lat-

Table 6-3 Contraindications for thrombolytic therapy

	Absolute Contraindication	Relative Contraindication
Major surgery, trauma or organ biopsy within 6 wk	X	
≥10 Minutes of chest compressions		X
Age ≥75 y		X
SBP ≥180 mm Hg, DBP ≥110 mm Hg		X
Cardiogenic shock		X
Remote stroke or recent transient ischemic attack		X
History of hemorrhagic or undefined stroke	X	
History of intracranial tumor, prior neurosurgery, or recent head trauma	X	
Melena, marked hematuria	X	
Occult fecal blood		X
Concurrent warfarin therapy		X
History of bleeding diathesis	X	

Table 6-4 GISSI-1: SK vs. placebo for AMI (15)

Mortality	Streptokinase (n=5860)	Placebo (n=5852)	*P*
≤3 h	9.2%	12%	0.0005
3–6 h	11.7%	14.1%	0.03
6–9 h	12.6%	14.1%	NS
9–12 h	15.8%	13.6%	NS
Overall mortality	10.7%	13.0%	0.0002

eral wall AMI), those without a prior history of AMI, and those in Killip class 1 through 3.

(5) The risks of major bleeding and anaphylactic shock were low: 0.3% and 0.1%, respectively.

2. Recombinant Tissue Plasminogen Activator—rtPA is an endogenous serum protease that forms a ternary complex with fibrin and plasminogen and catalyzes the conversion of plasminogen to plasmin. The enzymatic efficiency of fibrin-bound rtPA is markedly enhanced in comparison with that of soluble rtPA, resulting in a greater degree of clot-specific fibrinolysis and a lesser degree of systemic fibrinolysis. rtPA is converted in plasma from a nascent monomeric form to a less fibrin-specific dimeric form. Because rtPA is not a foreign antigen, the administration of rtPA poses no risk of anaphylactic shock. In the setting of relative hypotension, rtPA is therefore the preferred agent over SK or anisoylated plasminogen streptokinase activator complex (APSAC; see later discussion). Bleeding complications from rtPA are more likely caused by the lysis of fibrin plugs at local sites of vascular injury than by the modest reduction in plasma fibrinogen levels.

a. The Anglo-Scandinavian Study of Early Thrombolysis (ASSET)—This large study was designed as a PRCT of rtPA (100 mg over 3 hours) combined with an IV bolus of heparin (5000 U) followed by a continuous heparin infusion (1000 U/hour) for 21 hours versus heparin alone for the early management of suspected AMI (40). A total of 5011 patients with <5 hours of symptoms were randomly assigned to the two treatment groups in this study. The length of follow-up was 1 month.

(1) Combined therapy with rtPA and heparin was associated with a 26% reduction in total mortality and a 25% reduction in the incidence of cardiogenic shock during hospitalization, compared with heparin therapy alone (see Table 6-5).

(2) There were no significant differences in the rates of stroke, stroke-related mortality, postinfarction angina, heart failure, or reinfarction between the two treatment groups.

(3) Despite its theoretical clot specificity, rtPA therapy did not appear to be associated with fewer major bleeding complications (*i.e.*, hematemesis, melena, severe hemoptysis, or hematuria) than have been observed in trials of SK therapy.

(4) Subgroup analysis showed that the survival benefit from rtPA extended to both sexes and increased with increasing age.

3. Anisoylated Plasminogen Streptokinase Activator Complex—The anisoylated plasminogen streptokinase activator complex (APSAC) is a preformed complex of SK and human lys-plasminogen whose catalytic center is acylated with the goal of delaying enzymatic activity until the complex has bound a fibrin substrate. Spontaneous deacylation results in the resumption of fibrinolytic activity. Despite the acyl modification, systemic fibrinolysis remains significant with APSAC. Like its parent compound, APSAC may cause systemic hypotension and an allergic response. Compared with SK and rtPA, IV dosing of 30 U of APSAC requires less time (2- to 5-minute infusion), and its elimination half-life is much longer (90 minutes).

Table 6-5 ASSET: rtPA & heparin vs. heparin alone for AMI (40)

	rtPA/Heparin (n=2516)	Heparin (n=2495)	*P*
Total mortality	7.2%	9.8%	0.0011
Cardiogenic shock	3.8%	5.1%	<0.05
Stroke	1.1%	1.0%	NS
Reinfarction	3.9%	4.5%	NS
CHF	17.7%	18.4%	NS
Major bleeding	1.4%	0.4%	Not Reported

a. **The APSAC Intervention Mortality Study (AIMS)**—This study was designed as a PRCT of APSAC (30 U IV over 5 minutes) followed by intravenous heparin versus heparin therapy alone for management of patients presenting within 6 hours of onset of AMI (1).
   (1) The trial was terminated early when a planned interim data analysis found that therapy with APSAC was associated with a 47% reduction in mortality after only 30 days of follow-up. Preliminary 1-year mortality data showed a similar trend (see Table 6-6).
   (2) Subgroup analysis showed that the survival benefit of APSAC therapy extended to the elderly and was independent of time from onset of symptoms (0 to 4 hours versus 4 to 6 hours).
   (3) Although hematuria and hemoptysis occurred more frequently in the APSAC group, no excess of gastrointestinal bleeding, hypotension, or strokes was reported. The occurrence of anaphylaxis or purpuric rash in the APSAC group was rare (0.4% and 0.8%, respectively).

4. **Adjunctive Therapy and Comparison of Thrombolytic Agents**—The following sections focus on the role of aspirin, heparin, and Hirudin as adjunctive therapy to thrombolysis for patients with AMI. (See Chapters 3 and 5 for further discussion of the general role of these and other agents such as β-adrenergic receptor antagonists, calcium channel blockers, angiotensin-converting enzyme inhibitors, and nitrates for treatment of AMI.)
   a. **Aspirin**—During acute coronary thrombosis, platelet aggregation may occur in response to the paracrine influences of thromboxane A_2, adenosine diphosphate, and epinephrine. In addition, membrane-bound glycoprotein receptors may allow platelets to adhere directly to exposed fibrin and von Willebrand's substrates at sites of vascular injury. Aspirin is a unique derivative of salicylic acid that irreversibly inhibits the enzymatic function of cyclooxygenase by acetylating its catalytic serine residue. Inhibition of cyclooxygenase by aspirin produces, in a dose-dependent manner, two opposing vascular effects: a reduction in production of platelet thromboxane A_2 (a stimulator of platelet aggregation) and a reduction in production of of endothelial prostacyclin (a potent vasodilator). Compared with the transient effect of aspirin on endothelial prostacyclin production, inhibi-

Table 6-6 AIMS: APSAC & heparin vs. heparin alone for AMI (1)

	APSAC/Heparin (n=502)	Heparin (n=502)	*P*
Mortality—30 d	6.4%	12.2%	0.0016
Mortality—1 y	10.8%	19.4%	0.0006
Hematuria	0%	2.2%	0.001
Hemoptysis	1.4%	0.2%	0.07
Gastrointestinal bleeding	1.4%	1.6%	NS
Hypotension	1.6%	1.4%	NS
Stroke	0.4%	1.0%	NS

tion of platelet thromboxane A_2 is permanent because of the inability of platelets to restore their cyclooxygenase levels. Relatively low doses of aspirin (80 to 325 mg) are used to maximize the desired antiplatelet effect and minimize the unfavorable endothelial effect (41).

(1) ISIS-2 Collaborative Group Study—This large PRCT was designed to extend the encouraging results of GISSI-1 by studying the benefit of adding antiplatelet therapy to SK (23). A total of 17,187 patients were randomly assigned in a 2×2 placebo-controlled manner to receive SK (1.5 million U IV over 60 minutes) alone, aspirin (162 mg PO QD) alone, both, or neither. The entry criteria for ISIS-2 included patients with up to 24 hours of symptoms (median, 5 hours). The length of follow-up was 5 weeks.

(a) SK therapy alone and aspirin therapy alone were associated with a highly significant reduction in the primary end point of vascular death (*i.e.*, death from cardiac, cerebral, hemorrhagic, or other vascular cause). The combination of SK plus aspirin was significantly better than either agent alone; their effects appeared to be additive (see Table 6-7).

(b) The survival benefit of SK alone was greatest in those patients randomly assigned to receive the drug within 4 hours of symptom onset (odds reduction, 35±6%; $P<0.0001$), but was still significant in those who took the drug within 5 to 12 hours (odds reduction, 21±12%; $P=0.04$).

(c) Aspirin therapy alone reduced the incidence of nonfatal reinfarction by 50%. SK therapy alone was associated with a nonsignificant increase in the incidence of reinfarction, which was entirely avoided by the addition of aspirin.

(d) SK therapy alone or in combination with aspirin was associated with a small excess in confirmed intracerebral hemorrhage, all occurring early (days 0 or 1). However, SK therapy was also associated with a significant reduction in total strokes after day 1, so that the overall of risk of stroke for the entire follow-up period was not increased compared to placebo.

(e) The reductions in vascular mortality and all-cause mortality produced by SK and by aspirin remained highly significant ($P<0.001$ for each) after a median of 15 months of follow-up.

(2) A metaanalysis of 32 angiographic trials (19 PRCTs) of thrombolysis with either rtPA or SK in patients with AMI who presented within 6 hours after the onset of symptoms examined the effects of adjunctive therapy with aspirin on coronary reocclusion and recurrent ischemia (35). The studies using angiography assessed coronary artery patency at 90 minutes after initiation of thrombolysis and on predischarge days 8 through 14. Reocclusion was defined as the presence of occluded (TIMI grade 0 or 1) flow on the predischarge angiogram in an IRA that had previously been shown to be patent (TIMI grade 2 or 3) on the initial angiogram. Aspirin therapy was not randomized in any of the studies included in the analysis; all patients received heparin.

(a) Adjunctive therapy with aspirin in the presence of heparin was associated with a significant reduction in the rates of late reocclusion and recurrent ischemia after thrombolysis (see Table 6-8).

(b) The benefit of aspirin was almost identical in patients who received SK and those who received rtPA.

b. Heparin—Adjunctive therapy with heparin has been advocated based on its theoretical ability to reduce thrombin-mediated reocclusion of successfully recanalized coronary arteries. Heparin exerts its major anticoagulant effect by increasing the efficiency of antithrombin III–mediated inhibition of thrombin (factor IIa) and factor Xa, as well as factors IXa, XIa, and XIIa. At the high doses commonly used during coronary angioplasty, heparin

Table 6-7 ISIS-2: SK, aspirin, both, or neither for AMI (23)

	SK (n=8592)	Placebo (n=8595)	*P*	Aspirin (n=8587)	Placebo (n=8600)	*P*	Sk/Aspirin (n=4292)	Placebo (n=4300)	*P*
Vascular deaths	9.2%	12.0%	<0.00001	9.4%	11.8%	<0.0001	8.0%	13.2%	<0.0001
Reinfarction	2.8%	2.4%	NS	1.0%	2.0%	<0.0001	1.8%	2.9%	<0.001
Intracerebral hemorrhage	0.1%	0.0%	<0.01	0.06%	0.02%	NS	0.1%	0.0%	<0.01

Table 6-8 Metaanalysis: aspirin as adjunctive therapy to thrombolysis (35)

	ASA	No ASA	*P*
Reocclusion	11% (n=419)	25% (n=513)	<0.001
Recurrent ischemia	25% (n=2977)	41% (n=721)	<0.001

binds to heparin cofactor II and produces selective thrombin inhibition. High-molecular-weight fractions of heparin have an additional antiplatelet effect. SK therapy also results in a systemic anticoagulation lasting 12 to 24 hours or longer. This effect suggests that an additional benefit from adjunctive antithrombotic therapy may be difficult to demonstrate in patients undergoing thrombolysis with SK.

(1) The Heparin-Aspirin Reperfusion Trial (HART)—This study was designed as a PRCT comparing early IV heparin (5000 U IV bolus, followed by a continuous infusion) versus low-dose oral aspirin (80 mg QD without a loading dose) as adjunctive therapy in patients undergoing thrombolysis with rtPA (22). Patency of the IRA was evaluated by angiography 7 to 24 hours after initiation of thrombolysis and again on day 7.

(a) At the time of the first angiogram, the patency rate of the IRA was significantly higher in patients assigned to heparin therapy. The failure to demonstrate a higher early patency rate in the aspirin-treated group may be related to an inadequate initial dose of aspirin (see Table 6-9).

(b) After 7 days, there was a nonsignificant trend toward a greater patency rate of IRAs with aspirin.

(c) The risks of hemorrhagic events and recurrent ischemia were similar between the two groups.

(2) The European Cooperative Study Group (ECSG-6) Trial—This study was designed as a PRCT comparing early adjunctive heparin therapy (5000 U IV bolus, followed by continuous patency) versus placebo in patients already receiving rtPA (100 mg IV) and full-dose aspirin (250 mg IV or 300 mg oral bolus followed by a 75- to 125-mg oral dose every other day) for management of AMI (11). Patients were eligible if thrombolytic therapy could be started within 6 hours of onset of major symptoms.

(a) IRA patency (TIMI grades 3 or 4), as assessed by angiography 48 to 120 hours after initiation of thrombolytic therapy, was slightly better in the heparin-treated group (83.4% patency versus 74.4%). The relative risk of occlusion of the IRA was 0.66 (95% CI, 0.47 to 0.93) for heparin-treated patients.

(b) Heparin therapy was associated with nonsignificant trends toward smaller enzymatic infarct size and higher incidence of bleeding complications.

(c) Two additional small PRCTs of similar design to the ECSG-6 trial

Table 6-9 HART: Heparin vs. aspirin as adjunctive therapy to thrombolysis (22)

	Heparin (n=106)	ASA (n=99)	*P*
Patency at 7–24 h	82%	52%	<0.0001
Patency at 7 d	88%	95%	NS
Recurrent ischemia	8%	2%	NS
Intracranial hemorrhage	0%	1%	NS

failed to demonstrate any significant difference in IRA patency with adjunctive IV heparin therapy (9,31).

(3) The Studio sulla Calciparina nell'Angina e nella Trombosi Ventricolare nell'Infarto (SCATI) Trial—This study was designed as a PRCT comparing adjuvant heparin (12,500 U SQ BID) versus placebo in patients presenting within 24 hours of the onset of AMI (36). Patients admitted within 6 hours of symptom onset (61%) received SK. No other anticoagulants, aspirin, or other antiplatelet drugs were administered.

(a) Heparin therapy was associated with a barely significant reduction in mortality both in the two overall groups (5.8% versus 10.0%; *P*=0.03) and in the SK subgroups (4.6% versus 8.8%; *P*=0.05).

(b) There were no significant differences in the incidence of recurrent ischemia or nonfatal reinfarction between the two groups. Complications of heparin treatment were rare.

c. Combination Aspirin plus Heparin Adjunctive Therapy and Randomized Comparisons of Thrombolytic Agents—The combined use of full-dose aspirin plus heparin as adjunctive therapy to thrombolysis with various agents has been compared in several large mortality studies with delayed SQ heparin or early IV heparin (33).

(1) Gruppo Italiano per lo Studio della Sopravvivenza nell'Infarto Miocardico (GISSI-2)—This very large multicenter open trial with central randomization and a 2×2 factorial design was conducted to compare SK (1.5 million U IV over 30 to 60 minutes) versus rtPA (100 mg infused over 3 hours) and delayed heparin (12,500 U SQ BID, starting 12 hours after initiation of thrombolysis) versus usual therapy in patients presenting within 6 hours of onset of symptoms (15a). All patients received oral aspirin (300 to 325 mg QD). The length of follow-up was 35 days.

(a) There were no significant differences between the two thrombolytic agents with regard to the combined primary end point of death plus indices of severe LV damage (*i.e.*, clinical congestive heart failure, LV EF ≤35%) (see Table 6-10).

(b) The addition of SQ heparin had no effect on the combined primary end point.

(c) The rates of reinfarction, recurrent ischemia, and stroke were also similar in all groups. However, the incidence of major noncerebral bleeding was significantly higher in the SK and heparin treatment groups.

(d) When the results of GISSI-2 were combined with those of its international extension (The International Study Group) to give a total of 20,891 patients, the trend toward an increased incidence of stoke in the rtPA group reached statistical significance (1.3% versus 0.9%; RR, 1.41, 95% CI, 1.09 to 1.83) (27).

(2) ISIS-3—This very large multicenter open trial with central randomization and a 3×2 factorial design was conducted to compare the efficacy of SK (1.5 million U IV over 60 minutes) versus rtPA (0.60 million U/kg IV over 4 hours) versus APSAC (30 U over 3 minutes), and of SQ heparin for the first 7 days (12,500 U SQ BID starting at 4 hours) versus no heparin in patients presenting up to 24 hours (median, 4 hours) after the onset of suspected AMI (24). All patients received aspirin (162 mg daily), and the first dose was chewed for rapid and full antiplatelet effect. The length of follow-up was 35 days.

(a) There were no significant differences in the primary end point of overall mortality among the three thrombolytic agents (see Table 6-11).

(b) rtPA was associated with a lower incidence of reinfarction.

(c) SK was associated with lower incidences of noncerebral major bleeding, intracerebral hemorrhage, and total stroke.

Table 6-10 GISSI-2: rtPA vs. SK and heparin vs. no heparin for AMI (15a,27)

	rtPA (n=6182)	SK (n=6199)	RR (95% CI)	Heparin (n=6175)	No Heparin (n=6206)	RR (95% CI)
Combined primary end points	23.1%	22.5%	1.04 (0.95–1.13)	22.7%	22.9%	0.99 (0.91–1.08)
Reinfarction	1.9%	2.3%	0.80 (0.63–1.02)	1.9%	2.3%	0.84 (0.66–1.07)
Postinfarction angina	9.3%	10.0%	0.93 (0.82–1.04)	9.3%	10.0%	0.91 (0.81–1.03)
Major bleeding	0.5%	1.0%	0.57 (0.38–0.85)	1.0%	0.6%	1.88 (1.64–2.14)
Total stroke	1.1%	0.9%	1.30 (0.91–1.85)	1.0%	1.0%	0.97 (0.68–1.39)

(d) APSAC was associated with an excess of allergic reactions causing persistent symptoms.
(e) The addition of SQ heparin to full-dose aspirin was associated with slightly fewer deaths in the aspirin plus heparin group than in the aspirin alone group during the scheduled 7 days of heparin therapy. However, this small survival benefit was no longer evident by the end of the follow-up period (see Table 6-12).
(f) As in GISSI-2, the addition of delayed SQ heparin to aspirin was associated with a higher incidence of major noncerebral bleeding. In contrast to GISSI-2, the incidence of definite or probable intracerebral hemorrhage but not total stroke was higher in the heparin-treated group.
(g) The designs of both GISSI-2 and ISIS-3 have been criticized because of the erratic absorption of SQ heparin, the lack of an IV loading dose, and the delay before achieving therapeutic anticoagulation.

(3) **The Global Utilization of Streptokinase and Tissue Plasminogen Activator for Occluded Coronary Arteries (GUSTO-1) Trial**—To address the continued uncertainty about the efficacy of adjunctive heparin therapy in the setting of thrombolysis, this very large multicenter open trial with central randomization was conducted to compare the efficacy of four different thrombolytic strategies in patients presenting within 6 hours of onset of symptoms: SK (1.5 million U IV over 60 minutes) plus SQ heparin (12,500 U BID starting at 4 hours) versus SK plus IV heparin (5000 U IV bolus, followed by a continuous infusion) versus accelerated rtPA (15 mg IV bolus, followed by 1.25 mg/kg IV infusion with two-thirds given in the first 30 minutes and the remainder given over an additional 60 minutes, total dose not to exceed 100 mg) plus IV heparin versus a combination of SK (1 million U IV over 60 minutes) plus rtPA (1.0 mg/kg IV over 60 minutes) plus IV heparin (19). Prior angiographic studies had found excellent rates of

Table 6-11 ISIS-3: Comparison of thrombolytic agents for AMI (24)

	SK (n=13,780)	rtPA (n=13,746)	APSAC (n=13,773)	P (SK vs. rtPA)	*P* (SK vs. APSAC)
Total mortality	10.6%	10.3%	10.5%	NS	NS
Reinfarction	3.5%	2.9%	3.6%	<0.025	NS
Allergy	0.28%	0.09%	0.52%	<0.0005	<0.005
Intracerebral hemorrhage	0.24%	0.66%	0.55%	<0.000005	<0.00005
Total stroke	1.04%	1.39%	1.26%	<0.005	NS
Major bleeding	4.5%	5.2%	5.4%	<0.005	<0.0005

Table 6-12 ISIS-3: Aspirin +/- heparin as adjunctive therapy to thrombolysis (24)

	Aspirin Plus Heparin (n=20,656)	Aspirin Alone (n=20,643)	*P*
Total mortality—7d	7.4%	7.9%	0.03
Total mortality—35d	10.3%	10.6%	NS
Reinfarction	3.2%	3.5%	NS
Intracerebral hemorrhage	0.6%	0.4%	0.03
Total stroke	1.28%	1.18%	NS
Major bleeding	1.0%	0.8%	0.006

IRA patency with the accelerated rtPA regimen (30). The primary end point was 30-day mortality. Because there were no differences in 30-day mortality between the two SK groups (*P*=0.731), their results were combined in the statistical analysis presented here.

(a) Therapy with accelerated rtPA plus IV heparin was associated with a significant reduction in mortality compared with the two SK strategies (10 lives saved per 1000 patients treated; risk reduction, 14%; 95% CI, 5.9 to 21.3; *P*=0.001). Accelerated rtPA plus IV heparin was also superior to combination SK/rtPA plus IV heparin (*P*=0.04); the latter was no better than either of the SK strategies. The lack of a placebo arm for IV heparin still leaves unresolved the question of whether adjunctive IV heparin increases the survival benefit of accelerated rtPA alone (see Table 6-13).

(b) Compared with the SK and the combination strategies, accelerated rtPA plus IV heparin was also associated with reductions in the secondary end points of allergic reaction, anaphylaxis, congestive heart failure, and cardiogenic shock.

(c) Subgroup analysis showed that the benefit of accelerated rtPA plus IV heparin with respect to death or disabling stroke was greatest for patients younger than 75 years of age, for those presenting with anterior AMI, and for those presenting within 4 hours of symptom onset.

d. Recombinant Desulfatohirudin (CGP 39393)—Hirudin is a naturally occurring anticoagulant derived from the leech, *Hirudo medicinalis*. Recombinant desulfatohirudin (referred to as Hirudin herein) is a 65-amino-acid polypeptide that is identical to the natural substance except for the absence of a sulfate group on tyrosine-63. Hirudin is an irreversible inhibitor of all of the major actions of thrombin, including the cleavage of fibrinogen to fibrin, platelet activation, and the activation of thrombin's own positive amplification reactions. In animal models, Hirudin is superior to heparin in inhibiting platelet deposition and thrombus formation. Furthermore, in models of coronary thrombosis, Hirudin has been shown to both speed thrombolysis and prevent reocclusion (8). Although initial phase II trials have reported promising results (4,8,26), subsequent larger studies (GUSTO-2B and the Thrombolysis in Myocardial Infarction 9B Study [TIMI-9B]) have been less encouraging (5,17).

(1) The TIMI-9B trial was a large randomized comparison of IV heparin (5000 U as a bolus, followed by 1000 U/hour) versus IV Hirudin (0.1 mg/kg bolus, followed by 0.1 mg/kg/hour) as adjunctive therapy to thrombolysis. The study included 3002 patients with AMI who were treated with either SK or rtPA at the discretion of the treating physician. Either heparin or Hirudin was started within 60 minutes of thrombolysis and continued for 96 hours with a target activated partial thromboplastin time of 55 to 85 seconds. The primary end point of the study was any of the following events within 30 days: death, severe congestive heart failure, cardiogenic shock, or recurrent AMI. Major bleeding was defined as overt bleeding associated with ≥15% decrease in hematocrit or any intracranial or retroperitoneal bleeding.

(a) The primary end point occurred in 11.9% of patients in the heparin group versus 12.9% of patients in the Hirudin group (*P*=NS). There was a trend toward lower risk of recurrent AMI during hospitalization (OR, 0.65; 95% CI, 0.42 to 1.01), but the difference was not statistically significant (see Table 6-14).

(b) The risk of major bleeding was 5.3% for patients in the heparin group versus 4.6% for patients in the Hirudin group (*P*=NS).

(2) The GUSTO-2B Trial compared IV heparin (5000 U as a bolus, followed by 1000 U/hour infusion for 3 to 5 days) versus IV Hirudin (0.1 mg/kg bolus followed by 0.1 mg/kg/hour infusion for 3 to 5 days)

Table 6-13 GUSTO-1: IV or SQ heparin as adjunctive therapy to thrombolysis (19)

	A SK Plus SQ Heparin (n=9,796)	**B** SK Plus IV Heparin (n=10,377)	**C** rtPA Plus IV Heparin (n=10,344)	**D** SK/rtPA Plus IV Heparin (n=10,328)	**P** (**C** vs. **A+B**)
Total mortality—1d	2.8%	2.9%	2.3%	2.8%	0.005
Total mortality—30d	7.2%	7.4%	6.3%	7.0%	0.001
Death or disabling stroke	7.7%	7.9%	6.9%	7.6%	0.006
Intracerebral hemorrhage	0.49%	0.54%	0.72%	0.94%	0.03
Allergic reaction	5.7%	5.8%	1.6%	5.4%	<0.001
Anaphylaxis	0.7%	0.6%	0.2%	0.6%	<0.001
CHF	17.5%	16.8%	15.2%	16.8%	<0.001
Cardiogenic shock	6.9%	6.3%	5.1%	6.1%	<0.001
Reinfarction	3.4%	4.0%	4.0%	4.0%	NS
Recurrent ischemia	19.9%	19.6%	19.0%	18.8%	NS

among 12,142 patients with acute coronary syndromes; 4131 patients had ST-segment elevation. The target activated partial thromboplastin time was 60 to 85 seconds. Patients with ST-segment elevation were treated with SK or rtPA at the discretion of the attending physician. The primary composite end point was death or nonfatal MI within 30 days. Severe bleeding was defined as intracranial hemorrhage or bleeding that caused hemodynamic compromise requiring intervention. Moderate bleeding was defined as bleeding requiring transfusion but without hemodynamic compromise.

(a) The primary end point occurred in 9.8% of patients in the heparin group and 8.9% of patients in the Hirudin group (*P*=0.06). At 24 hours, the risk of death or MI was 1.3% with Hirudin versus 2.1% with heparin (*P*=0.001) (see Table 6-15).

(b) The risks of serious bleeding complications were similar (1.2% with Hirudin versus 1.1% with heparin; *P*=NS), but the risk of moderate bleeding was somewhat higher with Hirudin (8.8% with Hirudin versus 7.7% with heparin; *P*=0.03).

(c) Therefore, Hirudin may offer small advantage over heparin for patients with acute coronary syndromes (mainly a reduction in the risk of nonfatal AMI). Presence or absence of ST-segment elevation does not influence the benefit derived from Hirudin. The benefit is greatest during the first 24 hours of presentation but dissipates within 30 days.

E. Conclusions

1. For patients presenting with AMI, timely restoration of antegrade blood flow in the IRA can salvage myocardium and reduce morbidity and mortality. Acute reperfusion therapy should be implemented broadly and aggressively to achieve this goal. Patients presenting within 6 to 12 hours after symptom onset and who meet appropriate ECG criteria (ST-segment elevation, new left bundle branch block, or ST-segment depression in leads V_2 through V_4) derive a clear survival benefit from thrombolytic therapy. Whether this benefit extends to patients with more prolonged symptoms remains controversial.
2. Absolute contraindications to thrombolysis include major surgery, trauma, or organ biopsy within 6 weeks; history of hemorrhagic or undefined stroke; his-

Table 6-14 TIMI-9B: Hirudin vs. heparin as adjunctive therapy to thrombolysis (17)

	Heparin (n=1491)	Hirudin (n=1511)	*P*
Death	5.1%	6.1%	NS
Primary end point	11.9%	12.9%	NS
Need for any revascularization procedure	39.0%	40.5%	NS
Major bleeding	5.3%	4.6%	NS

Table 6-15 GUSTO-2B: Hirudin vs. heparin for acute coronary syndrome (5)

	Heparin (n=6073)	Hirudin (n=6069)	*P*
Death	4.7%	4.5%	NS
Primary end point among all patients	9.8%	8.9%	0.06
Primary end point among patients with ST elevation	11.3%	9.9%	NS
Primary end point among patients without ST elevation	9.1%	8.3%	NS
Risk of severe bleeding	1.1%	1.2%	NS
Risk of moderate bleeding	7.7%	8.8%	0.03

tory of intracranial tumor, prior neurosurgery, or recent head trauma; melena or marked hematuria; and history of bleeding diathesis. Relative contraindications to thrombolysis include ≥10 minutes of chest compressions; severe hypertension; cardiogenic shock; remote stroke or recent transient ischemic attack; occult fecal blood; and concurrent warfarin therapy. Advanced age, when considered alone, should not be an absolute contraindication to thrombolysis.

3. Each of the thrombolytic agents studied (SK, rtPA, and APSAC) has convincingly been shown to confer significant reductions in infarct-related morbidity and mortality. In general, most studies have found no significant differences between these various agents with respect to survival when administered with full-dose aspirin. The one exception is GUSTO-1, the results of which suggest that the thrombolytic strategy of accelerated rtPA plus IV heparin added to full-dose aspirin is superior to comparable SK strategies, especially for patients younger than 75 years of age, for those presenting with anterior AMI, and for those presenting within 4 hours of symptom onset. However, this additional survival benefit must be weighed against the higher risk of intracerebral hemorrhage associated with the accelerated rtPA strategy.
4. The ISIS-2 study clearly established a beneficial and independent effect of aspirin therapy on survival and on nonfatal reinfarction that was additive to the beneficial effect of SK therapy. Full-dose aspirin therapy (160 to 325 mg QD, first dose chewed and swallowed) should be administered as standard adjunctive therapy in all patients undergoing thrombolysis.
5. The role of IV heparin as an adjunct to thrombolysis has not completely been resolved despite the large numbers of patients studied in the GISSI-2, ISIS-3, and GUSTO-1 trials. There are no data to support an additional benefit of heparin in patients receiving SK or APSAC plus full-dose aspirin. For standard rtPA, IV heparin added to full-dose aspirin appears to provide a small additional benefit in terms of improved patency of the IRA. However, this additional benefit must be weighed against the higher risk of major bleeding associated with IV heparin and the higher risk of stroke with rtPA. Although GUSTO-1 demonstrated that a further reduction in mortality could be achieved with the thrombolytic strategy of accelerated rtPA plus IV heparin added to full-dose aspirin, the absence of a placebo arm for IV heparin therapy has left open the possibility that the additional survival benefit was independent of IV heparin. The ongoing First American Study of Infarct Survival (ASIS-1) will attempt to assess the independent benefit of IV heparin in patients receiving full-dose aspirin but not thrombolytic therapy for the management of AMI.
6. In the TIMI-9B study, Hirudin was similar to heparin in efficacy as an adjunct to thrombolytic therapy. In the GUSTO-2b study, Hirudin offered only a small benefit over heparin for acute coronary syndromes. The risk of bleeding appears to be similar with either agent. The precise role of Hirudin for treatment of AMI remains to be further defined.

Abbreviations used in Chapter 6

AMI = acute myocardial infarction
APSAC = anisoylated plasminogen streptokinase activator complex
ASA = aspirin
BID = twice daily
CHF = congestive heart failure
CI = confidence interval
DBP = diastolic blood pressure
ECG = electrocardiographic
IRA = infarct-related artery
IV = intravenous
LV = left ventricular

LVEDV = left ventricular end-diastolic volume
LV EF = left ventricular ejection fraction
LVESVI = left ventricular end-systolic volume index
N = number of patients in population
n = number of patients in sample
NRMI = National Registry of Myocardial Infarction
NS = not significant
OR = odds ratio
P = probability value
PRCT = prospective randomized controlled trial
PTCA = percutaneous transluminal coronary angioplasty
RR = relative risk
rtPA = recombinant tissue plasminogen activator
SBP = systolic blood pressure
SK = streptokinase
SQ = subcutaneous

References

1. AIMS Trial Study Group. Effect of intravenous APSAC on mortality after acute myocardial infarction: preliminary report of a placebo-controlled clinical trial. *Lancet* 1988;i:545.
2. American Heart Association. *1992 Heart and Strokes Facts.* American Heart Association, 1992, Dallas, TX.
3. Anderson. Current concepts: thrombolysis in acute myocardial infarction. *N Engl J Med* 1993;329:703.
4. Antman. Hirudin in acute myocardial infarction; safety report from the thrombolysis and Thrombin Inhibition in Myocardial Infarction (TIMI) 9A trial. *Circulation* 1994;90:1624.
5. Antman. Hirudin in acute myocardial infarction: thrombolysis and Thrombin Inhibition in Myocardial Infarction (TIMI) 9B trial. *Circulation* 1996;94:911.
6. Bates. Limitations of thrombolytic therapy for acute myocardial infarction complicated by congestive heart failure and cardiogenic shock. *J Am Coll Cardiol* 1991; 18:1077.
7. Becker. Cardiac rupture with thrombolytic therapy: impact of time to treatment in the Late Assessment of Thrombolytic Efficacy study. *J Am Coll Cardiol* 1995;25:1063.
8. Cannon. A pilot trial of recombinant desulfatohirudin compared with heparin in conjunction with tissue-type plasminogen activator and aspirin for acute myocardial infarction: results of the Thrombolysis in Myocardial Infarction (TIMI) 5 trial. *J Am Coll Cardiol* 1993;23:993.
9. Col. Infusion of heparin conjunct to streptokinase accelerates reperfusion of acute myocardial infarction: results of a double-blind randomized study (OSIRIS). *Circulation* 1992;86:I-259.
10. Collen. Towards improved thrombolytic therapy. *Lancet* 1993;342:34.
11. de Bono. Effect of early intravenous heparin on coronary patency, infarct size, and bleeding complications after alteplase thrombolysis: results of a randomised double blind European Cooperative Study Group trial. *Br Heart J* 1992;67:122.
12. DeWood. Prevalence of total coronary occlusion during the early hours of transmural myocardial infarction. *N Engl J Med* 1980;303:897.
13. Fibrinolytic Therapy Trialists (FTT) Collaborative Group. Indications for fibrinolytic therapy in suspected acute myocardial infarction: collaborative overview of early mortality and major morbidity results from all randomised trials of more than 1000 patients. *Lancet* 1994;343:311.
14. Fuster. The pathogenesis of coronary artery disease and the acute coronary syndrome. *N Engl J Med* 1992;326:242.
15. GISSI. Effectiveness of intravenous thrombolytic treatment in acute myocardial infarction. *Lancet* 1986;i:397.

15a. GISSI. A factorial randomised trial of alteplase versus streptokinase and heparin

versus no heparin among 12,490 patients with acute myocardial infarction. *Lancet* 1990;336:65.
16. GISSI. Long-term effects of intravenous thrombolysis in acute myocardial infarction: final report of the GISSI study. *Lancet* 1987;ii:871.
17. Global Use of Strategies to Open Occluded Coronary Arteries (GUSTO) IIb Investigators. A comparison of recombinant Hirudin with heparin for the treatment of acute coronary syndromes. *N Engl J Med* 1996;335:775.
18. GUSTO Angiographic Investigators. The effects of tissue plasminogen activator, streptokinase, or both on coronary-artery patency, ventricular function, and survival after acute myocardial infarction. *N Engl J Med* 1993;329:1615.
19. GUSTO Investigators. An international randomized trial comparing four thrombolytic strategies for acute myocardial infarction. *N Engl J Med* 1993;329:673.
20. Hackett. Intermittent coronary occlusion in acute myocardial infarction. *N Engl J Med* 1987;317:1055.
21. Honan. Cardiac rupture, mortality and the timing of thrombolytic therapy: a meta-analysis. *J Am Coll Cardiol* 1990;16:359.
22. Hsia. A comparison between heparin and low-dose aspirin as adjunctive therapy with tissue plasminogen activator for acute myocardial infarction. *N Engl J Med* 1990;323:1433.
23. ISIS-2. Randomized trial of intravenous streptokinase, oral aspirin, both, or neither among 17,187 cases of suspected acute myocardial infarction: ISIS-2. *Lancet* 1988;ii:349.
24. ISIS-3 (Third International Study of Infarct Survival) Collaborative Group. ISIS-3: a randomised comparison of streptokinase vs. tissue plasminogen activator vs. anistreplase and of aspirin plus heparin vs. aspirin alone among 41,299 cases of suspected acute myocardial infarction. *Lancet* 1992;339:753.
25. Krumholz. Cost effectiveness of thrombolytic therapy with streptokinase in elderly patients with suspected acute myocardial infarction. *N Engl J Med* 1992;327:7.
26. Lee. Initial experience with Hirudin and streptokinase in acute myocardial infarction: results of the Thrombolysis in Myocardial Infarction (TIMI) 6 trial. *Am J Cardiol* 1995;75:7.
27. Maggioni. The risk of stroke in patients with acute myocardial infarction after thrombolytic and antithrombotic treatment. *N Engl J Med* 1992;327:1.
28. McKay. Left ventricular remodeling after myocardial infarction: a corollary to infarct expansion. *Circulation* 1986;74:693.
29. Muller. Selection of patients with acute myocardial infarction for thrombolytic therapy. *Ann Intern Med* 1990;113:949.
30. Neuhaus. Improved thrombolysis with a modified dose regimen of recombinant tissue-type plasminogen activator. *J Am Coll Cardiol* 1989;14:1566.
31. O'Conner. *Duke University Clinical Cardiology Studies (DUCCS-1). Circulation* 1992;86:I–48.
32. Pfeffer. Effect of captopril on progressive ventricular dilatation after anterior myocardial infarction. *N Engl J Med* 1988;319:80.
33. Ridker. Are both aspirin and heparin justified as adjuncts to thrombolytic therapy for acute myocardial infarction. *Lancet* 1993;341:1574.
34. Rogers. Treatment of myocardial infarction in the United States (1990–1993). *Circulation* 1994;90:2103.
35. Roux. Effects of aspirin on coronary reocclusion and recurrent ischemia after thrombolysis: a meta-analysis. *J Am Coll Cardiol* 1992;19:671.
36. SCATI Group. Randomised controlled trial of subcutaneous calcium-heparin in acute myocardial infarction. *Lancet* 1989;ii:182.
37. Topol. A randomized trial of late reperfusion therapy for acute myocardial infarction. *Circulation* 1992;85:2090.
38. Topol. Thrombolytic therapy for elderly patients. *N Engl J Med* 1992;327:7.
39. Weaver. Time to thrombolytic treatment: factors affecting delay and their influence on outcome. *J Am Coll Cardiol* 1995;25(Suppl):3S.
40. Wilcox. Trial of tissue plasminogen activator for mortality reduction in acute myocardial infarction: Anglo-Scandinavian Study of Early Thrombolysis (ASSET). *Lancet* 1988;ii:525.
41. Willard. The use of aspirin in ischemic heart disease. *N Engl J Med* 1992;327:175.

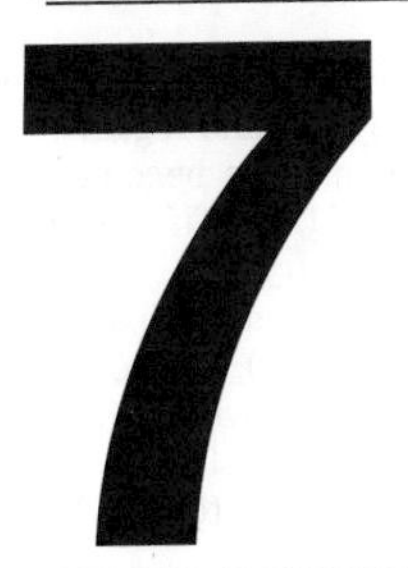

Percutaneous Transluminal Coronary Angioplasty

Marc L. Boom and
Patrick T. O'Gara

A. Introduction

1. Since the first use of percutaneous transluminal coronary angioplasty (PTCA) by Grüntzig in 1977, PTCA has become an increasingly common procedure (34). A number of large trials have recently been completed or are currently underway to examine the role of PTCA for chronic stable angina pectoris (CSAP), unstable angina pectoris (UA), or acute myocardial infarction (AMI).
2. This chapter examines the data supporting or refuting the use of PTCA for patients with CSAP, UA, or AMI. The reader is directed to the 1994 review by Landau for discussion of the technical aspects of the procedure and issues regarding the management of long-term complications (45).

B. PTCA for Patients With Chronic Stable Angina Pectoris

B. PTCA for Patients With Chronic Stable Angina Pectoris—The studies that have examined the role of PTCA for CSAP can be divided into observational studies, randomized comparisons of angioplasty versus medical treatment, and randomized comparisons of angioplasty versus coronary artery bypass graft surgery (CABG).

1. Observational Studies on PTCA for CSAP

a. In 1987, the long-term follow-up results of Grüntzig's first 169 patients treated with PTCA were reported posthumously (33). To be treated with angioplasty, patients had to have symptoms compatible with angina pectoris (100%), objective evidence of ischemia on exercise stress testing (97%), and proximal stenosis of short length at cardiac catheterization. Significant stenosis was defined as ≥50% reduction in the diameter of a coronary artery. Using these criteria, 98 patients with single-vessel disease and 71 patients with multivessel disease were selected. Nineteen of the patients had had previous CABG. The procedure was deemed technically successful if the narrowing was reduced by ≥20% and the final stenosis was ≤50%.

- **(1)** The procedure was technically successful in 79% of the patients. Of those, 67% were asymptomatic at a mean follow-up of 6 years. Although 97% had a positive stress test before the procedure, only 10% of those with a technically successful procedure had a positive stress test afterward.
- **(2)** Recurrent stenoses occurred in 30% of the patients, most within 6 months of the procedure. In addition, 15% of patients who had a late follow-up angiogram had restenosis between 6 months and 7 years after angioplasty.
- **(3)** Seventy-four percent of patients with a technically successful procedure were managed without surgery. However, 20% of these patients required repeat angioplasty.
- **(4)** All but two of the patients with multivessel disease had angioplasty of the culprit lesion only. Patients with multivessel disease experienced a lower primary success rate, a higher rate of death from cardiac causes, a higher rate of need for CABG, a higher rate of symptom recurrence, and a higher percentage of positive stress tests after the procedure.

b. The National Heart, Lung, and Blood Institute (NHLBI), which also coordinated the Coronary Artery Surgery Study (CASS) trial and registry, assembled a registry of patients treated with PTCA that has become another source of early observational data about PTCA (14,40). The NHLBI compared its 1977–1981 registry with its 1985–1986 registry.

(1) The 1985–1986 registry patients were older and more likely to have had multivessel disease (53% versus 25%; $P<0.001$), ejection fractions (EFs) less than 50% (19% versus 8%; $P<0.001$), previous MI (37% versus 21%; $P<0.001$), and previous CABG (13% versus 9%; $P<0.01$). The more recent registry patients were also more likely to have had complex coronary lesions.

(2) Despite these differences, the in-hospital outcome of the 1985–1986 group was better, with an angiographic success rate of 88%, compared with 67% for the earlier group ($P<0.001$). In-hospital mortality rates were similar for both cohorts at 1%, as were the rates of nonfatal MI.

2. Angioplasty Versus Medical Treatment for CSAP—The ACME (Angioplasty Compared to Medicine) trial was designed as a prospective randomized controlled trial (PRCT) of angioplasty versus medical therapy for treatment of single-vessel coronary artery disease (CAD). Only 4% (212 patients) of those who underwent angiography participated in the randomized study. The follow-up interval was 6 months, at which time all patients had a follow-up exercise tolerance treadmill test (ETT) and angiography (57).

a. Among the 100 patients treated with angioplasty, the technical success rate was 80%, with a reduction in mean percentage of stenosis from 76% to 36%.

b. At 6 months, patients in the PTCA group were more likely to be free of angina (64% versus 46%; $P<0.01$), better able to increase the total duration of exercise (2.1 versus 0.5 minutes; $P<0.0001$), and able to exercise longer without angina ($P<0.01$). In addition, patients in the PTCA group had a greater reduction in the frequency of anginal attacks (15 versus 7 fewer per month; $P=0.06$) and a larger improvement in the psychological well-being score ($P=0.03$). They also had a decreased need for nitrates, β-blockers, and calcium channel blockers ($P<0.01$ for each).

c. Complications of PTCA included 2 patients who required emergency CABG and 4 patients who had an AMI. In addition, 19 repeat PTCA procedures were performed in 16 patients, 5 additional patients required CABG, and 1 more patient had an MI during the 6-month follow-up period. None of the patients assigned to medical therapy required CABG, but 11 underwent PTCA. Three patients had MIs, and 1 patient died after PTCA. The difference in the rate of CABG was statistically significant ($P<0.01$), but the differences in the MI and the death rates were not.

d. Conclusions

(1) The efficacy of PTCA was comparable to that observed in the randomized CASS trial for surgical treatment of single-vessel disease. The percentage of PTCA-treated patients who were free of angina increased from 9% at baseline to 64% at the end of 6 months. In the CASS trial, the percentage of surgically treated patients who were free of angina increased from 20% at baseline to 55% at 1 year (13).

(2) PTCA is associated with a small initial increased risk of MI and emergency CABG. There is also a risk of restenosis requiring repeat angioplasty. Because survival is not improved by CABG in patients with single-vessel disease (according to data from the CASS trial), the authors concluded that the benefits of PTCA (including increased relief of symptoms, improved exercise tolerance, and decreased reliance on antianginal medications) must be weighed against the risks of the procedure (increased initial cost, increased initial risk of MI or need for emergency CABG, and need for repeat angioplasty).

3. Angioplasty Versus CABG for CSAP—A number of randomized trials comparing PTCA versus CABG in patients with stable angina (either single-vessel or multivessel CAD) are ongoing. Some of the studies have reached their primary end point; others have released only preliminary data. The major trials are listed in Table 7–1.

a. The Randomized Intervention Treatment of Angina (RITA) trial was designed as a 5-year PRCT of PTCA versus CABG for treatment of single or multivessel CAD. In 1993, preliminary results at a mean follow-up of 2.5 years were released (58). Only 3% (1011 patients) of those who were screened were enrolled in the study. Patients with angiographically proven CAD were screened for the trial if revascularization was thought to be necessary and if the investigators agreed that equivalent revascularization was possible with either CABG or PTCA. Exclusion criteria included left main CAD, previous PTCA or CABG, hemodynamically significant valve disease, and significant noncardiac disease deemed likely to limit long-term prognosis. The primary end point was defined as the combined 5-year incidence of death and MI. Secondary end points included the need for repeat PTCA or CABG, other major cardiovascular events (unstable angina, cardiac failure, arrhythmia, and stroke), Canadian Cardiovascular Society Classification (CCSC) of angina, physical activity level, breathlessness, ETT results, and left ventricular function. At baseline, 45% of the patients had single-vessel disease, 43% had two-vessel disease, and 12% had three-vessel disease. Results are summarized in Table 7–2.

(1) Angioplasty was deemed successful for 87% of the vessels. A successful dilation of all attempted vessels was possible for 81% of patients.

(2) There was no difference in the combined incidence of death or AMI (primary end point) between the two groups. There was also no significant difference in the incidence of stroke, the severity of breathlessness, the level of physical activity at 2 years, the degree of improvement in exercise testing, the EF, or the employment status.

(3) However, angioplasty patients were more likely to require repeat procedures, to have angina, and to require antianginal therapy at all points in the follow-up. CABG patients had a longer hospital stay, were more debilitated at 1 month, and were more likely to suffer cardiac failure or arrhythmia.

(4) In-hospital complications included a 4.5% incidence of emergency CABG in the PTCA group; the CABG group had a 0.6% risk of pulmonary embolism and a 4.9% incidence of wound-related complications. The incidence of unstable angina was greater with PTCA (2.7% versus 0%) but arrhythmia was more common with CABG (7.4% versus 1.4%).

(5) **Conclusions**—There was no significant difference in the combined risk of death or AMI between the two groups. However, CABG patients were more likely to be free of angina, less likely to require antianginal medications, and less likely to require subsequent PTCA or CABG. These advantages of CABG are balanced by a longer hospital

Table 7-1 Major Randomized Trials Comparing PTCA with CABG for CSAP

Trial	Acronym
Bypass angioplasty revascularization investigation	BARI
Coronary artery bypass revascularization intervention	CABRI
Emory angioplasty vs. surgery trial	EAST
Argentine randomized trial of coronary angioplasty vs. bypass surgery in multiple vessel disease	ERACI
German angioplasty bypass investigation	GABI
Randomized intervention treatment of angina	RITA

Table 7-2 RITA: CABG vs. PTCA for Single or Multivessel CAD (58)

	CABG	PTCA	*P*
Primary End Points	**8.6%**	**9.8%**	**0.47**
Death	3.6%	3.1%	—
Nonfatal MI	5.2%	6.7%	—
Secondary End Points			
Need for subsequent procedure			
Repeat arteriogram	7%	31%	<0.001
CABG	0.8%	19%	—
PTCA	4.2%	18%	—
Combined death, MI, CABG, or PTCA at 2 y	11%	38%	<0.001
Major cardiovascular events			
Unstable angina	1.0%	11.2%	—
Arrhythmia	10.0%	3.1%	—
Cardiac failure	4.4%	2.0%	—
Stroke	2.0%	1.8%	—
Angina			
6 mo	11%	31.6%	<0.001
2 y	21.5%	31.3%	0.007
Breathlessness (35% before treatment)	11%	11%	—
Physical activity (% moderate to vigorous)			
1 mo	38%	52%	—
1 y	65%	65%	—
Exercise testing (mean increase in exercise time)			
1 mo	1.6%	2.4%	0.0002
1 y	~3.4 min	~2.8 min	—
Ejection fraction (% change at 6 mo)	−0.1%	+0.3%	—
Other End Points			
Receiving antianginal drugs at 2 y	34%	61%	—
% unemployed at 2 y (47% at baseline)	23%	25%	—
Length of hospital stay	12 d	4 d	—

stay, a greater degree of short-term disability, and a higher risk of cardiac failure or arrhythmia.

b. The Emory Angioplasty versus Surgery Trial (EAST) was designed as a 3-year PRCT comparing PTCA versus CABG for treatment of multivessel CAD (41). Any patient with multivessel CAD who had not previously had PTCA or CABG was eligible. Only 16.5% of those screened were eligible, and only 7.7% (392 patients) agreed to participate. Exclusion criteria included angiographic factors (chronic occlusions of bypassable vessels lasting ≥8 weeks, ≥30% left main artery stenosis, more than two total occlusions, and EF ≤25%) and clinical factors (insufficient myocardium at risk to warrant CABG, AMI within 5 days, insufficient symptoms to warrant an invasive procedure, and the presence of a noncardiac illness threatening survival). The primary end point of the study was a composite end point consisting of death, Q-wave MI, and a large zone of ischemia on thallium ETT at 3 years (≥33% of the territory of the left anterior descending artery or ≥50% of the territory of the right coronary or left circumflex artery). Secondary end points included the degree of revascularization at 1 and 3 years, ventricular function, exercise performance, the need for subsequent PTCA or CABG, the quality of life, and overall cost. At baseline, 60% of patients had two-vessel disease, 40% had three-vessel disease, 72% had proximal left anterior descending artery disease, average EF was 61%, and 80% had CCSC III or IV angina. Results are summarized in Table 7–3.

(1) Angioplasty was deemed successful for 88% of vessels. A successful dilation of all attempted vessels was possible for 77% of patients.

(2) There was no significant difference in the primary end point between the two groups. There was also no difference between the two groups in terms of the incidence of stroke, the level of physical activity at 2 years, the EF, or the employment status.

(3) CABG patients were less likely to have angina, require antianginal therapy, or require subsequent procedures; more than half of the PTCA patients (54%) required subsequent CABG and/or repeat PTCA. In addition, CABG patients were more likely to be completely revascularized at all time points.

(4) There were more Q-wave MIs in the CABG group initially. However, by 3 years, there was no significant difference in the incidence of Q-wave MIs between the two groups. In addition, the higher incidence of Q-wave MIs in the CABG group did not significantly affect ventricular function.

(5) **Conclusions**—There was no significant difference in the primary end point (combined risk of death, Q-wave MI, or presence of a large ischemic defect) between the two groups. However, as in the RITA trial, CABG patients were more likely to be free of angina, less likely to require antianginal medications, and less likely to require subsequent PTCA or CABG.

c. The German Angioplasty Bypass Investigation (GABI) was designed as a 1-year PRCT of CABG versus PTCA for management of symptomatic multivessel CAD (36). Patients younger than 75 years of age with symptomatic multivessel CAD who had not had previous PTCA or CABG were eligible. Patients were highly selected, with only 4% (359 patients) of those screened participating in the trial. Revascularization of at least two major

Table 7-3 EAST: CABG vs. PTCA for Multivessel CAD (41)

	CABG	PTCA	*P*
Primary End Points	**27.3%**	**28.8%**	**0.81**
Death	6.2%	7.1%	0.72
Q-wave MI	19.6%	14.6%	0.21
Large ischemic defect on thallium	5.7%	9.6%	0.17
Secondary End Points			
% of Index segments revascularized			
Initial	99.1%	75.1%	<0.001
1 y	88.1%	58.8%	<0.001
3 y	86.7%	69.9%	<0.001
% with ≥80% of index segments revascularized			
Initial	99.0%	55.6%	<0.001
1 y	78.8%	36.1%	<0.001
3 y	75.3%	50.7%	<0.001
Ejection fraction	69%	69%	—
Need for subsequent procedure			
CABG	1%	22%	<0.001
PTCA	13%	41%	<0.001
CABG or PTCA	13%	54%	<0.001
Other End Points			
Class II, III, or IV angina	12%	20%	0.039
Need for antianginal medicine	51%	66%	0.005
Activity level moderate to strenuous	44.5%	47.0%	0.63
Employment status	38.5%	36.5%	0.89

coronary arteries supplying different myocardial regions had to be deemed clinically necessary and technically feasible. Exclusion criteria included total occlusion of a vessel, >30% left main CAD or left main equivalent lesions, more than 50% of the ventricular wall in jeopardy from disease of one vessel, lesion ≥2 cm in length, diffuse peripheral CAD, aneurysm, and AMI within the previous 4 weeks. The primary end point of the study was freedom from angina (<CCSC II) at 1 year after the intervention. Secondary end points included the combined incidence of death and AMI, procedure-related complications, and the need for further interventions. Results are summarized in Table 7–4.

(1) Angioplasty was successful for 92% of treated lesions. Complete revascularization was achieved for 86% of PTCA-treated patients.

(2) Initially, at 3 months, CABG patients were more likely to be free of angina (84% versus 60%; $P<0.001$). However, by 1 year, there was no significant difference between the two groups (74% versus 71%; probability value not given).

(3) As in the RITA and the EAST trials, PTCA-treated patients were much more likely to require repeat PTCA or CABG compared with CABG patients (44% versus 6%; $P<0.001$).

(4) On repeat angiography at 6 months, 13% of the vein grafts and 7% of internal mammary artery grafts did not function in the CABG group. In the PTCA group, 16% of the revascularized vessels were occluded or markedly stenosed.

(5) In-Hospital Complications and Adverse Events—CABG patients were more likely to suffer an acute Q-wave MI or develop pneumonia. PTCA patients were more likely to require an urgent CABG or repeat PTCA. The risks of death, pulmonary emboli, or stroke were similar (see Table 7–5).

(6) Conclusions—At 1 year, PTCA and CABG were equally effective in relieving angina. PTCA patients were more likely to require repeat PTCA or CABG, whereas CABG patients were more likely to suffer an AMI at the time of the procedure and to require a longer hospitalization.

d. The Bypass Angioplasty Revascularization Investigation (BARI) study was a 5-year PRCT that tested the hypothesis that initial therapy with PTCA was comparable to CABG for management of patients with multivessel CAD (9). Patients with angiographically proven multivessel CAD, sufficiently severe angina or objective evidence of ischemia, and lesions deemed technically suitable for revascularization by either procedure were enrolled. Exclusion criteria included left main or diffuse CAD, UA or AMI

Table 7-4 GABI: CABG vs. PTCA for Symptomatic Multivessel CAD (36)

	CABG	PTCA	*P*
Primary End Point			
Free of angina (CCS class<II) at 3 mo	84%	60%	<0.001
Free of angina (CCS class<II) at 12 mo	74%	71%	—
Secondary End Points			
Death of AMI	13.6%	6.0%	0.017
Need for further interventions			
CABG	1%	21%	<0.001
PTCA	5%	26%	<0.001
CABG or PTCA	6%	44%	<0.001
Other End Points			
Median hospital stay	19 d	5 d	—
Use of antianginal agents	78%	88%	0.041

Table 7-5 GABI: In-Hospital Complications

Complication/Event	CABG	PTCA	*P*
Death	2.5%	1.1%	0.431
Acute Q-wave MI	8.1%	2.3%	0.022
Need for urgent repeat PTCA	0.6%	2.8%	0.217
Need for urgent CABG	1.2%	8.5%	0.002
Stroke	1.2%	0%	0.227
Pulmonary embolism	0.6%	0%	0.477
Pneumonia	10.6%	1.1%	<0.001

Modified with permission from Hamm (36).

requiring emergency revascularization, and noncardiac illness expected to limit survival. Only 7.3% (1929 patients) of those who were screened participated in the randomized study. The primary end points were cumulative survival and survival free of Q-wave MI at 5 years. Secondary end points included outcome during hospitalization, cumulative rate of Q-wave MI at 5 years, need for subsequent revascularization, and survival in selected subgroups. At baseline, there were an average of 3.5 clinically significant coronary lesions per patient, and the mean left ventricular EF was 57%; 41% had triple-vessel disease and 30% had UA. Results are summarized in Table 7–5.

(1) In the 892 patients who underwent CABG as assigned, an average of 3.1 coronary arteries were bypassed; all intended vessels were grafted in 91% of patients. Among the 904 patients who underwent PTCA as assigned, an average of 1.9 of 3.5 clinically important lesions were successfully dilated (54%).

(2) There was no statistically significant difference in the rates of cumulative survival or survival free of Q-wave MI between the treatment groups. However, the difference in cumulative survival between the two groups was 2.9%, with a 95% CI of −0.2% to 6.0%, so it is possible that the survival rate with CABG may actually be superior by as much as 6% (65).

(3) Patients who underwent CABG had more frequent in-hospital Q-wave MIs and longer hospital stays; those who underwent PTCA had a greater need for repeat procedures both during the index hospitalization and at 5 years.

(4) Subgroup analysis of patients with CSAP, UA, two-vessel CAD, or three-vessel CAD at baseline did not demonstrate any statistically significant differences in survival between the CABG and PTCA groups. However, among diabetic patients who were being treated with insulin or oral hypoglycemic agents at baseline, the 5-year survival rate was significantly better for the CABG group than for the PTCA group.

(5) **Conclusions**—This large and well-conducted PRCT failed to establish with certainty that an initial strategy of PTCA is equivalent to CABG in patients with multivessel CAD and clinically severe angina (both CSAP and UAP) or objective evidence of ischemia. However, although CABG may be considered the established therapy for this patient group, PTCA appears to be an acceptable alternative. As in the GABI, RITA, and EAST trials, patients in the CABG group were more likely to suffer an acute Q-wave MI at the time of the procedure and to require longer hospitalizations, and patients in the PTCA group were more likely to require repeat revascularization. Subgroup analysis suggested that survival at 5 years was greater for treated diabetics managed with the initial CABG strategy.

e. Conclusions Regarding PTCA for Patients with CSAP

(1) For clinical situations in which CABG appears to have proven survival advantage compared with medical therapy (*i.e.*, triple-vessel CAD,

Table 7-6 BARI: CABG vs. PTCA for Multivessel CAD (9)

	CABG	PTCA	*P*
Primary End Point			
Survival	89.3%	86.3%	0.19
Survival free of Q-wave MI	80.4%	78.7%	0.84
Secondary End Points			
Outcome during index hospitalization			
Death	1.3%	1.1%	—
Q-wave MI	4.6%	2.1%	<0.004
Death or Q-wave MI	5.8%	3.0%	<0.01
Emergency CABG	0.1%	6.3%	<0.001
Emergency PTCA	0%	2.1%	<0.001
Stroke	0.8%	0.2%	—
Median hospital stay after treatment	7 d	3 d	<0.001
Q-wave MI	11.7%	10.9%	0.45
Need for subsequent procedure	8%	54%	—
PTCA	7%	23%	—
CABG	1%	31%	—
CABG or PTCA	—	11%	—
Multiple revascularizations	3%	19%	—
Subgroup Analysis			
Survival			
Stable angina (CCS class 3 or 4)	91%	85.5%	—
Unstable angina or non–Q-wave MI	88.8%	86.1%	—
Double-vessel CAD	89.7%	87.6%	—
Triple-vessel CAD	88.6%	84.7%	—
History of diabetes			
None or not treated	91.4%	91.1%	—
Treated	80.6%	65.5%	0.003

left main CAD, low EF), CABG should be the procedure of choice. In selected patients with multivessel disease (preserved EF, no left main CAD, no diabetes), PTCA appears to be an acceptable alternative to CABG. In other situations in which CABG does not appear to improve survival (*i.e.*, one- or two-vessel disease) but a revascularization procedure is deemed necessary, patient preference should guide the choice between PTCA and CABG, carefully weighing the risks and benefits of each procedure.

(2) PTCA and CABG are both effective in relieving anginal symptoms. Some studies found that patients treated with CABG were more likely to be free of angina and less likely to require antianginal medications. Other studies found the two procedures to be equally effective in relieving anginal symptoms at 1 year.

(3) Patients treated with PTCA are more likely to require repeat PTCA or subsequent CABG. Patients treated with CABG are more likely to suffer an AMI after the procedure and to require a longer hospital stay.

C. PTCA for Patients With Unstable Angina Pectoris—Three large PRCTs have examined the role of PTCA for management of patients with UA.

1. The Thrombolysis in Myocardial Ischemia (TIMI) IIIB study was a 1-year PRCT that randomly assigned patients in a 2 × 2 factorial design to receive tissue plasminogen activator (tPA) versus placebo and an early invasive strategy (early coronary arteriography followed by revascularization if the anatomy is suitable) versus an early conservative strategy (early coronary arteriography followed by revascularization if initial medical therapy fails) (67). All patients were treated with bed rest, antiischemic medications, aspirin, and heparin. Patients in the early invasive strategy underwent PTCA of single or multiple vessels at the time of angiography or as soon as possible. CABG was reserved for patients who had significant left main CAD or triple-vessel disease plus depressed left ventricular function; CABG was also used for patients with recurrent UA who were not suitable candidates for PTCA or in whom PTCA had failed. The study randomly assigned 1473 patients between the ages of 21 to 76 years who had 5 minutes to 6 hours of rest angina within 24 hours of enrollment that was thought to be caused by UA or non–Q-wave MI. Exclusion criteria included AMI within the preceding 21 days, coronary arteriography within the preceding 30 days, PTCA within the preceding 6 months, prior CABG, presence of pulmonary edema, and coexistent severe illness. The primary end point was death, postrandomization nonfatal MI, or an unsatisfactory symptom-limited ETT at 6 weeks. Secondary end points included length of initial hospitalization, rate of rehospitalization by 6 weeks, number of days of rehospitalization, need for antianginal medication, and severity of angina (CCSC level). After 6 weeks, patients were managed entirely at the discretion of their treating physicians, and follow-up contacts were made at 1 year to determine their long-term outcome. Results are summarized in Tables 7–7 and 7–8.

a. Overall, patients with UA or non–Q-wave MI had low mortality and reinfarction rates at 6 weeks, with no difference in the primary end point between the early invasive versus early conservative strategies.

b. The early invasive strategy significantly reduced the length of hospitalization as well as the need for antianginal medications.

c. Subgroup analysis suggested that the early conservative strategy may be associated with an improved primary end point in patients older than 65 years of age.

d. The use of tPA did not improve outcome but was associated with a higher

Table 7-7 TIMI IIIB: Early Invasive vs. Conservative Strategies for UAP (67)

	Early Invasive	Early Conservative	*P*
Primary End Point (6 wk)	**16.2%**	**18.1%**	**0.33**
Death	2.4%	2.5%	0.78
Nonfatal MI	5.1%	5.7%	0.78
Positive ETT	8.6%	10.0%	0.78
Secondary End Points (6 wk)			
Average length of initial hospitalization	10.2 d	10.9 d	0.01
No. patients rehospitalized	7.8%	14.1%	<0.001
No. days of rehospitalization	365 d	930 d	<0.001
No. antianginal medications			
0	19.3%	17.0%	0.02
1	37%	31%	0.02
2	25.5%	28.3%	0.02
3	18.3%	23.7%	0.02
CCS classification			
No angina	76%	71.4%	0.13
Class I or II	16.4%	19.1%	0.13
Class III or IV	7.6%	9.5%	0.13
Subgroup Analysis (Death or MI)			
Unstable angina at entry	7.2%	6.9%	0.80
Non–Q-wave MI at entry	7.2%	9.9%	0.30
Age ≥65 y	7.9%	14.8%	0.02
Age <65 y	6.9%	4.6%	0.11

risk of postrandomization MI (7.4% versus 4.9%; P=0.04) and intracranial hemorrhage (4 cases versus 0 cases; P=0.06).

e. At 1-year, the incidence of death or nonfatal MI remained similar between the two groups (1) (see Table 7–8). The early invasive strategy continued to be associated with fewer readmissions. There was no difference in the proportion of patients needing repeat revascularization procedures between 6 weeks and 1 year.

f. **Conclusions**—Early invasive strategy for patients with UA or non–Q-wave MI was associated with a requirement for slightly more PTCA procedures at both 6 weeks and 1 year than early conservative strategy. The incidence of the combined primary end point of death or nonfatal MI did not differ at 6 weeks or 1 year, but fewer patients in the early invasive strategy group required rehospitalization. The difference in cost incurred by the dif-

Table 7-8 TIMI IIIB: 1-Year Follow-Up Results

	Early Invasive	Early Conservative	*P*
Primary End Point (1 y)	**10.8%**	**12.2%**	**0.42**
Death	4.1%	4.4%	0.79
Nonfatal MI	8.3%	9.3%	0.51
Secondary End Points (1 y)			
No. patients rehospitalized	26%	33%	<0.005
No. days of rehospitalization	2743 d	2943 d	0.711
No antianginal medications			
0	30%	25%	0.146
1	36%	36%	0.146
2	22%	25%	0.146
3	11%	14%	0.146
CCS classification			
No angina	71%	69%	0.732
Class I or II	21%	22%	0.732
Class III or IV	8%	9%	0.732
Catheterization and Revascularization			
Catheterization			
By 6 wk	98%	64%	<0.001
By 1 y	99%	73%	<0.001
PTCA			
By 6 wk	38%	26%	<0.001
New, 6 wk–1 y	2%	8%	<0.001
Repeat, 6 wk–1 y	16%	17%	0.555
By 1 y	39%	32%	<0.001
CABG			
By 6 wk	25%	23%	0.169
New, 6 wk–1 y	7%	9%	0.205
Repeat, 6 wk–1 y	0%	0%	—
By 1 y	30%	30%	0.50
PTCA or CABG			
By 6 wk	61%	48%	<0.001
New, 6 wk–1 y	6%	19%	<0.001
Repeat, 6 wk–1 y	10%	10%	0.998
By 1 y	64%	58%	<0.001
Subgroup Analysis (Death or MI)			
Unstable angina at entry	11.1%	14%	0.35
Non–Q-wave MI at entry	10.7%	11.5%	0.74

ferences in these secondary end points is likely to be minimal. Therefore, either strategy is appropriate, and the choice should be guided by physician and patient preferences.

2. As discussed previously, the BARI study compared PTCA with CABG as an initial strategy for management of patients with multivessel CAD and severe angina or objective evidence of ischemia. For the overall group as well as for the subgroup with UA (65% of the entire cohort), there were no differences in cumulative 5-year survival or survival free of Q-wave MI between the two interventions (see section B3d for details).
3. **The Evaluation of c7E3 for the Prevention of Ischemic Complications (EPIC) Study**—The EPIC study was a 6-month PRCT that evaluated the role of c7E3 for prevention of ischemic complications in high-risk patients undergoing PTCA or directional atherectomy (*i.e.*, those with UA, early postinfarction angina, recent or evolving MI, or high-risk angiographic morphology) (25,73). c7E3 is a monoclonal-antibody antigen-binding Fab fragment directed against the platelet glycoprotein IIb/IIIa receptor, the final common pathway for platelet aggregation. All patients received aspirin (325 mg PO QD) and IV heparin during the procedure. The study randomly assigned 2099 patients to receive placebo (bolus plus infusion), c7E3 bolus plus 12-hour placebo infusion, or c7E3 bolus plus 12-hour c7E3 infusion. Exclusion criteria included any bleeding tendency, age greater than 80 years, stroke within the past 2 years, and major surgery up to 6 weeks before study entry. The primary end point at 30 days was the combined risk of death, MI, CABG, repeat PTCA, and need for an endoluminal stent or intraaortic balloon pump. The primary end point at 6 months was the composite of death, nonfatal MI, and the need for another revascularization procedure.
   a. By 30 days, c7E3 therapy (bolus and infusion) had reduced the rate of occurrence of primary end points by 35% compared with placebo (see Table 7–9). No statistically significant difference was observed with c7E3 bolus alone. However, during the first 48 hours after the procedure, the bolus appeared to delay the onset of ischemic events that required urgent revascularization. Bleeding was more common with c7E3 than with placebo (25).
   b. At 6 months, there was a persistent 23% reduction in the primary end point with c7E3 (bolus and infusion), compared with placebo (see Table 7–10). Most of this benefit resulted from a 26% reduction in the need for repeat revascularization after an initially successful coronary intervention. Pa-

Table 7-9 EPIC (30-d Outcome): c7E3 vs. Placebo for PTCA or Atherectomy (30)

30-Day Acute Phase Study	Placebo	c7E3 Fab Bolus	c7E3 Fab Bolus and Infusion	*P* for Dose Response
Primary End Point	**12.8%**	**11.4%**	**8.3%**	**0.009**
Death	1.7%	1.3%	1.7%	0.96
Nonfatal MI	8.6%	6.2%	5.2%	0.013
Nonfatal Q-wave MI	2.3%	1.0%	0.8%	0.020
Emergency PTCA	4.5%	3.6%	0.8%	<0.001
Emergency CABG	3.6%	2.3%	2.4%	0.177
Stent placement	0.6%	1.7%	0.6%	0.98
Balloon-pump insertion	0.1%	0.1%	0.1%	0.99
Secondary End Points				
Major bleeding	7%	11%	14%	0.001
Transfusions				
Red cells	7%	13%	15%	<0.001
Platelets	3%	4%	6%	<0.001

tients who had received c7E3 bolus and placebo infusion had an intermediate outcome which was not statistically better than that of patients who had received placebo bolus and placebo infusion (25).

c. Subgroup analysis comparing the outcome of patients with UA versus CSAP revealed significant reductions in composite events for both subgroups. However, the reduction in need for repeat coronary interventions was significant only for the CSAP group.

d. Conclusions—For high-risk patients undergoing PTCA, c7E3 (IV bolus followed by 12-hour infusion) appears to reduce the long-term risk of major ischemic events (death, MI, need for urgent revascularization) but increases the risk of bleeding.

4. Conclusions Regarding PTCA for Patients With UA

a. In selected patients with multivessel CAD and severe UA (but preserved EF, no left main disease, and no diabetes), there are no significant differences in long-term survival after PTCA or CABG therapy. However, patients treated with PTCA are more likely to require repeat PTCA or subsequent CABG, whereas patients treated with CABG are more likely to suffer an AMI after the procedure and to require a longer hospital stay.

b. UA can be appropriately managed with either an early invasive strategy or an early conservative strategy. Early invasive strategy is associated with a slightly increased rate of revascularization; early conservative strategy is associated with a slightly increased frequency of rehospitalization.

Table 7-10 EPIC (6-m Outcome): c7E3 vs. Placebo for PTCA or Atherectomy (30)

6-Month Follow-Up Study	Placebo	c7E3 Fab Bolus	c7E3 Fab Bolus and Infusion	*P* Pairwise†
Events of all patients enrolled	**35.1%**	**32.6%**	**27%**	**0.001**
Death	3.4%	2.6%	3.1%	0.832
Nonfatal MI	10.5%	8.0%	6.9%	0.016
CABG	10.9%	9.9%	9.4%	0.343
PTCA	20.9%	19.9%	14.14%	0.001
CABG or PTCA	29.4%	26.6%	22.7%	0.004
Target vessel repeat revascularization	22.3%	21.0%	16.5%	0.007
Events of all patients after 48 h	**25.4%**	**24.3%**	**19.2%**	**0.007**
Death	2.7%	2.3%	3.0%	0.660
Nonfatal MI	2.6%	2.4%	2.5%	0.866
CABG	7.6%	7.7%	7.0%	0.705
PTCA	16.5%	17.1%	11.6%	0.011
CABG or PTCA	23.0%	22.5%	18.0%	0.025
Target vessel repeat revascularization*	19.0%	18.6%	15.7%	0.135
Events of all patients with no event at 30 d	**19.3%**	**20.3%**	**15.3%**	**0.071**
Death	1.7%	1.3%	1.5%	0.795
Nonfatal MI	2.0%	1.9%	1.7%	0.723
CABG	5.6%	6.0%	4.7%	0.445
PTCA	12.6%	14.3%	10.1%	0.182
CABG or PTCA	17.5%	18.8%	14.5%	0.161
Target vessel repeat revascularization*	16.9%	16.6%	14.4%	0.265
Subgroup Analysis				
Unstable angina at entry				
Composite event	33.4%	29.0%	25.8%	0.037
Target vessel repeat revascularization	20.3%	16.9%	15.4%	0.134
Stable angina				
Composite event	36.2%	35.4%	28.0%	0.013
Target vessel repeat revascularization	21.3%	22.1%	13.5%	0.003

*Analysis of patients with initial successful PTCA. The after-48-h and after-30-d analyses include only patients who did not experience an end point in the preceding time interval.
†Pairwise comparison of bolus and infusion compared with placebo.

c. c7E3, an antagonist of the platelet glycoprotein IIb/IIIa receptor, may reduce the risk of major ischemic complications caused by restenosis in high-risk patients undergoing PTCA. However, it increases the risk of bleeding.

D. PTCA for Patients With an AMI—The use of PTCA for management of AMI has been reviewed by Landau (44). Angioplasty serves several potential roles in the management of AMI (44). PTCA has been used as salvage therapy after failed thrombolysis (rescue or salvage PTCA), to reduce residual stenosis after successful thrombolysis (routine PTCA), and as primary therapy in lieu of thrombolysis (primary PTCA). Several studies have also suggested that patients with cardiogenic shock represent a distinct, high-risk subset who may benefit from PTCA.

1. In 1995, Michels conducted a metaanalysis of 23 trials examining the use of PTCA for management of AMI. Table 7–11 presents the odds ratios and 95% confidence intervals from this metaanalysis (50).

2. PTCA After Failed Thrombolysis in AMI (Salvage or Rescue PTCA)—Although thrombolytic therapy is very effective, only 50% to 90% of infarct-related arteries achieve complete (TIMI grade 3) reperfusion within 90 minutes of thrombolysis, an outcome which has been shown to be an independent predictor of improved in-hospital survival (52,68,70). Therefore, for patients who fail thrombolysis, the concept of rescue angioplasty is attractive for restoring the patency of the infarct-related artery, salvaging myocardial function, and improving survival (44). Two trials and a metaanalysis addressed the role of immediate salvage PTCA (within 8 hours of onset of chest pain), and one trial addressed the role of late salvage PTCA (6 to 24 hours after onset of chest pain) salvage PTCA (5,22,23,50,72).

a. Immediate Rescue Angioplasty

(1) In a small randomized trial involving 28 patients with an AMI who had failed thrombolysis, one death was observed with rescue angioplasty, compared with four deaths with conservative medical therapy (5).

(2) The Randomized Evaluation of Salvage Angioplasty with Combined Utilization of Endpoints (RESCUE) trial was a PRCT designed to assess the role of immediate salvage PTCA in patients with an AMI (20,22). One hundred fifty-one patients with a first anterior MI that was refractory to thrombolysis (defined angiographically as an occluded infarct-related vessel within 8 hours of onset of chest pain) were randomly assigned to receive either conservative medical therapy or standard therapy plus rescue PTCA.

Table 7-11 Role of PTCA for Management of AMI: Metaanalysis (50)

Category of Trial	6-Wk Risk of Death*	6-Wk Risk of Death or Non-Fatal Reinfarction*	1-Y Risk of Death*
Rescue vs. no PTCA for failed thrombolysis	0.38 (0.13–1.06)	0.44 (0.16–1.21)	0.17 (0.02–1.15)
Immediate routine vs. no routine PTCA	1.09 (0.73–1.61)	0.89 (0.65–1.21)	1.05 (0.75–1.48)
Early routine vs. no routine PTCA	1.08 (0.84–1.39)	1.06 (0.89–1.25)	0.93 (0.74–1.17)
Delayed routine vs. no routine PTCA	1.33 (0.49–3.63)	1.78 (0.99–3.19)	6.79 (1.32–35.03)
Immediate routine vs. delayed routine PTCA	1.46 (0.71–2.97)	1.61 (0.91–2.86)	1.31 (0.68–2.51)
Primary PTCA vs thrombolysis	0.56 (0.33–0.94)	0.53 (0.35–0.80)	0.91 (0.42–2.00)

Modified with permission from Michels (50).
*Odds ratios and 95% confidence intervals.

(a) The combined end point of death or severe heart failure was significantly lower with rescue PTCA (6% versus 17%; *P*=0.05).

(b) At 30 days, there was no difference in the resting EF; however, the EF with exercise was higher for the rescue PTCA group (43% versus 38%; *P*=0.04).

(3) In a metaanalysis of these two studies, rescue PTCA appeared to improve both short- and long-term survival after failed thrombolysis, compared with no PTCA (see previous table). However, the 95% confidence limits for the odds ratios were wide and encompassed values greater than 1 (50).

b. The role of late rescue PTCA (range, 7 to 48 hours after symptom onset; mean, 25 hours) was addressed in the Thrombolysis and Angioplasty in Myocardial Infarction-6 (TAMI-6) trial (72). Patients presenting with an AMI at 6 to 24 hours after onset of symptoms were randomly assigned to receive either tPA or placebo. All patients were catheterized within 24 hours, and patients with an occluded infarct-related artery were randomly assigned to rescue angioplasty versus no angioplasty. The patency rate of the infarct-related artery at 6 months was similar in the two groups. There were also no differences in the EF, the mortality rate, the need for hospital readmission, or the risk of reinfarction.

c. Conclusions Regarding the Role of Rescue PTCA for Patients With an AMI Who Fail Thrombolysis

(1) Although the data on the role of rescue angioplasty for patients with an AMI who fail thrombolysis are limited, immediate rescue angioplasty may be indicated for those with large anterior AMIs who are suspected not to have achieved reperfusion within 2 hours of initiation of thrombolytic therapy. However, further studies are needed before definitive conclusions can be made regarding the benefit of immediate rescue PTCA.

(2) On the other hand, even if rescue PTCA were conclusively beneficial, the role of rescue PTCA may be limited by the current difficulty in promptly and definitively identifying those who are failing thrombolysis. Simple clinical measurements such as relief of chest pain, presence of reperfusion arrhythmias, and resolution of ST-segment elevations have been demonstrated by Califf to be unreliable in predicting reperfusion status after thrombolysis (11).

(3) Furthermore, even if the ability to identify thrombolytic failure were improved, there are additional reasons that salvage PTCA may not prove to beneficial (44).

(a) First, rescue PTCA typically occurs more than 3 hours after the onset of chest pain, when extensive myocardial necrosis may already have occurred. It is unlikely that this situation will improve, because unavoidable time delay is associated with presentation to the hospital, infusion of thrombolytic therapy, recognition of failed thrombolysis, and initiation of rescue PTCA.

(b) Second, rescue PTCA is ineffective in 10% to 15% of patients, and reocclusion occurs in 15% to 20% of those with initially successful procedures (12). Furthermore, unsuccessful rescue PTCA is associated with a high rate of mortality, as high as 44% in one older study (10).

(c) Finally, for many (30% to 60%) of the patients whose infarct-related artery remains occluded shortly after thrombolysis, reperfusion may eventually occur spontaneously during the next 24 hours. This spontaneous reperfusion may improve survival without the attendant risks of rescue angioplasty (46,60).

3. Routine PTCA After Thrombolysis in AMI—The role of routine PTCA after successful thrombolysis for an AMI has been addressed in numerous studies. The use of routine PTCA after thrombolysis can be subdivided into immediate routine PTCA (during the first several hours after onset of symptoms), early routine PTCA (hours to days after the onset of symptoms), or late routine PTCA (≥4 days from the onset of symptoms) (44,50). Numerous studies have evaluated the role of immediate (2,12,26,62,64,68,70,71), early (35,56,66,69,72, 75), or late routine PTCA after thrombolysis (3,7,21).

a. **Immediate Routine PTCA After Thrombolysis for AMI**—Four studies compared immediate routine PTCA versus no routine PTCA after thrombolysis; two compared immediate versus delayed routine PTCA after thrombolysis; and one trial compared immediate versus delayed versus no routine PTCA after thrombolysis (2,12,26,62,64,68,70,71). In the aggregate, there is no evidence that immediate routine PTCA within hours of clinically successful thrombolysis for AMI offers any additional benefit compared with thrombolysis alone. In fact, immediate routine PTCA may increase the incidence of bleeding, recurrent ischemia, need for emergent CABG, or death. Representative studies are summarized in Table 7–12.
b. **Early Routine PTCA After Thrombolysis for AMI**—Numerous studies have examined the role of early routine PTCA (within hours to days) after thrombolysis for AMI (35,56,66,69,72,75). In the aggregate, there is no evidence that early routine PTCA within hours to 3 days after thrombolysis of-

Table 7-12 Studies Evaluating Immediate Routine PTCA after Thrombolysis

Study (Reference)	Design	Findings
TIMI IIA (62, 68)	389 Patients with AMI randomly assigned to immediate routine PTCA vs. early routine PTCA (18–48 h) after thrombolysis with tPA.	1. No difference in EF. 2. Immediate PTCA patients were more likely to require CABG or experience bleeding complications.
TAMI (70)	197 Patients with AMI randomly assigned to immediate routine PTCA (0–90 min) vs. late routine PTCA (7–10 d) after thrombolysis with tPA.	1. No difference in the incidence of reocclusion (11% with immediate vs. 13% with late PTCA). 2. Neither group had a significant improvement in left ventricular function at 1 wk. 3. Late PTCA patients were more likely to require emergency PTCA for recurrent ischemia (16% vs. 5%, P=0.01).
ECSG VI (2, 64)	367 Patients with AMI randomly assigned to immediate routine PTCA vs. no routine PTCA after thrombolysis with tPA.	1. Immediate PTCA increased the number of patients with a patent infarct-related artery but was also associated with a high rate of early reocclusion and early recurrent ischemia. 2. Trial was stopped early because the mortality rate was higher with immediate PTCA at 2 wk (7% vs. 3%) and at 1 y (9.3% vs. 5.4%). 3. No difference in size of infarct estimated by enzymes or by EF.

fers any additional benefit over successful thrombolysis alone. Representative studies are summarized in Table 7–13.

c. **Late Routine PTCA After Successful Thrombolysis for AMI**—Three studies have examined the role of late routine use of PTCA (≥4 days) after thrombolytic therapy for AMI (3,7,21). In the aggregate, there is no evidence that late routine PTCA offers any additional benefit over thrombolysis alone. In fact, in a metaanalysis of these studies, there was a trend toward increased risk of adverse events with PTCA (3,7,21,50). A representative study is summarized in Table 7–14.

4. **Primary PTCA in Lieu of Thrombolysis for AMI**

a. Numerous studies have compared the efficacy of primary PTCA versus thrombolysis for patients with AMI (6,16,18,28,29,32,50,53,61,76). In Michels' metaanalysis of these trials, primary PTCA patients had an improved rate of survival (OR, 0.56; 95% CI, 0.33 to 0.94) and had a lower combined risk of death or nonfatal reinfarction at 6 weeks (OR, 0.53; 95% CI, 0.35 to 0.80). The infarct-related artery was successfully recanalized by primary PTCA in 95% of patients. However, these angioplasties were performed at highly specialized centers by very skilled operators. The outcome of primary PTCA may be less impressive when it is performed by less experienced operators (6,16,18,28,29,32,53,61,76). Landau also points out that only 18% of US hospitals have cardiac catheterization laboratories and even fewer have the capability of performing emergency PTCA (44).

b. For the purpose of illustration, the Primary Angioplasty in Myocardial Infarction trial (PAMI) is described as a representative of these studies. In PAMI, the largest PRCT to date on this subject, 395 patients with an AMI were randomly assigned to receive immediate primary PTCA versus tPA (32).

(1) The combined end point of reinfarction or death occurred less often with primary PTCA than with tPA during the hospitalization (5.1% versus 5.1%, respectively; P=0.02) and also at 6 months (8.5% versus 16.8%, respectively; P=0.02).

(2) The overall in-hospital mortality rate was not significantly different between the two groups (2.6% for PTCA versus 6.5% for tPA; P=0.06). However, for patients in the "not low risk" subgroup (age >65 years, anterior MI, tachycardia on presentation), the mortality rate was significantly lower with primary PTCA (10%, versus 2% for tPA; P=0.01).

(3) There was no significant difference in EF between the two groups at 6 weeks. The rate of intracranial hemorrhage after tPA therapy was higher in this study than in other US trials.

c. **Conclusions**—Primary PTCA is a promising therapy for AMI and appears

Table 7-13 Studies Evaluating Early Routine PTCA after Thrombolysis

Study (Reference)	Design	Findings
SWIFT (66)	800 Patients with AMI randomly assigned to early vs. no routine PTCA after thrombolysis.	1. No significant difference in mortality, reinfarction rate, or EF at 12 mo.
TIMI IIB (69)	3262 Patients with AMI randomly assigned to early (18–48 hours) vs. no routine PTCA after thrombolysis with tPA.	1. No significant difference in the primary end point of reinfarction or death within 42 d (10.9% with PTCA vs. 9.7% with conservative therapy). 2. No significant difference in EF at discharge or at 6 wk.

Table 7-14 Study Evaluating Late Routine PTCA after Successful Thrombolysis

Study (Reference)	Design	Findings
Barbash (3)	201 Patients with AMI randomly assigned to late (mean of 5 d after tPA) vs. no routine PTCA after thrombolysis.	1. No significant difference in EF, rate of reinfarction, or mortality at 10 mo. 2. If only those who died after the time of the scheduled protocol catheterization were considered, 5 of 94 patients in the late PTCA group died compared to 0 of 100 in the conservative group (*P*=0.02).

to be superior to thrombolysis. However, most hospitals are not able to offer rapid, around-the-clock access to angioplasty. Therefore, it is likely that in most centers thrombolysis will continue to be the treatment of choice for AMI.

5. **PTCA for AMI Complicated by Cardiogenic Shock**—Numerous observational and retrospective studies have addressed the role of PTCA for AMI complicated by cardiogenic shock (8,17,19,24,27,37–39,47–49,51,54,63,74). The use of PTCA for this subset of patients with AMI is attractive because the prognosis is dismal for these patients when treated with conventional therapy. Despite major advances in the management of patients with an AMI, the mortality in the subgroup with cardiogenic shock has remained at about 80% for the past 40 years (30,31,55). In contrast, several observational and retrospective studies suggest that the survival rate may be improved if these patients are treated with early CABG (15,43,59). Angioplasty may also offer similar benefit in these patients.
   - **a.** One representative study on this issue is a retrospective analysis by Lee that included 87 patients with cardiogenic shock complicating AMI; 59 were treated with conventional therapy and 24 were treated with conventional therapy plus angioplasty. Conventional therapy consisted of some combination of sympathomimetics, vasodilators, cardiac glycosides, antiarrhythmic agents, and intraaortic balloon pump counterpulsation (47).
     - **(1)** The percentage of patients alive at 30 days was significantly higher in the PTCA group than in the conventional therapy group (50% versus 17%; *P*=0.006).
     - **(2)** Furthermore, among the patients in the PTCA group, those whose angioplasty was successful were more likely to survive than those whose angioplasty was unsuccessful (77% versus 18%; *P*=0.006).
   - **b.** Numerous other studies have demonstrated that for patients in cardiogenic shock from an AMI, the mortality rate is significantly lower if the PTCA is successful than if it is unsuccessful (8,17,19,24,27,37–39,47–49, 51,54,63,74). This data is summarized in Table 7–15.
   - **c.** A large number of retrospective and observational studies suggest that PTCA may improve survival in patients with cardiogenic shock caused by an AMI. However, no randomized trial has yet been conducted. In addition, some of these studies may suffer from selection bias, because many do not clearly define their criteria for treating patients with conventional therapy versus angioplasty. For example, in one study, 84% of the PTCA patients but only 39% of the conventional therapy patients received intraaortic balloon pump counterpulsation (51). Similarly, in the SHOCK registry, which included 20 retrospective and 231 prospectively registered patients with cardiogenic shock at 19 participating centers in the United States and Bel-

Table 7-15 Studies Evaluating PTCA for Cardiogenic Shock Complicating AMI

Primary Author (Reference)	N	Reperfusion Rate	Mortality With Successful PTCA	Mortality With Unsuccessful PTCA
Brown (8)	28	61%	42%	82%
Disler (17)	7	71%	40%	100%
Ellis (19)	61	—	14%	68%
Eltchaninoff (24)	33	76%	24%	75%
Gachioch (27)	68	73%	39%	93%
Heuser (37)	10	60%	17%	75%
Hibbard (38)	45	62%	29%	71%
Hochman (39)	55	69%	61%	73%
Lee (47)	24	54%	23%	82%
Lee (48)	69	71%	31%	80%
Meyer (49)	25	88%	41%	100%
Moosvi (51)	38	78%	44%	93%
O'Neill (54)	27	88%	25%	67%
Shani (63)	9	66%	17%	100%
Verna (74)	7	100%	14%	—

Modified with permission from Bates (4) and O'Neill (55).

gium, the patients selected to undergo cardiac catheterization were significantly younger and had a lower mortality rate than those not selected (51% versus 85%; $P<0.0001$), even when revascularization was not actually performed (58%) (39). Finally, in at least one study, many patients did not meet the commonly accepted definition of cardiogenic shock based on hemodynamic variables (42,47).

E. Summary

1. A number of large trials have recently been completed or are underway which examine the role of PTCA for CSAP, UA, or AMI. For patients with CSAP, PTCA and CABG are both effective in relieving anginal symptoms. Some studies found that patients treated with CABG were more likely to be free of angina and less likely to require antianginal medications. Other studies found the two procedures to be equally effective in relieving anginal symptoms at 1 year. However, patients treated with PTCA are more likely to require repeat PTCA or subsequent CABG. On the other hand, patients treated with CABG are more likely to suffer an AMI after the procedure and to require a longer hospital stay. For clinical situations in which CABG appears to have proven survival advantage compared with medical therapy (three-vessel disease, left main CAD, low EF), CABG should be the procedure of choice, because no study has demonstrated a survival benefit with PTCA for patients with CSAP. In other situations in which CABG does not appear to improve survival (one- or two-vessel disease) but a revascularization procedure is deemed necessary, patient preference should guide the choice between PTCA and CABG.
2. UA can be appropriately managed with either an early invasive strategy (coronary arteriography followed by revascularization if the anatomy is suitable) or an early conservative strategy (coronary arteriography followed by revascularization if initial medical therapy fails). Early invasive strategy resulted in slightly more revascularization procedures than early conservative strategy; early conservative strategy is associated with an increased rate of rehospitalization. For selected patients with multivessel CAD and severe UA (but preserved EF, no left main CAD, no diabetes), revascularization by either PTCA or CABG is appropriate. Patients treated with PTCA are more likely to require repeat PTCA or subsequent CABG; patients treated with CABG are more likely to suffer an AMI after the procedure and to require a longer hospital stay. Use of c7E3, a monoclonal-

antibody Fab fragment directed against the platelet glycoprotein IIb/IIIa receptor, may reduce the risk of major ischemic events caused by restenosis in high-risk patients undergoing PTCA, but it increases the overall risk of bleeding.

3. The data on the role of rescue angioplasty for patients with an AMI who fail thrombolysis are limited. Nevertheless, immediate rescue angioplasty may be indicated for those with large anterior AMIs who are suspected not to have achieved reperfusion within 6 to 8 hours of onset on chest pain. Further studies are needed before definitive conclusions can be made regarding the benefit of immediate rescue PTCA. On the other hand, even if rescue PTCA were conclusively beneficial, its role may be limited by difficulty in promptly and definitively identifying those who are failing thrombolysis.
4. There is no evidence that routine PTCA after successful thrombolysis offers any additional benefit compared with thrombolysis alone, whether it is performed immediately, early, or late in the course of the AMI. In fact, routine PTCA may increase the incidence of bleeding, recurrent ischemia, need for emergent CABG, and death.
5. Primary PTCA is a promising therapy for AMI and appears to be superior to thrombolysis in the few trials reported to date. However, most hospitals are not capable of offering a rapid, around-the-clock access to angioplasty. It is therefore likely that thrombolysis will continue to be the treatment of choice for AMI in most centers.
6. A large number of retrospective and observational studies suggest that PTCA may improve survival in patients with cardiogenic shock due to an AMI. However, to date, no randomized trial has been conducted.

Abbreviations used in Chapter 7

AMI = acute myocardial infarction
CABG = coronary arterial bypass graft
CAD = coronary artery disease
CCSC = Canadian Cardiovascular Society Classification
CI = confidence interval
CSAP = chronic stable angina pectoris
ECSG = European Cooperative Study Group
EF = ejection fraction
ETT = exercise tolerance treadmill test
Fab = antigen-binding fragment (of immunoglobulins)
MI = myocardial infarction
N = number of patients in population
n = number of patients in sample
NHLBI = National Heart, Lung, and Blood Institute
PO = per os
PRCT = prospective randomized controlled trial
PTCA = percutaneous transluminal coronary angioplasty
QD = daily
SWIFT = Should We Intervene Following Thrombolysis
TAMI = Thrombolysis in Acute Myocardial Infarction
TIMI = Thrombolysis in Myocardial Infarction
tPA = tissue plasminogen activator
UA = unstable angina pectoris
vs. = versus

References

1. Anderson. One-year results of the Thrombolysis in Myocardial Infarction (TIMI) IIIB clinical trial: a randomized comparison of tissue-type plasminogen activator

versus placebo and early invasive versus early conservative strategies in unstable angina and non–Q wave myocardial infarction. *J Am Coll Cardiol* 1995;26:1643.

2. Arnold. Recombinant tissue-type plasminogen activator and immediate angioplasty in acute myocardial infarction: one-year follow-up. *Circulation* 1992;86:111.
3. Barbash. Randomized controlled trial of late in-hospital angiography and angioplasty versus conservative management after treatment with recombinant tissue-type plasminogen activator in acute myocardial infarction. *Am J Cardiol* 1990; 66:538.
4. Bates. Limitations of thrombolytic therapy for acute myocardial infarction complicated by congestive heart failure and cardiogenic shock. *J Am Coll Cardiol* 1991; 18:1077.
5. Belenkie. Rescue angioplasty during myocardial infarction has a beneficial effect on mortality: a tenable hypothesis. *Can J Cardiol* 1992;8:357.
6. Boer. Coronary angioplasty results in a lower rate of recurrent infarction and death when compared with streptokinase in patients with a myocardial infarction. *Circulation* 1993;88(Suppl I):I.
7. Brand. Randomized trial of deferred angioplasty after thrombolysis for acute myocardial infarction. *Coron Artery Dis* 1992;3:393.
8. Brown. Percutaneous myocardial reperfusion (PMR) reduces mortality in acute myocardial infarction (MI) complicated by cardiogenic shock. *Circulation* 1985; 72(Suppl III):III. Abstract.
9. Bypass Angioplasty Revascularization Investigation (BARI) Investigators. Comparison of coronary bypass surgery with angioplasty in patients with multivessel disease. *N Engl J Med* 1996;335:217.
10. Califf. Characteristics and outcome of patients in whom reperfusion with intravenous tissue plasminogen activator fails: results of the TAMI I trial. *Circulation* 1988;77:1090.
11. Califf. Failure of simple clinical measurements to predict perfusion status after intravenous thrombolysis. *Ann Intern Med* 1988;108:658.
12. Califf. Evaluation of combining thrombolytic therapy and timing of cardiac catheterization in acute myocardial infarction: Results of Thrombolysis and Angioplasty in Myocardial Infarction—Phase 5 randomized trial. *Circulation* 1991;83: 1543.
13. CASS Principal Investigators. Coronary Artery Surgery Study (CASS): a randomized trial of coronary artery bypass surgery. Survival data. *Circulation* 1983;68: 939.
14. Detre. Percutaneous transluminal coronary angioplasty in 1985–1986 and 1977–1981: the National Heart, Lung, and Blood Institute Registry. *N Engl J Med* 1988; 318:265.
15. DeWood. Intraaortic balloon counterpulsation with and without reperfusion for myocardial infarction shock. *Circulation* 1980;61:1105.
16. DeWood. Direct PTCA versus intravenous rtPA in acute myocardial infarction: preliminary results from a prospective randomized trial. *Circulation* 1989;80(Suppl II):II.
17. Disler. Cardiogenic shock in evolving myocardial infarction: treatment by angioplasty and streptokinase. *Heart Lung* 1987;16:649.
18. Elizaga. Primary coronary angioplasty versus systemic thrombolysis in acute anterior myocardial infarction: in-hospital results from a prospective randomized trial. *Circulation* 1993;88(Suppl I):I.
19. Ellis. Implications for patient triage from survival and left ventricular functional recovery analyses in 500 patients treated with coronary angioplasty for acute myocardial infarction. *J Am Coll Cardiol* 1989;13:1251.
20. Ellis. Present status of rescue coronary angioplasty: current polarization of opinion and randomized trials. *J Am Coll Cardiol* 1992;19:681.
21. Ellis. Randomized trial of late elective angioplasty versus conservative management for patients with residual stenoses after thrombolytic treatment of myocardial infarction. *Circulation* 1992;86:1400.
22. Ellis. Final results of the randomized RESCUE study evaluating PTCA after failed thrombolysis for patients with anterior infarction. *Circulation* 1993;88(Suppl I):I.

23. Ellis. Randomized comparison of rescue angioplasty with conservative management of patients with early failure of thrombolysis for acute anterior myocardial infarction. *Circulation* 1994;90:2280.
24. Eltchaninoff. Coronary angioplasty improves both early and 1 year survival in acute myocardial infarction complicated by cardiogenic shock. *J Am Coll Cardiol* 1991;17:167A. Abstract.
25. EPIC Investigators. Use of a monoclonal antibody directed against the platelet glycoprotein IIb/IIIa receptor in high-risk coronary angioplasty. *N Engl J Med* 1994; 330:956.
26. Erbel. Long-term results of thrombolytic therapy with and without percutaneous transluminal coronary angioplasty. *J Am Coll Cardiol* 1989;14:276.
27. Gachioch. Cardiogenic shock complicating acute myocardial infarction: the use of coronary angioplasty and the integration of the new support devices into patient management. *J Am Coll Cardiol* 1992;19:647.
28. Gibbons. Immediate angioplasty compared with the administration of a thrombolytic agent followed by conservative treatment for myocardial infarction. *N Engl J Med* 1993;328:685.
29. Gibbons. Randomized trial comparing immediate angioplasty to thrombolysis followed by conservative treatment for myocardial infarction. *N Engl J Med* 1993; 328:673.
30. Goldberg. Cardiogenic shock after acute myocardial infarction: incidence and mortality from a community-wide perspective, 1975 to 1988. *N Engl J Med* 1991; 325:1117.
31. Griffith. The treatment of shock associated with myocardial infarction. *Circulation* 1954;9:527.
32. Grines. A comparison of immediate angioplasty with thrombolytic therapy for acute myocardial infarction. *N Engl J Med* 1993;328:673.
33. Grüntzig. Long-term follow-up after percutaneous transluminal coronary angioplasty: the early Zurich experience. *N Engl J Med* 1987;316:1127.
34. Grüntzig. Transluminal dilatation of coronary-artery stenosis. *Lancet* 1978;1:263.
35. Guerci. A randomized trial of intravenous tissue plasminogen activator for acute myocardial infarction with subsequent randomization to elective coronary angioplasty. *N Engl J Med* 1987;317:1613.
36. Hamm. A randomized study of coronary angioplasty compared with bypass surgery in patients with symptomatic multivessel coronary disease. *N Engl J Med* 1994;331:1037.
37. Heuser. Coronary angioplasty in the treatment of cardiogenic shock: the therapy of choice. *J Am Coll Cardiol* 1986;7:219A. Abstract.
38. Hibbard. Percutaneous transluminal coronary angioplasty in patients with cardiogenic shock. *J Am Coll Cardiol* 1992;19:639.
39. Hochman. Current spectrum of cardiogenic shock and effect of early revascularization on mortality: results of an international registry. *Circulation* 1995;91:873.
40. Kent. Long term follow-up of the NHLBI-PTCA registry. *Circulation* 1986;74(suppl II):II.
41. King. A randomized trial comparing coronary angioplasty with coronary bypass surgery. *N Engl J Med* 1994;331:1044.
42. Klein. Optimal therapy for cardiogenic shock: the emerging role of coronary angioplasty. *J Am Coll Cardiol* 1992;19:654.
43. Laks. Surgical treatment of cardiogenic shock after myocardial infarction. *Circulation* 1986;74(Suppl III):III.
44. Landau. Coronary angioplasty in the patient with acute myocardial infarction. *Am J Med* 1994;96:536.
45. Landau. Percutaneous transluminal coronary angioplasty. *N Engl J Med* 1994; 330:981.
46. LATE Study Group. Late assessment of thrombolytic efficacy with alteplase 6–24 hours after onset of acute myocardial infarction. *Lancet* 1993;342:759.
47. Lee. Percutaneous transluminal coronary angioplasty improves survival in acute myocardial infarction complicated by cardiogenic shock. *Circulation* 1988;78: 1345.

48. Lee. Multicenter registry of angioplasty therapy of cardiogenic shock: initial and long-term survival. *J Am Coll Cardiol* 1991;17:599.
49. Meyer. Traitment de choc cardiogenique primaire par aniplastie tranluminale coronarienne a la phase aigue de l infarctus. *Arch Mal Coeur Vaiss* 1990;83:329.
50. Michels. Does PTCA in acute myocardial infarction affect mortality and reinfarction rates? A quantitative overview (meta-analysis) of the randomized clinical trials. *Circulation* 1995;91:476.
51. Moosvi. Early revascularization improves survival in cardiogenic shock complicating acute myocardial infarction. *J Am Coll Cardiol* 1992;19:907.
52. Neuhaus. Improved thrombolysis in acute myocardial infarction with front-loaded administration of alteplase: results of the rt-PA–APSAC Patency Study (TAPS). *J Am Coll Cardiol* 1992;19:885.
53. O Neill. A prospective randomized clinical trial of intracoronary streptokinase versus coronary angioplasty for acute myocardial infarction. *N Engl J Med* 1986;314: 812.
54. O Neill. Improvement in left ventricular function after thrombolytic therapy and angioplasty: results of the TAMI study. *Circulation* 1987;76(Suppl IV):IV. Abstract.
55. O Neill. Angioplasty therapy of cardiogenic shock: are randomized trials necessary? *J Am Coll Cardiol* 1992;19:915.
56. Ozbek. Comparison of invasive and conservative strategies after treatment with streptokinase in acute myocardial infarction: results of a randomized trial (SIAM). *J Am Coll Cardiol* 1990;15:63A. Abstract.
57. Parisi. A comparison of angioplasty with medical therapy in the treatment of single vessel coronary artery disease. *N Engl J Med* 1992;326:10.
58. Participants. Coronary angioplasty versus coronary artery bypass surgery: the Randomized Intervention Treatment of Angina (RITA) trial. *Lancet* 1993;341:573.
59. Phillips. Reperfusion protocol and results in 738 patients with evolving myocardial infarction. *Ann Thorac Surg* 1986;41:119.
60. PRIMI. Randomized double-blind trial of recombinant urokinase against streptokinase in acute myocardial infarction. *Lancet* 1989;1:863.
61. Ribeiro. Randomized trial of direct coronary angioplasty versus intravenous streptokinase in acute myocardial infarction. *J Am Coll Cardiol* 1993;22:376.
62. Rogers. Comparison of immediate invasive, delayed invasive, and conservative strategies after tissue-type plasminogen activator: results of the Thrombolysis in Myocardial Infarction (TIMI) Phase II-A Trial. *Circulation* 1990;81:1457.
63. Shani. Percutaneous transluminal coronary angioplasty in cardiogenic shock. *J Am Coll Cardiol* 1986;7:149A. Abstract.
64. Simoons. Thrombolysis with tissue plasminogen activator in acute myocardial infarction: no additional benefit from immediate percutaneous coronary angioplasty. *Lancet* 1988;1:197.
65. Simoons. Myocardial revascularization: bypass surgery or angioplasty? *N Engl J Med* 1996;335:275.
66. SWIFT (Should We Intervene Following Thrombolysis?) Trial Study Group. SWIFT trial of delayed elective intervention v conservative treatment after thrombolysis with anistreplase in acute myocardial infarction. *Br Med J* 1991;302:555.
67. TIMI IIIB Investigators. Effects of tissue plasminogen activator and a comparison of early invasive and conservative strategies in unstable angina and non–Q-wave myocardial infarction. *Circulation* 1994;89:1545.
68. TIMI Research Group. Immediate vs. delayed catheterization and angioplasty following thrombolytic therapy for acute myocardial infarction: TIMI IIA results. *JAMA* 1988;260:2849.
69. TIMI Study Group. Comparison of invasive and conservative strategies after treatment with intravenous tissue plasminogen activator in acute myocardial infarction: results of the Thrombolysis in Myocardial Infarction (TIMI) phase II trial. *N Engl J Med* 1989;320:618.
70. Topol. A randomized trial of immediate versus delayed elective angioplasty after intravenous tissue plasminogen activator in acute myocardial infarction. *N Engl J Med* 1987;317:581.

71. Topol. A randomized, placebo-controlled trial of intravenous recombinant tissue-type plasminogen activator and emergency coronary angioplasty in patients with acute myocardial infarction. *Circulation* 1987;75:420.
72. Topol. A randomized trial of late reperfusion therapy for acute myocardial infarction. *Circulation* 1992;85:2090.
73. Topol. Randomised trial of coronary intervention with antibody against platelet IIb/IIIa integrin for reduction of clinical restenosis: results at six months. *Lancet* 1995;343:881.
74. Verna. Emergency coronary angioplasty in patients with severe left ventricular dysfunction or cardiogenic shock after acute myocardial infarction. *Eur Heart J* 1989;10:958.
75. Williams. One-year results of the Thrombolysis in Myocardial Infarction (TIMI) phase II trial. *Circulation* 1992;85:533.
76. Zijlstra. A comparison of immediate coronary angioplasty with intravenous streptokinase in acute myocardial infarction. *N Engl J Med* 1993;328:680.

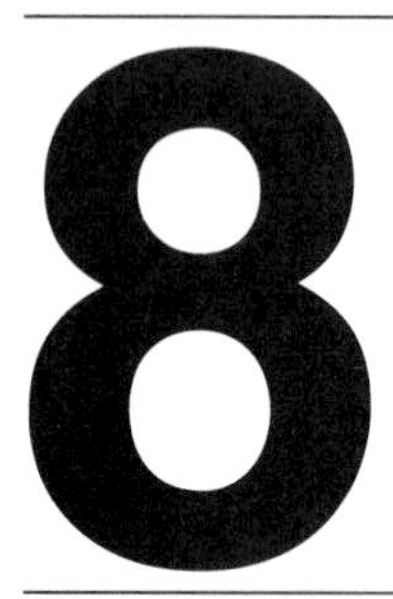

Coronary Artery Bypass Grafting for Stable Angina Pectoris

Marc L. Boom and
Patrick T. O'Gara

A. Introduction

1. The successful use of saphenous vein grafts (SVGs) for coronary artery bypass grafting (CABG) was first reported in 1968 by Favalaro (31). This procedure quickly gained popularity because up to 90% of patients experienced significant relief from angina after CABG. Although significant symptomatic benefit after CABG was readily demonstrated, very little was known initially about its effect on survival.
2. In the 1970s, three large prospective randomized controlled trials (PRCTs) were initiated to compare the relative benefits of CABG and conventional medical therapy. Much of the information available on the benefits of CABG comes from these trials. This chapter focuses on the results of these trials, compares them with the results of more recent registry studies, and attempts to formulate guidelines for identifying appropriate candidates for CABG.
3. In order to assess accurately the benefit of surgical versus medical treatment of coronary artery disease (CAD), it is necessary to understand the natural history of medically treated CAD, which is well described in the Coronary Artery Surgery Study (CASS) registry, the Duke University data bank, and elsewhere (41,62). For illustration, the mortality rates obtained from the CASS registry are summarized here (62). The CASS registry included 24,959 patients from 15 participating centers. The registry survival study analyzed the data on 20,088 patients with no history of cardiac surgery who were enrolled from 1975 to 1979. Angiographic data were obtained on all patients. Significant stenosis was defined as >50% reduction in the internal diameter of the left main coronary artery or >70% reduction in the internal diameter of other coronary arteries. Left ventricular (LV) ejection fraction (EF) was assessed in 97% of patients.
   a. In general, the 4-year survival rate was inversely correlated with the number of diseased coronary arteries. Among those with three-vessel disease, patients with left main CAD had poorer survival, compared with those without left main CAD.
   b. In addition, the 4-year survival rate was inversely correlated with LV function. The authors concluded that poor LV function may be the most important predictor of death.
   c. The survival rates in the CASS registry were similar to those obtained in the Duke University data bank and the European study and were slightly worse than those reported in the Veterans Administration (VA) study (28,41,83). Table 8–1 summarizes the major findings of the CASS registry studies.

B. The VA Cooperative Study of Surgery for Coronary Arterial Occlusive Disease

1. The VA study was the first PRCT to compare surgical versus medical therapy for patients with CAD. Although it was initially designed to evaluate the Vineberg operation, in which the left internal mammary artery (IMA) is implanted into a surgically created tunnel in the myocardium of the left ventricle, it soon became apparent that CABG was a more promising procedure and the study was redesigned to compare CABG versus medical therapy. Although the original study

Table 8-1 CASS Registry: Survival in Patients with Medically Treated CAD (62)

Variable	4-Y Survival Rate	Comments
No CAD	97%	
One-vessel CAD	92%	
Two-vessel CAD	84%	No significant difference in survival with or without left main disease
Left main disease	80%	
No left main disease	84%	
Three-vessel CAD	68%	Poorer survival for those with left main disease
Left main disease	60%	
No left main disease	70%	
Ejection fraction		These results pertain to those with at least one-vessel CAD, but not left main disease
>50%	92%	
35–49%	83%	
<35%	58%	
LV score		For each EF or LV score category, survival decreased with increasing number of vessels diseased
5–11	90%	
12–16	71%	
17–30	53%	

*LV score was calculated by dividing the ventriculogram into five segments and assigning a score of 1 to 6 (1 = normal, 6 = aneurysm) to each segment based on its contractility.

began in 1970, the evaluation of CABG started in 1972, and the period from 1972 to 1974 is considered to be the definitive period for this study (84).

2. This randomized study compared surgical therapy versus medical therapy among 686 patients with stable angina pectoris (65,73).

a. Entry criteria included (a) history of stable angina for longer than 6 months with at least a 3-month trial of medical management; (b) one of three electrocardiographic (ECG) or treadmill findings (old myocardial infarction [MI] on ECG, abnormal T waves or ST segments consistent with ischemia on the resting ECG, or positive exercise stress test); and (c) at least one major coronary artery with ≥50% reduction in lumen diameter that was amenable to bypass surgery.

b. Exclusion criteria included female gender, MI within the past 6 months, persistent diastolic hypertension (≥100 mm Hg) despite treatment, other cardiac disease (marked cardiac enlargement, ventricular aneurysm, or valvular heart disease), other significant systemic disease, previous surgery for angina, unstable angina, or congestive heart failure in the previous 3 weeks.

c. Subgroup Analysis (89)

(1) Angiographically defined risk groups were identified on the basis of the number of vessels diseased and LV function. High angiographic risk was defined as three-vessel disease and impaired LV function. All other combinations were defined as low angiographic risk.

(2) In addition, clinical risk terciles were determined using four clinical risk variables measured at baseline: New York Heart Association classification, history of hypertension, history of MI, and ST-segment depression on the resting ECG.

3. Results of the VA Study

a. Patients With Left Main CAD—It was quickly apparent that the subgroup of patients with left main CAD benefited from surgical intervention. At that point, participants in the study were informed of the results and offered surgical treatment. A preliminary report confirming this benefit was released in 1976 (85); subsequent reports were published in 1982 and 1985 (86,87).

(1) The cumulative survival rate in patients with left main CAD who underwent surgery was significantly better than in patients who received medical therapy; the 42-month survival rate was 88% for surgery versus 65% for medical therapy (*P*=0.016).
(2) When patients with left main CAD were stratified into high, middle, and low clinical risk terciles, the benefit of surgery was greatest in the high-risk tercile and lowest in the low-risk tercile.
(3) There was a statistically nonsignificant trend toward greater survival with surgery in the subgroups with impaired LV function or angiographic high-risk features (impaired LV function and significant right CAD).
(4) For patients with left main equivalent (LMEQ) lesions (disease of the proximal left anterior descending artery and the proximal left circumflex artery), no difference in survival was found between the two treatment groups.

b. **Patients Without Left Main CAD**—In 1977, the results for patients without left main CAD became available. No statistically significant difference in survival was found at 36 months, either for the group as a whole or for various subgroups (65). A subsequent analysis reported a 5-year survival benefit for patients in the tercile with high clinical risk (22). In 1984, the 11-year follow-up results were released (89). The major findings are summarized here and in Table 8–2.
(1) When the 686 patients (including those with left main CAD) were considered as a whole, the 7-year survival rate was significantly improved with surgery (77% versus 70%; *P*=0.043), but this benefit disappeared by 11 years.

Table 8-2 VA Cooperative Study: CABG vs. Medical Therapy (65,89)

	7-Y Survival Rate			11-Y Survival Rate		
Variable	Surgical	Medical	*P*	Surgical	Medical	*P*
All patients	77%	70%	0.043	58%	57%	0.45
All patients without left main disease	77%	72%	0.267	58%	58%	0.813
Number of vessels						
One	88%	83%	0.522	70%	65%	0.589
Two	73%	81%	0.213	55%	69%	0.045
Three	75%	63%	0.061	56%	50%	0.161
LV Function						
Normal	80%	84%	0.350	64%	71%	0.249
Impaired	74%	63%	0.049	53%	49%	0.249
Angiographic risk						
High	76%	52%	0.002	50%	38%	0.026
Low	77%	82%	0.156	68%	61%	0.105
Clinical risk tercile						
High	72%	52%	0.003	49%	36%	0.015
Middle	79%	71%	0.345	62%	61%	0.737
Low	81%	88%	0.093	63%	73%	0.066
High angiographic risk						
High clinical risk	76%	36%	0.002	54%	24%	0.005
Middle clinical risk	79%	49%	0.069	43%	40%	0.345
Low clinical risk	77%	50%	0.818	52%	62%	0.586
Low angiographic risk						
High clinical risk	71%	67%	0.531	46%	46%	0.732
Middle clinical risk	78%	82%	0.569	68%	73%	0.521
Low clinical risk	81%	90%	0.079	66%	76%	0.092

(2) When only those with three-vessel disease were considered, there was a statistically nonsignificant trend toward improved survival with surgery. No benefit was observed in patients with one-vessel disease, and a marginally significant disadvantage of surgical treatment was noted in patients with two-vessel disease.

(3) When only those with depressed LV function were considered, a marginally significant difference favoring surgery was detected at 7 years (74% versus 63%; *P*=0.049), but this benefit disappeared by 11 years.

(4) Patients in the group with high angiographic risk (three-vessel disease and impaired LV function) had a large survival benefit with surgery at 7 years (76% versus 52%; *P*=0.002) and a smaller but still significant benefit at 11 years (50% versus 38%; *P*=0.026). There was no significant difference in survival for patients in the group at low angiographic risk. When patients in the group with high angiographic risk were further stratified according to clinical risk terciles, a benefit of surgery was observed only for those in the tercile with high clinical risk (54% versus 24% at 11 years; *P*=0.005).

(5) Patients in the tercile with high clinical risk had a large survival benefit with surgery at 7 years (72% versus 51%; *P*=0.003) and a smaller but still significant benefit at 11 years (49% versus 36%; *P*=0.026). There was no significant difference in survival for patients in other terciles.

(6) CABG was associated with a statistically nonsignificant trend toward poorer survival in subgroups with normal LV function and in the tercile with low clinical and low angiographic risk.

c. Finally, in 1992, the 18-year follow-up results were released. By this time, no significant difference in survival was observed in the overall group or in any subgroup, including those with left main CAD (90).

4. Conclusions from the VA Study (24,86,90)

a. For the group as a whole, surgery significantly improved the 7-year survival rate, but this advantage disappeared by 11 years. Most of this benefit was observed in those with left main CAD, especially those in the high-risk tercile.

b. Surgery did not significantly improve the overall survival rate in the majority of patients without left main CAD. Exceptions are those in the group with high angiographic risk (three-vessel disease and impaired LV function) and those in the tercile with high clinical risk tercile, who did derive significant survival benefit from CABG at both 7 and 11 years.

C. The European Coronary Surgery Study (28,29,30,94)

1. The European Coronary Surgery Study was a PRCT of surgical versus medical therapy which was intended to have a 5-year follow-up period (29,30). The study group consisted of 768 men. The entry criteria included age <65 years, history of angina pectoris for at least 3 months, LV EF ≥50%, and at least two coronary arteries with ≥50% stenosis.

2. Results

a. After two interim reports, the final report of the European study was released in 1982 (28–30) (see Table 8–3).

(1) In the overall group, CABG significantly improved the rate of survival at 5 and 8 years.

(2) CABG was especially beneficial for the subgroup with three-vessel disease and for those with proximal left anterior descending artery (LAD) disease. In the subgroup with left main CAD, the difference in survival was not statistically significant. No difference in survival was noted for those with two-vessel disease.

(3) Other subgroups that benefited from CABG included patients with peripheral arterial disease, those with resting ECG changes, or those with ≥1.5 mm ST depression during stress testing. Older age was another predictor of benefit from CABG.

b. In 1988, the 12-year follow-up report was released (94).

(1) The observed survival benefit of CABG for the overall group was still present at 12 years (71% survival with surgery versus 67% with med-

Table 8-3 European Coronary Surgery Study: CABG vs. Medical Therapy (28-30)

Variable	5-Y Survival			8-Y Survival		
	Surgical	Medical	*P*	Surgical	Medical	*P*
All patients	92%	84%	0.00025	89%	80%	0.0013
Left main disease	86%	68%	0.11	82%	64%	0.12
Two-vessel disease	91%	88%	<0.20	85%	87%	>0.20
With proximal LAD involvement	91%	84%	0.15	Not stated in paper		
No proximal LAD involvement	91%	95%	>0.20	Not stated in paper		
Three-vessel disease	94%	82%	0.0003	92%	77%	0.00015
Proximal LAD disease						
Present	93%	82%	0.0004	88%	79%	0.003
Absent	93%	92%	>0.20	92%	88%	>0.20
ST depression on stress test						
>1.5 mm	92%	79%	0.0003	90%	77%	0.0003
0–1 mm	95%	90%	>0.20	88%	85%	>0.20
Peripheral arterial disease						
Present	89%	66%	0.0361	85%	57%	0.0229
Absent	93%	85%	0.0015	90%	81%	0.0040

ical therapy; P=0.04), but the magnitude of this benefit was smaller than at 8 years.

(2) Proximal LAD disease was again a strong predictor of both poor prognosis and benefit from CABG (76% survival at 10 years with surgery versus 65% with medical treatment; P=0.007). Similarly, older age, presence of resting ECG changes, positive exercise test, and history of peripheral arterial disease were again predictors of benefit from CABG.

(3) In addition, history of hypertension emerged as another important variable; the survival benefit of CABG was noted only for those without a prior history of hypertension. This was in direct contrast to the VA study, in which hypertension was one of the factors that placed a patient in the group at high clinical risk, a group that derived considerable benefit from CABG.

c. Conclusions from the European Coronary Surgery Study

(1) A significant improvement in survival was detected up to 12 years after CABG.

(2) CABG was especially beneficial for older patients and for the subgroups with three-vessel disease, proximal LAD disease, peripheral arterial disease, resting ECG changes, or ≥1.5 mm ST depression during stress testing.

D. The National Heart, Lung, and Blood Institute's CASS Trial (1,17,72)

1. The CASS study was a PRCT that compared medical therapy versus early CABG followed by medical therapy. Of the 2099 eligible patients from 15 clinical sites in the CASS registry, 780 entered the trial (1,51).

a. The entry criteria included the presence of one or more vessels with ≥70% reduction in diameter that were amenable to CABG. Symptomatic patients had class I or II angina according to the Canadian Cardiovascular Society (CCS) classification and asymptomatic patients had a well-documented MI within 6 months of enrollment.

b. Exclusion criteria included prior CABG, age >65 years, geographic or language barriers, EF <35%, overt heart failure or cardiogenic shock, CCS class III or IV angina, or ≥70% left main CAD.
c. Patients were first divided into three groups and treatments were then randomized within each group. Group A patients had angina and EF ≥50%; group B patients had angina and EF of 35% to 50%; and group C consisted of asymptomatic post-MI patients.

2. **Results** (see Table 8–4)
   a. At 5 years, there was no significant difference in survival between the two treatment arms (17). However, by 7 years of follow-up, CABG had significantly improved the survival rate in the subgroup of patients with depressed LV function. Almost all of this benefit was observed in those with depressed LV function and three-vessel disease (72).
   b. The 10-year follow-up results were released in 1990 (1).
      (1) Overall, there were no significant differences in the 5- or 10-year survival rates between the two treatment arms.
      (2) Patients in group A (mild angina with normal EF) who received medical treatment had a longer event-free survival time than those who were treated surgically. There was no difference in mortality between the two treatment arms.
      (3) For patients in group B (mild angina with depressed EF), CABG substantially reduced the mortality rate. Patients with three-vessel disease and depressed EF had the greatest benefit from surgery. There was also a trend toward improved survival for patients with depressed EF and one- or two-vessel disease. When all patients in the study with depressed EF were examined (including those in group C),

Table 8-4 CASS Trial: Early CABG vs. Medical Therapy (1,17,72)

	5-Y Survival			10-Y Survival		
Variable	Surgical	Medical	*P*	Surgical	Medical	*P*
All patients	95%	92%	0.34	82%	79%	0.25
Group A (angina and normal EF)	96%	94%	0.79	82%	86%	0.30
Group B (angina and low EF)	96%	85%	0.057	80%	59%	0.01
Group C (asymptomatic after MI)	90%	88%	0.79	81%	69%	0.12
EF ≥0.50	96%	95%	0.55	83%	84%	0.75
One-vessel disease	96%	95%	0.74	87%	85%	0.67
Two-vessel disease	96%	96%	0.13	84%	85%	0.87
Three-vessel disease	94%	94%	0.91	78%	84%	0.37
EF <0.50	92%	83%	0.085	79%	61%	0.01
One-vessel disease	100%	82%	0.95	88%	56%	0.14
Two-vessel disease	93%	86%	0.85	82%	65%	0.14
Three-vessel disease	90%	81%	0.063	85%	58%	0.08
Vessels diseased						
One	96%	93%	0.42	82%	85%	0.44
Two	96%	93%	0.52	79%	83%	0.43
Three	93%	90%	0.18	75%	76%	0.70
LAD 50%–70%	96%	91%	?	81%	81%	0.72
LAD ≥70%	94%	92%	?	82%	78%	0.26
One-vessel disease	96%	93%	?	91%	82%	0.34
Two-vessel disease	95%	94%	?	82%	78%	0.27
Three-vessel disease	91%	88%	?	75%	74%	0.96

a similar survival benefit of CABG was observed.

(4) When patients were stratified according to the number of diseased vessels (independent of the EF), benefit of CABG could not be demonstrated for one-, two-, or three-vessel disease. Similarly, there was no demonstrable benefit of CABG in those with LAD disease even in association with three-vessel disease.

3. Conclusions from the CASS Study (1)

a. CABG significantly improved survival in patients with mild angina and LV dysfunction, particularly those with three-vessel disease.

b. For patients with mild angina and normal LV function, a strategy of initial medical therapy does not place the patient at risk of increased mortality.

E. Summary of the Major Randomized Trials

1. Some of the key similarities and differences among the three major randomized studies are highlighted in Table 8–5.

2. In 1994, a metaanalysis of CABG trials was performed (98), using the data from three major randomized trials and four smaller studies (17,52,61,67,89,94).

a. Trials were selected in which patients with stable coronary heart disease (stable angina not severe enough to require surgery for symptom control, or MI) were randomly assigned to either initial medical management or initial CABG and were observed for at least 10 years. The metaanalysis used the original data from each of the trials. Therefore, the authors were able to standardize the data. Significant stenosis was defined as >50% occlusion. Because the primary angiographic data were available, the authors were able to adapt the CASS data to fit the 50% criterion. Depressed LV function was defined as EF <50%. An intention-to-treat analysis was used for all mortality comparisons.

Table 8-5 Summary of Major PRCTs Evaluating the Role of CABG for CAD

	VA Study	European Study	CASS
Design			
Time period	1972–1974	1973–1976	1975–1979
No. patients	686	768	780
Sex	100% Male	100% Male	90% Male
Age (y)	≤67	≤65	≤65
Severity of angina	Mild to severe	Mild to moderate	None to mild
No. diseased vessels	≥1	≥2	≥1
Disease threshold	≥50%	≥50%	≥70%
Left main disease threshold	≥50%	≥50%	50%–69%
Ejection fraction	All values	≥50%	≥35%
Patient characteristics			
Ejection fraction	Impaired in 55%	All with EF ≥0.50	0.35–0.49: 20.5% ≥0.50: 73.7% Not measured: 5.8%
Vessels diseased			
One	16%	0%	19%
Two	34%	43%	31%
Three	50%	57%	51%
Left main	16%	8%	1.8%
Operative mortality	5.8%	3.3%	1.4%
Medical nonadherence	5-y: 17.4% 11.2-y: 38%	5-y: 24% 12-y: 36%	5 y: 23.5% 10-y: 40%
5-Y surgical nonadherence	6%	7%	8%

Adapted from Table 1 in Nwasokwa (68) and Table 1 in Takaro (85).

b. The metaanalysis included 2649 patients from seven trials who were enrolled between 1972 and 1984. Of those patients randomly assigned to CABG, 94% underwent surgery. Of those assigned to medical therapy, 37% eventually underwent surgery as well. The crossover rates within the three large studies were similar.

c. Results

(1) The 30-day surgical mortality rate was 3.2%.

(2) CABG significantly lowered the overall mortality rate at 5, 7, and 10 years (see Table 8–6).

(3) In subgroup analysis, all patients with three-vessel or left main CAD benefited from surgery (see Table 8–7).

(4) All patients with proximal LAD disease benefited from surgery, regardless of how many vessels were diseased. Patients without proximal LAD disease benefited only if they had three-vessel or left main CAD.

(5) Patients benefited from CABG regardless of LV function. However, because the baseline mortality rate was higher for patients with impaired LV function (25% versus 13%), the absolute benefit of CABG was greater for those with low EFs.

(6) For patients in the tercile at low clinical risk (VA study definition), there was a nonsignificant trend toward greater mortality with CABG. However, the benefit of CABG increased as the risk tercile increased. Similarly, the benefit of CABG was higher for those with CCS class III or IV angina, although those with CCS class 0, I, or II angina also benefited from surgery.

F. The Role of CABG in High-Risk Subgroups—These studies demonstrate that CABG can improve survival in certain high-risk subgroups of patients with CAD. The following sections consider these high-risk subgroups and compare the results of the three large randomized trials, the metaanalysis, and other observational studies. This topic is discussed in greater detail in a review by Nwasokwa (68).

1. Left Ventricular Function—LV function is possibly the most important independent predictor of mortality in medically managed patients with CAD (62,74). The survival benefit of CABG for patients with depressed LV function was demonstrated in two of the randomized studies (a nonsignificant trend in the VA trial, significant in CASS) and several nonrandomized studies. The European study included only patients with EF >50% (1,2,23,74,99). The metaanalysis showed the benefit to be equivalent regardless of LV function (98).

a. The results of the nonrandomized trials suggest that the survival benefit of CABG increases as the LV function decreases. For example, in one CASS registry study, the 6-year survival rate for patients with LV EF of 26% to 30% was 49% for medically treated patients, compared with 66% for CABG patients (P=0.0749) (2). For patients with LV EF of 3% to 25%, the benefit of CABG was even more pronounced (38% survival at 7 years for medically treated patients versus 62% for CABG patients; P=0.0056).

b. In the VA study, patients with left main CAD derived greater survival benefit from CABG if the LV function was also depressed (85). A CASS registry study found a survival benefit for all patients with left main CAD, with survival benefit increasing with worsening LV function (18).

c. In another CASS registry study, patients with three-vessel disease and CCS class III or IV angina derived greater benefit from CABG if the LV function

Table 8-6 Metaanalysis of CABG vs. Medical Therapy for CAD (98)

Time	Medical Therapy	CABG	*P*	Risk Reduction
5 Y	15.8%	10.2%	<0.0001	39%
7 Y	21.7%	15.8%	<0.001	32%
10 Y	30.5%	26.4%	0.03	17%

Table 8-7 Subgroup Analysis of Survival Benefit from CABG

Subgroup	5-Y Mortality Reduction	*P*
Vessels diseased		
One	46%	NS
Two	16%	NS
Three	42%	<0.001
Left main	68%	0.004
Proximal LAD disease		
One or two vessels	42%	0.05
Three vessels	39%	0.009
Left main	70%	0.02
Overall	32%	0.001
No LAD disease		
One or two vessels	None	NS
Three vessels	53%	0.02
Left main	73%	0.03
Overall	34%	0.05
LV function		
Normal	39%	<0.001
Abnormal	41%	0.02
Exercise test result		
Normal	22%	NS
Abnormal	48%	<0.001
Severity of angina		
Class 0, I, II	37%	0.005
Class III, IV	43%	0.001
Risk strata by risk score*		
Lowest tercile	None	NS
Middle tercile	37%	0.05
Highest tercile	50%	0.001

Adapted from Table 4 in Yusuf (98).
*Terciles defined as in the VA study.

was also depressed (45). In yet another CASS registry study, patients with proximal two-vessel disease derived survival benefit from CABG if the LV function was depressed but not if it was normal (63).

d. **Conclusion**—Depressed LV function probably increases the benefit of CABG in most patients with CAD. For patients with other factors already favoring surgery, the presence of LV dysfunction tends to magnify the potential benefit of CABG.

2. Number of Diseased Vessels

a. Three-Vessel Disease

(1) In the VA study, patients with three-vessel disease benefited from CABG only if they had poor LV function and were in the tercile at high clinical risk (89,23). Similarly, in the CASS trial, patients with three-vessel disease benefited from CABG if they also had depressed LV function (EF 34% to 50%) Patients with three-vessel disease and normal LV function did not benefit from CABG in terms of survival (72). Furthermore, in a nonrandomized CASS registry study, patients with three-vessel disease benefited from CABG only if they had CCS class III or IV angina, and not if they had CCS class I or II angina (45).

(2) However, in the European study, CABG improved survival in all patients with three-vessel disease. All patients in this study had EF ≥50% (30,94). At first glance, the results of the European study seem to be at odds with those of the other randomized studies. However, differences in study design may account for some of the discrepancies among the three trials. For example, 43% of the patients in the European study had CCS class III or IV angina, whereas the randomized CASS trial included only patients with CCS class 0, I, or II angina. Furthermore, patients in the VA study had a higher perioperative mortality rate, which prevents direct comparison with the European study.

(3) The 1994 metaanalysis demonstrated a survival benefit for all surgically treated patients with three-vessel disease (98).

(4) **Conclusion**—Most, if not all, patients with three-vessel disease probably benefit from surgery. The effect is most pronounced in patients with other high-risk characteristics, such as low EF or severe angina.

b. Two-Vessel Disease

(1) In the VA study, there was a slight survival disadvantage for surgically treated patients with two-vessel disease (89).

(2) In the European study, there was no significant benefit of CABG for patients with two-vessel disease despite the fact that 61% of these patients had proximal LAD stenosis (94). All patients in the study had LV EF >50%. Similarly, in the CASS randomized trial, there was no demonstrable benefit of CABG in any subgroup of patients with two-vessel disease (17).

(3) In contrast, a nonrandomized CASS registry study did show survival benefit in certain subgroups of patients with two-vessel disease (63). These subgroups included (a) patients with CCS class III or IV angina, at least one proximal lesion, and moderate LV dysfunction, and (b) patients with CCS class III or IV angina and severe LV dysfunction.

(4) The 1994 metaanalysis revealed a benefit only in the subgroup of patients with proximal LAD involvement (98).

(5) **Conclusion**—CABG improves survival only in highly selected patients with two-vessel disease.

c. Single-Vessel Disease

(1) Only the European Coronary Surgery study has shown a survival benefit for CABG in patients with single-vessel disease. The benefit was only observed in the subgroup with isolated proximal LAD disease (see below).

(2) In the metaanalysis, patients with isolated proximal LAD stenosis derived some survival benefit from surgery (98).

(3) **Conclusion**—Only a very small minority of patients with single-vessel disease derived survival benefit from surgery.

3. Location of CAD

a. Left Main CAD

(1) Left main CAD is important because it threatens the blood supply to the entire myocardial territory of the LAD and the left circumflex artery (68). Patients with left main CAD who are managed medically have a relatively poor prognosis (typically 41% to 65% survived at 4 years) (21,62,86). The VA study serves as the definitive study of patients with left main stenosis. The 42-month survival rate was 88% for surgery and 65% for medical treatment (P=0.016). The benefit was most pronounced for patients with impaired LV function and for those in the group at high clinical risk (86). The metaanalysis supports the results of the VA study (98).

(2) The 1981 CASS registry study reported similar findings. Most patients with left main CAD benefited from CABG, particularly those with severe left main stenosis, impaired LV function, or significant right coronary artery stenosis. However, not all patients with left main CAD benefited from CABG. In general, those with normal LV function, less severe left main stenosis, and balanced coronary circulation did not derive survival benefit from surgery (18).

(3) **Conclusion**—Most patients with left main CAD derive survival benefit with surgery. The benefit is greatest in those with LV dysfunction or concomitant right coronary artery disease.

b. **Left Main Equivalent Disease**—LMEQ disease refers to stenoses of both the proximal LAD artery (before the first major septal perforator) and the proximal left circumflex artery (before any obtuse marginals). This pattern of stenoses is worrisome because it threatens the same myocardial territory as does left main CAD.
   (1) In a Duke data bank study, the 5-year survival rates for medically treated patients were 39% for those with left main CAD, 51% for LMEQ disease, 66% for non-LMEQ three-vessel disease, and 86% for non-LMEQ two-vessel disease involving the LAD and left circumflex arteries (11). Similarly, both the VA study and a CASS registry survival study found the mortality rate of patients with LMEQ disease to be between the mortality rates for non-LMEQ three-vessel disease and for left main CAD (62,86).
   (2) In a CASS registry study that examined 903 patients with LMEQ disease, the 5-year survival rates were 85% for those who received CABG and 55% for those who received medical therapy ($P<0.001$) (19). Similar results were reported in another nonrandomized study (92).
   (3) **Conclusion**—CABG significantly improves survival in patients with LMEQ disease, but LMEQ disease is not prognostically equivalent to left main CAD.

c. **Proximal LAD Disease**—Disease of the proximal part of the LAD artery (before the first septal perforator) is the most important type of single-vessel disease (68). A Duke data bank study found that 5-year survival rates for patients with isolated LAD disease was 98% if the lesion was distal to the first septal perforator but only 90% if the lesion was proximal to the first septal perforator ($P=0.01$) (12). Another observational study found that 5-year mortality rates were much higher if the right coronary artery was diseased in addition to the proximal LAD artery (80).
   (1) The European study specifically examined the issue of proximal LAD disease (28,30). When all patients with proximal LAD disease were considered, a survival benefit of CABG was detected at 5, 8, and 10 years (76% survival at 10 years with surgery versus 65% with medical treatment; $P=0.007$). The corresponding survival rates were 81% and 83% for patients without proximal LAD disease.
   (2) The randomized CASS trial also addressed this question, but CABG did not improve survival in this subgroup of patients (1).
   (3) The metaanalysis found that all patients with proximal LAD disease, including those with one- or two-vessel CAD, experienced a survival benefit with CABG. In contrast, patients without proximal LAD disease derived a survival benefit only if they had three-vessel or left main CAD (98).
   (4) **Conclusion**—Proximal LAD disease represents a strong risk factor for premature death, and it is likely that most patients with proximal LAD disease derive survival benefit from CABG.

4. **Severity of CAD**—The severity of stenosis can be difficult to assess because angiographic measurements can be imprecise (68). Nevertheless, the benefit of CABG appears to increase with increasing severity of stenosis. In a 1978 Duke database study, patients with ≥70% left main stenosis had poorer survival at 1, 2, and 3 years, compared with patients with 50% to 70% left main stenosis (21). In a 1981 CASS registry study that examined 1492 patients with left main CAD, the 3-year survival rate with medical treatment decreased as the severity of left main CAD increased. In contrast, the survival rate with CABG was essentially constant across all severities of stenosis. Correspondingly, the benefit of CABG was greatest for patients with increasing severity of stenosis (18) (see Table 8–8).

5. **Severity of Angina**
   a. If the degree of LV dysfunction and the severity of CAD are comparable, medically treated patients with angina have twice the annual mortality rate of those without angina (5.4% versus 2.7%; $P<0.05$) (20).

Table 8-8 Severity of Left Main Artery Stenosis and Survival Benefit from CABG (18)

% of Left Main Stenosis	Percent Survival	
	Medical Therapy	CABG
50–59	73%	90%
60–69	54%	87%
70–79	63%	90%
≥80	49%	86%

- **b.** In a 1985 CASS registry study that examined 4209 patients stratified according to the severity of angina, CABG improved survival in patients with CCS class III or IV angina and three-vessel disease. In contrast, CABG did not improve survival in patients with CCS class I or II angina, even in those with LV dysfunction and three-vessel disease (45).
- **c.** In the metaanalysis, the severity of angina did not have any impact on the benefit of surgery (98).
- **d.** **Conclusion**—Patients with more severe angina probably derive greater survival benefit from CABG, compared with patients with less severe angina.

6. Stress Testing

- **a.** Several studies have demonstrated that an abnormal stress test is a predictor of high mortality with medical therapy. In a 1984 CASS registry study of medically treated patients, patients with ≥1 mm ST depression and exercise limit at Bruce stage 1 (high-risk group) had an annual mortality rate of 5%, compared with those with <1 mm ST depression and exercise limit at Bruce stage 3 or higher (low-risk group), who had an annual mortality rate of less than 1% (95). Similarly, in a study of patients with three-vessel disease and normal LV function, a subgroup of patients with ST depression ≥1 mm, decreased EF during exercise, and exercise tolerance ≤120 W had a higher mortality rate with medical management than those without these features (8).
- **b.** In the European study, patients with >1.5 mm ST depression on stress testing had an 8-year survival rate of 90% with surgery versus 77% with medical management ($P<0.0003$) (30). Patients with ≤1 mm ST depression on stress testing had 8-year survival rates of 88% and 85%, respectively ($P>0.20$). Similarly, a 1986 CASS registry study demonstrated that the degree of ST depression during stress testing correlated with the likelihood of deriving survival benefit from CABG (96).
- **c.** In the randomized CASS trial, stratification of patients by exercise capacity and ECG findings during stress testing did not identify any subgroup who derived a survival benefit from CABG. However, CABG did improve survival in the subset of patients with exercise-induced angina (79).
- **d.** In the metaanalysis, the reduction in mortality at 5 years with CABG was 48% for patients with an abnormal stress test, compared with 22% for those with a normal stress test (98).
- **e.** **Conclusion**—Patients with an abnormal exercise test are more likely to benefit from CABG than those with a normal exercise test.

7. Clinical and Demographic Risk Factors

- **a.** **Age**—Older age adversely affects survival in medically treated patients with CAD (18,35,94). On the other hand, older age also increases the likelihood of perioperative death (64,44).
  - **(1)** For patients older than 47 years of age in the European study, the 10-year survival rate was 79% for both treatment groups. In comparison, for patients older than 53 years of age, the 10-year survival rate was 56% with medical therapy versus 72% with CABG ($P=0.01$) (94).

(2) Because none of the randomized trials included patients older than 65 years of age, only observational data are available for this age group. In a CASS registry study, CABG improved survival for patients of all age groups up to 74 years. CABG also improved survival in patients older than 74 years, but the difference was not statistically significant (35) (see Table 8–9).

(3) **Conclusion**—Although older patients have a higher risk of perioperative death, CABG appears to improve survival in all age groups.

b. **Gender**—Of the three large randomized trials, only CASS included women, and women represented only 10% of that study population (17). Therefore, data on the survival benefit of CABG for women with CAD is extremely limited and must be inferred from other studies (68).

(1) Data from numerous studies suggest that perioperative mortality is higher for women than for men (7,24,26,33,34,38,39,49,55,69,75,78,97).

(2) Studies also show that mortality during and after an MI is twice as high for women as it is for men (37,46).

(3) **Conclusion**—Very little information is available about the effect of gender on the potential survival benefit of CABG.

c. **Peripheral Vascular Disease**

(1) In the European study, the subgroup of patients with peripheral vascular disease had a greater survival benefit from CABG than those without peripheral vascular disease (94). The extent of CAD did not differ significantly between those with and without peripheral vascular disease.

(2) **Conclusion**—The presence of peripheral vascular disease may identify a subgroup of patients who derive increased benefit from CABG. The reason for this is unclear, although it is possible that peripheral vascular disease may be a marker of more aggressive CAD or of small-vessel disease (68).

d. **Baseline ECG Abnormalities**

(1) In the VA study, which stratified patients into risk terciles using resting ST depression and other clinical variables, those in the tercile at highest risk benefited most from surgery (22).

(2) Similarly, in the European study, a survival benefit was found in patients with both normal and abnormal ECGs, but the benefit was greater for those with ≥0.5 mm ST depression, T-wave inversion, or abnormal Q waves (94).

(3) **Conclusion**—Patients with baseline ECG abnormalities are more likely to obtain survival benefit from CABG than those with a normal baseline ECG.

G. **Perioperative Mortality**—In the three major randomized trials, the perioperative mortality rates for CABG ranged from 1.4% to 5.8% (17,30,89). In more recent studies, the perioperative mortality rates have been in the range of 1% to 2.5% for elective operations (76). However, the total perioperative mortality rate for CABG has increased since the 1970s because the number of emergency operations and number of high-risk patients undergoing CABG have substantially increased (35,66).

Table 8-9 Age and Survival Benefit from CABG (35)

	6-Y Survival Rate		
Age Group (y)	Medical Therapy	CABG	*P*
65–69	67%	81%	<0.0001
70–74	51%	77%	<0.0001
≥75	56%	75%	<0.14

1. Based on data from 500 patients, the Montreal Heart Institute developed a scoring system in 1983 to predict the risk of death for patients undergoing CABG or valve procedures (70). The predictors of perioperative death were LV dysfunction, unstable angina, recent MI, congestive heart failure, age greater than 65 years, emergency surgery, reoperation, and severe obesity. Other studies have found similar risk factors for perioperative death (40,42,47,53,58,71).
2. In a 1994 Australian study involving 12,003 CABG patients from a single surgical unit, the predictors of perioperative mortality included older age, female gender, depressed LV function, unstable angina, and prolonged bypass time (44). A very strong relation between mortality and perfusion time was demonstrated. The mortality rate was 0.63% for patients with a mean bypass time of 48 minutes, compared with 10.3% for those with a mean bypass time of 100 minutes. The overall mortality rate in the study was 0.99%.
3. In 1992, a clinical severity score for predicting perioperative outcome was developed based on data from 5051 CABG patients (43). This retrospective analysis used univariate and logistic regression to identify risk factors associated with perioperative mortality and morbidity.
   a. The risk factors are listed in Table 8–10. The first nine factors were predictive of mortality, while the last four factors were predictive of morbidity. A scoring system was developed using these 13 factors.
   b. The score was then prospectively validated on a cohort of 4069 patients for prediction of mortality. The maximum possible score was 31, but the maximum observed score was 18. For mortality, the threshold score with the highest sensitivity and specificity was 6. Approximate predicted and observed mortality rates are listed in Table 8–11 by clinical severity score. This model did not validate prospectively for morbidity.
4. **Effect of Gender**—One issue that deserves special mention is the effect of gender on perioperative mortality for CABG. This issue has been reviewed at length by Findlay (32).
   a. Excess mortality among women undergoing CABG, compared with men, has been known since at least 1975 (7). Two large studies reported perioperative mortality odds ratios of 1.79 to 2.13 for women compared with men (44,97). Numerous other studies have confirmed this finding (24,33,34,38, 39,48,49,55,69,75,78), including the Society of Thoracic Surgeons National

Table 8-10 Predictors of Perioperative Mortality and Morbidity for CABG (43)

Preoperative Factors	Score
Emergency operation	6
Serum creatinine	
≥1.6 but ≤1.8 mg/dl	1
≥1.9 mg/dl	4
Severe LV dysfunction	3
Reoperation	3
Operative mitral valve insufficiency	3
Age	
≥65 and ≤74 y	1
Age ≥75 y	2
Prior vascular surgery	2
COPD	2
Anemia (hematocrit ≤0.34)	2
Operative aortic valve stenosis	1
Weight ≤65 kg	1
Diabetes mellitus	1
Cerebrovascular disease	1

Table 8-11 System for Prediction of Perioperative Mortality for CABG (43)

Clinical Severity Score	Predicted Mortality	Observed Mortality
0	<1%	<1%
1–3	1%	1–2%
4–5	2%	2–3%
6	6%	4%
7–9	10%	7%
≥10	22%	28%

Cardiac Surgery Database study (26), a registry of 80,881 patients who underwent CABG in 1989 and 1990.

b. Although the adverse risk of female gender is well established, the reason for this finding is still unclear. Numerous hypotheses have been proposed and are summarized in the following sections.

(1) A large number of studies have shown that women are more likely to have other baseline characteristics that may increase the operative risk. In general, compared with men, women undergoing CABG tend to be older and smaller; are more likely to have diabetes, hypertension, angina, or unstable symptoms; and more often require emergency surgery. On the other hand, they are less likely to have LV dysfunction or severe CAD, compared with men (32,33,55,69,75,97).

(2) Several authors have suggested that, after matching for body surface area, gender is not an important predictor of mortality. For example, a CASS study found a direct relation between physical size and coronary artery diameter and an inverse relation between these variables and operative mortality (33). Furthermore, in a study of 3055 CABG patients, coronary arterial luminal diameter was directly related to body surface area and inversely related to the mortality risk in both men and women. In fact, mortality was no longer associated with gender after patients were matched by body surface area (69). In another study, gender also did not predict operative mortality after matching for body surface area (55).

(3) A small Swedish study suggested that the excess mortality among women may be caused by a higher incidence of small-vessel disease in women (77).

(4) In the Society of Thoracic Surgeons National Cardiac Surgery Database, women were less likely to receive IMA grafts (38% versus 52%). The operative mortality is significantly lower with the use of IMA grafts in both men and women (27).

(5) A higher rate of SVG closure has been observed in women than in men (7,24,55,93).

(6) Finally, several studies have suggested that a referral and treatment bias against women exists. (3,82,91) However, some studies have suggested other explanations for the delay in referral of women for CABG (6,60).

c. Despite the fact that women have a higher operative mortality, most studies have found no difference in long-term survival after CABG between men and women (25,38,50,54,55). Rahimtoola reported a small difference in the 18-year survival rate between men and women (42% versus 37%). The difference was most pronounced in women with three-vessel disease and LV dysfunction, whose 10-year survival rate was 53%, compared with 65% for men with similar conditions (75).

5. The various factors associated with increased mortality after CABG are summarized in Table 8–12. SVGs are included because patients who receive IMA grafts have a lower mortality rate than patients who receive only SVGs (27).

H. Limitations of the Available Data

1. Both PRCTs and large nonrandomized observational studies offer information on the benefits of CABG for patients with CAD, and both have advantages and disadvantages. The best information probably comes from a synthesis of data from these two sources (13).
   a. In general, PRCTs have important strengths, including minimization of the effects of known and unknown confounding variables. On the other hand, the crossover rate to CABG for patients assigned to medical therapy was approximately 40% by 10 to 12 years in all three studies. As a result, these trials are best regarded as a comparison between the two different initial management strategies: immediate surgery versus initial medical management with surgery reserved for failure of medical therapy. Furthermore, these studies examined only highly selected groups of patients. Many important groups were excluded or under represented, such as women, minorities, patients older than 65 years of age, and patients with moderate to severe angina, new-onset angina, recent MI, or severe LV dysfunction (68). One editorial estimated that only 4% to 13% of patients referred for cardiac catheterization would have been eligible for one of these trials (14). Therefore, the results are not necessarily generalizable to the entire population. Furthermore, because of the difficulty and expense, randomized studies tend to be smaller than registry studies and therefore do not always have the power to detect small but significant differences in outcome. Finally, these studies were begun 20 to 25 years ago and do not represent the current state of medical and surgical practice (see later discussion).
   b. The main advantage of registry studies is the ability to evaluate very large numbers of patients who are more representative of the general population with CAD. In addition, registry data better reflect the changes in medical and surgical practice with time. However, because these patients are not randomly assigned to the treatments under study, the data are subject to significant selection bias and do not adequately control for differences in the distribution of confounding variables such as LV function, severity of CAD, and severity of angina (2,13,18). Whenever possible, statistical analysis was used to adjust for these variables.
2. As stated previously, one of the main limitations of the randomized trials is that they were conducted at a time when medical and surgical treatments were different than they are today. Numerous advances have been made in both surgical and medical management of CAD since the time of these trials.
   a. Perhaps the most striking and important advance is the use of IMA for bypass grafting.
      (1) The IMA grafts are associated with a higher patency rate, a lower perioperative mortality rate, and a higher long-term survival rate. The 10-year patency rate for SVGs ranges from 40% to 60% (9,16,56). There is a 2% per year vein-graft attrition rate in the first seven postoperative years and a 5% per year attrition rate in years 7 through 12 (16). In con-

Table 8-12 Factors Associated with Increased Mortality after CABG

Cardiac Factors	Operative Factors	Comorbid Conditions	Other Factors
Unstable angina	Reoperation	Severe obesity	Female gender
LV dysfunction	Emergency surgery	Poor renal function	Age
Recent MI	Prolonged pump time	Diabetes	Weight ≤65 kg
Congestive heart failure	Saphenous vein grafts	COPD	
Valvular heart disease		Anemia	
		Cerebrovascular disease	

trast, the IMA graft has a 10-year patency rate of 90% (4,59,81,88). One study found a 100% patency rate in 15 patients at 15 to 21 years (5).

(2) In addition, the perioperative mortality rates are lower with IMA grafts than with SVG. In 1994, the Society of Thoracic Surgeons National Cardiac Surgery Database reported a 2% mortality rate for 18,614 patients who received at least one IMA graft, compared with a 4.5% mortality rate for 19,964 patients who received only SVGs (27).

(3) The use of IMA grafts is also associated with higher long-term survival. In an observational study comparing 2306 patients who received an IMA graft (alone or combined with SVGs) versus 3625 patients who received SVGs only, the 10-year survival rate was significantly better for the former group. The risks of late MI, hospitalization for cardiac events, and cardiac reoperation were all lower for patients receiving IMA grafts (57). In a CASS registry study, the 7-year survival rate was 90% for those who received an IMA graft, compared with 80% for those who did not (15). In a recent observational study that compared 100 consecutive patients who received an IMA graft with 100 consecutive patients who received an SVG for LAD disease, the 18-year survival rate was superior for those who received an IMA graft (10).

b. Another important advance has been the advent of percutaneous transluminal coronary angioplasty. This topic is discussed in detail in chapter 7.

c. Other improvements in surgical techniques, myocardial protection, cardiac anesthesia, and postoperative intensive care have resulted in lower perioperative mortality.

d. Furthermore, advances in medical therapy have improved long-term management of all patients with CAD, including post-CABG patients. These advances include the use of platelet inhibitors, β-blockers, angiotensin-converting enzyme inhibitors, and lipid-lowering agents, when appropriate.

e. There is some evidence to suggest that the advances in surgical technique have had more of an impact on survival than advances in medical therapy for patients with CAD. An observational study using the Duke database compared the hazard ratios of medical versus surgical treatment in 1970, 1977, and 1984 and found that the relative benefit of surgery over medical therapy became more pronounced over time (13).

I. Conclusion

1. There is compelling evidence that CABG improves survival in selected patients with CAD. By integrating the results of the major randomized trials, the meta-analysis, and various observational studies, it is possible to identify preoperative factors that predict survival benefit from CABG. These are summarized in Table 8–13. Other clinical factors such as stress test findings, severity of stenosis, severity of angina, baseline ECG findings, and comorbid conditions may modify the level of benefit derived from surgery.

2. The operative mortality rate in the three major randomized studies ranged from 1.4% to 5.8%. Predictors of perioperative death include unstable angina, LV dysfunction, recent MI, congestive heart failure, valvular heart disease, reoperation, emergency surgery, prolonged bypass pump time, severe obesity, poor renal function, chronic obstructive pulmonary disease, anemia, stroke, female gender, older age, and weight <65 kg.

Table 8-13 Summary: Survival Benefit from CABG

Variable	Survival Benefit
Three-vessel disease	Most, if not all, patients benefit
With low EF	Yes
With class III or IV angina	Yes
Two-vessel disease	Only highly selected patients benefit
With proximal LAD disease	Yes
With class III/IV angina, one proximal lesion, and moderate LV dysfunction	Yes
With class III/IV angina and severe LV dysfunction	Yes
One-vessel disease	Generally no benefit
With proximal LAD disease	Possible benefit
Left ventricular function	
Normal	Only selected patients benefit
Abnormal	Majority of patients benefit
Location of CAD	
Left main disease	Almost all patients benefit
Left main equivalent disease	Almost all patients benefit, but less than with left main disease
Proximal LAD disease	Most benefit

Abbreviations used in Chapter 8

CABG = coronary arterial bypass graft
CASS = Coronary Artery Surgery Study
CAD = coronary artery disease
CCS = Canadian Cardiovascular Society
ECG = electrocardiogram, electrocardiographic
EF = ejection fraction
IMA = internal mammary artery
LAD = left anterior descending
LMEQ = left main equivalent
LV = left ventricular
MI = myocardial infarction
NS = not significant
P = probability value
PRCT = prospective randomized controlled trial
SVG = saphenous vein graft
VA = Veterans Administration

References

1. Alderman. Ten-year follow-up of survival and myocardial infarction in the randomized Coronary Artery Surgery Study. *Circulation* 1990;82:1629.
2. Alderman. Results of coronary artery surgery in patients with poor left ventricular function (CASS). *Circulation* 1983;68:785.
3. Ayanian. Differences in the use of procedures between women and men hospitalized for coronary heart disease. *N Engl J Med* 1991;325:221.
4. Barner. Late patency of the internal mammary artery as a coronary bypass conduit. *Ann Thorac Surg* 1982;34:408.

5. Barner. Fifteen-to twenty-one-year angiographic assessment of internal thoracic artery as a bypass conduit. *Ann Thorac Surg* 1994;57:1526.
6. Bickell. Referral patterns for coronary artery disease treatment: gender bias or good clinical judgment? *Ann Intern Med* 1992;116:791.
7. Bolooki. Results of direct coronary artery surgery in women. *J Thorac Cardiovasc Surg* 1975;69:271.
8. Bonow. Exercise-induced ischemia in mildly symptomatic patients with coronary artery disease and preserved left ventricular function: identification of subgroups at risk of death with medical therapy. *N Engl J Med* 1984;311:1339.
9. Bourassa. Progression of atherosclerosis in coronary arteries and bypass grafts: ten years later. *Am J Cardiol* 1984;53:102C.
10. Boylan. Surgical treatment of isolated left anterior descending artery coronary stenosis: comparison of left internal mammary artery and venous autograft at 18 to 20 years of follow-up. *J Thorac Cardiovasc Surg* 1994;107:657.
11. Califf. "Left main equivalent" coronary artery disease: its clinical presentation and prognostic significance with nonsurgical therapy. *Am J Cardiol* 1984;53:1489.
12. Califf. Outcome in one-vessel coronary artery disease. *Circulation* 1983;67:283.
13. Califf. The evolution of medical and surgical therapy for coronary artery disease: a 15-year perspective. *JAMA* 1989;261:2077.
14. Califf. Beyond randomized clinical trials: applying clinical experience in the treatment of patients with coronary artery disease. *Circulation* 1986;74:1191. Editorial.
15. Cameron. Clinical implications of internal mammary artery bypass grafts: the Coronary Artery Surgery Study experience. *Circulation* 1988;77:815.
16. Campeau. The relation of risk factors to the development of atherosclerosis in saphenous-vein bypass grafts and the progression of disease in the native circulation: a study 10 years after aortocoronary bypass surgery. *N Engl J Med* 1984; 311:1329.
17. CASS Principal Investigators. Coronary Artery Surgery Study (CASS): a randomized trial of coronary artery bypass surgery. Survival data. *Circulation* 1983;68: 939.
18. Chaitman. Effect of coronary bypass surgery on survival patterns in subsets of patients with left main coronary artery disease: report of the Collaborative Study in Coronary Artery Surgery (CASS). *Am J Cardiol* 1981;48:765.
19. Chaitman. The role of coronary bypass surgery for "left main equivalent" coronary disease: the Coronary Artery Surgery Study registry. *Circulation* 1986;74(Suppl III):17.
20. Cohn. Prognostic importance of anginal symptoms in angiographically defined coronary artery disease. *Am J Cardiol* 1981;47:233.
21. Conley. The prognostic spectrum of left main stenosis. *Circulation* 1978;57:947.
22. Detre. The VA Cooperative Study Group for Surgery for Coronary Arterial Occlusive Disease: effect of bypass surgery on survival of patients in low- and high-risk subgroups delineated by the use of simple clinical variables. *Circulation* 1981;63: 1329.
23. Detre. Veterans Administration Cooperative Study of medical versus surgical treatment for stable angina: progress report. Section 4: Long-term survival results in medically and surgically randomized patients. *Prog Cardiovasc Dis* 1985;28:235.
24. Douglas. Reduced efficacy of coronary bypass surgery in women. *Circulation* 1981;64(Suppl 2):II-11.
25. Eaker. Comparison of the long-term, postsurgical survival of women and men in the Coronary Artery Bypass Surgery study (CASS). *Am Heart J* 1989;117:71.
26. Edwards. Coronary artery bypass grafting: the Society of Thoracic Surgeons National Database experience. *Ann Thorac Surg* 1994;57:12.
27. Edwards. Impact of internal mammary artery conduits on operative mortality of coronary revascularization. *Ann Thorac Surg* 1994;57:20.
28. European Coronary Surgery Study Group. Prospective randomised study of coronary artery bypass surgery in stable angina pectoris. *Lancet* 1980;2:491.
29. European Coronary Surgery Study Group. Coronary-artery bypass surgery in stable angina pectoris: survival at two years. *Lancet* 1979;i:889.

30. European Coronary Surgery Study Group. Long-term results of prospective randomised study of coronary artery bypass surgery in stable angina pectoris. *Lancet* 1982;2:1173.
31. Favalaro. Saphenous vein autograft replacement of several segmental coronary artery occlusions: operative technique. *Ann Thorac Surg* 1968;5:334.
32. Findlay. Coronary bypass surgery in women. *Curr Opin Cardiol* 1994;9:650.
33. Fisher. Association of sex, physical size, and operative mortality after coronary bypass in the Coronary Artery Surgery Study (CASS). *J Thorac Cardiovasc Surg* 1982; 84:334.
34. Gardner. Coronary artery bypass grafting in women. *Ann Thorac Surg* 1985;201: 780.
35. Gersh. Comparison of coronary artery bypass surgery and medical therapy in patients 65 years of age or older: a nonrandomized study from the Coronary Artery Surgery Study (CASS) registry. *N Engl J Med* 1985;313:217.
36. Gersh. The changing patient population and results of coronary bypass surgery. *Curr Opin Cardiol* 1988;3:894.
37. Gruppo Italiano per lo Studio della Streptochinasi nell'Infarto Miocardico (GISSI). Effectiveness of intravenous thrombolytic treatment in acute myocardial infarction. *Lancet* 1986;1:397.
38. Hall. Coronary artery bypass: long-term follow-up of 22,284 consecutive patients. *Circulation* 1983;68:20.
39. Hannan. Gender differences in mortality rates for coronary artery bypass patients. *Am Heart J* 1992;123:866.
40. Hannan. Adult open-heart surgery in New York state: an analysis of risk factors and hospital mortality rates. *JAMA* 1991;264:2768.
41. Harris. Survival in medically treated coronary artery disease. *Circulation* 1979;60: 1259.
42. Higgins. Risk stratification and outcome assessment of the adult cardiac surgical patient. *Semin Thorac Cardiovasc Surg* 1991;3:111.
43. Higgins. Stratification of morbidity and mortality outcome by preoperative risk factors in coronary artery bypass patients: a clinical severity score. *JAMA* 1992; 267:2344.
44. Iyer. Mortality and myocardial infarction after coronary artery surgery: a review of 12,003 patients. *Med J Aust* 1994;159:166.
45. Kaiser. Survival following coronary artery bypass grafting in patients with severe angina pectoris (CASS): an observational study. *J Thorac Cardiovasc Surg* 1985; 89:513.
46. Kannel. Prognosis after initial myocardial infarction: the Framingham study. *Am J Cardiol* 1979;44:53.
47. Kennedy. Multivariate discriminant analysis of the clinical and angiographic predictors of operative mortality from the Collaborative Study in Coronary Artery Surgery (CASS). *J Thorac Cardiovasc Surg* 1980;80:876.
48. Kennedy. Clinical and angiographic predictors of operative mortality from the Collaborative Study in Coronary Artery Surgery (CASS). *Circulation* 1981;63:793.
49. Khan. Increased mortality of women in coronary artery bypass surgery: evidence for referral bias. *Ann Intern Med* 1990;112:561.
50. Killen. Coronary artery bypass in women: long-term survival. *Ann Thorac Surg* 1982; 34:559.
51. Killip. The National Heart, Lung, and Blood Institute Coronary Artery Surgery Study (CASS). *Circulation* 1981;63(Suppl 1):I-1.
52. Kloster. Coronary bypass for stable angina. *N Engl J Med* 1979;300:149.
53. Kouchoukos. Coronary bypass surgery: analysis of factors affecting hospital mortality. *Circulation* 1980;62:84.
54. Lawrie. Long-term results of coronary bypass surgery. *Ann Surg* 1991;213:377.
55. Loop. Coronary artery surgery in women compared with men: analyses of risks and long-term results. *J Am Coll Cardiol* 1983;1:383.
56. Loop. New arteries for old. *Circulation* 1989;79(Suppl I):I-40.
57. Loop. Influence of the internal mammary artery graft on 10-year survival and other cardiac events. *N Engl J Med* 1986;314:1.

58. Lytle. Fifteen hundred coronary reoperations: results and determinants of early and late survival. *J Thorac Cardiovasc Surg* 1987;93:847.
59. Lytle. Long-term (5 to 12 years) serial studies of internal mammary artery and saphenous vein coronary bypass grafts. *J Thorac Cardiovasc Surg* 1985;89:248.
60. Mark. Absence of sex bias in the referral of patients for cardiac catheterization. *N Engl J Med* 1994;330:1101.
61. Mathur. Prospective randomized study of the surgical therapy of stable angina. *Cardiovasc Clin* 1977;8:131.
62. Mock. Survival of medically treated patients in the Coronary Artery Surgery Study (CASS) registry. *Circulation* 1982;66:562.
63. Mock. Comparison of effects of medical and surgical therapy on survival in severe angina pectoris and two-vessel coronary artery disease with and without left ventricular dysfunction: a Coronary Artery Surgery Study registry study. *Am J Cardiol* 1988;61:1198.
64. Mohan. Coronary artery bypass grafting in the elderly: a review of studies on patients older than 64, 69, or 74 years. *Cardiology* 1992;80:215.
65. Murphy. Treatment of chronic stable angina: a preliminary report of survival data of the randomized Veterans Administration Cooperative Study. *N Engl J Med* 1977; 297:621.
66. Naunheim. The changing profile of the patient undergoing coronary artery bypass surgery. *J Am Coll Cardiol* 1988;11:494.
67. Norris. Coronary surgery after recurrent myocardial infarction: progress of a trial comparing surgical with nonsurgical management for asymptomatic patients with advanced coronary disease. *Circulation* 1981;63:785.
68. Nwasokwa. Bypass surgery for chronic stable angina: predictors of survival benefit and strategy for patient selection. *Ann Intern Med* 1991;114:1035.
69. O'Connor. Differences between men and women in hospital mortality associated with coronary artery bypass graft surgery. *Circulation* 1993;88:2104.
70. Paiement. A simple classification of the risk in cardiac surgery. *Can J Anesth* 1983;30:61.
71. Parsonnet. A method of uniform stratification of risk for evaluating the results of surgery in acquired adult heart disease. *Circulation* 1989;79(Suppl I):I-3.
72. Passamani. A randomized trial of coronary artery bypass surgery: survival of patients with low ejection fraction. *N Engl J Med* 1985;312:1665.
73. Peduzzi. Veterans Administration Cooperative Study of medical versus surgical treatment for stable angina: progress report. Section 2: Design and baseline characteristics. *Prog Cardiovasc Dis* 1985;28:219.
74. Pigott. Late results of surgical and medical therapy for patients with coronary artery disease and depressed left ventricular function. *J Am Coll Cardiol* 1985;5: 1036.
75. Rahimtoola. Survival at 15 to 18 years after coronary bypass surgery for angina in women. *Circulation* 1993;88:71.
76. Rahimtoola. Coronary bypass surgery for chronic angina, 1981: a perspective. *Circulation* 1982;65:225.
77. Ramström. Multiarterial coronary artery bypass grafting with special reference to small vessel disease and results in women. *Eur Heart J* 1993;14:634.
78. Richardson. Reduced efficacy of coronary artery bypass grafting in women. *Ann Thorac Surg* 1986;42:S16.
79. Ryan. Exercise testing in the Coronary Artery Surgery Study randomized population. *Circulation* 1985;72:V31.
80. Samaha. Natural history of left anterior descending artery obstruction: significance of location of stenoses in medically treated patients. *Clin Cardiol* 1985;8: 415.
81. Singh. Long-term fate of the internal mammary artery saphenous vein grafts. *J Thorac Cardiovasc Surg* 1983;86:359.
82. Steingart. Sex differences in the management of coronary artery disease. *N Engl J Med* 1991;325:226.
83. Takaro. Cooperative study of surgery for coronary arterial occlusive disease: results of a randomized study of medical and surgical management of angina pectoris. *World J Surg* 1978;2:797.

84. Takaro. Veterans Administration Cooperative Study of medical versus surgical treatment for stable angina: progress report. Section 1: Historic perspective. *Prog Cardiovasc Dis* 1985;23:213.
85. Takaro. The VA Cooperative Randomized Study of surgery for coronary arterial occlusive disease: II. Subgroup with significant left main lesions. *Circulation* 1976; 54(Suppl III):107.
86. Takaro. Veterans Administration Cooperative Study of medical versus surgical treatment for stable angina: progress report. Section 3: Left main coronary artery disease. *Prog Cardiovasc Dis* 1985;28:229.
87. Takaro. Survival in subgroups of patients with left main coronary artery disease: Veterans Administration Cooperative Study of Surgery for Coronary Artery Occlusive Disease. *Circulation* 1982;66:14.
88. Tector. The internal mammary artery graft: its longevity after coronary bypass. *JAMA* 1981;246:2181.
89. The Veterans Administration Coronary Artery Bypass Surgery Cooperative Study Group. Eleven-year survival in the Veterans Administration randomized trial of coronary artery bypass surgery for stable angina. *N Engl J Med* 1984;311:1333.
90. The Veterans Administration Coronary Artery Bypass Surgery Cooperative Study Group. Eighteen-year follow-up in the Veterans Affairs Cooperative Study of Coronary Artery Bypass Surgery for stable angina. *Circulation* 1992;86:121.
91. Tobin. Sex bias in considering coronary bypass surgery. *Ann Intern Med* 1987; 107:19.
92. Tyras. Left main equivalent: results of medical and surgical therapy. *Circulation* 1981; 64:II-7.
93. Tyras. Myocardial revascularization in women. *Ann Thorac Surg* 1978;25:448.
94. Varnauskas. Twelve-year follow-up of survival in the randomized European Coronary Surgery Study. *N Engl J Med* 1988;319:332.
95. Weiner. Prognostic importance of a clinical profile and exercise test in medically treated patients with coronary artery disease. *J Am Coll Cardiol* 1984;3:772.
96. Weiner. The role of exercise testing in identifying patients with improved survival after coronary artery bypass surgery. *J Am Coll Cardiol* 1986;8:741.
97. Weintraub. Changing clinical characteristics of coronary surgery patients: differences between men and women. *Circulation* 1993;88:79.
98. Yusuf. Effect of coronary artery bypass graft surgery on survival: overview of 10-year results from randomised trials by the Coronary Artery Bypass Graft Surgery Trialists Collaboration. *Lancet* 1994;344:563.
99. Zubiate. Myocardial revascularization for patients with an ejection fraction of 0.2 or less. *West J Med* 1984;140:745.

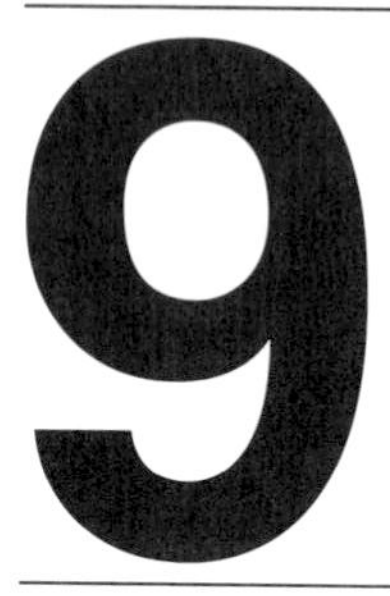

Management of Acute Asthma

David G. Morris and B. Taylor Thompson

A. Introduction

1. Definition of Asthma

a. Asthma is a chronic, intermittent, inflammatory disease of the airways that is characterized by exacerbations of coughing, wheezing, chest tightness, and difficulty in breathing. It is usually reversible, but can be severe and is sometimes fatal (43).

b. Status asthmaticus is an extreme form of asthma that is incompletely responsive to aggressive initial therapy. It can occur in any patient with underlying asthma, including those with previously mild disease.

c. Airway obstruction from asthma is differentiated from that caused by chronic obstructive pulmonary disease (COPD) by being completely or almost completely reversible with treatment. Most asthmatics are asymptomatic between flares, and many have no demonstrable airflow obstruction at those times. In contrast, COPD is defined by a fixed, structural bronchiolar obstruction to airflow that is not reversible with optimal treatment. However, chronic, severe asthma may be associated with structural changes in the airways that also result in fixed obstruction. Furthermore, some patients with COPD may also have a reversible component of airway obstruction (so-called chronic asthmatic bronchitis).

2. Epidemiology and Economics of Asthma

a. Asthma is common. Approximately 4% to 5% of the US population is affected. Deaths attributable to asthma appear to be increasing in frequency in the United States, especially among the medically underserved and the ethnic minority populations (9,20,69).

b. Asthma is expensive. Exacerbations of asthma frequently lead to emergency department visits and hospitalizations. The estimated cost of asthma in 1990 was $6.2 billion, with 25% of the total expense being directly related to hospitalization (69).

B. Pathogenesis of Asthma

1. **Inflammation**—Asthma results primarily from submucosal inflammation and associated smooth muscle hyperirritability of the airways. Inflammation may be precipitated by an exposure to allergens, certain dusts, chemical agents, or other unidentified factors. There are several mediators of inflammation. Inflammatory cells, including eosinophils, monocytes, and lymphocytes, have been observed in bronchial biopsies from asthmatics, even from those with mild disease (3,8). In addition, the level of immunoglobulin E (IgE) is elevated in asthmatic patients, suggesting that there is chronic activation of IgE-based humoral immunity (10). Finally, during acute exacerbations of asthma, the levels of leukotrienes and their metabolites are elevated in urine, bronchoalveolar lavage fluid, and plasma (15).

2. **Neural Activity**—The airways enjoy rich autonomic innervation. Animal data suggest that the activation of inflammatory cells and the release of inflammatory mediators (*e.g.*, leukotrienes, bradykinin) alter the depolarization thresholds of intrinsic neurons (C fibers) in the bronchi and the bronchioles. A partial depolarization of these neurons may cause increased irritability of the airways.

Minor additional stimulation of the neurons may lead to bronchial smooth muscle contraction and airway obstruction (67). In addition, a defective transduction of endogenous epinephrine and norepinephrine could play a role in persistent bronchospasm. A defective β_2-adrenergic receptor has been identified in few asthmatic patients (53). The clinical significance of these findings and the roles of acetylcholine and other neurotransmitters (*e.g.*, substance P, neurokinin A) remain the subject of active investigation (3,67).

3. **Infection**—Viral respiratory tract infections are common precipitants of asthma exacerbations. A British study revealed that colds were reported in 80% of adults with asthma at the onset of wheezing and breathlessness. Seventy-two percent of asthmatic patients had a significant (≥25 L/minute) decline in peak expiratory flow rate (PEFR) during nonbacterial infections. Causative agents can include rhinoviruses, coronaviruses, influenza B, respiratory syncytial virus, and parainfluenza viruses (5,21,29,44). Bacterial or chlamydial bronchitis also can precipitate bronchospasm but is much less common. Bronchial hyperirritability may persist for several weeks after infection and may be a result of persistent low-grade inflammation. Whether a single episode of a viral infection can induce a persistent inflammatory reaction in the airways and chronic asthma is controversial.

C. Clinical Diagnosis and Evaluation of Asthma

1. History

a. **Differential Diagnosis of Acute Asthma**—In order to avoid inappropriate therapy, the initial evaluation of a patient with wheezing must include a consideration of the differential diagnosis of asthma. Alternative diagnoses include pneumonia, bronchitis, pulmonary edema, anaphylaxis, aspiration of oral or gastric contents, upper airway obstruction (*i.e.*, tracheal tumors), chemical inhalation, airway burns, and laryngospasm (stridor can be mistaken clinically for wheezing). Rarely, laryngeal tumors, recurrent pulmonary embolism, pulmonary vasculitis, allergic aspergillosis, or eosinophilic pneumonia may mimic asthma (11,36,56). New-onset asthma in an adult is uncommon, and underlying illnesses such as COPD, pneumonia, or congestive heart failure should be strongly considered in these patients.

b. **Classification of Asthma**—As summarized in Table 9–1, asthma is classified into three general categories (mild, moderate, and severe) based on clinical characteristics (43).

c. **Evaluation of Short-Term Prognosis**—Certain key historical information obtained before initiation of therapy provides prognostic information and serves as an objective marker of severe asthma.

   (1) A prior history of intubation or life-threatening asthma is a poor prognostic factor. Multiple studies verify that prior intubation is both a predictor of future intubation and a marker for near-fatal or fatal asthma. In a case-control study, Rea reviewed the records of all patients who died from asthma in New Zealand in 1981 and 1982. Historical data were obtained from family members and case records. Controls were matched for severity and included two groups: randomly selected ambulatory asthmatics and asthmatic patients admitted to the hospital during the same time period. The two features that were more common among those who died were a previous episode of a life-threatening asthma exacerbation and psychosocial problems. A life-threatening exacerbation was defined as an episode in which the patient's consciousness had been disturbed or appreciable hypercapnia had occurred (51). These findings were validated by Molfino in a 1991 study of survivors of respiratory arrest in near-fatal asthma (40).

   (2) A history of steroid use is a poor prognostic factor. It is unlikely that the use of steroids independently contributes to an adverse outcome, but it probably serves as a marker for more severe asthma (43).

   (3) Rapid clinical progression is a poor prognostic factor.

Table 9-1 Clinical classification of asthma severity (62)

Asthma Severity	Clinical Features Before Treatment	Pulmonary Function	Regular Medications Needed for Control
Mild	Intermittent brief symptoms <1–2 times per week Nocturnal asthma symptoms <2 times per month Asymptomatic between exacerbations	PEFR >80% predicted at baseline PEFR variability† <20% PEFR normal after bronchodilator therapy	Intermittent inhaled short-acting β_2-agonist taken as needed
Moderate	Exacerbations >1–2 times per week Nocturnal asthma symptoms >2 times per month Symptoms requiring inhaled β_2-agonist almost daily	PEFR 60%–80% predicted at baseline PEFR variability† 20%–30% PEFR normal after bronchodilator therapy	Daily inhaled anti-inflammatory agent Possibly a daily long-acting bronchodilator, especially for nocturnal symtpoms
Severe	Frequent exacerbations Continuous symptoms Frequent nocturnal asthma symptoms Physical activities limited by asthma Hospitalization for asthma in previous year Previous life-threatening exacerbation	PEFR <60% predicted at baseline PEFR variability† >30% PEFR below normal despite optimal therapy	Daily inhaled anti-inflammatory agent at high doses Daily long-acting bronchodilator, especially for nocturnal symptoms Frequent use of systemic corticosteroids

Used with permission from National Heart, Lung, and Blood Institute (43, 62).

*An individual should usually be assigned to the most severe grade in which any feature occurs.

†PEFR variability is the percent difference between the "best" and "worst" PEFR measurements over 24 h. % PEFR variability = $(PEFR_{best} - PEFR_{worst})/PEFR_{best} \times 100$

(a) Patients who develop rapidly progressive symptoms are at increased risk for hypercapnia, respiratory failure, and eventual intubation. Even in patients who have had symptoms for many days, a rapid clinical deterioration in the hours before arrival at the hospital is common in patients with near-fatal outcomes (40). Late presentation may also be a marker for poor patient awareness of the severity of illness, indicating a need for increased asthma education and close outpatient follow-up (51,61).

(b) The sensitivity to airways obstruction or hypoxemia varies from patient to patient. In a study of 82 asthmatics, Rubinfeld was able to document an absence of subjective dyspnea in 15% of patients despite a 50% reduction in the forced expiratory volume at 1 second (FEV_1). (55) McFadden showed that among asthmatics recovering from a recent flare, the FEV_1 remained at only 40% to 50% of the predicted value despite complete resolution of symptoms (37). Finally, in a study by Kikuchi, patients with a history of near-fatal asthma had a dramatic reduction in their sensitivity to both increased resistive work of breathing and hypoxemia despite good control of their asthma (28). These findings support a physiologic basis for recurrent near-fatal asthma based on insensitivity to both bronchospasm and hypoxemia. All of these studies emphasize the need for objective end points in monitoring asthma.

(4) Nocturnal awakening is a frequent harbinger of severe asthma exacerbations. The circadian pattern of nocturnal decline in PEFR is well-documented in normal and asthmatic subjects. The cause of this phenomenon is unclear, and it has been shown to persist despite elimination of circadian declines in serum cortisol levels with cortisol infusion (59). Normal adults show a 16% to 18% variability between the maximum and minimum measured PEFR (49). This variability is exaggerated in asthmatic patients and increases during an exacerbation.

(5) Recent colds or ongoing exposure to allergens may predict relapse.

(6) An inadequate outpatient regimen is a poor prognostic factor. Undertreatment with inhaled steroids, overutilization of β_2-agonists, poor inhaler technique, and poor patient understanding of outpatient therapy are all risk factors for an adverse outcome (20,43,61).

(7) Inadequate access to health care increases the risk of relapse. Poor medical follow-up and medical disenfranchisement lead to frequent emergency room visits and poor control of disease (20,43,61).

2. **Physical Examination**—The physical examination is important for evaluation of patients with acute and resolving asthma. Nevertheless, a variety of studies have documented its relative insensitivity for detection of significant derangements in pulmonary airflow.

   a. In a 1973 study of asthmatics, McFadden found that retractions (use of the sternocleidomastoid muscles during respiration) occurred only during very severe asthma flares and correlated with a PEFR of <40 L/minute (or approximately 8% to 10% of predicted value) and an FEV_1 of <1 L (37).

   b. Hollerman published a critical summary of the clinical utility of the physical examination in predicting airflow obstruction in patients with chronic bronchitis or asthma. Physical examination findings were compared with the gold standard of spirometric measurements. All studies included in the analysis used a reduced ratio of FEV_1 to forced vital capacity (FVC) to objectively determine obstruction, although the precise criteria differed somewhat among studies. As shown in Table 9–2, wheezing, rhonchi, and accessory muscle use were shown to be most specific, but no sign was exceptionally sensitive (24).

   c. Although the presence of classic signs, especially wheezing, is a good pre-

Table 9-2 Sensitivity and specificity of physical exam findings in asthma (24)

Sign	LR+*	LR−†	Sensitivity	Specificity
Wheezing	36	0.85	15%	99.6%
Rhonchi	5.9	0.95	8%	99%
Accessory muscle use	—	0.70	24%	100%
Pulsus paradoxus >15 mm Hg	3.7	0.62	45%	88%
Hyperresonance	4.8	0.73	32%	94%
Forced expiratory time				
>9 s	4.8	—	—	—
6–9 s	2.7	—	—	—
<6 s	0.45	—	—	—

Adapted with permission from Hollerman (24).
*Likelihood ratio in the case of a positive test.
†Likelihood ratio in the case of a negative test.

dictor of obstruction, the absence of these signs can be deceiving. For example, a suddenly quiet chest in a severe asthmatic may be an harbinger of respiratory failure, resulting either from severe airflow reduction or tension pneumothorax.

3. **Ancillary Studies**
   a. **Pulmonary Function Studies**
      (1) **Peak Expiratory Flow Rate**
         (a) The National Asthma Education Program of the National Heart, Lung, and Blood Institute recommends that PEFR should be the objective parameter to follow when assessing airflow disruption and therapy (62). The PEFR is easily measured with an inexpensive, handheld spirometer. When full patient effort is employed, PEFR correlates well with the FEV_1 measured during formal pulmonary function studies (45,62). The PEFR has been shown in multiple studies to be an excellent predictor of response to acute asthma therapy and a useful predictor of early relapse (see section E1 of this chapter). The predicted average PEFRs for normal men and women are shown in Table 9–3 (32).
         (b) Physician estimates of PEFR are unreliable. Shim evaluated the ability of experienced pulmonary physicians to predict the PEFR based on clinical examination and found that only 44% of their estimates were within 20% of the actual PEFR measured simultaneously by another pulmonary physician. The correlation coefficient was 0.66 (57). Patients' perceptions of airways obstruction may also be unreliable (see section C1c3b). Therefore, PEFR must be measured repeatedly to assess the efficacy of treatment and to gauge clinical improvement.
         (c) PEFR is also useful in outpatient care. Each patient should establish a personal best PEFR at a time when asthma is well-controlled. A significant deviation from this personal best may indicate worsening disease, and the patient should promptly consult a physician for appropriate adjustment of medications (62). When a patient requires admission, the measured PEFR should be compared with the personal best value (rather than the values in normative tables) to assess progress.
      (2) **Spirometry**—A typical asthmatic shows an obstructive ventilatory defect characterized by a reduced FEV_1, a reduced FEV_1/FVC ratio, and a reduced PEFR. Unlike patients with emphysema, in whom inspiratory flow rates may be normal, asthmatics often have a reduced inspiratory flow rate as well. In addition, inspection of the flow-volume loop is critical in excluding upper airway obstruction that may

Table 9-3 Normal peak expiratory flow rates by age, sex, and height (32)

Predicted PEFR (L/min)				
Age (y)	Height			
Normal Men	**65″**	**70″**	**75″**	**80″**
20	602	649	693	740
30	577	622	664	710
40	552	596	636	680
50	527	569	607	649
60	502	542	578	618
70	477	515	550	587
Normal Women				
20	390	423	460	496
30	380	413	448	483
40	370	402	436	470
50	360	391	424	457
60	350	380	412	445
70	340	369	400	432

Adapted with permission from Leiner (32)

masquerade as asthma. A plateau in either the expiratory or inspiratory portion of the flow-volume loop is seen in such patients. Nevertheless in the acute phase of asthma, FEV_1 is no better at predicting outcome than PEFR (45).

(3) Measurement of the diffusion capacity for carbon monoxide (DLCO) and plethysmography (lung volume determinations) are useful in evaluation of lung function and should eventually be performed as part of full pulmonary function studies on all asthmatics. These tests help exclude coexistent emphysema or interstitial lung disease; the DLCO is reduced in those conditions but is normal in patients with pure asthma. However, these tests serve no purpose during acute management of asthma.

b. Chest Roentgenogram

(1) Patients should receive initial treatment for bronchospasm immediately on arrival at the emergency department. This should not be delayed to perform radiologic studies, especially in patients with a prior history of asthma. Slow response to treatment, fever, leukocytosis, purulent sputum, signs of pneumomediastinum, and spontaneous pneumothorax are indications for radiologic assessment. In a study by Findley, only 1% of radiographic films obtained in 90 episodes of acute asthma revealed a new infiltrate; 55% were normal, 33% showed hyperinflation, and 7% showed mild interstitial abnormalities (18). There was no correlation between chest film findings and requirement for hospital admission. Although this was a small study, it supports the general clinical experience that chest radiologic studies contribute little to the initial management of patients with uncomplicated asthma.

(2) Radiologic studies are useful in the evaluation new-onset wheezing. Patients without a prior history of asthma should undergo radiologic evaluation to rule out significant underlying cardiopulmonary diseases such as congestive heart failure or pneumonia.

c. Arterial Blood Gas Analysis—Arterial blood gas testing provides confirmatory evidence of respiratory failure. The presence of hypercapnia is primarily restricted to patients with FEV_1 <20% to 25% of predicted or PEFR <200 L/minute (2,38,46). In a study of 89 emergency room visits, Martin showed that no patient with a PEFR ≥25% of predicted had an arterial partial pressure of carbon dioxide ($PaCO_2$) >45 mm Hg or a pH <7.35 (35). Therefore, bedside spirometry should be performed initially and used as a guide for arterial blood gas analysis.

d. Other Laboratory Tests—In patients with purulent sputum, a complete blood count may be drawn before the initiation of glucocorticoid therapy to help evaluate for the possible presence of infection.

D. Management of Acute Asthma Exacerbations

1. Oxygen

a. Supplemental oxygen is recommended in all asthmatics if oximetry is not available (62). If oxygen saturation is known to be normal, it is optional. Hypoxemia is usually mild and is caused by ventilation-perfusion mismatch throughout the lungs (38). In a study by McFadden, an arterial partial pressure of oxygen (PaO_2) <55 mm Hg was found in only 5% of patients with acute asthma (16,38). Patients who are profoundly hypoxemic usually have significant ventilatory failure as well.

b. Oxygen-induced carbon dioxide retention is not a major problem in most patients with asthma. Hypercapnia in the patient with acute asthma reflects decreasing minute ventilation as a result of mechanical ventilatory failure rather than loss of central ventilatory drive.

2. β-Agonist Therapy

a. Nebulizers Versus Metered-Dose Inhalers (MDIs)

(1) Inhaled β_2-agonists are the cornerstone of the management of acute asthma. Many prospective, double-blind randomized placebo-controlled trials (DBRPCTs) have examined the effectiveness of various routes of medication delivery. In adults, β_2-agonist delivery by MDI with a spacer device is as efficacious as nebulizer therapy. However, optimal patient technique and proper education are critical. MDIs offer the advantage of more efficient drug delivery as a result of smaller particle size with better distribution to the distal airways. In a double-blind randomized clinical trial of 80 consecutive patients with moderately severe asthma (initial FEV_1, 36±12% of predicted), Colacone studied the efficacy of MDIs with a holding chamber versus small-volume nebulizers. The MDI dose of 0.4 mg (four puffs) of albuterol every 30 minutes delivered through a holding chamber was compared with a nebulized dose of 2.5 mg (0.5 ml) of albuterol given every 30 minutes. Spirometry was performed after each dose, and treatments were continued until no further change in FEV_1 was observed. The study had a power of 80% to detect a difference of 0.2 L in FEV_1 between groups. Patients were excluded if they were younger than 18 years old; were unable to perform spirometry; had known coronary disease, pneumonia, frequent ventricular ectopy, or unstable angina; were pregnant or nursing; or had received β_2-agonists in the emergency department before being enrolled in the trial. Most patients in both groups achieved maximal bronchodilation after two doses of either nebulized or aerosolized albuterol. All but 2 patients (both of whom were assigned to the nebulizer group) achieved maximal bronchodilation after four doses. There was no significant difference in the rates at which patients achieved maximal bronchodilation between the two groups. The dose-response was sixfold higher in the MDI group, indicating improved drug delivery (13). Similar results have been reported by several other groups using different spacer devices and other β_2-agonists (64). There appears to be no difference in the incidence of side effects (tachycardia, tremulousness, hypertension) between the two treatment modalities. Because MDI therapy is much more difficult to perform successfully in an acutely ill child, nebulizer therapy remains the treatment of choice in children (48).

(2) According to the National Asthma Education Program guidelines, patients should continue to receive β_2-agonists by inhalation every 1 to 2 hours until PEFRs normalize or return to baseline. Discharge from the hospital is reasonable after doses can be separated by 3 to 4 hours without exacerbation of symptoms (62).

b. **Parenteral Versus Inhaled β_2-Agonists**—Several studies have compared the effectiveness of inhalation versus intravenous or subcutaneous administration of β_2-adrenergic agonists. Most have focused on terbutaline, although albuterol has also been studied. In the best designed trial available, Van Renterghem compared IV terbutaline (6 mg/kg) versus inhaled terbutaline (0.1 mg/kg) in a double-blind randomized clinical trial of 23 patients; the PEFR response was equivalent in both groups (68). Similar results were found with albuterol (salbutamol) therapy (6). However, significant side effects have been observed with the use of parenteral β_2-agonists, including lactic acidosis, marked hypokalemia, and cardiac tachyarrhythmias (30). Given the lack of advantage of parenteral β_2-agonists, inhalational therapy is recommended. Parenteral administration should be considered only in patients who fail to respond to inhalational therapy, with the understanding that there is no convincing evidence of additional benefit (30).

c. **Side Effects of β_2-Agonist Therapy**

(1) **Electrolyte Abnormalities**—Hypokalemia and hypomagnesemia are frequently observed in patients treated with high-dose β_2-agonist therapy. Stimulation of the β_2-adrenergic receptor causes translocation of these ions into the intracellular space. There is no known clinical significance to these mild and transient electrolyte derangements (7). There have been no reports of electrolyte-induced arrhythmias in patients treated with frequent doses of inhaled β_2-agonists.

(2) **Excess Mortality Associated With β_2-Agonists**—Several reports have emphasized a possible link between excessive use of inhaled β_2-agonists (especially fenoterol) and increased risk of death from asthma (60). However, there is no evidence that the use of β_2-agonists acutely is associated with significant mortality or morbidity (40), and these agents remain essential in the care of patients with acute asthma.

3. **Epinephrine Therapy**—Studies have shown epinephrine to be effective when used as either initial or second-line therapy in adults with acute asthma (1,54).

a. In an emergency department study of patients with acute asthma, 48 patients younger than 45 years old were randomly assigned to receive nebulized metaproterenol (2.5 mg every 20 minutes for three doses), aminophylline IV (5.6 mg/kg load, followed by an infusion of 0.9 mg/kg/hour), or subcutaneous epinephrine (0.3 mg every 20 minutes for three doses). The FEV_1 improved significantly in patients treated with either metaproterenol (0.79 L improvement) or epinephrine (0.76 L improvement), in contrast to the minimal improvement seen in patients treated with aminophylline (0.23 L improvement; P=0.001). Although no significant difference was noted between the patients treated with epinephrine and those treated with metaproterenol, the power of the study was not adequate to make definitive statements about this issue (54).

b. In another emergency department DBRPCT with crossover, Appel compared nebulized metaproterenol (15 mg every 30 minutes for three doses) versus subcutaneous epinephrine (0.3 mg every 30 minutes for three doses) in 100 patients with asthma. Patients were treated initially with three doses of one agent, then with three doses of the other agent. As judged by improved PEFR (defined as an increase by 20% over baseline and an absolute PEFR $>$120 L/minute after 120 minutes), both epinephrine and metaproterenol were effective bronchodilators for most patients. After three doses, 89% of the patients treated initially with epinephrine improved, as did 61% of those treated initially with metaproterenol. When the latter patients were switched to epinephrine, an additional 13 patients improved. However, when patients who had been treated initially with epinephrine were switched to metaproterenol, only 1 additional patient improved ($P<0.01$). Although subjective side effects were slightly more frequent in the epinephrine-treated group, they were mild and self-limited. No significant cardiac or hemodynamic side effects were seen, but patients with a diagnosis of hypertension or coronary disease were excluded by the study criteria. In addition, the participants were relatively young, with a mean age of 36 years for men, 34 years for women (1).

c. Although these trials suggest that epinephrine may be more efficacious than inhaled agents for initial therapy, they excluded patients who may have been at high risk for development adverse side effects (*e.g.*, those with coronary artery disease or hypertension). Patients who receive epinephrine as secondary treatment appear to benefit equally as much as those who receive epinephrine initially. Concerns about potential adverse effects in older patients, including reports of coronary vasospasm with myocardial infarction, ventricular tachycardia, severe hypertension, and local vasospasm, have limited the use of epinephrine as first-line treatment. The incidence of side effects has not been extensively or prospectively evaluated in an unselected population.

d. The current data justify the use of epinephrine for those patients who fail to respond to maximal inhalational therapy and who are at low risk for cardiac side effects. Epinephrine is effective at 0.3 mg SQ every 20 minutes for three doses. Continuous IV epinephrine (0.25-2.0 mg/minute) is used occasionally in refractory status asthmaticus, but its added efficacy in adults has not been studied.

4. Steroid Therapy

a. Parenteral Corticosteroids in Acute Asthma

(1) Many prospective randomized trials have evaluated the role of corticosteroids in the treatment of asthma. The effects of corticosteroids on asthma have been studied in all patients presenting to emergency departments with bronchospasm and in patients with asthma that is refractory to conventional β_2-agonist therapy. The length of follow-up, the dose and route of administration of the steroid, and the end points of the trial varied significantly. Some studies showed benefit, but others did not. The consensus of most investigators and clinicians is that there is a steroid-induced improvement of acute asthma that occurs approximately 6 to 12 hours after initial administration of a corticosteroid drug (10 to 15 mg/kg/24 hours of hydrocortisone, 2 to 3 mg/kg/24 hours of methylprednisolone, or 40 to 60 mg of methylprednisolone QID which is continued for 2 to 4 days) (39).

(2) The most illustrative studies exploring the efficacy and dosing of parenteral steroids are the trials of Fanta (17) and Haskell (22), which are outlined in Table 9–4. The study by Fanta is the best placebo-controlled trial. It appropriately excluded patients who showed an initial brisk response to β_2-agonist therapy. This allowed a separate, delayed corticosteroid effect to be seen. The Haskell trial also excluded patients who showed a dramatic β_2-adrenergic response and had an adequate follow-up period to observe a steroid effect. It is also the only trial to date that has compared low-dose and high-dose therapy after excluding early responders. However, as with many trials in this area, data are expressed differently in the two studies, and different medications were used. The results shown were extrapolated from published reports and converted into comparable terms.

(3) Although an initial large bolus of corticosteroids (*e.g.*, 125 mg methylprednisolone) is widely used, no study has evaluated the necessity or the additional benefit of this practice.

b. Oral Corticosteroids in Acute Asthma

(1) Multiple trials have evaluated the oral versus the IV routes of steroid administration. The best trial to date is the study of Ratto (50). In this

Table 9-4 Efficacy of corticosteroids in acute asthma

Author (Reference)	Design	Dose of Methylprednisolone	Mean FEV_1 Before Treatment	Mean FEV_1 After Treatment	*P*
Fanta (17)	DBRPCT (N=20)	None (placebo)	0.89±0.06 L*	1.28±0.28 L	NS
		0.4 mg/kg bolus, then 0.1 mg/kg/h × 24 h	0.89±0.06 L*	1.64±0.11 L	<0.001
Haskell (22)	DBRCT (N=25)	15 mg IV q 6 h	27±3.9% predicted†	55% predicted†	NS
		40 mg IV q6 h	27±5% predicted†	62% predicted†	<0.01‡
		125 mg IV q 6 h	25±6% predicted†	65% predicted†	<0.01‡

*Mean value of all patients before randomization; no significant postrandomization differences were seen.
†Values estimated from graph. No absolute values were published.
‡*P* value is calculated for the comparison to the 15 mg dosing.

study, 77 patients admitted to an inpatient pulmonary service with status asthmaticus were separated into four groups. Each group received a different dose of methylprednisolone, either orally or intravenously. All patients received maximal β_2-agonist therapy. Results are shown in Table 9–5. The trial was not blinded, but objective end points were used. Although patients were initially randomly assigned to separate groups, the data from the oral treatment groups were pooled and compared with the pooled data from the IV treatment group. Dose-dependent effects for each route were not assessed.

(2) These results, which are consistent with those from smaller trials, suggest that oral glucocorticoids are adequate for the treatment of status asthmaticus and are equivalent in efficacy to IV therapy. The dosage guidelines for oral glucocorticoids are identical to the guidelines for IV therapy.

(3) The benefit of glucocorticoids for asthma is best demonstrated when a study includes only patients who have failed initial β_2-agonist therapy. Nevertheless, the use of steroids may decrease the rate of early relapse in all asthmatics regardless of initial response to inhaled adrenergic agents. Chapman treated 122 asthmatics with placebo versus prednisone (40 mg for 2 days, followed by a taper of 5 mg/day). In this study, 3 of the 48 patients treated with prednisone relapsed, compared with 11 of the 45 patients treated with placebo ($P<0.05$). Compared with those who did not relapse, the patients who relapsed had significantly worse pulmonary function on the day of discharge and 1 day after discharge. Objective spirometric data were not reported over the full course of follow-up for patients in either group (12). These data suggest a possible broader applicability of glucocorticoid therapy after emergency department care.

c. Tapering Corticosteroids After Treatment

(1) The method of tapering corticosteroids is controversial. In a DBRPCT of 43 hospitalized asthmatic patients, Lederle assigned patients to either a 1-week or a 7-week taper of oral corticosteroids. All patients received full-dose corticosteroid therapy (at least 60 mg of prednisone per day) for 8 days before beginning the taper. Patients continued with standard therapy including inhaled β_2-agonists, theophylline, and inhaled corticosteroids at standard doses. Patients were observed for 12 weeks. No statistically significant difference in the relapse rate or mean spirometry values was observed between the two groups (exacerbation rates were 41% with 7-week taper and 52% with 1-week taper). However, side effects occurred more frequently with the 7-week taper. The study is somewhat limited by the small number of enrolled patients. The study had a 90% chance of detecting a 50% or greater difference in the relapse rates. In addition, many patients had a significant history of tobacco abuse, making the coexistence of COPD a possibility (31). The data suggest, however, that in most patients with uncomplicated asthma corticosteroids can be tapered

Table 9-5 Relative efficacy of oral and parenteral corticosteroids (50)

Route of Administration	Dose of Methylprednisolone	FEV_1 Before Treatment	FEV_1 After Treatment	*P* (Oral vs. IV)
Oral	80 mg BID to QID*	26±2% predicted	58±4% predicted	NS
Intravenous	500–1000 mg QID*	27±2% predicted	55±3% predicted	NS

*Data pooled from both groups.

rapidly over 1 week to 10 days. Those with refractory disease may require more gradual tapering and frequent clinical follow-up. A standard regimen consists of a decrease of 10 mg every fourth day, with discontinuation after 4 days of 10 mg of prednisone (39). Empirical variations abound, and tapering regimens are often individualized.

5. Methylxanthine Therapy

a. Used alone, aminophylline provides much less clinical improvement in the patient with acute asthma than other currently available therapies. It should be used, if at all, only in combination with more potent or more rapidly-acting medications such as inhaled β_2-agonists, subcutaneous adrenergic agents, and corticosteroids. In a metaanalysis of the 13 best clinical trials of aminophylline therapy in acute asthma, Littenberg was unable to recommend for or against the use of aminophylline in conjunction with β_2-agonists and steroids (33).

b. The best single study of aminophylline in the emergency department setting is that by Murphy, performed at Cook County Hospital in Chicago. The study evaluated 44 patients who failed to achieve a PEFR of >40% of the predicted value after one nebulized dose of metaproterenol. Participants were randomly assigned in a double-blind fashion to receive a 125 mg IV bolus of methylprednisolone and either aminophylline or placebo. Aminophylline was given as a bolus with maintenance drip, and serum levels in both placebo and aminophylline groups were monitored. Aminophylline levels on admission in both groups were comparable and low. The study had a power of 90% to detect a 25% difference in the improvement of PEFR. At 5 hours, there was no statistically significant difference in the PEFR between the two groups. The aminophylline-treated group had a higher incidence of tremor, nausea or vomiting, and palpitations (42). Although other studies have been performed, design issues or end points chosen by the investigators weaken their conclusions. Some investigators found a decreased rate of hospitalization with aminophylline therapy; however, no significant spirometric differences were documented, and confounding variables may well account for these findings (71).

c. Aminophylline may provide some benefit in acutely ill asthmatics who require admission. In a recent trial, Huang (25) showed a more rapid rate of improvement in FEV_1 within the first 3 hours of hospitalization in patients with acute asthma who received aminophylline, compared with patients who received placebo (29%±23% versus 10%±10%, respectively; P=0.023). However, this DBRPCT was small (21 patients), and the difference in the rate of improvement of FEV_1 was heavily influenced by the inclusion of 2 patients with dramatic early bronchodilation. The results were barely statistically significant, and the confidence intervals were wide. Therefore, the additive benefit of aminophylline is still open for debate.

d. Despite equivocal evidence from clinical trials, aminophylline therapy is recommended for hospitalized patients as part of the National Asthma Education Program guidelines for the management of acute asthma (62). The recommended dosing is a 6 mg/kg load for patients not previously treated with methylxanthines, with a maintenance drip of 0.6 mg/kg/hour to keep levels between 10 and 15 mg/dl. The infusion rate should be adjusted based on serum levels and on other factors that influence methylxanthine metabolism, such as congestive heart failure, liver disease, cigarette smoking, and medications (erythromycin, cimetidine, ciprofloxacin). When converting to oral therapy, sustained-release theophylline preparations should be used in divided doses equivalent to 80% of the total aminophylline dose given over 24 hours (42).

6. Magnesium Therapy

a. The role of magnesium therapy, as an adjunct to conventional therapy with β_2-agonists and corticosteroids, is controversial. The initial enthusiasm developed after a report by Okayama in which 10 ambulatory asthmatic patients with relatively mild disease were studied. Treatment with magnesium sulfate (0.5 mmol/minute for 20 minutes) had a bronchodilatory effect similar to the effect of an additional albuterol inhalation, with FEV_1 doubling after therapy (FEV_1 after treatment was 118%±1% of baseline). This report stimulated further studies examining the potential additive role of IV magnesium in patients who respond poorly to initial conventional therapy (47).

b. Subsequent studies focused on the utility of IV magnesium for emergency treatment of acute asthma flares. The first report by Skobeloff examined 38 patients with an initial PEFR <200 L/minute. All patients received two inhaled β_2-agonist treatments as well as IV aminophylline and corticosteroid therapy. Patients whose PEFR failed to double or to exceed 200 L/minute were eligible for the study. In a double-blind fashion, patients were randomly assigned to receive either placebo or magnesium sulfate (1.2 g infused over 20 minutes). The treatment group had an increase in PEFR from 225 to 297 L/minute. In contrast, the mean PEFR rose from 208 to only 216 L/minute with placebo (P=0.043). The authors also noted a significantly higher rate of discharge from the emergency department among patients receiving magnesium therapy (15 in the treatment group versus 4 in the placebo group). Decision for discharge was made by a blinded observer. Neither the placebo group nor the treatment group received further inhalation treatments before completion of the study. This study validated the findings of Okayama and suggested a role for magnesium in the emergency treatment of asthmatic patients who fail to have a complete response to initial conventional therapy (58).

c. The major remaining question regarding magnesium therapy was whether it offered any significant advantages over repeated inhaled β_2-agonist therapy. This was addressed in a well designed DBRPCT by Tiffany. This study was similar in design to that of Skobeloff. It included only patients with initial PEFRs <200 L/minute and whose PEFRs failed to double or increase by more than 200 L/minute after two treatments with nebulized albuterol. Forty-eight patients were entered and separated into three groups: group 1 was treated with 10 g of magnesium sulfate (2 g over 20 minutes, then 2 g/hour for 4 hours); group 2 with 2 g of magnesium sulfate (2 g over 20 minutes, then placebo); and group 3 with placebo only. After entry into the trial, all patients received a third treatment of nebulized albuterol, methylprednisolone (125 mg IV), and aminophylline (infusion to maintain serum concentrations at approximately 15 mg/L). Despite the fact that the study had a power of 80% to detect a difference in PEFR of 26 L/minute and a difference in FEV_1 of 0.19 L/minute, magnesium sulfate improved neither of these parameters significantly. The addition of a third nebulized β_2-agonist treatment appeared to have efficacy similar to that of IV infusion of magnesium sulfate. The study failed to show any significant synergy between inhaled β_2-agonists and magnesium (63).

d. The additive role of magnesium for particular subgroups (*e.g.*, intubated patients with status asthmaticus) has not yet been studied. The effect of a prolonged infusion of magnesium in patients with refractory bronchospasm is also not known. Nevertheless, because there is no convincing evidence for additive benefit, magnesium cannot be recommended as standard therapy for acute asthma at the present time. It remains optional for patients with severe bronchospasm who have incomplete response to conventional therapy.

7. Anticholinergic Agents

a. The role of anticholinergic agents as substitutes for β_2-agonists in acute asthma is controversial, and there are only few well-designed clinical trials on which to base recommendations. Only one trial, which compared glycopyrrolate and metaproterenol in an emergency department setting, demonstrated an equivalent bronchodilator response with anticholinergic agents and β_2-agonists (19). In this double-blind trial, Gilman randomly assigned 46 patients with acute asthma (aged 18 to 45 years) with an FEV_1 >0.8 L to receive either glycopyrrolate (2 mg nebulized q 2 hours) or metaproterenol (15 mg nebulized q 2 hours) over a 6-hour study period. No other medications were given during the study period. The study had a 24% dropout rate (11 of 46 patients), with 10 patients failing to respond adequately to therapy. A similar number of patients dropped out in both groups. The initial respiratory mechanics did not differ significantly between patients who were treated and those who dropped out. Both treatment groups showed bronchodilation after each dose of medication, with no statistically significant difference between the groups at any time point. Side effects were less common with glycopyrrolate therapy. No power calculations were provided. This study suggests that glycopyrrolate may be equivalent to metaproterenol therapy, with fewer adverse effects. However, baseline spirometric data were not provided in the published report, making conclusions about the severity of asthma in this study population impossible. The high dropout rate is also of concern, although the authors found no objective difference in the pretreatment spirometric measurements of patients who dropped out, nor any apparent differences in their response to treatment (19). However, atropine sulfate, when given alone as a nebulized solution, is not as effective as nebulized metaproterenol sulfate (27).

b. Inhaled anticholinergic agents may offer further bronchodilation when added to inhaled β_2-agonists, however. In one study, nebulized ipratropium bromide (0.5 mg) offered significant benefit when simultaneously added to nebulized fenoterol (a β_2-agonist more potent than albuterol but not available in the United States) (52). However, although statistically significant, the absolute differences in FEV_1 were small (see Table 9–6) and the clinical significance of these findings is unclear. Nebulized ipratropium bromide has only recently become available in the United States.

c. Based on current data, the addition of nebulized anticholinergic agents to the standard inhaled β_2-agonist therapy remains optional. Few adverse effects are noted, and there may be some added benefit. In addition to increasing bronchodilation, addition of these agents may prolong the bronchodilatory effect achieved by albuterol, when compared with the use of albuterol alone (23). Caution should be exercised in older patients with a history of glaucoma, urinary retention, or other adverse effects in response to anticholinergic agents.

8. Cromolyn Sodium and Nedocromil Sulfate—These agents are useful in the management of chronic asthma but have not been studied in adult patients with acute asthma exacerbations. Therefore, no recommendations can be made.

9. Intravenous Fluids—Although traditionally a part of asthma management, the benefit of IV hydration to loosen secretions has not been rigorously studied. Hydration is recommended by the National Asthma Education Program only if the patient appears clinically dehydrated.

10. Mucolytics—Mucolytic agents such as acetylcysteine (Mucosil) may exacerbate bronchospasm and should not be used in patients who are acutely ill with asthma (62).

Table 9-6 Efficacy of anticholinergic therapy in acute asthma (52)

	Ipratropium	Fenoterol	Fenoterol and Ipratropium
Pretreatment FEV_1	1.21±0.64 L	1.09±0.62 L	1.22±0.66 L
FEV_1 at 45 min	1.42±0.78 L	1.46±0.80 L	1.75±0.88 L
FEV_1 at 90 min*	1.45±0.76 L	1.47±0.83 L	1.70±0.90 L

*$P<0.001$ for FEV_1 at 90 min for the combination vs. ipratropium alone, $P<0.05$ for FEV_1 at 90 min for the combination vs. fenoterol alone.

11. **Empiric Antibiotics**—Asthma that is precipitated by an infection is typically caused by a nonbacterial pathogen. Bronchospasm is probably the result of airway inflammation and should be treated in the same fashion as other asthma flares. Berman examined transtracheal aspirates from 27 asthmatic adults during a flare of disease and found very low bacterial recovery with no significant differences between the patients and asymptomatic controls (4). Therefore, empiric antibiotics, in the absence of convincing evidence of bacterial superinfection, are not indicated.
12. **Mechanical Ventilation**
    a. The indications for mechanical ventilation for patients with acute asthma are summarized in the following sections.
        (1) Respiratory or cardiac arrest is an obvious indication for prompt mechanical ventilation.
        (2) Mental status change is a marker for potentially fatal asthma. Obtundation is typically a result of both hypoxemia and hypercapnia. Although aggressive inhalational or parenteral therapy (or both) may be tried initially, preparations should be made for intensive care unit monitoring. Mechanical ventilation should be instituted if immediate results are not observed
        (3) Excessive fatigue is a marker for impending respiratory failure. No specific guidelines can be given regarding when the clinician should intervene in this situation. However, patients should be intubated before becoming moribund (30).
        (4) Elevated $PaCO_2$ with acute respiratory acidosis is an indication for mechanical ventilation if refractory to initial therapy. However, the finding of hypercapnia with respiratory acidosis before initiation of therapy is not an indication for intubation. In a study of 61 episodes of asthma with hypercapnia (mean $PaCO_2$, 54 mm Hg), only 8% of patients required mechanical ventilation after aggressive initial treatment with inhaled bronchodilators. Even among patients with an initial $PaCO_2$ of 50 to 126 mm Hg, only 20% ultimately required intubation (41).

    b. **Methods of Endotracheal Intubation**—Authors differ on recommendations regarding nasal versus oral intubation (30). Nasal intubation is readily accomplished in awake patients during spontaneous respiration. However, a nasal endotracheal tube has a somewhat smaller caliber and may complicate subsequent ventilator management. The choice of nasal versus oral intubation is principally one of personal preference, and no studies are available that document the superiority of one method over the other.
    c. **Principles of Mechanical Ventilation in the Patient With Acute Asthma**
        (1) **Assure Adequate Oxygenation**—Oxygenation should be maintained at $PaO_2 \geq 70$ mm Hg and continuously monitored (14).
        (2) **Minimize Barotrauma**—Barotrauma is a significant cause of morbidity and mortality among intubated patients with asthma, affecting as many as 19% to 27% of patients (34,70). Studies suggest that the incidence of barotrauma is correlated with the severity of air trapping behind airways that collapse or occlude during exhalation. Inadequate expiratory time leads to excessive alveolar distention with each subsequent breath, causing dynamic hyperinflation or a self-imposed peak end-expiratory pressure (auto-PEEP) (34). Dynamic hyperinflation increases intrathoracic pressure, resulting in poor venous return and decreased cardiac output. This leads to hypotension and decreased systemic oxygen delivery (65). Dynamic hyperinflation can also physically disrupt alveolar septae and pleurae, leading to pneumothorax and pneumomediastinum. The details of measurement of dynamic hyperinflation and its effects on hemodynamic monitoring are beyond the scope of this chapter and are fully detailed elsewhere

(66). Nevertheless, several methods of ventilation reduce dynamic hyperinflation and are important to review.

(a) **Prolonged Expiratory Time**—During mechanical ventilation, a sedated and paralyzed patient is ventilated at a fixed rate. This leads to a given cycle length for each breath. The proportions of time spent in each phase of respiration—that is, the inspiratory time (I-time) and the expiratory time (E-time)—are predetermined. When respiratory rate is increased, the respiratory cycle length is shortened, resulting in decreased I-time and decreased E-time. By increasing the respiratory rate with a fixed tidal volume and PEEP, Tuxen was able to show the dramatic effect of E-time on the severity of dynamic hyperinflation. In a study of 9 patients with severe airflow obstruction, an increase in the respiratory rate from 10 to 16 breaths per minute resulted in a doubling of dynamic hyperinflation (66). Generally, maintenance of a tidal volume of approximately 10 ml/kg is recommended (30). The respiratory rate should be adjusted to the lowest possible level while maintaining adequate oxygenation and ventilation.

(b) **Rapid Inspiratory Flow Rates**—Rapid inspiratory flow rates allow more time in the respiratory cycle for exhalation. Peak pressures become a concern at extremely high flow rates. Flow rates should be adjusted to match the patient's normal flow rates, usually between 60 and 100 L/minute (30).

(c) **Permissive Hypercapnia**—In an observational study of 34 episodes of mechanical ventilation for severe bronchospasm, Darioli maintained peak airway pressures of <50 cm H_2O, and patients were allowed to remain hypercapneic (mean $PaCO_2$, 100 mm Hg) until the bronchospasm improved. In 6 patients, resolution required more than 24 hours but no adverse effects were seen. Barotrauma occurred in fewer than 10% of the patients (14). Some authors suggest the use of IV buffer solutions to correct respiratory acidosis (30). No controlled trials have been performed to confirm the efficacy of these measures.

(3) **Minimize or Eliminate PEEP**—PEEP has convincingly been shown by Tuxen to increase functional residual capacity during mechanical ventilation. Despite reducing dynamic hyperinflation, PEEP increases lung volume. Increased lung volume leads to an increase in intrathoracic pressure as measured by an esophageal balloon. This increased intrathoracic pressure results in decreased venous return and possibly increased pulmonary vascular resistance, leading to decreased cardiac output and decreased tissue perfusion. The effect of PEEP on arterial oxygenation in an uncomplicated asthmatic is negligible (65).

(4) **Sedate and Paralyze**—Sedation minimizes the need for high inspiratory pressures during mechanical ventilation. Adequate relaxation often requires use of a paralytic agent as well. Occasionally, isoflurane anesthesia is required. Leatherman provides an excellent review of the methods and complications of prolonged sedation and neuromuscular blockade (60).

(5) Experimental approaches including the use of helium-oxygen combinations, extracorporeal membrane oxygenation, and extracorporeal carbon dioxide removal are detailed elsewhere (60).

E. Factors Predictive of Relapse After Initial Treatment and Discharge

1. Spirometry

a. Objective improvement in spirometric parameters is the most reliable predictor of successful hospital discharge with the lowest likelihood of relapse. This applies whether the patient is being discharged from an emergency department or from an inpatient setting.

b. Nowak studied the clinical outcomes of 109 asthmatic patients treated in the emergency room based on spirometric parameters. Patients were all treated initially with terbutaline (0.25 mg SQ), and spirometric measurements were recorded before and after treatment. Spirometry included FEV_1, which was known to the attending physician, and PEFR, which was not revealed. Decisions to admit patients were made independently by emergency physicians using clinical criteria (physical examination, arterial blood gas analysis, and FEV_1). Additional treatment was at the discretion of the attending physician. Patients were divided into three groups: group 1 consisted of patients who were admitted; group 2 were patients who were discharged but on follow-up questionnaire were found to have worsened symptomatically or to have required unexpected medical care after discharge; group 3 consisted of patients who were successfully discharged without subsequent clinical deterioration. A statistically significant difference was found in the posttreatment PEFR and FEV_1 values among all groups. Posttreatment spirometrics correlated with relapse and the need for hospitalization. For hospitalized patients, the PEFR after treatment was 184±82.7 L/minute, compared with 247.6±94.8 L/minute for the relapse group and 336±87.2 L/minute for the nonrelapse group ($P<0.05$ for all groups). A predictive model based on pretreatment and posttreatment spirometry was developed, and data for PEFR are shown in Table 9–7 (45). This model has not been prospectively validated, and there is significant room for confounding error because the decision to admit was based at least in part on the FEV_1.

c. In a study by Fischl, a predictive index was developed using the outcome data of patients presenting to an emergency room for treatment of acute asthma (18a). Of the 205 patients, 45 were hospitalized (admitted group) and 160 were discharged. Forty of the discharged patients experienced a relapse within 10 days (discharged/relapse group); 120 were successfully discharged without a relapse (discharged/no relapse group). Seven factors were predictive of relapse: heart rate >120/minute, respiratory rate >30/minute, pulsus paradoxus >18 mm Hg, PEFR <120 L/minute, moderate to severe dyspnea, accessory muscle use, and wheezing. These factors were used to develop a predictive index ranging in value from 0 to 7. The index score was 5.1 for the admitted group, 4.9 for the discharged/relapse group, and 1.6 for the discharged/no relapse group. The index score of the discharged/no relapse group was significantly different from those of the other two groups ($P<0.001$). An index of 4 or higher had an accuracy of 95% for predicting relapse.

d. Similar studies evaluating predictors of successful discharge after inpatient therapy (as opposed to discharge from an emergency room) have not been performed. Some expert panels recommend a PEFR that is at least 70% to 80% of either the predicted value or the patient's personal best. A PEFR variability of less than 20% is also recommended (24,43).

2. Resolution of Clinical Signs and Symptoms

Table 9-7 PEFR as a predictor of successful discharge (45)

Absolute PEFR (L/min)		Number (%) Patients in Each Group		
Pretreatment	Posttreatment	Groups 1 and 2	Group 3	Total
<100	<300	22 (92%)	2 (8%)	24
>100	<300	25 (66%)	13 (34%)	38
<100	>300	0 (0%)	5 (100%)	5
>100	>300	6 (16%)	32 (84%)	38

Adapted with permission from Nowak (45).

a. Although many clinical risk indices have been constructed to determine the risk of relapse, all are flawed by an inherent unreliability of symptoms and clinical signs as predictors of the severity of airflow obstruction. In a study of 22 asthmatic patients, McFadden found that PEFRs remained at approximately 50% of predicted values despite complete symptomatic recovery (37).

b. In a study of 102 emergency room patients whose discharge decision was based solely on clinical criteria without the use of spirometric data, the mean FEV_1 at discharge was only 57% of predicted, and 25% of patients had a relapse within 10 days, with 6% returning to the emergency department and requiring admission. Patients who had a relapse had significantly less improvement of FEV_1 and a lower FEV_1 on discharge ($P<0.05$). No other clinical or laboratory parameter, including pulsus paradoxus, accessory muscle use, arterial carbon dioxide, or oxygen tension, was sufficiently reliable to substitute for the FEV_1. PEFR was not measured in this study (26).

3. Social Factors—Careful discharge planning that ensures patient comprehension of the therapeutic plan, adequate follow-up, and access to medications is critical to minimize relapse. Brief hospitalization may be necessary if environmental triggers are temporary but cannot immediately be separated from the patient (*e.g.*, during household renovation or fumigation).

F. Summary

1. Asthma is a chronic inflammatory disease with exacerbations and remissions. Exacerbations may be life-threatening. Prompt recognition and treatment are essential. Treatment is multifaceted and directed at both reversal of acute bronchospasm and control of underlying inflammation. Inhaled β_2-agonists provide brisk but relatively short-acting bronchodilation (<3 hours). Corticosteroid therapy provides control of inflammation. The clinical effects of corticosteroids are often delayed 6 to 12 hours after administration.

2. Although critical in the initial assessment of the asthmatic, the patient's history and physical examination are insensitive for assessment of the degree of airway obstruction. Objective measurement of airflow is pivotal in management of the acute asthma flare. FEV_1 and PEFR are equally reliable indices of obstruction, and either can be employed routinely. Airflow measurements should be taken after each treatment with β_2-agonists. Patients with initial PEFRs <100 L/minute and those with PEFRs <300 L/minute after treatment usually require hospital admission. Even among patients with a posttreatment PEFRs >300 L/minute, up to 16% may require admission or experience a worsening of symptoms after discharge. PEFR should be measured at least twice daily (morning and evening) in hospitalized patients after initial stabilization. The variability between the maximum and minimum PEFR should be <30%, and absolute PEFR should be 70% to 80% of predicted (or of the patient's personal best) before discharge.

3. Specific historical features predict worse outcomes. These include prior intubation, hospitalization within the previous year for asthma, prior or current steroid use, rapid symptom progression, frequent nocturnal symptoms, ongoing exposure to triggers, undertreatment with inhaled corticosteroids, poor compliance with or understanding of the medical regimen, medical disenfranchisement, and psychosocial problems.

4. Arterial blood gas testing should be considered for patients with PEFRs <200 L/minute or <25% of predicted. A complete blood count may be helpful if associated infection is clinically suspected. Blood for this analysis should be drawn before initiation of steroid therapy. The applicability of the chest roentgenogram is limited unless underlying illness or complications are suspected.

5. Inhaled β_2-agonists remain the cornerstone of acute therapy. These can be delivered either by small-volume nebulizer or by MDI through a spacer device. Delivery by MDI is more efficient based on dose-response but requires careful attention to patient technique. Four puffs of an albuterol MDI (0.4 mg) are roughly equivalent in efficacy to one nebulized dose (2.5 mg) of albuterol. For hospitalized patients, inhaled adrenergic agents should be repeated at least every 1 to 2 hours until peak flow normalizes. They should be tapered to every 4 hours before discharge from the hospital.

6. Parenteral epinephrine is useful in the management of asthma that is refractory to initial therapy with inhaled β_2-agonists. Side effects related to both its α-adrenergic and its nonselective β-adrenergic properties limit its general applicability. The dose is 0.3 mg SQ every 20 minutes for three doses or until peak flow normalizes.
7. Corticosteroids are useful in the treatment of asthma. They are especially useful for patients who fail to respond adequately to inhalational therapy. Both oral and IV routes are efficacious. A dose of 40 to 60 mg of methylprednisolone IV every 6 hours or 80 mg of prednisone orally every 12 hours is appropriate for inpatient care. There are no data to support or refute the addition of an initial steroid bolus. After normalization of PEFR, steroids can be tapered over 7 to 10 days in most patients. Steroid therapy may reduce the incidence of relapse even in patients who respond well to β_2-agonist treatment and should be considered in all patients who present with an acute asthma exacerbation. Use of inhaled corticosteroids should be initiated before discontinuation of the oral medication.
8. Methylxanthines appear to offer little additive benefit in the acute management of patients with asthma. For those being treated with theophylline on an outpatient basis, a therapeutic level (10 to 15 mg/dl) should be maintained while the patient is hospitalized. Initiation of aminophylline therapy in all patients with an acute asthma flare is recommended by the National Asthma Education Program (49), but this recommendation is not strongly supported by published studies.
9. For patients with a routine asthma exacerbation, magnesium therapy offers no additional benefit compared with aggressive therapy with inhaled β_2-agonists. It has not been studied in severe, refractory bronchospasm.
10. Ipratropium bromide may provide additional bronchodilation and should be considered for use in combination with β_2-agonists.
11. IV fluids are indicated for dehydrated patients. Mucolytic agents should not be used.
12. Intubation and mechanical ventilation are indicated for patients with cardiopulmonary arrest, severe hypercapnia and respiratory acidosis, mental status change, or refractory hypoxemia. Low respiratory rates should be used in order to avoid dynamic hyperinflation. Inspiratory flow rates should be optimized while keeping peak airway pressures at <50 cm H_2O. In general, use of PEEP should be minimized. Hypercapnia can be tolerated with maintenance of serum pH at >7.20 with buffer infusion.
13. Asthma is a dynamic disease. Therapy continues to evolve as our understanding of the disease progresses. New antiinflammatory agents directed at leukotriene mediators of bronchoconstriction and inflammation have been developed and are undergoing clinical testing. The management of the patient with acute asthma will continue to change as our therapeutic choices expand.

Abbreviations used in Chapter 9

BID = twice daily
COPD = chronic obstructive pulmonary disease
DBRPCT = double-blind randomized placebo-controlled trial
DLCO = diffusion capacity for carbon monoxide
FEV_1 = forced expiratory volume in 1 second
FVC = forced vital capacity
IgE = immunoglobulin E
IV = intravenous

LR− = likelihood ratio in the case of a negative test
LR+ = likelihood ratio in the case of a positive test
MDI = metered-dose inhaler
N = number of patients in population
n = number of patients in sample
NS = not statistically significant
P = probability value
$PaCO_2$ = arterial partial pressure of carbon dioxide
PaO_2 = arterial partial pressure of oxygen
PEEP = peak end-expiratory pressure
PEFR = peak expiratory flow rate
QID = four times daily
SQ = subcutaneous
vs. = versus

References

1. Appel. Epinephrine improves expiratory flow rates in patients with asthma who do not respond to inhaled metaproterenol sulfate. *J Allergy Clin Immunol* 1989; 84:90.
2. Banner. Rapid prediction of need for hospitalization in acute asthma. *JAMA* 1976; 235:1337.
3. Barnes. A new approach to the treatment of asthma. *N Engl J Med* 1989;321:1517.
4. Berman. Transtracheal aspiration studies in asthmatic patients in relapse with infective asthma and in subjects without respiratory disease. *J Allergy Clin Immunol* 1983;72:206.
5. Bjornsdottir. Respiratory infections and asthma. *Med Clin North Am* 1992;76:895.
6. Bloomfield. Comparison of salbutamol given intravenously and by intermittent positive-pressure breathing in life-threatening asthma. *Br Med J* 1979;1:848.
7. Bodenhamer. Frequently nebulized β_2-agonists for asthma: effects on serum electrolytes. *Ann Emerg Med* 1992;21:1337.
8. Bosquet. Eosinophilic inflammation in asthma. *N Engl J Med* 1990;323:1033.
9. Burr. Epidemiology of asthma. *Monographs in Asthma* 1993;31:80.
10. Burrows. Association of asthma with serum IgE levels and skin-test reactivity to allergens. *N Engl J Med* 1989;320:271.
11. Cabanes. Bronchial hyperresponsiveness to methacholine in patients with impaired left ventricular function. *N Engl J Med* 1989;320:1317.
12. Chapman. Effect of a short course of prednisone in the prevention of early relapse after the emergency room treatment of acute asthma. *N Engl J Med* 1991;324:788.
13. Colacone. A comparison of albuterol administered by metered dose inhaler (and holding chamber) or wet nebulizer in acute asthma. *Chest* 1993;104:835.
14. Darioli. Mechanical controlled hypoventilation in status asthmaticus. *Am Rev Respir Dis* 1984;129:385.
15. Drazen. Recovery of leukotriene E_4 from the urine of patients with airway obstruction. *Am Rev Respir Dis* 1992;146:104.
16. Fanta. Key decisions in the initial phase of acute asthmatic episodes. *Contemporary Internal Medicine* 1992;4:75. Review.
17. Fanta. Glucocorticoids in acute asthma. *Am J Med* 1983;74:845.
18. Findley. The value of chest roentgenograms in acute asthma in adults. *Chest* 1981;80:535.

18a. Fischl. An index predicting relapse and need for hospitalization in patients with acute bronchial asthma. *N Engl J Med* 1981;305:783.

19. Gilman. Comparison of aerosolized glycopyrrolate and metaproterenol in acute asthma. *Chest* 1990;98:1095.
20. Haas. The impact of socioeconomic status on the intensity of ambulatory treatment and health outcomes after hospital discharge for adults with asthma. *J Gen Intern Med* 1994;9:121.

21. Hahn. Association of *Chlamydia pneumoniae* (strain TWAR) infection with wheezing, asthmatic bronchitis, and adult-onset asthma. *JAMA* 1991;266:225.
22. Haskell. A double-blind, randomized clinical trial of methylprednisolone in status asthmaticus. *Arch Intern Med* 1983;143:1324.
23. Higgins. Should ipratropium bromide be added to beta-agonists in treatment of acute severe asthma. *Chest* 1988;94:718.
24. Hollerman. Does the clinical examination predict airflow limitation? *JAMA* 1995; 273:313. Review.
25. Huang. Does aminophylline benefit adults admitted to the hospital for an acute exacerbation of asthma? *Ann Intern Med* 1993;119:1155.
26. Kelsen. Emergency room assessment and treatment of patients with acute asthma. *Am J Med* 1978;64:622.
27. Karpel. A comparison of atropine sulfate and metaproterenol sulfate in the emergency treatment of asthma. *Am Rev Respir Dis* 1986;133:727.
28. Kikuchi. Chemosensitivity and perception of dyspnea in patients with a history of near-fatal asthma. *N Engl J Med* 1994;330:1329.
29. Kondo. Progressive bronchial obstruction during the acute stage of respiratory tract infection in asthmatic children. *Chest* 1994;106:100.
30. Leatherman. Life-threatening Asthma. *Clin Chest Med* 1994;15:453. Review.
31. Lederle. Tapering of corticosteroid therapy following exacerbation of asthma. *Arch Intern Med* 1987;147:2201.
32. Leiner. Expiratory peak flow rate: standard values for normal subjects. Use as a clinical test of ventilatory function. *Am Rev Respir Dis* 1963;88:644.
33. Littenberg. Aminophylline treatment in severe, acute asthma. *JAMA* 1988;259: 1678. Review.
34. Mansel. Mechanical ventilation in patients with acute severe asthma. *Am J Med* 1990;89:42.
35. Martin. Use of peak expiratory flow rates to eliminate unnecessary arterial blood gases in acute asthma. *Ann Emerg Med* 1982;11:70.
36. McFadden. Asthma. In: Isselbacher KJ, Braunwald E, Wilson JD, Martin JB, Fauci AS, Kaspor DL, eds, *Harrison's Principles of Internal Medicine*, ed 13. New York: McGraw-Hill, 1994:1167.
37. McFadden. Acute bronchial asthma. *N Engl J Med* 1973;288:221.
38. McFadden. Arterial-blood gas tension is asthma. *N Engl J Med* 1968;278:1027.
39. McFadden. Dosages of corticosteroids in asthma. *Am Rev Respir Dis* 1993; 147:1306.
40. Molfino. Respiratory arrest in near-fatal asthma. *N Engl J Med* 1991;324:285.
41. Mountain. Clinical features and outcome in patients with acute asthma presenting with hypercapnia. *Am Rev Respir Dis* 1988;138:535.
42. Murphy. Aminophylline in the treatment of acute asthma when β_2-adrenergics and steroids are provided. *Arch Intern Med* 1993;153:1784.
43. National Heart, Lung, and Blood Institute. *International Consensus Report on Diagnosis and Treatment of Asthma*. Publication No. 92-3091. Bethesda, MD: National Institutes of Health, 1992:1. Review.
44. Nicholson. Respiratory viruses and exacerbations of asthma in adults. *Br Med J* 1993;307:982.
45. Nowak. Comparison of peak expiratory flow and FEV_1 admission criteria for acute bronchial asthma. *Ann Emerg Med* 1982;11:64.
46. Nowak. Arterial blood gases and pulmonary function testing in acute bronchial asthma. *JAMA* 1983;249:2043.
47. Okayama. Bronchodilating effect of intravenous magnesium sulfate in bronchial asthma. *JAMA* 1987;257:1076.
48. Papo. A prospective, randomized study of continuous versus intermittent nebulized albuterol for severe status asthmaticus in children. *Crit Care Med* 1993;21: 1479.
49. Quakenboss. The normal range of diurnal changes in peak expiratory flow rates. *Am Rev Respir Dis* 1991;143:323.
50. Ratto. Are intravenous corticosteroids required in status asthmaticus? *JAMA* 1988; 260:527.

51. Rea. A case-control study of deaths from asthma. *Thorax* 1986;41:833.
52. Rebuck. Nebulized anticholinergic and sympathomimetic treatment of asthma and chronic obstructive pulmonary disease in the emergency room. *Am J Med* 1987; 82:59.
53. Reihsaus. Mutations in the gene encoding for the β_2-adrenergic receptor in normal and asthmatic subjects. *Am J Respir Cell Mol Biol* 1993;8:334.
54. Rossing. Emergency therapy of asthma: comparison of the acute effects of parenteral and inhaled sympathomimetics and infused aminophylline. *Am Rev Respir Dis* 1980;122:365.
55. Rubinfeld. Perception of asthma. *Lancet* 1976;1:882.
56. Sasaki. Bronchial hyperresponsiveness in patients with chronic congestive heart failure. *Chest* 1990;97:534.
57. Shim. Evaluation of the severity of asthma: patients versus physicians. *Am J Med* 1980;68:11.
58. Skobeloff. Intravenous magnesium sulfate for the treatment of acute asthma in the emergency department. *JAMA* 1989;262:1210.
59. Soutar. Nocturnal and morning asthma: relationship to plasma corticosteroids and response to cortisol infusion. *Thorax* 1975;30:436.
60. Spitzer. The use of β-agonists and the risk of death and near death from asthma. *N Engl J Med* 1992;326:501.
61. Strunk. Identification of the fatality-prone subject with asthma. *J Allergy Clin Immunol* 1989;83:477.
62. The National Asthma Education Program. *Guidelines for the Diagnosis and Management of Asthma.* Publication 91-3042. Bethesda, MD: National Institutes of Health, 1991:19. Review.
63. Tiffany. Magnesium bolus or infusion fails to improve expiratory flow in acute asthma exacerbations. *Chest* 1993;104:831.
64. Turner. Equivalence of continuous flow nebulizer and metered-dose inhaler with reservoir bag for treatment of acute airflow obstruction. *Chest* 1988;93:476.
65. Tuxen. Detrimental effects of positive end-expiratory pressure during controlled mechanical ventilation of patients with severe airflow obstruction. *Am Rev Respir Dis* 1989;140:5.
66. Tuxen. The effects of ventilatory pattern on hyperinflation, airway pressures, and circulation in mechanical ventilation of patients with severe air-flow obstruction. *Am Rev Respir Dis* 1987;136:872.
67. Undem. Neural-immunologic interactions in asthma. *Hospital Practice* 1994;February 15:43.
68. Van Renterghem. Intravenous versus nebulized terbutaline in patients with acute severe asthma: a double-blind randomized study. *Ann Allergy* 1987;59:313.
69. Weiss. An economic evaluation of asthma in the United States. *N Engl J Med* 1992; 326:862.
70. Williams. Risk factors for morbidity in mechanically ventilated patients with acute severe asthma. *Am Rev Respir Dis* 1992;146:607.
71. Wrenn. Aminophylline therapy for acute bronchospastic disease in the emergency room. *Ann Intern Med* 1991;115:241.

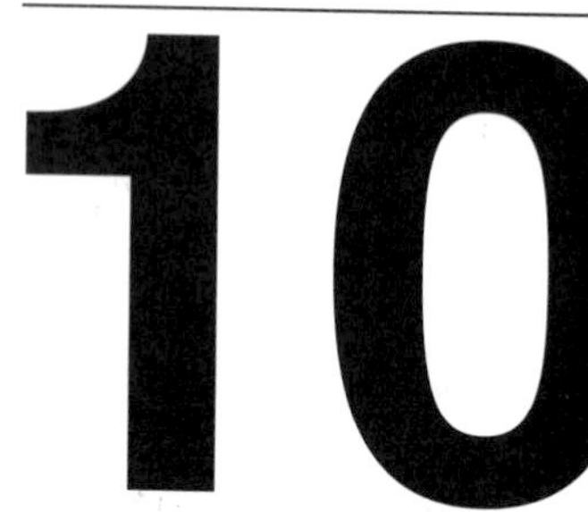

Chronic Obstructive Pulmonary Disease

David G. Morris, Les A. Szekely, and B. Taylor Thompson

A. Introduction

1. The term chronic obstructive pulmonary disease (COPD) can be applied to many conditions that are characterized by chronic airflow obstruction, including emphysema, chronic bronchitis, asthmatic bronchitis, and bronchiectasis. However, most clinicians reserve the use of this term for emphysema and chronic bronchitis. COPD is a broad term and should be considered a composite of these entities, with much overlap in clinical, physiologic, and pathologic features.
2. **Definition of Emphysema**—Emphysema is characterized by abnormal enlargement of the alveoli and destruction of the alveolar walls without obvious fibrosis (109). The abnormal airspace enlargement and destruction of lung units occur distal to the terminal bronchioles. Although predictable clinical manifestations may develop as a result of these structural abnormalities, emphysema, strictly defined, is a pathologic diagnosis. Nevertheless, the diagnosis can be inferred on clinical grounds, strongly suggested with pulmonary function testing, and diagnosed in some patients with high-resolution computed tomography (CT).
3. **Definition of Chronic Bronchitis**—Chronic bronchitis is characterized by chronic or recurrent excess mucus secretion into the bronchial tree (35). Historically, the diagnosis of chronic bronchitis requires that chronic cough with sputum production be present for at least 3 months per year for 2 or more years. The characteristic histologic features of chronic bronchitis are discussed in more detail in later sections. In contrast to emphysema, chronic bronchitis is principally a clinical rather than a histopathologic diagnosis. If the patient does not have significant airflow obstruction, the condition is called simple bronchitis and the prognosis is good. On the other hand, patients with chronic bronchitis who exhibit airflow limitation are at risk for premature morbidity and mortality.
4. **Clinical Course**—A typical patient with COPD follows a course of slow, progressive deterioration in respiratory function. This decline is frequently punctuated by COPD flares, or more abrupt deteriorations in respiratory function. These flares are characterized by worsening respiratory mechanics, increased dyspnea, sputum production, and further impairment of gas exchange. Although severe exacerbations can be fatal, successful management of COPD exacerbations usually returns the patient to baseline function.
5. **Epidemiology**—COPD is the fifth leading cause of death and affects 13 million people in the United States (16). From the time of initial diagnosis, the 10-year mortality rate exceeds 50% (46). Tobacco smoke exposure accounts for 80% to 90% of the cases of COPD in United States (30). Less common causes include severe chronic asthma and genetic disorders such as α_1-antitrypsin (AAT) deficiency. Other risk factors for development of various forms of COPD include advanced age, lower socioeconomic status, family history of COPD, exposure to air pollution, and occupational exposure (54,70).
6. **Pathology and Pathophysiology of Respiratory Dysfunction with COPD**
   a. **Emphysema**—The pathologic findings of emphysema include abnormal airspace enlargement and destruction of lung units distal to the terminal

bronchioles. Emphysema can be subdivided into distal acinar, centriacinar, and panacinar emphysema depending on the extent of acinar involvement. The pathogenesis of COPD remains unknown, although the elastase-antielastase theory remains the leading hypothesis. This hypothesis proposes that an imbalance between proteases and antiproteases leads to the destruction of the pulmonary interstitium. The best model for this hypothesis is the inherited AAT deficiency. Eriksson demonstrated that emphysema could be caused by congenital deficiencies of serum AAT (43). AAT is an antiprotease that protects the pulmonary interstitium from proteolytic digestion by elastases and proteases, which are secreted by intrapulmonary inflammatory cells. AAT is synthesized and secreted by hepatocytes. AAT enters the lung interstitium by transudation from the circulation. AAT is pleomorphic; more than 80 genotypes have been identified. A descriptive nomenclature has been established based on the electrophoretic mobility of AAT (F, fast; M, medium; S, slow; and Z, ultra-slow). The classic deficiency, PiZZ, occurs in 1 of every 6000 people (105). Patients who are homozygous for AAT deficiency have low serum levels of functional AAT. Irrespective of cigarette use, some of these patients develop lower lobe pulmonary emphysema at a relatively early age. IV replacement of AAT has been proposed as a means of preventing the development of emphysema in these individuals. Studies are underway to evaluate the long-term efficacy of AAT replacement therapy. It is unknown whether heterozygotes are also at increased risk of developing premature COPD. Heterozygotes (PiMZ) who are relatives of homozygous patients do have a slight increase in the incidence of COPD (80). On the other hand, PiMZ patients who were identified as part of a population survey did not have differing lung function from controls (23,81). Ingredients in tobacco smoke have been shown to oxidize and thereby inactivate AAT (60). This may be one mechanism whereby smokers with normal serum levels of AAT develop emphysema. However, only 10% to 15% of smokers develop clinically significant emphysema (12,25). Furthermore, it has been estimated that almost two-thirds of the homozygotes for AAT deficiency (PiZZ) have well preserved pulmonary function. Therefore, the elastase-antielastase theory does not fully account for the pathogenesis of COPD, and many questions in regard to the pathophysiology remain.

b. **Respiratory Muscle Dysfunction**—Mechanical changes in the muscles of respiration may also contribute to respiratory dysfunction in patients with COPD. Obstruction to airflow causes air trapping and hyperinflation of the lung, which leads to progressive flattening of the diaphragm and an unfavorable ratio of nerve stimulation to muscle tension development. In addition, a more horizontal rather than vertical insertion of the muscle into the costal margins results in decreased mechanical advantage during inspiration (37).

c. **Chronic Bronchitis**—Histologically, the bronchial mucosa is infiltrated with inflammatory cells and shows goblet cell metaplasia. Often, associated airway edema and varying degrees of fibrosis are present. Several cellular mechanisms appear to be important in the development and maintenance of chronic inflammation and subsequent fibrosis. These include epithelial cell–cytokine interactions, eicosanoids, and neurogenic mechanisms (71,99,103,115).

d. **Other Contributions to Obstruction**—The other mechanisms for airway obstruction in COPD are decreased driving pressure for expiratory flow due to loss of lung recoil; increased airway collapsibility due to loss of elastic parenchymal elements; bronchospasm; and increased airway resistance due to edema, inflammation, and secretions (14).

B. Etiology of COPD Exacerbations—For the purpose of discussion, the causes of COPD exacerbations can be divided in intrapulmonary causes (those occurring within the lung parenchyma and airways) and extrapulmonary causes (those occurring outside the lung parenchyma), as shown in Table 10-1.

1. Intrapulmonary Causes of COPD Exacerbations

a. **Acute Bronchitis**—Acute bronchitis is a major cause of clinical deterioration

Table 10-1 Precipitants of COPD exacerbations

Intrapulmonary	Extrapulmonary
Acute Bronchitis	Decreased Ventilatory Drive
Pneumonia	Decreased Respiratory Muscle Strength
Bronchospasm	Increased Metabolic Demands
Pulmonary Edema	Decreased Chest Wall Compliance
Pulmonary Embolism	Decreased Atmospheric Oxygen Tension
Pneumothorax	Cardiac Arrhythmia

in patients with underlying lung disease. Table 10-2 summarizes the relative importance of each class of pathogens in acute bronchitis for patients with COPD.

(1) Bacterial Bronchitis—Many studies have evaluated the causes of bacterial infection in patients with COPD. Most of them have focused primarily on the sputum Gram stain and culture to identify the putative pathogen. However, the inherent difficulty in differentiating a colonizing organism of the upper airway tract from a true pathogen limits the utility of these studies. Two studies have made an effort to avoid this problem by using a protected specimen brush (PSB) (45) or transtracheal aspirate (102). These studies are summarized in Table 10-3 and are described further in the following sections.

(a) In a study of 54 patients with COPD exacerbations requiring mechanical ventilation, Fagon performed bronchoscopy with PSB. All patients in this study had been intubated for <24 hours at the time of bronchoscopy. Those who had been treated with antibiotics within 10 days of the bronchoscopy and patients whose chest radiograph demonstrated an infiltrate were excluded. The PSB technique theoretically avoids upper airway contamination and allows direct quantitation of bacterial growth in the distal airway. Bacterial pathogens were recovered in 50% of the patients studied. Because the study included only those who required mechanical ventilation, the findings may not be generalizable to patients with less severe exacerbations (45).

(b) In a study of 87 patients with acute COPD exacerbation, Schreiner used transtracheal aspiration to identify lower respiratory tract pathogens (102). Although this technique does not sample the distal airways, when performed correctly it does avoid supraglottic contamination. A COPD exacerbation was defined as increased dyspnea and coughing, increased quantity and purulence of sputum, and a rise in body temperature >37.8°C. Patients found to have pneumonia, bronchiectasis, or asthma were excluded. In this study, bacteria could be isolated from 87% of the patients with acute flares.

Table 10-2 Prevalence of infectious agents associated with COPD exacerbations

	Prevalence	Reference
Bacteria	50–87%	(13, 45, 102)
Viruses	20–30%	(107)
Chlamydia pneumonia	<1%	(15)
Mycoplasma pneumoniae	<1%	(107)

Table 10-3 Major bacterial pathogens in COPD exacerbations

	Fagon 1990 (45) (n=54)	Schreiner 1978 (102) (n=87)
Method of diagnosis	Protected specimen brushing	Transtracheal aspirates
Any isolated bacteria	50%	87%
H. influenzae	14%	30%
S. pneumoniae	16%	26%
M. catarrhalis	7%	2%
*H. parainfluenzae**	25%	—

*Not known to be pathogenic.

(c) In both studies, the most common bacterial pathogens were *Streptococcus pneumoniae* and *Hemophilus influenzae*. *Moraxella catarrhalis* was also common. *H influenzae* and *M catarrhalis* are of particular interest because they frequently produce a β-lactamase (51,86,89). Although generally not thought to be a pathogen, *Hemophilus parainfluenzae* was also frequently isolated from the lower respiratory tract in one study (45). Nevertheless, its role in the pathogenesis of a COPD exacerbation has yet to be established.

(2) Viral Bronchitis—Several studies have evaluated the role of viral pathogens in the pathogenesis of COPD exacerbations.

(a) Smith monitored 150 patients for an average of 3.1 years; they had a total of 1000 acute respiratory illnesses (107). Eighty percent of the patients had a clinical diagnosis of COPD. Patients were seen every 3 months and at the development of any respiratory illness. Patients were screened with nasal washes, throat swabs, and antibody titers against viral pathogens and *Mycoplasma pneumoniae* at each visit. No bacterial pathogens were sought. The average number of acute respiratory illnesses per year was 2.19. There was no significant difference in the incidence of infection in patients with severe COPD compared with those with only mild or no disease. However, patients with more severe COPD were more likely than those with mild disease to experience cough and increased sputum production with viral infections. The most frequently found nonbacterial pathogens were rhinoviruses (4.8% of symptomatic infections), influenza viruses (4.9%), parainfluenza viruses (2.8%), and coronaviruses (1.7%). Respiratory syncytial virus, herpes simplex virus, adenoviruses, and *M pneumoniae* each caused symptomatic infection in $<1\%$ of acute respiratory illnesses. Only 20% of acute respiratory illnesses could be positively correlated with acute viral infection despite aggressive serologic and culture evaluation. No viral precipitant was identified in 80% of the exacerbations.

(b) Several other studies have shown the percentage of COPD exacerbations mediated by viral infection to be between 14% and 65% (27,28,40,53,69,75). However, these studies were limited by either a short duration of follow-up or a limited number of patients.

(c) Serologically documented viral infection is frequently asymptomatic in both healthy patients and those with COPD.

(3) Interaction Between Viral and Bacterial Pathogens—Few studies have carefully tested the commonly held concept that a bacterial superinfection frequently follows a viral infection. The most rigorous epidemiologic study was conducted by Smith. In an extension of the study previously outlined (107), 150 patients (120 with COPD and 30 controls) were monitored for 7 years. Patients were screened at regular intervals for asymptomatic bacterial, viral, and mycoplasma infections. Only those who had a negative sputum culture before development of the viral infection were included in the analysis, to avoid confounding by positive cultures resulting from chronic colonization. Within 7 days of an influenza infection, an infection with *S pneumoniae* occurred at 2.43 times the expected frequency ($P = 0.037$). Similarly, within 7 days of an influenza infection, an infection with *H influenzae* occurred at 2.06 times the expected frequency ($P = 0.056$). However, there was no significant association between other viral infections (rhinovirus or herpes simplex virus) and *S pneumoniae* or *H influenzae* infection (108). These data suggest that infections by influenza but not other viruses increase the risk of subsequent bacterial superinfection.

b. Pneumonia

(1) Clinical experience suggests that pneumonia occurs frequently in patients with COPD. Impaired mucociliary clearance and colonization by pathogenic organisms appear to promote the development of pneumonia in patients with underlying COPD. Nevertheless, the relative incidence of pneumonia among COPD patients compared with those without COPD has not been rigorously defined (50).

(2) The diagnosis of pneumonia in patients with COPD is often challenging and relies heavily on radiographic demonstration of an infiltrate. Roentgenographic features can be obscured or distorted by abnormal underlying pulmonary parenchyma.

(3) Chronic airway colonization by a potentially pathogenic organism often makes interpretation of sputum Gram stain and culture difficult. Several methods have been proposed to increase the diagnostic certainty of pneumonia in patients with COPD, including blood cultures, pleural fluid cultures, bronchoscopy with PSB, transtracheal aspiration, and transthoracic lung puncture. The diagnostic modalities, microbiology, and treatment of community-acquired pneumonia are fully discussed in Chapter 28.

c. Bronchospasm—Like patients with asthma, those with COPD may develop acute narrowing of the small airways as a result of bronchospasm. The degree to which this narrowing is caused by reversible factors such as smooth muscle constriction, mucus plugging, and airway inflammation is not always clear before treatment. Nevertheless, bronchospasm increases the resistive work of breathing and may precipitate respiratory failure in patients with compromised pulmonary mechanics (37).

d. Pulmonary Edema—Interstitial or alveolar edema may impair gas exchange and unfavorably affect lung mechanics (37). Pulmonary edema suggests the presence of another disorder, such as myocardial dysfunction, renal failure, or diffuse lung injury, in addition to chronic lung disease.

e. Pulmonary Embolism—has been reported to occur in as many as 50% of patients with severe COPD who ultimately come to autopsy. Premortem diagnosis of pulmonary embolism is often difficult in patients with COPD, and these estimates of prevalence are probably skewed because only autopsied patients were included in the study. Nevertheless, a high index of suspicion should be maintained in patients with COPD who suffer a clinical decompensation without a clear cause (57).

2. Extrapulmonary Causes of COPD Exacerbations

a. Decreased Respiratory Drive

(1) The neurologic stimulus to breathe is generated by the central nervous system and correlates with the strength of initial diaphragmatic contraction. A commonly used measure of respiratory drive is the P100, the inspiratory force generated against a closed airway at 0.1 seconds after initiation of inspiratory effort. During acute respiratory failure, the P100 and respiratory rate are typically high in patients with COPD, suggesting that the respiratory drive is preserved (5,6,37,84). A normal or decreased respiratory rate during an exacerbation of COPD, therefore, implies that another disorder is present, such as brainstem pathology, metabolic abnormality, or intoxication with drugs or alcohol.

(2) Hypothyroidism may cause an abnormal ventilatory response to both hypoxic and hypercapnic stimuli. In a study of 17 profoundly hypothyroid patients with no underlying lung disease, the hypoxic ventilatory drive normalized after thyroid hormone was fully replaced, but the hypercapnic response remained abnormal. The resting minute ventilation and arterial carbon dioxide tension ($PaCO_2$) were normal, suggesting that hypothyroidism alone was insufficient to cause respiratory failure (120). The mechanism of the abnormal ventilatory response in hypothyroidism is unknown.

(3) Although oxygen therapy has been blamed for leading to carbon dioxide retention by removal of the hypoxic drive in patients with COPD, there is no experimental evidence to support a progressive, persistent decline in respiratory drive in patients with COPD who are placed on oxygen therapy (5,37). The mechanisms of oxygen-induced hypercapnia in COPD are discussed more fully in later sections.

b. Decreased respiratory muscle strength is a frequent cause of respiratory failure in patients with COPD who are confronted with an acute or subacute increase in the work of breathing. Its causes are often multifactorial.

(1) Metabolic and electrolyte abnormalities are commonly observed in patients with a COPD flare. However, it is unclear whether these metabolic abnormalities cause the respiratory failure or result from it.

(a) Hypophosphatemia—Aubier measured the transdiaphragmatic pressure in 8 artificially ventilated patients with hypophosphatemia before and after phosphorus repletion. Two of the patients had COPD and the rest had respiratory failure from pneumonia. The transdiaphragmatic pressure doubled after serum phosphorus levels were normalized (7). Others have reported similar findings in less well-designed studies (87).

(b) Hypocalcemia—In animals, hypocalcemia appears to selectively impair diaphragmatic contractility. The degree of impairment was proportional to the degree of hypocalcemia. Restoration of normal serum calcium levels resulted in normalization of diaphragmatic strength (8).

(c) Hypomagnesemia—The effects of hypomagnesemia on respiratory function have not been studied extensively. A single double-blind randomized placebo-controlled trial (DBRPCT) has studied the effects of magnesium repletion on respiratory muscle power in patients with and without hypomagnesemia. Thirty-three patients were studied, 6 of whom had COPD. IV magnesium replacement resulted in a statistically significant increase in maximal inspiratory force from functional residual capacity in patients with hypomagnesemia. No significant change was observed in patients without hypomagnesemia (38).

(d) Hypoxemia—accelerates respiratory muscle failure under conditions of high mechanical load. A reduction of the partial pressure of oxygen in arterial blood (PaO_2) to approximately 50 mm Hg causes a reduction of 43% to 88% in the time to respiratory failure in normal volunteers. At a constant mechanical load, respiratory failure occurs more quickly under hypoxic conditions because of decreased muscle endurance. Cellular hypoxia results in lactic acidosis, causing further respiratory stimulation, which can hasten respiratory failure (61).

(2) Underlying neuromuscular diseases such as Guillain-Barré syndrome, amylotrophic lateral sclerosis, myasthenia gravis, polymyositis, and the muscular dystrophies can all result in decreased respiratory muscle strength. These conditions may coexist with COPD and should be considered in patients who show progressive respiratory deterioration without other identifiable causes (101).

c. **Increased Metabolic Demands**—$PaCO_2$ is a function of alveolar minute ventilation and the rate of carbon dioxide production. Under normal circumstances, any increase in the rate of carbon dioxide production is countered by an increase in alveolar ventilation to maintain a normal $PaCO_2$. Since the ability to adjust the alveolar minute ventilation may be severely limited in patients with COPD, an increase in the rate of carbon dioxide production may cause a dramatic rise in $PaCO_2$. Hyperthyroidism, sepsis, fever, hyperalimentation, and severe burns are examples of clinical situations in which the rate of carbon dioxide production may be increased (37).

d. A decrease in chest wall compliance leads to a decrease in tidal volume (V_T). For COPD patients with an increased dead space, a decrease in V_T may cause an increase in the proportion of each breath that ventilates dead space, leading to an increase in $PaCO_2$. Chest wall pain, ascites, upper abdominal surgery, and peritoneal dialysis are examples of situations that can cause decreased chest wall compliance and contribute to respiratory failure.

e. **High Altitude**—Typically, airline cabins are pressurized to the equivalent of an altitude of 5000 to 8000 ft. In general, a drop of 30 to 35 mm Hg should be anticipated in all patients traveling by air. At this altitude, the PaO_2 of a normal individual falls to 65 to 68 mm Hg. Persons with adequate pulmonary reserve typically hyperventilate, lowering the $PaCO_2$ and thereby limiting the fall in PaO_2. However, for patients with limited pulmonary reserve or significant hypoxemia at sea level, the PaO_2 may fall to 30 to 40 mm Hg. Supplemental oxygen should be provided for patients whose PaO_2 would be expected to fall below 55 mm Hg (39,49,106).

f. **Cardiac Dysrhythmias**—Hudson documented a very high incidence of cardiac rhythm disturbances in patients with COPD who were admitted with acute respiratory failure (58,104). Cardiac dysrhythmias may cause a decrease in cardiac output and may lead to further clinical deterioration, especially in those with impaired ventricular function.

C. Clinical Presentation and Diagnosis

1. History and Physical Examination

a. The symptoms may vary depending on the relative degree of emphysema versus chronic bronchitis.

(1) For patients with predominant emphysema, the lungs are overexpanded as a result of the destruction of the alveolar walls. These patients struggle with the mechanical limitation imposed by the overinflated respiratory system. Patients typically experience chronic dyspnea, but cough and wheezing are generally less pronounced than in patients with predominant chronic bronchitis.

(2) For patients with predominant chronic bronchitis, airway obstruction is the principal pathologic derangement. Chronic productive cough and intermittent wheezing are chief complaints. In practice, most patients have features of both chronic bronchitis and emphysema.

b. When the syndromes are fully developed, a myriad of classic physical findings occur in both chronic bronchitis and emphysema. There is rarely any diagnostic uncertainty with advanced disease. However, with early disease, diagnosis by clinical features alone may be difficult.

(1) The characteristic features found in the emphysematous patient include asthenia, tachypnea, a widely rounded chest, sternocleidomastoid hypertrophy, and pursed-lip breathing. Patients are typically not cyanotic. Frequently, patients unconsciously assume a tripod position with both elbows braced against their knees or other surfaces in order to use the upper extremity musculature to augment chest excursion. This is the classic pink puffer.

(2) The characteristic features found in the chronic bronchitic include obesity, cyanosis, peripheral edema, chronic cough, sputum produc-

tion, and wheezing. Generally, these patients do not appear dyspneic despite the presence of chronic cyanosis. Patients with advanced disease often show signs of cor pulmonale with severe peripheral edema.

c. Holleman recently published a critical review of all studies examining the diagnostic utility of specific clinical features for determining the presence or absence of chronic airway obstruction (56). Table 10-4 summarizes the clinical features that most reliably predict the presence of airflow limitation in patients with COPD. The most helpful findings were wheezing, barrel chest, decreased cardiac dullness (*i.e.*, a resonant percussion note in the fourth intercostal space just lateral to the left sternal margin), hyperresonant lungs, rhonchi, and an inability to blow out a lighted match at 10 cm (Snider test). When present, these features argued strongly for the presence of airflow obstruction. However, they were relatively insensitive for the presence of airflow obstruction on spirometric testing.

2. Radiographic Features

a. Standard Chest Radiograph—In a study of 189 patients, Burki compared standard anteroposterior and lateral radiographs with pulmonary function studies performed within 24 hours of each other. Data were gathered from consecutive patients referred to the pulmonary function laboratory regardless of the diagnosis. Three radiographic features correlated well with the presence of spirometric airflow obstruction (defined as a ratio of the forced expiratory volume in 1 second to the forced vital capacity [FEV_1/FVC] <75% of predicted) and were useful in the diagnosis of COPD (24).

(1) The degree of peripheral lucency, the curvature of the diaphragm, and

Table 10-4 Clinical features in the diagnosis of COPD

Clinical Features	Sensitivity	Specificity	Likelihood Ratio Positive	Likelihood Ratio Negative
Tobacco use: ever vs. never	92%	49%	1.8	0.16
>70 vs <70 pack-years	40%	95%	8.0	0.63
History of wheezing	51%	84%	3.8	0.66
Sputum >60 ml each day	20%	95%	4	0.84
Coughing	51%	71%	1.8	0.69
Exertional dyspnea	27%	88%	2.2	0.83
Wheezes present	15%	99.6%	36	0.85
Barrel chest	10%	99%	10	0.90
Decreased cardiac dullness	13%	99%	10	0.88
Diminished breath sounds	37%	90%	3.7	0.7
Snider test	61%	91%	7.1	0.43
Subxyphoid cardiac impulse	8%	98%	4.6	0.94
Hyperresonance	32%	94%	4.8	0.73
Rhonchi	8%	99%	5.9	0.95

Adapted from JAMA 1995, 273 (4), p. 313. Copyright 1995, American Medical Association (56).

Table 10-5 Sensitivity and specificity of radiographic findings in COPD (24)

Radiographic Finding	Sensitivity	Specificity
Right dome of diaphragm at or below the 7th rib	30%–40%	97%
Retrosternal space >4.4 cm	32%	85%–93%
Cardiac diameter <11.5 cm	23%–39%	88%–95%

the thickness of hilar bronchi were neither sensitive nor specific when compared with spirometry in this study. These authors suggest that plain chest roentgenograms are useful in the diagnosis of COPD if they are abnormal. Nevertheless, significant disease can be undetected by plain chest radiographs.

(2) Others have found that the most dependable piece of evidence on plain radiograph is flattening of the diaphragmatic domes. Nicklaus in a roentgenologic-pathologic correlation study, found that diaphragmatic flattening was the most accurate indicator of the presence of morphologic emphysema (88).

b. High-Resolution Chest Computed Tomography—High-resolution CT has been compared with spirometry and appears to be useful in the diagnosis of emphysema. In addition, expiratory views may provide radiographic evidence of air trapping. Nevertheless, the high cost and limited availability of high-resolution CT makes it unlikely that it will become a standard diagnostic tool (79).

3. Spirometry

a. All patients with suspected obstructive lung disease ultimately require spirometric confirmation of obstruction. In general, obstruction is considered significant if the FEV_1 and the FEV_1/FVC are below the fifth percentile for height, race, gender, and age (3). Typically, in most adults, this results in an FEV_1 <70% of predicted and an FEV_1/FVC <0.70.

b. The $PaCO_2$ does not increase above normal levels until the FEV_1 falls below 1.2 L; however, the correlation between FEV_1 and $PaCO_2$ below this threshold is poor (91,92).

4. Arterial blood gas analysis is recommended in all patients with COPD exacerbations who require hospital admission. Significant hypoxia, hypercapnia, and respiratory acidosis may be present despite relatively minor perturbations in spirometric parameters (42a).

D. Management of Acute COPD Exacerbations

1. Bronchodilators

a. β_2 Agonist Therapy—Numerous studies have demonstrated that β_2-agonists are effective bronchodilators during an acute COPD flare as well as during chronic stable disease (41,64,65). During an acute flare of COPD, three puffs of metaproterenol through a spacer device resulted in a 33% increase in FEV_1 in one study (64). However, the response to β_2-agonist therapy varies among patients, presumably because of the variable degree of reversible bronchospasm. The dosages and characteristics of commonly available β_2-agonists are outlined in Table 10-6.

b. Anticholinergic agents reduce parasympathetic stimuli transmitted by the vagus nerve to the bronchial smooth muscle. Atropine, a tertiary amine, is the oldest member of this family of compounds. The use of these agents is limited by their systemic side effects, which are caused by systemic absorption. Ipratropium bromide (Atrovent), a quaternary amine, is minimally absorbed from the respiratory and gastrointestinal tract and therefore has virtually no systemic toxicity. Several studies have compared the relative efficacy of ipratropium bromide and β_2-agonists both during COPD flares and in chronic stable disease.

(1) Ipratropium bromide and metaproterenol appear to be equally effective for acute COPD flares. In a prospective randomized controlled trial involving 32 patients with acute COPD exacerbations, Karpel compared ipratropium bromide (0.05 mg, three puffs) versus metaproterenol (1.95 mg, three puffs) administered through a metered-dose inhaler (MDI) with a spacer device. Significant bronchodilation was observed in both groups; the FEV_1 improved by 41% among patients treated with ipratropium bromide and by 33% among patients treated with metaproterenol (P = NS). No additional bronchodilation was observed when patients were crossed over to the other agent 90 minutes later (64). Similar findings were

Table 10-6 Commonly used inhaled β_2-agonists

Generic Name	Trade Name	mg/puff	Typical Dose	Duration of Action	Typical Dose for Acute Flare
Albuterol	Proventil, Ventolin	0.09	2 puffs q 4–6 h	3–4 h	4 puffs q 2–4 h
Metaproterenol	Alupent, Metaprel	0.65	2 puffs q 4–6 h	1–2.5 h	4 puffs q 2–4 h
Terbutaline	Brethaire	0.20	2 puffs q 4–6 h	3–4 h	Rarely used acutely
Pirbuterol	Maxair	0.20	2 puffs q 4–6 h	3–5 h	Rarely used acutely
Salmeterol	Serevent	0.02	2 puffs q 12 h	>12 h	Not used acutely

observed in several studies of patients with chronic stable COPD (41, 65).

(2) In clinical practice, both ipratropium bromide and β_2-agonists are administered to patients with COPD exacerbations. However, there are no data to support this practice.

c. Mode of Delivery of Inhalational Medications

(1) **β_2 Agonists**—Many studies have demonstrated that the delivery of β_2-agonists through an MDI with a spacer device is as effective as delivery through a continuous flow nebulizer (47,62,112). MDIs are also effective for patients on mechanical ventilation, although losses of drug in the ventilator tubing and endotracheal tube necessitate a doubling of conventional doses (47).

(2) Nebulized ipratropium bromide has recently become available in the United States. Studies in patients with stable COPD indicated that 0.4 mg of nebulized ipratropium provides maximal bronchodilation. These studies also indicated that two puffs of an ipratropium MDI is equivalent to approximately 0.1 mg of nebulized ipratropium in stable patients and is only 73% as effective as the maximal nebulized dose (52). Studies of nebulized ipratropium in acute COPD flare have not yet been published. Based on the data in patients with stable disease, nebulized ipratropium may provide some benefit beyond ipratropium delivered by MDI.

2. Corticosteroids

a. In a DBRPCT of 44 patients who were admitted to the hospital with acute flares of COPD and did not require mechanical ventilation, Albert randomly assigned patients to receive either 0.5 mg/kg of methylprednisolone or placebo in addition to standard therapy. Standard therapy consisted of inhaled isoproterenol, antibiotics, and aminophylline for 72 hours. Patients treated with methylprednisolone had a mean change in FEV_1 of 40%, compared with 18% in patients receiving placebo ($P < 0.001$). The effect of the methylprednisolone was not seen until 24 hours after entry, but it persisted until the study was terminated at 72 hours. No significant change in FVC was seen (1). This study has been criticized for its statistical analysis, however (48).

b. In a DBRPCT of 96 emergency room patients, Emerman studied the efficacy of a single bolus of methylprednisolone administered early in the course of a COPD exacerbation in reducing the rate of hospitalization (42). Patients received aminophylline, hourly β_2-agonists, and either placebo or 100 mg of IV methylprednisolone. Patients were monitored with spirometry. After 5 hours, a decision to admit or discharge the patients was made by a physician who was unaware of the previous treatment. No difference was found in spirometry or admission rate at 5 hours.

c. Corticosteroids given orally reduced the rate of relapse within 48 hours of discharge in patients with frequent COPD flares who presented to an emergency department. Murata studied 30 patients in a retrospective case-control study. Only patients with two or more relapses within the previous 4-year period were included. A relapse was defined as a return to the emergency department within 2 weeks of the initial visit. Patients and controls were matched for all other treatment variables. At 48 hours, the cumulative relapse rate for patients treated with corticosteroids was 8.9%, compared with 33% for those not receiving steroids ($P = 0.005$) (83).

d. Corticosteroids are frequently used to treat patients with COPD flares who require hospitalization. However, this practice is only marginally supported by published data. There appears to be a reduced rate of relapse among patients with a history of frequent early relapses who are treated with steroids in the emergency department setting. Corticosteroids have been associated with an improvement in FEV_1, although the effect on spirometric parameters is delayed for 24 to 36 hours. No data are available concerning the efficacy of corticosteroids in patients requiring mechanical ventilation. Either a new, large trial or reanalysis of existing data is needed to unequivocally prove the benefits of steroids in acute flares of COPD. It may be that a subgroup of COPD patients with an inflammatory asthma component to their disease is the group that benefits most from corticosteroids, although this is also unproven.

e. The latest American Thoracic Society (ATS) consensus document states that corticosteroids can be useful if there is an asthmatic component in a COPD patient. However, the statement notes that there is limited information supporting the use of IV or oral steroids in the management of COPD exacerbations (29).

3. **Antibiotics**—As noted previously, bacteria appear to play a prominent role in exacerbations of COPD. Antibiotics have been evaluated both as prophylactic agents to reduce the frequency of disease flares and as a means of abbreviating the duration of a particular flare. Based on multiple published reports, empiric treatment with antibiotics that cover the principal pathogens in patients with flares of COPD is appropriate and probably prevents some patients from progressing to more severe illness. Representative studies are summarized in Table 10-7. In each study, antibiotics were directed at three principal pathogens: *H influenzae, S pneumoniae,* and *M catarrhalis* (2,4,95).

   a. The studies by Anthonisen (4) and Allegra (2) have focused principally on outpatients with COPD exacerbations; those with pneumonia were excluded. In both trials, patients were assessed by blinded observers and clinical improvement was scored according to predefined clinical parameters (the so-called Winnepeg criteria: shortness of breath, sputum purulence, and sputum production). Spirometry was not used because it was thought by the investigators to be less clinically useful and poorly reflective of the patient's overall clinical status. In each study, a significantly more rapid clinical improvement was observed with antibiotic therapy. In the Anthonisen trial (4), patients with the most severe flares had the best response to antibiotics.

   b. The Pines study examined only hospitalized patients but did not rigorously exclude those with pneumonia. As with the other studies, there was a significant improvement in patients treated with antibiotics (95).

4. **Oxygen Therapy**—Many patients with acute flares of COPD present with significant hypoxemia.

   a. Under all circumstance, a primary goal of therapy should be to maintain an arterial PaO_2 >55 to 60 mm Hg. Typically, in an uncomplicated patient, nasal prong oxygen at a flow rate of 1 to 6 L/minute is adequate (4a,21,29). Flow rates are adjusted according to oxygen saturation, pH, and $PaCO_2$. Other complicating conditions such as pneumonia, pneumothorax, or pulmonary embolism should be considered and excluded.

   b. Acute hypoxemia may precipitate cardiac ischemia or tachyarrhythmia. Chronic hypoxemia may cause polycythemia, pulmonary hypertension, mental status changes, or cor pulmonale (34).

5. **Methylxanthines**—Although previously a mainstay in the treatment of COPD flare, the role of methylxanthines in the treatment of COPD flare has recently come into question.

   a. In a DBRPCT involving 28 patients with acute exacerbations of COPD, Rice compared IV aminophylline plus standard therapy versus standard therapy alone. Patients received either aminophylline or placebo in addition to inhaled β_2-agonists, methylprednisolone (0.5 mg/kg IV q 6 hours), ampicillin (500 mg IV q 6 hours), and oxygen as needed. Questionnaires regarding subjective dyspnea and medication side effects were completed by patients. Spirometry and arterial blood gas analyses were also performed. The study had a power of 95% to detect a difference in FEV_1 of 115 ml or larger. No significant difference in spirometry or oxygen tension was observed between the two groups. In fact, there was a trend toward an increased rate of side effects with aminophylline (P = NS). The investigators concluded that aminophylline adds no significant benefit for treatment of

Table 10-7 Efficacy of antibiotics in COPD exacerbations

Reference	Year	Antibiotic	Design	N	End Points	Placebo	Treatment	*P*
Pines (95)	1968	Ampicillin + streptomycin vs. placebo	DBRPCT	30	Clinical improvement, decreased sputum purulence, decreased fever	20%	67%	<0.05
Anthonisen (4)	1987	Trimethoprim-sulfamethoxazole or ampicillin or doxycycline vs. placebo	DBRPCT	362	Symptom resolution in 21 days	55%	68%	<0.05
Allegra (2)	1991	Amoxacillin-clavulinic acid vs. placebo	DBRPCT	369	Clinical improvement	50%	86%	<0.01

COPD flare but may cause an increased rate of nausea, vomiting, and tremor (97). The 1995 ATS consensus statement recommends the addition of theophylline if aerosol therapy cannot be given or proves inadequate; however, there are no well controlled studies to substantiate these recommendations (29).

b. However, for patients with chronic stable COPD, studies do suggest a beneficial effect of aminophylline on diaphragmatic function, myocardial function, airway inflammation, and mucociliary clearance (73,85,94,119). Furthermore, some authors have noted an additive bronchodilator effect of theophylline when combined with a β_2-agonist (63). Although the use of theophylline in the outpatient setting appears to be reasonable, its utility for acute COPD flares remains to be proved.

6. Mechanical Ventilation—is necessary if there are signs of impending respiratory arrest. Bone demonstrated that the degree of initial acidosis and hypoxemia are predictive of patients who will ultimately require mechanical assistance (17).

a. Mechanical ventilation is required only in a small minority of patients with COPD exacerbations. In this subset of patients, however, it may be lifesaving.

(1) Absolute indications for mechanical ventilation include respiratory arrest, severe obtundation, uncontrollable agitation, refractory hypoxemia, or refractory acidosis. Relative indications include severe respiratory muscle fatigue, as indicated by progressive hypopnea and paradoxical respiratory muscle movements; increasing somnolence; or progressive hypoxemia or respiratory acidosis despite maximal therapy.

(2) Principles of Ventilator Management in Acute Flares of COPD

(a) Minute ventilation requirements are usually normal to moderately increased in patients with COPD. A smaller V_T may be associated with fewer complications. Initial V_T settings of 7 to 8 ml/kg prevent development of a sudden respiratory alkalosis and may minimize the development of self-controlled positive end-expiratory pressure (auto-PEEP) (21). V_T and respiratory rate should be adjusted based on subsequent arterial blood gas analysis and clinical assessment.

(b) Auto-PEEP, or dynamic hyperinflation, is the consequence of air trapping that occurs distal to bronchioles that collapse during expiration, or if there is insufficient time during exhalation to return to functional residual capacity. The degree of auto-PEEP should be monitored in mechanically ventilated patients with COPD in an effort to minimize alveolar overdistention, reduce the incidence of barotrauma, and decrease the work of breathing (21). Auto-PEEP is measured by occluding the exhalation port at the very end of expiration and observing the change in airway pressure. If positive airway pressure exists at the end of exhalation in a relaxed patient, then auto-PEEP is present. Treating bronchospasm, decreasing V_T, increasing expiratory time, and reducing the respiratory rate may all reduce auto-PEEP.

b. Noninvasive positive-pressure ventilation (NIPPV) has been shown to prevent the need for invasive mechanical ventilation in selected patients with acute COPD flare (68,77,116). In a prospective, randomized trial of 85 patients, Brochard assigned hypoxemic, tachypneic, hypercapnic, and mildly acidotic patients with acute flares of COPD to one of two groups. The first group received standard care, which consisted of β_2-agonists, corticosteroids, and/or aminophylline, subcutaneous heparin, antibiotics, and nasal prong oxygen ($\leq$ 5 L/minute to achieve oxygen saturation >90%); the second group received standard therapy plus NIPPV. NIPPV was provided through a specially designed face mask with positive pressure applied during inspiration only. In general, an inspiratory pressure of 20 cm H_2O was used. Patients with respiratory arrest, tracheostomy, or other significant underlying medical causes for decompensation or who had received sedation were excluded. Patients were maintained on NIPPV for a minimum of 6 hours and a maximum of 22 hours per day. The duration of NIPPV was individualized according to the patient's clinical condition and arterial blood gas analysis. Predetermined criteria for invasive mechanical ventilation were established, and patients were intubated only if these criteria were strictly met. Eleven (26%) of 43 patients who received NIPPV ultimately required intubation, compared with 31 (74%) of 42 patients who received only standard care ($P<0.001$). The length of hospital stay and the in-hospital mortality rate were significantly reduced with NIPPV. The in-hospital mortality rate and the length of hospital stay were similar among those requiring invasive mechanical ventilation in both groups, suggesting that the primary benefit of NIPPV was in reducing the need for mechanical ventilation (22). Based on the results of this study and others (68,77,116), NIPPV appears to be a reasonable alternative to endotracheal intubation in selected patients who present with severe COPD flares.

7. **Nutrition**—Thirty percent to 50% of COPD patients have a body weight that is below 90% of their ideal (59). During acute respiratory failure, decreased levels of albumin, prealbumin, and transferrin have been associated with increased mortality. The mechanism for this chronic malnutrition has not been completely elucidated, but is thought to be multifactorial. Increased basal metabolic rate, poor oral intake, and possibly abnormal gastrointestinal function may play a role (37). Early initiation of nutritional supplementation, preferably by the enteral route, is advisable in all patients who appear to be clinically malnourished. As discussed previously, hypomagnesemia, hypocalcemia, and hypophosphatemia should be corrected.
8. **Chest Physical Therapy**—has not been shown to be beneficial in patients with routine exacerbations of COPD with scant secretions. In fact, several studies have demonstrated an acute decline in FEV_1 and PaO_2 after vigorous chest physical therapy. Connors studied 22 hospitalized, nonintubated patients with a variety of decompensated medical pulmonary disorders, including pneumonia, bronchiectasis, atelectasis, acute bronchitis, aspiration, pulmonary edema, and COPD. For patients with little or no mucous secretions, chest physical therapy (postural drainage, percussion, and chest compression), was associated with a fall in mean PaO_2 of 16.8 mm Hg ($P<0.05$) and a further fall of 5.3 mm Hg ($P<0.01$) 30 minutes after treatment. Even for patients with copious sputum production, no significant improvement in oxygenation was observed after chest physical therapy (31). In a small study involving mechanically ventilated patients without copious secretions, chest physical therapy failed to demonstrate any improvement in arterial oxygenation or the alveolar-arterial oxygen gradient. Improvement in chest radiographic abnormalities was noted in patients with copious secretions or atelectasis, but no significant change in clinical status could be demonstrated (66). Chest physical therapy is therefore indicated only in carefully selected patients with persistent atelectasis or copious secretions. When chest physical therapy is administered, supplemental oxygen and bronchodilators should be available.
9. **Respiratory Stimulants**—In general, respiratory stimulants should not be used to treat hypercapnia in patients with acute flares of COPD. Respiratory drive is increased in patients suffering acute hypercapnic respiratory failure (6,7,84). Furthermore, several physiologic studies in patients with oxygen-induced hypercapnia indicated normal ventilatory drive, which leaves little physiologic justification for use of these agents (5,100). A single well-designed trial of respiratory stimulants in oxygen-induced hypercapnia showed that hypercapnia and acidosis progressed in 36.8% of patients treated with placebo, compared with only 17.5% of patients treated with doxapram for 2 hours ($P<0.01$). However, there was no difference in the rate of intubation or other important clinical end points between the two groups. The authors argue that respiratory stimulants may buy time until other therapeutic maneuvers can reverse the cause of hypercapnia, but they could not assess the efficacy of these agents in reducing the need for mechanical ventilation (82).

10. Experimental approaches including infusions of dopamine and digoxin have been studied in patients with acute respiratory failure complicating COPD. Both agents may significantly increase the transdiaphragmatic pressure generated by supramaximal phrenic nerve stimulation in humans (9,10). The clinical utility of these agents has not yet been studied prospectively and is likely to be limited to a small subset of mechanically ventilated patients with refractory ventilatory failure.

E. Complications of COPD

1. Respiratory failure is a serious but relatively infrequent complication of COPD exacerbation. Acute respiratory failure is characterized by progressive deterioration in respiratory function resulting in hypercapnia, hypoxemia, and acute respiratory acidosis. Patients typically exhibit respiratory distress, tachypnea, and respiratory fatigue. In advanced respiratory failure, diaphoresis, accessory muscle use, paradoxical abdominal muscle movement, and mental status changes signal impending respiratory arrest.
   a. The cause of hypercapnia is multifactorial in COPD. Many patients have chronic elevations in $PaCO_2$ related to ventilation-perfusion (V/Q) mismatch, abnormal ventilatory control, abnormal respiratory muscle function, and abnormal breathing patterns. Full discussion of chronic hypercapnia in COPD is beyond the scope of this chapter, and the subject is well reviewed by Weinberger (113). Although no absolute $PaCO_2$ can be cited as diagnostic of acute respiratory failure, a significant increase in $PaCO_2$ over baseline in a patient with respiratory distress should raise concern. If hypercapnia leads to an acute decline in pH or mental status changes, mechanical ventilation should be considered.
   b. Oxygen-induced hypercapnia was studied by Aubier in patients with acute COPD flares. Patients with acute respiratory failure complicating COPD were given 100% oxygen, and minute ventilation and blood gases were assessed. A transient 18% decrease in minute ventilation occurred but resolved after 15 minutes of treatment with 100% oxygen. The $PaCO_2$, however, continued to rise (mean$\pm$SD, 23$\pm$5 mm Hg) despite resolution of the hypoventilation. This persistent increase in $PaCO_2$ appeared to be caused by an increase in dead space ventilation. Therefore, oxygen-induced hypercapnia may result from changes in pulmonary blood flow and V/Q mismatching caused by hyperoxia (11). A similar observation has been made in patients with stable COPD (100).
   c. Severe hypoxemia is the most serious complication of acute respiratory failure in COPD and must be corrected immediately. Supplemental oxygen should be administered to achieve a PaO_2 >60 mm Hg. Hypoxemia is principally a result of V/Q mismatch and can be corrected, typically with a modest amount of supplemental oxygen. Requirements of >35% inspired oxygen concentration (FiO_2) should prompt investigation for other underlying pathology such as pneumonia or pulmonary embolism (4a).
   d. Acute respiratory acidosis is the result of increased $PaCO_2$ with generation of carbonic acid. Acutely, this is buffered by plasma buffers and results in a decline in pH of 0.08 for every increase of 10 mm Hg in $PaCO_2$. Renal compensation during chronic hypercapnia results in a decline in pH of 0.03 for every 10 mm Hg increase in $PaCO_2$. Analysis of pH therefore provides a useful indicator of the acuity of hypercapnia in respiratory failure. As mentioned previously, progressive respiratory acidosis despite maximal medical support should prompt preparation for or initiation of mechanical ventilatory support.
2. Pulmonary hypertension and cor pulmonale are manifestations of long-standing COPD (74). However, both may become worse during flares of COPD as a result of hypoxic pulmonary vasoconstriction (67). Refractory right-sided heart failure is frequently a cause of death in mechanically ventilated patients with COPD. Inotropic agents are generally ineffective, and treatment must be directed at correcting the gas exchange abnormality, if possible. Similarly, angiotensin-converting enzyme inhibitors and calcium channel blockers have been disappointing in their

ability to improve right ventricular hemodynamics. Treatment of cor pulmonale with diuretics is reasonable, but the failing right ventricle is often dependent on adequate filling pressures to maintain cardiac output. Despite the presence of peripheral edema, overzealous diuresis can cause hypotension and azotemia. Nitric oxide has recently been shown to provide significant hemodynamic improvement in mechanically ventilated patients with pulmonary hypertension secondary to adult respiratory distress syndrome (98). No trials of this intervention have yet been published in patients with acute respiratory failure secondary to COPD exacerbation.

3. Cardiac dysrhythmias are common in patients with COPD. In 148 consecutive hospitalized patients with a history of COPD and a PaO_2 <50 mm Hg, the prevalence of major supraventricular or ventricular arrhythmias was 36%. Development of a ventricular arrhythmia carried a very poor prognosis, with a 2-year mortality rate of 100%. Ectopic atrial pacemaker, atrial tachycardia, and multifocal atrial tachycardia were the most frequent major supraventricular dysrhythmias, each occurring in 10% to 15% of admissions (58). Ventricular rhythm disturbances were most closely associated with the degree of hypoxemia; 86% of ventricular dysrhythmias occurred at PaO_2 levels <37 mm Hg (104).

4. Pneumothorax can occur spontaneously in patients with bullous emphysema. Patients who are mechanically ventilated are at particularly high risk for development of pneumothorax. The clinician must maintain a high index of suspicion, and frequent radiographic screening is advisable.

F. Prognostic Factors

1. Survival

a. After an episode of hospitalization for COPD flare, the patient's prognosis depends on the severity of the underlying lung disease. Martin studied a carefully selected cohort of 36 COPD patients after hospitalization. Patients with pneumonia or asthma were excluded. The 2-year survival rate was 72%, comparable to the rate in stable outpatients with similar degrees of airway obstruction (72). The baseline postbronchodilator FEV_1 and age appeared to be the best predictors of mortality. Other predictors included hypercapnia at rest, tachycardia, cor pulmonale, and excessive weight loss. Other studies have reported that patients with hyperreactive airways or clinical features compatible with asthmatic bronchitis tend to have better survival (26,96,110).

b. For patients surviving mechanical ventilation for a COPD exacerbation, Menzies found that the 1-year survival rate correlated positively with the premorbid level of physical activity and serum albumin concentration and inversely with the severity of dyspnea. Although cor pulmonale, hypercarbia, and a history of left ventricular failure were more common among patients who died, they did not reach statistical significance. The overall 1-year survival rate for all patients requiring mechanical ventilation for COPD flare was 32%. Among patients with poor exercise tolerance at baseline (*i.e.*, housebound or chair-confined) and an FEV_1 <25% of the predicted value, only 20% survived 1 year after intubation for a COPD flare. On the other hand, 90% of patients with good baseline exercise tolerance and an FEV_1 >40% of predicted survived at least 1 year (78).

2. Ability to Wean From Mechanical Ventilation

a. Ventilator dependence is an uncommon but feared complication of mechanical ventilation. The rate of long-term ventilator dependence among mechanically ventilated COPD patients is highly variable among institutions. In a retrospective analysis by Menzies, 3 of 95 patients survived 1 year and remained ventilator dependent; the other patients either died or were eventually weaned (78).

b. Based on a retrospective analysis of 95 patients with COPD and acute respiratory failure requiring mechanical ventilation, Menzies developed a model for predicting successful weaning. The premorbid level of activity and the FEV_1 were the best predictors for the ability to wean from mechanical ventilation. Patients with poor premorbid activity and an FEV_1 <25% of the predicted value had a 47% chance of weaning from mechanical ventilation within 4 months. On the other hand, 100% of patients with good premorbid function and an FEV_1 >40% of predicted were successfully weaned (78).

c. Optimal weaning strategies remain controversial. Two recent studies have shown that intermittent mandatory ventilation (IMV) prolongs weaning and probably should not be used as a weaning technique. Intermittent T-piece (or continuous positive airway pressure) trials and pressure-support weaning appear to be superior to the IMV weaning technique (21,118).

G. Miscellaneous

1. Pulmonary rehabilitation is commonly prescribed to patients with COPD and includes chest physiotherapy, psychosocial support, and exercise conditioning. Pulmonary rehabilitation has not been shown to improve or slow the expected decline in pulmonary function. However, it decreases dyspnea, anxiety, depression, and the frequency of subsequent hospital admissions. It also increases exercise capacity and may improve the quality of life (55).

2. Long-Term Outpatient Oxygen Therapy—The Medical Research Council (MRC) study and the Nocturnal Oxygen Therapy Trial (NOTT) are the two major trials that have evaluated the benefit of long-term oxygen therapy in COPD patients with hypoxemia. In the MRC study, patients who received 15 hours of continuous oxygen therapy had improved survival compared with those who received no supplemental oxygen. The NOTT study compared 24 versus 12 hours of oxygen therapy and found that patients assigned to continuous oxygen therapy had significantly better survival (76,90). Indications for oxygen therapy include resting room air PaO_2 <55 mm Hg or oxygen saturation <89% on two occasions; PaO_2 55 to 59 mm Hg but with evidence of pulmonary hypertension, cor pulmonale, psychologic impairment, or hematocrit >55%; PaO_2 >60 mm Hg at rest but PaO_2 <55 mm Hg or oxygen saturation <89% with exercise or sleep.

3. Surgical Options

a. In a subset of COPD patients with large bullae, bullectomy may be indicated if it causes incapacitating dyspnea and compression of adjacent normal lung (32,35,114). However, no well-controlled, randomized studies exist.

b. Volume reduction surgery for emphysema by means of multiple wedge resections was first performed by Brantigan more than 35 years ago (18–20). There was some modest success with subjective improvement, but the procedure never gained widespread acceptance because of a 16% early mortality rate. Recently, Cooper reexplored the role of volume reduction surgery and published the results for 20 patients who underwent bilateral volume reduction surgery. He reported significant postoperative improvements in FEV_1, 6-minute walk test, dyspnea indices, and quality-of-life measures with minimal complications (33). These results have sparked a nationwide interest in volume reduction surgery, but many questions remain unanswered, including the indications, contraindications, and long-term outcomes associated with volume reduction surgery and the physiologic changes to be expected after surgery.

c. Lung transplantation is the ultimate option for treatment of severe COPD. Single-lung transplantation has been shown to improve the FEV_1 by 20% to 50% with additional improvements in exercise tolerance (93,111,117).

H. Summary

1. Bronchodilators are important in the management of patients with an acute COPD flare. Both β_2-agonists and anticholinergic agents are effective. In practice, these drugs are often used in combination although there is little evidence that combined therapy is superior to either agent alone.

2. Corticosteroids are frequently used to treat COPD flares based on the results of a single placebo-controlled study that has been criticized on statistical grounds. Further studies or reanalysis of existing data is necessary before the use of high-dose corticosteroids can be unequivocally supported, although a recent ATS consensus conference advocates their use (29). Corticosteroids administered in the emergency department and continued after discharge may reduce the rate of short-term relapse.

3. Empiric antibiotic therapy is useful in treatment of acute COPD flares. Antimicrobial therapy should be directed against *H influenzae*, *M catarrhalis*, and *S pneumoniae* and should be selected on the basis of local resistance patterns.
4. Supplemental oxygen should be administered to maintain a PaO_2 >60 mm Hg. Methylxanthines offer no additional benefit when added to standard therapy for a COPD flare.
5. The selective use of NIPPV reduces the length of hospital stay and improves survival in patients with a COPD flare. Invasive mechanical ventilation may still be necessary in a minority of patients with COPD flares.
6. Chest physical therapy is not generally useful unless patients who have atelectasis or copious secretions. In fact, chest physical therapy may increase bronchospasm and worsen hypoxemia in patients without significant secretions.

Abbreviations used in Chapter 10

AAT = α_1-antitrypsin
ATS = American Thoracic Society
auto-PEEP = self-induced positive end-expiratory pressure
COPD = chronic obstructive pulmonary disease
CT = computed tomography
DBRPCT = double-blind randomized placebo-controlled trial
FEV_1 = forced expiratory volume in 1 second
FiO_2 = fractional concentration of inspired oxygen
FVC = forced vital capacity
IMV = intermittent mandatory ventilation
IV = intravenous
MDI = metered-dose inhaler
NIPPV = noninvasive positive-pressure mechanical ventilation
NS = results not reaching statistical significance
$PaCO_2$ = partial pressure of carbon dioxide in arterial blood
PaO_2 = partial pressure of oxygen in arterial blood
PSB = protected specimen brush
q = every
SD = standard deviation
V/Q = ventilation-perfusion
V_T = tidal volume

References

1. Albert. Controlled clinical trial of methylprednisolone in patients with chronic bronchitis and acute respiratory insufficiency. *Ann Intern Med* 1980;92:753.
2. Allegra. Ruolo degli antibiotici nel trattamento delle riacutizza della bronchite cronica. Italian Journal of Chest Disease 1991;144:138. Cited in Ball. Epidemiology and treatment of chronic bronchitis and its exacerbations. *Chest* 1995;2 (Suppl):43S.
3. American Thoracic Society. Lung function testing: selection of reference values and interpretative strategies. *Am J Respir Dis* 1991;144:1202.
4. Anthonisen. Antibiotic therapy in exacerbations of chronic obstructive pulmonary disease. *Ann Intern Med* 1987;106:196.

4a. Anthonisen. Long-term oxygen therapy. *Ann Intern Med* 1983;99:519. Review.

5. Aubier. Effects of the administration of O_2 on ventilation and blood gases in patients with chronic obstructive pulmonary disease during acute respiratory failure. *Am Rev Respir Dis* 1980;122:747.
6. Aubier. Central respiratory drive in acute respiratory failure of patients with chronic obstructive pulmonary disease. *Am Rev Respir Dis* 1980;122:191.

7. Aubier. Effect of hypophosphatemia on diaphragmatic contractility in patients with acute respiratory failure. *N Engl J Med* 1985;313:420.
8. Aubier. Effects of hypocalcemia on diaphragmatic strength generation. *J Appl Physiol* 1985;58:2054.
9. Aubier. Dopamine effects on diaphragmatic strength during acute respiratory failure in chronic obstructive pulmonary disease. *Ann Intern Med* 1989;110:17.
10. Aubier. Effects of digoxin on diaphragmatic strength generation in patients with chronic obstructive pulmonary disease during acute respiratory failure. *Am Rev Respir Dis* 1987;135:544.
11. Aubier. Effects of the administration of O_2 on ventilation and blood gases in patients with chronic obstructive pulmonary disease during acute respiratory failure. *Am Rev Respir Dis* 1980;122:747.
12. Auerbach. Relation of smoking and age to emphysema: whole lung section study. *N Engl J Med* 1972;286:853.
13. Ball. Epidemiology and treatment of chronic bronchitis and its exacerbations. *Chest* 1995;108(Suppl):43S.
14. Bates D, ed. Respiratory Function in Disease, ed 3. Philadelphia: WB Saunders, 1989, p. 172.
15. Beaty. *Chlamydia pneumoniae*, strain TWAR, infection in patients with chronic obstructive pulmonary disease. *Am Rev Respir Dis* 1991;144:1408.
16. Benson. Current estimates from the National Health Interview Survey 1992. *Vital Health Stat* 1994;189:1.
17. Bone. Controlled oxygen administration in acute respiratory failure in chronic obstructive pulmonary disease. *Am J Med* 1978;65:896.
18. Brantigan. Surgical treatment of pulmonary emphysema. *Am Surg* 1957;23:789.
19. Brantigan. A surgical approach to pulmonary emphysema. *Am Rev Respir Dis* 1959;80:194.
20. Brantigan. The surgical approach to pulmonary emphysema. *Dis Chest* 1961; 39:485.
21. Brochard. Comparison of three methods of gradual withdrawal from ventilatory support during weaning from mechanical ventilation. *Am J Respir Crit Care Med* 1994;150:896.
22. Brochard. Noninvasive ventilation for acute exacerbations of chronic obstructive pulmonary disease. *N Engl J Med* 1995;333:817.
23. Bruce. Collaboration study to assess the risk of lung disease in PiMZ phenotype subjects. *Am Rev Respir Dis* 1984;130:386.
24. Burki. Correlation of pulmonary function with the chest roentgenogram in chronic airway obstruction. *Am Rev Respir Dis* 1980;121:217.
25. Burrows. Quantitative relationship between cigarette smoking and ventilatory function. *Am Rev Respir Dis* 1977;115:195.
26. Burrows. The course and prognosis of different forms of chronic airway obstruction in a sample from the general population. *N Engl J Med* 1987;317:1307.
27. Buscho. Infections with viruses and *Mycoplasma pneumoniae* during exacerbations of chronic bronchitis. *J Infect Dis* 1978;137:377.
28. Carilli. A virologic study of chronic bronchitis. *N Engl J Med* 1964;270:123.
29. Celli. Standards for the diagnosis and care of patients with chronic obstructive pulmonary disease. *Am J Respir Crit Care Med* 1995;152:S77.
30. *Chronic Obstructive Lung Disease: The Health Consequences of Smoking. A Report of the Surgeon General.* Public Health Service Publication 84-50205. Rockville, MD: US Department of Health and Human Services, 1984. Review.
31. Connors. Chest physical therapy: the immediate effect on oxygenation in acutely ill patients. *Chest* 1980;78:559.
32. Conolly. The current status of surgery for bullous emphysema. *J Thorac Cardiovasc Surg* 1989;97:351.
33. Cooper. Bilateral pneumonectomy (volume reduction) for chronic obstructive pulmonary disease. *J Thorac Cardiovasc Surg* 1995;109:106.
34. Curtis. Emergent assessment and management of acute respiratory failure in COPD. *Clin Chest Med* 1994;3:481. Review.

35. Dantzker. Standards for the diagnosis and care of patients with chronic obstructive pulmonary disease (COPD) and asthma. *Am Rev Respir Dis* 1987;136:225.
36. Delarue. Surgical treatment for pulmonary emphysema. *Can J Surg* 1977, 20:222.
37. Derenne. Acute respiratory failure of chronic obstructive pulmonary disease. *Am Rev Respir Dis* 1988;138:1006. Review.
38. Dhingra. Hypomagnesemia and respiratory muscle power. *Am Rev Respir Dis* 1984;129:497.
39. Dillard. Hypoxemia during air travel in patients with chronic obstructive pulmonary disease. *Ann Intern Med* 1989;111:362.
40. Eadie. Virologic studies in chronic bronchitis. *Br Med J* 1966;2:671.
41. Easton. A comparison of the bronchodilating effects of a beta-2 adrenergic agent (albuterol) and an anticholinergic agent (ipratropium bromide), given by aerosol alone or in sequence. *N Engl J Med* 1986;315:735.
42. Emerman. A randomized controlled trial of methylprednisolone in the emergency treatment of acute exacerbations of COPD. *Chest* 1989;95:563.
42a. Emerman. Relationship between arterial blood gases and spirometry in acute exacerbations of chronic obstructive pulmonary disease. *Ann Emer Med* 1989;18:523.
43. Eriksson. Studies in alpha-1-antitrypsin deficiency. *Acta Med Scand* 1965;177:1.
44. Esteban. A comparison of four methods of weaning patients from mechanical ventilation. *N Engl J Med* 1995;332:345.
45. Fagon. Characterization of distal bronchial microflora during acute exacerbation of chronic bronchitis. *Am Rev Respir Dis* 1990;142:1004.
46. Ferguson. Management of chronic obstructive pulmonary disease. *N Engl J Med* 1993;328:1017. Review.
47. Fernandez. Bronchodilators in patients with chronic obstructive pulmonary disease on mechanical ventilation. *Am Rev Respir Dis* 1990;141:164.
48. Glenny. Steroids in COPD: the scripture according to Albert. *Chest* 1987;91:289.
49. Gong. Hypoxia: altitude simulation test. *Am Rev Respir Dis* 1984;130:980.
50. Griffith. Pneumonia in chronic obstructive lung disease. *Infect Dis Clin North Am* 1991;5:467. Review.
51. Groeneveld. *Haemophilus influenzae* infections in patients with chronic obstructive pulmonary disease despite specific antibodies in serum and sputum. *Am Rev Respir Dis* 1990;141:1316.
52. Gross. Dose response to ipratropium as a nebulized solution in patients with chronic obstructive pulmonary disease. *Am Rev Respir Dis* 1989;139:1188.
53. Gump. Role of infection in chronic bronchitis. *Am Rev Respir Dis* 1976;113:465.
54. Higgins. Risk of chronic obstructive lung disease: a collaborative assessment of validity of the Tecumseh index of risk. *Am Rev Respir Dis* 1984;130:380.
55. Hodgkins. Pulmonary rehabilitation. *Clin Chest Med* 1990;11:447.
56. Holleman. Does the clinical examination predict airflow limitation? *JAMA* 1995; 273:313. Review.
57. Hudson. Emergent assessment and management of acute respiratory failure in COPD. *Clin Chest Med* 1994;15:481. Review.
58. Hudson. Arrhythmias associated with acute respiratory failure in patients with chronic airway obstruction. *Chest* 1973;63:661.
59. Hunter. The nutritional status of patients with chronic obstructive pulmonary disease. *Am Rev Respir Dis* 1981;124:376.
60. Janoff. The role of oxidative processes in emphysema. *Am Rev Respir Dis* 1983; 127:S31.
61. Jardim. The failing inspiratory muscles under normoxic and hypoxic conditions. *Am Rev Respir Dis* 1981;124:274.
62. Jasper. Cost-benefit comparison of aerosol bronchodilator delivery methods in hospitalized patients. *Chest* 1987;91:614.
63. Jenne. Theophylline as a bronchodilator in COPD and its combination with inhaled β-adrenergic drugs. *Chest* 1987;92(Suppl):7S.
64. Karpel. A comparison of the effects of ipratropium bromide and metaproterenol sulfate in acute exacerbations of COPD. *Chest* 1990;98:835.
65. Karpel. Bronchodilator responses to anticholinergic and beta-adrenergic agents in acute and stable COPD. *Chest* 1991;99:871.

66. Kirilloff. Does chest physical therapy work? *Chest* 1985;88:436. Review.
67. Klinger. Right ventricular dysfunction in chronic obstructive pulmonary disease. *Chest* 1991;99:715. Review.
68. Kramer. Randomized, prospective trial of noninvasive positive pressure ventilation in acute respiratory failure. *Am J Respir Crit Care Med* 1995;151:1799.
69. Lamy. Respiratory viral infections in hospital patients with chronic bronchitis. *Chest* 1973;63:336.
70. Lebowitz. Tucson epidemiologic study of obstructive lung diseases: methodology and prevalence of disease. *Am J Epidemiol* 1975;102:137.
71. Levine. Bronchial epithelial cell–cytokine interactions in airway inflammation. In: Shelhamer, moderator. Airway inflammation. *Ann Intern Med* 1995;123:288.
72. Martin. The prognosis of patients with chronic obstructive pulmonary disease after hospitalization for acute respiratory failure. *Chest* 1982;82:310.
73. Matthay. Favorable cardiovascular effects of theophylline in COPD. *Chest* 1987;92(Suppl):22S.
74. Matthay. Cardiovascular-pulmonary interaction in chronic obstructive pulmonary disease with special reference to the pathogenesis and management of cor pulmonale. *Med Clin North Am* 1990;74:571.
75. McNamara. Viral and *Mycoplasma pneumoniae* infections in exacerbations of chronic lung disease. *Am Rev Respir Dis* 1969;100:19.
76. Medical Research Council Working Party. Long term domiciliary oxygen therapy in chronic hypoxic cor pulmonale complicating chronic bronchitis and emphysema. *Lancet* 1981;1:681.
77. Meduri. Noninvasive positive pressure ventilation via face mask. *Chest* 1996;109:179.
78. Menzies. Determinants of weaning and survival among patients with COPD who require mechanical ventilation for acute respiratory failure. *Chest* 1989;95:398.
79. Miniati. Radiologic evaluation of emphysema in patients with chronic obstructive pulmonary disease. *Am J Respir Crit Care Med* 1995;151:1359.
80. Mittman. The PiMZ phenotype: Is it a significant risk factor for the development of chronic obstructive lung disease? *Am Rev Respir Dis* 1978;118:649.
81. Morse. Relation of protease inhibitors phenotypes to obstructive lung disease in a community. *N Engl J Med* 1977;296:190.
82. Moser. Respiratory stimulation with intravenous doxapram in respiratory failure. *N Engl J Med* 1973;288:427.
83. Murata. Intravenous and oral corticosteroids for the prevention of relapse after treatment of decompensated COPD: effect on patients with a history of multiple relapses. *Chest* 1990;98:845.
84. Murciano. Comparison of esophageal, tracheal, and mouth occlusion pressure in patients with chronic obstructive pulmonary disease during acute respiratory failure. *Am Rev Respir Dis* 1982;126:837.
85. Murciano. A randomized, controlled trial of theophylline in patients with severe chronic obstructive pulmonary disease. *N Engl J Med* 1989;320:1521.
86. Murphy. Bacterial infection in chronic obstructive pulmonary disease. *Am Rev Respir Dis* 1992;146:1067. Review.
87. Newman. Acute respiratory failure associated with hypophosphatemia. *N Engl J Med* 1977;296:1101.
88. Nicklaus. The accuracy of the roentgenologic diagnosis of chronic pulmonary emphysema. *Am Rev Respir Dis* 1966;93:889.
89. Nicotra. *Branhamella catarrhalis* as a lower respiratory tract pathogen in patients with chronic lung disease. *Arch Intern Med* 1986;146:890.
90. Nocturnal Oxygen Therapy Trial Group. Continuous or nocturnal oxygen therapy in hypoxemic chronic obstructive lung disease: a clinical trial. *Ann Intern Med* 1980;93:391.
91. Parot. Concomitant changes in function tests, breathing pattern and $PaCO_2$ in patients with chronic obstructive pulmonary disease. *Bull Eur Physiopathol Respir* 1982;18:145.
92. Parot. Hypoxemia, hypercapnia and breathing pattern in patients with chronic obstructive pulmonary disease. *Am Rev Respir Dis* 1982;126:822.

93. Patterson. Lung transplant for COPD. *Med Clin North Am* 1990;11:547.
94. Pauwels. The effects of theophylline on airway inflammation. *Chest* 1987;92 (Suppl):32S.
95. Pines. Antibiotic regimens in severe and acute purulent exacerbations of chronic bronchitis. *Br Med J* 1968;2:735.
96. Postma. Prognosis of chronic obstructive pulmonary disease: the Dutch experience. *Am Rev Respir Dis* 1989;140(Suppl):S100.
97. Rice. Aminophylline for acute exacerbations of chronic obstructive pulmonary disease. *Ann Intern Med* 1987;107:305.
98. Rossaint. Inhaled nitric oxide for the adult respiratory distress syndrome. *N Engl J Med* 1993;328:399.
99. Rossi. Human ciliated bronchial epithelial cells: expression of the HLA-DR antigens and of the HLA-DR alpha gene, modulation of the HLA-DR antigens by gamma-interferon and antigen-presenting function in the mixed leukocyte reaction. *Am J Respir Cell Mol Biol* 1990;3:431.
100. Sassoon. Hyperoxic-induced hypercapnia in stable chronic obstructive pulmonary disease. *Am Rev Respir Dis* 1987;135:907.
101. Schmidt. Acute on chronic respiratory failure. *JAMA* 1989;261:3444. Review.
102. Schreiner. Bacteriological findings in the transtracheal aspirate from patients with acute exacerbations of chronic bronchitis. *Infection* 1978;2:54.
103. Shelhamer. The perpetuation of airway inflammation. In: Shelhamer, moderator, Airway inflammation. *Ann Intern Med* 1995;123:288.
104. Sideris. Type of cardiac dysrhythmias in respiratory failure. *Am Heart J* 1975;89:32.
105. Silverman. Variability of pulmonary function in alpha-1-antitrypsin deficiency: clinical correlates. *Ann Intern Med* 1989;111:982.
106. Smeets. Travel for technology-dependent patients with respiratory disease. *Thorax* 1994;49:77.
107. Smith. Association of viral and *Mycoplasma pneumoniae* infections with acute respiratory illness in patients with chronic obstructive pulmonary diseases. *Am Rev Respir Dis* 1980;121:225.
108. Smith. Interactions between viruses and bacteria in patients with chronic bronchitis. *J Infect Dis* 1976;134:552.
109. Snider. The definition of emphysema. *Am Rev Respir Dis* 1985;132:182.
110. Traver. Predictors of mortality in chronic obstructive pulmonary disease. *Am Rev Respir Dis* 1979;119:895.
111. Trulock. Single lung transplant for severe chronic obstructive pulmonary disease. *Chest* 1989;96:738.
112. Turner. Equivalence of continuous flow nebulizer and metered-dose inhaler with reservoir bag for treatment of acute airflow obstruction. *Chest* 1988;93:476.
113. Weinberger. Hypercapnia. *N Engl J Med* 1989;321:1223.
114. Wesley. Evaluation and surgery of bullous emphysema. *J Thorac Cardiovasc Surg* 1972;63:945.
115. Wu. Modulation of eicosanoid production by the airway epithelium. In: Shelhamer, moderator. Airway inflammation. *Ann Intern Med* 1995;123:288.
116. Wysocki. Noninvasive pressure support ventilation in patients with acute respiratory failure. *Chest* 1995;107:761.
117. Yacoubm. Single lung transplantation for obstructive airway disease. *Transplant Proc* 1991;23:1213.
118. Yang. A prospective study of indexes predicting the outcome of trials of weaning from mechanical ventilation. *N Engl J Med* 1991;324:1445.
119. Ziment. Theophylline and mucociliary clearance. *Chest* 1987;92(Suppl):38S.
120. Zwillich. Ventilatory control in myxedema and hypothyroidism. *N Engl J Med* 1975;292:662.

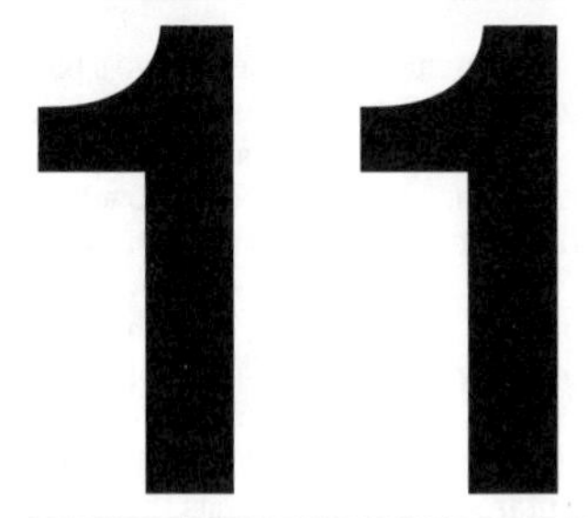

Pulmonary Embolism

Burton W. Lee and
B. Taylor Thompson

A. Introduction

1. Natural History of Venous Thromboembolism

a. **Epidemiology**—Although precise data do not exist, the incidence of pulmonary embolism (PE) has been estimated to be about 500,000 per year in the United States, and 2% to 10% of these patients die primarily as a consequence of PE (7,21,33,40). Among these, 75% to 90% die within the first few hours of the embolic event. In the remaining 10% to 25%, death is probably caused by recurrent emboli, usually within the first 2 weeks after the initial embolic event (7,40).

b. More than 90% of pulmonary emboli originate from the veins of the lower extremity. Other sources include the inferior vena cava, the renal veins, the chambers of the right side of the heart, and the veins of the upper extremity. The lower extremity clots usually start in a calf vein near a venous valve. These distal clots are an uncommon source of clinically significant embolism and almost never cause fatal embolism. However, 20% to 25% of these clots propagate to the iliofemoral system, which becomes the source of emboli for most patients with PE (31). Serial testing with impedance plethysmography (IPG) or ultrasound can identify those patients with isolated calf vein deep vein thrombosis (DVT) who develop proximal extension. In Moser's study of 36 patients with DVT, 8 of the 15 patients with proximal DVT had evidence of PE on ventilation-perfusion (V/Q) scan during 3 months of follow-up. In contrast, none of the 21 patients with calf DVT had evidence of PE (39).

c. **Hemodynamic Consequences of PE**

(1) When necessary, the pulmonary circulation has a large capacity to recruit previously underperfused vessels. For example, during exercise, such recruitment allows the increase in cardiac output to be accommodated with only a modest rise in the mean pulmonary artery (PA) pressure. As long as the elevation of PA pressure remains in the range in which right ventricular (RV) function can be preserved, similar recruitment of pulmonary vessels allows most patients with PE to remain hemodynamically stable.

(2) However, with a massive embolus, the recruitment of vessels may no longer compensate for the extensive loss of pulmonary vasculature. The sudden increase in pulmonary vascular resistance (PVR) may cause pulmonary hypertension, RV dysfunction, and decreased cardiac output. Under these circumstances, hypotension, tachycardia, shortness of breath, and jugular venous distention may be observed (33). Furthermore, in patients with preexisting lung disease, even a small embolus may produce severe pulmonary hypertension and acute RV failure because of the limited ability to recruit pulmonary vessels.

d. **Pulmonary Consequences of PE**—The pulmonary consequences of PE include increased alveolar dead space, pneumoconstriction, hyperventilation, atelectesis, pulmonary infarction, and hypoxia.

(1) By obstructing a pulmonary vessel, the embolus decreases blood flow to that region, creating a zone of high V/Q ratio or alveolar dead space. An increase in dead space causes regional hypocapnia, which may stimulate pneumoconstriction. The release of vasoactive mediators (*e.g.*, serotonin) from the embolus may also contribute to vasoconstriction (24).

(2) Hyperventilation is common but the mechanism remains unclear. Stimulation of the J receptors may be partly responsible. Atelectesis is also frequently observed because lack of perfusion leads to depletion of surfactant, which in turn causes alveolar collapse. The lung tissue is generally resistant to infarction because it has three sources of oxygen: the airways, the pulmonary circulation, and the bronchial circulation. Therefore, only about 10% of patients with PE experience pulmonary infarction (40).

(3) Several mechanisms may explain the frequent observation of hypoxia in patients with PE.

(a) **Redistribution of Blood Flow**—Assuming that the cardiac output remains unchanged, pulmonary blood flow must be redistributed to areas of the lung that are unaffected by PE. Therefore, blood flow must increase in some areas of the lung in which the ventilation remains normal (6). Initially in the course of acute PE, these low V/Q areas may be the primary cause of hypoxemia (25).

(b) **Intrapulmonary Shunts**—Later in the course of acute PE, intrapulmonary shunts become an important cause of hypoxemia (25). As previously described, the local loss of surfactant as a result of PE promotes atelectesis, creating areas of intrapulmonary shunts.

(c) **Intracardiac Shunting**—If a pulmonary embolus causes the pressures on the right side of the heart to exceed that of the left side, right-to-left shunting may occur through a patent foramen ovale (33,40).

(d) **Decreased Cardiac Output**—As described previously, massive PE may cause pulmonary hypertension, RV failure, and decreased cardiac output. The body compensates for the decrease in oxygen delivery by extracting more oxygen per liter of delivered blood. This increase in oxygen extraction causes a decrease in the mixed venous oxygen content, which in turn contributes to hypoxemia (25,33,40).

e. With time, heparin and the body's own fibrinolytic system recannulate most of the vessels obstructed by emboli. For example, 90% of patients with DVTs have a normal IPG study by 12 months (26). Similarly, in patients with PE, 76% of the V/Q scan defects resolve with anticoagulation (42). Therefore, in properly treated patients, chronic pulmonary hypertension should be uncommon.

2. **Prognosis**—The data from the Prospective Investigation of Pulmonary Embolism Diagnosis (PIOPED) study provide valuable information on the prognosis of patients with PE. As part of the study, the clinical course of PE was prospectively evaluated in 399 patients for 1 year. Standard anticoagulation was used in 73%, inferior vena cava (IVC) filter in 10%, thrombolytic therapy in 6%, embolectomy in 0.25%, and no therapy in 6% (7).

a. The rate of recurrent PE was 8.3% by 1 year. About half of the recurrences happened within 1 week of entry into the study.

b. The in-hospital and overall mortality rates were 9.5% and 23.8%, respectively. However, only 2.5% of patients died directly as a result of PE. The most common causes of death were cancer, infection, and cardiac disease. The major predictors of mortality were age >60 years, history of congestive heart failure, chronic lung disease, and cancer. Among those who died from PE, 90% had recurrent emboli and 90% died within 2 weeks of entry into the study.

B. Clinical Manifestations of Pulmonary Embolism

1. **Total Clot Burden and Baseline Cardiopulmonary Status**—Clinical manifestations of PE vary with total clot burden. Smaller clots usually cause nonspecific pulmonary manifestations such as pleuritic chest pain, shortness of breath, cough, or hemoptysis. Not infrequently, small emboli cause no noticeable symptoms or signs. In contrast, a larger embolus may cause hypoxia, hemodynamic collapse, and RV failure. In addition to the clot burden, the patient's baseline cardiopulmonary status also influences the clinical manifestations of PE. For example, in a previously healthy person, a large embolus may cause minimal clinical manifestations, but in a patient with severe chronic obstructive pulmonary disease, even a small embolus may cause significant symptoms and signs.
2. **Clinical Manifestations of PE in the PIOPED Study**—As part of the PIOPED study, the clinical manifestations of PE were evaluated in 365 patients who had no prior history of cardiopulmonary disease. PE was confirmed in 117 patients and excluded in 248 patients. The prevalence of various risk factors, symptoms, signs, laboratory abnormalities, radiographic changes, and electrocardiographic (ECG) findings were evaluated (52).
   a. **Risk Factors**—The most common risk factors for PE were history of immobilization (56%), surgery (54%), cancer (23%), thrombophlebitis (14%), and lower extremity trauma (10%). History of immobilization and surgery were statistically more prevalent in patients with PE than in those without PE (52). In another study, Svendsen confirmed cancer as an important risk factor for PE in a large autopsy series involving 21,530 patients. PE was found in 10.5% of patients with cancer but in only 8.4% of patients without cancer ($P<0.0005$). The autopsy rate was about 80% of all in-hospital deaths. The highest risk of PE was associated with ovarian, biliary, gastric, colonic, and pancreatic malignancies (55). In a separate analysis of the PIOPED data, female patients undergoing surgery while taking oral contraceptives had an increased risk of PE. Estrogen use alone was not a significant risk factor (44).
   b. **Symptoms and Signs**—Shortness of breath (73%), pleuritic chest pain (66%), cough (37%), leg swelling (28%), leg pain (26%), hemoptysis (13%), and palpitations (10%) were the most common symptoms in patients with PE. However, none of these symptoms was statistically more prevalent in patients with PE than those without PE (52). Tachypnea (70%), rales (51%), tachycardia (30%), fourth heart sound (S_4) (24%), and increased pulmonic component of the second heart sound (P_2) (23%) were the most common signs in patients with PE. Rales, S_4, and increased P_2 were statistically more prevalent in patients with PE than in those without PE. However, because of so much overlap in the two groups, no clinical sign reliably differentiated patients with PE from those without PE (52).
   c. **Arterial Blood Gas Analysis**
      (1) There was no statistically significant difference in the arterial partial pressure of oxygen (PaO_2) on room air or in the alveolar-arterial difference in partial pressure of oxygen ($P(A\text{-}a)O_2$ gradient) between patients with and without PE. Twenty-six percent of patients with documented acute PE had a room air PaO_2 >80 mm Hg, and 6% had a normal $P(A\text{-}a)O_2$ gradient. However, the room air PaO_2 was not measured in many patients who required oxygen therapy, which may have biased this finding (52) (see Table 11–1).
      (2) In another study involving retrospective analysis of arterial blood gas samples from 78 patients with angiographically documented PE, 95% had an abnormal $P(A\text{-}a)O_2$ gradient (8). Therefore, a normal $P(A\text{-}a)O_2$ gradient makes PE unlikely but does not exclude the possibility.
   d. **Chest Radiography**—Atelectesis or pulmonary parenchymal abnormality (68%), pleural effusion (48%), pleural-based opacity (35%), elevated hemidiaphragm (24%), decreased pulmonary vascularity (21%), prominent central pulmonary artery (15%), and cardiomegaly (12%) were the most common radiographic findings in patients with PE. Westermark's sign, the

Table 11-1 Arterial blood gas findings in PE (52)

	PE (n=88)	No PE (n=202)	*P*
Room air PaO_2	70 mm Hg	72 mm Hg	NS
$P(A\text{-}a)O_2$ gradient	37 mm Hg	35 mm Hg	NS

combination of prominent central pulmonary vessels with decreased peripheral pulmonary vessels, was observed in only 7% of patients with PE. Atelectesis or pulmonary parenchymal disease, pleural effusion, pleural-based opacity, and decreased pulmonary vascularity were statistically more prevalent in patients with PE than in those without PE. In contrast, pulmonary edema was less prevalent in patients with PE. However, because of so much overlap in the two groups, no radiographic finding reliably differentiated patients with PE from those without PE (52) (see Table 11–2).

e. **Electrocardiogram**—Ninety percent of patients with PE were in sinus rhythm, and 30% had a normal ECG. Nonspecific ST-segment and T-wave changes were the most common abnormalities in patients with PE (49%). Less than 6% of patients had evidence of "right-sided changes" such as P pulmonale, RV hypertrophy, right-axis deviation, or right bundle branch block. Similarly, atrial fibrillation (4%), atrial premature contractions (4%), and ventricular premature contractions (4%) were uncommon manifestations of PE (52).

3. Since patients in the PIOPED study were specifically recruited because their symptoms and signs suggested the possibility of PE, the fact that symptoms, signs, and laboratory findings were so similar between patients with and without PE should not be surprising. Ninety-seven percent of patients with PE experienced dyspnea, tachypnea, or pleuritic chest pain in the study (52). Not infrequently, however, PE may be clinically silent. For example, in a study by Moser, 38% of patients with DVT (but no clinical evidence of PE) had a V/Q scan suggestive of PE (41). Because these patients would not have been entered into the PIOPED study, the true prevalence of various symptoms, signs, and laboratory abnormalities may have been overestimated in the PIOPED study.

C. Diagnosis of Pulmonary Embolism

1. **Clinical Suspicion and V/Q Scan**—The role of clinical suspicion and V/Q scanning for diagnosis of PE has been best evaluated in the PIOPED study. This prospective study involved 1493 patients who had completed a V/Q scan within 24 hours of presentation for suspected PE. Among these patients, 933 were randomly selected to undergo mandatory pulmonary angiography if the V/Q scan was abnormal. Remaining patients underwent angiography at the discretion of

Table 11-2 Chest radiographic findings in PE (52)

	PE (n=117)	No PE (n=247)	*P*
Atelectesis or pulmonary parenchymal abnormality	68%	48%	<0.001
Pleural effusion	48%	31%	<0.01
Pleural-based opacity	35%	21%	<0.01
Elevated diaphragm	24%	19%	NS
Decreased pulmonary vascularity	21%	12%	<0.05
Prominent central pulmonary artery	15%	11%	NS
Cardiomegaly	12%	11%	NS
Westermark's sign	7%	2%	NS
Pulmonary edema	4%	13%	<0.05

the patient's physician. The patient's symptoms, signs, chest film, arterial blood gas analysis, and ECG were used to reach a clinical impression, in most cases before a V/Q scan or angiogram was obtained. PE was confirmed or excluded by angiography or by 12 months of follow-up. Among the 933 patients assigned to mandatory angiography, the procedure was performed in only 81% of patients. The remaining 19% did not undergo angiography because their V/Q scan was normal (7.4%) or because they dropped out of the study (11.5%) (43).

a. **Clinical Suspicion Alone**—Ten percent of patients were assigned high clinical probability for PE. However, PE was confirmed in only 68% of these patients. Similarly, 26% of patients were assigned low clinical probability, yet PE was confirmed in 9% of these patients. The rest of the patients were assigned an intermediate clinical probability. Therefore, the clinical suspicion was useful, but it was not accurate enough to reliably confirm or exclude PE in most cases (43). Similarly, in an autopsy series involving 21,529 patients, 9% of whom had PE on postmortem examination, clinical suspicion of embolus was present before death in only 16% of those with PE (32).
b. **V/Q Scan Alone**—The V/Q scan was introduced as a noninvasive tool for diagnosing PE. Technetium-labeled albumin and radioactive xenon are used for perfusion and ventilation scans, respectively. In the setting of normal ventilation, a perfusion defect is consistent with PE. Among the 755 patients who completed both a V/Q scan and a pulmonary angiography in the PIOPED study, only 41% of patients with angiographically confirmed PE had a high-probability V/Q scan, but 48% of patients with a negative angiography result had a high- or intermediate-probability V/Q scan. Overall, the V/Q scan was neither sensitive nor specific enough to be used alone for diagnosis of PE (43) (see Table 11–3).
c. **Clinical Suspicion Combined with V/Q Scan**—The percentage of patients with angiographically confirmed PE for various combinations of V/Q scan results and clinical suspicion are summarized in Table 11-4. If the clinical suspicion and the V/Q scan both indicated high probability, 96% of the patients had PE on angiography. On the other hand, when the clinical suspicion and the V/Q scan were both of low probability, 96% of the patients did not have PE on angiography. Finally, if the V/Q scan was normal or near-normal, the risk of PE was very low, regardless of clinical suspicion. However, fewer than 27% of the patients in the study met one of these three conditions (43) (see Table 11–4).

2. **D-Dimer Assay**—Degradation of crosslinked fibrin by plasmin creates a

Table 11-3 Utility of V/Q scan alone for diagnosis of PE (43)

V/Q Scan Probability	Sensitivity	Specificity
High	41%	97%
High or intermediate	82%	52%
High, intermediate, or low	98%	10%

Table 11-4 Utility of clinical suspicion and V/Q scan for diagnosis of PE (43)

	Clinical Suspicion for PE		
V/Q Scan Probability of PE	High	Intermediate	Low
High	96%	88%	56%
Intermediate	66%	28%	16%
Low	40%	16%	4%
Normal or near-normal scan	0%	6%	2%

unique epitope, the D-dimer. D-dimer may be elevated in various clinical settings, such as PE, DVT, myocardial infarction, or disseminated intravascular coagulation. The enzyme-linked immunosorbent assay (ELISA) for D-dimer is quantitative and more sensitive than the latex agglutination test. However, the ELISA technique is labor intensive and subject to longer turnaround time. All of the major trials that have evaluated the role of D-dimer in the diagnosis of PE used the ELISA assay (3,17,23). Two representative studies are discussed here.

a. Bounameaux prospectively evaluated the role of D-dimer in 171 consecutive patients referred for V/Q scan for suspected PE. Before the V/Q scan, each patient was assigned a prescan probability of PE based on history, physical examination, chest film, and ECG results. A postscan clinical probability was assigned using all available information including the V/Q scan result. Pulmonary angiography was performed for inconclusive cases. D-dimer determinations were made on day 0, day 3, and day 7, but the results were blinded. Diagnosis of PE was made in 55 patients by a high-probability V/Q scan (44%), a positive angiography result (29%), high postscan clinical probability (13%), or a positive test for DVT (14%). Positive D-dimer was defined as >500 µg/L (3).

(1) D-dimer was significantly higher in patients with PE than those without PE ($P<0.0001$). Only one patient with a D-dimer <500 µg/L had PE. The sensitivity and the specificity of D-dimer were 98% and 39%, respectively, and the NPV and PPV were 98% and 44%, respectively. Therefore, D-dimer was useful in excluding PE, but it could not reliably confirm PE (see Table 11–5).

(2) When the analysis was limited to those with inconclusive V/Q scans, no patient with a D-dimer level <500 µg/L had PE. The sensitivity and the NPV were both 100% in this population; the specificity and the PPV were 35% and 36%, respectively. Therefore, PE was essentially excluded when the D-dimer was <500 µg/L, and angiography was not necessary (see Table 11–6).

b. Goldhaber confirmed these findings in a series of 173 patients undergoing pulmonary angiography for suspected PE. D-dimer had a sensitivity and specificity of 93.3% and 25.0%, respectively; the NPV and PPV were 91.4% and 30.4%, respectively. Only 3 of the 35 patients with a D-dimer <500 mg/L had angiographic evidence of PE. However, in two of these three patients, PE may have been old. Therefore, the NPV may have been as high as 97.1% (17).

c. Bounameaux recently pooled the data from nine published papers reporting the utility of the D-dimer assay for diagnosis of PE. Among the 908 patients in these trials, the prevalence of PE was 38%. The weighted sensitivity and the NPV of the D-dimer assay as measured by the ELISA technique

Table 11-5 Utility of D-dimer assay for diagnosis of PE (3)

	PE	No PE	*P*
Median D-dimer value	2552 µg/L	666 µg/L	<0.0001
D-dimer <500 µg/L	1 patient	45 patients	—
D-dimer >500 µg/L	54 patients	70 patients	—

Table 11-6 Utility of D-dimer assay among those with inconclusive V/Q scans (3)

	PE	No PE	*P*
Median D-dimer value	1912 µg/L	767 µg/L	<0.0001
D-dimer <500 µg/L	0 patients	29 patients	—
D-dimer >500 µg/L	31 patients	55 patients	—

were 96.8% and 94.2%, respectively (4). Therefore, the ELISA assay for D-dimer may be useful in identifying patients who are unlikely to have PE. Given its high sensitivity and high NPV, some investigators have suggested that further diagnostic evaluation may be unnecessary when the D-dimer concentration is <500 μg/L, even if the diagnosis of PE remains inconclusive after a V/Q scan. However, this strategy awaits further prospective validation.

3. **Pulmonary Angiogram**—Pulmonary angiography remains the gold standard for diagnosis of PE. However, 3% of the angiograms in the PIOPED study were nondiagnostic. Furthermore, autopsy later revealed the presence of PE in 1% of patients whose angiograms had been interpreted as negative (43). The rates of death and major nonfatal complications associated with the procedure were 0.5% and 1%, respectively. Major complication was defined as any of the following: respiratory failure requiring cardiopulmonary resuscitation or intubation, renal failure requiring dialysis, or bleeding requiring transfusion of two or more units of packed red blood cells. Another 5% of patients suffered minor complications (53).
4. **Echocardiogram**—The role of echocardiography for diagnosis of PE is undefined. However, it can be useful to detect RV dysfunction, pulmonary hypertension, or the presence of a clot on the right side of the heart. It can also exclude other disorders that may mimic PE (14).
5. **Tests for DVT**—Hull advocated the use of serial IPG in patients with nondiagnostic V/Q scans. This strategy is based on the fact that detection of DVT would lead to anticoagulation therapy whether or not PE was simultaneously present. Hull reported a prospective cohort study involving 1564 consecutive patients with suspected PE. All patients were evaluated with V/Q scan and IPG. These patients were divided into four groups: (a) the normal V/Q scan cohort (negative control group), (b) the high-probability V/Q scan cohort (positive control group), (c) a cohort with nondiagnostic V/Q scans and adequate cardiopulmonary reserve, and (d) a cohort with nondiagnostic V/Q scans but inadequate cardiopulmonary reserve. The cardiopulmonary reserve was considered adequate if the patient did not experience congestive heart failure, RV failure, hypotension, syncope, or tachyarrhythmia. Furthermore, the forced expiratory volume at 1 second (FEV_1) had to be >1 L, the forced vital capacity >1.5 L, the PaO_2 >50 mm Hg, and the arterial partial pressure of carbon dioxide ($PaCO_2$) <45 mm Hg. The negative control group was observed without treatment or further diagnostic testing. The positive control group was treated with anticoagulation without further diagnostic testing. Patients with nondiagnostic V/Q scans and adequate cardiopulmonary reserve were evaluated by serial IPG over 14 days. If the results of serial IPG were negative, the patients were observed without treatment or further diagnostic testing (study group). If serial IPG results were positive, they were treated with anticoagulation. Patients were monitored for 3 months. Patients with inadequate cardiopulmonary reserve and nondiagnostic V/Q scans were excluded from the study (27) (see Table 11-7).
    a. The outcome was similar in all three groups of patients. In the study group, only 1.9% developed DVT or PE on follow-up, and only 1 patient died from PE. In the negative control group, 0.7% developed DVT or PE and no patient died from PE. In the positive control group, 5.5% had recurrent DVT or PE, and 1 patient died from PE (27).

Table 11-7 Outcome of patients followed with indeterminate V/Q scans (27)

	Study Group (n=627)	Negative Control (n=586)	Positive Control (n=150)
% with DVT or PE at 3 mo	1.9%	0.7%	5.5%
Number of deaths from PE	1	0	1

b. Among the 1564 patients in the study, 711 had nondiagnostic V/Q scans. Most of these patients would normally have required angiography. However, with the use of this noninvasive strategy, 627 patients (88%) avoided angiography (27).

c. In all likelihood, most of the patients in the study group did not have PE. Furthermore, because all of these patients had adequate cardiopulmonary reserve, the few who did have PE may have been able to tolerate the embolus without major consequences.

D. Treatment of Pulmonary Embolism

1. Standard Therapy for PE—The goal of therapy is to prevent recurrent embolization or further propagation of clot. Patients are typically placed on bed rest to promote adherence of clot to the vessel wall, but the value of this practice is unknown. The recommendation from the latest American College of Chest Physicians (ACCP) Consensus Conference on Antithrombotic Therapy is to administer heparin for 5 to 10 days. Warfarin may be begun on day 1 or 2 of heparin therapy and continued for minimum of 3 months (30).

a. Efficacy of Heparin—Barritt compared heparin versus placebo in a prospective randomized controlled trial (PRCT) involving 35 patients with suspected PE. Because neither angiography nor V/Q scan was available at the time of the study, it is not clear how many of these patients actually had PE. Nevertheless, heparin significantly decreased the risk of death in this group. The combined risk of dying from PE or experiencing a nonfatal recurrence was also substantially reduced with heparin (2) (see Table 11–8).

b. Failure to achieve an early anticoagulated state—that is, a partial thromboplastin time (PTT) >1.5 times control within 1 day—has been associated with an increase in the risk of recurrent embolism (5,28).

(1) In a retrospective analysis of the data from a PRCT comparing IV versus subcutaneous heparin therapy in patients with proximal DVT, almost all of the patients with recurrent venous thromboembolism had subtherapeutic levels of PTT (28).

(2) A double-blind PRCT compared acenocoumarol (dosed as described below) plus heparin (5000 U as a bolus, followed by 1250 U/hour initially, then adjusted to keep the PTT between 60 and 90 seconds for about 7 days) versus acenocoumarol alone (6 mg on day 1, 4 mg on day 2, then adjusted to keep the INR between 2.0 and 3.0) in patients with proximal DVT. The rate of clot extension or recurrence of venous thromboembolism was substantially lower with heparin during 6 months of follow-up (5). The rate of symptomatic clot extension or recurrence of venous thromboembolism was 6.7% with acenocoumarol plus heparin, compared with 20% with acenocoumarol alone. The rate of asymptomatic clot extension or silent PE was 8.2% with acenocoumarol plus heparin, compared with 39.6% with acenocoumarol alone. Presumably, early achievement of adequate anticoagulation with heparin therapy was responsible for the reduction in the rate of extension of clot or recurrence of thromboembolism. The rates of hemorrhagic complications were similar between the two groups. There were too few deaths for meaningful comparison between groups.

(3) In several studies, the average dose of heparin required to maintain adequate anticoagulation (1.5 to 2.5 times control) was about 1300

Table 11-8 Heparin vs. placebo for suspected acute PE (2)

	Heparin (n=16)	Placebo (n=19)	*P*
Death from PE or nonfatal recurrence of PE	0%	52%	0.0005
Death from PE	0%	26%	0.036

U/hour (12,28–30). Therapeutic anticoagulation can be achieved earlier and more successfully with protocol-based dosing of heparin than with physician-directed adjustment (11,34,46). For example, a weight-based heparin dosing regimen appears to be superior to a nonweight-based regimen. In a PRCT involving 115 patients with DVT, PE, unstable angina, or acute arterial insufficiency, Raschke compared weight-based dosing of heparin (80 U/kg as a bolus, followed by 18 U/kg/hour) versus a standard nonweight-based dosing regimen (5000 U as a bolus, followed by 1000 U/hour) (45). PTT was checked every 6 hours, with a therapeutic goal of 1.5 to 2.3 times control (see Table 11–9).

(a) The time to achieve PTT >1.5 times control and the time to achieve therapeutic PTT (1.5 to 2.3 times control) were significantly reduced with the use of the weight-based regimen. Ninety-seven percent of patients receiving the weight-based dosing regimen had a therapeutic PTT within 24 hours (>1.5 times control), compared with only 77% of those receiving the standard dosing regimen (*P*=0.002).

(b) Among patients with DVT or PE, the risk of recurrent venous thromboembolism was also significantly reduced with the use of the weight-based regimen (*P*=0.02).

(c) The risk of developing thrombocytopenia or bleeding was low and was not different between the two groups.

c. The recommendation of the ACCP Consensus Conference is to use continuous IV heparin for 5 to 10 days (30). For patients with submassive DVT or PE, 5 days of heparin appears to be equivalent in efficacy and safety to 10 days of therapy (12,29). The study by Hull is described for illustration (29). In this study, 199 patients with proximal DVT were randomly assigned in a double-blind fashion to receive either 5 days or 10 days of heparin therapy (5000 U as a bolus, followed by continuous IV infusion of 1250 to 1666 U/hour initially). The dose of heparin was then adjusted every 4 to 6 hours until the desired level of anticoagulation was achieved (PTT goal, 1.8 to 2.8 times control). Patients assigned to 5 days of heparin therapy received a placebo infusion on days 6 through 10. Warfarin was started on day 1 for patients assigned to 5 days of heparin therapy and on day 6 for those assigned to 10 days of heparin therapy. Warfarin was continued for 12 weeks with an INR goal of 2.0 to 3.0. Patients were monitored for 12 weeks (29) (see Table 11–10).

(1) There was no significant difference in the risk of recurrent venous thromboembolism between the two groups. Likewise, there was no significant difference in the rate of bleeding complications or in the mean blood transfusion requirement. Therefore, 5 days of heparin therapy with warfarin beginning on day 1 appears to be a safe and effective treatment strategy for many patients with venous thromboembolism.

Table 11-9 Standard vs. weight-based dosing regimens of heparin (45)

	Standard Dosing of Heparin (n=53)	Weight-Based Dosing of Heparin (n=62)	P
Time to achieve PTT > 1.5	20.2 hours	8.2 hours	<0.001
% with PTT > 1.5 within 24 hours	77%	97%	0.002
Time to achieve therapeutic PTT (1.5–2.3)	22.3 hours	14.1 hours	0.003
Risk of recurrent venous thromboembolism	25%	5%	0.02

Table 11-10 10 vs. 5 days of IV heparin for acute DVT (29)

	10 Days of Heparin (n=100)	5 Days of Heparin (n=99)	*P*
Recurrent venous thromboembolism	7.0%	7.1%	NS
Rate of bleeding complications	12.0%	9.1%	NS
Mean blood transfusion requirement	1.75 units	2.44 units	NS
Mortality rate	2.0%	8.1%	NS

(2) Although the difference was not statistically significant, the mortality rate was lower with the standard 10-day therapy. Therefore, further evaluation is required before the 5-day strategy can be recommended for patients with massive iliofemoral thrombosis or PE (30).

d. Warfarin

(1) Warfarin may be started on day 1 of heparin therapy with an INR goal of 2.0 to 3.0 (12,29). The ACCP Consensus Conference guidelines recommend that heparin and warfarin overlap for 4 to 5 days because of the initial, theoretical procoagulant effect of warfarin (30).

(2) In general, the duration of warfarin therapy should be at least 3 months, because patients treated for 3 months had better resolution of their thromboembolic disease and a lower rate of recurrence than those treated for 4 weeks (*P*=0.04) in one study (46). However, that was criticized because only 71% of the initial venous thromboembolic events and fewer than half of the recurrent events were objectively confirmed. The results are summarized in Table 11-11.

(3) In a multicenter, nonblinded PRCT involving 897 patients with their first episode of venous thromboembolism, 6 weeks versus 6 months of warfarin therapy were compared (48). Patients requiring permanent anticoagulation (*i.e.*, those with protein C deficiency or mechanical heart valves) were excluded. Patients were initially treated for at least 5 days with heparin (unfractionated or low-molecular-weight) and then randomly assigned to receive either 6 weeks or 6 months of warfarin (INR goal, 2.0 to 2.85) (see Table 11–12).

(a) The 2-year risk of recurrent venous thromboembolism was substantially lower with 6 months of therapy (*P*<0.001).

(b) Even for those with temporary risk factors (*i.e.*, surgery), there was a trend favoring the 6-month group.

(c) The overall risk of major bleeding was low and was not different between the two groups. The risk of fatal recurrence was also low (0.6%) and was not different between the two groups.

(4) Patients with persistent risk factors and those with multiple episodes of thromboembolism may require indefinite anticoagulation (30). Some investigators also advocate indefinite anticoagulation for patients with persistently abnormal IPG results on follow-up (40).

2. Thrombolytic Therapy for PE

a. Thrombolysis Versus Heparin—In theory, thrombolysis offers several advantages over heparin for treatment of acute PE. By rapidly lysing the clot, it may decrease the risk of death, improve the severity of symptoms, and prevent the development of chronic pulmonary hypertension. In addi-

Table 11-11 4 vs. 12 weeks of warfarin for venous thromboembolism (46)

	4 Weeks (n=358)	12 Weeks (n=354)	*P*
Reccurent venous thromboembolism	7.8%	4.0%	0.04

Table 11-12 6 weeks vs. 6 months of warfarin for venous thromboembolism (48)

	6 Weeks (n=443)	6 Months (n=454)	*P*
2-year risk of recurrent venous thromboembolism	18.1%	9.5%	<0.001
2-year risk of recurrent venous thromboembolism for patients with temporary risk factors	8.6%	4.8%	NS

tion, by dissolving the deep venous clots, it may prevent recurrent embolism and long-term postphlebitic complications. So far, none of these benefits has convincingly been demonstrated in a randomized trial. However, several studies have shown that thrombolysis causes more rapid improvement of hemodynamic, angiographic, V/Q scan, or echocardiographic abnormalities and more complete restoration of pulmonary microcirculation (9,16,47,49). Representative studies are described here. Whether these laboratory improvements translate into reduction of morbidity or mortality remains to be proved (1).

(1) Traditionally, angiographic documentation of PE was a prerequisite for thrombolysis. However, the risk of bleeding appears to be higher in patients who undergo pulmonary angiography before thrombolysis. Because of this observation, some authors recommend using thrombolysis based on the results of noninvasive testing whenever possible (16,36,54). Because intrapulmonary infusion does not offer any advantages over IV administration, these drugs should be given peripherally (56).

(2) The earliest and the largest trial to evaluate the efficacy of thrombolysis for PE was the Urokinase Pulmonary Embolism Trial (UPET). This PRCT compared heparin plus urokinase (4400 U/kg as a bolus, followed by 4400 U/kg/hour for 12 hours) versus heparin alone in 160 patients with acute PE (47) (see Table 11–13).

- **(a)** Urokinase plus heparin caused more rapid resolution of angiographic and hemodynamic abnormalities than did heparin alone. These benefits were short lived, however, because the V/Q scan findings were similar at 5 days.
- **(b)** There were no significant differences in the rates of recurrent embolism, death, or resolution of symptoms. However, the risk of major bleeding was significantly higher with urokinase plus heparin than with heparin alone.

(3) Goldhaber demonstrated that thrombolysis caused more rapid restoration of pulmonary perfusion and RV function, compared with heparin alone. This PRCT compared heparin plus tPA (100 mg over 2 hours) versus heparin alone (5000 U as a bolus plus 1000 U/hour initially) in 101 hemodynamically stable patients with acute PE. Pulmonary perfusion scans were performed at baseline and at 24 hours. Echocardiography was performed at baseline, 3 hours, and 24 hours (16) (see Table 11–14).

Table 11-13 Urokinase plus heparin vs. heparin alone for acute PE (47)

	Urokinase Plus-Heparin (n=82)	Heparin Alone (n=78)	*P*
Risk of recurrent PE	17%	23%	NS
Mortality rate	7%	9%	NS
Risk of major bleeding	45%	23%	<0.05

(a) Thrombolysis improved the RV wall motion abnormalities ($P<0.005$) and lung perfusion defects ($P<0.0001$) faster than heparin. In addition, there were nonsignificant trends toward improved survival and a lower rate of recurrent embolism at 14 days with tPA.

(b) However, the study may have been biased in favor of tPA, because the dose of heparin used in the control group may have been insufficient for adequate anticoagulation (12,28–30). In fact, the study did not report the percentage of heparin-treated patients who reached target levels of PTT within the first 24 hours. As described previously, failure to achieve an early anticoagulated state (*i.e.*, PTT >1.5 times control within 1 day) has been associated with an increase in the risk of recurrent embolism (5,28).

b. Long-Term Benefits of Thrombolysis

(1) Sharma compared heparin plus thrombolysis versus heparin alone in a PRCT involving 23 patients with angiographically proven PE and no prior history of cardiopulmonary disease. Either streptokinase or urokinase was used for thrombolysis. Hemodynamic measurements were made at baseline and at 4 hours after therapy. After an average follow-up of 7 years, these measurements were repeated at rest and with supine leg exercises. At follow-up, the resting PVRs and mean PA pressures were persistently elevated in patients treated with heparin alone. Furthermore, PVRs and mean PA pressures substantially increased with exercise. In contrast, PVRs and mean PA pressures were normal both at rest and with exercise in patients treated with thrombolysis (50).

(2) Schwarz described a 15-month follow-up study of 7 consecutive patients with DVT and angiographically documented massive PE who were treated with heparin and urokinase (250,000 U as a bolus, then 2000 U/kg/hour until the PA pressures returned to normal). Massive PE was defined as >50% obstruction of the pulmonary artery tree on angiography. At 15 months, all patients underwent pulmonary angiography, PA line monitoring, lower extremity venography, and exercise testing (49).

(a) Urokinase decreased the mean PA pressure, increased the mean PaO_2, and improved the angiographic score compared with baseline. Furthermore, 6 of the 7 patients had normal angiograms and 4 had normal lower extremity venograms at 15 months (see Table 11–15).

(b) At 15 months, the pulmonary hemodynamic measurements at rest were indistinguishable from those of a comparison population of normal volunteers. With heavy exercise, patients with PE had slightly lower cardiac indices than normal volunteers (see Table 11–16).

Table 11-14 tPA plus heparin vs. heparin alone for acute PE (16)

	tPA + Heparin (n=46)	Heparin Alone (n=55)	*P*
Improvement of RV wall motion abnormality at 24 h	39%	17%	0.005
Worsening of RV wall motion abnormality at 24 h	2%	17%	0.005
% of lung not perfused at baseline	43%	36%	NS
% of lung not perfused at 24 h	28%	34%	<0.0001
14-day risk of recurrent PE	0%	9%	NS
14-day risk of death due to PE	0%	4%	NS

Table 11-15 Long-term follow-up of patients thrombolysed for massive PE (49)

	Mean PA Pressure	PaO_2	Walsh Angiogram Score
Day 0	37 mm Hg	57 mm Hg	15 points
Day 6	13 mm Hg	89 mm Hg	—
15 Mo	15 mm Hg	—	1 point

Table 11-16 Hemodynamic results in patients thrombolysed for massive PE (49)

	Normal Volunteers (n=8)		Patients with PE (n=7)	
	At Rest	100-W Exercise	At Rest	100-W Exercise
Mean PA pressure (mm Hg)	15	22	15	25
Mean cardiac index ($L/min/m^2$)	3.9	8.1	3.6	6.5
Mean PVR ($dyn\text{-}s/cm^5$)	170	118	156	163

c. Choice of Thrombolytic Agents

(1) It is unclear whether one thrombolytic agent for PE is significantly superior to another (13,38).

(a) Goldhaber compared tPA (100 mg over 2 hours IV) versus urokinase (4400 U/kg as a bolus, followed by 4400 U/kg/hour for 24 hours) in 45 patients with angiographically documented PE. Patients underwent V/Q scan at baseline and at 24 hours. Angiography with hemodynamic measurements was performed at baseline and at 2 hours (13). At 2 hours, there was better angiographic resolution of clot with tPA. However, by 24 hours, there was no significant difference in the V/Q scan findings between the two groups. There was no difference in the mortality rate, but the rate of major bleeding was higher with urokinase than with tPA (see Table 11–17).

(b) In a similar PRCT involving 63 patients with acute massive PE, tPA was associated with faster improvement of PVR, compared with urokinase. At 2 hours, PVR decreased by 36% with tPA compared with 18% with urokinase (P=0.0009). However, there was no significant difference between the two groups at 12 hours (38).

(2) Recently, Goldhaber compared tPA (100 mg over 2 hours) versus rapid infusion of urokinase (1 million U as a bolus, followed by 2 million U over 2 hours) in 90 patients with angiographically documented PE. Patients underwent V/Q scan at baseline and at 24 hours. Angiography with hemodynamic measurements was performed at baseline and at 2 hours (15) (see Table 11–18).

Table 11-17 tPA vs. 24-hour infusion of urokinase for acute PE (13)

	tPA (n=22)	Urokinase (n=23)	*P*
Improvement of angiographic appearance at 2 h	82%	48%	0.008
Bleeding with more than 10-point hematocrit drop	18%	48%	NS
Mortality rate	9.1%	8.7%	NS

Table 11-18 tPA vs. 2-hour infusion of urokinase for acute PE (38)

	tPA (n=44)	Urokinase (n=46)	*P*
Improvement of angiographic appearance at 2 h	79%	67%	NS
Bleeding with more than 10-point hematocrit drop	16%	11%	NS
Mortality rate	4.5%	2.2%	NS

(a) In contrast to the previous studies, there were no significant differences in angiographic appearance at 2 hours or in the V/Q scan findings at 24 hours.

(b) The mortality rate and the rate of bleeding were also similar between the two groups.

d. Based on these and other studies, some investigators have proposed that bolus infusion of a thrombolytic agent may achieve more rapid lysis of clot and cause fewer hemorrhagic complications than slower infusion (10,35). Two separate trials used a similar study design to compare bolus versus standard infusion of tPA in patients with acute PE (18,19,51).

(1) Sors compared the hemodynamic effects of bolus infusion (0.6 mg/kg, but not more than 50 mg, over 15 minutes) versus standard infusion of tPA (100 mg over 2 hours) in a double-blind PRCT involving 53 patients with angiographically confirmed acute, massive PE. Patients assigned to receive a bolus infusion also received a placebo infusion over 2 hours, and the patients assigned to standard infusion also received a placebo bolus over 15 minutes. Hemodynamic measurements were performed at baseline and at 0.5, 1, 2, 4, and 12 hours. V/Q scans were performed at baseline and at 20 to 28 hours. Major bleeding was defined as any bleeding associated with intracranial hemorrhage, a decrease of >15 percentage points in hematocrit, or death. Important bleeding was defined as retroperitoneal or gastrointestinal bleeding, gross hematuria, or a decrease of >10 percentage points in hematocrit (51) (see Table 11–19).

(a) There was no significant difference in the V/Q scan findings between the two groups. Percent improvement of PVR from baseline was also statistically similar at all time points. However the rate of improvement was somewhat faster with the standard infusion than with the bolus infusion (*P*=0.0007). In part, this difference may have occurred because initiation of heparin therapy was delayed by 3 to 4 hours after completion of the bolus infusion, whereas heparin was started appropriately after completion of the standard infusion.

Table 11-19 Bolus vs. standard infusion of tPA for acute PE (51)

	Bolus Infusion of tPA (n=36)	Standard Infusion of tPA (n=17)	*P*
% of patients with RV failure at baseline	42%	71%	NS
PVR at baseline	15.2	16.2	NS
PVR at 1 h	29% decrease	36% decrease	NS
PVR at 12 h	43%	49%	NS
Rate of major bleeding	8%	6%	NS
Rate of important bleeding	0%	12%	NS

(b) There were no deaths or central nervous system bleeding events in either group. There was no difference in the rate of major bleeding, but the rate of important bleeding was nonsignificantly lower with the bolus infusion.

(c) Although the difference was not statistically significant, considerably fewer patients in the bolus group had RV failure at baseline than in the standard group. Therefore, the study may have been biased in favor of the bolus group as a result of uneven randomization.

(2) Goldhaber conducted a similar comparison in a double-blind PRCT involving 90 patients with acute PE diagnosed by high-probability V/Q scan or angiography (18). Patients were randomly assigned to receive either a bolus infusion (0.6 mg/kg, but not more than 50 mg, over 15 minutes) or a standard infusion of tPA (100 mg over 2 hours). Patients assigned to bolus infusion also received a placebo infusion over 2 hours, and the patients assigned to standard infusion also received a placebo bolus over 15 minutes. V/Q scans were performed at baseline and at 20 to 28 hours. In 60 patients, angiograms were performed at baseline and at 2 hours. In 30 patients, echocardiograms were performed at baseline, 3 hours, and 20 to 28 hours. In 48 patients, the fibrinogen and fibrin split products were measured. Major and important bleeding events were defined as in the study by Sors (51) (see Table 11–20).

(a) The study was terminated early because there was a nonsignificant trend toward higher mortality with the bolus therapy, compared with the standard therapy. However, the study may have been biased against bolus therapy. As in the previous study by Sors, initiation of heparin therapy was delayed by a few hours after completion of the bolus infusion. The PTT at 4 hours was 42 seconds in the bolus group and 66 seconds in the standard group (P=0.005). In addition, the follow-up angiograms at 2 hours were qualitatively worse compared with baseline in 6 patients assigned to bolus therapy but in no patients assigned to standard therapy.

(b) There were no significant differences in follow-up V/Q scans, echocardiograms, or mean angiographic scores between the two groups. However, as mentioned, the follow-up angiogram at 2 hours was qualitatively worse in 6 patients who received bolus but no patients assigned to standard therapy.

(c) As expected, bolus therapy was associated with higher mean fibrinogen levels (P=0.007) and lower mean fibrin degradation product levels (P=0.013) at 2, 6, and 12 hours. The rates of major and important bleeding were nonsignificantly lower in the bolus group than in the standard group. Similarly, the rate of all adverse events (deaths, nonfatal recurrent PE, major bleeding, and important bleeding) was nonsignificantly lower with bolus infusion than with standard infusion.

(3) Therefore, bolus infusion of a reduced dose of tPA was statistically similar in efficacy and safety to the standard 2-hour infusion of 100 mg of tPA in both studies. However, there was a nonsignificant trend toward higher mortality with bolus infusion, which caused premature termination of one study. On the other hand, initiation of heparin therapy was delayed for several hours in patients assigned to bolus infusion, and this may have biased the two studies against bolus infusion.

e. Summary of Thrombolysis for Acute PE

(1) Despite numerous trials, the precise role of thrombolysis for acute PE remains controversial. Some experts recommend thrombolysis for all patients with acute PE (16). However, most investigators limit the use of thrombolysis to patients with massive PE. There is no uniformly accepted definition of massive PE, but it usually includes those with

Table 11-20 Bolus vs. standard infusion of tPA for acute PE (18)

	Bolus Infusion of tPA (n=60)	Standard Infusion of of tPA (n=27)	*P*
Deaths	8.3%	3.7%	NS
Nonfatal recurrent PE	1.7%	3.7%	NS
Rate of major bleeding	3.3%	7.4%	NS
Rate of important bleeding	10%	15%	NS
All adverse events (deaths, nonfatal recurrent PE, major bleeding, and important bleeding)	17%	26%	NS
Mean PTT at 2 h	42 s	66 s	0.005
% of patients with worse angiographic appearance at 2 h	10%	0%	NS

hemodynamic instability, severe hypoxia, >40% to 50% occlusion of the pulmonary artery, or occlusion of two or more lobar arteries (33,40). This recommendation is based on the observation that massive PE is more likely to be associated with hemodynamic instability, hypoxia, and RV dysfunction. Because thrombolysis appears to improve these parameters, it may be indicated for massive PE. However, validation of this strategy is lacking. Furthermore, a clinically significant mortality or morbidity benefit has yet to be demonstrated with thrombolysis for PE.

(2) United States Food and Drug Administration–approved and alternate doses of commonly used thrombolytic agents for PE are summarized in Table 11-21.

(3) At the conclusion of thrombolytic infusion, PTT should be checked every 4 hours until PTT falls to less than 2 times control. At that time, heparin may be initiated with or without a 5000-U bolus, followed by a continuous infusion. The dose of heparin should subsequently be adjusted to keep PTT at 1.5 to 2.5 times control.

3. Other Therapeutic Options

a. Embolectomy—The precise role of embolectomy in acute PE is controversial. Traditionally, it has been reserved for patients with massive PE who deteriorate despite thrombolysis. It probably also has a role in patients for whom thrombolysis is contraindicated. There are no PRCTs comparing embolectomy versus thrombolysis for acute massive PE. In uncontrolled series, the perioperative mortality rate for embolectomy was between 29% and 37%. Among those who had suffered a cardiac arrest before embolectomy, the perioperative mortality rate was significantly higher at 58% to 64% (20,37). On the other hand, among those who survived the operation, 70% to 71% had no evidence of long-term cardiopulmonary limitation (21,37).

b. IVC Filter—An IVC filter is indicated if a patient with DVT or PE is unable to receive anticoagulation. It is also useful for patients who develop DVT

Table 11-21 Summary of thrombolytic agents used for treatment of acute PE

	FDA-Approved Doses		
	Bolus	Maintenance	Alternate Doses
Streptokinase	250,000 U over 30 min	100,000 U/h for 24 h	1,500,000 U over 1 h
Urokinase	4400 U/kg over 20 min	4400 U/kg/h for 12–24 h	3,000,000 U over 2 h
tPA	100 mg over 2 h	—	0.6 mg/kg over 2–15 min

or PE despite adequate anticoagulation. Less commonly, it is sometimes used for patients with massive PE for whom another embolus to the lung would be fatal. In an uncontrolled series, the risk of recurrent PE was only 2% with the Kimray-Greenfield IVC filter (22).

E. Summary

1. Although clinical suspicion is useful in diagnosis of PE, it is not accurate enough to reliably confirm or exclude PE in most cases. However, if the clinical suspicion and the V/Q scan both indicate high probability, 96% of these patients have PE. On the other hand, if the clinical suspicion and the V/Q scan are both of low probability, 96% of patients do not have PE. If the V/Q scan is normal or near-normal, the risk of PE is very low regardless of clinical suspicion. However, fewer than 27% of patients in the PIOPED study met one of these three conditions. Patients who do not meet these conditions require further diagnostic testing.
2. Pulmonary angiography remains the gold standard for diagnosis of PE. A negative angiography result essentially excludes clinically significant PE. The ELISA assay for D-dimer may be useful in identifying patients who are unlikely to have PE. Given its high sensitivity and NPV, some investigators have suggested that further diagnostic evaluation may be unnecessary when the D-dimer concentration is less than 500 μg/L, even if the diagnosis of PE remains inconclusive after a V/Q scan. However, this strategy awaits further prospective validation. Because D-dimer is not specific, it cannot be used to confirm PE. Serial IPG may also be a useful diagnostic tool in patients with nondiagnostic V/Q scans and no prior cardiopulmonary disease. If serial IPG is negative for DVT, patients with adequate cardiopulmonary reserve may be followed safely without the need for treatment or further diagnostic testing.
3. Treatment of patients with PE should probably include bed rest, but the value of bed rest and its optimal duration are unknown. Heparin should be administered for 5 to 10 days with a PTT goal of 1.5 to 2.5 times control. Therapeutic anticoagulation can be achieved earlier and more successfully with protocol-based dosing of heparin than with physician-directed adjustment. Warfarin should be administered for 3 to 6 months with an INR goal of 2.0 to 3.0. Some authors recommend that heparin and warfarin overlap for 2 to 5 days. Patients with persistent risk factors and those with multiple episodes of thromboembolism may require indefinite anticoagulation.
4. Traditionally, thrombolysis has been reserved for patients with acute massive PE with hemodynamic instability. However, some experts recommend thrombolysis for all patients with acute PE. Several studies have shown that thrombolysis causes more rapid improvement of hemodynamic, angiographic, V/Q scan, or echocardiographic abnormalities than does heparin alone. Some of these benefits are sustained at long-term follow-up. However, thrombolysis is associated with a higher risk of bleeding complications. Furthermore, it is unclear whether these laboratory improvements translate into clinically significant reduction of morbidity or mortality. The choice of thrombolytic drug and the optimal dosage of each agent remain controversial.
5. Embolectomy for acute PE is usually reserved for patients with massive PE who deteriorate despite thrombolysis. It may also have a role in patients for whom thrombolysis is contraindicated. IVC filter is indicated for patients with DVT or PE who are unable to receive anticoagulation. It is also useful for patients who develop DVT or PE despite adequate anticoagulation.

Abbreviations used in Chapter 11

ACCP = American College of Chest Physicians
DVT = deep venous thrombosis
ELISA = enzyme-linked immunosorbent assay

INR = international normalized ratio
IPG = impedance plethysmography
IV = intravenous
IVC = inferior vena cava
NPV = negative predictive value
NS = not significant
P = probability value
P_2 = pulmonic second sound
$P(A\text{-}a)O_2$ gradient = alveolar-arterial difference in partial pressure of oxygen
PA = pulmonary artery
$PaCO_2$ = partial pressure of arterial carbon dioxide
PaO_2 = partial pressure of arterial oxygen
PE = pulmonary embolism
PPV = positive predictive value
PRCT = prospective randomized controlled trial
PTT = partial thromboplastin time
PVR = pulmonary vascular resistance
q = every
RV = right ventricle
S_4 = fourth heart sound
tPA = tissue plasminogen activator
V/Q = ventilation-perfusion

References

1. Anderson. Thrombolytic therapy for the treatment of acute pulmonary embolism. *Can Med J* 1992;146:1317.
2. Barritt. Anticoagulant drugs in the treatment of pulmonary embolism: a controlled trial. *Lancet* 1960;1:1309.
3. Bounameaux. Measurement of D-dimer in plasma as diagnostic aid in suspected pulmonary embolism. *Lancet* 1991;337:196.
4. Bounameaux. Plasma measurement of D-dimer as diagnostic aid in suspected venous thromboembolism: an overview. *Thromb Haemost* 1994;71:1.
5. Brandjes. Acenocoumarol and heparin compared with acenocoumarol alone in the initial treatment of proximal-vein thrombosis. *N Engl J Med* 1992;327:1485.
6. Burton. Observations on the mechanism of hypoxaemia in acute minor pulmonary embolism. *Br Med J* 1984;289:276.
7. Carson. The clinical course of pulmonary embolism. *N Engl J Med* 1992;326:1240.
8. Cvitanic. Improved use of arterial blood gas analysis in suspected pulmonary embolism. *Chest* 1989;95:48.
9. Dalla-Volta. PAIMS 2: alteplase combined with heparin versus heparin in the treatment of acute pulmonary embolism. Plasminogen Activator Italian Multicenter Study 2. *J Am Coll Cardiol* 1992;20:520.
10. Diehl. Effectiveness and safety of bolus administration of alteplase in massive pulmonary embolism. *Am J Cardiol* 1992;70:1477.
11. Elliott. Physician-guided treatment compared with a heparin protocol for deep vein thrombosis. *Arch Intern Med* 1994;154:999.
12. Gallus. Safety and efficacy of warfarin started early after submassive venous thrombosis or pulmonary embolism. *Lancet* 1986;2:1293.
13. Goldhaber. Randomized controlled trial of recombinant tissue plasminogen activator versus urokinase in the treatment of acute pulmonary embolism. *Lancet* 1988;2:691.
14. Goldhaber. Diagnosis, treatment, and prevention of pulmonary embolism: Report of the WHO/International Society and Federation of Cardiology Task Force. *JAMA* 1992;268:1727.
15. Goldhaber. Recombinant tissue-type plasminogen activator versus a novel dosing regimen of urokinase in acute pulmonary embolism: a randomized controlled multicenter trial. *J Am Coll Cardiol* 1992;20:24.

16. Goldhaber. Alteplace vs heparin in acute PE. *Lancet* 1993;341:507.
17. Goldhaber. Quantitative plasma D-dimer levels among patients undergoing pulmonary angiography for suspected pulmonary embolism. *JAMA* 1993;270:2819.
18. Goldhaber. Reduced dose bolus alteplase vs conventional alteplase infusion for pulmonary embolism thrombolysis: an international multicenter randomized trial. *Chest* 1994;106:718.
19. Goldhaber. Two trials of reduced bolus alteplase in the treatment of pulmonary embolism: an overview. *Chest* 1994;106:725.
20. Gray. Pulmonary embolectomy for acute massive pulmonary embolism: an analysis of 71 cases. *Br Heart J* 1988;60:196.
21. Gray. Pulmonary embolectomy: its place in the management of pulmonary embolism. *Lancet* 1988;1:1441.
22. Greenfield. Greenfield vena caval filter experience. *Arch Surg* 1981;1:1451.
23. Heit. Plasma D-dimer levels and diagnosis of pulmonary embolism. *JAMA* 1994;271:1401.
24. Huet. Cardiopulmonary effects of ketanserin infusion in human pulmonary embolism. *Am Rev Respir Dis* 1987;135:114.
25. Huet. Hypoxemia in acute pulmonary embolism. *Chest* 1985;88:829.
26. Huisman. Utility of impedance plethysmography in the diagnosis of recurrent deep vein thrombosis. *Arch Intern Med* 1988;148:681.
27. Hull. A noninvasive strategy for the treatment of patients with suspected pulmonary embolism. *Arch Intern Med* 1994;154:289.
28. Hull. Continuous intravenous heparin compared with intermittent subcutaneous heparin in the initial treatment of proximal-vein thrombosis. *N Engl J Med* 1986;315:1109.
29. Hull. Heparin for 5 days as compared with 10 days in the initial treatment of proximal venous thrombosis. *N Engl J Med* 1990;322:1260.
30. Hyers. Antithrombotic therapy for venous thromboembolic disease. *Chest* 1992;102:408S.
31. Kakkar. Natural history of postoperative deep vein thrombosis. *Lancet* 1969;2:230.
32. Karwinski. Comparison of clinical and postmortem diagnosis of pulmonary embolism. *J Clin Pathol* 1989;42:135.
33. Kelley. Massive pulmonary embolism. *Clin Chest Med* 1994;15:547.
34. Kershaw. Computer-assisted dosing of heparin. *Arch Intern Med* 1994;154:1005.
35. Levine. A randomized trial of a single bolus dosage regimen of recombinant TPA in patients with acute pulmonary embolism. *Chest* 1990;98:1473.
36. Meneveau. Safety of thrombolytic therapy in elderly patients with massive pulmonary embolism: a comparison with nonelderly patients. *J Am Coll Cardiol* 1993;22:1075.
37. Meyer. Pulmonary embolectomy: a 20 year experience at one center. *Ann Thorac Surg* 1991;51:232.
38. Meyer. Effects of intravenous urokinase versus alteplase on total pulmonary resistance in acute massive pulmonary embolism: a European multicenter double-blind trial. *J Am Coll Cardiol* 1992;19:239.
39. Moser. Is embolic risk conditioned by location of deep venous thrombosis. *Ann Intern Med* 1981;94:439.
40. Moser. Venous thromboembolism. *Am Rev Respir Dis* 1990;141:235.
41. Moser. Frequent asymptomatic pulmonary embolism in patients with deep venous thrombosis. *JAMA* 1994;271:223.
42. National Heart. Urokinase pulmonary embolism trial: phase I results. *JAMA* 1970;214:2163.
43. PIOPED Investigators. Value of the ventilation/perfusion scan in acute pulmonary embolism: results of the Prospective Investigation of Pulmonary Embolism Diagnosis (PIOPED). *JAMA* 1990;263:2753.
44. Quinn. A prospective investigation of pulmonary embolism in women and men. *JAMA* 1992;268:1689.
45. Raschke. Weight based heparin dosing nomogram compared with a standard nomogram: a randomized controlled trial. *Ann Intern Med* 1993;119:874.

46. Research Committee of the British Thoracic Society. Optimum duration of anticoagulation for deep-vein thrombosis and pulmonary embolism. *Lancet* 1992;340: 873.
47. Sasahara. The urokinase pulmonary embolism trial: a national cooperative study. *Circulation* 1973;47:II.
48. Schulman. A comparison of six weeks with six months of oral anticoagulant therapy after a first episode of venous thromboembolism. *N Engl J Med* 1995;332:1661.
49. Schwarz. Sustained improvement of pulmonary hemodynamics in patients at rest and during exercise after thrombolytic treatment of massive PE. *Circulation* 1985; 71:117.
50. Sharma. Longterm hemodynamic benefit of thrombolytic therapy in pulmonary embolic disease. *JAMA* 1990;15:65A.
51. Sors. Hemodynamic effects of bolus vs 2-h infusion of alteplase in acute massive pulmonary embolism: a randomized controlled multicenter trial. *Chest* 1994;106: 712.
52. Stein. Clinical, laboratory, roentgenographic, and electrocardiographic findings in patients with acute pulmonary embolism and no pre-existing cardiac or pulmonary disease. *Chest* 1991;100:598.
53. Stein. Complications and validity of pulmonary angiography in acute pulmonary embolism. *Circulation* 1992;85:462.
54. Stein. Risks for major bleeding from thrombolytic therapy in patients with acute pulmonary embolism. *Ann Intern Med* 1994;121:313.
55. Svendsen. Prevalence of pulmonary embolism at necropsy in patients with cancer. *J Clin Pathol* 1989;42:805.
56. Verstraete. Intravenous and intrapulmonary recombinant tissue-type plasminogen activator in the treatment of acute massive pulmonary embolism. *Circulation* 1988;77:353.

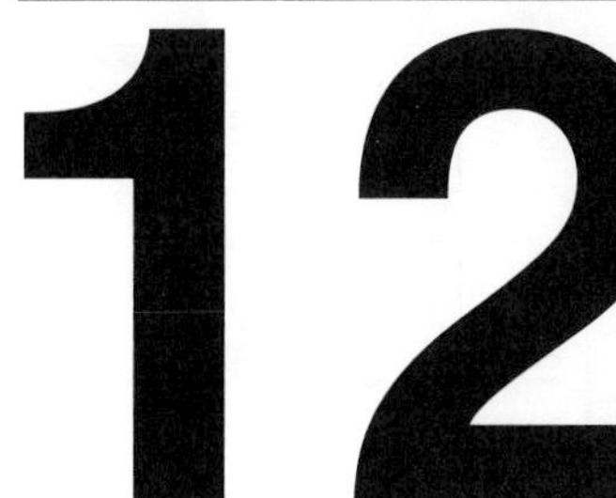

Pleural Effusions

R. Scott Harris and
B. Taylor Thompson

A. Introduction

1. During inspiration and expiration, the pleura allows for smooth movement of the lung relative to the chest wall and evenly distributes the expanding forces of the chest wall and diaphragm. The pleural space normally contains a small amount of fluid, about 0.1 to 0.2 ml/kg based on animal studies (111). A pleural effusion may occur when there is either increased formation or impaired removal of fluid from the pleural space. Increased formation of fluid can result from increased permeability of pleural capillaries, increased hydrostatic pressure within the pleural capillaries, or leakage of fluid from the thoracic duct, esophagus, blood vessels, or abdomen into the pleural space. The pleural fluid drains through the parietal pleural lymphatic system into the thoracic duct and eventually into the vena cava. Any obstruction along this route may impair drainage and cause a pleural effusion. In addition, Agostoni suggested that mesothelial cell active solute transport may also be important in removal of pleural fluid (2). In animal studies, the rate of production of pleural fluid in each pleural space has been calculated to be 0.1 to 0.4 ml/kg/hour, or about 300 to 1200 ml/day in an average adult (91,92). The pleural lymphatic system is estimated to be able to accommodate a rate of pleural fluid production that is up to 30 times greater than normal. Therefore, in order for pleural fluid to accumulate, the rate of fluid production must be greatly increased or the lymphatic or mesothelial cell drainage system significantly impaired, or both.
2. The pleural fluid arises from the systemic circulation; the pulmonary circulation does not participate in the formation of pleural fluid. It is a capillary filtrate formed in the parietal pleura from the intercostal arteries and in the visceral pleura from the bronchial arteries. The fluid formed flows in a downward direction from the lung apex to the base. It gains access to the lymphatic system through stomas in the parietal pleura that are approximately 10 to 12 mm in diameter and large enough to accommodate erythrocytes (12). The fluid then passes sequentially through the intercostal lymphatic vessels to parasternal and periaortic lymph nodes, to the thoracic duct, and finally to the vena cava. In addition to lymphatic drainage, mesothelial cell active solute transport may participate in pleural fluid removal (2).
3. In large reported series, 50% to 95% of effusions are caused by left atrial hypertension resulting from congestive heart failure (CHF), pneumonia, malignancy, or pulmonary embolus (15,28,44,71,81,93,104,105,127). The relative frequency of a given diagnosis, particularly with respect to tuberculosis (TB), varies depending on the country in which the study was performed and the extent to which a given diagnosis was sought by the investigators. In addition, many studies have excluded patients with undiagnosed effusions, effusions that were too small for thoracentesis, or effusions resulting from multiple causes (see Table 12–1).
4. The relative frequency of various causes of pleural effusions for patients infected with the human immunodeficiency virus (HIV) is different from that for non–HIV-infected patients. In Cadranel's series of 61 HIV-infected patients with pleural effusions, 35 effusions (57%) were caused by a malignancy and 26 (43%) were caused by an infection (18). Kaposi's sarcoma and lymphoma accounted

Table 12-1 Etiology of pleural effusions in selected studies

Location and Year (Reference)	S. America, 1995 (28)	S. Africa, 1995 (15)	Israel, 1990 (81)	Germany, 1987 (44)	Spain		United States		
					1991 (127)	1993 (104)	1972 (71)	1984 (93)	1990 (105)
No. patients excluded	67	29	0	0	11	15	18	7	3
No. patients in study	180	393	51	70	253	297	150	495	59
CHF	17%	21%	37%	41%	22%	10%	26%	16%	25%
Malignancy	30%	18%	29%	33%	26%	44%	29%	15%	44%
Infection, not TB	24%	16%	2%	10%	13%	16%	17%	19%	7%
Pulmonary embolus	—	2%	—	—	4%	6%	3%	1%	5%
Tuberculosis	12%	30%	2%	1%	26%	14%	9%	—	—
Cirrhosis	10%	—	2%	3%	1%	3%	3%	1%	2%
Collagen vascular disease	6%	—	—	—	2%	—	1%	1%	2%
Renal disease	—	5%	2%	—	1%	2%	2%	2%	3%
Undiagnosed	—	—	10%	11%	—	—	—	17%	—

for 91% and 6% of the malignancies, respectively. Aerobic bacteria, TB, and cryptococci accounted for 42%, 35%, and 15% of the infections, respectively.

B. Radiologic Tests for Evaluation of Pleural Effusions

1. Chest Radiograph

a. Collins demonstrated on cadavers that at least 175 ml of fluid had to be injected into the pleural space before the costophrenic angle (CPA) became blunted on a posteroanterior chest radiograph (25). In some cases, more than 500 ml could be injected without CPA blunting. However, CPA blunting on the posteroanterior film may occur in the absence of any pleural fluid. In this situation, a lateral decubitus film can confirm that a blunted CPA is indeed caused by free-flowing pleural fluid (86). In Collins' study, the injected fluid caused the appearance of a raised hemidiaphragm on lateral chest films; there was no comment on the presence or absence of blunting of the posterior sulcus.

b. Laterality of Pleural Effusions—The location of a pleural effusion can help narrow the differential diagnosis. CHF tends to cause bilateral pleural effusions; pericardial disease, pancreatitis, and Boerhaave's syndrome tend to cause left-sided effusions; and cirrhosis and Meig's syndrome tend to cause right-sided effusions (45,53,80,64,136). These observations are summarized in Table 12-2.

c. Massive Pleural Effusions—In a study by Maher, 46 patients with pleural effusions occupying an entire hemithorax were evaluated. Sixty-seven percent of these massive effusions were caused by a malignancy. Lung and breast tumors accounted for 50% and 25% of the malignancies, respectively. Nonmalignant causes of massive pleural effusions were equally divided among cirrhosis, CHF, empyema, TB, and hemothorax (76).

2. Ultrasonography

2. Ultrasonography—Ultrasound is a sensitive tool for locating pleural fluid; it reportedly can reveal as little as 3 to 5 ml of loculated fluid (41). In 80 patients with pleural fluid confirmed by aspiration, ultrasound was 84% sensitive for <50 ml and 99% sensitive for >50 ml of fluid (41). In one study by Kohan, ultrasound was superior to a lateral decubitus film for successful guidance of thoracentesis of small effusions (defined as those in which less than half of the hemidiaphragm was obliterated) (56). This study was a prospective, randomized trial at two community teaching hospitals involving 205 patients. All patients had a lateral decubitus film taken and then were randomly assigned to ultrasonography or no ultrasonography. For those assigned to ultrasound, a skin mark was placed as a target for thoracentesis. Thoracentesis was performed by clinicians and house officers. The effusions were subclassified as free-flowing or loculated. Ultrasound was superior to decubitus films for obtaining adequate fluid samples in small effusions ($P<0.01$), irrespective of whether the fluid was loculated ($P<0.01$) or free-flowing ($P<0.05$). However, there was no significant difference for large effusions. Moreover, ultrasound did not reduce the need for multiple attempts nor the risk of complications in any subgroup, including those with small effusions.

3. Chest Computed Tomography

Table 12-2 Laterality of pleural effusions by diagnosis

Diagnosis	Distribution of Effusion			Reference
	Right	Left	Bilateral	
CHF	19%	9%	73%	(136)
Pericardial disease	3%	60%	37%	(136)
Cirrhosis	67%	17%	17%	(64)
Meig's syndrome	71%	14%	14%	(80)
Pancreatitis	0%	100%	0%	(53)
Boerhaave's syndrome	0%	100%	0%	(45)

a. For patients with a pleural effusion, chest computed tomography (CT) may be used to better evaluate the lung parenchyma, identify the cause of the effusion (*e.g.*, pneumonia, malignancy), discriminate pleural from parenchymal disease, and confirm the position of chest tubes in relation to fluid collections. Chest CT is particularly helpful in distinguishing lung abscess from an empyema. In a study involving 58 empyemas and 12 abscesses, CT scan correctly distinguished between the two processes in 100% of the cases (123). The following radiographic criteria were characteristic of an empyema ($P<0.001$): (a) a thin wall, (b) uniform wall thickness, (c) smooth luminal and exterior margins, (d) separation of parietal and visceral pleura (split pleura sign), (e) lung compression, (f) obtuse angle with the chest wall, and (g) lenticular shape. However, these features were not observed in all cases; for equivocal cases, a contrast-enhanced CT scan can often better differentiate parenchymal from pleural lesions (11).

b. **Mesothelioma**—Chest CT can be a sensitive test for evaluation of suspected or confirmed mesothelioma. In a study by Kawashima, a CT evaluation of 50 patients with confirmed untreated mesothelioma revealed pleural thickening in 92%, thickening of interlobar fissures in 86%, pleural calcifications in 20%, pleural effusions in 74%, contractions of the involved hemithorax in 42%, contralateral mediastinal shift in 14%, and extrapleural disease in 6% (52). Although CT appears sensitive for detection of mesothelioma, a study by Law questions its advantage over plain chest films (61). In this study, a CT evaluation of 32 patients with mesothelioma was more sensitive for detection of pleural effusions than the standard chest film (no lateral decubitus view), but they both were equally sensitive for detection of disease of the lateral chest wall, lung, or mediastinum. Because the disease in most cases was extensive at presentation, the increased sensitivity of CT was thought not to be a significant advantage. In addition, CT was insensitive for detection of diaphragmatic involvement by tumor, producing many false-negative findings.

C. Thoracentesis for Evaluation of Pleural Effusions

1. Thoracentesis is the primary procedure for evaluation of pleural effusions. The diagnostic yield must be balanced against the risk of the procedure. There are no good data on how much fluid must be present before the benefit of finding a significant abnormality outweighs the risk of the procedure. Based on his experience, Light suggested that thoracentesis can be performed safely and successfully if the lateral decubitus film demonstrates $\geq$10 mm of layering fluid (72).

2. **Clinical Utility of Thoracentesis**—A prospective study by Collins was performed at a university hospital to evaluate the clinical usefulness and safety of thoracentesis (26). Among 129 thoracenteses performed on 86 patients, 78 patients had fluids that could be analyzed. Thoracentesis made a definitive diagnosis in 14 (18%), a presumptive diagnosis in 44 (56%), and no diagnosis in 20 (26%). Fourteen of the 20 nondiagnostic fluid results were still thought to be clinically useful, making 92% of the thoracenteses clinically useful. Of the 129 thoracenteses, pneumothorax occurred in 15 (12%) and a chest tube was required in 5 (4%). Major subjective complications were anxiety in 21% and local pain in 20%. Other reported complications, such as splenic rupture, abdominal hemorrhage, pulmonary edema, air embolism, death, catheter fragment left in the pleural space, and tumor seeding of the pleural tract, did not occur in this study. The authors concluded that thoracentesis is a useful diagnostic test but it can be associated with a significant number of complications as well as patient discomfort. In a recent review, Bartter concluded that most new pleural effusions should be evaluated unless the effusion is very small, is obviously caused by CHF, or occurs shortly after thoracoabdominal surgery or post partum (6). There are no absolute contraindications to thoracentesis, but relative contraindications include bleeding diathesis, systemic anticoagulation, a small volume of fluid, mechanical ventilation, an uncooperative patient, and cutaneous disease at the needle entry site (16).

3. **Fluid Appearance and Odor**—There are little data on the appearance and odor of pleural fluid as a diagnostic aid. Sahn stated that the following charac-

teristics of pleural fluid are helpful in diagnosis: (a) a bloody effusion in the absence of trauma is most likely caused by malignancy; (b) a whitish pleural effusion suggests chyle, cholesterol, or empyema; (c) anchovy-colored fluid results when an amebic liver abscess ruptures into the pleural space; (d) a putrid odor suggests an anaerobic empyema; (e) a viscous effusion suggests a malignant mesothelioma caused by increased levels of hyaluronic acid; (f) yellow-green fluid or debris suggests rheumatoid pleurisy; (g) food particles suggest esophageal rupture; and (h) an ammonia odor suggests urinothorax (110). For patients with a narrow-bore feeding tube, pleural fluid that resembles the enteral feeding solution suggests that the tube may have been misplaced into and through the lung parenchyma (85). Finally, a black color of the pleural fluid suggests infection by *Aspergillus niger* (84). The sensitivity and specificity of these characteristics are unknown.

4. **Pleural Pressure**
   - **a.** Pleural pressure measurements during thoracentesis has been proposed as a useful diagnostic aid. In a study by Light, 52 patients with effusions had pleural pressures monitored during thoracentesis (68). Thoracentesis continued until one of three conditions were met: (a) mean pleural pressure fell to less than -20 cm H_20; (b) no more fluid could be obtained; or (c) the patient developed symptoms of chest pain, cough, or dyspnea. Elastance was calculated as the change in pleural fluid pressure divided by the volume of fluid removed. Patients with pleural pressure <-5 cm H_2O or elastance >15 cm H_2O/L had either malignancy or trapped lung. Trapped lung is a fibrous peel over the visceral pleura that prevents the underlying lung from reexpanding. In contrast, those with bacterial or tuberculous empyemas had pleural pressures >0 cm H_2O and elastance <12 cm H_2O/L. If malignancy is reasonably excluded by cytology, pleural biopsy, thoracoscopy, and bronchoscopy, Light proposed that a diagnosis of trapped lung can be made when the initial pleural pressure is <-5 cm H_2O and rapidly falls during thoracentesis.
   - **b.** Light also recommended discontinuing thoracentesis when the pleural pressure falls to less than -20 cm H_2O. This is based on the observation that pulmonary edema can be induced in animals if the pleural pressures are reduced beyond this limit. Nevertheless, in Light's study just described, 1 patient developed pulmonary edema despite staying above this pleural pressure limit (68). If pleural pressures are not monitored during thoracentesis, Light recommends that no more than 1000 ml of fluid (near the mean amount removed in the study) be removed per day in order to avoid the risk of developing pulmonary edema. However, these recommendations have not been critically evaluated.

D. Diagnosis of Transudate Versus Exudate

1. Historically, pleural effusions have been divided into transudates or exudates as a way of distinguishing effusions that form because of an abnormal balance of oncotic and hydrostatic pressures (transudate) from those that form because of an abnormal filtration barrier (exudate). In general, transudative effusions are not caused by abnormalities of the pleura and directs diagnostic attention away from the pleural space. The major causes of transudative and exudative effusions are listed in Table 12-3. In the original study by which Light established his criteria for distinguishing transudates from exudates, clinical criteria were used as the gold standard. Subsequently, it was discovered that pleural effusions associated with pulmonary emboli, malignancy, sarcoidosis, or diuretic-treated CHF can be either transudative or exudative. Pulmonary emboli typically cause an exudative effusion, but up to 35% may be transudative (17). Malignant effusions are typically exudative, but up to 10% may be transudative (110). Despite these overlaps, Light's criteria remain useful for separating transudates from exudates and have been validated by numerous studies (see later discussion).
2. **Light's Criteria for Distinguishing Transudates From Exudates**—Light prospectively evaluated 150 patients with pleural effusions over an 18-month

Table 12-3 Differential diagnosis of pleural effusions

Transudates	Exudates
Congestive heart failure	Infection
Cirrhosis	Malignancy
Nephrotic syndrome	Pulmonary embolism
Hypoalbuminemia	Pancreatic disease
Superior vena cava obstruction	Abdominal or diaphragmatic abscess
Fontan procedure	Abdominal surgery
Urinothorax	Esophageal sclerotherapy
Peritoneal dialysis	Esophageal rupture
Glomerulonephritis	Rheumatoid pleurisy
Myxedema	Lupus pleuritis
Atelectesis	Sjögren's syndrome
Constrictive pericarditis	Churg-Strauss syndrome
Malignancy (<10% are transudates)	Wegener's granulomatosis
Pulmonary embolism (≤35% are transudates)	Drugs
Sarcoidosis	Asbestosis
	Postpericardiectomy or postmyocardial infarction
	Meig's syndrome
	Pericarditis
	Uremia
	Trapped lung
	Radiation therapy
	Yellow nail syndrome
	Lymphangiomyomatosis
	Hepatitis
	Hemothorax
	Chylothorax
	Diuretic-treated congestive heart failure

period to determine what tests could reliably distinguish a transudate from an exudate, using clinical criteria as his gold standard (71). The study excluded 33 effusions for which a diagnosis could not be confirmed by these criteria. Of the 150 effusions in the analysis, 47 were transudates and 103 were exudates. All patients had the pleural fluid analyzed for protein, lactate dehydrogenase (LDH), and cell count. Serum protein and LDH levels were determined within 30 minutes of the pleural sampling.

a. **Cell Count**—A pleural fluid red blood cell (RBC) count >100,000 was suggestive of an exudate, although fewer than 20% of exudates had a RBC count that high and about 10% of transudates had RBC counts between 10,000 and 100,000. Similarly, a leukocyte count >10,000 was almost always caused by an exudate, but more than 40% of exudates had leukocyte counts <2500. There was too much overlap in these values for cell counts to be clinically useful under most circumstances.
b. **Protein and LDH**—The authors then examined the utility of measurements of pleural protein, pleural LDH, the effusion-to-serum ratio of protein, and the effusion-to-serum ratio of LDH. No single criterion accurately distinguished transudate from exudate. Instead, the authors found the presence of any one of the following three conditions to be indicative of an exudate: pleural LDH >200 IU/L (or more than two-thirds of the upper limit of normal), effusion-to-serum protein ratio >0.5, and effusion-to-serum LDH ratio >0.6. Using these criteria, all but one exudate and one transudate were correctly classified. Although the analysis of pleural fluid was

performed prospectively, it should be noted that Light's criteria were determined retrospectively.

c. Peterman retrospectively evaluated 320 pleural fluid specimens to determine the clinical utility of distinguishing an exudative effusion from a transudative effusion using Light's criteria (93). Eighty-three specimens were transudates and 237 were exudates by Light's criteria. When 725 further tests were performed on the 83 transudative specimens, only 9 positive findings were noted, and at least 7 of the 9 were false-positive findings. In contrast, when 1997 further tests were performed on the 237 exudative specimens, 88 true-positive findings were noted. The authors concluded that further diagnostic testing is warranted for exudates but not for transudates. These results also suggest that Light's criteria are accurate for differentiation of transudates from exudates.

d. Table 12-4 summarizes the reported diagnostic utility of Light's criteria in various studies. All of the studies used clinical criteria as the gold standard for distinguishing transudates from exudates.

3. Other Criteria for Distinguishing Transudates From Exudates—One limitation of Light's criteria is that exudate-range protein levels may be found in some effusions caused by CHF, which may lead to unnecessary tests and procedures for these patients. Therefore, several other criteria have been proposed for more accurate separation of transudates from exudates, including the serum-effusion albumin gradient, the pleural cholesterol level, the effusion-to-serum cholesterol ratio, and the effusion-to-serum bilirubin ratio.

a. Albumin—Roth evaluated the serum-effusion albumin gradient as a way of distinguishing transudates from exudates (105). The study included 61 consecutive patients admitted to a military hospital who underwent diagnostic or therapeutic thoracentesis. In all cases, the diagnosis was determined by preset criteria through chart review. After analysis of the first 27 specimens, a serum-effusion albumin gradient <1.2 g/dl was noted to be indicative of an exudate. This value was then prospectively applied to the next 32 specimens. Fifty-nine patients were analyzed, 41 with exudates and 18 with transudates.

(1) Light's criteria correctly classified all of the exudates but misclassified five of the transudates as exudates. All 5 misclassified patients had CHF, and 4 of the 5 had been treated with diuretics before thoracentesis.

(2) In contrast to Light's criteria, the serum-effusion albumin gradient correctly classified these 5 patients. However, it classified two exudates as transudates, both of which were found to have been caused by a malignancy. The sensitivity and specificity of these criteria are shown in Table 12-5.

(3) In summary, the albumin gradient appears to be more specific but slightly less sensitive than Light's criteria, but neither of these differences achieved statistical significance. Moreover, a test that is less sensitive for exudates may not be desirable, because potentially ma-

Table 12-4 Diagnostic utility of Light's criteria in various studies

Study	Sensitivity	Specificity	Accuracy	PPV	NPV	Reference
Light	99%	98%	—	99%	98%	(71)
Burgess	98%	83%	93%	93%	96%	(15)
Roth	100%	72%	—	—	—	(105)
Valdez	95%	78%	90%	92%	83%	(127)
Romero	98%	77%	95%	—	—	(104)
Costa	98%	82%	—	—	—	(28)
Meisel	90%	82%	86%	87%	—	(81)

Table 12-5 Diagnostic utility of Light's criteria vs. albumin gradient (105)

	Sensitivity	Specificity
Light's criteria	100%	72%
Serum-effusion albumin gradient	95%	100%

lignant effusions may be missed. The authors also cautioned that CHF was diagnosed clinically in this study and that other causes for the effusion could not be entirely excluded.

b. **Bilirubin**—Meisel proposed using an effusion-to-serum bilirubin ratio of >0.6 as an indicator of an exudate (81). When this criterion was applied in a prospective manner to 51 patients, the sensitivity and specificity were 96% and 83%, respectively. In comparison, the sensitivity and specificity of Light's criteria were 90% and 82%, respectively. Although the authors concluded that the bilirubin ratio can be applied with the same accuracy as Light's criteria, these results must be interpreted with caution given the small number of patients in the study. Furthermore, in a direct comparison of various criteria for separating transudates from exudates, Light's criteria was found to be more reliable than any other criteria including the bilirubin ratio (15). This study is described in more detail in a later section.

c. **Cholesterol**—Valdez proposed using a pleural cholesterol value of >55 mg/dl or an effusion-to-serum cholesterol ratio of >0.3 to indicate an exudate (127). Over a 1-year period, 283 patients with pleural effusions were studied. Thirty patients were excluded because either no cause for the effusion could be determined or more than one cause was present. The findings of the study are presented in Table 12-6. The two cholesterol criteria appear to be more specific but less sensitive. However, as was the case with the albumin gradient, a test that is less sensitive for exudates may not be desirable because potentially malignant effusions may be missed.

d. **Pleural Fluid Cholesterol and LDH Without Serum Values**—Costa described a method of measuring only pleural fluid cholesterol and LDH, without simultaneous serum values (28). He found that the presence of a cholesterol level of >45 mg/dl or an LDH value of >200 IU/L, or both, identified exudates with a sensitivity of 99% and a specificity of 98% in 180 pleural effusions. This analysis may offer an advantage over Light's criteria in that it requires only pleural values, but it has not been as extensively validated.

4. **Comparison of Various Criteria for Distinguishing Exudates from Transudates**—Burgess conducted the only direct comparison of all of the major criteria for separating exudates from transudates (15). Over a 1-year period, 500 pleural effusions were analyzed. After discharge of the patient, the medical records were reviewed to determine whether a reliable diagnosis could be made. A reliable diagnosis was believed possible in 393 cases (270 exudates and 123 transudates). Among the various criteria, Light's criteria were found to be the most accurate. The results of this study are summarized in Table 12-7.

5. **Effect of Diuresis on Pleural Effusions**

a. Two studies have examined the effect of diuresis on pleural effusions, with slightly differing results (22,116). The study by Chakko involved 8 patients

Table 12-6 Diagnostic utility of Light's criteria vs. cholesterol level (127)

	Sensitivity	Specificity	PPV	NPV
Pleural cholesterol >55 mg/dl	91%	100%	100%	79%
Effusion to serum ratio >0.3	92%	88%	95%	80%
Light's criteria	95%	78%	92%	83%

Table 12-7 Comparison of major diagnostic criteria for transudates vs. exudates

Criteria	Accuracy	Sensitivity	Specificity	PPV	NPV
Light's criteria	93%	98%	83%	93%	96%
Albumin gradient 1.2 g/dl	89%	87%	92%	96%	77%
Cholesterol 60 mg/dl	70%	54%	92%	93%	50%
Cholesterol ratio 0.3	87%	89%	81%	91%	78%
Bilirubin ratio 0.6	75%	81%	61%	81%	60%

Modified with permission from Burgess (15).

with CHF confirmed by echocardiography (22). An initial thoracentesis was performed within 36 hours of enrollment and was repeated 4 to 8 days after diuresis. Patients lost a mean of 5.8 kg. On initial thoracentesis, all patients had a transudate by Light's criteria. However, on repeat thoracentesis (after diuresis), three effusions had become exudative by Light's criteria. Between the two thoracenteses, there were statistically significant increases in the pleural fluid protein, the effusion-to-serum protein ratio, the pleural fluid LDH, and the effusion-to-serum LDH ratio ($P<0.01$ for all changes).

b. The second study, by Shinto, examined 12 patients with CHF confirmed by echocardiography (116). After initial thoracentesis, patients were treated with diuresis, and a second thoracentesis was performed 12 to 48 hours later. Patients lost a mean of 4.5 kg. As in the study by Chakko, there were statistically significant increases in the pleural fluid protein, the effusion-to-serum protein ratio, the pleural fluid LDH, and the effusion-to-serum LDH ratio ($P<0.05$ for all changes). However, only 1 of the 12 patients had an effusion that changed from a transudate to exudate by Light's criteria. The shorter time interval between thoracenteses may account for the lower rate of conversion from transudate to exudate. Because Light's criteria can misclassify a CHF-induced effusion as an exudate in the setting of diuresis, the serum-effusion albumin gradient, the pleural fluid cholesterol, or the effusion-to-serum cholesterol ratio may offer better specificity in this situation.

E. Evaluation of Parapneumonic Effusions

1. Pneumonia is associated with a pleural effusion in 36% to 57% of cases (5, 69,124). A parapneumonic effusion is considered uncomplicated if it resolves with antibiotic therapy alone and complicated if it loculates or forms an empyema when left undrained. Parapneumonic effusions probably form when polymorphonuclear leukocytes (PMNs) are activated by bacteria and cause endothelial damage, resulting in increased pleural fluid formation (the capillary leak/exudative stage). If the infection continues, PMNs and bacteria can enter the pleural space, causing a fall in glucose and pH and a rise in LDH. At this stage (the bacterial invasion/fibrinopurulent stage), the fibrinolytic activity decreases and large amounts of plasma proteins leak into the pleural space, causing fibrin to be deposited on the pleural surface. In addition, fibroblast proliferation and collagen and glycosaminoglycan deposition lead to compartmentalization of the pleural space. When left untreated, the effusion may progress to the final stage, empyema, in which frank pus fills the pleural space and becomes difficult to drain by chest tube. The pleural surfaces may become encased in a thick fibrous peel, which can restrict lung expansion and inhibit drainage of pleural fluid. It has been the goal of numerous studies to predict which parapneumonic effusions are likely to develop into an empyema and which are likely to remain uncomplicated. Theoretically, if the former effusions could be identified and drained early, surgery could be avoided.
2. **Criteria for Tube Thoracostomy**

a. **Light's Criteria for Tube Thoracostomy**—Light prospectively evaluated the incidence and course of parapneumonic effusions in 203 patients with acute bacterial pneumonia (69). A pleural effusion was noted on a lateral decubitus film in 90 patients (44%), 10 of whom required chest tube drainage and therefore were considered to have had a complicated parapneumonic effusion. No clinical characteristic reliably separated complicated from uncomplicated effusions. However, a pleural fluid pH <7.00 or a pleural fluid glucose level <40 mg/dl, or both, were predictive of a complicated effusion; all patients in this study who met these criteria required a tube thoracostomy. In contrast, all patients with a pH >7.20 and a pleural fluid LDH <1000 mg/dl had an uncomplicated parapneumonic effusion. Based on these findings, the authors recommended tube thoracostomy if pleural fluid pH is <7.00 or pleural fluid glucose is <40 mg/dl but antibiotic therapy alone if pleural fluid pH is >7.20 and pleural fluid LDH is <1000 mg/dl. Some patients not meeting either set of criteria eventually required a tube thoracostomy, but others resolved with antibiotics alone. Therefore, the authors suggested that these patients be considered for tube thoracostomy on an individual basis. If tube thoracostomy is deferred, serial thoracenteses may be considered to ensure that the pH does not fall and the LDH does not rise significantly.

b. Ten major studies have analyzed the pleural fluid LDH, pH, and glucose in patients with a parapneumonic effusion, including that of Light (9,35,37, 57,66,69,74,96,97,99). Despite these studies, there has been no general consensus on what level of LDH, pH, or glucose most reliably separates complicated from uncomplicated effusions. In an attempt to arrive at a consensus, a metaanalysis of these studies was performed by Heffner (46). The metaanalysis excluded three of the studies because the diagnosis of pneumonia was insufficiently supported. From the remaining seven studies involving 274 patients, 251 pleural fluid pH data points, 135 glucose data points, and 114 LDH data points were obtained. A parapneumonic effusion was considered an empyema if the complicated effusion had the physical characteristics of pus. Receiver operating characteristic (ROC) curves were used to compare the usefulness of each test for predicting the outcome of the effusion.

   (1) The pleural fluid pH was the best predictor of a complicated effusion, as determined by the area under the ROC curve. This was also true after empyemas were excluded from the analysis.

   (2) The authors developed decision thresholds for pH based on the prior probability of developing a complicated effusion. A tube thoracostomy was recommended for low-risk patients with pleural fluid pH <7.21 or high-risk patients with pleural fluid pH <7.29. A low-risk patient was defined as a young patient without comorbid conditions who presented with a pneumococcal pneumonia. A high-risk patient was defined as an elderly patient with comorbid lung disease who presented with an anaerobic pneumonia.

c. **Loculated Parapneumonic Effusions**—Many studies of parapneumonic effusions have excluded patients with loculated effusions, including Light's study (69). Himelman evaluated the utility of Light's criteria for tube thoracostomy in patients with loculated pleural effusions (48). Forty-eight patients with ultrasound-guided thoracentesis were evaluated retrospectively for radiologic findings, pleural fluid chemistries, and outcome. In 30% of cases, chest CT or ultrasound detected loculations when the lateral decubitus film did not. Light's criteria were unreliable for diagnosis of complicated versus uncomplicated effusion if the effusion was loculated or if the patient had been treated with antibiotics before thoracentesis. Multiple internal pleural echoes on ultrasonography or evidence of loculation, cavitation, or pleural gas on chest CT scan were suggestive of exudates and more reliably predicted the presence of a complicated pleural effusion than Light's criteria for tube thoracostomy. However, no radiologic finding was specific for an empyema. Only nonloculated empyemas were successfully managed without chest tubes.

3. **Light's Classification System**—The correct management of parapneumonic effusions is still not entirely known. Treatment goals are to restore the patient's health as quickly as possible using the least invasive intervention. The treatment options, in order of increasing complexity and risk, are (a) antibiotics alone, (b) antibiotics plus drainage by thoracentesis, (c) small-bore chest tube (8 to 16F), (d) large-bore chest tube (>16F), (e) instillation of thrombolytic agents through small or large chest tubes (see section L3), (f) thoracoscopy, (g) open drainage, or (h) decortication (see section L4). How and when to apply these interventions is still debated. Light created the treatment guidelines shown in Table 12-8, some based on his own data, some based on others' uncontrolled data, and some from his own experience and bias (70). In this scheme, parapneumonic effusions are divided into seven classes.

F. Specific Chemistry and Hematology Tests

1. **pH and Glucose**

   a. The pleural pH and glucose levels usually rise and fall together (98). For most causes of pleural acidosis, the low pH is caused by lactic acid produc-

Table 12-8 Light's classification scheme for parapneumonic effusion & empyema

Class	Category	Features of Pleural Fluid	Intervention
1	Nonsignificant parapneumonic effusion	<10 mm thick on lateral decubitus film	Antibiotics; (no thoracentesis indicated)
2	Typical parapneumonic effusion	>10 mm thick on lateral decubitus film; glucose >40 mg/dl; pH >7.20; Gram stain and culture negative	Antibiotics
3	Borderline complicated parapneumonic effusion	pH between 7.0 and 7.2 and/or LDH>1000; glucose>40 mg/dl; Gram stain and culture negative	Antibiotics; serial thoracentesis; if loculated, small chest tube (8–16F) plus thrombolytic agents
4	Simple complicated parapneumonic effusion	pH<7.0 and/or glucose <40 mg/dl and/or Gram stain or culture positive; no loculations; no frank pus	Antibiotics; small chest tube (8–16F)
5	Complex complicated parapneumonic effusion	Same as class 4 but multiloculated	Antibiotics; thrombolytic agents via small or large chest tubes
6	Simple empyema	Frank pus; free-flowing or one locule	Antibiotics; large (28F) chest tube; decortication if cavity after 7 days
7	Complex empyema	Same as class 6 but multiloculated	Antibiotics; large (28F) chest tubes; thrombolytic agents (thoracoscopy, decortication, or open procedure often required)

Modified with permission from Light (70).

tion by the leukocytes in the pleural space. Even for esophageal rupture, the acidosis results not from the leakage of gastric acid into the pleural space but from the metabolism of glucose by PMNs. For example, pleural acidosis induced by experimental esophageal rupture in rabbits can be prevented if they are made neutropenic but not with distal esophageal ligation or antibiotic therapy (38). Alternatively, transport of glucose into and carbon dioxide out of the pleural space may be impaired in some patients with pleural fluid acidosis (39). This mechanism may be particularly important for rheumatoid effusions.

b. The pleural pH and glucose, but particularly the pH, are helpful in narrowing the differential diagnosis of an effusion (125). In a study involving 183 patients with pleural effusions (36 transudates and 147 exudates), all 46 patients with pleural fluid acidosis (*i.e.*, pH <7.30) had an exudative effusion (37). Six conditions were associated with pleural pH <7.30 in this study: empyema, malignancy, collagen vascular disease, TB, esophageal rupture, and hemothorax. Other studies have added systemic acidosis, urinothorax, paragonimiasis, and rheumatoid effusion to this list (72). Some of the lowest glucose and pH levels are found in effusions caused by rheumatoid arthritis, probably because of impaired influx of glucose into the pleural space and impaired egress of the metabolic products of glucose metabolism (108). In the original report by Carr, 10 of 11 patients with a rheumatoid effusion had a pleural glucose level ≤17 mg/dl; the other patient had a pleural glucose level of 58 mg/dl (21). In another retrospective review of 18 rheumatoid effusions, 82% of patients had a pleural glucose level ≤38 mg/dl (73). The authors combined the data from other reports and found 77% of patients to have a pleural glucose level ≤30 mg/dl.

c. Parapneumonic Effusions—The pH and glucose levels as predictors of outcome for parapneumonic effusions were described in a previous section (see section E).

d. Malignant Effusions—Rodriguez-Panadero evaluated the prognostic value of pleural pH and glucose in patients with a malignant effusion (102). When the pleural pH was <7.30 and the glucose was <60 mg/dl, 90% (9 of 10 patients) had a positive pleural cytology for malignancy. In addition, with decreasing pleural pH, pleurodesis was less likely to be successful, presumably owing to more extensive pleural disease and the failure of the pleural surfaces to be apposed. For example, when the pleural pH was <7.30, more than 50% of the pleurodeses were unsuccessful. In another study involving 50 patients with carcinomatous pleural metastases diagnosed by thoracoscopy, low pleural pH and low glucose were predictors of poorer prognosis (103). The mean survival time was 1.4 months when the pleural glucose level was <60 mg/dl, compared with 5.9 months when the pleural glucose level was >60 mg/dl. Similarly, the mean survival time was 1.9 months when the pleural pH was <7.35, compared with 6.4 months when the pleural pH was >7.35.

2. Amylase—An increased level of amylase in the pleural fluid can help narrow the differential diagnosis to one of three conditions: pancreatic disease, malignancy, or esophageal rupture (67). Light noted that pleural fluid amylase was elevated in four of five pancreatic pleural effusions, usually to a value markedly higher than the normal serum value. Amylase was also elevated in 4 of 43 malignant pleural effusions (67). Kramer, in another study, noted that pleural fluid amylase level was elevated in 33 malignant pleural effusions (59). In most cases, the effusion-to-serum amylase ratio was >1. Lung and gynecologic tumors were the most common malignancies associated with an elevated pleural amylase level.

3. Creatinine—Stark reported three cases of urinothorax associated with high levels of creatinine in the pleural fluid (121). In 71 control patients, the creatinine was not elevated above serum values, suggesting that an effusion-to-serum creatinine ratio >1 may have some specificity for urinothorax. However, the sensitivity is unknown.

4. **Adenosine Deaminase**—Valdez evaluated the utility of measuring the pleural fluid levels of adenosine deaminase (ADA), lysozyme (LYS), and interferon gamma (IFN) for detection of TB (128). In addition, the effusion-to-serum ratios of adenosine deaminase and lysozyme were calculated. Patients were classified according to their type of lesion into one of six groups: tuberculous pleurisy (91 patients), neoplastic (110 patients), parapneumonic (58 patients), empyema (10 patients), transudate (88 patients), and miscellaneous (48 patients).
   a. The clinical utility of these five criteria for detecting TB are summarized in Table 12-9.
   b. Based on these findings, the authors concluded that pleural ADA is a useful test for distinguishing tuberculous from nontuberculous effusions. It should be noted, however, that the PPV and the NPV assumed a 20% to 25% prevalence of TB in the study population. If the prevalence were only 5%, the PPV would decline to as low as 51%.
5. **Lipid Studies**
   a. **Pseudochylothorax Versus Chylothorax**—Pseudochylothorax is caused by accumulation of cholesterol and lecithin-globulin complexes in the pleural space, which give the pleural fluid a milky appearance. This typically occurs in the setting of a chronic exudative effusion that persists for more than 1 year, most commonly as a result of rheumatoid arthritis or TB. Chylothorax usually results from disruption of the thoracic duct and accumulation of chylomicrons in the pleural space. It too can cause a milky appearance because of a high lipid content, in this case caused by triglycerides rather than cholesterol. However, as discussed later, not all chylous or pseudochylous effusions have a milky appearance (120). Chylothorax is most often caused by lymphoma or surgical trauma. The common causes of chylothorax are summarized in Table 12-10, which is a compilation of 191 cases from eight series spanning the years 1964 to 1986 (129).
   b. **Diagnosis of Chylothorax**—In a prospective study involving 141 patients with a pleural effusion, Staats performed lipoprotein analysis and measured the pleural levels of cholesterol and triglycerides (120). Thirty-eight patients (27%) had a chylothorax, defined as the presence of chylomicrons on lipoprotein analysis. Only 50% of the chylous effusions were described as chylous based on the gross appearance of the fluid before the results of fluid tests were known. The triglyceride levels were significantly higher in chylous (median, 249 mg/dl; range, 49 to 2270 mg/dl) than in nonchylous effusions (median, 33 mg/dl; range, 13 to 107 mg/dl). In contrast, the cholesterol levels did not differ significantly between the two groups. When the triglyceride level was >110 mg/dl, the effusion was highly suggestive of a chylous effusion, but for values between 50 and 110 mg/dl, there was a significant overlap between the two groups. For equivocal cases, therefore, lipoprotein analysis would be necessary to distinguish between chylous and nonchylous effusions.

Table 12-9 Diagnostic utility of various criteria for tuberculous effusion

Parameter	Number of Samples	Sensitivity	Specificity	PPV	NPV
ADA >47 U/L	405	100%	95%	85%	100%
P/S ADA >1.5	276	86%	89%	63%	97%
LYS >15 g/ml	276	86%	62%	32%	95%
P/S LYS >1.1	276	67%	90%	60%	93%
IFN >140 pg/ml	145	94%	92%	78%	98%

Modified with permission from Valdez (128).

Table 12-10 Major causes of chylothorax

Causes	Number of Cases (%)
Nontraumatic	**138 (72)**
Malignant	87 (45)
Lymphoma	70 (37)
Other	17 (9)
Nonmalignant	51 (27)
Idiopathic	26 (14)
Miscellaneous*	15 (8)
Traumatic	**53 (28)**
Surgical	48 (25)
Nonsurgical	5 (3)

Modified with permission from Valentine (129).
*Miscellaneous causes include benign tumors, lymphangioleiomyomatosis, lymphagiomatosis, intestinal lymphangiectasis, protein-losing enteropathy, regional ileitis, reticular hyperplasia, pleuritis, cirrhosis, thoracic aortic aneurysm, and SLE.

6. **Red Blood Cells**—In Light's prospective series of 182 patients with a pleural effusion, a pleural RBC count >100,000 was highly suggestive of malignancy, pulmonary infarction, or trauma (65). A bloody effusion is considered a hemothorax when the ratio of hematocrit in pleural fluid to that in peripheral blood is ≥50% (72). Most hemothoraces are caused by blunt or penetrating trauma (77). If hemothorax occurs spontaneously, malignancy, coagulopathy, thoracic aortic aneurysm with dissection, pulmonary arteriovenous malformation, remote trauma, hemopneumothorax, infection (particularly TB), endometriosis, and exostosis should be considered (77). An RBC count and a hematocrit should be obtained on any pleural fluid that appears bloody, because the gross appearance of the fluid is a poor estimate of these values. Only about 30,000 RBCs per milliliter (hematocrit of approximately 0.25%) may impart a pink color to the fluid (72).
7. **Leukocytes**—The total leukocyte count is not very helpful in narrowing the differential diagnosis of a pleural effusion because it is highly variable, irrespective of the cause (65). On the other hand, the differential leukocyte count may be helpful.
   a. **Polymorphonuclear Leukocytes**—In Light's prospective series, a predominance of PMNs in the effusion correlated with the presence of acute inflammation caused by pneumonia, pulmonary infarction, pancreatitis, or another inflammatory condition (65). When there was not a predominance of PMNs in an effusion caused by an inflammatory condition, the effusion typically had been present for >5 days before thoracentesis. Nevertheless, the finding of PMN predominance did not rule out a malignancy or TB.
   b. **Lymphocytes**—Of the 102 exudative effusions in Light's study, 31 were lymphocyte-predominant, defined as >50% lymphocytes; of these 31 lymphocytic effusions, 30 were caused by either TB or malignancy (65). In another study involving 140 patients, 75 pleural effusions were lymphocyte-predominant, defined as >80% lymphocytes; these effusions resulted from probable TB in 31 patients (confirmed in 29), probable malignancy in 24 (confirmed in 18), and other causes in 20 (94). Although the majority of lymphocyte-predominant effusions are caused by TB or malignancy, the specificity appears to be low.
   c. **Mesothelial Cells**—The presence of mesothelial cells in the pleural fluid may be helpful diagnostically because this finding is rarely associated with a tuberculous effusion. In Light's study, all 14 patients with a tuberculous effusion had <1% mesothelial cells (65). In an older study by Spriggs, only

1 of the 65 tuberculous effusions had >0.1% mesothelial cells, and no tuberculous effusion had >0.25% mesothelial cells (119).

d. Eosinophils

(1) Eosinophilic pleural effusion may be caused by air entering the pleural space, as with prior chest surgery, thoracentesis, pneumothorax, or thoracic trauma (1). The mechanism is unknown.

(2) In an extensive review of the literature by Adelman, 343 cases of eosinophilic pleural effusion (>10% eosinophils) were identified (1). Fifty-two percent were related to asbestos, and 39% remained unexplained despite 2 to 3 years of follow-up for most patients. Effusions were considered to be related to asbestos (a) if there was history of direct or indirect exposure to asbestos, (b) if the effusion was transient, (c) if there was a lack of evidence of any other disease, and (d) if no malignancy was detected within 3 years. Given the high percentage of asbestos-related pleural effusions, the authors hypothesized that some of the unexplained effusions may also have been caused by benign asbestos-related pleural disease. The other striking finding was the low incidence of malignancy or TB in patients with eosinophilic pleural effusions: only 5% and 1.3%, respectively. The authors used estimates of prior probability of disease and Bayes' theorem to show that the finding of an eosinophilic pleural effusion lowers the probability of TB by a factor of 10 and the likelihood of malignancy by a factor of 2. However, it increases the likelihood that a diagnosis will not be found by a factor of 3.

(3) Eosinophils have also been reported in effusions caused by Churg-Strauss syndrome or paragonimiasis. In a case report, a man with Churg-Strauss syndrome had peripheral eosinophilia and 95% eosinophils in the pleural fluid (31). In a series of 17 patients with paragonimiasis, 12 had pleural effusions and many had up to 70% eosinophils in the pleural fluid. However, the exact number of patients with an eosinophilic effusion was not reported (51).

G. Immunology

1. Antinuclear Antibodies

a. In one report, 11 of 13 patients with lupus pleuritis had pleural antinuclear antibody (ANA) titers ≥1:160; for 9 patients, the effusion-to-serum ANA ratio was ≥1 (40). In a control group of 67 patients with pleural effusions not caused by lupus, all had a negative pleural ANA titer. The presence of LE cells confirmed the diagnosis in 7 of 8 patients tested.

b. In a more recent study, 82 patients with pleural effusions were tested for ANA using a newer test (54). Eight patients were found to have lupus pleuritis on chart review. Six of 8 patients with lupus pleuritis had a positive pleural ANA titer, and all but 1 had a high titer with a homogeneous staining pattern. Eight of 74 patients without clinical evidence of lupus also had a positive pleural ANA titer. The majority had a speckled pattern, but high titers were noted in 3. This study underscores the low specificity of the pleural ANA test. However, a homogeneous staining pattern and a high titer may be more specific for lupus.

2. Immune Complexes and Complement—Halla examined the utility of immune complexes and complement levels in the pleural fluid of 12 patients with rheumatoid arthritis, 9 with systemic lupus erythematosus (SLE), and 39 with other diseases (43). Low complement levels were found to distinguish rheumatoid and lupus effusions from controls but did not differentiate rheumatoid from lupus effusions. Immune complexes were found to be substantially higher in pleural fluid compared with serum in rheumatoid effusions; in contrast, the pleural fluid and serum levels were similar in lupus.

3. Bacterial Antigens—The utility of counterimmunoelectrophoresis (CIE) for bacterial antigens in the pleural fluid was examined in 87 patients by Lampe (60). CIE was positive for pneumococcus in all 21 culture-positive specimens and in 15 culture-negative specimens. For *Staphylococcus aureus*, CIE was positive in 12 of 14 culture-positive specimens and in 5 culture-negative specimens. For *Haemophilus influenzae*, CIE was positive in the single culture-positive specimen and in 3 culture-negative specimens. CIE for *H influenzae* was also positive in one specimen which grew *Escherichia coli*. Therefore, CIE may be more sensitive than culture. Alternatively, some of the culture-negative but CIE-positive specimens may represent false-positive tests.

4. **Cryptococcal Antigen**—Pleural fluid cryptococcal antigen was elevated in two cases reported by Young, one with localized pulmonary infection and the other with disseminated infection (139). This may prove to be a useful test, because the cultures are positive in only 42% of the infected effusions. However, the sensitivity and specificity of this test are unknown.
5. **Carcinoembryonic Antigen**
   a. The utility of measuring the carcinoembryonic antigen (CEA) level in pleural fluid was evaluated by McKenna in 34 malignant and 39 nonmalignant effusions (79). When abnormal CEA was defined as >20 mg/ml, it had a sensitivity of 91% and a specificity of 92% for adenocarcinoma in the pleural fluid. The specificity rose to 98% when abnormal CEA was defined as >55 mg/ml.
   b. Shimokata evaluated the utility of measuring the levels of CEA, cancer antigen CA15-3, and CA19-9 in 40 carcinomatous and 41 tuberculous effusions (115). The sensitivity and specificity for carcinoma were 77% and 100% respectively for CEA; 38% and 100% for CA15-3; and 61% and 95% for CA19-9.
6. **Monoclonal Antibody Panels**—Using cytologic smears from 262 serous effusions caused by a variety of benign and neoplastic (breast, ovary, and lung) conditions, Cappellari tested the utility of a monoclonal antibody panel directed against epithelial tumor cells (19). The cytology alone was 84% sensitive for malignancy, but when the information on the panel was added, the sensitivity rose to 98%. The specificity was 100%. In 30 patients with biopsy-proven metastatic breast cancer involving the pleura, Guzman tested a panel of monoclonal antibodies to CEA, epithelial membrane antigen (EMA), and human leukocyte antigen (HLA) and compared the results with those of conventional cytology (42). The cytology was positive in 43%, suspicious in 20%, and negative in 37%. However, all cases were positive by immunocytochemical analysis; 100% had a positive response to EMA, and 70% had a positive response to CEA. All mesothelial cells reacted with HLA, but some tumor cells did not. When tested on tissue specimens, monoclonal antibody panels against vimentin, keratin, human milk fat globule, CEA, and others were useful in distinguishing mesothelioma from adenocarcinoma (137,138). Other studies (36) suggest that monoclonal antibody panels against various tumor markers may help to distinguish among lymphoma, carcinoma, mesothelioma, and normal cells in pleural fluid. Nevertheless, larger studies are needed before these panels can be recommended for routine use.

H. Cytology

1. Malignancy causes approximately one quarter of all pleural effusions diagnosed in the hospital setting (62). An exudative effusion that remains unexplained after thoracentesis and pleural biopsy has a 33% to 70% chance of being caused by a malignancy (6). In Chernow's study involving 96 patients with a carcinomatous pleural effusion, the most common primary sites were lung (33%), breast (21%), ovary (9%), and stomach (7%) (24). The 6-month mortality rate was 84% in the series.
2. **Pleural Fluid Cytology Versus Biopsy**—Three studies have compared pleural fluid cytology versus biopsy for evaluation of a potentially malignant effusion. In all three studies, the cytologic examination offered a somewhat higher diagnostic yield but the two methods were complementary. The percentages of patients diagnosed by cytology, biopsy, or both are summarized in Table 12-11 (34,100,112).
3. **Repeat Cytology**—If the initial pleural fluid cytology result is negative, a repeat cytologic examination can increase the diagnostic yield somewhat, albeit

Table 12-11 Diagnostic utility of cytology & biopsy in malignant effusion

	Prakash (100) (n=281)	Frist (34) (n=44)	Salyer (112) (n=95)
Diagnosed with biopsy	43%	36%	58%
Diagnosed with cytology	58%	98%	73%
Diagnosed with either biopsy or cytology	65%	100%	90%

to a small degree. Prakash found that a second thoracentesis for cytology increased the diagnostic yield from 54% to 58% (100). Similarly, Light found that a second thoracentesis for cytology increased the diagnostic yield from 63% to 70% (65).

4. **Mesothelioma**—In a study involving 414 patients, 23 of whom had mesothelioma, cytology was positive in 48% and needle biopsy was positive in 39% (100). However, differentiation of mesothelioma from carcinoma was a difficult problem in more than one-third of the cases; in 61%, thoracotomy was necessary for diagnosis because of uncertainty in the cytologic examination.
5. **SLE and Rheumatoid Arthritis**—Cytologic examination can be helpful in identifying pleural effusions caused by SLE or rheumatoid arthritis. Three features are characteristic of rheumatoid effusions: (a) a background of granular necrotic debris which stains blue with the Papanicolau technique; (b) numerous macrophages, some being spindle-shaped; and (c) occasional multinucleated histiocytes. The presence of all of these features in the appropriate setting is thought to be diagnostic of a rheumatoid effusion (89). The finding of LE cells in the pleural fluid is highly specific for SLE-induced pleural effusion. However, the sensitivity of this finding is unknown.

I. Microbiology

1. **Bacterial Empyema**
   a. Alfageme reported the microbiologic causes of empyema in 82 patients from Spain (3). Of the 74 patients for whom a Gram stain was performed, 45 (61%) had a positive result; all but 3 patients with a positive Gram stain had a positive pleural fluid culture. Of the 29 patients with a negative Gram stain, 25 had a positive pleural fluid culture. Overall, 76 patients (93%) had a positive pleural fluid culture; 62% had aerobic organisms, 15% had anaerobic organisms, and 16% had both aerobic and anaerobic organisms. In addition, 3 patients had TB and 1 patient had fungus. Gram-positive cocci were the most common organisms in single-isolate cultures, with *Streptococcus pneumoniae* (8%) and *S aureus* (7%) leading the list. Other isolates included aerobic gram-negative bacilli, anaerobic gram-negative bacilli, and anaerobic gram-positive cocci.
   b. In the United States, Brook examined the microbiologic causes of 197 (pediatric and adult) culture-positive empyemas (13). The results were similar to those of Alfageme; 127 (64%) had aerobic organisms, 25 (13%) had anaerobic organisms, and 45 (13%) had both aerobic and anaerobic organisms. The common aerobic organisms were *S pneumoniae, S aureus, E coli, Klebsiella* species, and *H influenzae.* The common anaerobes were pigmented *Prevotella* and *Porphyromonas* species, *Bacteroides fragilis* group, anaerobic cocci, and *Fusobacterium* species. When a single organism was isolated, it was most commonly *S aureus, S pneumoniae, Bacteroides fragilis, Fusobacterium* species, or *Peptostreptococcus* species.
2. **Tuberculous Effusion**
   a. In Seibert's series of 1738 patients with TB from Mobile County, Alabama, 70 had tuberculous pleural effusions, constituting about 5% of all tuberculous disease in Mobile County (114). Of the 50 patients whose pleural fluid was cultured, 58% were positive for *M tuberculosis.* Of the 18 patients

whose pleural biopsies were cultured, 67% were positive. For comparison, sputum was positive for *M tuberculosis* in 50% of the cases. Not surprisingly, if an infiltrate was present on chest film, the sputum was more often positive for *M tuberculosis* than if only a pleural effusion was present (89% versus 11%). The presence or absence of an infiltrate on chest film did not influence the diagnostic yield of the pleural fluid culture or the pleural biopsy culture.

b. In Epstein's series of 26 patients with tuberculous pleural disease, 9% had positive acid-fast smears, 35% had positive pleural fluid cultures, and 39% had positive pleural biopsy cultures (30). Similarly, in Bueno's series of 107 patients with tuberculous pleural effusions (26% of all patients in the series), none had positive acid-fast smears, 13% had positive pleural fluid cultures, and 39% had positive pleural biopsy cultures (14). Addition of a pathologic examination of the biopsy specimen raised the diagnostic yield to 86%.

3. Fungal Pleural Effusions

a. Aspergillus—*Aspergillus fumigatus* is a rare cause of pleural infection. When it does occur, it is usually in patients with previously damaged lungs. For example, in a report of 6 patients with pleural aspergillosis, Hillerdal found that 5 had been treated previously for TB with therapeutic pneumothoraces (47). Similarly, in Krakowka's report of 10 patients with pleural aspergillosis, all had active or prior history of TB; some had been treated with therapeutic pneumothoraces or a lung resection (58). The pleural fluid culture was positive in 7 of the 10 patients, and fungal hyphae were seen during microscopy in 2 additional patients. One patient was not diagnosed until autopsy.

b. Coccidioides—Pleural effusion occurs in about 7% of patients with primary coccidioidomycosis (75). Often, the effusion occupies more than 50% of the hemithorax. There is usually a parenchymal infiltrate with the effusion. Culture of the pleural fluid is positive in 20%, but culture of the pleural biopsy specimen is almost always positive (72). In 1% to 5% of patients with chronic cavitary coccidioidomycosis, a cavity ruptures into the pleural space and causes a hydropneumothorax (72).

c. Other Fungi—Blastomycosis causes a pleural effusion in about 10% of patients (55). The pleural biopsy may reveal noncaseating granulomas. Clinically, the disease may resemble TB. Pleural effusions caused by cryptococcosis usually occur in the setting of disseminated disease and pulmonary parenchymal abnormality (139). In addition, many patients have the acquired immunodeficiency syndrome (AIDS) (133).w Histoplasmosis rarely causes a pleural effusion. In a retrospective review of 259 patients with histoplasmosis, only 1 had a pleural effusion (27).

4. Viral Pleural Effusions—In Fine's series of 59 patients with nonbacterial pneumonias (based on serologic criteria for mycoplasma, viral, or cold-agglutinin–positive pneumonia), 12 patients (20%) had evidence of a pleural effusion on chest film (33). For 4 patients, pleural fluid was demonstrated only on a lateral decubitus film.

J. Other Diagnostic Tests

1. Pleural Biopsy

a. Indications—For any undiagnosed pleural effusion, the American Thoracic Society recommends a pleural biopsy if malignancy or TB is suspected (117). This recommendation is based on a retrospective study involving 211 patients observed for 12 to 72 months (95). The study included all patients who underwent a pleural biopsy (three or more specimens per biopsy with a Cope or Abrams needle) over a 6-year period at one of three community hospitals in Rochester, New York. The specimens were examined histologically and cultured for *M tuberculosis* and for fungi.

(1) Biopsy revealed malignancy in 54 cases (26%), granulomatous disease in 10 cases (5%), normal findings in 143 cases (68%), and insufficient tissue in 4 cases (2%). Of the 143 patients with normal pleural biopsies, neoplasm or TB was eventually established in 30 and excluded in 101. No diagnosis was made in 12.

(2) Overall, the sensitivity was 65% for a malignancy and 90% for TB. The PPV was 98% and the NPV was 77%. One patient with nontuberculous granulomatous pleuritis had a false-positive result, making the specificity 99%. Therefore, pleural biopsy appears to be highly specific for malignancy or TB and more sensitive for TB than for malignancy.

(3) The sensitivity and the specificity of the pleural biopsy from this and other studies are summarized in Table 12-12 (14,49,83,95,113).

b. A closed pleural needle biopsy is thought to be inadequate for diagnosis of mesothelioma because a large piece of tissue is typically necessary. However, in a retrospective chart review of 20 patients with histologically proven mesothelioma, the diagnosis was made in 5 of 7 closed pleural needle biopsies, in 5 of 6 CT-guided pleural needle biopsies, and in 10 of 10 open pleural biopsies (7). The authors concluded that closed pleural biopsy, with or without CT guidance, is a reasonable first step for evaluation of mesothelioma.

c. Number of Biopsies—In a study involving 55 patients, Mungall found that multiple samples (usually 5; range, 2 to 10) taken from the same biopsy site improved the diagnostic yield of closed pleural needle biopsy (88). In a study involving 27 patients, Tomlinson found no significant advantage of using two biopsy sites if at least three samples were taken from one site (126).

2. Bronchoscopy

a. In the absence of another accepted indication for bronchoscopy or an abnormal chest film (in addition to the effusion), bronchoscopy is not routinely indicated in patients with unexplained pleural effusions. In a study by Feinsilver, bronchoscopy was performed in 45 patients with pleural effusions who did not have another indication for bronchoscopy such as a lung mass or atelectasis (32). Twenty-eight patients had unexplained pleural effusions and 17 had malignant pleural effusions by cytology with an unknown primary. Bronchoscopy revealed a diagnosis in only 3 patients, 1 in the unexplained pleural effusion group and 2 in the malignant effusion group.

b. In another study, 140 patients with pleural effusions underwent invasive pleural evaluation (thoracentesis plus pleural biopsy) as well as bronchoscopic examination (23). The patients were divided into groups depending on whether they had hemoptysis and whether the chest film was abnormal (in addition to the effusion). Thirty-nine patients had nonmalignant effusions, 95 had malignant effusions, and 6 had effusions that remained unexplained.

(1) Bronchoscopy was most helpful when there was another indication for the procedure, such as hemoptysis or an abnormal chest film. Of the 82

Table 12-12 Sensitivity & specificity of pleural biopsy for TB and malignancy

	Sensitivity		Specificity	
Author and Year (Reference)	TB	Malignancy	TB	Malignancy
Bueno, 1990 (14)	86%	79%	100%	100%
Poe, 1984 (95)	90%	65%	99%	100%
Scerbo, 1971 (113)	71%	39%	100%	100%
Mestitz, 1958 (83)	80%	54%	100%	95%
Hoff, 1975 (49)	57%	48%	98%	98%

patients without hemoptysis, a final diagnosis was made in 70% after invasive pleural evaluation, compared with 13% after bronchoscopic examination; of the 58 patients with hemoptysis, bronchoscopy made the diagnosis in 81%, and invasive evaluation of the pleura in 19%.

(2) Of the 74 patients with an otherwise normal chest film, invasive pleural evaluation was diagnostic in 61%, versus 16% with bronchoscopy. Finally, of the 59 patients with collapse, infiltrate, cavitary lesion, or nodular mass on chest film, bronchoscopy was diagnostic in 73% versus 36% with invasive pleural evaluation.

3. Thoracoscopy and Thoracotomy

a. About 25% of pleural effusions remain unexplained despite extensive investigation, including thoracentesis and pleural biopsy (82). In these cases, thoracoscopy or thoracotomy is indicated for further evaluation. Thoracoscopy is rapidly replacing thoracotomy as a diagnostic and therapeutic tool. Several studies have demonstrated that thoracoscopy requires equal or less operating time, shortens the length of hospital stay, reduces postoperative narcotic requirements, decreases the risk of perioperative complications, and causes less postoperative pleural drainage than thoracotomy (8,20,106,134). When performed for lung biopsy, thoracoscopy provides equal diagnostic accuracy. The overall mortality is approximately 1.4% for thoracoscopy, versus 2.2% for thoracotomy. One disadvantage of thoracoscopy is that conversion to a thoracotomy is required in about 18% of cases. This is particularly true when the procedure is performed for a therapeutic reason; when performed for lung biopsy, conversion to a thoracotomy is essentially never required.

b. The diagnostic yield of thoracoscopy for unexplained pleural effusions was prospectively evaluated by Menzies (82). Of the 102 patients undergoing thoracoscopy after thoracentesis and closed pleural needle biopsy had failed to reveal a diagnosis, a definitive diagnosis was made by thoracoscopy in 95 patients (93%); 42 had malignant and 53 had benign pleural disease. Overall, thoracoscopy was 91% sensitive, 100% specific, 96% accurate; the NPV for malignancy was 93%. There were no deaths associated with the procedure, but major and minor complications occurred in 2% and 6%, respectively. In an older study that included 215 patients, thoracoscopy was 97% sensitive for malignancy, compared with a 41% sensitivity of pleural fluid cytology plus needle biopsy done the day before thoracoscopy (10).

c. Thoracoscopy may also have a role in management of loculated parapneumonic effusions and as an alternative to decortication for empyemas. In a series of 12 patients with an empyema managed by thoracoscopy, irrigation was required for an average of 14 days, chest tubes were required for an average of 20 days, and the average length of hospital stay was 4.8 weeks (50). However, there have been no randomized controlled trials comparing these techniques.

K. Outcome of Exudative Effusions Without a Diagnosis

1. Unexplained Effusion After Needle Biopsy—Patients with an unexplained exudative effusion are considered to have nonspecific pleuritis if no diagnosis can be made after pleural biopsy. When these patients are observed in the long term, malignancy or TB is eventually diagnosed in 40% (113). Repeat closed pleural needle biopsies increase the yield of a positive result, but the yield diminishes rapidly after two consecutive biopsies. In a retrospective chart review of 119 patients with nonspecific pleuritis, Leslie identified several risk factors which correlated with the likelihood of subsequently being diagnosed with granulomatous or carcinomatous pleurisy: (a) weight loss, (b) fever, (c) positive skin reaction to purified-protein derivative, (d) pleural fluid lymphocytosis >95%, and (e) effusion occupying more than half a hemithorax (63). When one of these risk factors was present, the likelihood of eventually being diagnosed with TB or malignancy was 74%; with two or more risk factors, it was

90%. In contrast, when no risk factor was present, the likelihood of TB or malignancy was only 6%.

2. **Unexplained Effusion After Thoracotomy**—Among patients undergoing thoracotomy for further evaluation of an unexplained pleural effusion, the diagnosis may remain unknown in up to one third (29). Ryan evaluated the outcome of patients whose exudative pleural effusions were unexplained despite clinical evaluation, examination of the pleural fluid, and thoracotomy (107). Most of these patients had also undergone closed pleural needle biopsy. Thoracotomy included gross examination of the pleura, the lung, and the mediastinum as well as microscopic examination of appropriate tissue. Among 2071 patients with pleural effusions identified over an 11-year period, the cause was unexplained in 51 despite thoracotomy. The effusions were present for a mean of 15.7 weeks (range, 1 week to 2 years) before thoracotomy. Follow-up information was obtained in all cases. Two patients died soon after thoracotomy without a diagnosis. The cause of the effusion became apparent some time after thoracotomy in 18 patients (35%): 13 had malignancy (lymphoma in 6, mesothelioma in 4, and other tumors in 3); 3 had collagen-vascular disease; 1 had mitral stenosis; and 1 had yellow-nail syndrome. For the remaining 31 patients (61%), the cause of the effusion was never found despite 1.5 to 15 years of follow-up. None of these 31 patients had a recurrence after thoracotomy, which suggests that thoracotomy may have been therapeutic. Therefore, the majority (61%) of pleural effusions that remain unexplained after thoracotomy appeared to have a benign course. However, a malignancy was discovered eventually in 26% of these patients, most commonly a lymphoma.

L. Therapy for Parapneumonic or Malignant Effusions

1. Chest Tubes

a. When a chest tube is inserted for a complicated parapneumonic effusion or empyema, the largest tolerated tube should be used to avoid obstruction by clot, debris, or fibrin. Once a decision is made to insert a chest tube for an empyema, it should be placed without delay. In Ashbaugh's study, which included 122 patients with an empyema, delay in insertion of a chest tube by 3 days or longer (from the time of diagnosis) was associated with an increase in mortality from 3.4% to 16% (4). After the chest tube is placed, there is little information to guide further management of these patients. If there is no significant improvement within 24 to 48 hours after chest tube placement, most experts recommend obtaining either anteroposterior (AP) and lateral chest films or a chest CT to check the positions of the drainage tubes. Stark compared the utility of AP chest film, AP and lateral chest films, and CT scan for checking the tube position in 26 patients with empyema, 21 of whom had malpositioned chest tubes (122). The AP films alone were inadequate, identifying only 1 of the 21 malpositioned tubes. The AP and lateral films together identified 8 of 9 malpositioned tubes in whom both views of the chest were obtained. The chest CT scan identified 21 of 21 malpositioned tubes. Therefore, CT scan is the best test, but AP plus lateral chest films may suffice in most cases. CT scan can also provide other useful information, such as the presence of loculation, the patency of the airways, the character and size of lymph nodes, and parenchymal abnormalities such as lung nodules, cavities, abscess, or pneumonia. If the fluid collections are inadequately drained, further management options include insertion of a new chest tube, instillation of fibrinolytic agents into the pleural space, and exploration of the pleural space by thoracoscopy or thoracotomy. There are no well-designed studies that compare these management options.

b. The predictors of outcome for patients with a complicated parapneumonic effusion have not been well delineated. Van Way evaluated the effectiveness of chest tube drainage for three categories of complicated parapneumonic effusions: class I patients had pleural pH <7.2 and negative pleural fluid cultures; class II patients had positive pleural fluid cultures but no loculations; and class III patients had multiple loculations or trapped lung (130). The study enrolled 80 patients: 12 in class I, 28 in class II, and 40 in class III. For class I patients, 10 (83%) of the 12 were managed successfully with a single chest tube that was removed 4 to 7 days after insertion. For class II patients, all 28 (100%) were managed successfully with one or more chest tubes (mean number, 1.3). For class III patients, 18 of 40 were treated with multiple chest tubes, but 22 underwent early thoracotomy for manual disruption of loculations, followed by chest tube drainage. Of the 18 patients initially managed with chest tubes, 10 eventually required decortication; of the 22 patients managed with early thoracotomy, 5 eventually required decortication. These results suggest that early thoracotomy may be better than chest tube drainage for patients with multiple loculations. However, this study was retrospective and nonrandomized. In addition, fibrinolytic agents were not used in the study.

2. Pleurodesis and Pleurectomy

a. For patients with recurrent symptomatic pleural effusions, typically caused by a malignancy, pleurodesis or pleurectomy can offer relief by preventing reaccumulation of fluid. As an operative procedure, pleurectomy has all of the risks associated with general anesthesia and thoracotomy. In contrast, pleurodesis can be performed with local anesthesia. A sclerosing agent such as talc or tetracycline is instilled through a thoracostomy tube with the goal of obliterating the pleural space by having the two pleural surfaces bind together. Pleurectomy can be reserved for patients with failed pleurodesis or trapped lung and for those who need a thoracotomy for another purpose (78). In a review of 1168 patients treated with pleurodesis for malignant pleural effusion, the overall complete response rate was 64% (132). The most common adverse effects were pain in 23% and fever in 19%. However, the success rate with each agent varied widely, ranging from 0% for etoposide to 93% for talc. *Corynebacterium parvum*, tetracyclines, and bleomycin had success rates of 76%, 67%, and 54%, respectively. Of the tetracyclines, doxycycline and minocycline had the best success rates at 72% and 86%, respectively. Talc, although the most effective agent in this study, is usually given by insufflation through a thoracoscope and therefore requires a surgical procedure. Instillation of talc slurry through a thoracotomy tube has been reported, with a 100% success rate in two studies which included a total of 43 patients (118,135). However, 3 patients developed acute respiratory distress syndrome after receiving large quantities of talc slurry through a thoracostomy tube (101).

b. It is common practice to wait until the pleural drainage decreases to <150 ml/day before attempting pleurodesis. In theory, this is to ensure that the two pleural surfaces are apposed before the sclerosing agent is instilled. However, there are no data to support this practice (118). In a study involving 25 patients awaiting pleurodesis for a malignant effusion, Villanueva randomly assigned one group to receive treatment with tetracycline pleurodesis when the lung appeared fully expanded on chest film (regardless of the amount of pleural drainage) and another group to receive treatment when the pleural drainage was <150 ml/day and the lung appeared fully expanded on chest film (131). The success rate was 80% in both groups, suggesting that the amount of drainage may not be as important as whether or not the lung is fully expanded.

3. Fibrinolytic Agents—Numerous studies have described successful management of loculated complicated parapneumonic effusions with intrapleural administration of fibrinolytic agents (urokinase, streptokinase, tissue plasminogen activator) through small-bore (10 to 16F) chest tubes. Many of these studies have been criticized because they were small or uncontrolled. The largest report, also an uncontrolled study, included 118 patients: 79 with empyemas, 27 with sterile loculated parapneumonic effusions, 10 with sterile hemothoraces, and 2 with sterile postoperative exudative effusions (87). Forty-one patients had failed large-bore thoracostomy drainage. The mean duration of the effusion was 13 days (range, 1 to 175 days). Ultrasound, chest CT, or fluoroscopy was used to guide the placement of chest tubes as needed. Urokinase (100,000 to 250,000 U/ml in 20- to 240-ml aliquots) was instilled into the pleural space through a chest tube, allowed to dwell for 1 to 4 hours before drainage, and repeated up to four times per day until there was less than 20 ml/day of pleural drainage. The authors chose urokinase over streptokinase because of its nonantigenic and nonpyrogenic properties; there are no systemic fibrinolytic effects with either agent after instillation into the pleural space. With this strategy, 111 effusions (94%) were successfully drained; an average of 5 instillations for a mean total dose of 466,000 U of urokinase were used. The mean duration of chest tube drainage was 6.3 days, and 53 patients required more than one chest tube. Of the 7 patients in whom this treatment was unsuccessful, 2 died of sepsis with incomplete drainage and 5 required decortication (2 died postoperatively). The authors concluded that intrapleural instillation of urokinase through a small-bore chest tube is safe and effective for management of complicated parapneumonic effusions, empyemas, and hemothoraces. However, this approach is very labor intensive, and care must be taken to ensure that there is ongoing drainage.

4. Decortication

a. With ongoing intense inflammation in the pleural space, a feared complication of empyema is the formation of a fibrous peel as a result of fibrin deposition. Decortication is the removal of this fibrous peel from the visceral pleural surface, which eliminates the source of ongoing inflammation and allows any trapped lung to expand. The traditional indication for decortication is a complicated parapneumonic effusion that has not responded to chest tube drainage and fibrinolytic therapy. In a nonrandomized study involving 84 patients with an empyema managed by open drainage (19 patients) or with decortication (65 patients), patients managed with decortication had shorter hospital stays, required fewer days of chest tube drainage, and had a lower mortality rate (6.2% versus 21%) (4).

b. The timing of decortication has been a subject of debate. One reason for performing a decortication is to prevent the normal lung from becoming trapped by the noncompliant fibrous peel. However, some reports suggest that, given time, the fibrous peels and the accompanying lung restriction may resolve. Neff performed serial CT scans (at 4, 8, and 12 weeks after chest tube removal) to examine the natural history of pleural peels in 10 patients with empyemas managed with chest tube drainage (90). At 12 weeks, the pleura was essentially normal in 4 patients and demonstrated only small areas of thickening in 6 patients. In another study, Sahn performed serial pulmonary function tests (at 3, 6, and 9 months) on 11 patients with empyemas managed with chest tube drainage and antibiotics (109). By 9 months, the restrictive pulmonary defects had completely resolved for all patients. Based on these results, many experts suggest that decortication be reserved for symptomatic patients with nonresolving pleural peels or persistent restrictive defects on pulmonary function testing.

5. Open Drainage—Open drainage is reserved for patients who would typically require a decortication but are too ill to tolerate the procedure. There are two types of open drainage procedures. The simplest involves resection of several ribs over the empyema and insertion of one or more large-bore tubes into the pleural cavity. The tubes are irrigated daily, and the drainage is collected into a colostomy bag. A more complicated procedure is the Eloesser flap drainage, which involves removal of several ribs over the empyema and retention of a skin and muscle flap to line the tract between the pleural space and the surface of the chest. Both procedures allow gradual obliteration of the empyema cavity with granulation tissue. The major disadvantage of these procedures is the slow healing process. In one series involving 33 patients with empyemas treated with open drainage, a median of 142 days was required for healing of the drainage site (5).

M. Summary

1. In the United States, pleural effusions are most commonly caused by CHF, malignancy, pneumonia, or pulmonary embolus. TB is a common cause of pleural effusion in other parts of the world. For HIV-infected patients, malignancy (Kaposi's sarcoma and lymphoma) and infections (aerobic bacteria, TB, and cryptococcus) dominate the list.
2. In general, thoracentesis should be considered for all new, unexplained pleural effusions. There are no absolute contraindications, but relative contraindications include bleeding diathesis, systemic anticoagulation, a small volume of fluid, mechanical ventilation, an uncooperative patient, and cutaneous disease at the needle entry site. Light empirically suggested that thoracentesis can be performed safely and successfully if the lateral decubitus film demonstrates ≥10 mm of layering fluid.
3. According to Light's criteria, the presence of any one of the following is consistent with an exudate: pleural LDH >200 IU/L (or more than two-thirds of the upper limit of normal), effusion-to-serum protein ratio >0.5, and effusion-to-serum LDH ratio <0.6. In general, further diagnostic tests are warranted for exudates but not for transudates. Compared with various other criteria for identifying exudates (serum-effusion albumin gradient <1.2 g/dl, pleural cholesterol >55 mg/dl, effusion-to-serum cholesterol ratio >0.3, and effusion-to-serum bilirubin ratio >0.6), Light's criteria appear to be the most accurate. However, in the setting of diuretic therapy, an effusion caused by CHF can be mistaken for an exudate by this criteria. For these patients, the serum-effusion albumin gradient may be a useful complementary test to the standard Light criteria.
4. A parapneumonic effusion is considered uncomplicated if it resolves with antibiotics alone and complicated if it loculates or forms an empyema when left undrained. Although numerous studies have analyzed the fluid characteristics of parapneumonic effusions, there is still no consensus on what level of LDH, pH, or glucose most reliably separates complicated from uncomplicated effusions. A metaanalysis of these studies suggests the following criteria for tube thoracostomy: pleural pH <7.22 for low-risk patients and pH <7.29 for high-risk patients. A low-risk patient is defined as a young patient with a pneumococcal pneumonia and no comorbid conditions; a high-risk patient is defined as an elderly patient with an anaerobic pneumonia and comorbid lung disease. Nevertheless, the most widely known criteria for tube thoracostomy are those of Light, by which a chest tube is recommended if the pleural pH is <7.00 or if the glucose is <40 mg/dl. Antibiotic therapy alone is recommended when the pleural pH is >7.20 and the LDH is <1000 mg/dl. For patients not meeting either criterion, tube thoracostomy is recommended on an individualized basis. Light's criteria for tube thoracostomy may be unreliable if the effusion is loculated or if the patient had been treated with antibiotics before thoracentesis. More recently, Light has created a classification system for guiding therapy based on fluid characteristics and the presence or absence of loculations, but this has not yet been validated.
5. For a complicated effusion, once the decision to insert a chest tube is made, it should be placed without delay. Delay in insertion of a chest tube was associated with an increase in mortality in one study. If there is no significant improvement within 24 to 48 hours of chest tube placement, AP and lateral chest films or chest CT scan may be considered to check the position of the chest tubes in relation to the fluid collections. If the fluid collections remain inadequately drained, further management options include insertion of more chest tubes, instillation of fibrinolytic agents through the chest tube, or exploration of the pleural space by thoracoscopy or thoracotomy. For refractory cases, decortication or open drainage may be considered. There are no well-designed studies that rigorously compare these management options.
6. Malignancy causes approximately one quarter of all pleural effusions diagnosed in the hospital setting. The most common primary sites are lung, breast, ovary, and stomach. Cytologic examination of the pleural fluid offers a somewhat higher diagnostic yield compared with closed pleural needle biopsy (58%

to 98% versus 36% to 58%), but the two methods are complementary. If the initial pleural fluid cytology is negative, a repeat cytologic examination can increase the diagnostic yield, albeit to a small degree. The sensitivity of pleural biopsy varies from 57% to 90% for TB and from 39% to 79% for malignancy. Obtaining multiple samples (usually 5) from the same biopsy site improves the diagnostic yield of this test. However, biopsy of more than one site does not appear to improve the yield.

7. In the absence of another accepted indication for bronchoscopy or an abnormal chest film (in addition to the effusion), bronchoscopy is not routinely indicated in patients with unexplained pleural effusions.
8. Pleurodesis or pleurectomy can offer relief for patients with recurrent symptomatic pleural effusions. As an operative procedure, pleurectomy has all of the risks associated with general anesthesia and thoracotomy. In contrast, pleurodesis can be performed with local anesthesia. A sclerosing agent such as talc or tetracycline is instilled through a thoracostomy tube with the goal of obliterating the pleural space. Ideally, the lung should be fully expanded and the two pleural surfaces should be apposed before the sclerosing agent is instilled. Most commonly, a tetracycline or talc is used. Of the tetracyclines, doxycycline and minocycline have the best success rates at 72% and 86%, respectively. According to some reports, talc may be the most effective sclerosing agent, but it is usually given by insufflation through a thoracoscope and therefore requires a surgical procedure. Instillation of talc slurry through a thoracotomy tube has also been used with good success, but acute respiratory distress syndrome has been reported after its use.
9. About 25% of pleural effusions remain unexplained despite extensive investigation, including thoracentesis and closed pleural needle biopsy. For these patients, thoracoscopy or thoracotomy may be indicated. Patients whose exudative effusions remain unexplained despite pleural biopsy are considered to have nonspecific pleuritis. With long-term follow-up, malignancy or TB is eventually diagnosed in 40% of these patients. Repeat closed pleural needle biopsies are somewhat useful, but the diagnostic yield diminishes rapidly after two biopsies. When thoracotomy is performed for further evaluation, the effusion may remain unexplained in up to one third; in most of these patients, the effusion appears to have a benign course, but a malignancy, most commonly a lymphoma, is eventually found in about 25%.

Abbreviations used in Chapter 12

AIDS = acquired immunodeficiency syndrome
ADA = adenosine deaminase
ANA = antinuclear antibody
AP = anteroposterior
CEA = carcinoembryonic antigen
CHF = congestive heart failure
CPA = costophrenic angle
CIE = counterimmunoelectrophoresis
CT = computed tomography
EMA = epithelial membrane antigen
HIV = human immunodeficiency virus
HLA = human leukocyte antigen
IFN = interferon
LDH = lactate dehydrogenase
LYS = lysozyme
NPV = negative predictive value
P = probability value
PMN = polymorphonuclear leukocyte

PPV = positive predictive value
P/S ADA = effusion-to-serum adenosine deaminase
P/S LYS = effusion-to-serum lysozyme
RBC = red blood cells
ROC = receiver operating characteristic
SLE = systemic lupus erythematosus
TB = tuberculosis

References

1. Adelman. Diagnostic utility of pleural fluid eosinophilia. *Am J Med* 1984;77:915. Review.
2. Agostoni. Solute-coupled liquid absorption from the pleural space. *Respir Physiol* 1990;81:19.
3. Alfageme. Empyema of the thorax in adults: etiology, microbiologic findings, and management. *Chest* 1993;103:839.
4. Ashbaugh. Empyema thoracis: factors influencing morbidity and mortality. *Chest* 1991;99:1162.
5. Bartlett. Anaerobic infections of the lung and pleural space. *Am Rev Respir Dis* 1974;110:56.
6. Bartter. The evaluation of pleural effusion. *Chest* 1994;106:1209. Review.
7. Beauchamp. The role of closed pleural needle biopsy in the diagnosis of malignant mesothelioma of the pleura. *Chest* 1992;102:1110.
8. Bensard. Comparison of video thoracoscopic lung biopsy to open lung biopsy in the diagnosis of interstitial lung disease. *Chest* 1993;103:765.
9. Berger. Immediate drainage is not required for all patients with complicated parapneumonic effusions. *Chest* 1990;97:731.
10. Boutin. Thoracoscopy in malignant pleural effusions. *Am Rev Respir Dis* 1981; 124:588.
11. Bressler. Bolus contrast medium enhancement for distinguishing pleural from parenchymal lung disease: CT features. *J Comput Assist Tomogr* 1987;11:436.
12. Broaddus. Disorders of the pleura: general principles and diagnostic approach. In: Murray J, ed. *Textbook of Respiratory Medicine*. Philadelphia: WB Saunders, 1988:2145.
13. Brook. Aerobic and anaerobic microbiology of empyema: a retrospective review in two military hospitals. *Chest* 1993;103:1502.
14. Bueno. Cytologic and bacteriologic analysis of fluid and pleural biopsy specimens with a Cope's needle. *Arch Intern Med* 1990;150:1190.
15. Burgess. Comparative analysis of the biochemical parameters used to distinguish between pleural transudates and exudates. *Chest* 1995;107:1604.
16. Burgher. Guidelines for thoracentesis and needle biopsy of the pleura. *Am J Respir Dis* 1989;140:257.
17. Bynum. Characteristics of pleural effusions associated with pulmonary embolism. *Arch Intern Med* 1976;136:159.
18. Cadranel. Causes of pleural effusion in 75 HIV-infected patients. *Chest* 1993;104: 655.
19. Cappellari. Use of a pool of monoclonal antibodies in diagnosing cells from serous cavities. *Tumori* 1993;79:211.
20. Carnochan. Efficacy of video assisted thoracoscopic lung biopsy: an historical comparison with open lung biopsy. *Thorax* 1994;49:361.
21. Carr. Pleurisy with effusion in rheumatoid arthritis, with reference to the low concentration of glucose in pleural fluid. *Am Rev Respir Dis* 1962;85:345.
22. Chakko. Treatment of congestive heart failure: its effect on pleural fluid chemistry. *Chest* 1989;95:798.
23. Chang. The role of fiberoptic bronchoscopy in evaluating the causes of pleural effusions. *Arch Intern Med* 1989;149:855.

24. Chernow. Carcinomatous involvement of the pleura: an analysis of 96 patients. *Am J Med* 1977;63:695.
25. Collins. Minimal detectable pleural effusions. *Radiology* 1972;105:51.
26. Collins. Thoracocentesis: clinical value, complications, technical problems, and patient experience. *Chest* 1987;91:817.
27. Connell. Radiographic manifestations of pulmonary histoplasmosis: a 10-year review. *Radiology* 1976;121:281.
28. Costa. Measurement of pleural fluid cholesterol and lactate dehydrogenase: a simple and accurate set of indicators for separating exudates from transudates. *Chest* 1995;108:1260.
29. Douglass. Diagnostic thoracotomy in the study of idiopathic pleural effusion. *Am Rev Tuberculosis* 1956;74:954.
30. Epstein. Tuberculous pleural effusions. *Chest* 1987;91:106.
31. Erzurum. Pleural effusion in Churg-Strauss syndrome. *Chest* 1989;95:1357.
32. Feinsilver. Fiberoptic bronchoscopy and pleural effusion of unknown origin. *Chest* 1986;90:516.
33. Fine. Frequency of pleural effusions in mycoplasma and viral pneumonias. *N Engl J Med* 1970;283:790.
34. Frist. Comparison of the diagnostic values of biopsies of the pleura and cytologic evaluation of pleural fluids. *Am J Clin Pathol* 1979;72:48.
35. Funahashi. PO_2, pCO_2 and pH in pleural effusions of various types. *Chest* 1971; 60:693.
36. Ghosh. Immunocytochemical staining of cells in pleural and peritoneal effusions with a panel of monoclonal antibodies. *J Clin Pathol* 1983;36:1154.
37. Good. The diagnostic value of pleural fluid pH. *Chest* 1980;78:55.
38. Good. The pathogenesis of the low pleural fluid pH in esophageal rupture. *Am Rev Respir Dis* 1983;127:702.
39. Good. The pathogenesis of low glucose, low pH malignant effusions. *Am Rev Respir Dis* 1985;131:737.
40. Good. Lupus pleuritis: clinical features and pleural fluid characteristics with special reference to pleural fluid antinuclear antibodies. *Chest* 1983;84:714.
41. Gryminski. The diagnosis of pleural effusion by ultrasonic and radiologic techniques. *Chest* 1976;70:33.
42. Guzman. The value of the immunoperoxidase slide assay in the diagnosis of malignant pleural effusions in breast cancer. *Acta Cytol* 1988;32:188.
43. Halla. Immune complexes and other laboratory features of pleural effusions. *Ann Intern Med* 1980;92:748.
44. Hamm. Cholesterol in pleural effusions: a diagnostic aid. *Chest* 1987;92:296.
45. Han. Perforation of the esophagus: correlation of site and cause with plain film findings. *Am J Roentgenol* 1985;145:537.
46. Heffner. Pleural fluid chemical analysis in parapneumonic effusions. *Am J Respir Crit Care Med* 1995;151:1700.
47. Hillerdal. Pulmonary aspergillus infection invading the pleura. *Thorax* 1981;36: 745.
48. Himelman. The prognostic value of loculations in parapneumonic pleural effusions. *Chest* 1986;90:852.
49. Hoff. Diagnostic reliability of needle biopsy of the parietal pleura. *Am J Clin Pathol* 1975;64:200.
50. Hutter. The management of empyema thoracis by thoracoscopy and irrigation. *Ann Thorac Surg* 1985;39:517.
51. Johnson. Paragonimiasis in Indochinese refugees. *Am Rev Respir Dis* 1983;128: 534.
52. Kawashima. Malignant pleural mesothelioma: CT manifestations in 50 cases. *Am J Radiol* 1990;155:965.
53. Kaye. Pleuropulmonary complications of pancreatitis. *Thorax* 1968;23:297.
54. Khare. Antinuclear antibodies in pleural fluid. *Chest* 1994;106:866.
55. Kinasewitz. The spectrum and significance of pleural disease in blastomycosis. *Chest* 1985;86:580.

56. Kohan. Value of chest ultrasonography versus decubitus roentgenography for thoracentesis. *Am Rev Respir Dis* 1986;133:1124.
57. Kokkola. Oxygen and carbon dioxide tensions and the pH of pleural effusions. Scand J Respir Dis Suppl 1974;89:195.
58. Krakowka. Infection of the pleura by *Aspergillus fumigatus*. *Thorax* 1970;25:245.
59. Kramer. High amylase levels in neoplasm-related pleural effusion. *Ann Intern Med* 1989;110:567.
60. Lampe. Detection of bacterial antigen in pleural fluid by counterimmunoelectrophoresis. *J Pediatr* 1976;88:557.
61. Law. Computed tomography in the assessment of malignant mesothelioma of the pleura. *Clin Radiol* 1982;33:67.
62. Leff. Pleural effusion from malignancy. *Ann Intern Med* 1978;74:532.
63. Leslie. Clinical characteristics of the patient with nonspecific pleuritis. *Chest* 1988;94:603.
64. Lieberman. Pathogenesis and treatment of hydrothorax complicating cirrhosis and ascites. *Ann Intern Med* 1966;64:341.
65. Light. Cells in pleural fluid. *Arch Intern Med* 1973;132:854.
66. Light. Diagnostic significance of pleural fluid pH and pCO_2. *Chest* 1973;64:591.
67. Light. Glucose and amylase in pleural effusions. *JAMA* 1973;225:257.
68. Light. Observations on pleural fluid pressures as fluid is withdrawn during thoracentesis. *Am Rev Respir Dis* 1980;121:799.
69. Light. Parapneumonic effusions. *Am J Med* 1980;69:507.
70. Light. A new classification of parapneumonic effusions and empyema. *Chest* 1995;108:299.
71. Light. Pleural effusions: the diagnostic separation of transudates and exudates. *Ann Intern Med* 1972;77:507.
72. Light. *Pleural Diseases*, ed 2. Philadelphia: Lea & Febiger, 1990. Review.
73. Lillington. Rheumatoid pleurisy with effusion. *Arch Intern Med* 1971;128:764.
74. Limthongkul. Diagnostic and prognostic significance of pleural fluid pH and pCO_2 in the exudative phase of parapneumonic effusions. *J Med Assoc Thai* 1983;66:762.
75. Lonky. Acute coccidioidal pleural effusion. *Am Rev Respir Dis* 1976;114:681.
76. Maher. Massive pleural effusion: malignant and nonmalignant causes in 46 patients. *Am Rev Respir Dis* 1972;105:458.
77. Martinez. Spontaneous hemothorax: report of 6 cases and review of the literature. *Medicine (Baltimore)* 1992;71:354.
78. Martini. Indications for pleurectomy in malignant effusions. *Cancer* 1975;35:734.
79. McKenna. Diagnostic value of carcinoembryonic antigen in exudative pleural effusions. *Chest* 1980;78:587.
80. Meigs. Fibroma of the ovary with ascites and hydrothorax. *Am J Obstet Gynecol* 1937;33:249.
81. Meisel. Pleural fluid to serum bilirubin concentration ratio for the separation of transudates from exudates. *Chest* 1990;98:141.
82. Menzies. Thoracoscopy for the diagnosis of pleural disease. *Ann Intern Med* 1991;114:271.
83. Mestitz. Pleural biopsy in the diagnosis of pleural effusion. Lancet 1958;2:1349.
84. Metzger. Pulmonary oxalosis caused by *Aspergillus niger*. *Am Rev Respir Dis* 1984;129:501.
85. Miller. Pleuropulmonary Complications of Enteral Tube Feedings. *Chest* 1985;88:230.
86. Moskowitz. Roentgen visualization of minute pleural effusion. *Radiology* 1973;109:33.
87. Moulton. Treatment of complicated pleural fluid collections with image-guided drainage and intracavitary urokinase. *Chest* 1995;108:1252.
88. Mungall. Multiple pleural biopsy with the Abrams needle. *Thorax* 1980;35:600.
89. Naylor. The pathognomonic cytologic picture of rheumatoid pleuritis: the 1989 Maurice Goldblatt Cytology Award Lecture. *Acta Cytol* 1990;34:465.

90. Neff. CT follow-up of empyemas: pleural peels resolve after percutaneous catheter drainage. *Radiology* 1990;176:195.
91. Negrini. Fluid exchanges across the parietal, peritoneal, and pleural mesothelia. *J Appl Physiol* 1993;74:1779.
92. Negrini. Contribution of lymphatic myogenic activity and respiratory movements to pleural lymph flow. *J Appl Physiol* 1994;76:2267.
93. Peterman. Evaluating pleural effusions: a two-stage laboratory approach. *JAMA* 1984;252:1051.
94. Pettersson. Diagnostic value of total and differential leukocyte counts in pleural effusions. *Acta Med Scand* 1981;210:129.
95. Poe. Sensitivity, specificity, and predictive values of closed pleural biopsy. *Arch Intern Med* 1984;144:325.
96. Poe. Utility of pleural fluid analysis in predicting tube thoracostomy/decortication in parapneumonic effusions. *Chest* 1991;100:963.
97. Potts. Pleural fluid pH in parapneumonic effusions. *Chest* 1976;70:328.
98. Potts. The acidosis of low-glucose pleural effusions. *Am Rev Respir Dis* 1978; 117:665.
99. Potts. The glucose-pH relationship in parapneumonic effusions. *Arch Intern Med* 1978;138:1378.
100. Prakash. Comparison of needle biopsy with cytologic analysis for the evaluation of pleural effusion: analysis of 414 cases. *Mayo Clin Proc* 1985;60:158.
101. Rinaldo. Adult respiratory distress syndrome following intrapleural instillation of talc. *J Thorac Cardiovasc Surg* 1983;85:523.
102. Rodriguez-Panadero. Low glucose and pH levels in malignant pleural effusions. *Am Rev Respir Dis* 1989;139:663.
103. Rodriguez-Panadero. Survival time of patients with pleural metastatic carcinoma predicted by glucose and pH studies. *Chest* 1989;95:320.
104. Romero. Evaluation of different criteria for the separation of pleural transudates from exudates. *Chest* 1993;104:399.
105. Roth. The serum-effusion albumin gradient in the evaluation of pleural effusions. *Chest* 1990;98:546.
106. Rubin. Intrathoracic biopsies, pulmonary wedge excision, and management of pleural disease: is video-assisted closed chest surgery the approach of choice? *Am Surg* 1994;60:860.
107. Ryan. The outcome of patients with pleural effusion of indeterminate cause at thoracotomy. *Mayo Clin Proc* 1981;56:145.
108. Sahn. Rheumatoid pleurisy: observations on the development of low pleural fluid pH and glucose level. *Arch Intern Med* 1980;140:1237.
109. Sahn. Decortication is rarely necessary following empyema. *J Clin Res* 1981;29: 88A.
110. Sahn. Pleural fluid analysis: narrowing the differential diagnosis. *Semin Respir Med* 1987;9:22. Review.
111. Sahn. The pleura. *Am Rev Respir Dis* 1988;138:184. Review.
112. Salyer. Efficacy of pleural needle biopsy and pleural fluid cytopathology in the diagnosis of malignant neoplasm involving the pleura. *Chest* 1975;67:536.
113. Scerbo. A prospective study of closed pleural biopsies. *JAMA* 1971;218:377.
114. Seibert. Tuberculous pleural effusion: a twenty-year experience. *Chest* 1991;99:883.
115. Shimokata. Diagnostic value of cancer antigen 15-3 (CA15-3) detected by monoclonal antibodies (115D8 and DF3) in exudative pleural effusions. *Eur Respir J* 1988;1:341.
116. Shinto. Effects of diuresis on the characteristics of pleural fluid in patients with congestive heart failure. *Am J Med* 1990;88:230.
117. Sokolowski. Guidelines for thoracentesis and needle biopsy of the pleura. *Am Rev Respir Dis* 1989;140:257.
118. Sorensen. Treatment of malignant pleural effusion with drainage, with and without instillation of talc. *Eur J Respir Dis* 1984;65:131.
119. Spriggs. Absence of mesothelial cells from tuberculous pleural effusions. *Thorax* 1960;15:169.

120. Staats. The lipoprotein profile of chylous and nonchylous pleural effusions. *Mayo Clinic Proc* 1980;55:700.
121. Stark. Biochemical features of urinothorax. *Arch Intern Med* 1982;142:1509.
122. Stark. CT and radiographic assessment of tube thoracostomy. *Am J Roentgenol* 1983;141:253.
123. Stark. Differentiating lung abscess and empyema: radiography and computed tomography. *AJR Am J Roentgenol* 1983;141:163.
124. Taryle. The incidence and clinical correlates of parapneumonic effusions in pneumococcal pneumonia. *Chest* 1978;74:170.
125. Taryle. Acid generation by pleural fluid: possible role in the determination of pleural fluid pH. *J Lab Clin Med* 1979;93:1041.
126. Tomlinson. Closed pleural biopsy: a prospective study of dual biopsy sites. *Am Rev Respir Dis* 1986;133:56A.
127. Valdez. Cholesterol: a useful parameter for distinguishing between pleural exudates and transudates. *Chest* 1991;99:1097.
128. Valdez. Diagnosis of tuberculous pleurisy using the biologic parameters adenosine deaminase, lysozyme, and interferon gamma. *Chest* 1993;103:458.
129. Valentine. The management of chylothorax. *Chest* 1992;102:586. Review.
130. Van Way. The role of early limited thoracotomy in the treatment of empyema. *J Thorac Cardiovasc Surg* 1988;96:436.
131. Villanueva. Efficacy of short term versus long term tube thoracostomy drainage before tetracycline pleurodesis in the treatment of malignant pleural effusions. *Thorax* 1994;49:23.
132. Walker-Renard. Chemical pleurodesis for malignant pleural effusions. *Ann Intern Med* 1994;120:56. Review.
133. Wasser. Pulmonary cryptococcosis in AIDS. *Chest* 1987;92:692.
134. Weatherford. Thoracoscopy versus thoracotomy: indications and advantages. *Am Surg* 1995;61:83.
135. Webb. Iodized talc pleurodesis for the treatment of pleural effusions. *J Thorac Cardiovasc Surg* 1992;103:885.
136. Weiss. Laterality of pleural effusions in chronic congestive heart failure. *Am J Cardiol* 1984;53:951.
137. Wick. Malignant epithelioid pleural mesothelioma versus peripheral pulmonary adenocarcinoma: a histochemical, ultrastructural, and immunohistologic study of 103 cases. *Hum Pathol* 1990;21:759.
138. Wirth. Immunohistochemical evaluation of seven monoclonal antibodies for differentiation of pleural mesothelioma from lung adenocarcinoma. *Cancer* 1991; 67:655.
139. Young. Pleural effusions due to *Cryptococcus neoformans*: a review of the literature and report of two cases with cryptococcal antigen determinations. *Am Rev Respir Dis* 1980;121:743. Review

13 Acute Pancreatitis

Daniel C. Chung, David S. Stasior,
and Lawrence S. Friedman

A. Introduction

1. Epidemiology

a. Precise data on the incidence of acute pancreatitis in the US are not available. However, European studies have reported a rising incidence of acute pancreatitis over the past several decades. In the United Kingdom, the rate of hospital admissions for acute pancreatitis was 21 to 83 per million in the early 1970s but rose to 242 per million by the mid-1980s (10,85,93). Similarly, in Finland, the rate of hospital admissions for acute pancreatitis rose from 47 per 100,000 in 1970 to 73 per 100,000 in 1989 (40). The reason for this increased incidence is unclear, but it may be related in part to improved diagnostic capabilities. Over similar time periods, mortality from acute pancreatitis has fallen from 5.9% to 2.6% in Finland (40) and from 17.8% to 5.6% in Scotland (93).

b. In recent years, a rapid rise in the incidence of acute pancreatitis has been observed among persons infected with the human immunodeficiency virus (HIV), for whom the rate typically ranges from 4% to 5% (16,53). The increase in incidence is attributable primarily to the frequent exposure of these patients to potential pancreatic toxins such as 2′,3′-dideoxyinosine (ddI) or pentamidine (16).

2. Classification—The Marseilles Conference of 1984 classified pancreatitis simply into two types: acute and chronic. Acute pancreatitis was defined clinically as "abdominal pain accompanied by increased pancreatic enzymes in blood or urine, or both. Though it usually runs a benign course, severe attacks may lead to shock with renal and pulmonary insufficiency that may prove fatal. Acute pancreatitis may be a single episode or it may recur" (78). A more refined classification system was developed by 40 international experts in pancreatitis. In this system, acute pancreatitis is defined as "an acute inflammatory process of the pancreas, with variable involvement of other regional tissues or remote organ systems" (11). Severe pancreatitis is characterized by organ failure and/or local complications such as necrosis, abscess, or pseudocyst. Mild pancreatitis is characterized by minimal organ dysfunction and an uneventful recovery. Previously used terms such as phlegmon, hemorrhagic pancreatitis, and infected pseudocyst are considered ambiguous and their use is now discouraged.

3. Pathophysiology—In general, the local inflammatory damage and systemic complications of acute pancreatitis are a consequence of inappropriate release and activation of proteolytic enzymes that are normally synthesized and stored within the pancreatic acinar cells. Conversion of the proenzyme trypsinogen to trypsin is thought to be a key initiating event, leading to subsequent activation of additional proteases and lipases. The activation of these enzymes presumably damages the pancreas as well as the distant organs. Experimental animal models of pancreatitis suggest that lysosomal hydrolases, which inappropriately colocalize with zymogen granules in acinar cells, may be responsible for this activation (73).

B. Etiology of Acute Pancreatitis—Acute pancreatitis can be caused by a variety of factors which may be classified as obstructive, toxic, metabolic, traumatic, or idiosyncratic in nature. The precise mechanisms by which these varying causes lead to the final common pathway of pancreatic injury are unknown. Biliary tract stones and ethanol ingestion are the two most common causes of acute pancreatitis, accounting for approximately 70% to 80% of all cases (80). There are important epidemiologic distinctions: ethanol tends to be the most common cause among men in urban populations, whereas gallstone disease is the most common cause among older women.

1. **Gallstone Pancreatitis**—Approximately 40% to 50% of all cases of acute pancreatitis are caused by gallstones (18,27,45,51,57,85,87,94). The frequency of gallstones as the cause of acute pancreatitis may be as high as 60% in community hospitals, but as low as 10% to 20% in inner-city or veterans' hospitals. The association of gallstones with acute pancreatitis was first described by Opie in 1901, when he observed a biliary calculus lodged in the ampulla of Vater in a patient with severe acute pancreatitis (62). In 1974, Acosta screened the stool of patients with presumed gallstone pancreatitis and identified biliary stones in 34 of 36 patients, compared with 3 of 36 control patients without pancreatitis but with known gallstones (1). The overall mortality rate of untreated acute gallstone pancreatitis can reach 16% (2), and the risk of recurrent pancreatitis from residual stones varies from 36% to 63% (66). Evidence suggests that biliary sludge, a precursor of gallstones, may also be an important risk factor for acute pancreatitis. In a series of 82 patients with idiopathic acute pancreatitis, biliary sludge was the only abnormality documented by ultrasonography or microscopic crystal analysis of bile in 74% of the patients (46,72). Therefore, biliary disease, in the form of either biliary sludge or discrete stones, may be the most common cause of acute pancreatitis.
2. **Alcoholic Pancreatitis**
   - **a.** Ethanol is the most common toxin that causes pancreatitis; it accounts for up to 35% of all cases (18,27,45,51,57,85,87,94). The precise relation between the amount of ethanol consumed and the risk of developing pancreatitis is not clear. However, pancreatitis is rarely observed in casual drinkers and is seen in only 5% of alcoholics (25). It is suggested that consumption of >80 g of ethanol per day is necessary for the development of histologic changes in the pancreas (60).
   - **b.** The cumulative amount of alcohol consumed predicts the severity of pancreatitis; increased rates of complications and mortality were observed in patients with acute pancreatitis who had consumed either ≥5000 g of alcohol during the two previous months or ≥1000 g during the previous week before admission (41).
   - **c.** The mechanisms by which ethanol causes pancreatic injury are not clear. There are several leading theories: reflux of duodenal contents through a sphincter of Oddi made lax by ethanol, obstruction of the pancreatic duct with proteinaceous plugs caused by alcohol, and direct toxicity of ethanol on the pancreas (79).
3. **Drug-Induced Pancreatitis**—The list of medications and toxins that have been implicated in acute pancreatitis is long and has been reviewed by Steinberg (80). Some of the more common offenders deserve mention. In one study involving patients with Crohn's disease, pancreatitis developed in 5 (4.4%) of 113 patients treated with azathioprine within the first 21 days of treatment; in contrast, pancreatitis did not occur in those treated with sulfasalazine (132 patients), prednisone (146 patients), or placebo (178 patients) (84). The active metabolite of azathioprine, 6-mercaptopurine, can also cause pancreatitis, with a frequency of 3.25% among 400 patients treated for inflammatory bowel disease (34). Another cause of pancreatitis is the antiretroviral agent, ddI. In a retrospective analysis of 51 male patients with acquired immunodeficiency syndrome (AIDS) who were treated with ddI, 12 (23.5%) developed acute pancreatitis and 2 died from subsequent complications (53). The onset of pancreatitis was somewhat delayed at 14 weeks, suggesting that the toxicity may result from accumulation of a toxic metabolite rather than from a

hypersensitivity reaction, which would be expected to occur within the first several weeks.

4. **Post-ERCP Pancreatitis**—Asymptomatic hyperamylasemia is common after both diagnostic and therapeutic endoscopic retrograde cholangiopancreatography (ERCP). Symptomatic pancreatitis may also occur; most estimates place the frequency at 6% or lower, although it is as high as 39.5% by some reports (76). The variability in reported incidence is in part caused by the imprecise definition of post-ERCP pancreatitis. Hyperamylasemia occurs commonly after the procedure, but the level of serum amylase that defines pancreatitis is not standardized. Differences in study design, including whether the data are collected prospectively or retrospectively, probably also contribute to the variability in the reported incidence. A particularly high frequency of acute pancreatitis (24%) is observed in the subset of patients undergoing biliary manometry for suspected sphincter of Oddi dysfunction (77).
5. **Postoperative Pancreatitis**—Acute pancreatitis has been described after abdominal or thoracic surgery and is best studied after cardiac surgery. In a prospective study of 300 patients undergoing cardiac surgery with cardiopulmonary bypass, elevation of pancreatic enzymes above the upper limit of normal was seen in 80 patients; 23 had associated clinical symptoms consistent with a diagnosis of acute pancreatitis (28). Multivariate analysis identified four independent risk factors for acute pancreatitis: renal insufficiency, valvular surgery, postoperative hypotension, and administration of calcium chloride in doses of >800 mg per m^2 of body-surface area. Of the 19 deaths in the study, 2 (10.5%) were directly attributable to the complications of pancreatitis.
6. **Miscellaneous Causes of Pancreatitis**—Other, less common causes of acute pancreatitis are pancreatic or ampullary tumors; helminthic infection (*Ascaris*); pancreas divisum with stenosis of the minor papilla; hypertensive sphincter of Oddi; hypertriglyceridemia; hypercalcemia; various infections such as cytomegalovirus, mumps, coxsackievirus B, or tuberculosis; Crohn's disease; penetrating duodenal ulcer; and trauma. After all other causes of acute pancreatitis have been ruled out, as many as 30% of the cases may remain unexplained (18,27,45,51,57,85,87,94). As discussed previously, biliary sludge may account for up to two thirds of these cases.

C. Diagnosis

1. **Clinical Presentation**—Classically, patients with acute pancreatitis present with an abrupt onset of sharp epigastric pain associated with nausea and vomiting. The pain is typically constant rather than colicky, sharp, or knife-like and often radiates to the back. On physical examination, patients often display a slightly distended abdomen with diminished bowel sounds. Guarding is common, and peritoneal signs such as rebound tenderness are frequently noted. In severe cases associated with hemorrhage, ecchymoses may develop in the flanks or umbilical region (Grey-Turner's and Cullen's signs, respectively). Finally, skin nodules resulting from subcutaneous fat necrosis may develop in severe cases.
2. **Laboratory Tests**—The clinical presentation and physical examination of the patient presenting with acute pancreatitis can be nonspecific and consistent with a variety of acute abdominal conditions. Although the gold standard for the diagnosis of acute pancreatitis is pancreatic histology, such an aggressive approach is usually not indicated. The serum amylase determination has become the most widely used laboratory test for diagnosing acute pancreatitis; elevations greater than two to three times normal are usually considered diagnostic. Because the serum amylase is used so routinely and elevated levels are used as a diagnostic criterion, it is difficult to identify patients with acute pancreatitis in whom the serum amylase level is normal. Nevertheless, there have been reported cases of acute pancreatitis diagnosed at autopsy in patients who did not have significant hyperamylasemia (44).
   a. The most careful study to evaluate the sensitivity and specificity of hyperamylasemia for diagnosis of acute pancreatitis compared 39 patients who were referred to a gastroenterology service with ultrasonographic, com-

puted tomographic (CT), or surgical evidence of acute pancreatitis with 127 patients who presented to an emergency room with nonpancreatic abdominal pain (81). Using the upper limit of normal as the diagnostic threshold, the sensitivity of two different assays for amylase was 95% and the specificity was 86% to 89%. Using 1.5 times the upper limit of normal as the diagnostic threshold, the sensitivity remained unchanged but the specificity increased to 98% to 100%.

b. In contrast, in a prospective study involving 100 patients presenting with acute abdominal pain, acute pancreatitis was confirmed in only 5 of 32 patients with hyperamylasemia (>300 IU/L), yielding a specificity of only 71.6% (63). The relatively low specificity may be a reflection of the various nonpancreatic sources of amylase (*e.g.*, salivary glands, lungs, fallopian tubes) as well as conditions such as macroamylasemia.

c. Steinberg, using assays for tissue-specific pancreatic isoamylase, was not able to improve the sensitivity or specificity (92.3% and 85.1%, respectively) (81). However, using the upper limit of normal as the diagnostic threshold, an elevated serum lipase level had a sensitivity of 86.5% and a specificity of 99.0% for acute pancreatitis. The improved specificity of the lipase assay has been confirmed by other studies (86,91).

d. The lipase level can remain elevated for up to a week (33). In contrast, the amylase level falls within several days, limiting its usefulness primarily to the acute presentation.

3. Radiologic Tests

a. In suspected cases of gallstone pancreatitis, ultrasonography is useful for detection of cholelithiasis or choledocholithiasis. However, the presence of overlying bowel gas may preclude optimal visualization of the abdominal organs, especially in the setting of pancreatitis-associated ileus. Abdominal CT scan is the preferred modality for imaging of the pancreas under these conditions.

b. The use of abdominal CT scan has become routine in the evaluation of acute pancreatitis, and abnormal findings such as pancreatic enlargement, peripancreatic inflammatory changes, or peripancreatic fluid collections are seen almost universally. In complicated cases, CT scan is the preferred modality to detect pancreatic pseudocysts, abscesses, and necrosis. Dynamic pancreatography, a CT imaging technique in which intravenous contrast material is administered rapidly with a pressure injector, is particularly well suited for the detection of pancreatic necrosis. Nonenhancement of the pancreas correlates with necrosis at the time of surgery (9,42). The true sensitivity and specificity of dynamic pancreatography is not known, because histologic confirmation of pancreatic necrosis can be obtained only in selected cases that require surgical intervention or percutaneous needle aspiration.

D. Prognosis—The natural history of acute pancreatitis is variable and can range from mild disease with rapid recovery to severe necrotizing pancreatitis with sepsis, adult respiratory distress syndrome (ARDS), renal failure, and death. Numerous researchers have attempted to identify the risk factors that determine poor prognosis. The most widely known criteria for predicting the prognosis in acute pancreatitis were described by Ranson in 1974 and updated in 1982 (66,67). The initial study evaluated primarily patients with alcoholic pancreatitis, but the Ranson criteria were later revised to include those with gallstone pancreatitis. Other prognostic indices, including the modified Glasgow criteria and the Acute Physiology and Chronic Health Evaluation (APACHE-II) scores have proved useful in clinical studies. The Simplified Acute Physiology Score (SAPS) (23), the Multi Organ System Failure (MOSF) score (87), and the Medical Research Council (MRC) score (26) have not been studied extensively.

1. Ranson Criteria

a. Table 13-1 lists the 11 Ranson criteria, 5 of which are determined at the time of admission and 6 of which are assessed over the subsequent 48 hours. In a composite analysis of 450 patients with acute pancreatitis, Ran-

Table 13-1 The Ranson Criteria (66,67)

Ranson Criteria	Non-Gallstone Pancreatitis	Gallstone Pancreatitis
At admission		
Age (y)	>55	>70
Leukocyte count (cells/mm^3)	>16,000	>18,000
Glucose (mg/dl)	>200	>220
LDH (IU/L)	>350	>400
AST (IU/L)	>250	>250
Within 48 h		
Fall in hematocrit (%)	>10	>10
Rise in BUN (mg/dl)	>5	>2
Calcium (mg/dl)	<8	<8
PaO_2 (mm Hg)	<60	—
Base deficit (mEq/L)	>4	>5
Estimated fluid loss (L)	>6	>4

son found that patients with two or fewer risk factors had a very low mortality rate. The mortality rate increased with an increasing number of risk factors. The mortality rate was 0.9% for patients with one or two risk factors, 16% for those with three or four, 40% for those with five or six, and 100% for those with seven or more risk factors (66).

b. In the original description, these criteria were used to predict mortality, not morbidity. Subsequently, attempts have been made to use the criteria to predict the severity as well as the mortality. Although most such definitions include pancreatic necrosis, abscess, and pseudocyst formation, there is no consistent definition of severe pancreatitis.

(1) In a comprehensive review of seven studies evaluating >700 patients with acute pancreatitis, the presence of three or more positive Ranson criteria predicted "severe" pancreatitis. However, the sensitivity was only 72% (range, 40% to 88%), the specificity was 76% (43% to 99%), the PPV was 51% (31% to 95%), and the NPV was 89% (74% to 94%) (82).

(2) The largest study, which prospectively analyzed 290 episodes of acute pancreatitis, reported a sensitivity, specificity, PPV, and NPV of 75%, 68%, 37%, and 91%, respectively, for the Ranson criteria determined at 48 hours (45). When compared with a subjective "assessment by an expert clinician" at the time of admission, the Ranson criteria had a better sensitivity (75% versus 44%) but a lower specificity (68% versus 95%) and a lower PPV (37% versus 68%). When compared with the "expert clinical assessment" at 48 hours, the sensitivity of the clinical assessment was comparable to that of the Ranson criteria for predicting severe outcome.

2. Glasgow Criteria

a. The Glasgow criteria were first described in 1978 and have been modified several times. The most recent set of modified Glasgow (or Imrie) criteria, from 1984, are listed in Table 13-2 (8). These eight criteria are similar to the Ranson criteria and are also assessed over a period of 48 hours.

b. Steinberg analyzed six studies that used the Glasgow criteria to predict the severity of acute pancreatitis and estimated an overall sensitivity of 63% (range, 56% to 85%), a specificity of 84% (79% to 89%), a PPV of 52% (39% to 71%), and an NPV of 89% (85% to 94%) (82). The single largest prospective analysis of patients presenting with acute pancreatitis reported a sensitivity of 61%, a specificity of 89%, a PPV of 59%, and an NPV of 90% (45).

3. APACHE II Index

a. The most recent and by far the most complex index that has been used to

Table 13-2 The Modified Glasgow (Imrie) criteria (8)

Age (y)	>55
Leukocyte count (cells/mm^3)	>15,000
Glucose (mg/dl)	>180
BUN (mg/dl)	>96
PaO_2 (mm Hg)	<60
Calcium (mg/dl)	<8
Albumin (g/dl)	<3.2
LDH (IU/L)	>600

predict the severity of pancreatitis is the APACHE II score. This system is a simplified version of the original APACHE index; it measures 12 acute variables and also incorporates the patient's age and chronic health status into the index (43). The distinguishing feature of the APACHE II index is its applicability at any time point during the hospitalization, not just during the initial 48-hours. In addition, because the APACHE index factors in concurrent disease parameters such as the immune status, it is probably a better system for predicting prognosis in special groups of patients (*e.g.*, AIDS patients) (16).

b. For an APACHE II score >9, the single largest prospective analysis of patients presenting with acute pancreatitis reported a sensitivity of 75%, a specificity of 92%, a PPV of 71%, and an NPV of 93% (45).

4. **Comparison of the Ranson, modified Glasgow, and APACHE II Scoring Systems**—Several studies have compared these three indices for their accuracy in predicting the severity of acute pancreatitis (45,87,94). The results of these studies are summarized in Table 13-3.
5. **Pancreatic Necrosis**—Nonenhancement of the pancreas during dynamic CT scanning correlates with the finding of pancreatic necrosis at the time of surgery (9,42). However, the prognostic significance of pancreatic necrosis is un-

Table 13-3 Comparison of the major predictive indices for acute pancreatitis

	Sensitivity (%)	Specificity (%)	PPV (%)	NPV (%)	Accuracy (%)
Larvin (45)					
APACHE II score at 48 h	75	92	71	93	88
Ranson Criteria at 48 h	75	68	37	91	69
Modified Glasgow Score at 48 h	61	89	59	90	83
Clinical assessment at 48 h	66	95	76	92	89
Clinical assessment at admission	44	95	68	87	84
Wilson (94)					
APACHE II score at 48 h	82	74	50	93	76
Ranson Criteria at 48 h	87	71	49	94	75
Modified Glasgow score at 48 h	71	88	66	91	84
Tran (87)					
APACHE II score at 48 h	60	97	90	86	87
Ranson Criteria at 48 h	60	96	85	86	86
Modified Glasgow score at 48 h	58	89	68	84	80

clear. According to some reports, patients with pancreatic necrosis generally have a poorer outcome because of the high risk of secondary bacterial infections (4,5,92). For example, in a prospective study involving 88 patients with acute pancreatitis, the presence of pancreatic necrosis was associated with an increased rate of complications (82% versus 6%) and a higher mortality rate (23% versus 0%) (4), However, according to other reports, the presence of pancreatic necrosis predicted a severe outcome with a sensitivity of 79% to 83% but a specificity of only 42% to 65% (51,52). Because a severe outcome can occur in the absence of necrosis and recovery can be uneventful in the presence of necrosis, dynamic CT scanning may not offer a significant advantage over clinical or biochemical assessment for predicting outcome. Nevertheless, CT can provide useful information and guide decisions regarding the need for percutaneous aspiration or surgery, as discussed in a later section.

6. **Peritoneal Tap**—A diagnostic paracentesis that reveals ≥20 ml of fluid, dark "prune-juice" fluid, or fluid darker than pale straw after a 1-L lavage had a sensitivity of 53% for predicting a poor prognosis (54). Although this was better than the 34% sensitivity provided by subjective clinical assessment in the study, the prognostic value of paracentesis is certainly lower than that of the Ranson criteria. The major advantage of paracentesis is that it can provide prognostic information immediately at the time of presentation. Nevertheless, it is an invasive procedure which can cause bleeding, infection, or perforation of a viscus.
7. **Blood Tests**—Because pancreatitis is an acute inflammatory disorder, numerous blood tests that detect levels of various inflammatory markers have been analyzed. In one study, the C-reactive protein, a nonspecific inflammatory marker, compared favorably with the Glasgow and the Ranson scores in predicting severe pancreatitis, with a sensitivity and specificity of 83% and 85%, respectively (95). However, in another study, C-reactive protein had a sensitivity and specificity of only 53% and 55% (32). Trypsinogen activation peptide (TAP), which is released during the enzymatic conversion of trypsinogen to trypsin, can serve as a surrogate marker for trypsinogen activation. In an analysis of 55 patients with acute pancreatitis, immunoassay for urinary levels of TAP had a sensitivity and specificity of 80% and 90%, respectively (32). Measurement of serum polymorphonuclear leukocyte elastase had both a sensitivity and a specificity >90% for predicting severe acute pancreatitis (24). At this time, however, none of these tests is widely available.

E. **Management**—The management of acute pancreatitis is primarily supportive. The basic measures include bowel rest, IV fluid support, and narcotic analgesia. However, certain situations dictate the need for specific interventions, and these are discussed in the following sections.

1. **Nasogastric Suction**—Because delivery of gastric acid to the duodenum stimulates pancreatic exocrine secretion, removal of gastric contents through a nasogastric tube theoretically may allow the inflamed pancreas to rest. However, several prospective, randomized trials comparing nasogastric suction with no intervention failed to demonstrate an improved outcome with nasogastric suction (49,50,58,74) There was no increase in the complication rate in the group not receiving nasogastric suction, and in particular there was no increase in the frequency of ileus. Therefore, nasogastric suction should be reserved for patients with specific clinical indications, such as severe ileus, nausea, or vomiting.
2. **Histamine$_2$-Receptor Antagonists**—Another strategy for reducing the delivery of gastric acid to the duodenum is to use histamine$_2$ (H_2)-receptor antagonists. The first prospective, randomized clinical trial to address this issue was reported in 1982 (14). A total of 116 patients were analyzed, and no statistically significant differences were observed between the two groups. Subsequent studies have confirmed these findings (50). Therefore, the routine use of H_2-receptor antagonists is not recommended, in the absence of another specific indication.
3. **Antibiotics**
   a. Several randomized, controlled studies in the 1970s demonstrated no sig-

nificant benefit of prophylactic administration of ampicillin to patients with mostly mild to moderate alcoholic pancreatitis (19,29,35).

b. However, in a more recent randomized, prospective study involving 74 patients with CT-based evidence of severe necrotizing pancreatitis, the prophylactic use of imipenem (which has high pancreatic tissue penetration) significantly reduced the rate of pancreatic sepsis (12.2% versus 30.3%) compared with no antibiotic therapy (64). Although the mortality rate was also lower with imipenem (7.3% versus 12.1%), the difference was not statistically significant. If these findings can be confirmed, the use of prophylactic antibiotics may become standard therapy for those with acute pancreatitis and CT-based evidence of necrosis.

4. **Total Parenteral Nutrition**

a. **Mild Pancreatitis**—In a randomized, prospective trial involving 54 patients with mild acute pancreatitis (average Ranson score of 1), the administration of total parenteral nutrition (TPN) within 24 hours after admission offered no significant benefit (75). In fact, there was an increased rate of catheter-related sepsis (10.5% versus 1.5%) in the TPN group.

b. **Severe Pancreatitis**—In a prospective study comparing early (within 72 hours) versus late (after 72 hours) administration of TPN among patients with severe acute pancreatitis, early use of TPN was associated with reduced rates of complications (23.6% versus 95.6%) and mortality (13% versus 38%) (38). However, the randomization process may have been biased, making interpretation of these results difficult.

5. **Sonatostatin and Octreotide**

a. Both somatostatin and octreotide (a long-acting eight-amino-acid analog of somatostatin) decrease the amount of pancreatic exocrine secretion. Several prospective, randomized controlled studies involving a total of 375 patients failed to demonstrate any significant benefit of somatostatin (100 to 250 μg/hour by continuous infusion) in terms of reducing the rate of complications, the length of hospital stay, the narcotic requirement, or mortality in patients with acute pancreatitis (17,20,31,89).

b. Other studies have evaluated the benefit of somatostatin or octreotide for the prevention of post-ERCP pancreatitis. Initial reports suggested that these drugs may lower the frequency of post-ERCP pancreatitis, but larger prospective, randomized trials demonstrated no significant benefit. The first large trial involving 84 patients undergoing ERCP with or without sphincterotomy had to be terminated early because of a higher frequency of acute pancreatitis in the group treated with octreotide (35% versus 11%) (83). Subsequent studies showed no difference in outcome with the prophylactic use of somatostatin or octreotide (6,65).

6. **Protease Inhibitors**-Because uncontrolled activation of numerous pancreatic proteases is one of the key pathophysiologic mechanisms in acute pancreatitis, various protease inhibitors have been tested for treatment of this disease. The first protease inhibitor to be tested was aprotinin, an inhibitor of trypsin, plasmin, and kallikrein. Despite initially promising results (88), most controlled trials have failed to demonstrate a benefit (36,56). Similarly, two randomized double-blind trials tested gabexate mesylate (an inhibitor of trypsin, plasmin, kallikrein, and phospholipase A_2) but also found no clinical benefit (15,90). Finally, an attempt to replenish the normal complement of human antiproteases with fresh frozen plasma at low (2 U/day × 3 days) or high (8 U/day × 3 days) doses did not alter the course of acute pancreatitis in randomized, controlled trials (47,48).

7. **Peritoneal Lavage**—An initial report suggested that therapeutic continuous peritoneal lavage may reduce the rate of complications and the mortality rate in acute pancreatitis (68). However, a randomized, controlled trial of 3-day peritoneal lavage in 91 patients with severe acute pancreatitis failed to demonstrate any significant benefit in terms of mortality or morbidity (pseudocysts, abscesses) when compared with standard conservative treatment (55). A subsequent evaluation of 39 patients with severe pancreatitis compared 2-day ver-

sus 7-day lavage, including antibiotics in the lavage fluid (69). Ten patients were excluded. Among the remaining 29 patients, there was a decrease in the rate of pancreatic sepsis in the 7-day treatment group (21% versus 40%), but there was no overall difference in mortality. Because of the invasive nature of the procedure and the uncertain benefit, therapeutic paracentesis is in general not recommended.

8. **Surgery for Gallstone Pancreatitis**—Because gallstones represent a frequent, identifiable, and remediable cause of acute pancreatitis, much attention has been focused on management of gallstone pancreatitis. In most cases, the stone passes spontaneously and pancreatitis resolves with conservative management alone. A subsequent cholecystectomy is usually indicated to prevent a recurrence of pancreatitis. Several studies have addressed whether there is any benefit to early surgical intervention. In a 1988 prospective study, 165 patients with gallstone pancreatitis were randomly assigned to receive either early (within 48 hours) or delayed (after 48 hours) cholecystectomy (39). For patients with mild pancreatitis (three or fewer Ranson criteria), there was no significant difference in outcome between the two groups. However, for patients with severe pancreatitis (more than three Ranson criteria), early surgery was associated with a higher rate of complications (83% versus 18%) and a higher mortality rate (48% versus 11%).
9. **ERCP and Sphincterotomy**—ERCP and sphincterotomy is a less invasive alternative to surgery for the diagnosis and treatment of common bile duct stones. Several studies have evaluated this treatment modality.
   a. In the first study, 121 patients with presumed gallstone pancreatitis were randomly assigned to either ERCP with sphincterotomy within 72 hours or conventional conservative treatment (59). For patients with mild pancreatitis as judged by the Glasgow criteria, there was no significant benefit to urgent ERCP. However, for patients with severe pancreatitis, urgent ERCP reduced the rate of complications (24% versus 61%), the mortality rate (4% versus 18%), and the length of hospital stay (9.5 versus 17 days). The rates of cholangitis were similar in the two groups (10% versus 8%). Patients who had retained stones on ERCP were not analyzed separately, even though these presumably are the patients targeted by this intervention. Nevertheless, early endoscopic sphincterotomy appears to be safe and particularly beneficial for patients predicted to have severe pancreatitis as judged by the Glasgow criteria.
   b. In a second study from Hong Kong, 195 patients with any form of acute pancreatitis were randomly assigned to either ERCP within 24 hours or conservative treatment (27). Gallstone pancreatitis accounted for approximately two-thirds of the cases in both groups. If a stone was identified in the bile duct, an endoscopic sphincterotomy was performed. Early ERCP significantly reduced the rate of biliary sepsis (0 of 97 patients undergoing early ERCP versus 12 of 98 patients receiving conservative treatment). The rates of other complications were similar between the two groups. The mortality rate was also lower in the early ERCP group (5.2% versus 9.2%), but the difference was not statistically significant. When patients were analyzed based on the presence or absence of bile duct stones on ERCP, the only subgroup that benefited from ERCP were those with common bile duct stones who were predicted to have severe pancreatitis by the Ranson criteria.
   c. A more recent study from Germany randomized 238 patients with presumed gallstone pancreatitis but without evidence of obstructive jaundice or cholangitis to either ERCP and papillotomy within 72 hours or conservative treatment (29a). Stones were identified in 46% of the early ERCP group. 20% of the patients in the conservative treatment group developed jaundice or cholangitis and subsequently underwent ERCP; stones were identified in 59% of those patients. The overall rates of mortality and complications were similar in both groups, suggesting that ERCP can be deferred in patients with gallstone pancreatitis who do not present with evidence of obstructive jaundice.
   d. Endoscopic sphincterotomy is also an option for the treatment of biliary

sludge. In a nonrandomized study involving 21 patients with acute pancreatitis and biliary sludge, 6 were treated with cholecystectomy and 4 with papillotomy (46). Among the 10 patients who were treated surgically or endoscopically, only one recurrence of pancreatitis was documented during a mean follow-up period of 4 years. In contrast, among the 11 untreated patients, 8 experienced at least one recurrence of acute pancreatitis. In another nonrandomized study involving 34 patients with acute pancreatitis and biliary sludge, 13 with cholesterol monohydrate crystals were treated with ursodeoxycholic acid (10 mg/kg/day) (72). Eight of the 13 had no recurrence of biliary sludge or pancreatitis, and the remaining 5 patients underwent surgery, stopped treatment, or continued treatment despite recurrent symptoms. In the same study, 18 patients underwent cholecystectomy, and only 3 developed recurrent pancreatitis during a mean follow-up period of 36 months. There was no untreated control group. Collectively, these data suggest that treatment with ursodeoxycholic acid, endoscopic papillotomy, or cholecystectomy may be effective in preventing recurrent episodes of pancreatitis in patients with biliary sludge, but these conclusions require confirmation by randomized controlled trials.

F. **Management of Complications**—Table 13-4 lists both local and systemic complications of acute pancreatitis. The management of a critically ill patient with acute pancreatitis is primarily supportive. However, specific interventions may be indicated for those who develop pancreatic necrosis, pseudocysts, or abscesses.

1. **Pancreatic Necrosis**—As discussed previously, pancreatic necrosis may occur early in the course of acute pancreatitis and usually implies a severe form of the disease. There is no consensus regarding optimal management of patients with pancreatic necrosis.

a. **Infected Pancreatic Necrosis**—Bacterial superinfection complicates pancreatic necrosis in up to 71% of cases and is uniformly fatal without surgical débridement (12,71). CT-guided aspiration of the pancreas is a safe and accurate means of differentiating sterile from infected pancreatic necrosis. In one study, 50 negative aspirates were all confirmed to be sterile at surgery, and 41 of 42 positive aspirates were confirmed to be infected at surgery (30). Aggressive surgical débridement is indicated for patients with infected pancreatic necrosis; surgical options include pancreatic resection and necrosectomy. The risk of ongoing pancreatic necrosis has led some authorities to recommend postoperative follow-up with peritoneal lavage or planned reexploration (21). There are no randomized controlled studies that compare these strategies.

b. **Sterile Pancreatic Necrosis**—The optimal management of sterile pancreatic necrosis remains controversial. Some authorities advocate surgical debridement even in the absence of documented infection (71), and others recommend conservative management (12). In general, the need for surgery is more likely as the clinical severity of the illness increases, but well-designed, randomized, controlled studies are required.

Table 13-4 Complications of acute pancreatitis

Local	Systemic
Necrosis	ARDS
Infected necrosis	Renal failure
Ascites	Sepsis
Hemorrhage	Fat necrosis
Pseudocyst	
Abscess	
Bowel perforation or obstruction	
Fistula	

2. **Pseudocyst**—Pseudocysts occur as a late complication of acute pancreatitis in up to 8% of all cases, typically at least 2 weeks after presentation (37,51,70, 85,87). Up to 40% of acute pseudocysts resolve spontaneously (13), but the factors that predict spontaneous resolution are unknown. Some studies suggest that pseudocysts smaller than 4 to 6 cm in diameter can be observed, because they are less likely than larger pseudocysts to require an intervention (61,96). An intervention is urgently indicated in cases of superimposed infection, bleeding, or rupture; for less urgent symptoms such as pain or nausea, drainage procedures can usually be delayed for 6 weeks to permit maturation of the pseudocyst wall. Therapeutic options include percutaneous drainage, endoscopic cystgastrostomy, and surgical drainage. No randomized, controlled studies have compared these options. Percutaneous drainage is reasonable when the pseudocyst does not communicate with the pancreatic duct; in a study of 13 such pseudocysts that were drained percutaneously, none recurred (22). The experience with endoscopic cystgastrostomy is small but promising.
3. **Abscess**—Pancreatic abscess is usually a late complication of acute pancreatitis, occurring no sooner than 5 weeks after presentation (7). The literature on the management of pancreatic abscess is difficult to interpret, in part because of the changing definition of the term. Currently, a pancreatic abscess is defined as a "circumscribed intraabdominal collection of pus, usually in proximity to the pancreas, containing little or no pancreatic necrosis" (11). However, most studies fail to distinguish an abscess from phlegmon, necrosis, infected necrosis, or infected pseudocyst. Despite this ambiguity, it is clear that definitive therapy for a pancreatic abscess includes antibiotics and drainage. Traditionally, drainage has been performed surgically, but percutaneous drainage may be appropriate in selected patients with a solitary, easily accessible abscess who are not critically ill (3). However, no study has carefully compared percutaneous versus surgical options for drainage.

G. Summary

1. Biliary tract stones and ethanol are the two most common causes of acute pancreatitis, accounting for approximately 70% to 80% of all cases. Other causes of acute pancreatitis include various drugs; ERCP, surgery, or trauma; pancreatic or ampullary tumors; helminthic infection (*Ascaris*); pancreas divisum with stenosis of the minor papilla; hypertensive sphincter of Oddi; hypertriglyceridemia; hypercalcemia; various infections such as cytomegalovirus, mumps, coxsackievirus B, or tuberculosis; Crohn's disease; and penetrating duodenal ulcer.
2. The serum amylase level is the most widely used laboratory test for diagnosis of acute pancreatitis. In various studies, the sensitivity of hyperamylasemia for acute pancreatitis ranged from 92% to 95%, and the specificity from 72% to 100%, depending on the design of the study, the diagnostic threshold, and the type of assay used. Compared with an elevated amylase level, an elevated serum lipase level is more specific for acute pancreatitis.
3. The natural history of acute pancreatitis is variable and can range from mild disease with rapid recovery to severe necrotizing pancreatitis with sepsis, ARDS, renal failure, and death. Several indices have been proposed for predicting the prognosis in acute pancreatitis, including the Ranson criteria, the modified Glasgow scale, and the APACHE-II score. The presence of pancreatic necrosis may also be a poor prognostic factor.
4. The management of acute pancreatitis is primarily supportive. The basic measures include bowel rest, IV fluid support, and narcotic analgesia. There appears to be no significant benefit to routine use of nasogastric suction, H_2-receptor antagonists, octreotide, or ampicillin in the absence of another specific indication. However, the prophylactic use of imipenem may be beneficial for those with acute pancreatitis and CT-based evidence of pancreatic necrosis.
5. The use of TPN is controversial. For patients with mild pancreatitis, the early use of TPN offers no significant benefit and may increase the risk of catheter-related sepsis. For patients with severe pancreatitis, the early use of TPN reduced the rates of complications and mortality in one study, but the randomiza-

tion process may have been biased, making interpretation of the results difficult.

6. In most cases of acute gallstone pancreatitis, the stone passes spontaneously and pancreatitis resolves with conservative management alone. A delayed cholecystectomy is usually indicated to prevent a recurrence of pancreatitis. Early surgical intervention should be avoided because it may be associated with a higher rate of complications and a higher mortality rate.
7. ERCP and sphincterotomy is a less invasive alternative to surgery for management of gallstone pancreatitis. Early endoscopic sphincterotomy appears to be safe and particularly beneficial for patients with obstructive jaundice.
8. Bacterial superinfection may complicate pancreatic necrosis in up to 71% of cases and is uniformly fatal without surgical débridement. Surgical options include pancreatic resection and necrosectomy. The optimal management of sterile pancreatic necrosis remains controversial. Some authorities advocate surgical débridement even in the absence of documented infection, whereas others recommend conservative management. CT-guided aspiration of the pancreas is a safe and accurate method for differentiating sterile from infected pancreatic necrosis.
9. Pseudocysts can occur as a late complication of acute pancreatitis in up to 8% of patients. Some studies suggest that pseudocysts smaller than 4 to 6 cm in diameter can be observed, because they are less likely than larger pseudocysts to require an intervention. An intervention is urgently indicated in cases of superimposed infection, bleeding, or rupture; for less urgent symptoms such as pain or nausea, drainage procedures can usually be delayed for 6 weeks to permit maturation of the pseudocyst wall. Therapeutic options include percutaneous drainage, endoscopic cystgastrostomy, and surgical drainage.
10. Pancreatic abscess is usually a late complication of acute pancreatitis. Definitive therapy for a pancreatic abscess includes antibiotics and drainage. Traditionally, drainage has been performed surgically, but percutaneous drainage may be appropriate in selected patients with a solitary, easily accessible abscess who are not critically ill.

Abbreviations used in Chapter 13

AIDS = acquired immune deficiency syndrome
APACHE = Acute Physiology and Chronic Health Evaluation
ARDS = adult respiratory distress syndrome
CT = computed tomography
ddI = 2′,3′-dideoxyinosine
ERCP = endoscopic retrograde cholangiopancreatography
H_2 = $histamine_2$
HIV = human immunodeficiency virus
IV = intravenous
MOSF score = Multi Organ System Failure score
MRC = Medical Research Council
NPV = negative predictive value
PPV = positive predictive value
SAPS = Simplified Acute Physiology Score
TAP = trypsinogen activation peptide
TPN = total parenteral nutrition

References

1. Acosta. Gallstone migration as a cause of acute pancreatitis. *N Engl J Med* 1974;290: 484.

2. Acosta. Early surgery for acute gallstone pancreatitis: evaluation of a systematic approach. *Surgery* 1978;83:367.
3. Adams. Percutaneous catheter drainage of infected pancreatic and peripancreatic fluid collections. *Arch Surg* 1990;125:1554.
4. Balthazar. Acute pancreatitis: value of CT in establishing prognosis. *Radiology* 1990;174:331.
5. Beger. Bacterial contamination of pancreatic necrosis. *Gastroenterology* 1986;91: 433.
6. Binmoeller. Does the somatostatin analog octreotide protect against ERCP induced pancreatitis? *Gut* 1992;33:1129.
7. Bittner. Pancreatic abscess and infected pancreatic necrosis. *Dig Dis Sci* 1987;32: 1082.
8. Blamey. Prognostic factors in acute pancreatitis. *Gut* 1984;25:1340.
9. Block. Identification of pancreas necrosis in severe acute pancreatitis: imaging procedures versus clinical staging. *Gut* 1986;27:1035.
10. Bourke. Variation in annual incidence of primary acute pancreatitis in Nottingham, 1969–1974. *Lancet* 1975;2:967.
11. Bradley. A clinically based classification system for acute pancreatitis. *Arch Surg* 1993;128:586.
12. Bradley. A prospective longitudinal study of observation versus surgical intervention in the management of necrotizing pancreatitis. *Am J Surg* 1991;161:19.
13. Bradley. The natural history of pancreatic pseudocysts: a unified concept of management. *Am J Surg* 1979;137:135.
14. Broe. A clinical trial of cimetidine in acute pancreatitis. *Surg Gynecol Obstet* 1982; 154:13.
15. Buchler. Gabexate mesilate in human acute pancreatitis. German Pancreatitis Study Group. *Gastroenterology* 1993;104:1165.
16. Cappell. Acute pancreatitis in HIV-seropositive patients: a case control study of 44 patients. *Am J Med* 1995;98:243.
17. Choi. Somatostatin in the treatment of acute pancreatitis: a prospective randomised controlled trial. *Gut* 1989;30:223.
18. Corfield. Prediction of severity in acute pancreatitis: prospective comparison of three prognostic indices. *Lancet* 1985;2:403.
19. Craig. The use of ampicillin in acute pancreatitis. *Ann Intern Med* 1975;83:832.
20. D'Amico. The use of somatostatin in acute pancreatitis: results of a multicenter trial. *Hepatol Gastroenterol* 1990;37:92.
21. D'Egidio. Surgical strategies in the treatment of pancreatic necrosis and infection. *Br J Surgery* 1991;78:133.
22. D'Egidio. Percutaneous drainage of pancreatic pseudocysts: a prospective study. *World J Surg* 1991;16:141.
23. Dominguez-Munoz. Evaluation of the clinical usefulness of APACHE II and SAPS systems in the initial prognostic classification of acute pancreatitis: a multicenter study. *Pancreas* 1993;8:682.
24. Dominguez-Munoz. Clinical usefulness of polymorphonuclear elastase in predicting the severity of acute pancreatitis: results of a multicentre study. *Br J Surg* 1991; 78:1230.
25. Dreiling. The natural history of alcoholic pancreatitis: update 1985. *Mt Sinai J Med* 1985;52:340.
26. Elabute. The grading of sepsis. *Br J Surg* 1983;70:29.
27. Fan. Early treatment of acute biliary pancreatitis by endoscopic papillotomy. *N Engl J Med* 1993;328:228.
28. Fernandez-del Castillo. Risk factors for pancreatic cellular injury after cardiopulmonary bypass. *N Engl J Med* 1991;325:382.
29. Finch. A prospective study to determine the efficacy of antibiotics in acute pancreatitis. *Ann Surg* 1976;183:667.

29a. Fölsch. Early ERCP and papillotomy compared with conservative treatment for acute biliary pancreatitis. *New Eng J Med* 1997;336:237.

30. Gerzof. Early diagnosis of pancreatic infection by computed tomography-guided aspiration. *Gastroenterology* 1987;93:1315.

31. Gjorup. A double-blinded multicenter trial of somatostatin in the treatment of acute pancreatitis. *Surg Gynecol Obstet* 1992;175:397.
32. Gudgeon. Trypsinogen activation peptides assay in the early prediction of severity of acute pancreatitis. *Lancet* 1990;335:4.
33. Gwozdz. Comparative evaluation of the diagnosis of acute pancreatitis based on serum and urine enzyme assays. *Clin Chim Acta* 1990;187:243.
34. Haber. Nature and course of pancreatitis caused by 6-mercaptopurine in the treatment of inflammatory bowel disease. *Gastroenterology* 1986;91:982.
35. Howes. Evaluation of prophylactic antibiotics in acute pancreatitis. *J Surg Res* 1975; 18:197.
36. Imrie. A single-centre double-blind trial of Trasylol therapy in primary acute pancreatitis. *Br J Surg* 1978;65:337.
37. Imrie. Importance of cause in the outcome of pancreatic pseudocysts. *Am J Surg* 1988;156:159.
38. Kalfarentzos. Total parenteral nutrition in severe acute pancreatitis. *J Am Coll Nutr* 1991;10:156.
39. Kelly. Gallstone pancreatitis: a prospective randomized trial of the timing of surgery. *Surgery* 1988;104:600.
40. Jaakkola. Pancreatitis in Finland between 1970 and 1989. *Gut* 1993;34:1255.
41. Jaakkola. Amount of alcohol is an important determinant of the severity of acute alcoholic pancreatitis. *Surgery* 1994;115:31.
42. Kivisaari. A new method for the diagnosis of acute hemorrhagic-necrotizing pancreatitis using contrast-enhanced CT. *Gastrointest Radiol* 1984;9:27.
43. Knaus. APACHE II: a severity of disease classification system. *Crit Care Med* 1985; 12:975.
44. Lankisch. Undetected fatal acute pancreatitis: why is the disease so frequently overlooked? *Am J Gastroenterol* 1991;86:322.
45. Larvin. APACHE-II score for assessment and monitoring of acute pancreatitis. *Lancet* 1989;2:201.
46. Lee. Biliary sludge as a cause of acute pancreatitis. *N Engl J Med* 1992;326:589.
47. Leese. Multicentre clinical trial of low volume fresh frozen plasma therapy in acute pancreatitis. *Br J Surg* 1987,74:907.
48. Leese. A multicentre controlled clinical trial of high-volume fresh frozen plasma therapy in prognostically severe acute pancreatitis. *Ann R Coll Surg Engl* 1991; 73:207.
49. Levant. Nasogastric suction in the treatment of alcoholic pancreatitis. *JAMA* 1974; 229:51.
50. Loiudice. Treatment of acute alcoholic pancreatitis: the roles of cimetidine and nasogastric suction. *Am J Gastroenterol* 1984;79:553.
51. London. Contrast-enhanced abdominal computed tomography scanning and prediction of severity of acute pancreatitis: a prospective study. *Br J Surg* 1989; 76:268.
52. London. Rapid-bolus contrast-enhanced dynamic computed tomography in acute pancreatitis: a prospective study. *Br J Surg* 1991;78:1452.
53. Maxson. Acute pancreatitis as a common complication of 2′,3′-dideoxyinosine therapy in the acquired immunodeficiency syndrome. *Am J Gastroenterol* 1992; 87:708.
54. Mayer. The diagnostic and prognostic value of peritoneal lavage in patients with acute pancreatitis. *Surg Gynecol Obstet* 1985;160:507.
55. Mayer. Controlled clinical trial of peritoneal lavage for the treatment of severe acute pancreatitis. *N Engl J Med* 1985;312:399.
56. Medical Research Council Multicentre Trial. Morbidity of acute pancreatitis: the effect of aprotinin and glucagon. *Gut* 1980;21:334.
57. Millat. Predictability of clinicobiochemical scoring systems for early identification of severe gallstone-associated pancreatitis. *Am J Surg* 1992;164:32.
58. Naeije. Is nasogastric suction necessary in acute pancreatitis? *Br Med J* 1978;2:659.
59. Neoptolemos. Controlled trial of urgent endoscopic retrograde cholangiopancreatography and endoscopic sphincterotomy versus conservative treatment for acute pancreatitis due to gallstones. *Lancet* 1988;2:979.

60. Noronha. Alcohol and the pancreas I: clinical associations and histopathology of minimal pancreatic inflammation. *Am J Gastroenterol* 1981;76:114.
61. O'Malley. Pancreatic pseudocysts: cause, therapy, and results. *Am J Surg* 1985; 150:680.
62. Opie. The etiology of acute hemorrhagic pancreatitis. *Bull Johns Hopkins Hosp* 1901; 12:182.
63. Pace. Amylase isoenzymes in the acute abdomen: an adjunct in those patients with elevated total amylase. *Am J Gastroenterol* 1985;80:898.
64. Pederzoli. A randomized multicenter clinical trial of antibiotic prophylaxis of septic complications in acute necrotizing pancreatitis with imipenem. *Surg Gynecol Obstet* 1993;176:480.
65. Persson. Can somatostatin prevent injection pancreatitis after ERCP? *Hepatol Gastroenterol* 1992;39:259.
66. Ranson. Etiological and prognostic factors in human acute pancreatitis: a review. *Am J Gastroenterol* 1982;77:633.
67. Ranson. Prognostic signs and the role of operative management in acute pancreatitis. *Surg Gynecol Obstet* 1974;139:69.
68. Ranson. Prognostic signs and nonoperative peritoneal lavage in acute pancreatitis. *Surg Gynecol Obstet* 1976;143:209.
69. Ranson. Long peritoneal lavage decreases pancreatic sepsis in acute pancreatitis. *Ann Surg* 1989;211:708.
70. Ranson. The role of surgery in the management of acute pancreatitis. *Ann Surg* 1990;211:382.
71. Rattner. Early surgical debridement of symptomatic pancreatic necrosis is beneficial irrespective of infection. *Am J Surg* 1992;163:105.
72. Ros. Occult microlithiasis in "idiopathic" acute pancreatitis: prevention of relapses by cholecystectomy or ursodeoxycholic acid therapy. *Gastroenterology* 1991;101: 1701.
73. Saluja. Pancreatic duct obstruction in rabbits causes digestive zymogen and lysosomal enzyme colocalization. *J Clin Invest* 1989;84:1260.
74. Sarr. Prospective, randomized trial of nasogastric suction in patients with acute pancreatitis. *Surgery* 1986;100:500.
75. Sax. Early total parenteral nutrition in acute pancreatitis: lack of beneficial effects. *Am J Surg* 1987;153:117.
76. Sherman. ERCP- and endoscopic sphincterotomy-induced pancreatitis. *Pancreas* 1991;6:350.
77. Sherman. Sphincter of Oddi manometry: decreased risk of clinical pancreatitis with use of a modified aspirating catheter. *Gastrointest Endosc* 1990;36:462.
78. Singer. Revised classification of pancreatitis. *Gastroenterology* 1985;89:683.
79. Singh. Ethanol and the pancreas. *Gastroenterology* 1990;98:1051.
80. Steinberg. Acute pancreatitis. *N Engl J Med* 1994;330:1198.
81. Steinberg. Diagnostic assays in acute pancreatitis. *Ann Intern Med* 1985;102:576.
82. Steinberg. Predictors of severity of acute pancreatitis. *Gastroenterol Clin North Am* 1990;19:849.
83. Sternlieb. A multicenter, randomized, controlled trial to evaluate the effect of prophylactic octreotide on ERCP-induced pancreatitis. *Am J Gastroenterol* 1992;87: 1561.
84. Sturdevant. Azathioprine-related pancreatitis in patients with Crohn's disease. *Gastroenterology* 1979;77:883.
85. Thomson. Epidemiology and outcome of acute pancreatitis. *Br J Surg* 1987;74: 398.
86. Thomson. Diagnosis of acute pancreatitis: a proposed sequence of biochemical investigation. *Scand J Gastroenterol* 1987;22:719.
87. Tran. Evaluation of severity in patients with acute pancreatitis. *Am J Gastroenterol* 1992;87:604.
88. Trapnell. A controlled trial of Trasylol in the treatment of acute pancreatitis. *Br J Surg* 1974;61:177.
89. Usadel. Treatment of acute pancreatitis with somatostatin: results of the multicenter double-blind trial (APTS-study). *Dig Dis Sci* 1985;30:992.

90. Valderrama. Multicenter double-blind trial of gabexate mesylate (FOY) in unselected patients with acute pancreatitis. *Digestion* 1992;51:65.
91. Ventrucci. A rapid assay for serum immunoreactive lipase as a screening test for acute pancreatitis. *Pancreas* 1986;4:320.
92. Vesentini. Prospective comparison of C-reactive protein level, Ranson score and contrast-enhanced computed tomography in the prediction of septic complications of acute pancreatitis. *Br J Surg* 1993;80:755.
93. Wilson. Changing patterns of incidence and mortality from acute pancreatitis in Scotland, 1961–1985. *Br J Surg* 1990;77:731.
94. Wilson. Prediction of outcome in acute pancreatitis: a comparative study of APACHE II, clinical assessment and multiple factor scoring systems. *Br J Surg* 1990;77:1260.
95. Wilson. C-reactive protein, antiproteases and complement factors as objective markers of severity in acute pancreatitis. *Br J Surg* 1989, 76:177.
96. Yeo. The natural history of pancreatic pseudocysts documented by computed tomography. *Surg Gynecol Obstet* 1990;170:411.

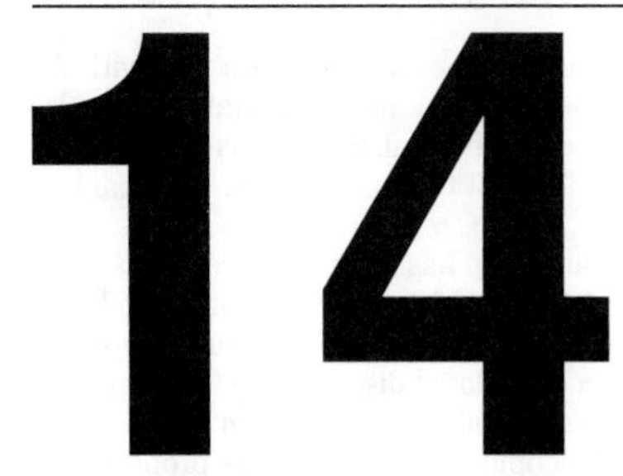

14 Variceal Bleeding: Primary Prophylaxis

Burton W. Lee and
Lawrence S. Friedman

A. Introduction

1. Epidemiology of Variceal Bleeding

a. Variceal upper gastrointestinal (UGI) bleeding is the seventh leading cause of death in United States (13). Although varices account for only 2% to 15% of the cases of UGI bleeding, more than 50% of the severe or persistent cases are caused by varices (3).

b. Among 2 million Americans with cirrhosis, at least 60% have varices. Among cirrhotic patients without varices, 10% develop them each year (3). Among cirrhotic patients with known varices, 25% to 40% ultimately bleed from them during their lifetimes (11).

c. The risk of death from a single episode of variceal bleeding is about 25% to 50% (7,11). This contrasts with a 10% mortality rate associated with UGI bleeding from all causes (3). Among patients who survive an acute episode of bleeding, about 70% eventually rebleed from varices. Half of the patients who rebleed do so within 6 weeks of the index event (3,40).

2. Portal Hypertension

a. Portal hypertension is defined as a portal venous pressure >10 mm Hg or a hepatic vein pressure gradient (HVPG) >5 mm Hg. HVPG is the difference between the wedged hepatic vein pressure (WHVP) and the free hepatic vein pressure. However, variceal bleeding is unlikely until the HVPG exceeds 12 mm Hg (20).

b. Differential Diagnosis of Portal Hypertension—Schistosomiasis and viral hepatitis are the two most common causes of portal hypertension worldwide. In Western countries, alcoholism and viral hepatitis are the most common causes. Major causes of portal hypertension are listed in Table 14-1 (39,40).

3. Predicting the Risk of Variceal Bleeding

—Because only 25% to 40% of cirrhotic patients with proven varices ultimately bleed from them, if all patients with varices were treated prophylactically, 60% to 75% would be treated unnecessarily (11). On the other hand, because an episode of variceal bleeding is associated with a 25% to 50% risk of death, investigators have tried to identify high-risk patients who may benefit from prophylactic therapy and low-risk patients who may be observed without any intervention.

Table 14-1 Major causes of portal hypertension (39,40)

Presinusoidal	Sinusoidal	Postsinusoidal
Portal vein thrombosis	Cirrhosis	Budd-Chiari syndrome
Malignancy		Venoocclusive disorder
Fibrosis		
Schistosomiasis		

a. **Portal Pressure**—Portal pressure does not correlate well with the risk of variceal bleeding. Furthermore, measurement of portal pressure is impractical for routine screening because it requires an invasive procedure. However, as previously stated, if the HVPG is <12 mm Hg, variceal bleeding is uncommon (20).

b. **Prognostic Index**—An Italian group has studied the relations between the risk of variceal bleeding and various biochemical, clinical, and endoscopic features in patients with cirrhosis. This prospective study involved 321 cirrhotic patients (42% with alcohol-related disease, 20% with hepatitis B, and 37% with cirrhosis of unknown origin) who had proven varices and no prior history of UGI bleeding. Endoscopic criteria were those proposed by Beppu: the size, color, and location of varices; presence and grade of red wale markings (longitudinal dilated venules) and cherry-red spots (small red spots about 2 mm in diameter); the presence or absence of hematocystic spots (larger round projections resembling blood blisters); esophagitis; and diffuse redness (2). Patients were observed for an average of 23 months (22).

(1) Bleeding occurred in 26% of patients. Six endoscopic and five clinical-biochemical features listed in Table 14-2 were significantly correlated with the risk of UGI bleeding in an univariate analysis. The age and sex of the patient, presence of encephalopathy, cause of cirrhosis, and serum level of aspartate aminotransferase (SGOT) did not correlate with the risk of bleeding (22).

(2) In a multivariate analysis, only 3 of the 11 factors listed correlated with the risk of variceal bleeding: the Child's class, the size of the varices, and the presence of red wale markings (22).

(a) A point system assigned relative weight to these features as shown in Table 14-3.

(b) The point system was then used to predict the risk of variceal bleeding. For example, the risk of variceal bleeding was only 1.6% per year for a patient with Child's class A cirrhosis, small varices, and no red wale markings. In contrast, the risk of bleeding was 68.9% for a patient with Child's class C cirrhosis, large varices, and any degree of red wale markings. This index was prospectively validated in 75 additional patients in the same study (see Table 14-4).

Table 14-2 Univariate predictors of UGI bleeding in patients with varices (22)

Endoscopic Features	Biochemical-Clinical Features
Presence of red wale markings	Child's class
Size of the varices	Presence of ascites
Presence of cherry-red spots	Elevated serum bilirubin
Superior location of the varices	Decreased serum albumin
Presence of diffuse redness	Elevated PT
Presence of hematocystic spots	

Table 14-3 Multivariate predictors of UGI bleeding in patients with varices (22)

Child's Class		Varices		Red Wale Markings	
A	6.5	Small	8.7	Absent	3.2
B	13.0	Medium	13.0	Mild	6.4
C	19.5	Large	17.4	Moderate	9.6
				Severe	12.8

Table 14-4 System for predicting UGI bleeding in patients with varices (22)

Risk	Points	No. of Patients	Risk of Bleeding Per Year
1	0–19.9	63	1.6%
2	20–25	76	11.0%
3	25.1–30.0	63	14.8%
4	30.1–35.0	56	23.3%
5	35.1–40.0	48	37.8%
6	>40.0	11	68.9%

B. β-Blockers for Primary Prophylaxis of Variceal Bleeding

1. β-Blockers lower the portal pressure and/or the portal blood flow by decreasing cardiac output and splanchnic blood flow (31). They are typically administered to decrease the heart rate by 25% or to lower the HVPG to <12 mm Hg. However, in about 20% of patients, the HVPG does not respond to β-blockers (11). Nonselective b-blockers may be more efficacious than β_1-selective agents (11,31).

2. Efficacy of β-Blockers in Primary Prophylaxis (23)

a. Many prospective randomized controlled trials (PRCTs) have examined the role of β-blockers in the primary prevention of variceal bleeding in cirrhotic patients (1,5,7,14,15,19,23,25,29,38). Follow-up has ranged from 12 to 34 months. Five studies compared β-blockers versus control (7,14,15, 19,25), three compared β-blockers versus sclerotherapy versus placebo (1,29,38), and one compared β-blockers versus placebo for primary and secondary prophylaxis (5). The results of these studies have been mixed.

(1) Risk of UGI Bleeding

(a) Four studies found no statistically significant benefit to β-blockade (19,25,29,38).

(b) One study found β-blockers to increase the risk of UGI bleeding (5).

(c) Four studies found β-blockers to decrease the risk of UGI bleeding (1,7,14,15).

(2) Risk of Death

(a) Eight studies found no significant benefit to β-blockade (1,5,7, 14,15,19,29,38).

(b) One study found β-blockers to improve the rate of survival (25).

(3) A metaanalysis of these nine studies favored β-blockers over control (23) (see Table 14-5).

(a) β-Blockers significantly decreased the risk of UGI bleeding (P<0.05).

(b) β-Blockers also decreased the risk of death, but this difference was not statistically significant.

b. A study representative of trials favoring β-blockers for primary prophylaxis of variceal bleeding is Conn's PRCT, which involved 102 cirrhotic patients with endoscopically confirmed varices and HVPG >12 mm Hg. No patient had a prior history of variceal bleeding; 78% had alcoholic liver disease, and 92% were in Child's class A or B. Before randomization, all patients underwent hemodynamic studies to determine the optimal dose of

Table 14-5 Metaanalysis of PRCTs evaluating the role of β-blockers (23)

	Control (n=507)	β Blockers (n=489)	Pooled Odds Ratio	*P*
Risk of UGI bleeding	25%	15%	0.54	<0.05
Risk of death	28%	19%	0.75	NS

propranolol to decrease the HVPG to <12 mm Hg or the resting heart rate to <55 beats per minute. Placebo was compared with propranolol (titrated to the previously determined dose). Mean follow-up was 16 months (7) (see Table 14-6).

(1) Propranolol significantly decreased the risk of variceal bleeding ($P<0.01$). The beneficial effect of propranolol was especially impressive for patients with large varices ($P<0.001$) and for those with alcoholic cirrhosis ($P<0.01$).

(2) However, the mortality rate did not differ significantly between the two groups.

(3) The risk of complications requiring cessation of therapy was also statistically similar between the two groups.

3. Summary of the Role of β-Blockers in Primary Prophylaxis (11,23)

a. Some, but not all, studies have found β-blockers to decrease the risk of UGI bleeding. In a metaanalysis, this benefit was statistically significant.

b. Most studies have not demonstrated a survival benefit with β-blockade.

C. Sclerotherapy for Primary Prophylaxis of Variceal Bleeding

1. Sclerotherapy can be performed by an intravariceal method of injection to cause thrombosis, by a paravariceal method to cause fibrosis, or by a combination of the two methods (39). Sodium morrhuate, sodium tetradecyl sulfate, ethanolamine, and ethanol are some of the commonly used sclerosants. No one agent appears to be better than another (21).

2. Efficacy of Sclerotherapy in Primary Prophylaxis

a. Numerous PRCTs have evaluated the role of sclerotherapy in the primary prophylaxis of variceal bleeding (1,8,9,17,24,26–29,33–36,38,41–43). Follow-up has ranged from 13 to 61 months. Most of the studies compared sclerotherapy versus no therapy (8,17,24,26–28,33–36,41—43), three compared β-blockers versus sclerotherapy (1,29,38), and one compared sclerotherapy for primary prophylaxis versus sclerotherapy for secondary prophylaxis (9). The results of these studies have also been mixed (11,23).

(1) Risk of UGI Bleeding

(a) Most of the studies found no statistically significant benefit to sclerotherapy (1,8,9,17,27–29,33,36,41,42).

(b) Four studies found sclerotherapy to decrease the risk of UGI bleeding (24,26,34,43).

(c) Two studies found sclerotherapy to increase the risk of UGI bleeding (35,38).

(2) Risk of Death

(a) Most of the studies found no statistically significant benefit to sclerotherapy (1,8,9,17,26,27,29,33–36,38,41).

(b) Three studies found sclerotherapy to decrease the risk of death (24,28,43). Two of these studies, however, did not use emergency sclerotherapy to manage acute variceal bleeding in the control group (24,43). Therefore, these studies may have been biased against the control group.

(c) One study found sclerotherapy to increase the risk of death (42).

Table 14-6 Conn's PRCT evaluating the role of β-blockers (7)

	Control (n=51)	Propranolol (n=51)	*P*
Risk of variceal bleeding	22%	4%	<0.01
Risk of death	22%	16%	NS
Risk of major complications	8%	16%	NS

(3) In a metaanalysis of these 17 trials, no meaningful conclusions were possible because there was too much heterogeneity of results among the studies (*P*<0.0001) (23).

b. A representative study favoring sclerotherapy for primary prophylaxis of variceal bleeding is described as an illustration. Witzel's PRCT involved 109 cirrhotic patients with endoscopically confirmed varices but no prior history of variceal bleeding. Intravariceal sclerotherapy every 1 month was compared to endoscopy without sclerotherapy every 2.5 months. Average follow-up was 25 months (43).

(1) Sclerotherapy significantly decreased the risk of variceal bleeding and improved survival.

(2) However, this study can be criticized because the rate of UGI bleeding in the control group was unusually high compared with rates reported in the literature. Furthermore, emergency sclerotherapy was withheld from actively bleeding control patients. Because sclerotherapy is known to be effective for acute variceal bleeding, this study may have been biased in favor of sclerotherapy (see Table 14-7).

c. Two representative studies that have found sclerotherapy to be harmful for prophylactic therapy are described.

(1) Santangelo's study found prophylactic sclerotherapy to increase the risk of UGI bleeding (35). This PRCT involved 101 cirrhotic patients with large varices on endoscopy but no prior history of variceal bleeding. Intravariceal sclerotherapy every 14 days was compared with observation by interview every 3 months. Average follow-up was 13 months.

(a) The study was terminated early at 22 months because sclerotherapy increased the risk of UGI bleeding.

(b) There was no significant difference in survival.

(c) Major complications of sclerotherapy included strictures (20%) and ulcers (65%) (see Table 14-8).

(2) The Veterans Administration Cooperative Variceal Sclerotherapy study found prophylactic sclerotherapy to increase the risk of death (42). To date, this has been the largest study to evaluate the role of sclerotherapy for primary prophylaxis of variceal bleeding in cirrhotic patients. This PRCT involved 281 male veterans with alcoholic cirrhosis and varices but no prior history of variceal bleeding. Patients with a prior history of sclerotherapy or β-blocker use were excluded. Sham sclerotherapy was compared with sclerotherapy per-

Table 14-7 Witzel's PRCT evaluating the role of sclerotherapy (43)

	Control (n=53)	Sclerotherapy (n=56)	*P*
Risk of variceal bleeding	57%	9%	<0.01
Risk of death	55%	21%	<0.01

Table 14-8 Santangelo's PRCT evaluating the role of sclerotherapy (35)

	Control (n=50)	Sclerotherapy (n=51)	*P*
Risk of variceal bleeding	8%	29%	<0.05
Risk of death	22%	23%	NS

formed on day 0, day 5, day 10, 1 month, 3 months, then every 3 months for 2 years.

(a) The study was terminated early because sclerotherapy increased the risk of death. Most of the difference in mortality occurred during the 2-year treatment period. However, the sclerotherapy group had a significantly higher proportion of patients with major comorbid illnesses. Therefore, this study may have been biased against sclerotherapy.

(b) Sclerotherapy also increased the risks of heartburn, dysphagia, esophageal ulcers, and esophageal strictures.

(c) During the 2-year treatment period, the risk of variceal bleeding was lower with sclerotherapy. However, there was no appreciable difference in the rate of all UGI bleeding. After the 2-year treatment period, both the risk of variceal bleeding and the risk of all UGI bleeding were lower with sclerotherapy (see Table 14-9).

3. Summary of the Role of Sclerotherapy in Primary Prophylaxis (11, 23)

a. Prophylactic sclerotherapy was not effective in decreasing the risk of UGI bleeding or the risk of death in most studies.

b. In some studies, sclerotherapy actually increased the risk of UGI bleeding, and in the largest study done to date, sclerotherapy significantly increased the risk of death.

c. Given these data, sclerotherapy for primary prophylaxis of variceal bleeding cannot be recommended.

4. Endoscopic band ligation is a relatively new procedure that uses an endoscopically introduced O-ring to strangle a varix. It has been shown to be useful for acute management and secondary prophylaxis of variceal bleeding (10,18,37). The details of these trials are fully discussed in Chapter 16. At this time, its role in primary prophylaxis of variceal bleeding is unknown, but studies are in progress.

D. Shunt Surgery for Primary Prophylaxis of Variceal Bleeding

1. Types of Shunt Operations

a. Nonselective Shunts

(1) End-to-Side Portacaval Shunts—In this operation, the portal vein is divided; the splanchnic end is connected to the side of the inferior vena cava (IVC), and the hepatic end becomes a stump. The operation results in a total shunt of the portal system into the systemic circulation. This procedure does not preserve blood flow to the liver and

Table 14-9 VA Cooperative Study evaluating the role of sclerotherapy (42)

	Sham (n=138)	Sclerotherapy (n=143)	*P*
Episodes of all UGI bleeding during treatment period	40	53	NS
Episodes of variceal bleeding during treatment period	19	10	0.007
Episodes of all UGI bleeding after treatment period	41	15	?
Episodes of variceal bleeding after treatment period	11	5	?
Risk of death at the end of 2 y of sclerotherapy	17%	32%	0.004
Risk of death at 37 mo among survivors of 2 y of therapy	36%	35%	NS
Patients with major comorbid illnesses	27%	47%	0.001
Average child's class score	8.0	8.2	NS

therefore increases the risk of hepatic encephalopathy to a greater extent than does selective portosystemic shunting. Furthermore, the sinusoids remain under high pressure and the patient remains at high risk for development of ascites. This operation is rarely performed today (39,40).

(2) Side-to-Side Portacaval Shunts—This operation is similar to the end-to-side portacaval shunt except that the side of the portal vein is connected to the side of the IVC. Variations of this theme include the portacaval H-graft, in which a graft connects the portal vein with the IVC, and the mesocaval H-graft, in which a graft connects the superior mesenteric vein with the IVC. Because the hepatic end of the portal vein is kept intact, these shunts are designed to preserve hepatic blood flow and relieve ascites (39,40).

b. Selective Shunts

(1) The most widely used selective shunt is the distal splenorenal (DSR) shunt. This operation is based on separation of the portal venous system into the esophagogastric compartment and the superior mesenteric compartment. Connection of the distal end of the splenic vein to the side of the left renal vein causes selective decompression of the esophagogastric compartment, while the superior mesenteric compartment remains under high pressure. Collateral connections between the two compartments are often ligated, whereas the spleen is left intact (39,40).

(2) When compared with portacaval shunts, the DSR shunt is designed to decrease the risk of encephalopathy by maintaining hepatopetal blood flow. However, with time, about 50% of patients with alcoholic cirrhosis lose portal blood flow. Meticulous ligation of collateral vessels between the spleen and pancreas (splenopancreatic disconnection) may lower the risk of hepatic encephalopathy. For unclear reasons, patients with nonalcoholic cirrhosis maintain better blood flow to the liver (4,12).

(3) This is a technically more demanding operation than the portacaval shunt. Therefore, it is usually limited to elective situations. Because the operation does not involve the porta hepatis, it is the preferred shunt operation in patients who may be future candidates for liver transplantation.

2. Efficacy of Shunt Surgery in the Primary Prophylaxis of Variceal Bleeding—Several studies have examined the role of shunt surgery in the primary prophylaxis of variceal bleeding in cirrhotic patients (6,16,30). Overall, these studies found that shunt surgery decreased the risk of variceal bleeding (6,30), increased the risk of encephalopathy (6,16,30), and did not improve survival (6,16,30). One study, however, found that shunt surgery increased the risk of death (16). Two of these studies are described for illustration.

a. Resnick's PRCT involved 93 patients with moderately advanced cirrhosis, varices, and a recent episode of acute liver decompensation. No patient had a prior history of GI bleeding that required a transfusion. Conventional medical therapy was compared with portacaval shunt (30).

(1) Using an intention-to-treat analysis, surgery significantly decreased the risk of variceal bleeding ($P<0.01$).

(2) There was a nonsignificant trend toward higher risk of encephalopathy with surgery.

(3) There was no difference in survival between the two groups (see Table 14-10).

b. Jackson's PRCT involved 112 cirrhotic patients with varices but no prior history of GI bleeding. More than 90% had alcoholic cirrhosis. Average follow-up was 42 months. Conventional medical therapy was compared with portacaval shunt. Fifty-eight patients were randomly assigned to medical therapy (Medical) and 54 were assigned to surgery. Thirty-seven of the lat-

Table 14-10 Resnick's PRCT evaluating the role of portacaval shunt surgery (30)

	Medical Therapy (n=45)	Surgery (n=48)	*P*	Comments
Variceal bleeding	26.7%	6.2%	<0.01	2 of the 3 surgical patients who bled died waiting for surgery
Hepatic encephalopathy	35.6%	50.0%	NS	4 of the 16 medical patients who experienced encephalopathy went on to surgery; if these 4 patients are excluded, *P* is <0.05
Mortality rate	42.2%	45.8%	NS	Death due to variceal bleeding was less frequent in the surgical group, but the risk of death due to hepatorenal syndrome was higher

ter group received a shunt operation (Surgery). The remaining 17 patients were randomly designated but did not go on to surgery (No Surgery) (16).

(1) The risk of variceal bleeding was similar among all three groups.

(2) There was a nonsignificant trend toward higher risk of encephalopathy with surgery (Medical versus Surgery). When the Medical and the No Surgery groups together were compared with the Surgery group, surgery significantly increased the risk of encephalopathy ($P<0.05$).

(3) The risk of death was significantly higher with surgery than with medical therapy ($P<0.02$). Because the operative mortality rate was only 13.5%, the difference in mortality cannot entirely be explained by perioperative death (see Table 14-11).

3. Summary of the Role of Shunt Surgery in the Primary Prophylaxis of Variceal Bleeding

a. Shunt surgery decreases the risk of UGI bleeding but appears to increase the risk of hepatic encephalopathy.

b. Shunt surgery does not improve survival. In one study, it increased the mortality rate.

c. Several studies have reported the utility of transjugular intrahepatic portosystemic shunts (TIPS) for secondary prophylaxis of variceal bleeding (4a,17a,32)). Its role for primary prophylaxis is unknown.

E. Summary of the Role of Primary Prophylaxis of Variceal Bleeding in Cirrhotic Patients

1. β-Blockers decreased the risk of UGI bleeding in some but not all studies. A

Table 14-11 Jackson's PRCT evaluating the role of portacaval shunt surgery (16)

	Medical Therapy (n=58)	No Surgery (n=17)	Surgery (n=37)	*P*
Variceal bleeding	19%	18%	16%	NS
Hepatic encephalopathy	21%	18%	38%	<0.05 (Medical + No surgery vs. Surgery)
Mortality rate	27.5%	29.4%	51.3%	<0.02 (Medical vs. Surgery)

metaanalysis of nine studies found β-blockers to decrease the risk of UGI bleeding significantly. However, survival was not convincingly improved.

2. Numerous PRCTs have evaluated sclerotherapy in the primary prophylaxis of variceal bleeding, but the results have been mixed. Sclerotherapy was not effective in decreasing the risk of UGI bleeding or the risk of death in most studies. In some studies, sclerotherapy increased the risk of UGI bleeding, and in the largest study done to date, it increased the risk of death significantly.
3. Several PRCTs have evaluated the role of shunt surgery in the primary prophylaxis of variceal bleeding. Overall, shunt surgery decreased the risk of variceal bleeding, increased the risk of encephalopathy, and did not improve survival. However, in one study, shunt surgery increased the risk of death, compared with medical therapy. On the basis of these data, neither sclerotherapy nor shunt surgery can be recommended for primary prophylaxis of variceal bleeding.

Abbreviations used in Chapter 14

DSR = distal splenorenal
HVPG = hepatic vein pressure gradient
IVC = inferior vena cava
P = probability value
PRCT = prospective randomized controlled trial
PT = prothrombin time
TIPS = transjugular intrahepatic portosystemic shunt
UGI = upper gastrointestinal
vs. = versus
WHVP = wedged hepatic vein pressure

References

1. Andreani. Preventive therapy of first gastrointestinal bleeding in patients with cirrhosis: results of a controlled trial comparing propranolol, endoscopic sclerotherapy and placebo. *Hepatology* 1990;12:1413.
2. Beppu. Prediction of variceal hemorrhage by esophageal endoscopy. *Gastrointest Endosc* 1981;27:213.
3. Brewer. Treatment of acute gastroesophageal variceal hemorrhage. *Med Clin North Am* 1993;77:993. Review.
4. Burroughs. Prevention of variceal rebleeding. *Gastroenterol Clin North Am* 1992; 21:119. Review.

4a. Cabrera. Transjugular intrahepatic portosystemic shunt versus sclerotherapy in the elective treatment of variceal hemorrhage. *Gastroenterology* 1996;110:832.

5. Colman. Propranolol in the prevention of variceal hemorrhage in alcoholic cirrhotic patients. *Hepatology* 1990;12:851. Abstract.
6. Conn. Prophylactic portacaval anastomosis: a tale of two studies. *Medicine (Baltimore)* 1972;51:27.
7. Conn. Propranolol in the prevention of the first hemorrhage from oesophageal varices: a multicenter, randomized clinical trial. *Hepatology* 1991;13:902.
8. De Franchis. Prophylactic sclerotherapy in high risk cirrhotics selected by endoscopic criteria: a multicenter randomized controlled trial. *Gastroenterology* 1991; 101:1087.
9. Fleig. A randomized trial comparing prophylactic and therapeutic endoscopic sclerotherapy in cirrhotic patients with large esophageal varices and no previous hemorrhage. *Hepatology* 1988;7:S128.
10. Gimson. Randomised trial of variceal banding ligation versus injection sclerotherapy for bleeding oesophageal varices. *Lancet* 1993;342(8868):391.

11. Grace. Prevention of initial variceal hemorrhage. *Gastroenterol Clin North Am* 1992; 21:149. Review.
12. Henderson. Endoscopic variceal sclerosis compared with distal splenorenal shunt to prevent recurrent variceal bleeding in cirrhosis: a prospective, randomized trial. *Ann Intern Med* 1990;112:262.
13. Henderson. Management of variceal bleeding in the 1990s. *Cleve Clin J Med* 1993; Nov-Dec:431. Review.
14. Ideo. Nadolol can prevent the first gastrointestinal bleeding in cirrhotics: a prospective, randomized study. *Hepatology* 1988;8:6.
15. Italian Multicenter Project for Propranolol in Prevention of Bleeding. Propranolol prevents first gastrointestinal bleeding in nonascitic cirrhotic patients: final report of a multicenter randomized trial. *J Hepatol* 1989;9:75.
16. Jackson. A clinical investigation of the portacaval shunt: survival analysis of the prophylactic operation. *Am J Surg* 1967;115:22.
17. Koch. Prophylactic sclerosing of esophageal varices: results of a prospective controlled study. *Endoscopy* 1986;18:40.
17a. Laberge. Two-year outcome following transjugular intrahepatic portosystemic shunt for variceal bleeding: results in 90 patients. *Gastroenterology* 1995;108:1143.
18. Laine. Endoscopic ligation compared with sclerotherapy for the treatment of bleeding esophageal varices. *Ann Intern Med* 1993;119:1.
19. Lebrec. Nadolol for prophylaxis of gastrointestinal bleeding in cirrhotic patients: a randomized trial. *J Hepatol* 1988;7:118.
20. Lebrec. Methods to evaluate portal hypertension. *Gastroenterol Clin North Am* 1992;21:41. Review.
21. Matloff. Treatment of acute variceal bleeding. *Gastroenterol Clin North Am* 1992; 21:103. Review.
22. North Italian Endoscopic Club for the Study and Treatment of Esophageal Varices. Prediction of the first variceal hemorrhage in patients with cirrhosis of the liver and esophageal varices: a prospective multicenter study. *N Engl J Med* 1988; 319:983.
23. Pagliaro. Prevention of first bleeding in cirrhosis: a meta-analysis of randomized trials of non-surgical treatment. *Ann Intern Med* 1992;117:59.
24. Paquet. Prophylactic endoscopic sclerosing treatment of the esophageal wall in varices: a prospective controlled randomized trial. *Endoscopy* 1982;14:4.
25. Pascal. Propranolol in the prevention of first upper gastrointestinal tract hemorrhage in patients with cirrhosis of the liver and esophageal varices. *N Engl J Med* 1987;317:856.
26. Piai. Prophylactic sclerotherapy of high risk esophageal varices: results of a multicentric prospective controlled trial. *Hepatology* 1988;8:1495.
27. Planas. Prophylactic sclerosis of esophageal varices: prospective trial. *J Hepatol* 1989;9:S73.
28. Potzi. Prophylactic endoscopic sclerotherapy of oesophageal varices in liver cirrhosis: a multicentre prospective controlled randomized trial in Vienna. *Gut* 1989; 30:873.
29. PROVA Study Group. Prophylaxis of first hemorrhage from oesophageal varices by sclerotherapy, propranolol or both in cirrhotic patients: a randomized multicenter trial. *Hepatology* 1991;14:1016.
30. Resnick. A controlled study of the prophylactic portacaval shunt: a final report. *Ann Intern Med* 1969;70:675.
31. Rodriguez-Perez. Pharmacologic treatment of portal hypertension. *Gastroenterol Clin North Am* 1992;21:15. Review.
32. Rossle. The transjugular intrahepatic portosystemic stent-shunt procedure for variceal bleeding. *N Engl J Med* 1994;330:165.
33. Russo. Prophylactic sclerotherapy in nonalcoholic liver cirrhosis: preliminary results of a prospective controlled randomized trial. *World J Surg* 1989;13:149.
34. Saggioro. Prophylactic sclerotherapy: a controlled study. *Dig Dis Sci* 1986;31: 504S. Abstract.

35. Santangelo. Prophylactic sclerotherapy of large esophageal varices. *N Engl J Med* 1988;318:814.
36. Sauerbruch. Prophylactic sclerotherapy before the first episode of variceal hemorrhage in patients with cirrhosis. *N Engl J Med* 1988;319:8.
37. Steigmann. Endoscopic sclerotherapy as compared with endoscopic ligation for bleeding esophageal varices. *N Engl J Med* 1992;326:1527.
38. Strauss. A randomized controlled trial for the prevention of the first upper gastrointestinal bleeding due to portal hypertension in cirrhosis: sclerotherapy or propranolol versus control groups. *Hepatology* 1988;8:1395. Abstract.
39. Terblanche. Controversies in the management of bleeding esophageal varices: part I. *N Engl J Med* 1989;320:1393. Review.
40. Terblanche. Controversies in the management of bleeding esophageal varices: part II. *N Engl J Med* 1989;320:1469. Review.
41. Triger. Prophylactic sclerotherapy for esophageal varices: long term results of a single center trial. *Hepatology* 1991;13:117.
42. VA Cooperative Variceal Sclerotherapy Group. Prophylactic sclerotherapy for esophageal varices in men with alcoholic liver disease. *N Engl J Med* 1991;324:1779.
43. Witzel. Prophylactic endoscopic sclerotherapy of esophageal varices. *Lancet* 1985;1:773.

15 Variceal Bleeding: Acute Management

Burton W. Lee and
Lawrence S. Friedman

A. General Approach to Acute Variceal Bleeding

1. Initial Management (4,22)

a. The first priority in the management of any patient with gastrointestinal (GI) bleeding is hemodynamic resuscitation and stabilization. IV access should be established, and the blood bank should set up packed red blood cells (PRBC), fresh frozen plasma, and platelets. Blood should also be sent for a complete blood count and determinations of creatinine, blood urea nitrogen, calcium, prothrombin time, and partial thromboplastin time. In patients with massive hematemesis, endotracheal intubation should be considered to protect against aspiration. Endotracheal intubation can also facilitate esophageal tamponade or sclerotherapy if they become necessary. In general, patients with acute variceal bleeding should be treated in an intensive care unit with cardiac monitoring.

b. IV fluids should be given to maintain hemodynamic stability and to achieve adequate urinary output. If necessary, blood products and vitamin K should be given to ensure adequate oxygen delivery and to restore hemostasis. However, excessive administration of fluid and blood products should be avoided so as not to worsen portal hypertension. In alcoholic patients, parenteral thiamine should be given before administration of dextrose solutions to avoid precipitating Wernicke's syndrome.

c. Measurement of vital signs is essential in estimating the amount of intravascular volume loss, as shown in Table 15-1. However, these estimates do not necessarily apply to patients with chronic or recurrent bleeding because of physiologic compensation.

d. A careful rectal examination including anoscopy should be performed to check for hemorrhoids, masses, and fissures. If the possibility of lower GI bleeding exists, rigid or flexible sigmoidoscopy should be performed to examine the colonic mucosa for inflammatory, infectious, ischemic, or neoplastic processes.

e. Nasogastric (NG) lavage should be performed to assess the severity of bleeding and to confirm that bleeding is from an upper gastrointestinal (UGI) source. Iced saline offers no advantages over room-temperature water. A negative NG aspirate does not exclude an UGI source, because NG lavage misses up to 16% of actively bleeding lesions detectable on en-

Table 15-1 Correlation between vital signs and the amount of acute blood loss

Physical Examination	Estimated Acute Volume Loss
Normal vital signs	0%–15%
Orthostasis >10 mm Hg	20%
Resting tachycardia	25%
Systolic blood pressure <100 mm Hg	>30%

doscopy (31). The presence of bile in the NG aspirate suggests, but does not guarantee, that the bleeding source is distal to the ligament of Treitz (17).

2. Further Management

a. Patients should be observed meticulously for alcohol withdrawal, aspiration pneumonia, sepsis, hepatorenal syndrome, congestive heart failure, and hepatic encephalopathy. Abdominal ultrasonography should be considered to exclude portal vein thrombosis, which may be a sign of hepatocellular carcinoma (36). About 30% to 60% of variceal bleeding episodes stop spontaneously, a fact that should be kept in mind when evaluating the efficacy of various therapies.

b. Early endoscopy is essential for diagnosis and management. About 30% of patients with cirrhosis and UGI bleeding do not have varices. Among the 70% who have varices, only one third are actively bleeding from them. Another third have stopped bleeding from varices, and the remaining third have varices but are bleeding from another source (36). Furthermore, urgent endoscopy permits therapeutic interventions such as sclerotherapy, which can control bleeding in about 90% of cases (35).

c. Many options exist in the specific management of acute variceal bleeding. For the sake of discussion, these can be divided into temporizing and definitive therapies. Temporizing therapies include administration of vasopressin with nitroglycerin (TNG), administration of somatostatin, and esophageal tamponade. These measures are often effective in controlling the acute bleeding, but most patients experience rebleeding unless more definitive therapy is administered. Definitive therapies include sclerotherapy, band ligation, portosystemic shunt surgery, transjugular intrahepatic portosystemic shunting, esophageal transection, and liver transplantation (see Table 15-2). Each option is discussed in greater detail in subsequent sections.

B. Pharmacotherapy for Management of Acute Variceal Bleeding

1. Currently, there are two major classes of drugs available for the treatment of portal hypertension, vasoconstrictors and vasodilators. Vasoconstrictors increase splanchnic vascular resistance and thereby decrease splanchnic blood flow. Examples include vasopressin, somatostatin, and β-blockers. Vasodilators, such as TNG, decrease the vascular resistance of the liver and the collateral vessels. TNG also lowers the systemic preload. Decrease in systemic preload decreases the mean blood pressure, which increases splanchnic resistance (28).

2. Vasopressin

a. Vasopressin is a nine-amino-acid peptide with a half-life of 10 to 20 minutes that binds to V_1 receptors on vascular smooth muscle cells. Its binding activates phospholipase C, which cleaves phosphatidylinositol triphosphate to generate diacyl glycerol and inositol triphosphate. These second-messenger molecules ultimately cause vascular smooth muscle contraction and thereby increase vascular resistance (28).

b. Use of vasopressin for the acute management of variceal bleeding is supported only weakly by the literature. Nevertheless, its routine use continues in many centers. Two studies are described for illustration.

Table 15-2 Management options for acute variceal bleeding

Temporizing Therapies	Definitive Therapies
Pharmacotherapy	Sclerotherapy
Vasopressin and nitroglycerin	Band ligation
Somatostatin	Surgical portosystemic shunts
Esophageal tamponade	Transjugular intrahepatic portosystemic shunts
	Esophageal transection
	Liver transplantation

(1) Merigan's prospective randomized controlled trial (PRCT) involved 30 cirrhotic patients with active variceal bleeding. Vasopressin (in the form of 20 U of extract of the posterior pituitary gland) was compared with 200 ml of 5% dextrose in water (D5W). One hour after the infusion, NG aspirates were examined. Bleeding was considered "controlled" if the aspirate was clear and "indeterminate" if the aspirate had cleared before initiation of therapy or if it showed incomplete clearing; the remaining cases were considered to have "failed" (23).

(a) Posterior pituitary extract controlled variceal bleeding better than placebo (*P*<0.01) but did not improve survival (see Table 15-3).

(b) However, this study may be criticized for several limitations. First, the cause of bleeding was not confirmed by endoscopy. Second, clinically important control of bleeding should have decreased the blood transfusion requirement, but this end point was not addressed by the study. Third, the efficacy of treatment was determined only 1 hour after the infusion by examination of the NG aspirate; the clinical relevance of this end point is questionable.

(2) Fogel's PRCT involved 33 patients with endoscopically confirmed active variceal bleeding. This was part of a larger study of 60 patients with UGI bleeding from any cause, but the variceal bleeding patients were randomized separately. In a double-blind fashion, placebo was compared with vasopressin (infused for 24 hours). Cessation of bleeding was defined as the absence of fresh blood in the NG aspirate (12) (see Table 15-4).

(a) Vasopressin was not effective in controlling variceal bleeding.

(b) The blood transfusion requirements were similar in the two groups.

(c) There was no difference in the mortality rates.

c. Lack of survival benefit with IV vasopressin has raised concerns about the negative side effects of the drug, which include bradycardia, hypertension, arrhythmias, and cardiac ischemia. In order to minimize these systemic side effects, some authors have advocated direct intraarterial infusion of vasopressin. However, in a PRCT, intraarterial infusion offered no advantages over IV administration (8). Another approach to minimizing the side effects of vasopressin has been to combine it with TNG.

Table 15-3 Merigan's PRCT of vasopressin vs. placebo (23)

	Vasopressin (n=15)	Placebo (n=15)	*P*
No. of bleeding episodes	29	24	—
Successful control of UGI bleeding	55.2%	0%	<0.01
Indeterminate control of UGI bleeding	24.1%	33.3%	?
Failed control of UGI bleeding	20.7%	66.7%	?
Death during hospitalization	93%	80%	?

Table 15-4 Fogel's PRCT of vasopressin vs. placebo (12)

	Vasopressin (n=14)	Placebo (n=19)	*P*
Cessation of GI bleeding by 24 hours	28.6%	36.8%	NS
In-hospital death rate	50.0%	42.1%	NS
No. of transfusions during hospitalization	14	17	NS

(1) Hemodynamic Effects of Vasopressin and Nitroglycerin—Westaby studied the hemodynamic effects of vasopressin and TNG in 12 cirrhotic patients with a history of recent variceal bleeding. All patients had indwelling pulmonary artery catheters and hepatic vein catheters to measure the heart rate, the mean arterial pressure, the right atrial pressure, the pulmonary capillary wedge pressure (PCWP), the systemic vascular resistance index (SVRI), the cardiac index, the left ventricular stroke work index (LVSWI), and the hepatic vein pressure gradient (HVPG). Patients were randomly assigned to receive either vasopressin (10 U as a bolus, followed by 0.4 U/minute) or TNG (1 g as a bolus, followed by 200 μg/minute). The same measurements were repeated during the drug infusion. Finally, TNG and vasopressin were administered simultaneously, and the hemodynamic measurements were measured for a third time (39).

(a) TNG decreased the mean arterial pressure ($P<0.005$), the PCWP (P=NS), the right atrial pressure ($P<0.02$), the LVSWI ($P<0.02$), and the HVPG ($P<0.01$). Therefore, it appeared to decrease the work of the heart and to lower the portal pressure (see Table 15-5).

(b) Vasopressin increased the PCWP ($P<0.01$), the right atrial pressure ($P<0.05$), and the LVSWI (P=NS) and decreased the mean arterial pressure (P=NS) and the HVPG ($P<0.001$). Therefore, vasopressin appeared to increase the work of the heart and to lower the portal pressure. Some investigators have noted the effect on the portal pressure to be less profound in actively bleeding patients compared with nonbleeding patients, but others have challenged this observation (28) (see Table 15-6).

(c) When TNG and vasopressin were administered concomitantly, the portal pressure was lowered even further. In addition, the

Table 15-5 Hemodynamic effects of sequentially adding TNG then vasopressin (39)

	Baseline	TNG	TNG and Vasopressin	*P* (Baseline vs. TNG)	*P* (Baseline vs. Combination)	*P* (TNG vs. Combination)
HR (bpm)	84	97	75	NS	NS	<0.02
MAP (mmHg)	95	79	94	<0.005	NS	<0.05
RAP (mmHg)	7.7	5.2	7.4	<0.02	NS	NS
PCWP (mmHg)	10.0	7.1	11.5	NS	NS	NS
SVRI (dynes/sec /cm^5/m^2)	1887	1784	1856	NS	NS	NS
CI (L/min/m^2)	4.11	3.29	3.74	<0.05	NS	NS
LVSWI (gm/m^2/beat)	53	33	50	<0.02	NS	<0.005
HVPG (mmHg)	16.4	13.3	11.6	<0.01	<0.005	NS

Table 15-6 Hemodynamic effects of sequentially adding vasopressin then TNG (39)

	Baseline	Vasopressin	Vasopressin and TNG	*P* (Baseline vs. Vasopressin)	*P* (Baseline vs. Combination)	*P* (Vasopressin vs. Combination)
HR (bpm)	85	79	90	NS	NS	<0.02
MAP (mmHg)	89	92	81	NS	<0.01	<0.02
RAP (mmHg)	5.8	8.3	4.7	<0.05	NS	<0.01
PCWP (mmHg)	8.0	13.5	7.8	<0.01	NS	<0.01
SVRI (dynes/sec /cm^5/m^2)	1969	1888	1900	N?S	NS	NS
CI (L/min/m^2)	3.54	3.64	3.32	NS	NS	NS
LVSWI (gm/m^2/beat)	47	50	39	NS	NS	<0.05
HVPG (mmHg)	20.7	14.0	11.8	<0.001	<0.01	NS

negative hemodynamic effects of vasopressin were ameliorated by TNG.

(2) Three controlled trials have tested the hypothesis that the combination of vasopressin and TNG is superior to vasopressin alone (3,13, 37). Two of these studies found the combination to cause fewer side effects than vasopressin alone (13,37). A representative study is described here. Gimson's PRCT involved 57 patients with endoscopically confirmed variceal bleeding. Vasopressin (20 U over 15 minutes, then 0.4 U/minute for 12 hours) was compared with vasopressin and TNG (40 to 400 μg/minute so as to keep systolic blood pressure at 100 mm Hg) (13).

(a) The addition of TNG increased the efficacy of vasopressin significantly ($P<0.05$). Most of the benefit was in reduction of the risk of major complications. Patients receiving both drugs had fewer complications that required cessation of therapy ($P<0.02$), allowing more patients to receive the treatment (see Table 15-7).

(b) Major complications included congestive heart failure, severe chest pain, and profound bradycardia.

(c) No survival benefit was observed.

d. Summary of the Role of Vasopressin in the Management of Acute Variceal Bleeding

(1) There is some evidence that IV vasopressin can temporarily control variceal bleeding in about 50% of cases. However, half of the patients who initially respond experience rebleeding. Intraarterial infusion of vasopressin does not offer any advantages over IV infusion. Concomitant administration of TNG and vasopressin decreases the rate of complications compared with vasopressin alone.

(2) Survival is not improved with any method of vasopressin administration.

(3) Vasopressin is not the ideal drug for the treatment of acute variceal bleeding. However, it may have some role in temporizing the bleeding episode until more definitive therapy can be delivered.

3. Somatostatin and Octreotide

a. Somatostatin is a 14-amino-acid peptide that is isolated from the brain, pancreas, and GI tract. Because of its short half-life (about 1 to 3 minutes), it must be given continuously. Although somatostatin has been shown to decrease the amount of collateral blood flow in cirrhotic patients, not all studies have demonstrated a decrease in portal pressure (28). Octreotide is a synthetic analog of somatostatin with a half-life of 1 to 2 hours. Its longer half-life makes it easier to use than somatostatin (34).

b. Somatostatin Versus Placebo—Of the two major placebo-controlled studies that have examined this issue (6,38), only one showed somatostatin to be superior (6). This PRCT involved 92 patients with 120 episodes of endoscopically confirmed variceal bleeding. All patients had a systolic blood

Table 15-7 PRCT of vasopressin vs. vasopressin and TNG (13)

	Vasopressin (n=30)	Vasopressin and Nitroglycerin (n=32)	*P*
No. of bleeding episodes	34	38	—
Cessation of bleeding by 12 h	44%	68%	<0.05
Mortality rate during hospitalization	30%	29%	NS
Major complications requiring cessation of therapy	21%	2.6%	<0.02

pressure <100 mm Hg or a heart rate >100 bpm. Patients who had been treated with balloon tamponade or sclerotherapy were excluded. The study also excluded patients who were receiving vasoactive medications and those who had been randomized within 30 days for a prior bleeding episode. Somatostatin (250 μg as a bolus, followed by 250 μg/hour for 5 days) was compared with placebo. Failure of therapy was declared if the patient died, if the patient required transfusion of >6 units of PRBCs in a 6-hour period, or if significant hematemesis or melena recurred within 5 days of therapy (6) (see Table 15-8).

(1) Somatostatin was superior to placebo in controlling variceal bleeding ($P<0.01$).

(2) The transfusion requirement was also lower with somatostatin ($P<0.045$).

(3) There was no difference in survival.

c. Somatostatin Versus Vasopressin

(1) Several PRCTs have compared somatostatin with vasopressin (1,16,18,28,30). A metaanalysis of these trials showed somatostatin to be superior to vasopressin in controlling acute variceal bleeding (28) (see Table 15-9).

(2) A representative study by Jenkins is described here. This PRCT involved 22 patients with endoscopically confirmed variceal bleeding. All patients had a systolic blood pressure <100 mm Hg or a heart rate >100 bpm for 2 or more hours. Vasopressin (starting at 0.4 U/minute for 6 hours, then 0.2 U/minute for 6 hours, then 0.1 U/minute for 6 hours, and then discontinued) was compared with somatostatin (250 μg as a bolus, followed by 250 μg/hour for 24 hours). Cessation of bleeding was defined as the absence of fresh blood in the NG aspirate and a stable hematocrit and vital signs for 18 to 24 hours (16) (see Table 15-10).

(a) Somatostatin was better than vasopressin for controlling the acute bleeding episode ($P=0.003$). All 10 patients receiving somatostatin stopped bleeding, but 30% experienced rebleeding before definitive therapy could be delivered.

(b) No major complications were observed with somatostatin.

(c) Mortality rates and transfusion requirements were not clearly described in the study.

d. Octreotide Versus Sclerotherapy—Sung described a PRCT involving 100 patients living in Hong Kong who had endoscopically confirmed acute variceal bleeding. Sclerotherapy was compared with octreotide (50 mg as a bolus, followed by 50 mg/hour for 48 hours). Both groups underwent

Table 15-8 PRCT of somatostatin vs. placebo (6)

	Somatostatin (n=61)	Placebo (n=59)	*P*
Failure to control bleeding	36%	59%	<0.01
Median No. of PRBC transfusions during the infusion of drug	3	6	<0.045
30-D mortality rate	15%	12%	NS

Table 15-9 Metaanalysis of PRCTs comparing somatostatin vs. vasopressin (28)

	Somatostatin	Vasopressin
Control of GI bleeding	72%	44%
Major side effects	3%	18%

Table 15-10 PRCT of vasopressin vs. somatostatin (16)

	Vasopressin (n=12)	Somatostatin (n=10)	*P*
Cessation of Bleeding	33%	100%	0.003

weekly sclerotherapy for secondary prophylaxis. Patients who failed initial therapy were treated with balloon tamponade. Two patients were excluded from the study (34) (see Table 15-11).

(1) Overall control of bleeding, the 48-hour mortality rates, and the 30-day mortality rates were similar between the two groups.

(2) No major complications were associated with octreotide.

e. Summary of the Role of Somatostatin and Octreotide in Acute Variceal Bleeding

(1) Somatostatin and octreotide appear to be more effective than placebo or vasopressin in controlling the acute bleeding episode. Octreotide is as effective as sclerotherapy, at least in a predominantly nonalcoholic population.

(2) Somatostatin and octreotide have fewer side effects than vasopressin.

(3) Survival benefit has not been clearly demonstrated with somatostatin or octreotide.

(4) Although more studies are needed before these drugs can be recommended for routine use, somatostatin and octreotide appear to be useful for initial management of acute variceal bleeding.

4. Pharmacotherapeutic options for treatment of acute variceal bleeding are summarized in Table 15-12.

C. Esophageal Balloon Tamponade for the Management of Acute Variceal Bleeding

1. Introduction

a. Types of Esophageal Tamponade Tubes—Esophageal tamponade tubes differ in the number of associated lumens and balloons. Gastric and esophageal lumens are used to suction the respective contents of these areas, whereas gastric and esophageal balloons mechanically compress varices in these respective areas. The Minnesota tube is preferred by most authors because it has both an esophageal and a gastric lumen for suction, which may decrease the risk of aspiration. However, there are no data to support this claim (4,22) (see Table 15-13).

b. Technique (4,22)

(1) The Minnesota tube is passed orally into the stomach. Prior history of gastric surgery is a relative contraindication to esophageal tamponade. Patients usually require intubation for airway protection.

(2) The gastric balloon is inflated with 100 cc of air to check for abdominal discomfort. If the patient is comfortable, the balloon can be inflated with a total of 400 cc of air. The tube is withdrawn until the bal-

Table 15-11 PRCT of sclerotherapy vs. octreotide (34)

	Sclerotherapy (n=49)	Octreotide (n=49)	*P*
Overall control of bleeding without recurrence at 48 h	74%	70%	NS
48-H mortality	8.2%	6.1%	NS
30-D mortality	41%	29%	NS

Table 15-12 Summary of pharmacotherapeutic options for acute variceal bleeding

	Morbidity Benefit	Mortality Benefit	Typical Dose
Vasopressin and nitroglycerin	Yes?	No	An optional 20-U IV bolus may be given. Start vasopressin at 0.4 U/min; the dose can be increased to 1.0 U/minute as needed to control hemorrhage Use IV nitroglycerin at 0–400 μg/min to keep the systolic blood pressure between 90–100 mm Hg Once bleeding has been controlled, taper vasopressin by 0.1 U every 6–12 h until off
Somatostatin or octreotide	Yes	No	Somatostatin 250 μg IV bolus then 250 μg/h IV for 30 h Octreotide 50 mg IV bolus followed by 50 mg/h IV for 48 h

Table 15-13 Types of esophageal balloon tamponade tubes

Type of Tube	Lumen	Balloon
Linton	Gastric and esophageal	Gastric only
Sangstaken-Blakemore	Gastric only	Gastric and esophageal
Minnesota	Gastric and esophageal	Gastric and esophageal

loon is lodged at the gastroesophageal junction. The balloon is then fixed at the mouth.

(3) A chest radiograph is obtained to confirm placement. Both ports should be connected to suction.

(4) If the patient is still bleeding, the esophageal balloon can be inflated to 25 to 40 mm Hg and maintained under constant manometric monitoring. Some authors inflate both balloons simultaneously rather than sequentially.

(5) The esophageal balloon cannot be used for more than 24 hours owing to the risk of pressure necrosis of the esophagus. Some authors recommend deflating the balloon for 1 hour every 8 hours.

2. Efficacy of Balloon Tamponade for Acute Variceal Bleeding

a. In an uncontrolled series, esophageal tamponade was effective in stopping acute variceal bleeding in 90.7% of patients. However, the rate of subsequent rebleeding was high, and permanent hemostasis was achieved in only 47.7% (26).

b. Tamponade Versus Vasopressin—Correia described a PRCT involving 37 patients with actively bleeding, endoscopically confirmed esophageal or gastric varices. Patients with coronary artery disease, a serum sodium level <125 mmol/L, moderate or severe ascites, or age >60 years were excluded from the study. Vasopressin (20 U as a bolus over 20 minutes and 0.6 U/minute for 4 hours, then adjusted to control bleeding) was compared with the Sengstaken–Blakemore tube. No nitrates were used with vasopressin. The esophageal balloon was inflated only if the gastric balloon failed to control the bleeding. Control of bleeding was defined as no fresh blood in the NG aspirate and a stable hematocrit for 12 hours (10) (see Table 15-14).

(1) Tamponade was no better than vasopressin for controlling the acute bleeding episode. In fact, the blood transfusion requirements were lower with vasopressin ($P<0.05$).

(2) There was a nonsignificant trend toward a higher mortality rate with esophageal tamponade.

c. Tamponade Versus Sclerotherapy—Paquet described a PRCT involving 43 patients with endoscopically confirmed bleeding varices. A Sengstaken–Blakemore tube (inserted immediately after endoscopy and used for 12 to 24 hours) was compared with endoscopic sclerotherapy (30 to 50 injections of polidocanol per session for 2 to 4 sessions at 6- to 7-day intervals). Control of bleeding was defined as no fresh blood in NG aspirate, stable vital signs, and a stable hematocrit for 24 hours. Definitive control was defined as ultimate control of bleeding at the end of the study. Rebleeding patients who were subsequently controlled with repeat tamponade tube therapy or sclerotherapy were included in the "definitive control" group (27) (see Table 15-15).

(1) The rates of initial and definitive control of bleeding were superior with sclerotherapy. The risk of recurrent bleeding was also lower with sclerotherapy, but this difference was not statistically significant.

(2) One-month and 6-month mortality rates were lower with sclerotherapy ($P<0.01$).

(3) The complication rates were similar with either procedure.

3. Summary of the Role of Balloon Tamponade in the Treatment of Acute Variceal Bleeding (4,22)

a. Balloon tamponade can be technically difficult and should be done only by an experienced person. There is a significant risk of esophageal rupture or aspiration pneumonia.

b. Although variceal bleeding can be controlled in about 90% of patients, most patients experience rebleeding when the balloon is deflated.

c. Balloon tamponade offers no advantages over IV vasopressin therapy, which is technically easier to administer. It is inferior to emergency sclerotherapy in controlling the acute bleeding episode and improving survival.

Table 15-14 PRCT of vasopressin vs. balloon tamponade (10)

	Vasopressin (n=17)	Tamponade (n=20)	*P*
Control of bleeding	65%	70%	NS
Deaths	12%	24%	NS
Blood transfusion requirement during the first 48 h	1580 ml	2980 ml	<0.05

Table 15-15 PRCT of balloon tamponade vs. sclerotherapy (27)

	Tamponade (n=22)	Sclerosis (n=21)	*P*
Initial control	73%	95%	NS
Recurrent bleeding	44%	20%	NS
Definitive control	55%	90%	<0.01
30-D mortality rate	27%	10%	<0.01
Cumulative 6-mo mortality rate	50%	14%	<0.01
Acute complication rate	10%	10%	NS

d. For these reasons, balloon tamponade has fallen out of favor in recent years and has become a second-line therapy. However, it remains useful when medical therapy fails, sclerotherapy is not available, or temporary resuscitation is necessary until more definitive therapy can be administered.

D. Endoscopic Sclerotherapy for the Management of Acute Variceal Bleeding

1. Sclerotherapy can be performed immediately during active bleeding, or it can be delayed until the patient has been stabilized temporarily with pharmacotherapy or balloon tamponade, or both. Many experts favor intervening after the patient has been stabilized, because sclerotherapy is technically more difficult in the setting of massive UGI bleeding (4).
2. **Efficacy of Endoscopic Sclerotherapy for the Treatment of Acute Variceal Hemorrhage**
   a. In an uncontrolled study, Terblanche found sclerotherapy to be highly effective in controlling acute variceal bleeding. This prospective study involved 66 patients with 93 episodes of endoscopically confirmed, massive variceal bleeding. All patients were refractory to vasopressin (20 U q 4 hours), and placement of a Sengstaken–Blakemore tube was required in all cases to control bleeding. Intravariceal sclerotherapy with ethanolamine was performed under general anesthesia with a rigid endoscope, a technique that is no longer used. Recurrent bleeding was treated in a similar fashion, but sclerotherapy was not repeated once the bleeding was controlled (35).
      (1) Seventy percent of the bleeding episodes were controlled with only one sclerotherapy session; 90% were controlled by the second treatment session.
      (2) Ultimately, 95% of the bleeding episodes were controlled. These figures are in sharp contrast with ultimate control rates of about 50% reported for pharmacotherapy or balloon tamponade.
   b. There have been six major PRCTs comparing sclerotherapy with standard therapy for acute variceal bleeding in cirrhotic patients (2,9,21,24,27,40).
      (1) The efficacy of sclerotherapy for the treatment of acute variceal hemorrhage can be evaluated in regard to three major parameters: control of the acute bleeding episode; reduction of the short-term rebleeding rate; and reduction of the short-term survival rate. Five of the six studies found sclerotherapy to be significantly superior to control for at least one of these parameters (2,21,24,27,40). One study found sclerotherapy to be no better than control in regard to all three parameters (9). No study found sclerotherapy to be inferior to control for any of the three parameters. Table 15-16 summarizes the conclusions of each study.
      (2) **Control of the Acute Bleeding Episode**—Three of the six studies found sclerotherapy to be superior to standard therapy for the control of acute variceal bleeding (24,27,40). However, in only one study was the difference statistically significant (40). Three studies did not directly evaluate this end point (2,9,21). A representative study demonstrating the superiority of sclerotherapy is described here (40). Westaby described a PRCT involving 50 patients with 64 episodes of acute variceal hemorrhage. All patients had active hemorrhage at the time of endoscopy. Intravariceal sclerotherapy (5% ethanolamine) was compared with vasopressin (20 U as a bolus, then 0.4 U/minute) plus TNG (titrated to keep the systolic blood pressure at about 100 mm Hg). Patients in both groups were enrolled into a long-term sclerotherapy program for secondary prophylaxis (see Table 15-17).
         (a) Sclerotherapy was superior to medical therapy for the acute control of bleeding ($P<0.05$).
         (b) However, the short-term risks of rebleeding or death were similar.
      (3) **Reduction of the Short-Term Rebleeding Rate**—Four of the six studies found sclerotherapy to be superior to medical therapy in reducing the short-term risk of rebleeding (2,21,24,27). In three of these

Table 15-16 Summary of major PRCTs comparing sclerotherapy vs. control

Author (Reference)	N	Control of the Acute Bleeding Episode	Reduction of the Short-Term Rebleeding Rate	Reduction of the Short-Term Term Survival Rate
Barsoum (2)	100	Not evaluated	Sclerotherapy better than control ($P<0.01$)	Not evaluated
Copenhagen (9)	187	Not evaluated	No difference	No difference
Larson (21)	82	Not evaluated	Sclerotherapy better than control ($P<0.01$)	No difference
Moreto (24)	43	Sclerotherapy better than control ($P>0.05$)	Sclerotherapy better than control ($P<0.05$)	No difference
Paquet (27)	43	Sclerotherapy better than control ($P>0.05$)	Sclerotherapy better than control ($P>0.05$)	Sclerotherapy better than control ($P<0.01$)
Westaby (40)	50	Sclerotherapy better than	No difference	No difference

Table 15-17 PRCT of medical therapy vs. sclerotherapy (40)

Episodes of Hemorrhage	Medical Therapy (n=31)	Sclerotherapy (n=33)	*P*
Control of hemorrhage at 12 h	65%	88%	<0.05
Short-term risk of rebleeding	31%	31%	NS
Short-term mortality rate	39%	27%	NS

four studies, the differences were statistically significant (2,21,24). Two studies found no difference between sclerotherapy and standard therapy (9,40). A representative study demonstrating the superiority of sclerotherapy is described here (21). Larson described a PRCT involving 82 patients with endoscopically confirmed acute variceal hemorrhage associated with hematemesis or melena. All bleeding episodes caused hemodynamic instability or were associated with a drop in the hematocrit of >6%. Standard medical therapy (IV fluids, blood transfusions, vasopressin, and balloon tamponade as needed) was compared with sclerotherapy plus standard therapy. Intravariceal injection of 3% sodium tetradecyl sulfate was used every 3 to 7 days, as needed. Rebleeding was defined as hematemesis or bright red blood in the NG aspirate, a drop in the hematocrit of >6% over 24 hours, hemodynamic instability, or a drop in the hematocrit of >3% over 24 hours after no bleeding for 48 hours. Patients were observed for 2 weeks.

(a) The risk of recurrent bleeding was significantly lower with sclerotherapy than with control therapy. Only 23% of sclerotherapy patients had a rebleeding episode, compared with 53% of the medically treated patients ($P<0.01$).

(b) The average blood transfusion requirement with sclerotherapy was 2.5 units, compared with 8.5 units with medical therapy ($P<0.03$).

(c) There was no difference in survival.

(4) Reduction of the Short-Term Mortality Rate—One study found sclerotherapy to be superior to standard therapy in improving survival (27). One study did not evaluate this end point (2). Other studies found no difference between the two groups (9,21,24,40). The study demonstrating a survival benefit of sclerotherapy is described here (27). Paquet described a PRCT involving 43 patients with endoscopically confirmed bleeding varices. Treatment with a Sengstaken–Blakemore tube (inserted immediately after endoscopy and used for 12 to 24 hours) was compared with sclerotherapy (30 to 50 injections of polidocanol per session for 2 to 4 sessions at 6- to 7-day intervals). Control of bleeding was defined as no fresh blood in the NG aspirate, stable vital signs, and a stable hematocrit for 24 hours. Definitive control was defined as ultimate control of bleeding at the end of the study. Rebleeding patients who were subsequently controlled with repeat tamponade tube therapy or repeat sclerotherapy were included in the "definitive control" group (27) (see Table 15-18).

(a) The rates of initial and definitive control of variceal bleeding were superior with sclerotherapy ($P<0.01$).

(b) The risk of recurrent bleeding was lower with sclerotherapy, but this difference was not statistically significant.

(c) One-month and 6-month mortality rates were lower with sclerotherapy ($P<0.01$).

(d) The complication rates were similar.

Table 15-18 PRCT of balloon tamponade vs. sclerotherapy (27)

	Tamponade (n=22)	Sclerotherapy (n=21)	*P*
Initial control	73%	95%	NS
Recurrent bleeding	44%	20%	NS
Definitive control	55%	90%	<0.01
30-D mortality rate	27%	10%	<0.01
Cumulative 6-mo mortality rate	50%	14%	<0.01
Acute complication rate	10%	10%	NS

(5) One study found no short-term benefit of sclerotherapy over standard therapy (9). This PRCT involved 187 patients with cirrhosis and endoscopically confirmed active variceal bleeding. Patients with an estimated life expectancy of <1 year were excluded. Placement of a Sengstaken–Blakemore tube for 24 hours was compared with "paravariceal" sclerotherapy (*i.e.*, injection between varices). Patients who continued to bleed despite balloon tamponade were treated with vasopressin. Sclerotherapy was performed every 1 to 2 weeks until varices were obliterated. Follow-up ranged from 9 to 52 months. The "initial period" was considered to be the first 40 days, and the "late period" was considered to be after the first 40 days. In contrast to the previously described studies, this trial did not show any short-term benefit of sclerotherapy (9) (see Table 15-19).

(a) Sclerotherapy did not offer any advantage in stopping the acute bleeding episode.

(b) There was no difference in the short-term risk of rebleeding.

(c) The overall mortality rates and the 2-day mortality rates were also similar.

(d) However, the study did demonstrate a significant benefit of chronic sclerotherapy for the secondary prevention of variceal bleeding. The risk of rebleeding in the late period was 31% for sclerotherapy, compared with 60% for medical therapy ($P<0.0006$) (see Chapter 16).

c. Sclerotherapy Versus Octreotide—A study involving predominantly nonalcoholic cirrhotic patients found octreotide to be as effective as sclerotherapy in controlling acute variceal hemorrhage (34). (See the previous discussion of octreotide for details.) More studies are needed to determine whether these findings can be generalized to predominantly alcoholic patients typical of Western populations.

3. Complications Associated With Sclerotherapy (see Table 15-20)

a. The risk of serious complications ranges from 10% to 30% (22).

Table 15-19 PRCT of standard therapy vs. sclerotherapy (9)

	Standard Therapy (n=94)	Sclerotherapy (n=93)	*P*
% of patients with recurrent hemorrhage during initial period	30%	37%	NS
% of patients with recurrent hemorrhage during late period	60%	31%	0.0006
Mortality rate at 2 d	23%	16%	NS
Overall mortality	78%	65%	NS

Table 15-20 Complications associated with sclerotherapy (11,22)

Local Complications	Pulmonary Complications	Systemic Complications
Ulcers (90%) Bleeding (43%–58%) Chest pain (50%) Strictures (2%–12%) Perforations (1%–4%) Mediastinitis (<5%)	Pleural effusion (50%) Aspiration (5%–7%) ARDS (<5%) Pneumothorax (Rare) Bronchoesophageal fistula (Rare)	Bacteremia Peritonitis (<5%) Sepsis (<5%) Fever (50%)

b. The risk of death directly attributable to the procedure ranges from 0.5% to 2% (22).

c. Almost 90% of patients develop superficial esophageal ulcers after sclerotherapy. These lesions usually do not cause symptoms or signs; in fact, they may be considered a desired effect of therapy. Deeper ulcers may cause bleeding, bowel necrosis, or mediastinitis, but these events are less common (22).

d. Bacteremia is common with sclerotherapy, but the risk of sepsis appears to be low. The role of antibiotic prophylaxis is controversial; it is recommended by the American Heart Association only for patients with risk factors for endocarditis (11).

4. Summary of the Role of Sclerotherapy for Acute Variceal Hemorrhage

a. Most studies found sclerotherapy to be better than vasopressin or esophageal tamponade for the treatment of acute variceal hemorrhage.

b. Complications associated with sclerotherapy occur in about 10% to 30% of cases. Death directly attributable to the procedure occurs in about 1% to 2% of patients.

E. Endoscopic Band Ligation for the Management of Acute Variceal Bleeding

1. Band ligation involves endoscopic introduction of an elastic O-ring to strangle a varix. Theoretically, since it does not involve needles or chemicals, band ligation should cause fewer systemic complications than sclerotherapy. Banding also appears to be technically less demanding than sclerotherapy (40).

2. Efficacy of Band Ligation for Acute Variceal Bleeding

a. There have been three major PRCTs comparing sclerotherapy with band ligation (14,19,32). The conclusions of these studies are summarized here (see Table 15-21).

(1) All three studies found band ligation to be as effective as sclerotherapy for control of acute hemorrhage.

(2) In two of the three studies, banding was associated with a lower risk of rebleeding, compared with sclerotherapy (14,32). However, the difference was statistically significant in only one study (14).

(3) Only one of the three studies found a survival benefit with banding, compared with sclerotherapy (32).

(4) The risk of complications was significantly lower with banding in two of the three studies (19,32).

(5) All three studies found fewer treatment sessions were necessary to eradicate the varices with banding than with sclerotherapy. These differences were statistically significant in two of the three studies (14,19).

b. For illustration, the latest of the three studies is described here. Gimson's PRCT involved 103 patients with recent history of variceal bleeding. About 40% of the patients were actively bleeding at the time of initial endoscopy, and the rest had bled within 10 days of enrollment into the study. Band ligation was compared to intravariceal sclerotherapy with ethanolamine. Patients were treated weekly until the varices were obliterated. Thereafter,

Table 15-21 Summary of major PRCTs comparing banding with sclerotherapy

	Gimson (14) (n=103)	Stiegmann (32) (n=130)	Laine (19) (n=77)
% actively bleeding patients	43%	21%	23%
Control of acute hemorrhage	No difference	No difference	No difference
Rate of rebleeding	Lower with banding ($P<0.05$)	Lower with banding (NS)	No difference
Survival rate	No difference	Improved with banding ($P=0.04$)	No difference
Rate of complications	No difference	Lower with banding ($P<0.001$)	Lower with banding ($P<0.01$)
Number of sessions required to eradicate varices	Fewer sessions required with banding ($P=0.006$)	Fewer sessions required with banding (NS)	Fewer sessions required with banding ($P<0.001$)

endoscopy was performed at 1, 3, 6, and 12 months to detect recurrence of varices. Average follow-up was about 10.8 months. Patients who had previously been treated with sclerotherapy and those with a life expectancy of <6 months were excluded from the study (see Table 15-22).

(1) Both band ligation and sclerotherapy were highly effective in controlling the acute bleeding episode. Control of hemorrhage was achieved in 91% and 92% of patients treated with banding and sclerotherapy, respectively.

(2) The risk of rebleeding during the study was significantly lower with banding ($P<0.05$).

(3) Fewer treatment sessions were required to completely eradicate the varices ($P=0.006$).

(4) There was no significant difference in the risk of complications or in the rate of survival between the two groups.

3. Summary of the Role of Band Ligation for the Emergency Management of Acute Variceal Bleeding

a. Band ligation controls acute variceal bleeding as well as sclerotherapy.

b. In one study, the long-term survival rate was better with band ligation than with sclerotherapy (19). In the other two studies, the survival rates were similar.

c. Fewer treatment sessions are required to completely eradicate varices with banding than with sclerotherapy. In addition, the risk of recurrent bleeding may be lower with banding than with sclerotherapy.

Table 15-22 Gimson's PRCT of banding vs. sclerotherapy (14)

	Banding (n=54)	Sclerotherapy (n=49)	*P*
Control of acute hemorrhage	91%	92%	NS
Rate of rebleeding	30%	53%	<0.05
Complete eradication of varices	59%	55%	NS
Number of treatment sessions for complete eradication	3.4	4.9	0.006

d. Complications may be less likely with banding.

F. Shunt Surgery for the Management of Acute Variceal Bleeding

1. Introduction

a. With the development of less invasive procedures such as sclerotherapy and banding, the use of emergency shunt surgery has declined (4,20). It is still advocated by some experts as first-line therapy (25), but most reserve it for the 10% to 15% of patients who remain refractory to sclerotherapy or other nonsurgical interventions. Patients who bleed despite aggressive sclerotherapy are at high risk of death. However, these same patients also tend to have the most advanced liver disease and consequently tolerate major operations poorly. Therefore, the exact role of emergency shunt surgery remains controversial (20).

b. Different types of surgical shunts are discussed in Chapter 14. In general, distal splenorenal (DSR) shunts are more difficult and more time-consuming to perform than portacaval shunts. For this reason, most surgeons avoid DSR shunts in emergency settings (20).

c. Compared with an elective procedure, emergency shunt surgery is associated with a higher mortality rate. These rates range from 19% to >50%, depending on patient selection criteria and whether the operation is used as primary or last-resort therapy (20).

2. Shunt Surgery Versus Medical Therapy for Acute Variceal Bleeding—Orloff has long been an advocate of early shunt surgery for the emergency treatment of variceal bleeding (25). He described a PRCT involving 43 patients with cirrhosis and bleeding esophageal varices. Emergency portacaval shunt (performed within 8 hours of admission as first-line therapy) was compared with standard medical therapy (including vasopressin or tamponade, as needed). The patients who received medical therapy and survived the index hospitalization underwent an elective shunt procedure 2 to 6 weeks later. All patients were observed for 3 years or longer (see Table 15-23).

a. Early shunt surgery resulted in better permanent control of the bleeding episode, compared with initial conservative therapy.

b. Shunt surgery also improved the short- and long-term survival rates ($P<0.01$). This benefit was observed despite the fact that the patients who underwent surgery tended to have more advanced liver disease.

3. Shunt Surgery Versus Sclerotherapy for Acute Variceal Bleeding—Cello described a PRCT involving 64 patients with Child's class C cirrhosis and endoscopically confirmed variceal bleeding who required transfusion of ≥6 units of blood. Intravariceal sclerotherapy (performed within 2 hours of randomization) was compared with portacaval shunt surgery (performed within 6 hours of randomization). Sclerotherapy was repeated on three more occasions during the index hospitalization, again 1 week after discharge, and then monthly until varices were obliterated. Average follow-up was 530 days (7).

a. Short-Term Outcome (see Table 15-24)

(1) Shunt surgery did not improve survival during the index hospitalization.

(2) Sclerotherapy was associated with a shorter hospital stay ($P<0.0007$)

Table 15-23 PRCT of medical therapy vs. shunt surgery (25)

	Medical Therapy (n=22)	Shunt Surgery (n=21)	*P*
Child's class C	27%	52%	?
In-hospital mortality rate	55%	19%	<0.01
3-Y mortality rate	73%	33%	<0.01
Permanent control of GI bleeding	45%	100%	<0.01

Table 15-24 PRCT of sclerotherapy vs. shunt surgery: short-term outcome

	Sclerotherapy (n=32)	Shunt Surgery (n=32)	*P*
In-hospital mortality rate	50%	56%	NS
Length of index hospitalizations	13.7 d	17.3 d	0.0007
Blood transfusion requirement during index hospitalization	12.2 units	20.1 units	0.0001

and lower blood transfusion requirements ($P<0.0001$), compared with shunt surgery.

b. Long-Term Outcome (see Table 15-25)

(1) Among survivors of the index hospitalization, shunt surgery decreased the risk of recurrent bleeding ($P<0.0001$). Furthermore, 44% of patients, who underwent sclerotherapy and survived the index hospitalization eventually required a shunt operation because of recurrent bleeding.

(2) The survival rates were similar in the two groups.

(3) Shunt surgery did not increase the risk of hepatic encephalopathy.

4. Summary of the Role of Emergency Shunt Surgery for the Management of Acute Variceal Bleeding

a. Emergency shunt surgery is more effective than vasopressin or balloon tamponade in controlling bleeding, and, when performed by an exceptionally skilled surgeon, it may improve survival.

b. However, in the short-term, emergency shunt surgery is not better than sclerotherapy, which is associated with a shorter hospital stay and lower blood transfusion requirements.

c. In the long-term, the risk of rebleeding is lower with shunt surgery than with sclerotherapy.

d. Overall mortality rates appear to be similar with sclerotherapy and shunt surgery.

G. Esophageal Transection for the Management of Acute Variceal Bleeding

1. Although there are many variations, the basic procedure for esophageal transection involves insertion of a staple gun into the esophagus through a small gastrotomy, transection of the esophagus and reconnection of the two ends. Transection is usually combined with varying degrees of devascularization (5,36). Although this operation is technically easier than a shunt operation and lies within the ability of general surgeons, it is rarely performed in the United States.

2. Esophageal Transection Versus Sclerotherapy—Burroughs described a PRCT involving 101 patients with hematemesis or melena and endoscopically confirmed variceal bleeding who did not respond to blood transfusions or vasoactive drugs. Patients with portal hypertension not caused by cirrhosis were

Table 15-25 PRCT of sclerotherapy vs. shunt surgery: long-term outcome

	Sclerotherapy (n=16)	Shunt Surgery (n=14)	*P*
% of patients with recurrent bleeding requiring hospitalization	75%	0%	0.0001
Blood transfusion requirement since index hospitalization	6.1 units	0.7 units	0.0001
Encephalopathy requiring hospitalization	1.6%	1.4%	NS
18-Mo mortality rate	72%	88%	NS

excluded. Staple transection of the esophagus was compared with sclerotherapy (intravariceal injection of 5% ethanolamine administered for recurrent or persistent bleeding, up to three times within 5 days of the first injection). Control of bleeding was defined as the absence of bleeding for 5 days (5) (see Table 15-26).

a. Transection controlled acute bleeding better than sclerotherapy (88% versus 62%, respectively). However, when the results of up to three sessions of sclerotherapy were compared with those of transection, the success rates were similar (88% versus 82%, respectively).

b. The transfusion requirement was lower with transection. However, the statistical significance of this finding was not reported.

c. The 6-week and 1-year mortality rates were similar in the two groups.

d. When the data were analyzed according to treatment received rather than by an intention-to-treat analysis, the 6-week risk of rebleeding was lower with transection than with one session of sclerotherapy. It may have been more meaningful to compare transection with chronic sclerotherapy, but this analysis was not done.

3. The Sugiura procedure (gastric devascularization) has been successful in Japan, where rebleeding rates as low as 6% and operative mortality rates of 13% have been reported. Most of the reported experiences have been with elective cases (4,33). In Western countries, where alcoholic liver disease predominates, operative mortality with this procedure has ranged from 50% to 100%, depending on patient selection (20). In addition, unlike esophageal transection, the Sugiura procedure is not simple. It therefore has been abandoned by most experts in Western countries.

4. Summary of the Role of Esophageal Transection in Acute Variceal Bleeding (4,20,22)

a. Some authors favor the use of esophageal transection as primary therapy for bleeding varices. It appears to be at least as effective as sclerotherapy in stopping the bleeding episode.

b. However, the operative mortality for emergency esophageal transection has ranged from 28% to 90%, depending on patient selection. Furthermore, the long-term risk of rebleeding is reported to be as high as 50% (5,20). Therefore, most authors have abandoned this procedure entirely in the emergency setting (5,20). It may still be useful for patients who are refractory to sclerotherapy and for those who are not candidates for emergency shunt surgery or liver transplantation.

c. The Sugiura procedure probably has no role in emergency management of alcohol-related cirrhotic patients with bleeding varices.

H. Other Treatment Options for the Management of Acute Variceal Bleeding

1. Transjugular Intrahepatic Portosystemic Shunts—An uncontrolled study reported the efficacy and safety of TIPS in 100 patients (29). However, only 10 of these patients were treated on an emergency basis, making meaningful conclusions impossible. Although this technique holds some promise, the efficacy of the procedure in controlling bleeding may be offset by the risk of hepatic encephalopathy and shunt stenosis or occlusion. Controlled studies are neces-

Table 15-26 PRCT of sclerotherapy vs. esophageal transection

	Sclerotherapy (n=50)	Transection (n=51)	*P*
Control of bleeding	62% (after 1 session)	88%	<0.01
	82% (up to 3 sessions)	88%	?
Blood transfusion requirement	380 units	291 units	?
6-Wk mortality rate	44%	35%	NS
12-Mo mortality rate	58%	55%	NS
6-Wk rebleeding rate	42% (after 1 session)	7%	<0.001

sary to define the role of TIPS in the emergency management of acute variceal bleeding. (See Chapter 16 for further discussion.)

2. **Liver Transplantation**—Liver transplantation is the only treatment option that is aimed at restoring normal liver function. With the advent of improved immunosuppressive techniques, the 5-year survival rate has been reported to be 60% to 70% (15). Transplantation should be considered for appropriate candidates who present with variceal bleeding. (See Chapter 16 for further details.)

I. Conclusions

1. Pharmacotherapy with vasopressin, somatostatin, or octreotide can be useful for the temporary control of acute variceal bleeding. When vasopressin is used, IV TNG should be administered in combination to decrease the risk of complications. Somatostatin also appears to cause fewer complications than vasopressin. Octreotide appears to be more promising than vasopressin or somatostatin but awaits further validation. Because drug therapy is associated with a high risk of rebleeding, more definitive therapy (*i.e.*, sclerotherapy or banding) should be performed as soon as possible.
2. Balloon tamponade has become a second-line therapy because it is associated with a high risk of rebleeding and complications. It also does not offer any advantages over drug therapy and is inferior to sclerotherapy. However, balloon tamponade can still be useful if drug therapy fails and when sclerotherapy is not immediately available.
3. As soon as possible, endoscopic sclerotherapy or banding should be attempted. Many studies have found sclerotherapy to be more effective than drug therapy or tamponade. Emergency sclerotherapy also appears to be more effective in the short run than emergency shunt surgery. The immediate bleeding episode can be controlled by repeated sclerotherapy in about 85% to 90% of cases.
4. Banding appears to be as effective as sclerotherapy, and it is probably safer. Acute variceal bleeding can be controlled with fewer sessions of banding than of sclerotherapy.
5. About 10% to 15% of cases remain refractory to two sessions of sclerotherapy. Treatment options in this group include shunt surgery, transection, and liver transplantation. TIPS holds some promise for the future, but further studies are necessary to define its role in the emergency management of acute variceal bleeding.
6. Although sclerotherapy is highly effective in the short-term control of acute variceal bleeding, a secondary prophylactic measure is needed to decrease the risk of recurrent bleeding. These treatment options include β-blockers, chronic sclerotherapy or banding, shunt surgery, TIPS, esophageal transection, and liver transplantation (see Chapter 16).

Abbreviations used in Chapter 15

ARDS = adult respiratory distress syndrome
bpm = beats per minute
CI = cardiac index
DSR = distal splenorenal
D5W = 5% dextrose in water
GI = gastrointestinal
HR = heart rate
HVPG = hepatic vein pressure gradient
IV = intravenous
LVSWI = left ventricular stroke work index
MAP = mean arterial pressure
NG = nasogastric
NS = not significant
P = probability value

PCWP = pulmonary capillary wedge pressure
PRBC = packed red blood cells
PRCT = prospective randomized controlled trial
q = every
RAP = right atrial pressure
SVRI = systemic vascular resistance index
TIPS = transjugular intrahepatic portosystemic shunt
TNG = nitroglycerin
UGI = upper gastrointestinal
vs. = versus
WHVP = wedged hepatic vein pressure

References

1. Bangarani. Effect of somatostatin in controlling bleeding from esophageal varices. *Ital J Surg Sci* 1987;17:21.
2. Barsoum. Tamponade and injection sclerotherapy in the management of bleeding esophageal varices. *Br J Surg* 1982;69:76.
3. Bosch. Association of transdermal nitroglycerin to vasopressin infusion in the treatment of variceal hemorrhage: a placebo controlled clinical trial. *Hepatology* 1989;10:962.
4. Brewer. Treatment of acute gastroesophageal variceal hemorrhage. *Med Clin North Am* 1993;77:993. Review.
5. Burroughs. A comparison of sclerotherapy with staple transection of the esophagus for the emergency control of bleeding from esophageal varices. *N Engl J Med* 1989;321:857.
6. Burroughs. Randomized, double-blind, placebo-controlled trial of somatostatin for variceal bleeding. *Gastroenterology* 1990;99:1388.
7. Cello. Endoscopic sclerotherapy versus portacaval shunt in patients with severe cirrhosis and acute variceal hemorrhage: long term follow-up. *N Engl J Med* 1987; 316:11.
8. Chojkier. A controlled comparison of continuous intraarterial and intravenous infusions of vasopressin in hemorrhage from esophageal varices. *Gastroenterology* 1979;77:540.
9. Copenhagen Esophageal Varices Sclerotherapy Project. Sclerotherapy after first variceal hemorrhage in cirrhosis. *N Engl J Med* 1984;311:1594.
10. Correia. Controlled trial of vasopressin and balloon tamponade in bleeding esophageal varices. *Hepatology* 1984;4:885.
11. Danaji. Prevention of bacterial endocarditis. *JAMA* 1990;264:2919.
12. Fogel. Continuous intravenous vasopressin in active upper gastrointestinal bleeding. *Ann Intern Med* 1982;96:565.
13. Gimson. A randomized trial of vasopressin and vasopressin plus nitroglycerin in the control of acute variceal hemorrhage. *Hepatology* 1986;6:410.
14. Gimson. Randomised trial of variceal banding ligation versus injection sclerotherapy for bleeding oesophageal varices. *Lancet* 1993;342(8868):391.
15. Henderson. Liver transplantation for portal hypertension. *Gastroenterol Clin North Am* 1992;21:197. Review.
16. Jenkins. A prospective randomized controlled clinical trial comparing somatostatin and vasopressin in controlling acute variceal hemorrhage. *Br Med J* 1985; 290:275.
17. Jensen. Diagnosis and treatment of severe hematochezia: the role of urgent colonoscopy after purge. *Gastroenterology* 1988;95:1569.
18. Kravetz. Comparison of intravenous somatostatin and vasopressin infusions in treatment of acute variceal hemorrhage. *Hepatology* 1984;4:442.
19. Laine. Endoscopic ligation compared with sclerotherapy for the treatment of bleeding esophageal varices. *Ann Intern Med* 1993;119:1.
20. Langer. Emergency surgical treatment of variceal hemorrhage. *Surg Clin North Am* 1990;70:307. Review.

21. Larson. Acute esophageal variceal sclerotherapy. *JAMA* 1986;255:497.
22. Matloff. Treatment of acute variceal bleeding. *Gastroenterol Clin North Am* 1992; 21:103. Review.
23. Merigan. Effect of intravenously administered posterior pituitary extract on hemorrhage from bleeding esophageal varices. *N Engl J Med* 1962;266:134.
24. Moreto. A randomized trial of tamponade or sclerotherapy as immediate treatment for bleeding esophageal varices. *Surg Gynecol Obstet* 1988;167:331.
25. Orloff. A prospective randomized trial of emergency portacaval shunt and medical therapy in unselected cirrhotic patients with bleeding varices. *Gastroenterology* 1986;90:1754. Abstract.
26. Panes. Efficacy of balloon tamponade in treatment of bleeding gastric and esophageal varices. *Dig Dis Sci* 1988;33:454.
27. Paquet. Endoscopic sclerosis and esophageal balloon tamponade in acute hemorrhage from esophagogastric varices: a prospective controlled randomized trial. *Hepatology* 1985;5:580.
28. Rodriguez-Perez. Pharmacologic treatment of portal hypertension. *Gastroenterol Clin North Am* 1992;21:15. Review.
29. Rossle. The transjugular intrahepatic portosystemic stent-shunt procedure for variceal bleeding. *N Engl J Med* 1994;330:165.
30. Saari. Comparison of somatostatin and vasopressin in bleeding esophageal varices. *Am J Gastroenterol* 1990;85:804.
31. Silverstein. The national ASGE survey on upper gastrointestinal bleeding II: Clinical prognostic factors. *Gastrointest Endosc* 1981;27:80.
32. Stiegmann. Endoscopic sclerotherapy as compared with endoscopic ligation for bleeding esophageal varices. *N Engl J Med* 1992;326:1527.
33. Sugiura. Esophageal transection with paraesophageal devascularizations (the Sugiura procedure) in the treatment of esophageal varices. *World J Surg* 1984;8:673.
34. Sung. Octreotide infusion or emergency sclerotherapy for variceal hemorrhage. *Lancet* 1993;342:637.
35. Terblanche. Acute bleeding varices: a five-year prospective evaluation of tamponade and sclerotherapy. *Ann Surg* 1981;194:521.
36. Terblanche. Controversies in the management of bleeding esophageal varices: part I. *N Engl J Med* 1989;320:1393. Review.
37. Tsai. Controlled trial of vasopressin plus nitroglycerin vs. vasopressin alone in the treatment of bleeding esophageal varices. *Hepatology* 1986;6:406.
38. Valenzuela. A multicenter, randomized, double-blind trial of somatostatin in the management of acute hemorrhage from esophageal varices. *Hepatology* 1989;10: 958.
39. Westaby. Hemodynamic response to intravenous vasopressin and nitroglycerin in portal hypertension. *Gut* 1988;29:372.
40. Westaby. Controlled clinical trial of injection sclerotherapy for active variceal bleeding. *Hepatology* 1989;9:274.

16 Variceal Bleeding: Secondary Prophylaxis

Burton W. Lee and
Lawrence S. Friedman

A. Once a patient has bled from varices, the risk of rebleeding is between 50% and 80% (32). Although most experts agree that some form of prophylactic therapy is necessary to decrease the risk of rebleeding, there is no consensus as to which therapy is optimal. Treatment options include pharmacotherapy, sclerotherapy, band ligation, shunt surgery, transjugular intrahepatic portosystemic shunt (TIPS), esophageal transection, and liver transplantation.

B. **β-Blockers for Secondary Prophylaxis of Variceal Bleeding**—Numerous prospective randomized controlled trials (PRCTs) have compared β-blockers versus no therapy for secondary prophylaxis of variceal bleeding. Some of these studies have favored β-blockers, but others have not (4).

1. An early study by Lebrec showed a significant benefit of propranolol compared with placebo. This PRCT involved 74 cirrhotic patients with recent gastrointestinal bleeding. Sixty-five patients had alcohol-related cirrhosis, and 5 had hepatitis B. Ascites, jaundice, and encephalopathy were absent, mild, or transient. On endoscopy, 56 cases were found to be caused by varices and 18 by gastritis. Patients were included in the study at a mean of 21 days from the bleeding. Most of the patients in the study had Child's class A cirrhosis. The study compared oral propranolol (given twice daily and titrated to decrease the resting heart rate by 25%) versus placebo. Follow-up was done every 2 months for the first year, then every 4 months for the second year. Data were analyzed according to the Kaplan–Meier method and by the log-rank test, which takes into account the follow-up duration of each patient. Only 20% of patients admitted for acute variceal bleeding were entered into the study (18) (see Table 16–1).
   - **a.** In this group of cirrhotic patients with stable liver function, propranolol significantly decreased the risk of rebleeding ($P<0.0001$). Rebleeding, when it occurred, usually did so within 3 months of the index episode.
   - **b.** Survival was also improved with propranolol ($P<0.02$), but the analysis excluded patients who were lost to follow-up. When these patients were included, the survival benefit was no longer statistically significant.
   - **c.** A separate analysis of patients with variceal bleeding did not alter the conclusions.
2. However, subsequent studies have not confirmed these findings. A representative study is described here. Burroughs described a PRCT involving 48 cirrhotic patients with previous endoscopically confirmed acute variceal bleeding. Placebo was compared with propranolol (titrated to decrease the heart rate by 25%). Patients were enrolled at an average of 12 days after the bleeding episode. Measurement of the hepatic vein pressure gradient (HVPG) was obtained for 10 patients in the propranolol group and 9 in the placebo group at baseline and 1 month after initiation of therapy. Patients were observed for 21 months. Ninety-two percent of all patients admitted for acute variceal bleeding during the study period were enrolled into the trial (2) (see Table 16–2).
   - **a.** Propranolol decreased the HVPG significantly. Despite this benefit, the risks of rebleeding and mortality were similar in the two groups.

Table 16-1 Lebrec's PRCT evaluating the role of propranolol (18)

	Propranolol (n=38)	Placebo (n=36)	*P*
No. varices/No. gastric erosions	28/10	28/8	?
% Lost to follow-up	21%	11%	?
% of patients free of any rebleeding at 2 y	79%	32%	<0.0001
% of patients free of variceal rebleeding at 2 y	86%	33%	<0.0001
% of patients free of rebleeding due to gastric erosions at 2 y	56%	25%	<0.05
2-Y survival rate excluding those lost to follow-up	90%	57%	<0.02
2-Y survival rate among variceal bleeding patients	91%	53%	<0.02

b. In contrast to Lebrec's study, this trial did not select for patients with stable liver function. Lebrec's patients were mostly in Child's class A or B, whereas many patients in this study had decompensated liver disease.

3. Summary of the Role of β-Blockers for the Secondary Prophylaxis of Variceal Bleeding

a. The data are conflicting regarding the value of β-blockers for secondary prophylaxis of variceal bleeding. Some studies have shown that β-blockers decrease the risk of rebleeding and improve the rate of survival, whereas others have not confirmed such benefit. Most authors do not recommend β-blockade as first-line therapy for secondary prophylaxis of variceal bleeding.

b. If there is a benefit to β-blockade, it may be limited to a subset of patients with alcoholic liver disease and stable liver function. β-Blockers do not appear to be useful in unselected patients.

c. In about 30% of patients, β-blockade does not significantly lower the portal pressure. There is no simple, noninvasive method by which to select patients who will respond favorably to β-blockade.

C. Sclerotherapy for Secondary Prophylaxis of Variceal Bleeding

1. Sclerotherapy is typically performed weekly for 3 to 4 weeks, then every 1 to 4 weeks until the varices are obliterated. Once eradicated, varices often recur, usually within 12 months of obliteration. Therefore, one popular schedule is to repeat endoscopy every 3 months for 1 year. If no varices are found, then endoscopy is performed every 6 months. If none is found after 2 years, endoscopy is performed yearly. Any recurrent varix found on endoscopy is treated promptly with repeat sclerotherapy (4,31).

2. Efficacy of Sclerotherapy for Secondary Prophylaxis of Variceal Bleeding

a. Sclerotherapy Versus No Therapy—Numerous trials have compared sclerotherapy with no elective therapy. A recent metaanalysis showed that sclerotherapy decreases the risks of rebleeding and mortality. The pooled

Table 16-2 Burrough's PRCT evaluating the role of propranolol (2)

	Propranolol (n=26)	Placebo (n=22)	*P*
Baseline HVPG (mm Hg)	18.1	18.7	NS
HVPG at 1 mo (mm Hg)	11.5	18.1	<0.01
% Rebleeding from varices	46.2%	50%	NS
Overall mortality	15.4%	22.7%	NS

relative risks of rebleeding and death were 0.56 ($P<0.05$) and 0.61 ($P<0.05$), respectively, favoring sclerotherapy in both parameters (4).

(1) As an example, Westaby described a PRCT involving 116 patients with endoscopically confirmed variceal bleeding. Only those patients surviving the first 48 hours of admission were entered into the study. Most patients had alcoholic liver disease, primary biliary cirrhosis, cryptogenic cirrhosis, or chronic active hepatitis. Emergency sclerotherapy followed by chronic sclerotherapy was compared with standard supportive measures. The initial bleeding event and the rebleeding events in the control group were not treated with sclerotherapy. Median length of follow-up was 37 months (36) (see Table 16–3).

(a) Sclerotherapy significantly decreased the risk of rebleeding ($P<0.01$).

(b) Sclerotherapy also significantly improved survival ($P<0.01$).

(2) Other studies have failed to confirm a survival benefit for sclerotherapy. An example is described here. Terblanche described a PRCT involving 75 patients with endoscopically confirmed massive variceal bleeding. Patients with persistent bleeding were managed with placement of a Sengstaken–Blakemore tube followed by emergency sclerotherapy. Medical management was compared with repeated sclerotherapy; all episodes of recurrent bleeding were managed with sclerotherapy. Sclerotherapy was performed with the use of a rigid endoscope under general anesthesia at 1 week, 1 month, and then every 3 months until the varices were obliterated. Twenty-five months into the study, the protocol was changed so that sclerotherapy was performed every 2 weeks until the varices were obliterated. Average follow-up was 5 years (29) (see Table 16–4).

(a) The percentage of patients who experienced recurrent bleeding (P=NS) and the number of episodes of recurrent bleeding ($P<0.004$) were lower with sclerotherapy. Furthermore, the bleeding episodes in the control group were more often severe or life-threatening.

(b) However, there was no difference in mortality between the two groups.

b. Sclerotherapy Versus β-Blockers—Numerous studies have compared sclerotherapy with β-blockers. In a metaanalysis of these studies, the

Table 16-3 Westaby's PRCT evaluating the role of sclerotherapy (36)

	Standard Therapy (n=60)	Sclerotherapy (n=56)	*P*
% of patients with recurrent bleeding	80%	55%	<0.01
No. of rebleeding episodes	125	66	<0.01
Mortality rate	53%	32%	<0.01

Table 16-4 Terblanche's PRCT evaluating the role of sclerotherapy (29)

	Control Group (n=38)	Sclerotherapy (n=37)	*P*
Number of recurrent bleeding	73	43	<0.004
% of patients with recurrent bleeding	77%	58%	NS
Number of patients surviving 1 mo	26	24	NS
Overall mortality rate	63%	62%	NS

pooled relative risk of rebleeding was 0.62 ($P<0.05$), favoring sclerotherapy. There was no difference in survival between the two groups. However, firm conclusions cannot be made because there was significant statistical heterogeneity ($P<0.04$) in these studies (4).

(1) The study described here serves as an example. Alexandrino's PRCT involved 65 patients with Child's class A or B cirrhosis with endoscopically proven variceal bleeding. Intravariceal sclerotherapy every 3 weeks was compared with propranolol (titrated to decrease the resting heart rate by 25%). Follow-up ranged from 17 to 57 months (1) (see Table 16–5).

(a) Sclerotherapy was more effective than propranolol in decreasing the risk of variceal rebleeding ($P<0.02$).

(b) However, the risk of rebleeding from any source and the rate of survival were statistically similar in the two groups.

(2) Other studies have not found a significant difference between propranolol and sclerotherapy. For example, Westaby described a PRCT involving 108 cirrhotic patients with endoscopically confirmed acute variceal bleeding. Only those who had stopped bleeding at the time of endoscopy were entered into the trial. All Child–Pugh class C patients as well as those who had contraindications to β-blockade were excluded. Propranolol (given BID to decrease the resting heart rate by 25%) was compared with sclerotherapy (given every week for 3 weeks, then every 3 to 4 weeks until the varices were obliterated). Surveillance endoscopy was performed in both groups. Rebleeding episodes in the sclerotherapy group were treated with emergency sclerotherapy. Patients randomly assigned to receive propranolol and who were actively bleeding at the time of endoscopy were treated with sclerotherapy, whereas those who had spontaneously stopped bleeding were continued on propranolol alone. An intention-to-treat analysis was used (38) (see Table 16–6).

(a) The risks of rebleeding and the survival rates were similar in the two groups.

(b) Twenty-seven percent of patients treated with propranolol crossed over to sclerotherapy because of severe or recurrent rebleeding. Therefore, an intention-to-treat analysis may have overlooked a potential advantage of sclerotherapy. However, exclusion of these patients from the analysis did not significantly alter the results.

(c) Since all patients in this study had well-compensated cirrhosis, they were the patients most likely to have benefited from β-blockade (18). However, a similar study involving unselected patients also failed to show any significant difference between propranolol and sclerotherapy (6).

c. Sclerotherapy Versus Sclerotherapy With β-Blockade—Although a metaanalysis showed no benefit from addition of β-blockers to chronic sclerotherapy, a significant statistical heterogeneity of results among the studies precluded firm conclusions (4).

Table 16-5 Alexandrino's PRCT of sclerotherapy vs. propranolol (1)

	Propranolol (n=34)	Sclerotherapy (n=31)	*P*
% of patients free of rebleeding from esophageal varices	25%	67%	<0.02
% of patients free of rebleeding from any source	16%	37%	NS
Cumulative survival rate	54%	69%	NS

Table 16-6 Westaby's PRCT of sclerotherapy vs. propranolol (38)

	Propranolol (n=52)	Sclerotherapy (n=56)	*P*
% of patients with recurrent bleeding	54%	45%	NS
Risk of rebleeding per patient per month	0.05	0.037	NS
3-Y cumulative survival rate	53%	66%	NS

(1) An example of a study favoring the addition of β-blockade to sclerotherapy is described here. Vinel described a PRCT involving 75 cirrhotic patients with endoscopically proven variceal bleeding. After initial control of bleeding, the study compared sclerotherapy versus sclerotherapy plus propranolol. Patients were observed until the varices were eradicated. Results have been reported in an abstract (35) (see Table 16–7).

(a) The addition of propranolol significantly decreased the number of episodes of variceal rebleeding ($P<0.01$).

(b) The effect of propranolol on survival was not reported.

(2) An example of a study that showed no advantage of adding propranolol to sclerotherapy is described here. Westaby described a PRCT involving 53 patients with endoscopically confirmed variceal bleeding. Most but not all patients had cirrhosis. The initial bleeding episode was stabilized, after which sclerotherapy was compared with sclerotherapy plus propranolol (titrated to decrease the heart rate by 25%). Sclerotherapy was performed weekly for 3 weeks, then every 1 to 3 weeks until the varices were obliterated (37) (see Table 16–8).

(a) There was no difference in the rate of rebleeding.

(b) The mortality rates were also similar between the two groups.

d. Summary of the Role of Sclerotherapy for Secondary Prophylaxis of Variceal Rebleeding

(1) Chronic sclerotherapy has emerged as the treatment of choice for secondary prophylaxis against variceal bleeding. It has become popular because it can be performed relatively easily by a large number of physicians; it avoids the risk of a major operation; and it does not contribute to the risk of hepatic encephalopathy.

Table 16-7 Vinel's PRCT of sclerotherapy vs. propranolol & sclerotherapy (35)

	Sclerotherapy Alone (n=36)	Sclerotherapy Plus Propranolol (n=39)	*P*
No. of episodes of rebleeding from any cause	17	8	NS
No. of episodes of rebleeding from varices	13	4	<0.01

Table 16-8 Westaby's PRCT of sclerotherapy vs. propranolol & sclerotherapy (37)

	Sclerotherapy Alone (n=27)	Sclerotherapy Plus Propranolol (n=26)	*P*
% of patients with an episode of rebleeding	30%	27%	NS
Cumulative risk of death	26%	35%	NS

(2) Most of the studies that compared sclerotherapy versus no elective therapy clearly documented a decrease in the risk of rebleeding with sclerotherapy. Some but not all studies also showed a survival benefit.

(3) Among studies that compared β-blockers versus sclerotherapy, some showed the two modalities to be equally effective, and others showed sclerotherapy to be superior. A metaanalysis favored sclerotherapy, but there was too much statistical heterogeneity to reach any firm conclusions. The addition of β-blockers to chronic sclerotherapy has not conclusively improved outcome.

(4) The efficacy of sclerotherapy is eventually limited by the fact that the underlying portal hypertension and liver dysfunction persist. Even if the esophageal varices are successfully obliterated, patients can still bleed from recurrent esophageal varices, gastric varices, or portal hypertensive gastropathy. About 40% of patients who successfully complete variceal obliteration eventually rebleed. In addition, surveillance endoscopy is required indefinitely. This can be expensive and time-consuming. Noncompliance of alcoholic patients may also limit the utility of this treatment.

D. Endoscopic Band Ligation for Secondary Prophylaxis of Variceal Bleeding–Banding is a relatively new procedure that uses an endoscopically introduced O-ring to strangle a varix. The technique does not involve needles or chemicals. Three major trials have compared banding versus sclerotherapy (7,16,27). The details of these trials are fully discussed in Chapter 15. Only the points relevant to secondary prophylaxis of variceal bleeding are reiterated here.

1. In the short term, the risks of recurrent bleeding or death with banding are similar to those with sclerotherapy.
2. In one study, banding was associated with improved survival compared with sclerotherapy (27). In the other two studies, survival rates were similar in the two groups (7,16).
3. Fewer treatment sessions were required to eradicate the varices with banding than with sclerotherapy (16).
4. The complication rate may be lower with banding (16,27).
5. Preliminary data suggest that banding may be safer and more effective than sclerotherapy. In some centers, it has replaced sclerotherapy.

E. Shunt Surgery for Secondary Prophylaxis of Variceal Bleeding

1. During the past decade, the number of portosystemic shunt operations has declined markedly because of the popularity of sclerotherapy and the growing availability of liver transplantation. The emergence of TIPS procedure may further challenge the role of surgical shunts in the future. Various types of shunt operations were discussed in detail in Chapter 14.
2. **Efficacy of Surgical Shunt Operations for the Secondary Prophylaxis of Variceal Bleeding**

a. **Shunt Surgery Versus No Treatment**—Four PRCTs have compared nonselective shunt operations with no treatment (15,21,22,25). As a whole, these studies showed that shunt surgery decreases the risk of rebleeding, worsens the risk of encephalopathy, and does not change the survival rate.

(1) The study by Reynolds serves as an example (22). This PRCT involved 89 patients with biopsy-confirmed alcoholic cirrhosis and endoscopically confirmed variceal bleeding. All patients had portal hypertension confirmed by catheterization. Candidates for surgery were randomly assigned to receive either medical (supportive) therapy or end-to-side portacaval shunts. Patients were observed for at least 5 years. Four patients randomly assigned to receive surgery did not receive the shunt, and 11 patients randomly assigned to receive medical therapy were ultimately treated with surgery. It is not clearly described whether an intention-to-treat analysis was used.

(a) The risk of rebleeding was lower with surgery than with medical therapy (11 versus 190 episodes, respectively). Although this difference is dramatic, no statistical values were reported.

(b) The risk of hepatic encephalopathy was reported to be significantly higher with surgery. However, the rate of encephalopathy in the medical group was not reported. Therefore, a decrease in the risk of rebleeding was balanced by an increase in the risk of encephalopathy with surgery.

(c) There was no significant difference in survival (Table 16–9).

(2) An important criticism of these studies is that the trials randomized only a small percentage of cirrhotic patients who presented with variceal bleeding (range, 9% to 30%). Second, 16% to 37% of patients assigned to the control group crossed over and underwent surgery, whereas 20% of patients assigned to surgery did not undergo surgery. Such a large percentage of crossover patients makes the interpretation of results more difficult (4,15,21,22,25).

b. Distal Splenorenal Shunts Versus Nonselective Shunts—The lack of survival benefit and increased risk of encephalopathy with nonselective shunts encouraged the development of the distal splenorenal (DSR) shunt. The DSR shunt was designed to decrease the risk of encephalopathy by maintaining hepatopetal blood flow while achieving selective portal decompression. Six PRCTs have compared DSR shunts with nonselective shunts, predominantly in alcoholic patients (5,8,9,17,19,20). Trials have ranged in size from 41 to 81 patients. The results of these studies have been mixed, and firm conclusions are not possible.

(1) Warren was the first to introduce the DSR shunt operation. A 10-year study from his group at Emory is described here. (19) This PRCT involved 55 biopsy-confirmed cirrhotic patients with variceal bleeding and documented hepatopetal blood flow on angiogram. Patients with significant ascites or any evidence of encephalopathy were excluded. The DSR shunt was compared with various nonselective shunts. An H-graft interposition shunt was the nonselective shunt used in most patients. Two patients randomly assigned to receive a DSR shunt instead received nonselective shunts, and 1 patient randomly assigned to receive a nonselective shunt received a DSR shunt instead. Minimum follow-up was 110 months. Data were analyzed according to treatment received. The study was terminated early because the DSR shunt was shown to be superior to nonselective shunts (see Table 16–10).

(a) The risks of both rebleeding and encephalopathy were lower with DSR shunts than nonselective shunts.

(b) There was no significant difference in overall survival. However, for nonalcoholic patients, the survival rate was better with the DSR shunt. This difference was attributed to a higher rate of shunt patency for nonalcoholic than alcoholic patients.

(c) This study has been criticized because H-graft interposition shunts may have a higher occlusion rate than other nonselective shunts (9). Furthermore, although portacaval shunts have been shown to decrease the risk of rebleeding, the efficacy of H-graft interposition shunts is less well established.

(2) Other studies have not confirmed Warren's findings. One study showing

Table 16-9 Reynold's PRCT evaluating the role of portacaval shunt surgery (22)

	End-To-Side Portacaval Shunt Surgery (n=45)	Medical Therapy (n=44)	*P*
No. of episodes of rebleeding	11	190	?
% of patients developing hepatic encephalopathy	49%	?	?
Overall mortality rate	58%	66%	NS

Table 16-10 Warren's PRCT of selective vs. nonselective shunt surgery (19)

	Nonselective Shunt (n=29)	DSR Shunt (n=26)	*P*
No. of episodes of rebleeding in 10 y	13	8	?
Risk of encephalopathy	75%	27%	<0.01
10-Y survival rate	28%	41%	NS
10-Y survival in nonalcoholic patients	29%	63%	?

opposite results from those of the Emory study is described here. Harley's PRCT involved 54 patients with biopsy-proven alcoholic cirrhosis and recurrent variceal bleeding. The DSR shunt was compared with the end-to-side portacaval shunt. Median follow-up was 31 months (9) (see Table 16–11).

(a) The risk of variceal rebleeding was actually higher with DSR shunts (30% versus 4%).

(b) The risk of hepatic encephalopathy and the rate of survival were similar.

(3) As illustrated by the two trials just described, the results of these six studies have been mixed. A metaanalysis was done to pool the data from these small studies (4).

(a) Three of the six studies found no significant difference in the risk of rebleeding (5,8,17). One study found this risk to be higher (9) and another study found it to be lower with the DSR shunt (19). One study did not report this end point (20). A metaanalysis of these studies revealed a similar risk of rebleeding with either procedure (4).

(b) Three of the six studies found a lower risk of encephalopathy with the DSR shunt (17,19,20), but the other three studies found no difference (5,8,9). In the metaanalysis, the pooled relative risk of hepatic encephalopathy was 2.0 in favor of DSR shunts, but this finding was not statistically significant (4).

c. DSR Shunt Surgery Versus Sclerotherapy—Four major randomized controlled studies have compared DSR shunts versus sclerotherapy for secondary prophylaxis of variceal rebleeding (10,23,26,33). A summary of the major findings in these studies is presented in Table 16-12.

(1) Risk of Rebleeding—All four studies found the DSR shunt to be better than sclerotherapy in decreasing the risk of rebleeding (10,23,26, 33). A representative study is described here. Spina described a PRCT involving 40 patients with biopsy-confirmed Child's class A or B cirrhosis and a history of endoscopically proven variceal hemorrhage. The DSR shunt was compared with sclerotherapy. Surgery was done by a single team, and splenopancreatic disconnection (meticulous lig-

Table 16-11 Harley's PRCT of selective vs. nonselective shunt surgery (9)

	End-to-Side Portacaval Shunt (n=27)	DSR Shunt (n=27)	*P*
Risk of upper GI rebleeding	33%	42%	?
Risk of variceal rebleeding	4%	30%	?
Risk of encephalopathy	32%	39%	NS
Perioperative mortality	6.4%	11.5%	NS
Cumulative 5-y survival	31%	43%	NS

Table 16-12 Summary of major trials comparing DSR shunts vs. sclerotherapy

Author (Reference)	Treatment With Lower Risk of Rebleeding	Treatment With Lower Risk of Encephalopathy	Treatment With Better Survival Rate
Rikkers (23)	DSR shunt surgery	Same	Same
Spina (26)	DSR shunt surgery	Same	Same
Teres (33)	DSR shunt surgery	Sclerotherapy	Same
Henderson (10)	DSR shunt surgery	Not addressed	Sclerotherapy

ation of collaterals between the spleen and pancreas) was performed if appropriate (26) (see Table 16–13).

(a) The DSR shunt was superior to sclerotherapy in decreasing the risk of rebleeding.

(b) There was no major difference in the risk of encephalopathy or the rate of survival.

(2) Risk of Hepatic Encephalopathy—The relative effects of shunt surgery and sclerotherapy on the risk of encephalopathy are more controversial. Two studies found the risk to be similar with either procedure (23,26). One study did not directly report this end point (10). However, Teres found DSR shunts to be associated with an increased risk of encephalopathy. This PRCT involved 112 Child's class A or B cirrhotic patients with endoscopically confirmed variceal bleeding. Patients were randomly assigned to receive either DSR shunts or sclerotherapy after they had been stable for 10 to 15 days. Sclerotherapy was performed weekly until varices were obliterated. Splenopancreatic disconnection was not performed (33) (see Table 16–14).

(a) A decreased risk of rebleeding was balanced by an increased risk of encephalopathy with the DSR shunt.

(b) The survival rates were similar in the two groups.

(c) The patients who received sclerotherapy patients had poorer liver function at baseline than those who received shunts. Therefore, the study may have been biased against sclerotherapy. On the other hand, splenopancreatic disconnection was not performed as part of the DSR shunt surgery, and so these patients may not have received the most optimal shunt.

(3) Survival Rate—Three of the four studies showed no difference in survival between the two procedures (23,26,33). However, one study found better rates of survival with sclerotherapy (10). This study is described here for illustration. Henderson's PRCT involved 72 patients with biopsy-confirmed cirrhosis, previous variceal hemorrhage, and no contraindication to sclerotherapy or DSR shunt surgery. No patient had been treated with chronic sclerotherapy. The DSR shunt was compared with sclerotherapy. Sclerotherapy was performed weekly, then biweekly, then monthly as determined by the response of

Table 16-13 Spina's PRCT of DSR shunt surgery vs. sclerotherapy (26)

	Sclerotherapy (n=20)	Shunt Surgery (n=20)	*P*
Risk of rebleeding	35%	5%	<0.05
Risk of encephalopathy requiring hospitalization	21%	25%	NS
2-Y survival rate	90%	95%	NS

Table 16-14 Teres' PRCT of DSR shunt surgery vs. sclerotherapy (33)

	Sclerotherapy (n=55)	Shunt Surgery (n=57)	*P*
Patients excluded	4	14	<0.02
Risk of variceal rebleeding	37.5%	14.3%	<0.02
Risk of hepatic encephalopathy	8%	24%	<0.05
2-Y survival rate	68%	71%	NS

the varices to treatment. Splenopancreatic decompression was added to the standard DSR shunt procedure, if appropriate. Failure of therapy was defined as death or refractory rebleeding. Patients with persistent bleeding despite chronic sclerotherapy were treated with shunt surgery. Median follow-up was 61 months. An intention-to-treat analysis was used (see Table 16–15).

(a) The risk of rebleeding was significantly lower with shunt surgery than sclerotherapy.

(b) The risk of hepatic encephalopathy was not specifically addressed in the study.

(c) Sclerotherapy was associated with a better survival rate than DSR shunt surgery. Interestingly, this study was performed at Emory University by the same people who popularized the DSR shunt. In addition, splenopancreatic disconnection was performed whenever appropriate, and intention-to-treat analysis was used. Therefore, this study appears to have been done carefully by competent surgeons using optimal technique. Nevertheless, shunt surgery was associated with a poorer 4-year survival rate.

(d) A subgroup analysis revealed a persistent survival advantage of sclerotherapy in alcoholic patients (P=0.01). No significant difference was found among nonalcoholic patients. Therefore, DSR shunts may be more favorable for nonalcoholic patients than for alcoholic patients.

3. Summary of the Role of Shunt Surgery for Secondary Prophylaxis of Variceal Bleeding

a. Shunt surgery is highly effective in decreasing the risk of rebleeding. Both the portacaval shunt and the DSR shunt decrease the risk of rebleeding better than repeated sclerotherapy.

b. However, portacaval shunt surgery is associated with a higher risk of encephalopathy than is sclerotherapy. The DSR shunt was designed to minimize the risk of encephalopathy, but whether it succeeds in this goal is still controversial. Despite numerous trials, no firm conclusions are possible, because the results have been mixed.

c. Survival benefit has not been demonstrated convincingly with any form of shunt surgery. In fact, one trial found survival to be better with sclerother-

Table 16-15 Henderson's PRCT of DSR shunt surgery vs. sclerotherapy (10)

	Sclerotherapy (n=37)	Shunt Surgery (n=35)	*P*
Alcoholic liver disease	62%	57%	NS
Child's class C	43%	43%	NS
Risk of recurrent bleeding	59%	3%	0.001
4-Y survival rate	65%	43%	0.02

apy than with DSR shunts, provided that sclerotherapy was backed by rescue shunt surgery. Therefore, most authors favor repeated sclerotherapy as the first-line prophylactic treatment against variceal rebleeding, reserving shunt surgery for those patients whose disease remains refractory to sclerotherapy. In the meantime, the role of surgical shunts is being further challenged by the growing availability of liver transplantation and the emergence of the TIPS procedure.

d. If a surgical shunt is to be performed, most authors prefer the DSR shunt because of the theoretically lower risk of encephalopathy; however, this point remains controversial. The DSR shunt operation is also preferred because it does not involve the porta hepatis and hence does not interfere with the prospect for future liver transplantation. Some recommend the addition of total splenopancreatic disconnection to the standard DSR shunt procedure to prolong the selectivity of the shunt, but the benefit of this modification remains unproven.

e. In patients with refractory ascites, a side-to-side portacaval shunt should be performed, because the DSR shunts do not provide adequate relief of ascites. Similarly, in an emergency situation, a portacaval shunt is preferred, because the DSR shunts are technically more demanding and time-consuming to perform. For unclear reasons, some authors have observed a poorer outcome with DSR shunts in alcoholic patients than in nonalcoholic patients.

F. TIPS for Secondary Prophylaxis of Variceal Bleeding

1. TIPS involves introduction of a catheter and a curved needle through a transjugular approach into a right hepatic vein. Under ultrasound guidance, the needle and catheter are advanced into an intrahepatic branch of the portal vein. An expandable tubular wire-mesh stent is introduced by means of a guidewire; the stent expands to an appropriate diameter to create a portosystemic shunt. The diameter of the shunt varies from 8 to 12 mm, and the goal is to reduce the HVPG to <12 mm Hg (24).

2. Theoretically TIPS has a number of advantages over other treatment methods.

a. Like surgical shunts, the TIPS is designed to relieve portal hypertension permanently. In this sense, it is more attractive than pharmacotherapy, esophageal transection, or sclerotherapy, because these therapies do not reduce the portal pressure reliably or permanently.

b. Unlike shunt surgery, TIPS does not involve a major operation nor does it require general anesthesia. It is therefore thought to be safer. It can also be done in 1 to 3 hours by an experienced interventional radiologist.

c. Furthermore, unlike surgical shunts, the diameter of a TIPS shunt can be modified by percutaneous catheterization. Also, shunt malfunctions or occlusions can be corrected relatively easily by another TIPS procedure.

d. Because TIPS does not involve an abdominal operation and the shunt is entirely intrahepatic, it does not interfere with future liver transplantation. For this reason, TIPS is being used as a temporary bridge to transplantation in many centers.

3. Efficacy of TIPS for Secondary Prophylaxis of Variceal Bleeding

a. A representative uncontrolled study reporting the efficacy and safety of TIPS in 100 cirrhotic patients with variceal bleeding is summarized below. Ten TIPS were placed to control acute bleeding, and 90 were placed electively. Before shunt placement, all patients received lactulose, and in patients with tense ascites, therapeutic paracentesis was performed. Most patients had failed sclerotherapy at other centers and had been referred for further management. Twenty-two percent had Child's class C cirrhosis. The diameter of the stent was adjusted to decrease the HVPG to <12 mm Hg. After the procedure, heparin was given for 1 month, except to patients with severe coagulopathy or thrombocytopenia. Mean follow-up was 12 months (24).

(1) TIPS was technically successful in 93% of cases. The procedure was completed in a mean of 1.2 hours. On average, the portal pressure was reduced by 57%, and the portal flow velocity increased 2.5-fold.

(2) Major complications occurred in 15% of patients and included intraabdominal hemorrhage, intrahepatic hemorrhage, biliary bleeding, and migration of the stent into the pulmonary artery. The 30-day mortality rate was 3%. Thirty-one percent of the patients had stent stenosis or occlusion. All shunt failures were easily treated with dilation, thrombolysis, or additional TIPS procedures.

(3) Eighty-two percent of patients were free of variceal rebleeding at 1 year.

(4) Hepatic encephalopathy occurred in 25% of patients.

(5) The 1-year survival rate was 85%.

b. In another uncontrolled study involving 90 patients who underwent a TIPS procedure for management of variceal bleeding (30 emergent and 60 elective procedures), the cumulative risk of rebleeding at 2 years was 32%, and the 2-year survival rate was 51% (15a). The shunt patency rate was only 53% at 2 years but 95% of the occlusions or stenosis responded successfully to percutaneous revision of the shunt.

c. A PRCT compared TIPS with sclerotherapy (weekly for the first month and every 1 to 3 months thereafter) among 63 consecutive cirrhotic patients with esophageal variceal bleeding. The mean duration of follow-up was 15 months. The overall risk of rebleeding was significantly lower with TIPS (23% versus 52%, $p<0.02$), but the risk of hepatic encephalopathy was significantly higher with TIPS (33% versus 13%, $p<0.05$). The 1-year survival rates were statistically similar (93% with TIPS versus 82% with sclerotherapy) (4a).

G. Esophageal Transection for Secondary Prophylaxis of Variceal Bleeding

1. Although there are numerous variations on the theme, the basic procedure involves insertion of a staple gun into the esophagus through a small gastrotomy, transection of the esophagus, and reconnection of the two ends. Although this operation is technically easier than a shunt operation and it lies within the ability of general surgeons, it is rarely performed in the United States (3,30). Esophageal transection is usually combined with varying degrees of devascularization of the distal esophagus and stomach. A particularly extensive operation popularized by Sugiura involves splenectomy, vagotomy, and devascularization of the stomach and distal esophagus (28). However, unlike standard esophageal transection, the Sugiura procedure is technically difficult and time-consuming (28). Some authors have expressed concern about this procedure because it may interfere with future plans for liver transplantation (34).

2. The perioperative mortality rate and the long-term survival rate associated with esophageal transection vary with several factors.

a. Elective Versus Emergency Operation—In one study from Taiwan, the overall operative mortality rate for esophageal transection was 26.4%. However, for elective cases it was 18.5%, and for emergency cases it was 44.4% (12).

b. Child's Class—In the same study, the operative mortality rates were 10%, 37.5%, and 73% for patients in Child's class A, B, or C, respectively (12). Similarly, in a Japanese study, the 10-year survival rates were 73.4%, 45.3%, and they were 14.1% for patients in Child's class A, B, or C, respectively (13).

c. Cause of Portal Hypertension—In the same Japanese study, the 10-year survival rates were 90.7%, 77.6%, and 33.0% for patients with extrahepatic portal obstruction, idiopathic portal hypertension, and cirrhosis, respectively (13).

3. Efficacy of Esophageal Transection for Secondary Prophylaxis of Variceal Bleeding

a. Firm conclusions regarding the role of esophageal transection for secondary prophylaxis of variceal bleeding are difficult for many reasons. First, most studies of esophageal transection have been done in non-Western nations where the proportion of patients with alcoholic cirrhosis is small. For example, the Suguira procedure has a reported long-term survival rate of 72% and a rebleeding rate of 5% among predominantly nonalcoholic patients in Japan (28). The generalizability of these results to predominantly alcoholic patients in Western countries is questionable. Second, most of the studies have been uncontrolled, and PRCTs have been relatively scarce. Furthermore, studies have used various techniques of transection and different degrees of devascularization, making direct comparison difficult.

b. One of the few PRCTs done in a Western country with adequate long-term follow-up is described here. This PRCT involved 97 patients with biopsy-proven Child's class A or B cirrhosis and first episode of endoscopically confirmed variceal bleeding. Alcohol was the cause of liver disease in 68% of the patients. All patients were initially treated with emergency sclerotherapy and, if stable for 5 days, were randomly assigned to receive either intravariceal sclerotherapy or esophageal transection with gastric devascularization. Recurrent bleeding was treated with sclerotherapy, regardless of treatment assignment. Average follow-up was 52 months. The data presented here are derived from an intention-to-treat analysis (34) (see Table 16–16).

(1) Transection was associated with a lower risk of variceal rebleeding, but the statistical significance was not reported.

(2) The risk of hepatic encephalopathy was not specifically addressed.

(3) Overall long-term mortality rates were similar in the two groups.

(4) The economic cost during the first year was substantially lower with sclerotherapy than with transection (P<0.0001). This difference persisted into the fifth year of follow-up, although it was no longer statistically significant by then.

4. Summary of the Role of Esophageal Transection for Secondary Prophylaxis of Variceal Bleeding

a. In one of the few PRCTs done in a Western country with adequate long-term follow-up, there was no significant advantage to esophageal transection compared with sclerotherapy, and transection was substantially more expensive than sclerotherapy.

b. Transection may be more useful in nonalcoholic than alcoholic patients.

H. Liver Transplantation for Secondary Prophylaxis of Variceal Bleeding—Liver transplantation is the only therapy that can eliminate portal hypertension and restore hepatic function.

1. Selection criteria for liver transplantation continue to evolve. In most centers, it is offered to patients with end-stage cirrhosis who have limited life expectancy. Sclerotherapy, esophageal transection, shunt surgery, and drug therapy do not convincingly improve survival. Patients with end-stage cirrhosis have reported 5-year survival rates of 13% to 35% with sclerotherapy (14). In contrast, the 5-year survival after liver transplantation is about 71% (11).

2. Although the risk of variceal bleeding generally increases with the severity of liver disease, not all patients with variceal bleeding have end-stage liver disease. Therefore, only a subset of patients with variceal bleeding are candidates for transplantation (11,23).

3. In addition to determining the medical necessity of liver transplantation, a preoperative evaluation is conducted to exclude patients with major contraindications to transplantation. Patients with a history of severe heart or lung disease,

Table 16-16 Triger's PRCT of esophageal transection vs. sclerotherapy (34)

	Sclerotherapy (n=51)	Transection (n=46)	*P*
% of patients with variceal rebleeding	49%	35%	?
Overall mortality rate	35%	33%	NS
Average economic costs during first year	£1094	£4369	<0.0001

sepsis, metastatic cancer, acquire immunodeficiency syndrome, or active alcohol or drug abuse are excluded at most centers. Patients must also have the ability to comply with the stringent immunosuppressive protocols. Patients who have had prior shunt surgery may undergo liver transplantation, but a portacaval shunt must be dismantled. A DSR shunt usually can be left intact (11,23).

4. Ideally, liver transplantation should be available to all patients with end-stage liver disease. However, in practice, the economic cost of the procedure, the extreme shortage of donor organs, and the risk of lifelong immunosuppression limit the application of this procedure to a relatively small number of patients (11).

I. Summary of Secondary Prophylaxis of Variceal Bleeding in Cirrhotic Patients

1. The data regarding the role of β-blockers for secondary prophylaxis of variceal bleeding are conflicting. If there is a benefit to β-blockade, it is limited to the subset of patients with alcoholic liver disease and stable liver function. β-Blockade does not appear to be useful for secondary prophylaxis in unselected patients. The addition of β-blockers to sclerotherapy has not shown convincing benefit.
2. Sclerotherapy decreases the risk of rebleeding without increasing the risk of hepatic encephalopathy or subjecting patients to the risks of a major operation. Sclerotherapy also does not interfere with future prospects for liver transplantation. Some but not all studies have shown a survival benefit to sclerotherapy when compared with no specific elective intervention or with DSR shunt surgery.
3. Endoscopic banding appears to be as effective as sclerotherapy in decreasing the risk of rebleeding. However, it is associated with fewer complications, and fewer treatment sessions are necessary to completely eradicate the varices. There is some evidence that banding may even improve survival compared with sclerotherapy.
4. Portacaval shunts effectively decrease the risk of rebleeding but increase the risk of hepatic encephalopathy without improving survival. They also complicate the prospect for future liver transplantation.
5. The DSR shunt was designed to decrease the risk of hepatic encephalopathy, but its advantage over the portacaval shunt is still uncertain. The DSR shunt is superior to sclerotherapy in decreasing the risk of rebleeding but has been associated with a higher mortality rate and a higher risk of hepatic encephalopathy in some studies.
6. Like surgical shunts, TIPS is superior to sclerotherapy in decreasing the risk of variceal rebleeding but is associated with a higher risk of hepatic encephalopathy. The rate of shunt occlusion or stenosis is also high but are usually amenable to percutaneous revision of the shunt.
7. Firm conclusions regarding the role of esophageal transection are not possible. Among alcoholic patients, esophageal transection does not offer any significant advantage over sclerotherapy.
8. No randomized controlled trials have compared liver transplantation with other treatment modalities. However, the 5-year survival rate after liver transplantation has been reported to be about 70%, which is substantially better than historically reported survival rates for Child's C cirrhotic patients treated with other modalities.
9. There is a consensus that once a patient has bled from varices, some form of therapy is necessary to decrease the risk of rebleeding; however, it is unclear which therapy is optimal. One possible scheme, outlined here, is to evaluate all patients who present with variceal bleeding for liver transplantation.
   a. Although there is some debate, most transplantation candidates with good hepatic reserve can be treated initially with sclerotherapy or banding. If they become refractory to such treatment, a procedure that serves as a bridge to transplantation should be performed. The DSR shunt, H-graft interposition shunt, or TIPS procedure can serve this purpose. If possible, portacaval shunts and esophageal transection should be avoided,

because they may complicate future plans for transplantation. Transplantation can be reconsidered if progressive liver dysfunction occurs during follow-up.

b. Suitable candidates with end-stage liver disease (Child's class C, and in some cases class B) should undergo transplantation. Patients who are not candidates for transplantation should be treated with sclerotherapy or banding. If they become refractory to such therapy, treatment options include nonselective shunt surgery, DSR shunt surgery, esophageal transection, and the TIPS procedure.

Abbreviations used in Chapter 16

BID = twice daily
£ = British pound
DSR = distal splenorenal
HVPG = hepatic vein pressure gradient
NS = not significant
P = probability value
PRCT = prospective randomized controlled trial
q = every
TIPS = transjugular intrahepatic portasystemic shunt

References

1. Alexandrino. Propranolol or endoscopic sclerotherapy in the prevention of recurrence of variceal bleeding: a prospective, randomized comparison of propranolol and sclerotherapy. *Hepatology* 1987;7:355.
2. Burroughs. Controlled trial of propranolol for the prevention of recurrent variceal hemorrhage in patients with cirrhosis. *N Engl J Med* 1983;309:1539.
3. Burroughs. A comparison of sclerotherapy with staple transection of the esophagus for the emergency control of bleeding from esophageal varices. *N Engl J Med* 1989;321:857.
4. Burroughs. Prevention of variceal rebleeding. *Gastroenterol Clin North Am* 1992; 21:119. Review.

4a. Cabrera. Transjugular intrahepatic portosystemic shunt versus sclerotherapy in the elective treatment of variceal hemorrhage. *Gastroenterology* 1996;110:832.

5. Fischer. Comparison of distal and proximal splenorenal shunts: a randomized prospective trial. *Ann Surg* 1981;194:531.
6. Fleig. Prevention of recurrent bleeding in cirrhotics with recent variceal hemorrhage: prospective, randomized comparison of propranolol and sclerotherapy. *Hepatology* 1987;7:355.
7. Gimson. Randomised trial of variceal banding ligation versus injection sclerotherapy for bleeding oesophageal varices. *Lancet* 1993;342(8868):391.
8. Grace. Distal splenorenal vs porta-systemic shunts after hemorrhage from varices: a randomized controlled trial. *Hepatology* 1988;8:1475.
9. Harley. Results of a randomized trial of end to side portacaval shunt and distal splenorenal shunt in alcoholic liver disease with variceal bleeding. *Gastroenterology* 1986;91:802.
10. Henderson. Endoscopic variceal sclerosis compared with distal splenorenal shunt to prevent recurrent variceal bleeding in cirrhosis: a prospective, randomized trial. *Ann Intern Med* 1990;112:262.
11. Henderson. Liver transplantation for portal hypertension. *Gastroenterol Clin North Am* 1992;21:197. Review.
12. Huang. Long-term results of esophageal transection and devascularization procedure in treatment of esophageal variceal bleeding. *J Formos Med Assoc* 1993;92:117.

13. Idezuki. Twenty-five year experience with esophageal transection for esophageal varices. *J Thorac Cardiovasc Surg* 1989;98:876.
14. Iwatsuki. Liver transplantation in the treatment of bleeding esophageal varices. *Surgery* 1987;104:697.
15. Jackson. A clinical investigation of the portacaval shunt: survival analysis of the therapeutic operation. *Ann Surg* 1971; 174:672.
15a. LaBerge. Two-year outcome following transjugular intrahepatic portosystemic shunt for variceal bleeding: results in 90 patients. *Gastroenterology* 1995;108:1143.
16. Laine. Endoscopic ligation compared with sclerotherapy for the treatment of bleeding esophageal varices. *Ann Intern Med* 1993;119:1.
17. Langer. Further report of a prospective randomised trial comparing distal splenorenal shunt with end to side portacaval shunt: an analysis of encephalopathy, survival and quality of life. *Gastroenterology* 1985;88:424.
18. Lebrec. A randomized controlled study of propranolol for prevention of recurrent gastrointestinal bleeding in patients with cirrhosis: a final report. *Hepatology* 1984; 4:355.
19. Millikan. The Emory prospective randomised trial: selective versus non-selective shunt to control variceal bleeding. Ten year follow-up. *Ann Surg* 1985;201:712.
20. Reichle. Prospective comparative clinical trial with distal splenorenal and mesocaval shunts. *Am J Surg* 1979;137:13.
21. Resnick. A controlled study of the therapeutic portacaval shunt. *Gastroenterology* 1974;6:843.
22. Reynolds. Results of a 12 year randomized portacaval shunt in patients with alcoholic liver disease and bleeding varices. *Gastroenterology* 1981;80:1005.
23. Rikkers. Shunt surgery versus endoscopic sclerotherapy for variceal hemorrhage: late results of a controlled trial. *Hepatology* 1989;10:577. Abstract.
24. Rossle. The transjugular intrahepatic portosystemic stent-shunt procedure for variceal bleeding. *N Engl J Med* 1994;330:165.
25. Rueff. A controlled study of therapeutic portacaval shunt in alcoholic cirrhosis. *Lancet* 1976;1:655.
26. Spina. Distal splenorenal shunt versus endoscopic sclerotherapy in the prevention of variceal rebleeding: first stage of a randomized, controlled trial. *Ann Surg* 1990;211:178.
27. Stiegmann. Endoscopic sclerotherapy as compared with endoscopic ligation for bleeding esophageal varices. *N Engl J Med* 1992;326:1527.
28. Sugiura. Esophageal transection with paraesophageal devascularizations (the Sugiura procedure) in the treatment of esophageal varices. *World J Surg* 1984;8:673.
29. Terblanche. Failure of repeated injection sclerotherapy to improve long-term survival after esophageal variceal bleeding. *Lancet* 1983;2:1328.
30. Terblanche. Controversies in the management of bleeding esophageal varices: part I. *N Engl J Med* 1989;320:1393. Review.
31. Terblanche. Controversies in the management of bleeding esophageal varices: part II. *N Engl J Med* 1989;320:1469. Review.
32. Terblanche. The treatment of esophageal varices. *Ann Rev Med* 1992;43:69. Review.
33. Teres. Sclerotherapy vs. distal splenorenal shunt in the elective treatment of variceal hemorrhage: a randomized controlled trial. *Hepatology* 1987;7:430.
34. Triger. A prospective trial of endoscopic sclerotherapy v. oesophageal transection and gastric devascularization in the long term management. *Gut* 1992;33:1553.
35. Vinel. Propranolol reduces the rebleeding rate during injection sclerotherapy: final results of a randomized study. *Gastroenterology* 1990;98:A644.
36. Westaby. Improved survival following injection sclerotherapy for esophageal varices: final analysis of a controlled trial. *Hepatology* 1985;5:827.
37. Westaby. Use of propranolol to reduce the rebleeding rate during injection sclerotherapy prior to variceal obliteration. *Hepatology* 1986;6:673.
38. Westaby. A controlled trial of oral propranolol compared with injection sclerotherapy for the long-term management of variceal bleeding. *Hepatology* 1990;11:353.

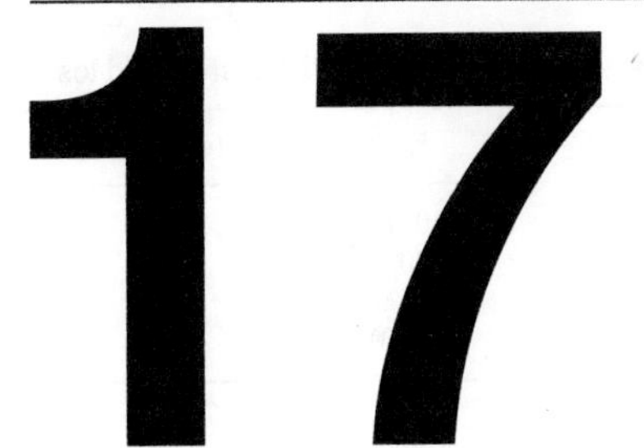

Nonvariceal Upper Gastrointestinal Bleeding

Burton W. Lee and
Lawrence S. Friedman

A. Introduction

1. Initial Approach to Patients with Upper Gastrointestinal Bleeding

a. The first priority in the management of any patient with gastrointestinal (GI) bleeding is hemodynamic resuscitation and stabilization. IV access should be established, and the blood bank should set up packed red blood cells (PRBC), fresh-frozen plasma, and platelets. Blood should also be sent for a complete blood count and determinations of creatinine, blood urea nitrogen, calcium, prothrombin time, and partial thromboplastin time. In patients with massive hematemesis, endotracheal intubation should be considered to protect against aspiration.

b. IV fluids should be administered to maintain hemodynamic stability and to achieve adequate urinary output. If necessary, blood products should be given to maintain adequate oxygen delivery. In alcoholic patients, parenteral thiamin should be given before administration of dextrose solutions to avoid precipitating Wernicke's syndrome.

c. Patients with GI bleeding are often allowed nothing by mouth (NPO), so that the food will not interfere with endoscopy or surgery. Furthermore, this practice may decrease the risk of aspiration in patients who are vomiting.

d. A brief history and a tailored physical examination should be performed.

(1) A prior history of use of aspirin or nonsteroidal antiinflammatory drugs (NSAIDs) raises the suspicion of gastritis or ulcers. A history of alcohol abuse suggests variceal bleeding, portal hypertensive gastropathy, or gastritis. Mallory–Weiss tear should be suspected in patients with the triad of alcoholism, hematemesis, and a history of vomiting. However, a history of prior retching may be absent in about half of the cases.

(2) In general, a history of hematemesis or melena suggests an upper gastrointestinal (UGI) source of bleeding (proximal to the ligament of Treitz), whereas hematochezia suggests a lower GI source. However, melena can also occur from sources in the small intestine or right colon, and severe UGI bleeding can result in hematochezia. Under experimental conditions, about 50 ml of blood introduced into the UGI tract was needed to cause melena, and 1000 ml was necessary to cause hematochezia (14).

(3) A careful rectal examination including anoscopy should be performed to check for hemorrhoids, masses, and fissures. If the possibility of lower GI bleeding exists, rigid or flexible sigmoidoscopy should be performed to examine the mucosa for inflammatory, infectious, ischemic, or neoplastic processes.

(4) Measurement of vital signs is essential in estimating the amount of intravascular volume loss, as shown in Table 17-1. However, these estimates do not necessarily apply to patients with chronic or recurrent bleeding, because of physiologic compensation.

e. Nasogastric (NG) lavage should be performed to assess the severity of bleeding and to confirm that bleeding is from a UGI source. Iced saline of-

Table 17-1 Correlation between vital signs and the amount of acute blood loss

Physical Examination	Estimated Acute Volume Loss
Normal vital signs	0–15%
Orthostasis >10 mm Hg	20%
Resting tachycardia	25%
Systolic blood pressure <100 mm Hg	>30%

fers no advantage over room-temperature saline. Aspiration of red blood suggests active bleeding, whereas aspiration of "coffee-grounds" blood suggests that bleeding has ceased. If the blood clears with saline lavage, it also suggests that the bleeding is no longer active. However, if no blood is detected, a UGI source is not excluded because NG lavage may miss up to 16% of actively bleeding lesions detectable on upper endoscopy (20). On the other hand, the presence of bile in the NG aspirate suggests but does not guarantee that the bleeding source is distal to the ligament of Treitz (8).

2. **Causes of UGI Bleeding**—The American Society for Gastrointestinal Endoscopy (ASGE) National Survey has provided the most reliable information on the causes of UGI bleeding (15). The ASGE survey was done prospectively, included a large number of patients, and was not limited to patients from academic centers. Over an 18-month period, 277 endoscopists submitted data on 2225 patients with UGI bleeding. Each patient's age, sex, presenting symptoms and signs, laboratory results, endoscopic findings, final diagnosis, transfusion requirements, need for surgery, complications, and mortality were recorded along with other variables (19).
   a. The most common causes of UGI bleeding were peptic ulcer disease (46%), gastritis (23%), and varices (10%).
   b. Other common causes included Mallory–Weiss tears (7%), esophagitis (6%), duodenitis (6%), and neoplasms (3%).
3. **Prognostic Factors**—UGI bleeding is a serious condition associated with a mortality rate of 10%. On the other hand, 70% to 85% of these patients stop bleeding spontaneously, and 25% do not require blood transfusions (5,19). Investigators have attempted to identify prognostic factors that separate patients at high risk of rebleeding or death from those with a more benign prognosis. This is important because the low-risk patients may be treated conservatively, whereas the higher risk patients may require endoscopic therapy or surgery. Some of the major prognostic factors identified in the ASGE survey are presented here.
   a. **Age**—The mortality rate among patients <60 years old was 8.7%, compared with 13.4% among patients >60 years old (20).
   b. **Comorbid Illnesses**—A patient's past medical conditions were placed into one of eight categories: cardiac, central nervous system, GI, hepatic, neoplastic, pulmonary, renal, and "stress." The last category included a variety of conditions such as acidosis, burns, diabetes, recent surgery, peritonitis, rheumatism, sepsis, and major trauma. The mortality rate varied from 2.6% in patients with no comorbid illnesses to 66.7% in patients who identified illnesses in six or more categories. In 70% of fatal cases, death was caused by deterioration of the underlying illness rather than by exsanguination (19,20).
   c. **Severity of Bleeding**—Markers of the severity of bleeding—such as the color of the NG aspirate, the color of stool, the blood transfusion requirement, and the hemodynamic status—all correlated with the risk of recurrent hemorrhage or death.
      (1) **Color of Nasogastric Aspirate and Stool**—The mortality rate progressively increased as the color of the NG aspirate went from clear (6.0%), to "coffee grounds" (9.7%), to red blood (17.9%). Similarly, the

mortality rate was 8.8% with brown or black stool, compared to 20.1% with red stool. Patients with both red stool and red NG aspirates had a mortality rate of 28.7% (20).

(2) **Blood Transfusion Requirements**—The mortality rate also varied with the transfusion requirement. For example, the mortality rate was 2.5% with no transfusion requirement, 6.7% with 1 to 3 units, 11.7% with 4 to 6 units, 15.4% with 7 to 9 units, and 34.2% with 10 or more units (20).

(3) **Hemodynamic Instability**—Bornman's prospective observational study of 177 patients with acute UGI bleeding demonstrated an important relation between the patient's hemodynamic status and the risk of rebleeding. In all patients, bleeding was caused by peptic ulcer disease. The risk of rebleeding was 2% in 114 patients with stable vital signs, 18% in 38 patients with tachycardia, and 48% in 25 patients with hypotension. Tachycardia was defined as a heart rate >100 bpm and hypotension as systolic blood pressure <100 mm Hg (2).

d. **Cause of Bleeding**—Bleeding caused by varices, neoplasms, or Rendu-Osler-Weber syndrome was associated with a poorer prognosis; the mortality rate in these patients ranged from 17% to 30%. In contrast, bleeding caused by peptic ulcer disease, Mallory–Weiss tear, duodenitis, or esophageal ulcer was associated with a better prognosis; the mortality rate in these patients ranged from 2% to 8% (20).

e. **Endoscopic Appearance**—The endoscopic characteristics of a lesion can predict the risk of rebleeding. Among all patients with UGI bleeding in the ASGE survey, those with an oozing or pumping lesion had a higher mortality rate (16.1% versus 6.7%), a higher rate of complications (16.7% versus 8.7%), higher blood transfusion requirements (≥5 units of blood in 37.6% versus 20.1%), and more frequent need for surgery (24.1% versus 11.4%) than patients without active bleeding (21). This issue has been studied further in patients with peptic ulcers. Table 17-2 summarizes the association between the endoscopic appearance of an ulcer and the risk of rebleeding or continuous bleeding. The data are derived from the control arms of some of the major prospective randomized controlled trials (PRCTs) to evaluate the efficacy of endoscopic therapy in patients with ulcers (13,15,16,18,22). The risks of rebleeding as estimated in review articles by Gupta (6) and Laine (14) are also shown in the two columns on the far right.

f. **Location of the Ulcer**—Ulcers located high on the lesser curvature can erode into the left gastric artery, and ulcers lying over the posteroinferior duodenal bulb can erode into the gastroduodenal artery. Because such erosions can produce catastrophic results, aggressive treatment of these lesions is recommended (6).

B. Endoscopic Therapies

1. Several endoscopic modalities are available to treat nonvariceal UGI bleeding (3,6).

a. **Thermal Contact Devices**—Heater probe devices deliver a pulse of thermal energy to the tip of the probe to cause hemostasis. Multipolar electrocoagulation devices deliver electrical energy to achieve a similar effect. With either device, firm pressure is applied on the bleeding site.

b. **Injection Therapy**—Endoscopic injection of ethanol, epinephrine, or polidocanol causes dehydration and fixation of underlying tissue and/or vasoconstriction and thrombosis of bleeding vessels. This is the simplest and least expensive therapeutic modality.

c. **Laser Therapy**—Laser treatment causes coagulation of bleeding vessels without the need for contact between the device and the bleeding tissue. It works rapidly, and the amount of thermal damage to the tissue is predictable. The most commonly used laser is the neodymium:yttrium-aluminum-garnet (Nd:YAG) laser. The major limitations of laser therapy are the high cost of the equipment and the lack of portability. It also requires a high degree of technical expertise.

Table 17-2 Endoscopic appearance of an ulcer and the rebleeding risk

Author (Reference)	Laine (13)	O'Brien (16)	Swain (22)	Panes (18)	MacLeod (15)	Gupta (6)	Laine (14)
No. of control patients	182	103	68	58	24	—	—
Active bleeding on endoscopy	—	62%	80%	54%	100%	90%–100%	55%
Risk of rebleeding or continued bleeding							
Nonbleeding pigmented protuberance	—	37%	48%	48%	—	40%–50%	43%
Adherent clot	14%	13%	23%	33%	—	20%–30%	22%
Oozing without visible vessel	—	—	17%	—	—	10%	—
Flat spot or clean base	2%–8%	—	0%	—	0%	1%–10%	5%–10%

2. **Efficacy of Endoscopic Therapy for Nonvariceal UGI Bleeding**—Although the diagnostic utility of endoscopy in patients with UGI bleeding has long been unquestioned, its therapeutic role has evolved more slowly (1). To date, >30 randomized trials have compared endoscopic therapy versus control in patients with nonvariceal UGI bleeding. Although the results of these studies have seemingly been conflicting, one should recall that 70% to 85% of patients with UGI bleeding stop spontaneously (5,14). Therefore, in order to demonstrate a clinically significant reduction in the rate of rebleeding, a study must collect a large number of patients or limit the population to those with the highest risk of rebleeding. In general, trials that have limited the study population to patients with active bleeding or pigmented protuberances have been able to confirm the utility of endoscopic therapy. In contrast, the results of studies that included patients with flat spots or clean bases have been less clear-cut.
   - **a.** To help resolve the controversy, Cook performed a metaanalysis of all available data on endoscopic therapy for acute nonvariceal UGI bleeding. Among the 298 sources identified as of 1992, Cook selected 30 PRCTs that evaluated the impact of endoscopic therapy on the risk of rebleeding, the need for surgery, and/or the rate of survival (see Table 17–3).
     - **(1)** When the data were analyzed for all endoscopic modalities combined, all major outcome measures were significantly improved with endoscopic therapy.
     - **(2)** However, there was significant statistical heterogeneity in the risk of rebleeding and in the need for surgery, which limits the confidence in the results of the metaanalysis (3).
   - **b. Thermal Contact Devices**
     - **(1)** Cook's metaanalysis included 13 studies that compared contact thermal modalities with no endoscopic treatment. As a group, heater probe or electrocoagulation devices significantly decreased the risk of rebleeding and the need for surgery. However, there was significant statistical heterogeneity in these results. The rate of survival was also improved with thermal modalities, but the difference was not statistically significant (3) (see Table 17–4).
     - **(2)** **Active UGI Bleeding**—Two studies by Laine demonstrated the efficacy of thermal contact devices in nonvariceal UGI bleeding. Laine performed a PRCT of multipolar electrocoagulation versus sham endoscopy in 44 patients with endoscopically confirmed active nonvariceal UGI bleeding. All patients had a bloody NG aspirate, melena, or

Table 17-3 Metaanalysis of all endoscopic modalities for UGI bleeding (3)

	OR of Treatment vs. Control (Value <1.0 Favors Treatment)	Statistical Heterogeneity	95% CI
Risk of rebleeding	0.38	Yes	0.32–0.45
Need for surgery	0.36	Yes	0.28–0.45
Risk of death	0.55	No	0.40–0.76

Table 17-4 Metaanalysis of thermal contact devices for UGI bleeding (3)

	OR of Treatment vs. Control (Value <1.0 Favors Treatment)	Statistical Heterogeneity	95% CI
Risk of rebleeding	0.32	Yes	0.22–0.41
Need for surgery	0.31	Yes	0.19–0.43
Risk of death	0.67	No	0.39–1.14

hematochezia that resulted in unstable vital signs; a blood transfusion requirement of >2 units of PRBCs over 12 hours; or a drop in hematocrit of >6% over 12 hours. Fifty-four percent of patients were bleeding from ulcers and 39% from Mallory-Weiss tears (11) (see Table 17–5).

(a) Endoscopic therapy was significantly superior to control in all outcome measures, including hemostasis, blood transfusion requirement, length of hospitalization, and the need for emergency surgery or other procedures.

(b) The mortality rate was also lower with therapy, but the difference was not statistically significant.

(3) Nonbleeding Visible Vessels (Pigmented Protuberances)—Laine performed another PRCT of multipolar electrocoagulation versus sham endoscopy in 75 consecutive patients with UGI bleeding from an endoscopically confirmed peptic ulcer with a nonbleeding visible vessel. All patients had a bloody NG aspirate, melena, or hematochezia that resulted in unstable vital signs; a blood transfusion requirement of >2 units of PRBCs over 12 hours; or a drop in hematocrit of >6% over 12 hours (12) (see Table 17–6).

(a) Endoscopic therapy was significantly superior to control in terms of the rate of rebleeding, the length of hospitalization, and the need for emergency surgery.

(b) The blood transfusion requirement was also lower with therapy, but the difference was not statistically significant.

(c) There were too few deaths to evaluate the impact on mortality.

c. Laser Therapy

(1) Cook's metaanalysis included 13 studies that compared laser therapy versus no endoscopic treatment. Laser therapy significantly decreased the risk of rebleeding, the need for surgery, and the mortality rate. There was statistical heterogeneity only for the risk of rebleeding (3) (see Table 17–7).

(2) For illustration, the data from two conflicting studies by Swain (22) and Krejs (10) are presented. Swain compared endoscopic laser ther-

Table 17-5 Electrocoagulation for active nonvariceal UGI bleeding (11)

	Multipolar Electrocoagulation (n=21)	Sham Endoscopy (n=23)	*P*
Hemostasis	90%	13%	<0.0001
Mean transfusion requirement	2.4 units	5.4 units	0.002
Length of hospitalization	4.4 d	7.2 d	0.02
Emergency surgery or procedures	14%	57%	0.01
Mortality	0%	13%	NS

Table 17-6 Electrocoagulation for ulcers with nonbleeding visible vessels (12)

	Multipolar Electrocoagulation (n=38)	Sham Endoscopy (n=37)	*P*
Rate of rebleeding	18%	41%	<0.05
Mean transfusion requirement	1.6 units	3.0 units	NS
Length of hospitalization	4.3 d	6.2 d	<0.05
Need for emergency surgery	8%	30%	<0.05
Mortality	2.6%	0%	NS

Table 17-7 Metaanalysis of endoscopic laser therapy for UGI bleeding (3)

	OR of Treatment vs. Control (Value <1.0 Favors Treatment)	Statistical Heterogeneity	95% CI
Risk of rebleeding	0.58	Yes	0.38–0.69
Need for surgery	0.58	No	0.40–0.80
Risk of death	0.49	No	0.30–0.81

apy versus control (supportive measures only) in 138 patients with ulcer-related UGI bleeding and stigmata of recent hemorrhage (79 patients with visible vessels, 26 patients with adherent clots, 33 patients with other stigmata). Patients with endoscopically inaccessible lesions were excluded. Patients were stratified according to endoscopic stigmata (see Table 17–8).

(a) Overall, endoscopic laser therapy was significantly superior to control in improving the rate of rebleeding, the need for surgery, and the rate of mortality.

(b) When analyzed according to the endoscopic appearance, laser therapy significantly improved the rate of rebleeding for patients with visible vessels but not for those with adherent clots or other stigmata (22).

(3) Krejs also compared laser therapy versus control in 174 patients with ulcer-related UGI bleeding. All patients were either actively bleeding (32 patients) or had stigmata of recent bleeding on endoscopy (29 with visible vessels, 142 with other stigmata). Patients with endoscopically inaccessible lesions were excluded. Patients were stratified by endoscopic stigmata (10).

(a) In contrast to Swain's study, there were no significant differences in outcome between laser therapy and control.

(b) The discrepancy in these two studies may be explained by the fact that Swain's study included "sicker" patients with higher risk of rebleeding or death. For example, 57% of patients were ac-

Table 17-8 Swain's PRCT evaluating the role of endoscopic laser therapy (22)

	Laser Therapy (n=70)	Control (n=68)	*P*
Overall risk of rebleeding	10%	40%	<0.001
Risk of rebleeding with visible vessels	15%	53%	<0.001
Risk of rebleeding with adherent clots	8%	18%	NS
Risk of rebleeding with other stigmata	0%	8%	NS
Risk of needing emergency surgery	10%	35%	<0.005
Risk of death	1%	12%	<0.05

Table 17-9 Krejs' PRCT evaluating the role of endoscopic laser therapy (10)

	Laser Therapy (n=85)	Control (n=89)	*P*
Overall risk of rebleeding	22%	20%	NS
Risk of needing emergency surgery	16%	17%	NS
Risk of death from bleeding	1%	1%	NS

tively bleeding or had visible vessels in Swain's study, compared with only 35% in Krejs' study.

(c) Furthermore, Krejs' study apparently excluded patients in intensive care units, who are those perhaps most likely to benefit from therapy (6). Lending support to this argument is the fact that the mortality rate in Swain's control group was 12%, compared with only 1% in Krejs' control group.

(4) Despite its probable efficacy, laser therapy requires a high degree of technical expertise; moreover, the equipment is generally not portable and is extremely expensive. For these reasons, laser therapy is currently not recommended as first-line therapy for UGI bleeding (14).

d. Injection Therapy

(1) Cook's metaanalysis included seven studies that compared injection therapy versus no endoscopic treatment. Overall, injection therapy decreased the risk of rebleeding and the need for surgery significantly. The mortality rate was also decreased with injection therapy, but the difference was not statistically significant. There was no statistical heterogeneity (3) (see Table 17–10).

(2) The study by Oxner is described for illustration. Oxner compared endoscopic injection versus control in a PRCT of 93 patients in nonacademic hospitals who had acute UGI bleeding caused by peptic ulcer disease. All patients had actively bleeding or nonbleeding visible vessels on endoscopy. Patients with endoscopically inaccessible lesions were not excluded. Epinephrine (1 to 2 ml of a 1:10,000 preparation) was injected around and into the vessel, after which ethanolamine (1 to 2 ml of a 5% solution) was injected into the vessel (17) (see Table 17–11).

(a) Injection therapy decreased the risk of rebleeding significantly.

(b) The need for emergency surgery, the blood transfusion requirement, and the risk of death were also lower with injection therapy, but the differences were not statistically significant.

(c) A subgroup analysis demonstrated that injection therapy was more effective and was associated with fewer complications when performed by more experienced endoscopists.

C. Other Therapeutic Measures

1. If possible, any modifiable factors that may have contributed to bleeding should be eliminated. These include use of aspirin, NSAIDs, anticoagulants, alcohol, and tobacco. Corticosteroids alone do not appear to increase the risk of ulcers or GI bleeding. However, in combination with NSAIDs, corticosteroids do significantly increase these risks (14). Patients at low risk of rebleeding by endoscopic criteria may be allowed to eat. Patients at higher risk of rebleeding should be kept NPO or on a clear liquid diet until it appears that further endoscopy or surgery will not be necessary (13,14).

2. Anti-ulcer medications such as omeprazole, sucralfate, antacids, and histamine$_2$ (H_2)–receptor blockers do not affect the course of an acute UGI bleeding episode significantly even if bleeding is a result of ulcers or gastritis (4). Furthermore, by coating the mucosa, antacids may interfere with visualization at endoscopy. Vasopressin (Pitressin) and somatostatin have also been used to

Table 17-10 Metaanalysis of endoscopic injection for UGI bleeding (3)

	OR of Treatment vs. Control (Value <1.0 Favors Treatment)	Statistical Heterogeneity	95% CI
Risk of rebleeding	0.23	No	0.12–0.45
Need for surgery	0.18	No	0.11–0.32
Risk of death	0.50	No	0.22–1.12

Table 17-11 Oxner's PRCT evaluating the role of endoscopic injection (17)

	Injection Therapy (n=48)	Control (n=45)	*P*
Risk of rebleeding	16.7%	46.7%	0.011
Risk of needing surgery	8.3%	17.8%	NS
Transfusion requirement	5 units	7.56 units	NS
Risk of death	8.3%	20.0%	NS

treat acute nonvariceal bleeding, but their efficacy has not been clearly demonstrated in this setting (14).

3. Any patient who presents with significant UGI bleeding should be managed in consultation with a surgeon. In the ASGE survey, the mortality rate was 11.7% for patients who had a blood transfusion requirement of 4 to 6 units, 15.4% for those requiring 7 to 9 units, and 34.2% for those requiring $10 units (20). Therefore, patients who require multiple blood transfusions should be considered for surgery. If the patient is not a surgical candidate, angiography with embolization may be considered.
4. If bleeding is caused by peptic ulcer disease or gastritis, the patient should be treated with an 8- to 12-week course of omeprazole, sucralfate, or H_2-receptor blockers to promote healing of the ulcer and to decrease the risk of recurrent hemorrhage (9). Furthermore, if *Helicobacter pylori* infection is associated with the lesion, combination antibiotics should be administered to increase the speed of healing and prevent ulcer relapse (7).

D. Summary

1. The most common causes of UGI bleeding are peptic ulcer disease, gastritis, and varices. Other causes include Mallory–Weiss tears, esophagitis, duodenitis, neoplasms, Rendu-Osler-Weber syndrome, and Dieulafoy's lesion.
2. The patient's age, cause of bleeding, presence of comorbid illnesses, severity of bleeding, and endoscopic stigmata are important prognostic factors in patients who present with UGI bleeding.
   - **a.** Patients who bleed from varices, neoplasms, or Rendu-Osler-Weber syndrome have a poorer prognosis than those who bleed from ulcers, gastritis, or Mallory–Weiss tears.
   - **b.** The number of comorbid conditions positively correlates with the risk of death. In fact, death is most often caused by deterioration of the underlying illness rather than exsanguination.
   - **c.** Evidence of severe bleeding, as suggested by bloody NG aspirates, hematochezia, hemodynamic instability, or a high blood transfusion requirement, also portends a poor prognosis.
   - **d.** In patients with peptic ulcers, endoscopic features such as active bleeding or nonbleeding visible vessels are associated with a high risk of rebleeding and death; other endoscopic features such as adherent clots, flat spots, oozing without a visible vessel, or a clean ulcer base are associated with a lower risk. Current practice is to endoscopically treat patients with actively bleeding ulcers or nonbleeding visible vessels but not to treat those with other stigmata.
3. Most patients who present with UGI bleeding require endoscopy but not endoscopic therapy. For patients with endoscopic stigmata associated with a high risk of rebleeding, endoscopic therapy appears to decrease the risk of rebleeding, the need for surgery, and the transfusion requirement. Survival benefit has not been clearly demonstrated but has been suggested by a metaanalysis of the published studies. Because no modality has been shown conclusively to be superior to another, the choice should be based on the availability of the equipment and the expertise of the endoscopist.

4. Medications such as antacids, sucralfate, H_2-receptor blockers, and omeprazole do not significantly alter the course of acute UGI bleeding. However, they may be helpful in the secondary prevention of recurrent bleeding and are indicated for the treatment of ulcer disease. Patients who remain refractory to endoscopic therapy should be considered for surgery, and nonsurgical candidates may be considered for angiography with embolization.

Abbreviations used in Chapter 17

ASGE = American Society for Gastrointestinal Endoscopy
bpm = beats per minute
CI = confidence interval
GI = gastrointestinal
H_2 = histamine$_2$
IV = intravenous
Nd:YAG laser = neodymium:yttrium-aluminum-garnet laser
NG = nasogastric
NPO = nothing by mouth
NSAID = nonsteroidal antiinflammatory drug
OR = odds ratio
P = probability value
PRBC = packed red blood cells
PRCT = prospective randomized controlled trial
UGI = upper gastrointestinal
vs. = versus

References

1. Therapeutic endoscopy and bleeding ulcers: NIH consensus. *JAMA* 1989;262:1369.
2. Bornman. Importance of hypovolemic shock and endoscopic signs in predicting hemorrhage from peptic ulceration: a prospective evaluation. *Br Med J* 1985;291 (6490):245.
3. Cook. Endoscopic therapy for acute nonvariceal upper gastrointestinal hemorrhage: a meta-analysis. *Gastroenterology* 1992;102:139.
4. Daneshmend. Omeprazole versus placebo for acute upper gastrointestinal bleeding: randomized double blind controlled study. *Br Med J* 1992;304(6820):143.
5. Fromm. Endoscopic coagulation for gastrointestinal bleeding. *N Engl J Med* 1987; 316(26):1652.
6. Gupta. Nonvariceal upper gastrointestinal bleeding. *Med Clin North Am* 1993;77: 973. Review.
7. Hentschell. Effect of ranitidine and amoxacillin plus metronidazole on the eradication of *H. pylori* and the recurrence of duodenal ulcer. *N Engl J Med* 1993;328: 308.
8. Jensen. Diagnosis and treatment of severe hematochezia: the role of urgent colonoscopy after purge. *Gastroenterology* 1988;95:1569.
9. Jensen. A controlled study of ranitidine for the prevention of recurrent hemorrhage from duodenal ulcer. *N Engl J Med* 1994;330:382.
10. Krejs. Laser photocoagulation for the treatment of acute peptic ulcer bleeding. *N Engl J Med* 1987;316:1618.
11. Laine. Multipolar electrocoagulation in the treatment of active upper gastrointestinal tract hemorrhage: a prospective controlled trial. *N Engl J Med* 1987;316(26): 1613.
12. Laine. Multipolar electrocoagulation in the treatment of peptic ulcers with nonbleeding vessels: a prospective, controlled trial. *Ann Intern Med* 1989;110:510.

13. Laine. Prospective evaluation of immediate versus delayed refeeding and prognostic value of endoscopy in patients with upper gastrointestinal hemorrhage. *Gastroenterology* 1992;102:314.
14. Laine. Bleeding peptic ulcer. *N Engl J Med* 1994;331(11):717. Review.
15. Macleod. Neodymium yttrium aluminum garnet laser photocoagulation for major hemorrhage from peptic ulcer and single vessels. *Br Med J* 1983;286:345.
16. O'Brien. Controlled trial of small bipolar probe in bleeding peptic ulcers. *Lancet* 1986;1:464.
17. Oxner. Endoscopic injection for bleeding peptic ulcers. *Lancet* 1992;339:996.
18. Panes. Controlled trial of endoscopic sclerosis in bleeding peptic ulcers. *Lancet* 1987;2:1282.
19. Silverstein. The national ASGE survey on upper gastrointestinal bleeding: I. Study design and baseline data. *Gastrointest Endosc* 1981;27:73.
20. Silverstein. The national ASGE survey on upper gastrointestinal bleeding: II. Clinical prognostic factors. *Gastrointest Endosc* 1981;27:80.
21. Silverstein. The national ASGE survey on upper gastrointestinal bleeding: III. Endoscopy in upper gastrointestinal bleeding. *Gastrointest Endosc* 1981;27:94.
22. Swain. Controlled trial of Nd:YAG laser photocoagulation in bleeding peptic ulcers. *Lancet* 1986;1:1113.

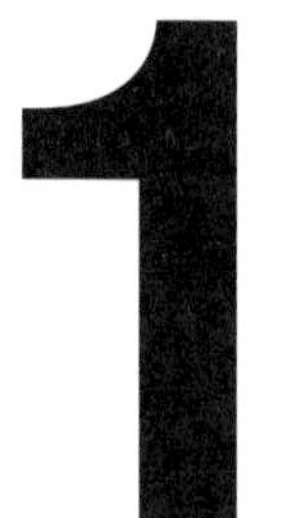
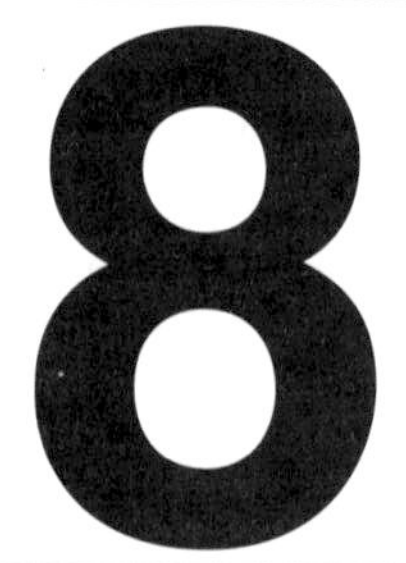

Acute Lower Gastrointestinal Bleeding

Burton W. Lee and
Lawrence S. Friedman

A. Introduction

1. A literature-based discussion of lower gastrointestinal (LGI) bleeding is more difficult than that of upper gastrointestinal (UGI) bleeding for a number of reasons. First, there is a paucity of good data regarding the efficacy of various management strategies for patients with LGI bleeding. Second, the available studies differ significantly in their design, making comparisons difficult. They vary in size, diagnostic strategies employed, degree to which patients with UGI or anorectal bleeding are excluded, inclusion or exclusion criteria, and indications for surgical intervention. Furthermore, most of the data generated in the preangiography and preendoscopy era are no longer relevant to modern practice. Even in the modern era, study of the LGI tract is considerably more cumbersome than that of the UGI tract, because lower endoscopy can be made more difficult by the presence of active hemorrhage. Because there is no simple LGI technique that is equivalent to the nasogastric (NG) lavage, differentiation of active bleeding from passage of old blood is also difficult. Finally, the diagnostic and therapeutic utilities of colonoscopy or angiography are strongly operator-dependent. Results indicating that one procedure is superior to another may not be generalizable to other clinical settings. Therefore, the management strategies recommended in the literature are based mostly on the authors' expert opinions rather than on rigorously tested principles (7,11,24,28, 31,32,37).
2. **Categorization of LGI Bleeding**—The management of patients with LGI bleeding depends largely on the rate and pattern of bleeding. Therefore, it is useful to categorize these patients into one of three groups, as suggested by Buchman and Buckley (7).
   a. **Occult GI Bleeding**—Patients with occult gastrointestinal (GI) bleeding have guaiac-positive stools but, by definition, no overt signs of GI bleeding, such as hematemesis, melena, hematochezia, or hemodynamic instability. These patients usually can undergo an outpatient evaluation with colonoscopy or the combination of barium enema and flexible sigmoidoscopy. Esophagogastroduodenoscopy or a UGI barium series with or without small bowel follow-through may also be necessary, depending on the clinical situation. Management of patients with occult GI bleeding is not discussed further in this chapter.
   b. **Slow LGI Bleeding**—Patients with slow LGI bleeding pass grossly recognizable blood per rectum but remain hemodynamically stable because physiologic compensatory mechanisms can keep up with the rate of blood loss.
   c. **Rapid LGI Bleeding**—These patients pass grossly recognizable blood per rectum but are hemodynamically unstable because the physiologic compensatory mechanisms are unable to keep up with the rate of blood loss.
3. **Etiology of LGI Bleeding**
   a. LGI bleeding is defined as bleeding distal to the ligament of Treitz. In most cases, bleeding is from the colon, but the small bowel can also be a source. In the United States, diverticulosis, angiodysplasia, neoplasms, and inter-

nal hemorrhoids are responsible for most cases of LGI bleeding. Major causes of LGI bleeding are listed in Table 18-1 (28).

b. Assigning relative frequencies to various causes of LGI bleeding is difficult. Among older patients, diverticulosis and angiodysplasia are common incidental findings. Therefore, detection of a nonbleeding angiodysplastic or diverticular lesion cannot be equated with identification of the true bleeding source. In addition, patient populations differ significantly from study to study. For example, studies that include patients with occult bleeding report different etiologic profiles than studies that limit the patient population to those with massive bleeding. Furthermore, the availability of diagnostic tests, the choice of diagnostic strategy, and the skill of the physicians performing the procedures all affect the relative frequency of each diagnosis. With these limitations kept in mind, representative data from some of the published series are summarized in Tables 18–2 and 18–3 (12,18,21).

B. Major Diagnostic Tools

1. Barium Enema—In general, barium enema has a limited role in the evaluation of acute LGI bleeding. It is unable to detect angiodysplasia, and diverticula that are detected may be incidental findings rather than the true source of bleeding. Furthermore, barium can interfere with plans for endoscopy or angiography. However, barium enema remains useful in nonacute settings, especially when colonoscopy is nondiagnostic or not readily available.

2. Nuclear Bleeding Scan

a. The most widely used bleeding scan is the technetium 99m (^{99m}Tc) scan. In this technique, the patient's own blood is withdrawn, labeled in vitro with radioactively labeled sodium pertechnetate, and then reinjected into the circulation. Sometimes, radioactively labeled sulfur colloid is injected simultaneously. Sulfur colloid has a short half-life in the circulation and detects active hemorrhage, whereas sodium pertechnetate stays in the circulation longer, so that delayed hemorrhage is not missed. The patient is scanned periodically for up to 24 hours to look for an area of pooled blood in the abdomen. Unlike colonoscopy or angiography, the nuclear bleeding scan is strictly a diagnostic tool (27).

(1) In theory, there are three major ways that a nuclear bleeding scan can be useful. First, it can be used for prognostic purposes. Because a positive scan is indicative of active or intermittent hemorrhage, it may identify patients who are most likely to rebleed, die, or require surgery. Second, it can be used to localize the site of bleeding. This information can be used to plan selective angiography and to direct the

Table 18-1 Major causes of LGI bleeding (7,11,28,31,32,37)

Diverticular disease
Angiodysplasia
Neoplasms
Anal fissures
Hemorrhoids
Inflammatory bowel disease
Ischemic colitis
Radiation enteritis
Aortoenteric fistula
Rendu-Osler-Weber syndrome
Meckel's diverticulum

Table 18-2 Major published series of LGI bleeding: summary of study design

	Jensen (18)	Leitman (21)	Farrands (12)
Summary of study design	Prospective study of 80 consecutive patients with severe ongoing hematochezia; "severe bleeding" was not defined precisely	Retrospective study of all 68 patients with massive active LGI bleeding requiring angiography; "massive GI bleeding" was not defined	Retrospective review of all 107 patients admitted for LGI bleeding to a British hospital over 4 y
Diagnostic tests used	Upper endoscopy 100%; colonoscopy 100%, angiography 28%	Angiography 100%; bleeding scan 41%	Upper endoscopy 100%; angiography 8.4%, colonoscopy 9.3%
Mean blood transfusion requirement	6.5 units	6 units in 24 hours	0–2 units in 78%; 3–4 units in 10%; 5–25 units in 11%
% needing surgery	24%	50%	6.5%
Mortality rate	Not stated	20%	1.8%

Table 18-3 Major published series of LGI bleeding: causes of bleeding

	Jensen (18) (n=80)	Leitman (21) (n=68)	Farrands (12) (n=107)
Diverticular disease	17%	26%	28%
Colonic angiodysplasia	30%	24%	6%
Colonic neoplasms	13%	9%	35%
Inflammatory bowel disease	—	4%	16%
Ischemic colitis	—	4%	3%
Other colonic lesions	14%	—	6%
Small bowel lesions	9%	6%	—
UGI lesions	11%	—	—
Hemorrhoids and anal fissures	—	1.5%	1.8%
No site found	6%	21%	1%

type of surgery performed. Finally, it can be used as a screening tool so that angiography can be used more efficiently. Because the bleeding scan is more sensitive than angiography, limiting angiography to patients with positive nuclear scans can decrease the number of nondiagnostic angiograms. In practice, the role of the nuclear bleeding scan is still controversial, mostly because of insufficient data. A sample of the available literature is presented here for illustration.

(2) Markisz described a retrospective review of 39 patients with LGI bleeding who underwent nuclear bleeding scans at a Boston teaching hospital. The average blood transfusion requirement was 4.4 units, the in-hospital mortality rate was 15%, and surgery or Gelfoam embolization was required in 28% of cases. Only 21 of the 39 patients underwent one or more confirmatory tests to validate the results of the bleeding scan. Colonoscopy, surgery, and angiography were performed 1, 7, and 19 times, respectively (25).

(a) Prognostic Value—A positive bleeding scan correlated with the blood transfusion requirement, the risk of death, and the need for surgery or embolization as shown in Table 18–4.

Table 18-4 Prognostic value of bleeding scans in LGI bleeding (25)

	Positive Scan (n=17)	Negative Scan (n=22)	*P*
Mean transfusion requirement	6.9 units	2.5 units	<0.01
Mortality rate	35%	0%	<0.05
Need for surgery or embolization	58%	4.5%	<0.01

(b) Localization—Twenty-one patients underwent one or more confirmatory tests. The accuracy of localization was verified by a confirmatory test in 10 of the 13 patients with positive bleeding scans, giving a PPV of 77%. A UGI site of hemorrhage was mistakenly identified as bleeding from the transverse colon in one case, and no bleeding sites were identified in 2 patients. Among the 8 patients with negative bleeding scans, a bleeding site was identified in 1 patient by additional confirmatory tests, giving an NPV of 88%.

(c) Utility As a Screening Tool for Angiography—Nineteen patients underwent angiography. Angiography was positive in 4 of the 11 patients with positive bleeding scans, giving a PPV of only 36%. However, angiography was negative in all 8 of the patients who had negative bleeding scans, giving an NPV of 100%. Therefore, the bleeding scan appears to be a reasonable screening tool for angiography.

(3) A similar study by Nicholson reported a PPV of 94% and an NPV of 92% for localization of the site of bleeding with nuclear scans. In addition, the bleeding scan accurately directed the type of surgery in all 15 patients who underwent surgery (29).

(4) In contrast, in a retrospective review of all 203 patients who had undergone a nuclear bleeding study for GI bleeding at three Canadian hospitals, Hunter was unable to confirm the value of the bleeding scan. A bleeding scan was positive in 52 patients, but confirmatory tests were done only in 22; in these, the bleeding scan was reported to be inaccurate in localizing the bleeding site in 13 patients. Even if all 30 nonconfirmed cases were assumed to be accurately localized, the scan would have been incorrect in 25% of cases. The authors questioned the utility of this test and urged that surgery not be based exclusively on the result of the bleeding scan (16). However, 6 of the 13 errors in localization were assumed to be inaccurate because they rebled after limited surgery. It is not clear whether this assumption was valid in all cases. Furthermore, five cases of UGI bleeding were mistaken for LGI bleeding, because the extravasated blood had moved downstream as a result of peristalsis. Careful upper endoscopy would have eliminated this error.

(5) Unless well-designed prospective studies become available, the role of nuclear bleeding scans in the management of patients with LGI bleeding will remain uncertain. The main advantage of this technique is that it is relatively simple and noninvasive. It identifies both active and intermittent bleeding and is more sensitive than angiography because it can detect bleeding rates of 0.1 to 0.5 ml/minute. The main disadvantage of the bleeding scan is that it lacks the spatial resolution of angiography and can only localize the site of bleeding to an approximate part of the abdomen. In addition, migration of extravasated blood as a result of peristalsis may be an important source of error in localizing the bleeding site (16,25,27,29).

3. Angiography

a. With angiography, the vascular system is accessed by a transfemoral approach and contrast dye is infused. An active bleeding rate of >0.5 ml/minute is required for detection by this method. The main advantage of angiography is its ability to localize and characterize the bleeding lesion precisely. In contrast to colonoscopy, bowel preparation is not necessary. In addition to its diagnostic utility, angiography offers the option of selective infusion of vasopressin (1,6,21). However, the technique is invasive and is associated with many complications, including dye allergies, renal failure, cardiac or bowel ischemia, laceration of cannulated vessels, and groin hematomas (11).

b. The diagnostic yield of angiography depends on the patient population, but the result is frequently negative even among patients with severe bleeding. For example, in Leitman's series of 68 patients with massive LGI bleeding, the average 24-hour blood transfusion requirement was 6 units, the surgery rate was 50%, and the mortality rate was 20%. In these patients, angiography was positive in only 40% of cases (21). In Browder's series of 50 patients with massive LGI bleeding, 70% required surgery, and all were either hypotensive or required transfusion of ≥4 units of blood within the first 2 hours of presentation. In this group of critically ill patients, angiography was positive in 72% of cases (6). If angiography is applied to patients with less severe bleeding, the diagnostic yield may be significantly lower. In a study reported by Jensen, the diagnostic yield of angiography was only 14%, and the rate of complications was 9% (18).

c. In Leitman's study, there were 12 patients with negative angiograms who required surgery; 6 of these patients had positive bleeding scans, indicating that the two tests may complement each other (21). As described previously, the nuclear bleeding scan can also be used as a screening tool to decrease the number of nondiagnostic angiograms.

4. Colonoscopy

a. If colonoscopy is performed under proper conditions, it is a highly accurate tool for identifying the cause of LGI bleeding. Furthermore, it offers the option of endoscopic therapy for many lesions. However, successful colonoscopy requires that the patient be hemodynamically stable and that the bowel be properly prepared. In the actively bleeding patient, colonoscopy may be difficult to perform because blood may obscure the visual field. Therefore, colonoscopy has traditionally been reserved for stable patients without evidence of ongoing bleeding (11).

b. More recently, several authors have demonstrated that emergency colonoscopy can be performed safely and effectively in patients with active, even severe LGI bleeding. The diagnostic yield was 80% or higher in most cases (8,18,35). The most widely quoted of these studies is by Jensen. In this study, the role of emergency colonoscopy was evaluated prospectively in 80 consecutive patients with severe ongoing hematochezia. The average blood transfusion requirement was 6.5 units, and 24% of patients required surgery. All patients had a negative NG lavage and negative results on rigid sigmoidoscopy. After oral purge, esophagogastroduodenoscopy and colonoscopy were performed within 24 hours of admission. Identification of the bleeding source required demonstration of active bleeding, an adherent clot over a lesion, or a visible vessel in an ulcer without other lesions. Several findings are worthy of note (18).

(1) Satisfactory examination to the cecum was possible in all 80 patients, and a bleeding source was identified in 94% of the cases. More than 60% of patients in the study had diverticulosis, but it was the source of bleeding only in 17%.

(2) The complication rate was only 4%, and complications in all cases resulted from fluid overload caused by the saline or sulfate purge. A different study using GoLYTELY, an isoosmotic purge solution, found no complications in 35 patients undergoing emergency colonoscopy for acute LGI bleeding (8).

(3) In comparison, the diagnostic yield of angiography was only 14%, with a complication rate of 9%. However, only 22 of the 80 patients underwent angiography.

(4) Eleven percent of patients were found to be bleeding from a UGI source, although all had negative results on NG lavage. However, when bile was present in the NG aspirate, no patient was found to be bleeding from an UGI source.

c. Caos also demonstrated that emergency colonoscopy identified the source of bleeding in 77% of the cases. Furthermore, 11 of the 12 patients were successfully treated with electrocautery (7 for angiodysplasia, 5 for polyps). All 7 patients requiring surgery underwent successful limited resections based on the colonoscopic findings (8).

C. General Approach to LGI Bleeding—The first priority in the management of a patient with LGI bleeding is hemodynamic resuscitation and stabilization. Therefore, the initial steps are no different from those applicable to patients with UGI bleeding (see Chapters 15 and 17). The following discussion concentrates on the features that are unique to the patient with LGI bleeding.

1. The patient's history can provide important diagnostic clues (11).

a. Age is an important diagnostic clue, because the two most common causes of LGI bleeding among older patients are angiodysplasia and diverticula. Among younger patients, hemorrhoids, anal fissures, inflammatory bowel disease, and Meckel's diverticulum are more common (11).

b. Abdominal pain suggests inflammatory bowel disease, ischemic bowel, or ruptured aortic aneurysm; painless bleeding is consistent with angiodysplasia or diverticula. The suspicion of ischemic colitis should be raised in elderly patients with a history of extensive vascular disease.

c. A history of constipation and weight loss suggests malignancy. Patients with hemorrhoids or anal fissures may complain of constipation, rectal pain, blood on the toilet tissue, or blood dripping into the toilet bowl at the end of the bowel movement.

d. Patients with chronic renal failure are at increased risk of bleeding from angiodysplasia. In Zuckerman's retrospective review of all consecutive patients with chronic renal failure undergoing upper endoscopy for UGI bleeding at Barnes Hospital, angiodysplasia of the stomach or duodenum was the most common cause of bleeding. Twenty-four percent of these patients were bleeding from angiodysplasia, compared with only 5% of patients without renal failure (42). Although the relation is less well documented, colonic and small bowel angiodysplasia have also been implicated as common sources of bleeding in patients with chronic renal failure (5,31).

2. NG lavage should be performed to exclude an UGI source of bleeding. However, if no blood is detected, a UGI source is not ruled out, because NG lavage may miss up to 16% of actively bleeding UGI lesions detectable on endoscopy (38). On the other hand, the presence of bile in the NG aspirate provides reassurance that the bleeding source is distal to the ligament of Treitz (18). If any doubt remains, esophagogastroduodenoscopy should be performed.

3. Localization

a. Hemodynamically Stable Patients in Whom Bleeding Stops—In most patients with LGI hemorrhage, bleeding stops spontaneously without further intervention. Because these patients are no longer actively bleeding, nuclear scans or angiography usually will not be helpful. Therefore, colonoscopy is the diagnostic procedure of choice in these patients (11). However, differentiating active bleeding from passage of old blood is difficult, because the colon can temporarily hide large amounts of blood. In addition, there is no simple LGI technique that is equivalent to the NG lavage to check quickly for active bleeding.

b. Hemodynamically Stable Patients in Whom Bleeding Continues—For stable patients who continue to bleed, there is controversy as to the best diagnostic strategy. Traditionally, colonoscopy has not been recommended in actively bleeding patients, because blood often obscures the visual field. Instead, selective angiography with or without a bleeding scan has been the standard at most centers. More recently, as discussed in a previous section, several investigators have reported encouraging results with colonoscopy that have challenged this traditional view (8,18,35). In light of these reports, colonoscopy is assuming an increasingly more prominent role in the evaluation of acute LGI bleeding. Nevertheless, emergency colonoscopy remains a challenging procedure and should be performed by experienced endoscopists. If colonoscopy is unsuccessful and the patient continues to bleed, angiography with or without a bleeding scan can be attempted. (See previous discussions on nuclear bleeding scans, angiography, and colonoscopy.) Because the utility of these procedures is operator dependent, management strategies, in the absence of compelling data, should be tailored to institutional strengths and preferences.

c. Unstable Patients

(1) In patients who continue to bleed despite conservative therapy, surgery may be required. If the bleeding site cannot be localized, emergency subtotal colectomy is usually performed. However, this procedure is associated with significant morbidity and mortality and does not guarantee that bleeding will not recur postoperatively (*e.g.*, from a small intestinal source that was missed on preoperative evaluation) (6). Therefore, every effort should be made to localize the bleeding site, so that a more limited operation can be performed. If the patient is hemodynamically unstable, localization is currently best achieved with angiography.

(2) Some investigators have tried to temporize the bleeding episode in these patients so that surgery can be performed electively rather than emergently. Intravascular infusion of vasopressin during angiography or endoscopic therapy during colonoscopy may be helpful for this purpose (1,6,10,15,17,19,21,36,37). Nevertheless, data from well-designed studies are still lacking. (See later discussions of diverticulosis and angiodysplasia.) Subtotal colectomy may be unavoidable in patients who continue to experience refractory massive LGI hemorrhage.

D. Management of Specific Causes of LGI Bleeding

1. Diverticulosis

a. In the United States, more than 50% of people older than 80 years of age have colonic diverticulosis. The pathogenesis of this condition has been linked to the lack of dietary fiber in the Western diet. Although it is a major cause of LGI bleeding in United States, only 3% to 5% of patients with diverticulosis experience acute bleeding in their lifetimes (11,26,32). Therefore, differentiating the incidental finding of diverticulosis from a true source of bleeding can sometimes be difficult (3).

b. Diverticular bleeding is usually painless and of sudden onset. In contrast, diverticulitis is usually painful but rarely causes GI bleeding. Because diverticular hemorrhage is arterial in origin, bleeding is often brisk. Although most diverticula are found in the sigmoid colon, about half of those that bleed are found in the right colon (9).

c. In 70% of cases, patients who present with diverticular hemorrhage stop bleeding spontaneously. In 10% to 25% of these patients, bleeding recurs. Once a patient rebleeds, the subsequent risk of rebleeding appears to be even higher. Therefore, surgery should be considered for these patients (26). Although the efficacy of such measures is unproven, the 75% to 90% of patients who do not rebleed can be treated conservatively with stool softeners and a high-fiber diet.

d. For patients who continue to bleed despite conservative therapy, selective infusion of vasopressin has been useful in some cases. In Browder's uncontrolled study of 50 patients with massive LGI bleeding, selective infusion of vasopressin was attempted in 22 patients. It successfully controlled bleeding in 20 patients (91%); however, 10 patients rebled within 3 days. Nevertheless, these 10 patients were able to undergo elective rather than emergency surgery (6). Athanasoulis described a similar uncontrolled study of 24 patients with massive rectal bleeding caused by diverticulosis. In all patients, there was clinical evidence of ongoing bleeding and extravasation of dye on angiography. Although all of these patients normally would have required surgery, 22 of the 24 patients were initially controlled with intraarterial vasopressin, and only 7 patients required urgent surgery (1). In contrast, in a study by Leitman, selective infusion of vasopressin was successful in <36% of cases. Only 6 of the 14 patients in this study were bleeding from diverticulosis, suggesting that nondiverticular bleeding may be less responsive to vasopressin than diverticular bleeding (21). Endoscopic therapy for diverticular bleeding has also been reported, but there are fewer data than for angiodysplasia (17).

2. Angiodysplasia

a. Angiodysplasia are common lesions found in about 25% of asymptomatic elderly Americans (2). Histologically, they consist of ectatic thin-walled venules and capillaries, which can progress to form a complex of dilated vascular channels and arteriovenous fistulas. They are thought to represent degenerative lesions of previously normal blood vessels and to result from repeated episodes of colonic distention. Boley has theorized that transient increases in the intraluminal pressure and the size of the colon cause temporary obstruction of venous outflow, leading to vascular dilation and arteriovenous communication. Consistent with this theory are the observations that these lesions tend to be multiple and that they commonly involve the right colon and cecum, where wall tensions are highest (2,4).

b. Because less than 10% of these lesions cause acute bleeding, prophylactic treatment of asymptomatic angiodysplasia is not warranted (11). When acute bleeding does occur, it tends to stop spontaneously, but the risk of rebleeding has been estimated to be as high as 85%. The true risk of rebleeding is still unknown (3,7,32). Angiodysplasia is also an important cause of occult GI bleeding (4,34).

c. The diagnosis of angiodysplasia requires angiography or colonoscopy. On angiography, slowly emptying intramural veins, vascular tufts, early filling veins, or extravasation of contrast dye can be observed. In the past, angiography was the gold standard for diagnosis of angiodysplasia, but colonoscopy is now assuming a greater role (11). Colonoscopy can detect smaller angiodysplastic lesions not detectable on angiography, but other conditions can mimic angiodysplasia (4,11,31). As for diverticulosis, the mere demonstration of a nonbleeding angiodysplastic lesion cannot be equated with identification of the bleeding site.

d. Therapeutic Options

(1) Medical Therapy—Initially based on the report of a female patient with Rendu-Osler-Weber syndrome who experienced epistaxis that varied with her menstrual cycle, hormonal therapy with estrogen-progesterone combination has been advocated by some authors. Uncontrolled studies have supported this practice (5,41). However, in a cohort study of 64 patients bleeding from angiodysplasia, the benefit of hormonal therapy was not confirmed. None of the patients in this study had chronic renal failure or Rendu-Osler-Weber syndrome (23). Some authors believe that the benefit of hormonal therapy may be limited to patients with vascular ectasias that are associated with chronic renal failure or Rendu-Osler-Weber syndrome (5,24,41).

(2) Vasopressin Infusion During Angiography—Selective intraarterial infusion of vasopressin may be useful in temporizing the bleeding episode in patients who continue to bleed despite conservative therapy (see earlier discussion of diverticulosis). However, unlike diverticular bleeding, bleeding from angiodysplasia is venous in origin. Therefore, some experts believe that vasopressin may be less effective for bleeding from angiodysplasia than for bleeding from diverticula (21).

(3) Endoscopic Therapy

(a) Many investigators have reported successful endoscopic therapy for LGI bleeding resulting from angiodysplasia. Endoscopic options currently include laser therapy, electrocautery, and heater probe devices. There are no data to suggest that one modality is better than another. However, the argon laser is favored over the neodymium:yttrium-aluminum-garnet (Nd:YAG) laser because it is associated with a lower risk of complications (10,15,19,36,37).

(b) Representative of the available data is Cello's uncontrolled study, in which 43 patients with GI bleeding caused by vascular ectasia were treated with argon or Nd:YAG laser therapy. During an average follow-up of 392 days, 49% did not rebleed. For patients who had only colonic angiodysplasia, 68% did not rebleed after laser therapy (10).

(4) Surgery may be required for patients who continue to bleed despite conservative therapy. Limited colonic resection directed by angiography or colonoscopy should be performed whenever possible. Occasionally, subtotal colectomy may be necessary for massive bleeding that cannot be localized.

3. Miscellaneous Causes

a. Aortoenteric Fistulas—The possibility of aortoenteric fistula should be considered in patients with GI bleeding and a history of an abdominal aortic aneurysm or aortic surgery. Most often, the fistula is to the third portion of the duodenum. Angiography is usually required for diagnosis. Immediate surgical correction is necessary (7,28).

b. Neoplasms—Neoplasms are common causes of LGI bleeding but infrequently result in severe bleeding. The most common neoplasms that cause LGI bleeding are polyps and adenocarcinoma of the colon. Metastatic disease, lymphoma, leiomyoma, and leiomyosarcoma can also cause GI bleeding. Diagnosis can usually be made by colonoscopy, but the detection of small bowel neoplasms may require enteroclysis, enteroscopy, or intraoperative endoscopy (7,13,22,28,33,40).

c. Radiation Colitis—Chronic radiation colitis can occur months to years after the initial exposure to radiation. The severity of radiation colitis depends on the pattern and total dose of radiation received. Radiation causes acute injury to blood vessels which can progress to obliterative endarteritis, in turn resulting in colonic inflammation, fibrosis, ulceration, and mucosal fissures. Clinically, patients experience abdominal pain and chronic, recurrent bleeding. Fistula formation and bowel obstruction from strictures are potential complications. The endoscopic appearance resembles that of ulcerative colitis; mucosal telangiectasias are often observed. Medical therapy with corticosteroids, sulfasalazine, or sucralfate enemas has been disappointing. Endoscopic laser therapy has been successful in decreasing the bleeding rate and blood transfusion requirement. Surgery may be necessary in refractory cases (14,20,28,30,39).

d. Meckel's Diverticulum—Meckel's diverticulum is a congenital anomaly affecting about 2% of the population. The diverticulum is found in the ileum, usually within 100 cm of the ileocecal valve. Most patients are asymptomatic, but the most frequent complications are bowel obstruction and GI bleeding. Although a common cause of GI bleeding in children, it is a rare cause in adults. Bleeding is from ulcers that result from acid production by heterotopic gastric mucosa, which is found in about 50% of patients with Meckel's diverticulum. The diagnosis can be established by angiography in actively bleeding patients or by ^{99m}Tc-pertechnetate scanning. ^{99m}Tc-pertechnetate accumulates in mucin-secreting cells of the gastric mucosa and in the right lower quadrant in a patient with a Meckel's diverticulum with heterotopic gastric mucosa. Surgical resection is the treatment of choice in symptomatic patients (28).

e. **Ischemic Colitis**—A diagnosis of ischemic colitis should be considered in elderly patients who present with LGI bleeding and a history of severe vascular or cardiac disease. Usually, symptoms also include abdominal pain, nausea, vomiting, and fever. Physical examination is usually unremarkable but may reveal peritoneal signs in advanced cases. The diagnosis can be confirmed by endoscopy, which may demonstrate a friable mucosa with edema, ulceration, and bleeding; the rectum is invariably spared because of its rich collateral circulation. Alternatively, barium enema may demonstrate characteristic thumbprinting. Surgery may be necessary in advanced cases in order to resect infarcted bowel, but most cases can be managed with supportive care. Broad-spectrum antibiotics are often administered to prevent sepsis, but their value has not been confirmed in controlled trials (28).

f. **Inflammatory Bowel Disease**—Patients with ulcerative colitis or Crohn's disease can present with acute GI bleeding, but severe bleeding is rare. Endoscopy with biopsy is usually diagnostic. Therapeutic options include oral or topical sulfasalazine or other aminosalicylates; parenteral, oral, or topical corticosteroids; and immunosuppressants. Surgical resection may be indicated in severe cases.

g. **GI Bleeding of Obscure Origin**—Despite extensive investigation, the cause of GI bleeding may remain obscure in about 5% to 10% of cases (3,18,24). Most of these patients prove to have colonic angiodysplasia, small bowel vascular anomalies, Meckel's diverticulum, or small bowel neoplasms (40). Enteroclysis, enteroscopy, intraoperative endoscopy, or a Meckel's scan may be helpful in this setting (13,22,33).

E. Summary

1. Literature-based discussion of LGI bleeding is difficult. Well-designed trials are scarce, and the available studies differ significantly in their design, making direct comparisons difficult. The management strategies recommended in the published literature are based mostly on the authors' expert opinions rather than on rigorously tested principles.
2. LGI bleeding should be categorized at presentation into one of three groups: occult, slow, or rapid. Patients with occult GI bleeding do not require hemodynamic resuscitation and can be evaluated electively on an outpatient basis. Other patients should be hemodynamically resuscitated and stabilized.
3. The most common causes of acute LGI bleeding are angiodysplasia and diverticula. Other causes include neoplastic lesions, inflammatory bowel disease, ischemic colitis, infectious colitis, radiation enteritis, Meckel's diverticulum, hemorrhoids, anal fissures, isolated ulcers, Rendu-Osler-Weber syndrome, and aortoenteric fistula. Despite extensive investigation, the cause of bleeding may not be identifiable in about 5% to 10% of cases. Further testing with a Meckel's scan, enteroclysis, enteroscopy, or intraoperative endoscopy may be helpful in some of these patients.
4. In all patients, careful NG lavage or esophagogastroduodenoscopy (or both) should be performed to exclude a UGI source of bleeding. After proper bowel preparation, stable patients without evidence of further bleeding should undergo colonoscopy. Many lesions can be treated endoscopically at that time. Biopsy of neoplastic lesions is also possible.
5. In actively bleeding patients, colonoscopy may be difficult because blood may obscure the visual field. However, recent studies have demonstrated that colonoscopy can be performed safely and effectively in most cases. If colonoscopy is not possible, a nuclear bleeding scan followed by selective angiography is recommended. Intraarterial infusion of vasopressin or endoscopic therapy may be considered for control of hemorrhage. However, the enthusiasm for

these procedures is based almost entirely on uncontrolled data at this time. For patients who fail conservative therapy, limited surgical resection guided by angiography or colonoscopy should be performed.

6. Unstable patients often require surgery. If possible, a limited surgical resection guided by angiography should be performed. Selective infusion of vasopressin or endoscopic therapy may be helpful in converting an emergency operation into an elective one. In some cases, subtotal colectomy may be unavoidable.

Abbreviations used in Chapter 18

GI = gastrointestinal
LGI = lower gastrointestinal
Nd:YAG laser = neodymium:yttrium-aluminum-garnet laser
NG = nasogastric
NPV = negative predictive value
P = probability value
PPV = positive predictive value
UGI = upper gastrointestinal

References

1. Athanasoulis. Mesenteric arterial infusions of vasopressin for hemorrhage from colonic diverticulosis. *Am J Surg* 1975;129:212.
2. Boley. On the nature and etiology of vascular ectasias of the colon: degenerative lesions of aging. *Gastroenterology* 1977;72:650.
3. Boley. Lower gastrointestinal bleeding in the elderly. *Am J Surg* 1979;137:57.
4. Boley. Vascular ectasias of the colon. *Dig Dis Sci* 1986;31:26s.
5. Bronner. Estrogen-progesterone therapy for bleeding gastrointestinal telangiectasias in chronic renal failure. *Ann Intern Med* 1986;105:371.
6. Browder. Impact of emergency angiography in massive lower gastrointestinal bleeding. *Ann Surg* 1986;204:530.
7. Buchman. Current management of patients with lower gastrointestinal bleeding. *Surg Clin North Am* 1987;67:651. Review.
8. Caos. Colonoscopy after GoLYTELY preparation in acute rectal bleeding. *J Clin Gastroenterol* 1986;8:46.
9. Casarella. Right-sided colonic diverticula as a cause of acute rectal hemorrhage. *N Engl J Med* 1972;286:450.
10. Cello. Endoscopic laser therapy treatment for gastrointestinal vascular ectasias. *Ann Intern Med* 1986;104:352.
11. DeMarkles. Acute lower gastrointestinal bleeding. *Med Clin North Am* 1993;77:1085. Review.
12. Farrands. Management of acute lower gastrointestinal hemorrhage in a surgical unit over a 4 year period. *J R Soc Med* 1987;80:79.
13. Flickinger. Intraoperative video panendoscopy for diagnosing sites of chronic intestinal bleeding. *Am J Surg* 1989;157:137.
14. Goldstein. Treatment of chronic radiation enteritis and colitis with salicylazosulfapyridine and systemic corticosteroids. *Am J Gastroenterol* 1976;65:201.
15. Gostout. Mucosal vascular malformations of the gastrointestinal tract: clinical observations and results of endoscopic neodymium:yttrium-aluminum-garnet laser therapy. *Mayo Clin Proc* 1988;63:993.
16. Hunter. Limited value of technetium 99m–labeled red cell scintigraphy in localization of lower gastrointestinal bleeding. *Am J Surg* 1990;159:504.
17. Jensen. Endoscopic heater probe coagulation of the bleeding colonic diverticulum. *Gastrointest Endosc* 1986;32:160.

18. Jensen. Diagnosis and treatment of severe hematochezia: the role of urgent colonoscopy after purge. *Gastroenterology* 1988;95:1569.
19. Jensen. Endoscopic diagnosis and treatment of bleeding colonic angiomas and radiation telangiectasias. *Perspectives in Colon and Rectal Surgery* 1989;2:99.
20. Ladas. Sucralfate enemas in the treatment of chronic postradiation proctitis. *Am J Gastroenterol* 1989;84:1587.
21. Leitman. Evaluation and management of massive lower gastrointestinal hemorrhage. *Ann Surg* 1989;209:175.
22. Lewis. Intraoperative enteroscopy versus small bowel enteroscopy in patients with obscure GI bleeding. *Am J Gastroenterol* 1991;86:171.
23. Lewis. Does hormonal therapy have any benefit for bleeding angiodysplasia. *J Clin Gastroenterol* 1992;15:99.
24. Lewis. Small intestinal bleeding. *Gastroenterol Clin North Am* 1994;23:67. Review.
25. Markisz. An evaluation of Tc-99m red blood cell scintigraphy for the detection and localization of gastrointestinal bleeding sites. *Gastroenterology* 1982;83:394.
26. McGuire. Massive hemorrhage from diverticulosis of the colon: guidelines for therapy based on bleeding patterns observed in fifty cases. *Ann Surg* 1972;175:847.
27. McKusick. Tc-99m red blood cells for detection of gastrointestinal bleeding: experience with 80 patients. *AJR Am J Roentgenol* 1981;137:1113.
28. Miller. Less frequent causes of lower gastrointestinal bleeding. *Gastroenterol Clin North Am* 1994;23:21. Review.
29. Nicholson. Localization of lower gastrointestinal bleeding using in vivo technetium-99m–labeled red blood cell scintigraphy. *Br J Surg* 1989;76:358.
30. O'Connor. Argon laser treatment of radiation proctitis. *Arch Surg* 1989;124:749.
31. Potter. Lower gastrointestinal bleeding. *Gastroenterol Clin North Am* 1988;17:341. Review.
32. Reinus. Vascular ectasias and diverticulosis. *Gastroenterol Clin North Am* 1994; 23:1. Review.
33. Rex. Enteroclysis in the evaluation of suspected small intestinal bleeding. *Gastroenterology* 1989;97:58.
34. Richter. Angiodysplasia: clinical presentation and colonoscopic diagnosis. *Dig Dis Sci* 1984;29:481.
35. Rossini. Emergency colonoscopy. *World J Surg* 1989;13:190.
36. Rutgeerts. Long term results of treatment of vascular malformations of the gastrointestinal tract by neodymium YAG laser photocoagulation. *Gut* 1985;26:586.
37. Schrock. Colonoscopic diagnosis and treatment of lower gastrointestinal bleeding. *Surg Clin North Am* 1989;69:1309. Review.
38. Silverstein. The national ASGE survey on upper gastrointestinal bleeding: II. Clinical prognostic factors. *Gastrointest Endosc* 1981;27:80.
39. Strockbine. Complications in 831 patients with squamous cell carcinoma of the intact uterine cervix treated with 3000 rads or more whole pelvis radiation. *AJR Am J Roentgenol* 1970;108:293.
40. Thompson. Specialist investigation of obscure gastrointestinal bleeding. *Gut* 1987; 28:47.
41. Van Cutsem. Estrogen-progesterone treatment of Osler-Weber-Rendu disease. *J Clin Gastroenterol* 1988;10:676.
42. Zuckerman. Upper gastrointestinal bleeding in patients with chronic renal failure. *Ann Intern Med* 1985;102:58

19

Acute Renal Failure

Ravi I. Thadhani and
Joseph V. Bonventre

A. Introduction

1. **Definition of Acute Renal Failure**—In the clinical setting, acute renal failure (ARF) is generally defined as a syndrome characterized by a deterioration in renal function, resulting in failure of the kidney to excrete nitrogenous waste products and to regulate fluid and electrolyte homeostasis. Oliguria (urine output <400 to 500 ml/day) is common but not universal in the course of ARF. The causes of ARF are usually divided into three categories: decrease in renal perfusion (prerenal azotemia); intrinsic renal parenchymal disease (renal azotemia); and obstruction of urinary outflow (postrenal azotemia).
2. A literature-based discussion of ARF is difficult because only a few of the studies on this topic have been prospective or randomized, and even those studies have included relatively small numbers of patients (73a). Most of the studies on ARF have been case series that lack an adequate control group and are subject to selection and information bias. In addition, the available studies often differ in their design, definition of ARF, and exclusion criteria, which has made comparison between studies difficult (11). For example, Novis analyzed 26 studies of postoperative renal failure and found that no two studies used the same definition for ARF (55).
3. **Incidence**—The incidence of ARF varies from study to study depending on the definition used and the population studied. The incidence of ARF among patients just arriving to the hospital appears to be lower than the incidence among those already in the hospital, which in turn is lower than the incidence among postoperative patients.
   a. **Incidence of ARF on Admission to a Hospital**—Among all patients admitted to a Veterans Administration hospital during a 17-month period in one study, 1% (100 patients) had a serum creatinine level of >2.0 mg/dl with a documented acute elevation of ≥0.5 mg/dl from baseline (36).
   b. **Incidence of ARF During Hospitalization**—In Hou's prospective study of 2262 consecutive patients admitted to the general medical and surgical units of a tertiary care center, the incidence of hospital-acquired ARF was 5% (29). If the episodes of ARF associated with volume contraction (excluding cardiac dysfunction and sepsis) or surgery are included in the analysis (together with those caused by contrast media, aminoglycoside antibiotics, and *cis*-platinum), 55% of the hospital-acquired cases of ARF had an iatrogenic cause. On the other hand, in Davidman's study of 4569 patients admitted to a tertiary care center over a 4-month period, only 1.3% had an iatrogenic cause (17).
   c. **Incidence of ARF After Surgery**—In a study of 734 patients with normal baseline renal function (all with preoperative serum creatinine <1.5 mg/dl) who underwent cardiopulmonary bypass surgery, 15% had a peak postoperative serum creatinine level of >1.5 mg/dl; 11% had a peak of 1.5 to 2.5 mg/dl, and 4% peaked at ≥2.5 mg/dl (84). In an analysis of 26 studies evaluating >10,000 postsurgical patients, the frequency of renal failure ranged from 1% to 84%, with the highest risk among those undergoing cardiovascular procedures (55).

d. **Incidence of ARF After Cardiopulmonary Arrest**—After cardiopulmonary resuscitation, the prevalence of ARF is as high as 30%. On the average, the patients who developed ARF required a longer duration of resuscitation (12±2 minutes versus 7±1 minutes; $P<0.01$) and received a higher total dose of epinephrine during the resuscitation (1.81±0.36 mg versus 0.90±0.18 mg; $P<0.02$), compared with those who did not develop ARF (46).

4. **Mortality Rate**—The mortality rate associated with ARF is estimated to be 40% to 70%. This figure has not changed over the past 20 years despite the advances in diagnosis and management of ARF (26). Several studies have addressed this issue.
   a. Turney compared two cohorts of patients who underwent dialysis in the periods 1960 to 1969 and 1980 to 1989, respectively, in the same hospital (76) (see Table 19–1). All patients had ARF caused by sepsis. Turney concluded that the mortality rate in patients with ARF remains high (without significant change over several decades) because the more recent patients are older and are more likely to have complicated underlying conditions such as multisystem organ failure.
   b. Woodrow evaluated the cause of death in 636 patients with ARF (serum creatinine >6.8 mg/dl) who died between 1956 and 1989 (82). As in the previous study, the mean age of patients had significantly increased over the period. The frequency of death caused by gastrointestinal bleeding or nonrecovery of renal function had declined, whereas deaths from cardiovascular instability or withdrawal of support had increased.
   c. Some of the most important causes of death in patients with ARF are the comorbid conditions that precipitated or were present at the time of ARF. For example, in a recent study by Liano involving 228 patients with acute tubular necrosis (ATN), no patient died because of uremia or hyperkalemia. Instead, the major causes of death in the 128 patients who died were original disease (40%), sepsis (14%), cardiovascular or respiratory complication (9%), and gastrointestinal hemorrhage (7%) (40).

5. **Predictors of Poor Outcome**
   a. **Comorbid Conditions**—Several comorbid conditions in the setting of ARF are associated with poor outcome. In particular, patients with sepsis or respiratory complications (*i.e.*, aspiration pneumonia, respiratory arrest or failure, the need for assisted ventilation, adult respiratory distress syndrome [ARDS]) are less likely to survive (9,14,40,72). Representative studies that have evaluated these associations are discussed in the following sections.
      (1) In Bullock's study of 462 patients with ARF, the mortality rate was estimated at 68% (9). Patients with concomitant pulmonary complications, such as aspiration pneumonia, respiratory arrest or failure, or ARDS, had an eight times greater chance of dying during their course of ARF than patients without these conditions. Other risk factors included older age, jaundice, and cardiovascular complications.
      (2) In a study of 151 patients with ARF from both medical and surgical units, Corwin demonstrated that sepsis, respiratory failure, and oli-

Table 19-1 Comparison of two cohorts requiring acute dialysis (76)

	1960–1969 Cohort (n=119)	1980–1989 Cohort (n=124)	*P*
Mean age	50.9	63.1	<0.0001
Ventilated patients	1.7	41.1%	<0.0001
Median APACHE II score	32	35	<0.0001
Survival	48.7%	36.6%	>0.05

guria were the major predictors of nonrecovery of renal function, and sepsis and nonrecovery of renal function were important predictors of death (14).

(3) Spiegel evaluated 43 consecutive critically ill patients requiring dialysis for ARF and found that ARDS ($P<0.05$), requirement for antibiotics ($P<0.01$), and ventilatory failure ($P<0.01$) were associated with nonrecovery of renal function (72). In addition, the need for ventilatory support at the initiation of dialysis was independently predictive of poor survival. For example, 100% (31/31) of the patients needing this intervention died, compared with 58% (7/12) of those not requiring ventilatory support ($P<0.001$).

(4) In the previously described study by Liano of patients with ATN, univariate analysis demonstrated that persistent hypotension ($P<0.001$), need for dialysis ($P<0.01$), and need for assisted respiration ($P<0.001$) were predictors of increased mortality (40).

b. Oliguric Versus Nonoliguric ARF—Several studies have found a lower mortality rate for patients with nonoliguric (>450 ml urine per 24 hours) than for those with oliguric (<400 to 450 ml urine per 24 hours) renal failure. A summary of these studies is presented in Table 19-2 (9,14,21,29,40, 61). This observation has stimulated interest in the use of diuretic agents in an attempt to convert oligo-anuric renal failure into nonoliguric renal failure. However, whether this practice improves outcome is doubtful, especially in light of evidence that patients who respond to diuretics probably have less severe renal damage at baseline compared with those who do not respond to diuretics (41).

c. Severity of ARF and Mortality—The severity of ARF also correlates with mortality. In Hou's study of 109 patients with ARF, the mortality rate was 15% for those with a mild increase in the serum creatinine (≥3.0 mg/dl from baseline) compared with 64% ($P<0.001$) for those with a more substantial increase (≥3.0 mg/dl from baseline) (29). In Kaufman's study of 100 patients with ARF, the mean peak serum creatinine level among the survivors was 4.1 mg/dl, compared with 7.1 mg/dl among those who died ($P<0.005$) (36). In Zanardo's study of patients with postoperative ARF, the mortality rate was 0.8%, 10%, and 44% among patients with peak serum creatinine levels of <1.5 mg/dl, 1.5 to 2.5 mg/dl, and >2.5 mg/dl, respectively ($P=0.0001$) (84).

6. Risk Factors for ARF—In Rasmussen's series of 143 patients with ATN developing in the hospital, current use of antihypertensives and a documented history of diastolic blood pressure >100 mm Hg and preexisting renal disease (baseline serum creatinine >1.7 mg/dl) were found on linear regression analysis to be important risk factors for the development of ARF (61). After correcting for both chronic hypertension and preexisting renal disease, age was not an independent risk factor in this study. This latter finding is also supported by two additional studies (29,40), but other studies suggest that age is indeed a risk factor for the development of ARF (21,72,76,84).

Table 19-2 Studies comparing nonoliguric and oliguric ARF

Author (Reference)	N	Mortality from Nonoliguric ARF	Mortality from Oliguric ARF	*P*
Rasmussen (61)	143	28%	78%	<0.001
Bullock (9)	462	58%	65%	<0.05
Corwin (14)	151	42%	83%	Not given
Hou (29)	109	17%	52%	<0.01
Liano (40)	228	42%	65%	<0.01
Feest (21)	125	23%	63%	<0.001

7. **Etiology of ARF**—As mentioned previously, the causes of ARF are traditionally divided into three categories: prerenal, renal, and postrenal. The relative frequency of each category of ARF varies depending on the population studied.
   a. For patients with ARF at the time of admission to the hospital, Kaufman found that the causes were prerenal in 70%, renal in 11%, postrenal in 17%, and unclassified in 2% (36). The prerenal causes included vomiting, poor oral intake, diarrhea, fever, gastrointestinal bleeding, glucosuria, use of angiotensin-converting enzyme inhibitors (ACEIs), use of diuretics, and congestive heart failure. The intrinsic renal causes included infections (infective endocarditis, xanthogranulomatous pyelonephritis, and septic shock), drugs (*cis*-platinum, rifampin, and glyburide), spontaneous cholesterol emboli, renal vein thrombosis, and progressive focal glomerulosclerosis. The postrenal causes included benign prostatic hyperplasia, prostatic carcinoma, bladder stones, and lymphoma. Among all patients who entered the hospital with ARF, 80% had a potentially reversible cause (36).
   b. For patients who develop ARF during the course of their hospitalization, usually more than one cause contributes to the renal dysfunction. In Davidman's series of 59 patients with hospital-acquired ARF who were evaluated by a nephrology consultation team, 47% had more than one cause of ARF (*e.g.*, administration of aminoglycoside antibiotics in the setting of hypotension) (17). Similarly, in Rasmussen's study of 143 patients with hospital-acquired ARF, 62% had more than one potential cause of ARF (61).
   c. In general, prerenal azotemia from cardiovascular disease, surgery, or volume depletion and renal azotemia from aminoglycosides, contrast agents, or ischemia account for the majority of cases of hospital-acquired ARF. The exact prevalence of each cause, however, differs from study to study. In Hou's prospective study of 109 patients with hospital-acquired ARF, the major causes of ARF were decreased renal perfusion (42%), postoperative renal insufficiency (18%), contrast agents (12%), and aminoglycosides (7%). Miscellaneous causes including hepatorenal syndrome, obstruction, vasculitis, *cis*-platinum, and no defined cause accounted for 21% of the cases (29). In Corwin's study of 151 patients with ARF (after excluding patients with prerenal azotemia), the major causes included ischemia (47%), drugs (19%), contrast agents (15%), and hemoglobin or myoglobin toxicity (9%) (14). In Feest's prospective study of 125 patients with severe ARF (serum creatinine >5.7 mg/dl), the major diagnoses included cardiovascular disease (13%); surgery (14%); obstetric complications (11%); prostatic obstruction (25%); various medical conditions including volume loss, hematologic causes, intrinsic renal causes, toxins, and combinations of insults (34%); and unknown factors (4%) (21). The major causes of ARF are considered in greater detail in the following sections.

B. Prerenal Azotemia

1. Prerenal azotemia results from inadequate perfusion of the kidney. If corrected rapidly, it usually leads to minimal, if any, renal injury. If renal hypoperfusion persists, ischemic ATN (and potentially cortical necrosis) may occur, at which point volume expansion or other means of improving renal perfusion may no longer be effective in restoring renal function. For example, Bickell conducted a prospective study of 598 young, otherwise healthy adults (mean age, about 31 years) with penetrating torso injuries and a prehospital systolic blood pressure ≤90 mm Hg (7). Patients were randomly assigned to receive either immediate fluid resuscitation (begun before arrival at the hospital; n=309) or delayed fluid resuscitation (begun intraoperatively; n=289). The time from arrival of aid at the scene to arrival of the patient in the operating room did not differ between the two groups (about 80 minutes). As expected, patients who received immediate resuscitation had a higher systolic blood pressure on arrival at the hospital (79 versus 72 mm Hg; P=0.02). The incidence of postoperative ARF, however, did not differ significantly between the two groups (P=0.11).
2. The major causes of prerenal ARF include true volume depletion (*e.g.*, vomit-

ing, diarrhea, nasogastric suction, hemorrhage, diuresis, excessive sweating, burns), other causes of low effective intravascular volume (*e.g.*, congestive heart failure, nephrotic syndrome, cirrhosis, sequestration of fluid as a result of pancreatitis or peritonitis), other causes of hemodynamic insufficiency or systemic hypotension (*e.g.*, sepsis, cardiogenic shock, massive pulmonary embolism), and drugs (*e.g.*, cyclosporine, nonsteroidal antiinflammatory drugs [NSAIDs], ACEIs, a-adrenergic agents) (see Table 19–3). Surgery can cause ARF by a combination of these mechanisms (*e.g.*, blood loss, fluid shifts, anesthesia, cross-clamping of the aorta) and is considered separately.

a. Patients with true volume depletion or low effective intravascular volume are prone to development of ARF because of renal hypoperfusion. In addition, all forms of shock or systemic hypotension cause renal hypoperfusion and thus prerenal azotemia. Although patients with an intraaortic balloon pump (IABP) can develop ARF by various mechanisms, the most common cause is hemodynamic instability, which is often the very reason the IABP was inserted. In three large series involving a total of 1586 patients requiring IABP support for cardiac pump failure, the incidence of ARF was <1% (24,35,48). If the pump is positioned properly, the risk of developing ARF as a result of the IABP itself is low.

b. Drugs—Countless drugs can cause prerenal ARF. Drugs with α-adrenergic agonist properties, such as vasopressor medications used in the treatment of septic shock (high-dose dopamine, norepinephrine) cause vasoconstriction of the renal arterioles and thereby decrease renal blood flow. Antihypertensive drugs may decrease renal blood flow by reducing systemic blood pressure. In addition to these more obvious examples, cyclosporine, ACEIs, and NSAIDs can also decrease renal perfusion.

(1) Cyclosporine—Cyclosporine causes functional prerenal azotemia by inducing vasoconstriction of the afferent arterioles, which reduces glomerular filtration pressure. Acute nephrotoxicity from cyclosporine is usually dose dependent and reversible by dose reduction (34).

(2) Angiotensin-Converting Enzyme Inhibitors

(a) Juxtaglomerular cells in the afferent arterioles synthesize and release renin in response to renal hypoperfusion and increased sympathetic activity. Renin converts angiotensinogen into angiotensin I (AT I). In turn, AT I is converted to AT II by a converting enzyme located primarily in the lung. AT II causes vasoconstriction of both the efferent and afferent arterioles, but because the efferent arteriole has a smaller basal diameter, the effect of AT II on this segment is greater than its effect on the afferent arteriole. Constriction of the efferent arterioles by AT II increases intraglomerular hydrostatic pressure, which in turn enhances

Table 19-3 Prerenal causes of acute renal failure

Category	Examples
True volume depletion	Vomiting, diarrhea, nasogastric suction, hemorrhage, diuresis
Other causes of low effective intravascular volume	Congestive heart failure, nephrotic syndrome, cirrhosis, sequestration of fluid due to pancreatitis or peritonitis
Other causes of systemic hypotension	Sepsis, cardiogenic shock, massive pulmonary embolism
Drugs	α-Adrenergic drugs, cyclosporine, ACEI, NSAIDs, FK506, Anesthesia
Surgery	Hemorrhage, fluid shifts, anesthesia, cross-clamping of the aorta

glomerular filtration, especially in states of reduced renal blood flow. Correspondingly, ACEIs, by decreasing the formation of AT II, may reduce the hydrostatic pressure within the glomerulus.

(b) In the original description of ACEI–induced ARF in patients with renal artery stenosis, Hricik evaluated the effect of captopril (75 to 225 mg/day) in 7 patients with bilateral renal artery stenosis and 4 patients with unilateral renal artery stenosis and a solitary kidney (30). The age of the patients ranged from 36 to 81 years, and all were taking a diuretic during the trial. The time from initiation of captopril to peak impairment of renal function ranged from 4 to 60 days. Discontinuation of captopril resulted in improvement of renal function in all patients who survived. The authors concluded that diuretics may have also contributed to the renal dysfunction.

(c) Mandal studied whether the risk of ARF is higher with the use of an ACEI alone or with the use of an ACEI plus a diuretic (45). Seventy-four patients with hypertension (n=57), congestive heart failure (n=36), or diabetes mellitus (n=12) were evaluated retrospectively, and the 41 patients who were taking ACEIs only were compared with the 33 patients taking an ACEI and a diuretic. ARF (rise in serum creatinine ≥0.5 mg/dl from baseline) developed in 2.4% of those receiving ACEIs only, compared with 33% of those receiving the combination therapy ($P<0.001$). Furthermore, after 8.7 months of therapy, patients who received the combination therapy had a higher mean serum creatinine level than those who received ACEIs alone (3.1 versus 1.2 mg/dl, respectively; $P<0.01$). Renal function recovered equally well in both groups, and volume infusion seems to have enhanced recovery. Through sodium wasting and volume depletion, diuretics appear to potentiate the effects of ACEIs and increase the risk of renal dysfunction.

(3) Nonsteroidal Antiinflammatory Drugs

(a) In states of renal hypoperfusion, the renin-angiotensin-aldosterone pathway is activated. As stated, AT II, a product of this pathway, promotes constriction of both the afferent and efferent glomerular arterioles. AT II is also a potent stimulus for renal production of prostaglandin E_2, which augments renal perfusion through its vasodilatory effect on the afferent arterioles. In the basal state prostaglandins play a minor role in maintaining perfusion, but in states of renal hypoperfusion prostaglandins are important in protecting renal blood flow. Prostaglandin E_2 helps to maintain renal perfusion in times of stress and to counteract the effects of vasoconstrictive catecholamines on the kidney (12). NSAIDs block the vasodilatory effect of prostaglandin E_2 on the afferent arterioles by inhibiting prostaglandin synthesis. Patients who develop NSAID-induced ARF usually have other concomitant factors that also contribute to renal injury or hypoperfusion. For example, in one study involving 27 patients with NSAID-induced ARF, 93% were taking other nephrotoxic medications or had another condition contributing to renal hypoperfusion at the time the NSAIDs were implicated (*e.g.*, shock, gastrointestinal bleeding, congestive heart failure, diuretics) (69). In addition to their renovascular effects, NSAIDs may also cause allergic interstitial nephritis, nephrotic syndrome, sodium retention, hyperkalemia (by decreasing renin and, subsequently, aldosterone production), and hyponatremia (12).

c. Postoperative ARF—Reduction in renal blood flow is also the major mechanism responsible for ARF after surgery. Anesthesia and blood loss contribute to renal hypoperfusion through volume depletion, fluid shifts, and systemic vasoconstriction. Prerenal azotemia (as well as ischemic ATN) is especially common after cardiac bypass surgery or abdominal aneurysm resection, in which the aorta is clamped above the renal vessels. In Zanardo's prospective study involving 775 consecutive patients who survived >24 hours after cardiac bypass surgery, patients with baseline renal dysfunction (serum creatinine >1.5 mg/dl) had significantly higher rates of death and perioperative complications than those with baseline serum creatinine <1.5 mg/dl (84). Compared with patients with normal baseline renal function, those with baseline renal dysfunction had higher rates of cardiovascular complications (18% versus 32%, respectively; *P*<0.05), neurologic complications (3% versus 20%; *P*<0.001), and death (3% versus 17%; *P*<0.001). Among those with normal baseline renal function, older age (*P*=0.0001), longer bypass time (*P*=0.0001), a low rate of diuresis during bypass (*P*=0.0001), and the need for IABP postoperatively (*P*=0.001) were predictive of postoperative renal dysfunction.

C. Postrenal Azotemia

1. Obstruction of the urinary tract is an important cause of ARF. Prompt relief of the obstruction leads to minimal, if any, permanent injury to the kidney. On the other hand, long-standing obstruction may lead to irreversible renal dysfunction. To cause ARF, obstruction must be bilateral (or unilateral in a patient with a single functional kidney), as may occur for example with enlargement of the prostate gland. The site of the obstruction may be intraluminal (*e.g.*, clots, stones, lack of peristalsis) or extraluminal (*e.g.*, prostatic hypertrophy, malignancy, fibrosis). Major causes of postrenal ARF are summarized in Table 19-4.
2. In a series of 50 cases of postrenal azotemia secondary to bilateral ureteral obstruction, the most common presenting symptoms were anuria (50%) and abdominal pain (34%) (54). In 76% of these patients, underlying malignancies were the cause of obstruction, the most common being cervical carcinoma (in 52% of women) and prostatic carcinoma (in 47% of men). The remaining 24% of the patients had a nonmalignant cause of ureteral obstruction, the most important being retroperitoneal fibrosis (66%). Only two patients had bilateral renal stones as the cause of ARF.
3. Immediate relief of the obstruction by surgical decompression, cystoscopic retrograde ureteral stenting, or percutaneous nephrostomy tube (PNT) insertion is the cornerstone of therapy for patients with ARF caused by obstruction. In patients who cannot undergo general anesthesia, PNT insertion remains an appropriate option because it can be performed under local anesthesia. In Watkinson's study of 50 patients with urinary tract obstruction, the insertion of a PNT prolonged survival and improved the quality of life in most patients. However, in the subset of patients with obstruction caused by a relapse of malignancy, PNT did not offer any benefit if there were no viable options for treatment of the relapse (78).

D. Renal Azotemia: Acute Tubular Necrosis—Syndromes that fall under the category of renal azotemia include ATN, acute interstitial nephritis, and acute glomerulonephritis (GN). The frequency of each type depends on the population studied, but after prerenal azotemia, ATN is probably the most common cause of ARF among hospitalized patients. ATN is characterized by an abrupt decline in the glomerular filtration rate that results from an acute ischemic or toxic insult to the kidney. The most common predisposing factor for ATN is persistent ischemia after

Table 19-4 Postrenal causes of acute renal failure

Primary Sites	Examples
Bladder and urethra	Neurogenic bladder, malignancy, clot, prostatic hyperplasia, urethral stricture
Ureters	Stones, clot, malignancy, retroperitoneal fibrosis

Table 19-5 Causes of acute tubular necrosis

Category	Examples
Ischemic	Similar to causes of prerenal ARF
Toxic	Aminoglycosides, amphotericin B, contrast agents, rhabdomyolysis, myeloma

prolonged prerenal azotemia. Tubular injury can also be caused by toxins such as aminoglycosides, contrast dyes, pigment, and multiple myeloma. Major causes of ATN are summarized in Table 19-5.

1. **Clinical Course of Ischemic or Toxic ATN**—Traditionally, the clinical course of ATN is divided into three phases: initial, maintenance, and recovery. During the initial phase, there is a reduction in glomerular filtration rate and a concomitant increase in serum concentrations of urea and creatinine. Oliguria may occur, but anuria (<100 ml/day) should suggest obstruction or cortical necrosis. Renal dysfunction may persist for varying lengths of time during the maintenance phase. The initial and maintenance phases are characterized by the presence of casts in the urine sediment and a urine osmolarity of <350 mOsm/L. Heralding recovery, there is a gradual increase in urine volume if the ARF was oliguric. Finally, a decrease in blood urea nitrogen (BUN) and serum creatinine become evident in the recovery phase. The duration of each phase is variable.
2. **Aminoglycosides**
   a. Aminoglycoside antibiotics are freely filtered at the glomerulus and subsequently excreted. In the proximal tubule, however, aminoglycosides bind to the brush-border phospholipids on the luminal surface. The drug is then pinocytosed into membrane vesicles and incorporated into proximal tubular lysosomes, where it exerts its toxicity. The most common clinical presentation of aminoglycoside toxicity is an asymptomatic rise in serum creatinine 7 to 10 days after the initiation of therapy. Patients are usually nonoliguric if there are no other factors compromising their hemodynamic status. After the drug is discontinued, renal dysfunction may persist and worsen for another 5 to 7 days owing to the accumulation of the drug in the renal cortex (12).
   b. **Risk Factors for Aminoglycoside Nephrotoxicity**—Two randomized, double-blind controlled trials found the following to be independent risk factors in the development of aminoglycoside nephrotoxicity (defined as ≥50% fall in the calculated creatinine clearance rate): preexisting liver disease (albumin <3.0 g/dl, total bilirubin >2.5 mg/dl, aspartate transaminase >38 IU/L, or alanine transaminase >34 IU/L, a history of hepatic insufficiency, or the presence of ascites); a higher initial 1-hour postdose aminoglycoside level (7.2±0.4 versus 5.3±0.1 g/ml); shock (systolic blood pressure <80 mm Hg with a urine output <500 ml/24 hours, or a subsequent fall in the systolic blood pressure by >50 mm Hg if the initial systolic blood pressure was >100 mm Hg); and female sex (50). Patients with a higher baseline creatinine clearance rate (70±5 versus 58±3 ml/minute) were also at an increased risk for nephrotoxicity in the study. The reason for this association is not clear, but the dose of aminoglycosides was adjusted for renal dysfunction, so that those with greater renal function received higher doses of the nephrotoxin. In addition, patients with higher creatinine clearance may have had a higher filtered load of the drug, resulting in a higher concentration of the nephrotoxin in the proximal tubules. Other studies have found that increased age, prior history of renal insufficiency, a recent course of aminoglycoside therapy, and concomitant administration of other nephrotoxins (*e.g.*, cephalothin, *cis*-platinum, amphotericin B) were also risk factors for aminoglycoside nephrotoxicity (12). An elevated trough level of gentamicin does not appear to be an independent risk factor

for nephrotoxicity, but it may suggest that aminoglycoside nephrotoxicity is developing (12).

c. The rate of cortical uptake of gentamicin is saturable. Therefore, less drug appears to accumulate in cells when the same amount is given as a single large dose than when it is given in multiple divided doses. Once- versus thrice-daily dosing of gentamicin was compared in a prospective randomized trial conducted by Prins (58) (see Table 19–6). Patients with various infections were randomly assigned to treatment with IV gentamicin (4 mg/kg) given once daily or divided into three doses per day. Acute Physiology and Chronic Health Evaluation II (APACHE-II) scores were similar between the two groups. Nephrotoxicity was defined as a rise in serum creatinine of 0.5 mg/dl above baseline. Patients with initial serum creatinine >3.4 mg/dl and those with neutropenia ($<1.0 \times 10^9$ leukocytes per liter) were excluded.

(1) A favorable clinical response (clinical improvement and a 15% decrease in the leukocyte count) was noted in 91% of the once-daily group and in 78% of the thrice-daily group. The mortality rates were similar in the two groups.

(2) Nephrotoxicity developed in 5% of the once-daily group compared with 24% of the thrice-daily group (P=0.016). In both groups, patients who developed nephrotoxicity tended to have been treated longer and to have had a lower mean creatinine clearance rate at the start of therapy. Not all patients were tested for ototoxicity, but the rates of ototoxicity between the two groups were also similar.

(3) Given an almost five-fold lower risk of nephrotoxicity and the fact that once-daily dosing is less labor-intensive and more cost-efficient, the authors recommended once-daily dosing of gentamicin for non-neutropenic patients with preserved renal function (serum creatinine <3.4 mg/dl).

3. Contrast Dyes—With the increasing use of contrast dyes for diagnostic tests and therapeutic interventions, contrast-induced nephrotoxicity has become a common clinical problem. Contrast dyes are thought to cause direct tubular toxicity, to contribute toward tubular obstruction, and to cause medullary ischemia through contrast-induced vasoconstriction.

a. Risk Factors for the Development of Contrast Nephropathy—Although the use of contrast dyes is generally safe, patients with diabetes mellitus or baseline renal dysfunction appear to be at an increased risk for contrast nephropathy (16,56). Other identified risk factors include multiple myeloma, older age, history of hypertension, presence of albuminuria, male sex, use of a large amount of contrast material, and use of ionic rather than nonionic contrast dye (5,65). Representative studies are described in the following sections.

(1) Baseline Renal Dysfunction—In a prospective study of 378 patients exposed to contrast dyes, 30% of those with a baseline serum creatinine level ≥1.5 mg/dl developed renal failure (defined as an increase in serum creatinine of ≥1.0 mg/dl), compared with only 2% of patients with a baseline serum creatinine level <1.5 mg/dl (16).

Table 19-6 Comparison of different aminoglycoside dosing regimens (58)

	Once-Daily Dosing (n=59)	Thrice-Daily Dosing (n=64)	*P*
Favorable clinical response	91%	78%	>0.05
Mortality from infection	2	2	>0.05
Nephrotoxicity	5%	24%	0.016
Ototoxicity	58%	55%	>0.05

(2) **Diabetes Mellitus**—At any given level of azotemia, a diabetic patient is more likely to experience contrast-induced nephropathy than a nondiabetic patient. In a prospective series of 220 patients with baseline azotemia (serum creatinine >1.7 mg/dl) who were exposed to contrast dyes, the incidence of ARF (>50% increase in serum creatinine from baseline) was 8.8% among diabetic patients but only 3.5% among nondiabetic patients (56). The risk of contrast-induced ARF among diabetic patients with preserved baseline renal function, however, does not appear to be increased over the risk in the general population.

(3) **Ionic Versus Nonionic Agents**—Before the study by Rudnick, smaller trials failed to demonstrate a difference in the incidence of nephrotoxicity after use of ionic versus nonionic agents. In Rudnick's prospective, randomized, double-blind, multicenter trial involving 1196 patients with and without renal insufficiency (defined as baseline serum creatinine >1.5 mg/dl), the overall risk of contrast nephropathy was 3% with the nonionic contrast dyes and 7% with the ionic contrast dyes ($P<0.002$). Among patients without baseline renal insufficiency, the incidence of contrast nephropathy was low and not significantly different between the two types of agents. Among patients with baseline renal insufficiency, however, the use of ionic contrast dye was associated with a 3.3 times higher risk of contrast nephropathy compared with the use of nonionic contrast dye. This study also confirmed that the presence of baseline renal dysfunction and a history of diabetes mellitus were independent risk factors for the development of contrast nephropathy (65).

(4) **Other Risk Factors**—In addition to baseline renal dysfunction, diabetes mellitus, and the use of ionic contrast dye, the other independent risk factors for the development of contrast nephropathy in Rudnick's study were male gender and the use of a large volume of contrast material (65). In a review of several studies evaluating the risk of contrast-induced nephropathy, albuminuria (≥2+), age >60 years, history of hypertension, and multiple myeloma were also found to be independent risk factors (5).

b. Prevention of Contrast-Induced Nephrotoxicity—As discussed previously, nonionic contrast dyes are preferred for high-risk patients because these agents are associated with a lower risk of contrast nephropathy (65). In addition, investigators have evaluated the roles of hydration, mannitol, and furosemide for reducing the frequency of contrast-induced ATN. The representative studies are described here.

(1) Anto studied the effect of mannitol plus hydration in 37 patients with baseline renal insufficiency (serum creatinine, 1.8 to 9.7 mg/dl) who underwent intravenous pyelography (IVP) (2). Each patient received 250 mls of 20% mannitol 60 minutes after the start of IVP, and the urine output was matched with an IV infusion of half-normal saline. The incidence of contrast nephropathy was compared with the incidence in an historical control group of patients with chronic renal insufficiency who had undergone IVP. Only 22% of the study patients developed ARF, compared with 70% of the historical control patients.

(2) In a prospective randomized controlled trial involving 78 patients with chronic renal insufficiency (mean serum creatinine, 2.1 ± 0.6 mg/dl) undergoing diagnostic cardiac angiography, Solomon compared the benefits of half-normal saline (1 ml/kg/hour for 12 hours before and after angiography), mannitol (25 g, 60 minutes before angiography), and furosemide (80 mg, 30 minutes before angiography) for prevention of contrast-induced ARF (defined as an increase in the baseline serum creatinine by ≥0.5 mg/dl) (71).

(a) ARF occurred in 11%, 28%, and 40% of patients assigned to saline, saline plus mannitol, or saline plus furosemide, respectively (P=0.05, comparing all three groups). Therefore, for high-risk patients, hydration with half-normal saline provided better protection against contrast nephropathy than did saline plus mannitol or saline plus furosemide.

(b) A potential criticism of the study is that IV hydration was not aggressively used to exactly match the hourly urine output in patients who were treated with furosemide or mannitol. Therefore, these patients may have been in a state of prerenal azotemia before being exposed to the contrast dye, which would have increased the risk of contrast nephropathy and biased the study against furosemide and mannitol. The authors defend against this criticism by demonstrating that the mean weight of these patients did not change significantly throughout the study.

4. Rhabdomyolysis

a. Background

(1) Rhabdomyolysis (RML) has been described in a variety of settings, including crush injuries, excessive exercise, protracted seizures, arterial embolism to a limb, heat-induced disorders, alcoholism, viral infections, and ingestion of drugs such as cocaine (6).

(2) Because the creatine that is released from damaged muscle is subsequently transformed into creatinine, patients with RML tend to have disproportionately high serum creatinine levels. RML is manifested by pigmenturia, hyperkalemia, hyperphosphatemia, and elevation of muscle enzymes, creatine kinase, and lactate dehydrogenase.

(3) Compartmental syndrome may occur when muscle injury leads to tissue swelling in a space confined by fascia. If swelling occurs to the point that intramuscular pressures exceed the arterial blood pressure, inflow of blood is impeded and further tissue ischemia and injury may occur (6).

(4) The development of ARF in association with RML has been attributed to a variety of mechanisms, including (a) direct toxic effects of myoglobin or decomposition products such as ferrihemate, (b) tubular obstruction by myoglobin or uric acid crystals, (c) renal ischemia caused by release of vasoconstrictive mediators, and (d) disseminated intravascular coagulation (28,64).

b. Risk Factors for the Development of ARF in Patients with Rhabdomyolysis—The risk of developing ARF is not uniform among patients with RML. Several studies identified various clinical risk factors that predicted development of renal dysfunction in patients with RML. These include hypotension, seizures, liver dysfunction, severity of muscle damage, disseminated intravascular coagulation, and dehydration (19,64,77). The representative studies are described here.

(1) Roth retrospectively evaluated the clinical factors associated with development of ARF in 39 patients with cocaine-induced RML (64). Compared with the 26 patients without ARF, the 13 patients who did develop ARF (serum creatinine >2 mg/dl) were more likely to have had complications such as systolic blood pressure ≤100 mm Hg (1/26 patients without ARF versus 6/13 patients with ARF; $P<0.001$), seizures (2/26 versus 4/13 patients, respectively; $P<0.025$), liver dysfunction (2/26 versus 11/13 patients; $P<0.001$), creatine kinase level >8000 U/L (13/26 versus 13/13 patients; $P<0.01$), and disseminated intravascular coagulation (0/26 versus 7/13 patients; $P<0.001$).

(2) In a retrospective study of 20 patients with RML and myoglobinuria (caused by drug overdose, seizure, trauma, or embolism), all patients were treated initially with crystalloid solutions followed by mannitol and bicarbonate therapy (25 g of mannitol and 100 mEq of bicarbonate in 1 L of 5% dextrose in water, administered at a rate of 250 ml/hour) (19). Nine patients who responded with adequate urine output and did not require dialysis (group 1) were compared with 11 refractory patients who required dialysis (group 2). The initial BUN, creatinine, and fractional excretion of sodium (FE_{Na}) did not differ between the two groups. On the other hand, compared with the patients in group 1, those in group 2 had evidence of hemoconcentration and more severe muscle injury, as evidenced by a higher initial hematocrit (42.5% versus 51.7%; $P<0.01$) and a higher peak creatine kinase level (15,926 versus 54,431 U/L; $P<0.001$), respectively.

(3) In an historical cohort study of 157 patients with a creatine kinase level >1000 U/L, ARF developed in 16.5% of patients (77). In comparing the 26 patients with ARF versus the 131 patients without ARF, 58% versus 11% ($P<0.001$), respectively, had creatine kinase levels >16,000 U/L; 39% versus 5% ($P<0.001$) were dehydrated (as evidenced by a hematocrit >50%, orthostatic changes in systolic blood pressure, FE_{Na} <1%, or pulmonary capillary wedge pressure <5 mm Hg, all resolving with fluid administration); and 35% versus 14% ($P<0.04$) had systolic blood pressure <90 mm Hg on admission. In addition, sepsis, burns, and drug ingestion were strongly associated with the development of renal failure.

c. Management of RML-induced ARF—Some uncontrolled series suggest that early, vigorous IV volume replacement may prevent ARF in patients with RML (5,37,62). In addition, according to animal studies, bicarbonate therapy (adjusted to maintain urine pH ≥6.0) and mannitol plus isotonic saline infusion (adjusted to maintain adequate urine output) may protect against the development of RML-induced ARF (63). However, such data is lacking in humans (6,38,63). Representative studies are described here.

(1) Intravenous Fluid Resuscitation—In a series of 200 cases of traumatic RML, patients who received a balanced salt solution (sodium, potassium, magnesium, chloride, and bicarbonate) within 12 hours after their injury were less likely to develop ARF (defined as serum creatinine persistently >2.25 mg/dl) than those who were treated after the first 12 hours (2.5% versus 21.7%, respectively; $P<0.00001$) (38). In addition, the mortality rate was lower among those treated within the first 12 hours than among patients whose treatment was delayed (0.8% versus 4.8%, respectively; $P<0.00001$). Patients who died had a higher peak creatine kinase level than those who survived.

(2) Combination of Intravenous Fluids, Bicarbonate and Mannitol—Ron described the management of 7 patients with severe crush injuries (peak creatine kinase >30,000 U/L) after collapse of a building (63). All 7 patients received on-site IV fluids, and by the time of arrival at the hospital each had received 1.5 to 3.0 L of lactated Ringer's solution. Mannitol (1 g/kg as a 20% solution) was administered as needed to achieve a urinary output >300 ml/hour. In addition, sodium bicarbonate (44 mEq in every other 500-ml bottle) was added to the standard IV solution and adjusted to keep the urine pH >6.5. Acetazolamide was administered as needed to prevent excessive alkalosis (plasma pH >7.45). During an average of 60 hours, a mean of 12 L of IV fluids, 685 mEq of sodium bicarbonate, and 160 g/day of mannitol were required to maintain the desired urine output and pH. Remarkably, none of the 7 patients developed ARF with this vigorous therapy. However, because there was no control group and all of the patients had received the same therapy, the efficacy of each individual intervention could not be assessed.

(3) In the absence of controlled trials in humans, the efficacy of volume replacement, bicarbonate therapy, or mannitol infusion for prevention of ARF in patients with RML remains inconclusive. Nevertheless, these prophylactic measures are warranted for patients with severe RML because the available data from human case series and animal studies support their use and there appear to be relatively few side effects when they are used in a monitored setting.

5. Multiple Myeloma

a. **Background**—Renal insufficiency complicates the clinical course of almost half of patients with multiple myeloma. Bence Jones proteinuria and hypercalcemia are responsible for >90% of the cases of ARF in patients with multiple myeloma (1). Large tubular casts made of precipitated Bence Jones proteins are described in the classic myeloma kidney. These proteins cause obstruction and direct damage to the proximal tubules. Neither the type (κ versus λ) nor the isoelectric point of the light chains has been conclusively associated with nephrotoxicity (39). Hypercalcemia, which is observed in 20T to 30% of patients with multiple myeloma at the time of diagnosis, may also contribute to the nephrotoxicity.

b. **Prognostic Factors in Patients with Myeloma-Related ARF**

(1) In a comparison of 27 patients with myeloma-related ARF who died within 1 year (group 1) with 10 similar patients who survived for ≥36 months (group 2), Pasquali identified hypercalcemia and infection within the first 2 months of diagnosis as the strongest predictors of poor survival. Lesser predictors of poor outcome were not having been treated with plasmapheresis and the severity of tubulointerstitial damage. For example, 70% of the patients in group 2 had received plasma exchange, compared with 33% of the patients in group 1 ($P<0.05$), and tubulointerstitial damage was observed in 11% of the patients in group 2, compared with 57% of the patients in group 1 ($P<0.05$) (57).

(2) In a study of 89 patients with renal failure and multiple myeloma, Alexanian found that myeloma control was much more important for prolonging survival than reversal of renal failure. When the data were controlled for the degree of hypercalcemia and dehydration, renal function did not necessarily improve more often in patients who responded favorably to antimyeloma therapy (1). Similar findings have been reported in a study of 21 patients by Johnson (33).

(3) The presence of cast formation has been correlated with irreversibility of myeloma-related renal dysfunction. Alexanian noted that reversal of renal insufficiency (*i.e.*, a decrease in serum creatinine by 0.7 to 1.4 mg/dl from the peak) occurred in 51% of patients with ARF or chronic renal failure of various causes all but that patients with Bence Jones proteinuria and renal insufficiency had a reversal rate of only 24%, perhaps because of severe cast nephropathy (1). In a study involving 16 myeloma patients undergoing a renal biopsy, the main determinant of the irreversibility of the renal failure was the severity of myeloma cast formation. Recovery of renal function occurred in 8 of 9 patients with ≤1+ myeloma casts on biopsy, compared with 2 of 7 patients with ≥2+ myeloma cast formation (33). Renal biopsy at presentation may then be useful for diagnostic and prognostic purposes, especially if plasma exchange is contemplated (see later discussion).

c. **Treatment of Renal Failure in Patients with Multiple Myeloma**

(1) Patients with multiple myeloma and ARF should promptly receive chemotherapy. As noted previously, antimyeloma therapy improves the overall prognosis in these patients but does not necessarily improve renal function (1). In addition, other potential contributors to nephrotoxicity such as hypovolemia, infection, and hypercalcemia should be aggressively managed.

(2) If renal function does not improve with these measures, a renal biopsy may be useful (33). If cast formation or tubulointerstitial changes are noted, plasmapheresis, in addition to chemotherapy, may be warranted (33,57). In theory, plasmapheresis may reduce the filtered load of the nephrotoxic light-chain proteins.

(a) As noted, treatment with plasmapheresis was predictive of longer survival in Pasquali's study.

(b) Johnson randomly assigned 21 patients with active myeloma and progressive renal failure (serum creatinine ≥3.0 mg/dl despite correction of hypovolemia and infection) to receive either forced diuresis (oral sodium bicarbonate and/or furosemide to maintain urine flow >100 ml/hour) plus chemotherapy (melphalan, 0.15 mg/kg/day and prednisone, 15 mg QID) or forced diuresis plus chemotherapy plus plasmapheresis (3 times per week for 1 to 4 weeks) (33). Patients were entered within a mean of 1.21 months from the time of diagnosis of the renal impairment. Of the 12 patients requiring hemodialysis, only 3, all treated with plasmapheresis and with ≤2+ cast formation on biopsy recovered from renal dysfunction. There was no difference in outcome among patients who did not require dialysis.

E. Renal Azotemia: Allergic Interstitial Nephritis

1. Background

a. The first cases of acute interstitial nephritis (AIN) were reported in patients with diphtheria and scarlet fever. AIN is now most often caused by medications such as antibiotics, diuretics, NSAIDs, oral hypoglycemic drugs, allopurinol, and cimetidine (10). AIN may also be caused by a number of other infectious agents (*e.g.*, *Legionella*, *Leptospira*, *Hantavirus*), systemic diseases (*e.g.*, sarcoidosis, systemic lupus erythematosus (SLE), Sjögren's syndrome, lymphoma, leukemia), pyelonephritis, and various idiopathic conditions associated with anterior uveitis (10) (see Table 19–7).

b. After the offending cause is removed or treated, the clinical and histologic abnormalities of AIN usually resolve. However, up to 35% of patients may require temporary dialysis (42). The occurrence of drug-related AIN is not usually dose dependent, but at least 1 to 2 weeks of exposure to a drug is usually necessary, supporting the theory of an immune-mediated mechanism of injury (22).

2. Clinical Features and Diagnosis of AIN

a. The two studies described here illustrate the clinical features of AIN (22,42).

(1) Galpin retrospectively described the clinical features of 14 patients with methicillin-induced AIN (22). All patients exhibited fever (>100.0°F) and eosinophilia (mean peak of 1930 cells/μL). Rash (primarily maculopapular) developed in 28% of patients. Eight patients became febrile for a second time after having initially defervesced, a scenario consistent with a drug reaction. Renal impairment (>1.0 mg/dl increase in serum creatinine from baseline) began an average of 11 days after the initiation of antibiotic therapy. There was no relation between the level of eosinophilia and the severity of renal failure. Hematuria was observed in 85% of patients, with 3 patients demonstrating gross hematuria. Nine patients whose urine was examined by Wright's stain had eosinophiluria (an average of >33% of total leukocytes in the urine).

(2) Linton described a series of 9 patients with drug-induced AIN (42). Fever and rash were present in 6 and 4 patients, respectively. Six patients had evidence of eosinophilia (>700 cells/μL) and eosinophiluria (>33% of total leukocytes in the urine). Hematuria was noted in 6 patients, with 2 patients demonstrating gross hematuria. Patients had

Table 19-7 Major causes of acute interstitial nephritis

Category	Examples
Drugs	β-Lactam antibiotics, sulfonamides, rifampin, NSAIDs, diuretics, oral hypoglycemic agents, allopurinol, cimetidine
Infections	Pyelonephritis, legionnaires' disease, leptospirosis
Miscellaneous	Sarcoidosis, SLE, Sjögren's syndrome, lymphoma, leukemia

been exposed to the drug for 5 to 26 days before developing signs of renal impairment.

b. The classic triad of fever, rash, and eosinophilia is helpful when it is present, but its absence does not exclude the diagnosis of AIN because it is found in only 10% to 40% of the cases (10,42). The triad appears to be more common with antibiotic-related AIN than with NSAID-related AIN. For example, in one reference, this triad was observed in up to 80% of the cases involving β-lactam antibiotics, compared with only 20% of those involving NSAIDs (25). In the absence of these classic clinical findings, the diagnosis of AIN is often difficult without a biopsy. Among the patients with ARF of uncertain origin, AIN is found to be the cause in 11% to 13% of the cases when biopsy is obtained (70,81).

c. Although modest proteinuria (1–2+) is most common with AIN, patients with NSAID-induced AIN may be associated with nephrotic-range proteinuria. As with patients with minimal-change disease, minimal glomerular changes with fusion of foot processes are observed on electron microscopy. Unlike patients with antibiotic-related AIN, whose renal dysfunction is usually reversible, patients with NSAID-related AIN may demonstrate only partial recovery of renal function (10).

3. Treatment of AIN—The efficacy of corticosteroids for the treatment of AIN has not been adequately evaluated in clinical trials. In addition, a major reservation against the routine use of corticosteroids for AIN is the possibility that the patient may harbor a subclinical infection. Nevertheless, small, nonrandomized studies have suggested that steroids may be of some benefit in patients with drug-induced AIN.

a. In Galpin's retrospective study of 14 patients with methicillin-induced AIN, prednisone (an average of 60 mg/day for a mean of 9.6 days) was administered to 8 patients (22). For those treated with prednisone, a new mean baseline serum creatinine of 1.43 mg/dl was reached in 9.6 days. In comparison, for those not treated with prednisone, a new mean baseline serum creatinine of 1.9 mg/dl was reached in 54 days.

b. In Linton's retrospective series of 9 patients with drug-induced AIN, 7 patients without spontaneous recovery of renal function received a regimen of prednisone similar to that just described. In these treated patients, renal function began to improve within 2 days of starting prednisone, and renal function returned to previous baseline levels within 10 days (42).

F. Renal Azotemia: Acute GN, RPGN, and Miscellaneous Diseases—Acute GN is defined as the sudden appearance of glomerular disease with microscopic or gross hematuria, proteinuria, and red blood cell casts, often in the setting of hypertension, peripheral edema, and decreasing renal function (43). In the absence of obvious red blood cell casts, the presence of dysmorphic red blood cells detected by phase-contrast microscopy is suggestive of active glomerular inflammation. The following discussion focuses on rapidly progressive glomerulonephritis (RPGN), a form of GN that is characterized by ≥50% loss of renal function within 3 months. This is in contrast with acute GN, which is usually characterized by a deterioration in renal function over days to weeks. In clinical practice, however, it is difficult to distinguish between these two forms of GN. Because of space limitations, only selected causes of RPGN are discussed in detail. In addition, certain conditions that mimic RPGN, such as cryoglobulinemia, hemolytic uremic syndrome, atheroembolism, and nephropathy associated with the human immunodeficiency virus (HIV), are discussed. Malignant hypertension, postinfectious GN, and SLE-associated nephritis are not discussed in detail.

1. Background

a. Classification—RPGN may be categorized according to its immunohistologic features: (a) granular deposition of immunoglobulin and complement; (b) linear deposition of immunoglobulins in the glomerular basement membrane (e.g. anti-GBM GN); and (c) scanty glomerular immunoglobulin deposition, or pauciimmune GN (*e.g.*, Wegener's granulomatosis [WG]). Among patients with all types of proliferative GN, the pauciimmune variety tends to be the most common (49% to 81%) and the anti-GBM form the least common (0% to 12%) (31).

b. Patients with pauciimmune GN can be further classified according to the results of assays for antineutrophil cytoplasmic autoantibodies (ANCA).

(1) The presence of cytoplasmic-staining ANCA, or C-ANCA (antibodies directed against p29, a 29-kDa serine proteinase), in the setting of severe hemoptysis suggests WG. The presence of perinuclear-staining ANCA or P-ANCA (antibodies directed against myeloperoxidase) suggests microscopic polyarteritis nodosa, but other diseases such as SLE and the acquired immunodeficiency syndrome (AIDS) can be associated with P-ANCA.

(2) Niles compared the serums of control patients with the serums of 123 patients with RPGN to determine the sensitivity and specificity of ANCA for pauciimmune necrotizing and crescentic GN (52). Using renal histology results from 42 patients as the gold standard, the sensitivity and specificity of ANCA by radioimmunoassay for this form of GN were 95% and >99%, respectively. Of the 18 patients with anti-GBM GN, 2 also had anti-p29 antibody (C-ANCA) and 6 also had antimyeloperoxidase antibodies (P-ANCA). Therefore, for patients with RPGN, both the sensitivity and specificity for detection of anti-p29 or antimyeloperoxidase antibodies by radioimmunoassay are >95% for pauciimmune GN, provided that the test for anti-GBM antibodies is negative. The enzyme-linked immunosorbent assay (ELISA), currently used in several laboratories, has a similar sensitivity and specificity to the radioimmunoassay. The predictive value of the ANCA assay can vary depending on the population being studied, as was recently noted in a prospective study (59a).

c. The development of sensitive and specific serologic tests has changed the approach to patients with acute GN. A diagnosis can often be made based on the patient's clinical presentation and the results of serologic testing.

(1) Clinical Presentation (31)

(a) In general, poststreptococcal GN and Henoch–Schönlein purpura (HSP) tend to occur in young children, membranoproliferative GN in older children, immunoglobulin A (IgA) nephropathy and anti-GBM GN in young adults, and idiopathic and arteritis-associated GN in older adults.

(b) Patient gender may provide further clues. SLE occurs predominantly in women, whereas IgA and anti-GBM GN tend to occur in men.

(c) Purpura is seen in Henoch–Schönlein purpura but is also reported with WG and polyarteritis nodosa.

(d) Severe hemoptysis should suggest anti-GBM GN, WG, or, less commonly, SLE.

(2) Serologic Testing (31)

(a) The presence of anti-GBM antibodies in the setting of severe hemoptysis strongly suggests anti-GBM GN. Goodpasture's syndrome specifically refers to patients with pulmonary hemorrhage and anti-GBM GN.

(b) The presence of C-ANCA in the setting of severe hemoptysis suggests WG.

(c) The presence of P-ANCA suggests microscopic polyarteritis nodosa.

(d) The presence of anti–deoxyribonuclease B (anti–DNase B) and anti–streptolysin-O antibodies suggests poststreptococcal GN.

(e) The presence of cryoglobulins and hepatitis C virus antibodies suggests cryoglobulinemic GN.

(f) The presence of antinuclear antibodies and antibodies to double-stranded DNA antibodies suggests SLE.

(g) Low serum complement levels are compatible with postinfectious GN, SLE nephritis, or membranoproliferative GN.

2. Wegener's Granulomatosis

a. WG is an idiopathic disorder characterized by granulomatous vasculitis involving the kidney and the upper and lower respiratory tract. In the past, the diagnosis was suggested when biopsy revealed granulomas and vasculitis. Currently, the diagnosis may be based on the detection of C-ANCA. In contrast to anti-GBM, C-ANCA has not conclusively been shown to have a pathogenic role.

b. Two large American reviews have described the clinical characteristics of patients with WG (see Table 19–8). Fauci evaluated 85 patients who were observed for >21 years; Hoffman evaluated 158 patients who were observed for 6 months to 24 years, including patients from the Fauci study (20,27). A summary of the major findings is presented here.

c. Treatment

(1) Immunosuppressive Medications—Standard therapy for WG consists of a combination of oral cyclophosphamide (2 mg/kg/day) and prednisone (1 mg/kg/day). Patients with fulminant disease may be given 3 to 5 mg/kg/day of cyclophosphamide (20,27). With this regimen, a complete remission was achieved in 93% and 75% of the patients in Fauci's and Hoffman's series, respectively (20,27). In Hoffman's series, the median time to discontinuation of steroids was 1 year; cyclophosphamide was continued for 1 year, then tapered by 25-mg increments every 2 to 3 months (27). In Fauci's series, 10 of the 11 patients who were started on azathioprine instead of cyclophosphamide did not achieve remission, but 8 of the 9 patients who were switched to azathioprine because of cyclophosphamide-related cystitis did remain in remission (20).

(2) Plasma Exchange—Plasma exchange removes presumed pathologic substances from patients' plasma and replaces it with fluid (usually albumin or fresh-frozen plasma) that is void of these substances. There has been only one small, randomized trial that evaluated the effect of plasma exchange in patients with WG (59). In this trial, which took 10 years to complete, 48 patients with impaired renal function caused by biopsy-proven focal necrotizing GN with crescents were randomly assigned to receive either chemotherapy (similar to the immunosuppressive regimen described in the previous section) or chemotherapy plus plasma exchange (4-L exchanges five times per

Table 19-8 Clinical characteristics of patients with WG (20,27)

Selected Sign, Symptom, or Laboratory Findings	Fauci	Hoffman
Mean age (y)	44	41
Pulmonary infiltrates at presentation	71%	45%
Hemoptysis at presentation	18%	12%
Cough at presentation	34%	19%
Overall incidence of lung disease	94%	85%
Evidence of renal disease at presentation	11%	18%
Overall incidence of renal disease	85%	77%
Fever at presentation	34%	23%
Overall incidence of fever	Not given	50%
Overall incidence of anemia (hematocrit <35%)	50%	73%
Overall incidence of thrombocytosis (>400 $\times 10^9$/L)	33%	65%
Mean leukocyte count at presentation (cells $\times 10^9$/L)	9.6	10.5

week, with a mean of 9 exchanges). Twenty-three patients had WG, 20 had microscopic polyarteritis nodosa, and 5 had idiopathic RPGN.

(a) Among those not requiring dialysis, there was no statistically significant difference in outcome between the two treatment groups.

(b) However, among the 19 patients requiring dialysis, more patients were taken off of dialysis in the group treated with plasma exchange plus chemotherapy than with chemotherapy alone (10/11 versus 3/8 patients, respectively; $P=0.041$). When the analysis is limited to only the 9 patients with WG who required dialysis, 4 out of 5 patients treated with plasma exchange could be taken off of dialysis, compared with 2 out of 4 patients treated with chemotherapy only. These numbers were too small to assign statistical significance to the difference.

3. Anti-GBM–Mediated Disease

a. Anti-GBM–mediated ARF is characterized by the presence of anti-GBM antibodies and RPGN with or without hemoptysis. In the setting of RPGN, the presence of anti-GBM antibodies (by ELISA) is highly sensitive and specific (>95%) for the diagnosis (37). Although a relatively rare disorder, anti-GBM–mediated RPGN is an important cause of ARF because of its poor prognosis in the absence of prompt diagnosis and therapy (37). The most common glomerular lesion is proliferative GN with crescent formation, and immunofluorescent staining reveals linear deposition of IgG along the GBM. The linear deposition of IgG may also be found on the alveolar basement membrane of the lung.

b. Clinical Features

(1) The presenting clinical symptoms and signs were reviewed by Kelly, who compiled the results from five studies involving a total of 129 patients with this syndrome (37) (see Table 19–9).

(2) The most common laboratory abnormality was anemia (hemoglobin <12 mg/dl), which was reported in 90% to 100% of patients. Other laboratory abnormalities and their frequencies were as follows: leukocyte count >10,000 cells/mm^3 (38% to 50%); azotemia (55% to 71%); proteinuria (76% to 100%); hematuria (83% to 94%); pyuria (36% to 71%); and red blood cell casts (6% to 100%).

(3) Chest radiograph may reveal diffuse alveolar filling in the presence of alveolar hemorrhage. Patients with anti-GBM GN who smoke may be predisposed to development of alveolar hemorrhage. In a series of 51 patients with newly diagnosed anti-GBM GN, all 37 current smokers developed pulmonary hemorrhage, compared with only 2 of the 10 nonsmokers ($P=0.24 \times 10^{-8}$) (18).

c. The therapy for anti-GBM–mediated RPGN consists of early administration of immunosuppressive drugs and plasma exchange. Before the advent of these therapies, mortality ranged from 75% to 90%, but the current rate of

Table 19-9 Clinical characteristics of anti-GBM disease (37)

Symptoms	Frequency	Signs	Frequency
Hemoptysis	82%–92%	Rales	35%–55%
Dyspnea	57%–72%	Pallor	51%–90%
Fatigue	38%–66%	Heart murmur	17%–28%
Cough	40%–66%	Hepatomegaly	2%–20%
Prior upper respiratory infection	19%–28%	Edema	6%–25%
Chills, fever	15%–24%	Hypertension	4%–17%
Weight loss	7%–14%	Fundoscopic changes	4%–14%
Gross hematuria	10%–41%	Skin rash	0%–8%

short-term survival is at least 80% (37). The only prospective randomized study to evaluate the benefit of plasma exchange for patients with anti-GBM GN was that of Johnson (32). Nine patients were treated with immunosuppressive therapy consisting of cyclophosphamide (2 mg/kg/day for 3 months, then 1 mg/kg/day) plus prednisone (2 mg/kg/day for 1 week, 1 mg/kg/day for 3 weeks, then tapered to an alternate-day regimen for the next 3 months), and 8 patients were managed with a similar immunosuppressive regimen plus plasma exchange (4-L exchanges every 3 days until the level of antibody was <5% binding or the patient was on stable dialysis for <30 days).

(1) Compared with the patients treated by immunosuppression alone, those treated with the combination of immunosuppression and plasma exchange had a more rapid rate of disappearance of the antibody, a higher likelihood of not requiring long-term dialysis (3/9 versus 6/8, respectively; *P* not given), and a lower mean creatinine level at the end of the study (9.2 versus 4.1 mg/dl, respectively; $P<0.05$).

(2) However, a high degree of crescent formation (>30%) and an elevated serum creatinine at entry (specific value not stated) were more important in predicting a poor prognosis than whether or not the patient was treated with plasma exchange. On the other hand, plasma exchange was beneficial for those with preserved renal function and a mild degree of crescent formation (32). This observation is consistent with other studies which suggest that the benefit of plasma exchange is minimal if the patient already has severe renal dysfunction (37).

4. Cryoglobulinemia—Cryoglobulins are a group of immunoglobulins that precipitate in serum when cooled. Three types of cryoglobulins have been identified: type I, a single monoclonal immunoglobulin; type II, polyclonal IgG bound to monoclonal IgM that acts as an antiglobulin and thus has rheumatoid factor activity; and type III, polyclonal IgG bound to polyclonal IgM, which also demonstrates rheumatoid activity. Only type II cryoglobulinemia has been strongly associated with GN (15). Hepatitis C virus has been associated with type II cryoglobulinemia with a prevalence of up to 98% to 100%. Treatment with α-interferon, which eradicates hepatitis C ribonucleic acid, has been shown to improve renal function (49). Corticosteroids and cyclophosphamide have also been used, but no randomized controlled trial has demonstrated their efficacy. Testing for hepatitis C and cryoglobulins is warranted in patients with RPGN, because 20% to 25% of patients with hepatitis C may present with an acute nephritic syndrome complicated by acute oliguric renal failure (15).

5. Hemolytic Uremic Syndrome and Thrombotic Thrombocytopenic Purpura

a. Hemolytic uremic syndrome (HUS) is defined by the classic triad of thrombocytopenia, nonimmune microangiopathic hemolytic anemia, and acute renal failure. Although not a GN *per se*, HUS often mimics RPGN and therefore should be considered in the differential diagnosis of RPGN. HUS has been associated with infectious agents including *Escherichia coli* O157:H7 and HIV, and with various drugs such as cyclosporine, mitomycin, ticlopidine, or quinine (51). Thrombotic thrombocytopenic purpura (TTP) is characterized by fever and central nervous system (CNS) abnormalities in addition to the three manifestations of HUS. HUS and TTP represent a continuum and should not be thought of as separate entities. The clinical abnormalities include microscopic hematuria, proteinuria (usually 1 or 2+), and oliguria. Other features of TTP-HUS include neutrophilic leukocytosis, CNS disturbances, bowel perforation, and normal clotting studies.

b. Treatment of TTP-HUS consists of supportive therapy and plasmapheresis. The major trials that have evaluated the therapeutic options for TTP-HUS are described here.

(1) In a 10-year series of 108 patients with TTP-HUS, Bell evaluated the outcome of two treatment strategies: individuals with only minimal symptoms and without CNS abnormalities received prednisone 200 mg/day with a rapid taper, whereas those with CNS abnormalities, severe anemia (hematocrit <20%), thrombocytopenia (<10 × 10^9 platelets per liter), and elevated lactate dehydrogenase levels (>600 U/L) received a similar steroid regimen plus plasmapheresis and plasma exchange. On the average, 24 units (range, 18 to 32) of fresh-frozen plasma were administered per session of plasmapheresis, and exchange was performed for a mean of 7 and 9 sessions for male and female patients, respectively. Each patient was observed for at least 1 year after recovery (4).

(a) The overall rate of survival was 91% in this series. The overall rate of relapse, however, was 64%, with 84% of the relapses occurring within 30 days of diagnosis. Among those with fewer symptoms and without CNS involvement, who were treated with prednisone only, the risk of relapse was substantially lower (7%).

(b) Splenectomy and platelet transfusions should be avoided in patients with TTP-HUS. All 6 patients who underwent splenectomy and 9 of 11 patients who received platelet therapy deteriorated rapidly.

(c) Given the high overall rate of survival of patients treated with plasma exchange in this study, the authors concluded that some form of plasma therapy was beneficial in the treatment of TTP-HUS. In addition, because the rate of relapse was so low among those treated with prednisone only, the authors recommended that corticosteroids also be included in the initial management of these patients. However, because patients who were assigned to receive prednisone had minimal symptoms to begin with, the low rate of relapse may have reflected a milder form of the disease more than a beneficial effect of prednisone.

(2) Rock prospectively studied 102 patients with TTP who were randomly assigned to receive either plasma exchange or plasma infusion (62). Patients with poor or nonexistent renal function were excluded from the study. The total volume of plasma received by patients undergoing plasma exchange was three times that received by patients undergoing plasma infusion. The rates of survival and of response to therapy (defined by an absolute platelet count >150 × 10^9/L and no new neurologic events) were compared. At day 9 of therapy, compared with the patients receiving plasma infusion, the patients treated with plasma exchange had a higher rate of response (24/51 versus 13/51 patients; P=0.025) and a lower mortality rate (2/51 versus 8/51 patients; P=0.035). At 6 months, a higher rate of response to therapy (40/51 versus 25/51 patients; P=0.002) and a lower rate of mortality (11/51 versus 19/51 patients; P=0.036) were still observed for patients treated with plasma exchange. Based on these findings, the authors concluded that plasma exchange was superior to plasma infusion.

(3) In the study just described, it was unclear whether the improved outcome in patients treated with plasma exchange occurred because plasma exchange effectively removed some toxic material from the plasma or simply because three times more plasma was administered with this treatment than with plasma infusion. The following study supports the latter of the two possibilities. In a case report of a patient with relapsing TTP, three interventions were compared: removal and infusion of plasma (*i.e.*, plasma exchange), infusion of plasma only, or removal of plasma and infusion of albumin plus saline (67). In contrast to the first two interventions, which increased the platelet count, removal of plasma followed by infusion of albumin plus saline was ineffective in increasing the platelet count. Therefore, infusion of normal plasma, rather than the removal of a toxic substance or infusion of a generic protein plus saline, appears to be the effective component of plasma therapy. Because this particular patient had relapsing TTP, further studies are needed to determine whether this observation can be generalized to those with acute TTP-HUS.

6. Atheroembolism

a. Either spontaneously or after local trauma, atheromatous plaque material containing cholesterol crystals may dislodge from the arterial wall and embolize to distal sites. Although anticoagulation has been associated with spontaneous atheroembolism, it occurs more commonly after invasive procedures such as cardiac catheterization or aortic aneurysm repair. When distal embolization affects the kidney, renal dysfunction may occur rapidly or over the course of several weeks. In either case, the clinical presentation of atheroembolism can mimic that of RPGN.

b. The largest case series of patients with histologically proven atheroembolism is described in the following sections. The study included a total of 52 patients who developed atheroembolism and ARF after angiography or cardiovascular surgery (74).

(1) Patients were typically elderly men (mean age, 69 years) with a history of hypertension (81%), coronary artery disease (73%), and peripheral vascular disease (69%). Fifty percent of the patients were current smokers.

(2) Within 30 days of the invasive procedure, 50% had cutaneous signs of atheroembolism (*e.g.*, livedo, blue toes), and 14% had eosinophilia. Urinalysis was often abnormal but nonspecific.

(3) Hemodynamically unstable patients died shortly after the invasive procedure, yet the renal function in surviving patients continued to decline over the course of 3 to 8 weeks. Patients who eventually required dialysis had a higher baseline serum creatinine than those who did not require dialysis (1.9 versus 1.5 mg/dl; P=0.02). Dialysis was initiated after a median of 29 days from the time of the invasive procedure.

(4) In comparison to those with multiple causes for renal insufficiency, patients with renal failure caused by atheroembolism alone were more likely to recover from the renal dysfunction: 5 (24%) of 21 versus 1 (3%) of 31 patients, respectively (P=0.03). They were also less likely to die within 6 months of the invasive procedure (58% versus 91%, respectively; P=0.002).

c. As noted previously, ARF caused by procedure-induced atheroembolism is characterized, in the absence of hemodynamic instability, by a decline in renal function over a period of 3 to 8 weeks. This time course is not consistent with ARF resulting from other iatrogenic causes, such as aminoglycoside antibiotics or contrast dyes, which usually presents earlier and often resolves within 2 to 3 weeks from onset. Therefore, if the time course of the renal failure is consistent with atheroembolism and other reversible causes of renal failure can be excluded, biopsy may be unnecessary, even in the absence of characteristic cutaneous manifestations. Regardless, current therapy for ARF caused by atheroembolism is primarily supportive. No systematic study has addressed the role of steroids in atheroembolic renal failure.

7. HIV-Associated Nephropathy

a. HIV-associated nephropathy (HIVAN) may also mimic RPGN. In 1983, HIVAN was defined as a clinical entity with typical histologic findings of focal (versus all glomeruli) segmental (versus the entire glomerulus) glomerulosclerosis, microcystic dilatation of renal tubules with pale eosinophilic casts, and tubuloreticular structures on electron microscopy. In addition, tubulointerstitial disease is common in HIVAN.

b. Clinical Features (73)

(1) The most common clinical presentation is asymptomatic proteinuria or proteinuria accompanied by pedal edema. Pedal edema often occurs abruptly. Patients are typically male and African-American or Haitian. HIVAN may occur early or late in the course of the HIV infection. Although hypoalbuminemia is observed, hypertension is uncommon. Ultrasonography typically reveals enlarged kidneys, an unusual finding in other chronic renal diseases such as heroin nephropathy.

(2) The clinical course is quite rapid, with end-stage renal disease occurring within 4 to 16 weeks from the time proteinuria is first noted. No medication, including azidothymidine (AZT), has been shown convincingly to alter this rapidly deteriorating course of HIVAN. In addition, dialysis does not significantly prolong survival in these patients (60,73).

c. HIVAN should not be the only diagnosis considered in patients with ARF and AIDS. For example, in Rao's prospective study of 78 patients with AIDS and renal abnormalities seen over a 4-year period, 30% developed ARF as a result of administration of nephrotoxic drugs (pentamidine, aminoglycosides, trimethoprim-sulfamethoxazole, NSAIDs, and contrast agents), sepsis, or other causes of hypotension (60). In this subgroup of patients with ARF not due to HIVAN, 5 of the 6 patients who underwent dialysis recovered renal function. This is in contrast to patients with HIVAN, in whom rapid irreversible progression to end-stage renal disease is common (60,73). Therefore, other causes of ARF, especially prerenal azotemia, should always be sought and excluded in these patients.

G. Diagnosis and Initial Approach to Patients with ARF

1. Initial Evaluation—The major goals in the initial management of patients with ARF are to determine the cause of the ARF and to search for the complications of ARF that may require prompt intervention.

a. History and Physical Examination—Careful history taking frequently reveals the cause of the renal dysfunction, such as prerenal azotemia from gastrointestinal hemorrhage, ATN caused by use of aminoglycosides, or obstruction resulting from a pelvic malignancy. Other important clues to the diagnosis include a history of medications, preexisting systemic diseases (*e.g.*, hypertension, diabetes), and symptoms associated with other organs (*e.g.*, lungs, heart). Physical examination should focus on evaluation of volume status, presence of other involved organs including the skin (*e.g.*, purpura, livedo), and symptoms of uremia (*e.g.*, pericarditis, asterixis). Bladder catheterization is useful to exclude obstruction (below the bladder) and to monitor urine production.

b. Laboratory Evaluation—Electrolytes, BUN, and creatinine levels can suggest the diagnosis of ARF. Anemia (in the absence of another obvious cause) and hyperphosphatemia suggest that the renal dysfunction has occurred over an extended period rather than over a few days. A markedly elevated lactate dehydrogenase level suggests renal infarction, and elevated creatine kinase levels suggest RML. In the absence of a prerenal or postrenal cause, evaluations of ANCA, anti-GBM, serum and urine electrophoresis, complement levels, antinuclear antibodies, anti–DNase B, anti–streptolysin-O, and blood cultures should considered. The electrocardiogram should be examined for evidence of hyperkalemia, pericarditis, and cardiac ischemia. A urine sample should examined for the presence of erythrocytes, leukocytes, eosinophils, and cellular casts. The urine electrolytes, osmolality, and creatinine levels should also be determined.

2. Analysis of Urine

a. Dipstick Urinalysis Versus Microscopic Urinalysis—The urine dipstick is a relatively easy and inexpensive means of screening for diagnostic clues. In a large prospective, blinded study, Bonnardeaux examined the sensitivity and specificity of dipstick analysis of 5486 urine samples using the nephrologist-performed urinalysis as the gold standard (8). All 2359 urine samples that were positive by dipstick and 456 of the 3127 that were negative by dipstick were submitted to one of two nephrologists for formal microscopic urinalysis. If the dipstick urinalysis was negative for protein, leukocytes, nitrites, glucose, and ketones, only 5.3% had abnormalities on microscopic evaluation. The sensitivity and the specificity of the dipstick test for blood were 75% and 89%, respectively. The corresponding values for the dipstick test for leukocytes were 81% and 64%, respectively. The urine samples that were positive by dipstick for glucose or ketones had lower sensitivities for detecting leukocytes; therefore, such urine samples should be examined microscopically. Furthermore, the correlation between the dipstick and microscopic analyses was poor for low-grade microscopic hematuria (*i.e.*, 1 to 10 erythrocytes per high-powered field). The clinical significance of dipstick-negative, microscopy-positive urine for erythrocytes has yet to be determined.

b. Whether or not the urine dipstick is used for initial screening, microscopic urinalysis is usually required to confirm the presence of erythrocytes, leukocytes, eosinophils, cellular casts, dysmorphic erythrocytes, or infectious organisms. This is regardless of the fact that certain cells and casts may be difficult to identify. The following findings can be helpful for diagnosis.

(1) Granular casts (>5 per high-powered field) can be seen in all forms of renal failure, but they are the principal findings in ATN.

(2) Red blood cell casts or dysmorphic erythrocytes suggest GN, but more commonly only red blood cells are identified, and thus the differential diagnosis expands to include catheter trauma, interstitial nephritis, TTP-HUS, and GN. In addition, many other causes of ARF secondary to tubulointerstitial processes, including ischemia, can result in hematuria and, rarely, in red blood cell casts.

(3) The presence of leukocytes usually suggest interstitial nephritis or pyelonephritis.

(4) The presence of urine eosinophils suggest AIN (see further discussion in a later section).

c. Urine Electrolytes—Clinicians have used the urine electrolyte and osmolality values for differentiating prerenal from renal azotemia. In prerenal azotemia, urine sodium (U_{Na}) and FE_{Na} are typically low because of avid reabsorption of sodium by normally functioning tubules. In renal azotemia, U_{Na} and FE_{Na} are typically high because of less avid reabsorption of sodium by damaged tubules. Similarly, in prerenal states, the urine osmolality (U_{osm}) is typically high because the medullary gradient is maintained; an increase in the level of the antidiuretic hormone causes an increase in water reabsorption by the collecting tubules and the urine becomes concentrated. In renal azotemia, the medullary gradient is disrupted and the antidiuretic hormone response is impaired, leading to urine that is isosthenuric. The utility of urinary indices for differentiating prerenal azotemia from ATN is well illustrated in the following study. Miller prospectively compared the urinary indices of patients with prerenal azotemia with those of patients with ATN (48). As demonstrated in Table 19–10, patients with prerenal azotemia tended to have U_{osm} >500 mOsm/kg, U_{Na} <20 mEq/L, and FE_{Na} <1.0; those with ATN tended to have U_{osm} <350 mOsm/kg, U_{Na} >40 mEq/L, and FE_{Na} >1.0%. However, as is also demonstrated in the table, these indices are not foolproof and must be interpreted in the clinical context.

Table 19-10 Urinary indices in acute renal failure (48)

Index	Prerenal Azotemia (n=30)	ATN (n=55)
U_{osm} >500 mOsm/kg	63%	10%
U_{osm} <350 mOsm/kg	8%	67%
U_{Na} <20 mEq/L	60%	4%
U_{Na} >40 mEq/L	0%	51%
FE_{Na} <1.0%	90%	17%

d. Urine Eosinophils

(1) Testing for urine eosinophils has traditionally been a screen for AIN. Initially, Wright's stain was the most commonly used method, but Hansel's stain appears to be more sensitive for this purpose (13,53). Nevertheless, the presence of urine eosinophils is neither highly sensitive nor specific for AIN. Ruffing evaluated the sensitivity and specificity of urine eosinophils (determined by both Wright's and Hansel's stain) for the diagnosis of AIN (66). The urine samples from 148 patients with pyuria but no clinical suspicion for AIN and 51 patients with pyuria in whom a consulting nephrologist suspected AIN were examined for the presence of eosinophils.

(a) Of the 51 patients with suspected AIN, 15 proved to have AIN and 36 proved to have other renal disorders. Only 6 of the 15 patients with AIN had urine eosinophils >1% (per 100 cells), compared with 10 of the 36 patients with other renal diagnoses. Therefore, in these 51 patients, the sensitivity and the specificity of eosinophiluria for AIN were 40% and 72%, respectively. The corresponding PPV and NPV were 38% and 74%, respectively.

(b) Of the 148 patients with no clinical suspicion for AIN, 100 patients had no specific diagnosis. Among these patients, 4 had urine eosinophils, yielding a specificity for urine eosinophils for AIN of 96%.

(c) Not all patients believed to have AIN had a renal biopsy to confirm the diagnosis. Rather, the authors relied solely on clinical information in some cases. Without the use of biopsy as the gold standard, the calculated sensitivity and specificity of the urine eosinophils as presented in this study should be viewed with some caution.

(2) Although the data are more limited, the presence of urine eosinophils has also been associated with ARF caused by atheroembolism. Wilson evaluated the presence of urine eosinophils in 9 patients who had biopsy-proven atheroembolism involving the kidney (80). Of the 9 patients, 8 had a positive Hansel's stain for eosinophiluria. For 6 of the 8 patients, more than 5% of the urinary leukocytes were eosinophils. However, 4 patients had other potential explanations for the eosinophiluria, such as IgA nephropathy or GN.

3. Establishment of Diagnosis of Prerenal, Renal, or Postrenal ARF—After careful history taking, physical examination, urinalysis, and selected laboratory tests, most patients can be divided into one of the three categories: prerenal, renal, and postrenal azotemia.

a. Prerenal Versus Renal Azotemia—Distinguishing between these forms of ARF may be difficult because often more than one insult is present and severe prerenal azotemia can lead to renal azotemia. A volume challenge is helpful to distinguish between these two forms of ARF if an obvious insult is not readily apparent and the patient can tolerate the fluid. This should be done with caution, preferably in a monitored setting, if signs and symptoms of intravascular volume excess are present.

b. Exclusion of Postrenal Azotemia—Ultrasonography, IVP, and computed tomography are useful for excluding obstruction of urinary flow as the cause of ARF. With a sensitivity that exceeds 90% for hydronephrosis, ultrasonography should usually be the first test for this purpose (44). No study has evaluated the benefit of obtaining ultrasound studies in all patients with ARF, but clinical discretion should suggest when this evaluation is necessary.

(1) In an evaluation of 80 patients with acute obstructive renal failure, only 4 did not demonstrate urinary tract dilatation on ultrasonography (44). The causes of obstruction in these four cases were uric acid stones (2 patients), trauma to the ureteral meatus, and infiltrative urothelial carcinoma extending into the ureteral meatus.

(2) If the clinical suspicion of obstruction is high but the ultrasonography is negative, computed tomography scanning (especially for imaging the retroperitoneal area), IVP, or ureteropyelography (retrograde and anterograde) may be helpful. This is especially true when tumor causes retroperitoneal encasement of the kidney and the collecting system, thus preventing dilatation of the calyces.

4. The Role of Biopsy for Diagnosis of ARF

a. Percutaneous renal biopsy is a relatively simple and safe procedure in the nonhypertensive patient without uremia. For patients with marked uremia or hypertension, however, renal biopsy is associated with a higher risk of retroperitoneal or perinephric hemorrhage. Biopsy is most useful when the kidneys are enlarged or of normal size. In contrast, small, atrophic kidneys usually demonstrate fibrosis and atrophy regardless of the cause of renal failure (83). If a patient with suspected renal azotemia demonstrates features atypical for ATN, a renal biopsy may be indicated. This point is illustrated by two studies that retrospectively evaluated the diagnostic yield of the renal biopsy in patients with ARF and features atypical for ATN (see Table 19–11). For all patients, prerenal and postrenal causes of ARF were clinically excluded before the biopsy (70,81).

H. Treatment of Patients With ARF—In most cases of prerenal azotemia, toxin induced nephropathy, or postrenal failure, correction of the volume status, removal or treatment of the offending cause, or relief of the obstruction is sufficient to reverse the renal dysfunction. Careful management of hyperkalemia, hyponatremia, hyperphosphatemia, metabolic acidosis, or volume overload is often necessary. In addition, the patient should be monitored closely for the development of infection, pericarditis, hemorrhage, or neurologic dysfunction. The specific treatment options for various causes of ARF (*e.g.*, plasma exchange for anti-GBM GN, corticosteroids for AIN) have already been discussed. The following is a discussion of the therapeutic options not previously presented in detail, namely, diuretics, dopamine, and dialysis.

1. Diuretics—As noted previously, the mortality rate appears to be lower for patients with nonoliguric (>450 ml urine/24 hours) renal failure than for those with oliguric (<400 to 450 ml urine/24 hours) renal failure (9,14,21,29,40,61). This observation has stimulated an interest in the use of diuretic agents in an attempt to convert oligo-anuric renal failure into nonoliguric renal failure. In experimental animals, diuretics prevent the formation of obstructing casts, preserve cellular energy stores, and improve renal hemodynamics by dilating the renal vasculature. If diuretics are administered early in the course of ATN (24 to 48 hours), patients may convert from an oliguric to a nonoliguric state. Whether this practice improves outcome is not known, especially in light of the evidence that the patients who respond to diuretics probably have less severe renal damage at baseline compared with those who do not respond to diuretics (41). Although some controlled studies suggest that diuretics reduce the need for acute dialysis, others do not, and all agree that mortality is not altered (41). In addition, no clinical evidence supports the use of diuretics once ATN is established. The place for diuretics may be early in the course of oliguric ARF if

Table 19-11 Renal biopsy findings in atypical acute renal failure (70,81)

	Wilson (n=650)	Solez (n=976)
Atypical cases with biopsy	84 (13%)	218 (22%)
ATN	17%	32%
Interstitial nephritis	11%	13%
Tubulointerstitial nephritis	0%	12%
Glomerulonephritis	53%	24%
Vascular disease	18%	30%

volume overload is also a concern. Thereafter, existing data suggest that diuretics offer no benefit but may actually be harmful (41).

2. **Dopamine**—Stimulation of the type 1 and 2 dopamine receptors in the renal arterioles by dopamine causes vasodilatation, which may lead to increases in renal blood flow and glomerular filtration rate. Although dopamine is commonly used in intensive care units for patients with or at risk for oliguria, the data in support of this practice are weak (41). Two representative studies are presented here.
   a. In a study of 37 consecutive patients who were randomly assigned to receive either dopamine or placebo after elective vascular abdominal surgery, Baldwin demonstrated no differences in renal function or in the rate of urine production between the two groups (3).
   b. In a randomized comparison of dopamine versus placebo in patients with chronic renal failure (serum creatinine >1.8 mg/dl), dopamine did not protect against the development of contrast-induced ARF after cardiac catheterization (79).
   c. In the absence of large, well-designed, randomized trials, the use of dopamine for oliguric ARF remains controversial. Some experts contend that although dopamine may offer some improvement in urine output, the benefit is outweighed by the risk of complications such as tachyarrhythmias, pulmonary shunting, and gut or digital necrosis (75). Others argue that despite some risks, low-dose dopamine (2.5 μg/kg/minute) has few side effects and may still be useful for selected patients with oliguric ARF (47).
3. **Dialysis**
   a. **Indications for Dialysis**—No controlled studies have explored the issue of when (*i.e.*, at what level of BUN) dialysis should be initiated (47). In clinical practice, the indications for dialysis include volume overload, hyperkalemia, metabolic acidosis, uremic pericarditis, or uremic encephalopathy.
   b. Once the decision is made to proceed with dialysis, several options are available, including continuous hemodialysis, intermittent hemodialysis, or peritoneal dialysis. The major advantages and disadvantages of these options are summarized in Table 19-12 (47).
   c. **Biocompatible Versus Cuprophane Membranes**—Unlike the biocompatible dialysis membranes, the use of cuprophane membranes (CM) is known to impair the phagocytic response of granulocytes and to activate the complement and the lipoxygenase pathways. In fact, the use of CM for dialysis has been associated with a delay in recovery from ARF and a decrease in the rate of survival (26,68). Representative studies that have compared the two membranes are described here.
      (1) In Schiffl's study of 52 patients with postoperative ARF, patients were stratified according to the APACHE-II score and then randomly assigned to receive dialysis with either CM or biocompatible membranes (68). The patients who were dialyzed with CM had a lower rate of survival (38% versus 65%; P=0.052), required more dialysis sessions (12 versus 9; P not given), and required longer time to recover from

Table 19-12 Comparisons of different modalities of dialysis (47)

	Provides Rapid Correction of Hyperkalemia	Requires Anti-coagulation	Produces Hemodynamic Instability	Provides Rapid Fluid Removal	Causes Loss of Albumin
Continuous hemodialysis	No	Yes	No	No	No
Intermittent hemodialysis	Yes	No	Yes	Yes	No
Peritoneal dialysis	No	No	No	No	Yes

ARF (22 versus 15 days; *P* not given). In addition, 71% of the deaths occurring in patients dialyzed with CM were caused by sepsis, compared with only 40% of the deaths in patients dialyzed with biocompatible membranes (P=0.016).

(2) In Hakim's study of 72 medical and surgical patients with ARF, patients were also randomly assigned to dialysis with either CM or biocompatible membranes (26). Baseline characteristics were similar in the two groups. After adjusting for the APACHE-II score, patients exposed to CM were less likely to recover from ARF (37% versus 62%; P=0.04), more likely to develop oliguria (75% versus 40%; P=0.047), and less likely to survive (37% versus 57%: P=0.11) than patients dialyzed with biocompatible membranes. Based on these studies, CM should not be used for dialysis in patients with ARF.

d. No controlled study has shown that intensive (daily) dialysis improves outcome compared with nonintensive dialysis for patients with ARF. For example, Gillum prospectively compared the outcome of patients with ARF managed with intensive dialysis (daily dialysis to maintain a serum BUN <60 mg/dl) versus nonintensive dialysis (dialysis to a BUN level of about 100 mg/dl) and found no difference in the overall rates of complications or survival between the two groups (23). Patients were not initiated on dialysis until the serum creatinine had reached 8 mg/dl. Therefore, the study did not address the role of early intensive dialysis in patients with ARF. Furthermore, this study may be criticized because patients were dialyzed with the use of CM, which, as previously described, have been associated with poorer outcome compared with biocompatible membranes (26,68).

I. Summary

1. A literature-based discussion of ARF is difficult because only a few of the studies on this topic have been prospective or randomized, and even those studies have included a relatively small number of patients. Most of the studies on ARF have been case series which lacked an adequate control group and were subject to selection and information bias. In addition, the available studies often differ in their design, definition of ARF, and exclusion criteria, which has made comparisons among various studies difficult.

2. The rate of mortality associated with ARF remains high despite advances in diagnosis and treatment. The cause of death in patients with ARF is often a comorbid condition that precipitated or was present at the time of ARF. Such conditions include sepsis, cardiovascular or respiratory complications, and gastrointestinal hemorrhage. This does not mean, however, that ARF does not contribute to the mortality. The uremic state contributes to septic, cardiovascular, and respiratory complications leading to mortality.

3. Prerenal azotemia results from inadequate perfusion to the kidney. The major causes of prerenal ARF are true volume depletion (*e.g.*, hemorrhage), other causes of low effective intravascular volume (*e.g.*, congestive heart failure), other causes of hemodynamic insufficiency or systemic hypotension (*e.g.*, sepsis), surgery (*e.g.*, blood loss, anesthesia), and drugs (*e.g.*, nonsteroidal anti-inflammatory drugs, ACEIs). After careful history taking and thorough physical examination, the cause of the ARF is usually obvious when it is prerenal. Urinary indices of U_{Na} <20 mEq/L, U_{osm} >500 mOsm/kg, and FE_{Na} <1.0% are consistent with prerenal azotemia. These indices are not foolproof, however, and they must be interpreted in the clinical context. If corrected rapidly, prerenal azotemia usually leads to minimal, if any, renal injury.

4. It is important to exclude obstruction as a cause of ARF, because delayed diagnosis may lead to permanent renal dysfunction. To cause ARF, obstruction must be bilateral (or unilateral in a patient with a single functional kidney). With a sensitivity that exceeds 90%, ultrasonography is usually the first test for excluding an obstruction. If the clinical suspicion remains high despite a negative result on ultrasound, a computed tomography scan or IVP may be helpful. An underlying malignancy (*e.g.*, cervical carcinoma in women, prostatic carcinoma or benign prostatic hypertrophy in men) can cause bilateral obstruction.

Immediate relief of the obstruction by surgical decompression, prostatectomy, cystoscopic retrograde ureteral stenting, or percutaneous nephrostomy tube (PNT) insertion is the cornerstone of therapy for these patients.

5. ATN is usually caused by ischemic (*e.g.*, prolonged episode of hypotension) or toxic (*e.g.*, aminoglycosides, contrast agents) injury to the kidney. Urinary indices of U_{Na} >40 mEq/L, U_{osm} <350 mOsm/kg, and FE_{Na} >1.0% are consistent with ATN. After careful history taking and thorough physical examination, the cause of ARF is usually obvious when it is ATN. Granular casts may also be observed with microscopic examination of the urine. Once identified, the offending cause of ATN should be removed (*e.g.*, by restoration of renal perfusion or discontinuation of gentamicin therapy) or treated (*e.g.*, sepsis).
6. AIN is most often caused by drugs, but infections and autoimmune diseases may also be responsible. The classic triad of fever, rash, and eosinophilia is helpful if present, but its absence does not exclude the diagnosis, because it is present in only 10% to 40% of cases. Similarly, the presence of urine eosinophils is helpful for diagnosis, but it is not a highly sensitive or specific test for AIN. After the offending cause is removed or treated, the clinical and histologic abnormalities of AIN usually resolve. In addition, small, nonrandomized studies have suggested that corticosteroids may hasten the recovery of renal function in these patients.
7. The diagnosis of RPGN can be narrowed by use of sensitive and specific serologic tests that differentiate between pauciimmune GN, anti-GBM GN, and immune-mediated disease. Patients with pauciimmune GN can be further classified according to the results of the assays for ANCA. The presence of red blood cell casts or dysmorphic red blood cells in the urine is suggestive of glomerular injury. HUS, cryoglobulinemia, atheroembolic disease, and HIVAN are among the disorders that may mimic RPGN. Renal biopsy is indicated if the diagnosis remains uncertain.
8. Management of patients with ARF involves correction of the electrolyte abnormalities and the volume status. In addition, patients should be followed closely for the development of complications such as infection, pericarditis, hemorrhage, or neurologic dysfunction. Diuretics have been used by some to convert oliguric renal failure into nonoliguric renal failure. However, no clinical evidence supports the use of diuretics once ATN is established. Similarly, in the absence of large, well-designed, randomized trials, the use of dopamine for oliguric ARF remains controversial. Some contend that although dopamine may offer improvement in urine output, the benefit is outweighed by the risk of complications (*e.g.*, tachyarrhythmias, pulmonary shunting, gut or digital necrosis) (75). Others argue that, despite some risks, low-dose dopamine has few side effects and may still be useful for selected patients with oliguric ARF.
9. No controlled studies have explored the issue of when (*i.e.*, at what level of BUN) dialysis should be initiated. In clinical practice, the indications for dialysis include volume overload, hyperkalemia, metabolic acidosis, uremic pericarditis, and mental status changes that are refractory to conventional medical therapy. The use of CM for dialysis has been associated with a delay in recovery from ARF and a decrease in the rate of survival (26,68). Therefore, CM should not be used for dialysis in patients with ARF. No controlled study has shown that intensive (daily) dialysis improves outcome compared with nonintensive dialysis for patients with ARF.

Abbreviations used in Chapter 19

AT I = angiotensin I
AT II = angiotensin II
ACEI = angiotensin-converting enzyme inhibitor
AIDS = acquired immunodeficiency syndrome

AIN = acute interstitial nephritis
ANCA = antineutrophil cytoplasmic autoantibodies
APACHE-II = Acute Physiology and Chronic Health Evaluation II
ARDS = adult respiratory distress syndrome
ARF = acute renal failure
ATN = acute tubular necrosis
AZT = azidothymidine
BUN = blood urea nitrogen
C-ANCA = cytoplasmic-staining ANCA
CM = cuprophane membranes
CNS = central nervous system
DNase = deoxyribonuclease
ELISA = enzyme-linked immunosorbent assay
FE_{Na} = fractional excretion of sodium
GBM = glomerular basement membrane
GFR = glomerular filtration rate
GN = glomerulonephritis
HIV = human immunodeficiency virus
HIVAN = human immunodeficiency virus–associated nephropathy
HUS = hemolytic uremic syndrome
IABP = intraaortic balloon pump
IgA = immunoglobulin A
IgG = immunoglobulin G
IgM = immunoglobulin M
IV = intravenous
IVP = intravenous pyelography
n = number of patients in sample
NPV = negative predictive value
NSAID = nonsteroidal antiinflammatory drug
P-ANCA = perinuclear-staining ANCA
PNT = percutaneous nephrostomy tube
PPV = positive predictive value
QID = four times daily
RML = rhabdomyolysis
RPGN = rapidly progressive glomerulonephritis
SLE = systemic lupus erythematosus
TTP = thrombotic thrombocytopenic purpura
U_{Na} = urinary concentration of sodium
U_{osm} = urine osmolality
WG = Wegener's granulomatosis

References

1. Alexanian. Renal failure in multiple myeloma. *Arch Intern Med* 1990;150:1693.
2. Anto. Infusion intravenous pyelography and renal function: effects of hypertonic mannitol in patients with chronic renal insufficiency. *Arch Intern Med* 1981;141:1652.
3. Baldwin. Effect of postoperative low-dose dopamine on renal function after elective major vascular surgery. *Ann Intern Med* 1994;120:744.
4. Bell. Improved survival in thrombotic thrombocytopenic purpura–hemolytic uremic syndrome. *N Engl J Med* 1991;325:398.
5. Berns. Nephrotoxicity of contrast media. *Kidney Int* 1989;36:730.
6. Better. Early management of shock and prophylaxis of acute renal failure in traumatic rhabdomyolysis. *N Engl J Med* 1990;322:825.
7. Bickell. Immediate versus delayed fluid resuscitation for hypotensive patients with penetrating torso injuries. *N Engl J Med* 1994;331:1105.

8. Bonnardeaux. A study on the reliability of dipstick urinalysis. *Clin Nephrol* 1994; 41:167.
9. Bullock. The assessment of risk factors in 462 patients with acute renal failure. *Am J Kidney Dis* 1985;5:97.
10. Cameron. Allergic interstitial nephritis: clinical features and pathogenesis. *Q J Med* 1988;250:97.
11. Chew. Outcome in acute renal failure. *Nephrol Dial Transplant* 1993;8:101.
12. Cooper. Nephrotoxicity of common drugs used in clinical practice. *Arch Intern Med* 1987;147:1213.
13. Corwin. The detection and interpretation of urinary eosinophils. *Arch Pathol Lab Med* 1989;113:1256.
14. Corwin. Prediction of outcome in acute renal failure. *Am J Nephrol* 1987;7:8.
15. D Amico. Cryoglobulinemic glomerulonephritis: a membranoproliferative glomerulonephritis induced by hepatitis C virus. *Am J Kidney Dis* 1995;25:361.
16. D Elia. Nephrotoxicity from angiographic contrast material. *Am J Med* 1982;72: 719.
17. Davidman. Iatrogenic renal disease. *Arch Intern Med* 1991;151:1809.
18. Donaghy. Cigarette smoking and lung hemorrhage in glomerulonephritis caused by autoantibodies to glomerular basement membrane. *Lancet* 1983;2:1390.
19. Eneas. The effect of infusion of mannitol–sodium bicarbonate on the clinical course of myoglobinuria. *Arch Intern Med* 1979;139:801.
20. Fauci. Wegener's granulomatosis: prospective clinical and therapeutic experience with 85 patients for 21 years. *Ann Intern Med* 1983;98:76.
21. Feest. Incidence of severe acute renal failure in adults: results of a community based study. *Br Med J* 1993;306:481.
22. Galpin. Acute interstitial nephritis due to methicillin. *Am J Med* 1978;65:756.
23. Gillum. The role of intensive dialysis in acute renal failure. *Clin Nephrol* 1986; 25:249.
24. Gol. Vascular complications related to percutaneous insertion of intraaortic balloon pumps. *Ann Thorac Surg* 1994;58:1476.
25. Grunfeld, Acute interstitial nephritis. In: Schrier, ed. *Diseases of the Kidney.* Boston:Little, Brown, 1993:1331.
26. Hakim. Effect of the dialysis membrane in the treatment of patients with acute renal failure. *N Engl J Med* 1994;331:1338.
27. Hoffman. Wegener granulomatosis: an analysis of 158 patients. *Ann Intern Med* 1992;116:488.
28. Honda. Acute renal failure and rhabdomyolysis. *Kidney Int* 1983, 23:888.
29. Hou. Hospital-acquired renal insufficiency: a prospective study. *Am J Med* 1983; 74:243.
30. Hricik. Captopril-induced functional renal insufficiency in patients with bilateral renal-artery stenosis or renal artery stenosis in a solitary kidney. *N Engl J Med* 1983;308:373.
31. Jennette. Diagnosis and management of glomerulonephritis and vasculitis presenting as acute renal failure. *Med Clin North Am* 1990;74:893.
32. Johnson. Therapy of anti–glomerular basement antibody disease: analysis of prognostic significance of clinical, pathologic, and treatment factors. *Medicine (Baltimore)* 1985;64:219.
33. Johnson. Treatment of renal failure associated with multiple myeloma. *Arch Intern Med* 1990;150:863.
34. Kahan. Drug therapy: cyclosporine. *N Engl J Med* 1989;321:1725.
35. Kantrowitz. Intraaortic balloon pumping 1967 through 1982: analysis of complications in 733 patients. *Am J Cardiol* 1986;57:976.
36. Kaufman. Community-acquired acute renal failure. *Am J Kidney Dis* 1991;17:191.
37. Kelly. Goodpasture syndrome: molecular and clinical advances. *Medicine (Baltimore)* 1994;73:171.
38. Knottenbelt. Traumatic rhabdomyolysis from severe beating: experience of volume diuresis in 200 patients. *J Trauma* 1994;37:214.
39. Kyle. Monoclonal proteins and renal disease. *Annu Rev Med* 1994;45:71.

40. Liano. Easy and early prognosis of acute tubular necrosis: a forward analysis of 228 cases. *Nephron* 1989;51:307.
41. Lieberthal. Treatment of acute tubular necrosis. *Semin Nephrol* 1990;10:571.
42. Linton. Acute interstitial nephritis due to drugs. *Ann Intern Med* 1980;93:735.
43. Madaio. The diagnosis of acute glomerulonephritis. *N Engl J Med* 1983;309:1299.
44. Maillet. Nondilated obstructive acute renal failure: diagnostic procedures and therapeutic management. *Radiology* 1986;160:659.
45. Mandal. Diuretics potentiate angiotensin converting enzyme inhibitor–induced acute renal failure. *Clin Nephrol* 1994;42:170.
46. Mattana. Prevalence and determinants of acute renal failure following cardiopulmonary resuscitation. *Arch Intern Med* 1993;153:235.
47. Mehta. Therapeutic alternatives to renal replacement for critically ill patients in acute renal failure. *Semin Nephrol* 1994;14:64.
48. Miller. Urinary diagnostic indices in acute renal failure. *Ann Intern Med* 1978;89:47.
49. Misiani. Interferon alpha-2a therapy in cryoglobulinemia associated with hepatitis C virus. *N Engl J Med* 1994;330:751.
50. Moore. Risk factors for the nephrotoxicity in patients treated with aminoglycosides. *Ann Intern Med* 1984;100:352.
51. Neild. Haemolytic-uraemic syndrome in practice. *Lancet* 1994;343:398.
52. Niles. Antigen-specific radioimmunoassay for anti-neutrophil cytoplasmic antibodies in the diagnosis of rapidly progressive glomerulonephritis. *J Am Soc Nephrol* 1991;2:27.
53. Nolan. Eosinophiluria: a new method of detection and definition of the clinical spectrum. *N Engl J Med* 1986;315:1516.
54. Norman. Acute renal failure secondary to bilateral ureteric obstruction: review of 50 cases. *Can Med Assoc J* 1982;1:601.
55. Novis. Association of preoperative risk factors with postoperative acute renal failure. *Anesth Analg* 1994;78:143.
56. Parfrey. Contrast material–induced renal failure in patients with diabetes, renal insufficiency, or both. *N Engl J Med* 1989;320:143.
57. Pasquali. Long term survival patients with acute and severe renal failure due to multiple myeloma. *Clin Nephrol* 1990;34:247.
58. Prins. Once versus thrice daily gentamicin in patients with serious infections. *Lancet* 1993;341:335.
59. Pusey. Plasma exchange in focal necrotizing glomerulonephritis without anti-GBM antibodies. *Kidney Int* 1991;40:757.
59a. Rao. A prospective study of antineutrophil cytoplasmic antibody (C-ANCA) and clinical criteria in diagnosing Wegener's granulomatosis. *Lancet* 1995;346:926.
60. Rao. The types of renal disease in the acquired immunodeficiency syndrome. *N Engl J Med* 1987;316:1062.
61. Rasmussen. Acute renal failure: Multivariate analysis of causes and risk factors. *Am J Med* 1982;73:211.
62. Rock. Comparison of plasma exchange with plasma infusion in the treatment of thrombotic thrombocytopenic purpura. *N Engl J Med* 1991;325:393.
63. Ron. Prevention of acute renal failure in traumatic rhabdomyolysis. *Arch Intern Med* 1984;144:277.
64. Roth. Acute rhabdomyolysis associated with cocaine intoxication. *N Engl J Med* 1988;319:673.
65. Rudnick. Nephrotoxicity of ionic and nonionic contrast media in 1196 patients: a randomized trial. *Kidney Int* 1995;47:254.
66. Ruffing. Eosinophils in urine revisited. *Clin Nephrol* 1994;41:163.
67. Ruggenenti. Thrombotic thrombocytopenic purpura: evidence that infusion rather than removal of plasma induces remission of the disease. *Am J Kidney Dis* 1993;21:314.
68. Schiffl. Biocompatible membranes in acute renal failure: prospective case-controlled study. *Lancet* 1994;344:570.
69. Shankel. Acute renal failure and glomerulopathy caused by nonsteroidal anti-inflammatory drugs. *Arch Intern Med* 1992;152:986.

70. Solez. The morphology of acute tubular necrosis in man: analysis of 57 renal biopsies and a comparison with the glycerol model. *Medicine (Baltimore)* 1979;58:362.
71. Solomon. Effects of saline, mannitol, and furosemide on acute decreases in renal function induced by radiocontrast agents. *N Engl J Med* 1994;331:1416.
72. Spiegel. Determinants of survival and recovery in acute renal failure patients dialyzed in intensive-care units. *Am J Nephrol* 1991;11:44.
73. Stone. Human immunodeficiency virus-associated nephropathy: current concepts. *Am J Med Sci* 1994;307:212.
73a. Thadhani. Acute renal failure. *N Engl J Med* 1996;334:1448.
74. Thadhani. Atheroembolic renal failure after invasive procedures: an analysis of 52 histologically-proven cases. *Medicine* 1995;74:350.
75. Thompson. Renal-dose dopamine: a siren song? *Lancet* 1994;344:7.
76. Turney. Why is mortality persistently high in acute renal failure. *Lancet* 1990; 335:971.
77. Ward. Factors predictive of acute renal failure in rhabdomyolysis. *Arch Intern Med* 1988;148:1553.
78. Watkinson. The role of percutaneous nephrostomy in malignant urinary tract obstruction. *Clin Radiol* 1993;47:32.
79. Weisberg. Dopamine and renal blood flow in radiocontrast-induced nephropathy in humans. *Renal Failure* 1993;15:61.
80. Wilson. Eosinophiluria in atheroembolic renal disease. *Am J Med* 1991;91:186.
81. Wilson. Value of renal biopsy in acute intrinsic renal failure. *Br Med J* 1976;2:459.
82. Woodrow. Cause of death in acute renal failure. *Nephrol Dial Transplant* 1992;7: 230.
83. Wrong. Management of the acute uremic emergency. *Br Med Bull* 1971;27:97.
84. Zanardo. Acute renal failure in the patient undergoing cardiac operation. *J Thorac Cardiovasc Surg* 1994;107:1489.

20 Hypertensive Crisis

Robert B. Fogel and
Cecil H. Coggins

A. Introduction

1. **Epidemiology**—According to recent estimates, fewer than 1% of 60 million Americans with hypertension develop hypertensive crisis (HC). Some have defined HC arbitrarily as elevation in the diastolic blood pressure (DBP) above 120 to 130 mm Hg (16). However, the absolute level of DBP does not determine the presence or absence of HC. Patients with baseline hypertension tolerate a much higher blood pressure (BP) without incurring end-organ damage than those who are normotensive at baseline. The mean age of patients with HC is 40 to 50 years, and the ratio of men to women is 2:1. In a retrospective review of patients presenting with HC in New York City, Shea found that the typical patient was young, did not have a primary care doctor, was noncompliant with antihypertensive therapy, and used illicit drugs or ethanol (72). Smoking also appears to be an independent risk factor for development of HC (44). However, not all studies have confirmed these risk factors (71). Although HC most commonly occurs in persons with essential hypertension, secondary hypertension is proportionately more common among patients with HC than among the general population. For example, among 123 patients who presented to Vanderbilt University between 1964 and 1977 with HC (DBP >125 mm Hg and grade III/IV retinopathy), 31% were found to have renovascular hypertension (26). Sinclair reported that secondary hypertension accounted for 8% of the 3800 hypertensive patients (median DBP, 115 mm Hg) monitored at a BP clinic (74).
2. **Definitions**—The 1984 Joint National Committee on Detection, Evaluation and Treatment of High Blood Pressure proposed the following operational classification of hypertensive crises (79):
   a. **Hypertensive Emergency**—With hypertensive emergency, there is evidence of acute end-organ damage in the setting of an elevated BP and the BP must be lowered within 1 hour of presentation to minimize further damage (30). Table 20-1 lists some of these conditions.
   b. **Hypertensive Urgency**—With hypertensive urgency, the DBP is >120 mm Hg but there is no evidence of immediate end-organ damage or there is hypertension in a setting of potential organ damage from elevated BP. Therefore, the BP should be controlled within 24 hours of presentation to reduce the potential risk of end-organ damage. These conditions are listed in Table 20-2 (3).
   c. **Accelerated or Malignant Hypertension**—These are older terms that classified HC on the basis of funduscopic findings. Accelerated hyperten-

Table 20-1 Conditions of hypertensive emergency (30)

Hypertensive Encephalopathy	Intracranial Hemorrhage
Pulmonary edema	Stroke
Acute myocardial infarction	Aortic dissection
Disseminated intravascular coagulation	Scleroderma renal crisis
Eclampsia	Renal failure

Table 20-2 Conditions of hypertensive urgency (3)

Conditions
Hypertension in a patient with unstable angina
Postoperative hypertension
Preeclampsia
Hypertension in a renal transplant patient
DBP >120 mm Hg with no evidence of end-organ damage and no impending complications

sion is defined as elevated BP and the presence of grade III retinopathy (exudates or hemorrhages, or both). Malignant hypertension is defined as severe hypertension and the presence of papilledema. However, both of these findings represent end-organ damage and would be classified as hypertensive emergencies according to the current nomenclature (61). The older terminology has fallen out of favor because severe HC can be associated with end-organ damage without severe fundoscopic findings. Furthermore, studies have shown that differentiating between accelerated and malignant hypertension does not offer prognostic information and does not appear to be clinically relevant in the era of effective antihypertensive therapy (2,85). In addition, differentiating accelerated from malignant hypertension is highly dependent on the examiner's ability to perform an adequate fundoscopic examination. For these reasons, hypertensive emergency and hypertensive urgency are the terms used in this chapter.

3. **Pathophysiology**—Most of our understanding of the pathophysiology of HC is derived from experimental animal models or from autopsy specimens. In experimental animal models in which the BP is increased by pharmacologic means, characteristic vascular lesions are seen in the arteriolar walls at a critical level of mean arterial pressure (MAP). The arteriolar changes consist of fibrinoid necrosis, hemorrhage, platelet/fibrin thrombi, and loss of autoregulation of blood flow. The critical MAP is determined in part by the type of animal used and the presence or absence of underlying hypertension (40,46). In these animal models, all of these changes are potentially reversible. Similar pathologic findings are observed in some organs at autopsy, most notably the kidney, where the classic onion-skin lesion is seen (60,77). In most animal models, there appears to be a secondary activation of the renin–angiotensin II system owing to decreased renal perfusion. There is also a subsequent increase in the levels of other hormones such as norepinephrine and antidiuretic hormone.
4. **Prognosis**
   a. The prognosis for patients with HC has clearly improved with the advent of effective antihypertensive therapy and dialysis. Among the 81 patients with HC described by Keith in 1939, the 1-year mortality rates were 35% for those with grade III retinopathy and 80% for those with grade IV retinopathy (48). In 1966, Breslin reported a 10-year survival rate of 17% and 7% for patients with grade III and IV retinopathy, respectively, compared with 81% and 51% for patients with grade I and II retinopathy, respectively (13). Other studies during this period reported similar findings, and the presence of renal insufficiency appeared to be a poor prognostic factor (12,49). The major causes of death were myocardial infarction (MI), stroke, uremia, and sudden death. However, in more modern series, the prognosis of patients with HC appears to have improved significantly. Of the 69 patients with hypertension and grade III/IV retinopathy reported in one study (published in 1979), the 5-year survival rate was 75% (37). Similarly, two studies of patients with grade III/IV retinopathy also reported an improved 5-year survival rate, as shown in Table 20-3 (47,85).

Table 20-3 Long-term outcome in patients with hypertensive crisis

	Webster (85) (n=128)	Kuwazoe (47) (n=69)
Median age at presentation	52	39
% with secondary hypertension	28	46
5-Y survival rate	90%	90%
Renal survival* (%)	NA	37

*Survival without the need for dialysis or renal transplantation.

b. Even in the modern era, the presence of impaired renal function appears to indicate a poor prognosis. In one study involving 33 patients with hypertensive emergency and relatively preserved renal function (initial serum creatinine <3.4 mg/dl), 85% had stable or improved renal function on long-term follow-up. In contrast, among 32 patients with hypertensive emergency and poor renal function (serum creatinine >3.4 mg/dl), all but 3 patients had further deterioration in renal function and 76% required dialysis (90).

5. **Clinical Manifestations**—The most common presenting symptoms are headache, visual changes, and chest pain. End-organ damage is manifested in various ways in different organ systems.
   a. **Neurologic Manifestations**—The potential neurologic manifestations of HC include retinopathy, encephalopathy, stroke, and hemorrhage. Hypertensive retinopathy is defined by the Keith–Wagener classification scheme, whereby grades III and IV retinopathy are characterized by hemorrhage, cotton wool exudates, and papilledema. Patients may complain of blurred vision and have decreased visual acuity on examination (20). Hypertensive encephalopathy is less common but indicates altered cerebral function in the setting of severe hypertension. Patients may experience headache, depressed level of consciousness, and vomiting. Less commonly, seizures or focal neurologic deficits may occur (37). The pathophysiology of hypertensive encephalopathy is debated, but the prevailing theory is one of breakthrough blood flow. In normal as well as most hypertensive individuals, constant cerebral blood flow can be maintained over a wide range of BPs because of cerebral autoregulation. However, with severe hypertension, the autoregulatory mechanism is unable to compensate for the degree of BP elevation and cerebral blood flow increases, leading to cerebral edema (31,34). Less commonly, focal infarct or hemorrhage may occur. Several studies using computed tomography and magnetic resonance imaging techniques have confirmed the presence of cerebral edema in patients with hypertensive encephalopathy (33,86). However, at least one well-designed autopsy study failed to find significant edema in patients with hypertensive encephalopathy (18).
   b. **Cardiac Manifestations**—The cardiovascular effects of severe hypertension include increased afterload, myocardial oxygen demand, and wall stress. The most common clinical manifestations include congestive heart failure, unstable angina pectoris, and MI.
   c. **Renal Manifestations**—Proteinuria is the earliest manifestation of renal injury in experimental models of severe hypertension. Hematuria and impaired creatinine clearance may follow. The rise in creatinine is caused by fibrinoid necrosis of the renal arterioles, decreased renal blood flow, and perhaps concomitant volume depletion from pressure natriuresis. Up to 50% of patients are hypokalemic from secondary activation of the renin-angiotensin-aldosterone axis. Pathologic findings include focal and segmental fibrinoid necrosis of the glomerular tuft, increased mesangial matrix, wrinkling of the glomerular basement membrane, and hyperplasia of the juxtaglomerular apparatus (65).

d. **Hematological Manifestations**—Clinically, microangiopathic hemolytic anemia or thrombocytopenia may be observed in patients with HC. In one study, 16 of 24 patients with malignant hypertension had evidence of microangiopathic hemolytic anemia (56). Occasionally, an elevated prothrombin time and the presence of fibrin split products may be observed and may mimic disseminated intravascular coagulation (32).

B. Etiology

1. **Essential Hypertension**—The most common cause of HC remains poorly controlled essential hypertension. African-Americans appear to be at particularly high risk. Other causes of HC are discussed in the following sections.
2. **Renal Disease**—Severe hypertension can be a complication of almost any renal disease, including acute glomerulonephritis, chronic pyelonephritis, immunoglobulin A nephropathy, and renovascular disease (23,26). Hypertensive emergency has also been described with cholesterol embolization syndrome and with renin-secreting tumors (70). Scleroderma renal crisis is characterized by sudden hypertension with rapid deterioration of renal function in a patient with underlying systemic sclerosis. For unclear reasons, scleroderma renal crisis is more common during the winter months (80).
3. **Pregnancy-Related Hypertension**—Preeclampsia is characterized by hypertension (BP >140/90 mm Hg, or a rise of >30 mm Hg in systolic BP or >15 mm Hg of DBP), proteinuria, and edema developing after 20 weeks of gestation. Eclampsia is defined by the presence of seizures in addition to the features of preeclampsia. Preeclampsia affects 7% of all pregnancies. Risk factors for preeclampsia include nulliparity, prior history of preeclampsia, diabetes mellitus, and African-American race (73). Both preeclampsia and eclampsia are associated with significant maternal and fetal morbidity and increased mortality. The exact pathophysiology of these syndromes is unclear, but pathologic examination of kidney and placental specimens reveals platelet clumping, endothelial damage, and severe vasoconstriction (69).
4. **Endocrine Hypertension**—Pheochromocytoma is the most common cause of endocrine-related HC. It is usually caused by a tumor in the adrenal medulla, or less commonly, in the sympathetic paraaortic ganglia. These tumors usually produce norepinephrine and are a rare cause of hypertension, accounting for 0.1% to 0.7% of cases (29). As with other causes of HC, headache and visual changes are common, but classic symptoms include diaphoresis, palpitations, anxiety, and tremor (87). Other endocrine causes of hypertension, such as Cushing's syndrome and hyperaldosteronism, only rarely cause HC.
5. **Drugs and Medications**
   a. Illicit drugs associated with hypertensive crises include cocaine, methamphetamine, lysergic acid diethylamide (LSD), and phencyclidine (PCP). They all appear in some fashion to stimulate the sympathetic nervous system (16,27).
   b. Monoamine oxidase (MAO) inhibitors, a class of antidepressant medications, decrease the degradation of dopamine and norepinephrine. If foods rich in tyramine (certain cheeses, wines, beers, and nuts) are ingested by a patient taking MAO inhibitors, massive release of norepinephrine may cause a catechol crisis, characterized by severe hypertension, flushing, nausea, vomiting, and end-organ damage (40).
   c. Some over-the-counter diet pills and cold medications containing phenylpropanolamine have caused HC, usually when taken in excess of the recommended dosage (7,52).
   d. Medication withdrawal is a fairly common precipitant of HC. In particular, abrupt discontinuation of b-adrenergic receptor blockers, angiotensin-converting enzyme inhibitors (ACEIs), or centrally acting antihypertensive agents may cause HC (62).

C. Management—A literature-based recommendation for the management of HC is difficult because of a paucity of well-designed studies that compare various therapeutic strategies. Therefore, the management guidelines described here are derived mostly from expert opinions rather than from clinical data. Nevertheless, it is clear that modern therapeutic interventions have greatly improved the prognosis of what was once an almost uniformly fatal illness. Two important issues to be addressed before initiation of therapy for HC are at what rate and to what extent the BP should be lowered. For reasons discussed later, complete normalization of BP is usually not necessary and should not be the goal of acute therapy (35).

1. **Hypertensive Urgency**—Although retrospective data suggest that immediate antihypertensive therapy improves the prognosis for those with true hypertensive emergencies, there is less convincing data for hypertensive urgencies. Therefore, in the absence of acute end-organ damage, oral antihypertensive medications should be the first line of therapy. The most commonly used oral agents are listed in Table 20-4.
   a. **Clonidine**—This centrally acting drug selectively stimulates the postsynaptic a-adrenergic receptors in the medulla oblongata and thereby diminishes the neuronal vasoconstrictor tone in the heart, kidneys, and peripheral vasculature. It decreases serum levels of catechols and suppresses plasma renin activity (39,42). Several case series that have evaluated the use of clonidine for patients with hypertensive urgencies are summarized in Table 20-5 (4,21,75). As these studies demonstrate, clonidine is an effective agent for rapidly lowering the BP in most patients. The most commonly observed adverse effects were dry mouth, sedation, and dizziness. Severe orthostatic hypotension was reported in one study.
   b. **Nifedipine**—This dihydropyridine calcium channel antagonist is the most extensively studied oral agent for acute management of HC. More than 20 studies support the use of oral, sublingual, or rectal nifedipine for management of HC. Some of the representative studies that have used nifedipine for management of HC are summarized in Table 20-6 (8–10,24,28). The studies by Beer (8) and Bertel (9,10) included placebo control periods but in a single-blind manner. The studies by Bertel (9,10) also documented no significant reduction in the cerebral blood flow with nifedipine therapy. Adverse

Table 20-4 Oral agents used in treatment of hypertensive urgency

Agent	Dose and Route	Onset	Peak	Duration	Side Effects
Clonidine	0.2 mg, then 0.1 mg PO q 1 h	30–60 min	2 h	8–12 h	Sedation, dry mouth, orthostasis
Nifedipine	5–20 mg PO or SL	5–15 min	15–30 min	3–6 h	Headache, tachycardia, orthostasis
Captopril	6.25–50 mg PO or SL	15 min	45–60 min	2–6 h	Tachycardia, renal failure, hypotension
Labetolol	200–400 mg PO	15–45 min	60 min	2–6 h	Orthostasis, bronchospasm

Table 20-5 Clonidine for management of hypertensive urgency

	Cohen (21) (n=15)	Anderson (4) (n=36)	Spitalewitz (75) (n=20)
Initial dose (mg)	0.1 or 0.2	0.2	0.2
Mean total dose (mg)	0.39	0.45	0.32
Initial MAP (mm Hg)	141	163	160
Mean decrease in MAP (mm Hg)	33	44	40
% responding to clonidine	80	94	100

Table 20-6 Nifedipine for management of hypertensive urgency

	Beer (8) (n=26)	Bertel (9,10) (n=25)	Ellrodt (28) (n=30)	Davidson (24) (n=19)
Dose and route (mg)	10–20 SL	10–20 PO	10–20 SL	10–20 SL
Initial MAP (mm Hg)	153	158	158±16	144±11
Mean decrease in MAP (mm Hg)	35	48	36	35
P	<0.001	<0.001	<0.001	<0.001

effects attributable to nifedipine were minimal, but it has rarely been associated with severe hypotension or syncope. No deaths have been reported among more than 500 patients described in the literature. Nifedipine produces a prompt, consistent, and usually predictable lowering of BP (43).

c. Captopril—The use of ACEIs for management of HC has been evaluated in several small series. The results of these studies are summarized in Table 20-7 (17,38,81). Several authors reported severe hypotension associated with the first dose of captopril, especially in volume-depleted patients. In addition, some authors noted captopril to be less effective when tested in an inner-city, largely African-American population (3).

d. Labetalol—The oral form of this combined α- and β-receptor antagonist has an a:b blocking ratio of 1:3. It has been studied in only few small series (25). The largest and most recent study was a randomized, double-blind dose-response evaluation involving 36 patients with hypertensive urgency. Patients were randomly assigned to receive 100, 200, or 300 mg of oral labetalol. At 2 hours, the desired result (DBP <100 mm Hg or a decrease in DBP of 30 mm Hg) was achieved in 68% of patients in the study without significant differences among the three doses. However, the antihypertensive effect of the 100-mg dose appeared to wane sooner, compared with the higher doses (36).

e. Several studies in the 1990s compared the effectiveness and safety of various oral antihypertensive agents. The representative comparative studies are summarized in Table 20-8 (5,6,45,64). These studies are limited by small sample size, varying dosing regimens, and different patient populations. Nevertheless, no study found a significant difference among the various agents, either in the percentage of patients who responded or in the magnitude of the overall BP response (41).

f. Conclusions

(1) Although the literature regarding the use of oral antihypertensive therapy for hypertensive urgency is clearly inadequate, a few useful conclusions may be drawn. Among the commonly used agents, the largest reported clinical experience has been with nifedipine, which remains the agent of choice for most patients with hypertensive urgency. Clonidine also has a long record of safety and efficacy. However, because of

Table 20-7 Captopril for management of hypertensive urgency

	Case (17) (n=20)	Tschellor (81) (n=6)	Heuger-Klevene (38) (n=13)
Dose and Route (mg)	10–50 PO	25 SL	25 SL
Initial MAP (mm Hg)	150	165	144
Mean decrease in MAP (mm Hg)	—	35	29
Mean decrease in DBP (mm Hg)	35	—	—

Table 20-8 Studies comparing various oral agents for hypertensive urgency

Reference	N	Drug	Dose/Route (mg)	Mean BP reduction (mm Hg)	Responders (%)
Jaker	28	Clonidine	0.1 (PO load)	51/30	79
(45)	23	Nifedipine	20 (PO)	47/29	96
Angeli	10	Captopril	25 (SL)	55/29	90
(5)	10	Nifedipine	10 (SL)	44/39	80
Atkin	18	Clonidine	0.2 (PO load)	57/32	83
(6)	18	Labetalol	200–800 (PO)	54/37	94
McDonald	10	Labetalol	200–400 (PO)	41/27	80
(64)	10	Nifedipine	10 (PO)	35/28	100

its relatively delayed onset of action, it may be less suited for use in the emergency department. The published experience with labetalol for hypertensive urgency is relatively limited, but it does appear to be a safe and an effective alternative. Captopril may also be useful, but, given the lack of data, it is currently not the agent of choice except in special circumstances. In addition, it seems reasonable to initiate therapy acutely with an agent that may be continued for long-term therapy.

(2) The benefit of immediate treatment of asymptomatic patients with severe hypertension but no end-organ damage has been called into question (55). Patients with hypertensive urgency are clearly vulnerable to the long-term consequences of hypertension, but they typically are not in immediate danger. Although acute therapy for hypertensive urgency is the standard of care at many centers, there are no data indicating that reduction of BP over hours is better than gradual reduction over days to weeks.

2. **Hypertensive Emergency**—For hypertensive patients with ongoing, acute end-organ damage, the BP should expeditiously be lowered to a safe level to prevent further damage, but this goal should be balanced by the need to maintain adequate organ perfusion. Although not examined in controlled trials, a reasonable goal is to lower the MAP by approximately 25% in the first few hours of therapy. Most authorities recommend the use of parental antihypertensive therapy with continuous BP monitoring in an intensive care unit. However the oral agent nifedipine has also been used successfully in this setting. The commonly used parenteral agents are listed in Table 20-9 (16,46,61).

   a. When nitroprusside became available for general use in United States in 1974, it rapidly became the agent of choice for treatment of almost all hypertensive emergencies (16,46,61,82). It is clearly the most potent and the most predictably effective of all available agents, and its onset of action is almost instantaneous. It is a balanced arterial and venous dilator and allows the BP to be titrated without precipitous change. It has little or no effect on the autonomic nervous system, central nervous system, gastrointestinal system, or cardiac smooth muscle, and patients do not develop tachyphylaxis to its effects (66). In a study by Ahearn, nitroprusside reduced the DBP to the goal of 90 to 100 mm Hg within 5 minutes in all 7 patients with a hypertensive emergency. All of these patients had been refractory to other agents (1). However, despite more than 20 years of extensive clinical experience with nitroprusside for hypertensive emergencies, no randomized study has directly compared it with other agents (22). Nitroprusside is converted by the red blood cells to cyanide, which is then metabolized to thiocyanate within the liver. Thiocyanate is excreted renally. Therefore, toxicity is most likely with prolonged use (>48 hours), especially in patients with renal insufficiency.

Table 20-9 Parenteral agents used for hypertensive emergency (16,46,61)

Agent	Dose/Route	Onset	Duration	Side Effects
Diazoxide	50–100 mg IV bolus as needed, or 15–30 mg/min IV	1–5 min	6–12 h	Hypotension, tachycardia, myocardial ischemia, vomiting
Nitroprusside	0.3–10 μg/kg/min IV	Immediate	2–3 min	Vomiting, thiocyanate toxicity
Nitroglycerin	5–100 μg/min IV	1–2 min	3–5 min	Headache, vomiting, tachyphylaxis
Hydralazine	10–20 mg IV bolus as needed	5–15 min	2–6 h	Hypotension, tachycardia, headache, vomiting
Labetalol	20–80 mg IV bolus as needed, or 2 mg/min IV	5–10 min	2–6 h	Hypotension, heart block, vomiting, bronchospasm
Phentolamine	5–10 mg IV bolus as needed	1–2 min	15–60 min	Hypotension, hypertension, tachycardia

b. Diazoxide, another potent direct arterial vasodilator, is effective in >90% of patients with hypertensive emergencies (50). In 1977, McDonald used IV diazoxide in 41 consecutive patients with HC and found it to be effective (DBP decreased >30 mm Hg) in 38 patients, without any severe adverse reactions. However, the use of diazoxide for HC has fallen out of favor for several reasons (63). Although its long half-life after bolus injection can be useful, it can also cause episodes of prolonged severe hypotension, which have been reported in up to 4.5% of patients (51).

c. Nitroglycerin, labetalol, hydralazine, and phentolamine are all useful in certain situations, as discussed in later sections. Although not yet approved for use in this country, IV nicardipine also appears to be safe and effective.

3. Management of Specific Hypertensive Situations

a. Stroke—Patients with acute stroke are often hypertensive on presentation. Although the initial instinct may be to reduce the BP, there are reasons to be cautious. Both in animal models and in patients with acute strokes, autoregulation of cerebral blood flow appears to be lost in periinfarct areas of the injured brain. Therefore, cerebral blood flow becomes directly proportional to the perfusion pressure (which is equal to the MAP minus the intracranial pressure). Because the intracranial pressure is often elevated as a result of edema or hemorrhage, lowering the BP may decrease cerebral blood flow and thereby worsen the neurologic deficit (53, 68). Wallace studied 334 consecutive patients with an acute stroke (excluding subarachnoid hemorrhage) and found 84% to be acutely hypertensive on presentation. Among patients with an ischemic stroke, the BP decreased spontaneously over 10 days, but those with a hemorrhagic stroke had a more variable course (84). Britton compared the outcome of acute stroke patients with and without accompanying severe hypertension (BP >200/115 mm Hg). The hypertensive patients were more likely to have baseline hypertension ($P<0.001$), but there was no significant difference in neurologic outcome between the two groups (15). No study has demonstrated improvement in neurologic outcome with acute lowering of BP in hypertensive patients with stroke. Therefore, most neurologists avoid treatment of hypertension associated with acute stroke unless there is evidence of other end-organ damage, hypertensive encephalopathy is present, or DBP is >130 mm Hg (78). If the hypertension is to be treated, an easily titratable drug with a short half-life (*e.g.*, nitroprusside) is typically chosen, and many would advocate the use of continuous intracranial pressure monitoring.

b. Aortic Dissection—For patients with an aortic dissection, the risk of progression is directly related to the BP as well as to the mechanical stress on the arterial wall, as measured by the slope of the rise in BP over time (dp/dt). Drugs that lower the BP but cause reflex tachycardia (*e.g.*, diazoxide, hydralazine) may increase the dp/dt and paradoxically extend the dissection. In general, nitroprusside lowers the BP without causing tachycardia, but by decreasing the afterload it may increase cardiac contractility and also increase dp/dt. For this reason, nitroprusside should be used in combination with an IV β-adrenergic receptor blocker such as propranolol, esmolol, or labetalol (54,89). However, there are no published data comparing the relative efficacy of these agents.

c. Acute Myocardial Infarction—The adverse effects of hypertension on myocardial oxygen demand and myocardial blood flow were described previously. Many agents can lower the BP during an acute MI, but those that cause reflex tachycardia may increase myocardial oxygen demand and therefore should be avoided. β-Adrenergic receptor blockers are clearly beneficial for patients with an acute MI and should be given whenever possible. Another commonly used agent is nitroglycerin. Although both nitroglycerin and nitroprusside may effectively reduce the BP, experimental studies favor nitroglycerin for patients with coronary ischemia. In a study that evaluated the effects of nitroglycerin and nitroprusside on regional myocardial blood flow in patients with coronary artery disease, both drugs decreased the MAP and the wedge pressure but nitroprusside reduced the myocardial blood flow to areas supplied by stenotic vessels (60). In contrast, nitroglycerin increased the regional myocardial blood flow to these same areas. Chiarello studied the effects of nitroprusside infusion in 10 patients with an acute MI and stable ST-segment elevation within the first 8 hours of onset of symptoms. Despite a consistent decrease in the MAP and the wedge pressure, nitroprusside increased the mean ST-segment elevation by 2.0 mm. When 5 of these patients were switched to IV nitroglycerin, a similar decrease in MAP and wedge pressure was observed, but the mean ST-segment elevation decreased by 1.4 mm (19).

d. Pregnancy-Related Hypertension—Although several antihypertensive drugs have been used for management of preeclampsia or eclampsia, delivery of the fetus remains the only definitive therapy. Magnesium sulfate is clearly indicated for treatment of eclamptic seizures, and it is an effective antihypertensive agent as well. The drug with the longest record of use for pregnancy-related hypertension is hydralazine. IV administration of 5 to 10 mg of hydralazine given every 20 minutes is highly effective in lowering the BP. However, it has been associated with precipitous falls in BP in up to 58% of treated patients. Hydralazine is also associated with fetal distress and has variable effects on placental blood flow (73). Experience with labetalol in pregnancy-related hypertension is rapidly increasing. It is effective for most patients but does not appear to reduce the amount of placental blood flow (58). Pickles used oral labetalol in 144 women with pregnancy-induced hypertension and found it to be safe and effective (67). When IV labetalol was compared with hydralazine in 110 patients with pregnancy-related hypertension, both drugs were highly effective in lowering the BP; 90% and 100% of patients responded to labetalol and hydralazine, respectively. There was no significant difference in maternal or fetal outcome between the two groups (59). Because of its long track record, hydralazine remains the agent of choice for most obstetricians, but labetalol appears to be an adequate alternative. The experience with other antihypertensive agents is limited, and all ACEIs are contraindicated in pregnancy.

e. **Pheochromocytoma**—Hypertension associated with pheochromocytoma is primarily caused by a-adrenergic stimulation, whereas palpitations, diaphoresis, and tachycardia are caused by β-adrenergic stimulation. Phentolamine is an α-adrenergic antagonist (5- to 10-mg IV boluses) that is recommended by some as the agent of choice for HC related to pheochromocytoma. Nitroprusside has also been used with much success, but no comparative studies exist (11,29,87). β-Adrenergic antagonists should be avoided at least until adequate a-adrenergic blockade has been achieved, because a paradoxical increase in BP may occur owing to blockade of β_2-vasodilatory receptors. Labetalol, a combined α- and β-adrenergic receptor antagonist, has been advocated by some authors (11,29). However, it should be used with caution, because paradoxical hypertension has been associated with its use in patients with pheochromocytoma (14).

f. **Scleroderma Renal Crisis**—Until the late 1970s, this syndrome was almost always associated with malignant hypertension, rapidly progressive renal failure, and early death. It is associated with elevated plasma renin activity and high levels of angiotensin II. Captopril, an ACEI, is the drug of choice for management of patients with this syndrome (57). In the largest reported series, Steen retrospectively evaluated the outcome of patients with scleroderma renal crisis at a university hospital. The 1-year survival rate for patients treated with an ACEI was 76%, compared with 15% for those not treated with an ACEI ($P<0.001$). The 5-year survival rates were 65% and 10%, respectively ($P<0.001$). Only 4 of 53 patients not treated with captopril survived without dialysis, compared with 31 of 55 patients treated with captopril (76).

D. Conclusions

1. HC remains a rare event, developing in fewer than 1% of 60 million Americans with hypertension. HC can be defined arbitrarily as an elevation in the DBP to >120 to 130 mm Hg. However, the absolute level of BP does not determine the presence or absence of HC. Patients with baseline hypertension tolerate a much higher BP without incurring end-organ damage than those who are normotensive at baseline. The prognosis for patients presenting with a hypertensive emergency has significantly improved over the years; a 90% 5-year survival rate can now reasonably be expected, and about 40% survive without the need for dialysis or renal transplantation. The prognosis for those with hypertensive urgency is even better.
2. With hypertensive urgency, the DBP is >120 mm Hg but there is no evidence of immediate end-organ damage. Although emergency treatment of an asymptomatic but severely hypertensive patient remains controversial, most centers advocate reducing the BP within 24 hours of presentation to reduce the potential risk of end-organ damage. In general, hypertensive urgency can be treated with oral medications. Nifedipine, clonidine, labetalol, and captopril are most often used.
3. Hypertensive emergency is defined by the presence of acute end-organ damage such as MI, pulmonary edema, aortic dissection, stroke, disseminated intravascular coagulation, or renal failure. Immediate therapy is recommended. For most hypertensive emergencies, nitroprusside allows rapid but safe reduction of BP. For some specific hypertensive situations, other agents may be preferred.
   a. In general, acute reduction of BP for hypertensive patients with acute stroke is not warranted.
   b. Nitroglycerin is preferred over nitroprusside for patients with acute ischemic coronary syndromes.
   c. A b-adrenergic receptor antagonist is often added for patients with acute aortic dissection or coronary ischemia.

d. Phentolamine is recommended by some as the agent of choice for management of HC associated with pheochromocytoma.
e. Captopril is the agent of choice for scleroderma renal crisis.
f. For pregnancy-related hypertension, hydralazine or labetalol appears to be safe and effective.

Abbreviations used in Chapter 20

BP = blood pressure
DBP = diastolic blood pressure
dp/dt = the slope of the curve indicating rise in BP over time
HC = hypertensive crisis
IV = intravenous
LSD = lysergic acid diethylamide
MAO = monoamine oxidase
MAP = mean arterial pressure
MI = myocardial infarction
P = probability value
PCP = phencyclidine
PO = per os
q = every
SL = sublingual

References

1. Ahearn. Treatment of malignant hypertension with sodium nitroprusside. *Arch Intern Med* 1974;133:187.
2. Ahmed. Lack of difference between malignant and accelerated hypertension. *Br Med J* 1986;292:235.
3. Anderson. Current concepts in treatment of hypertensive urgencies. *Am Heart J* 1986;111:211. Review.
4. Anderson. Oral clonidine loading in hypertensive urgencies. *JAMA* 1981;246:848.
5. Angeli. Comparison of sublingual captopril and nifedipine in immediate treatment of hypertensive emergencies. *Arch Intern Med* 1991;151:678.
6. Atkin. Oral labetalol versus oral clonidine in the emergency treatment of severe hypertension. *Am J Med Sci* 1992;303:9.
7. Backlin. Decongestant-induced hypertensive crisis. *Can Fam Physician* 1993;39:375.
8. Beer. Efficacy of sublingual nifedipine in the acute treatment of systematic hypertension. *Chest* 1981;79:572.
9. Bertel. Nifedipine in hypertensive emergencies. *Br Med J* 1983;286:19.
10. Bertel. Treatment of hypertensive emergencies with the calcium channel blocker nifedipine. *Am J Med* 1985;79(Suppl 4A):31.
11. Bravo. Pheochromocytoma. *Endocrinol Metab Clin North Am* 1993;22:329.
12. Breckenridge. Prognosis of treated hypertension. *Q J Med* 1970;155:411.
13. Breslin. Prognostic importance of ophthalmoscopic findings in essential hypertension. *JAMA* 1966;195:91.
14. Briggs. Hypertensive response to labetalol in pheochromocytoma. *Lancet* 1978:1045.
15. Britton. Very high blood pressure in acute stroke. *J Intern Med* 1990;228:611.
16. Calhoun. Treatment of hypertensive crisis. *N Engl J Med* 1990;323:1177. Review.
17. Case. Acute and chronic treatment of severe and malignant hypertension with oral angiotensin-converting enzyme inhibitor captopril. *Circulation* 1981;64:765.
18. Chester. Hypertensive encephalopathy: a clinicopathologic study of 20 cases. *Neurology* 1978;28:929.

19. Chiariello. Comparison between the effects of nitroprusside and nitroglycerin on ischemic injury during acute myocardial infarction. *Circulation* 1976;54:766.
20. Coggins. Management of hypertensive emergencies. In Earle Wilkins (Ed.). *Emergency Medicine: Scientific Foundations and Current Practice*, 3rd edition. Williams & Wilkins, Baltimore, 1989;8:133. Review.
21. Cohen. Oral clonidine loading for rapid control of hypertension. *Clin Pharmacol Ther* 1978;24:11.
22. Cohn. Diagnosis and treatment: Drugs five years later. Nitroprusside. *Ann Intern Med* 1979;91:752.
23. Danielsen. Arterial hypertension in chronic glomerulopnephritis: an analysis of 310 cases. *Clin Nephrol* 1983;19:284.
24. Davidson. Oral nifedipine for the treatment of patients with severe hypertension. *Am J Med* 1985;79(Suppl 4A):26.
25. Davies. Rapid reduction of blood pressure with acute oral labetalol. *J Clin Pharmacol* 1982;13:705.
26. Davis. Prevalence of renovascular hypertension in patients with grade III or IV hypertensive retinopathy. *N Engl J Med* 1979;301:1273.
27. Eastman. Hypertensive crisis and death associated with phencyclidine poisoning. *JAMA* 1975;231:1270.
28. Ellrodt. Efficacy and safety of sublingual nifedipine in the hypertensive emergencies. *Am J Med* 1985;79(Suppl 4A):19.
29. Falterman. Pheochromocytoma: clinical diagnosis and management. *South Med J* 1982;75:321.
30. Ferguson. Hypertensive emergencies and urgencies. *JAMA* 1986;255:1607. Review.
31. Finnerty. Hypertensive encephalopathy. *Am J Med* 1972;52:672.
32. Gavras. Abnormalities of coagulation and the development of malignant phase hypertension. *Kidney Int* 1975;8:S252.
33. Gibby. Reversal of white matter edema in hypertensive encephalopathy. *AJNR Am J Neuroradiol* 1989;16:S78.
34. Gifford. Hypertensive encephalopathy: mechanisms, clinical features, and treatment. *Prog Cardiovasc Dis* 1974;17:115.
35. Gifford. Management of hypertensive crises. *JAMA* 1991;266:829.
36. Gonzalez. Dose-response evaluation of oral labetalol in patients presenting to the emergency department with accelerated hypertension. *Ann Emerg Med* 1991;20: 333.
37. Reserved.
38. Heuger-Klevene. Captopril in hypertensive crisis. *Lancet* 1985;2(8457):732.
39. Houston. Clonidine hydrochloride: review of pharmacologic and clinical aspects. *Prog Cardiovasc Dis* 1981;23:337. Review.
40. Houston. Hypertensive emergencies and urgencies: pathophysiology and clinical aspects. *Am Heart J* 1986;111:205.
41. Houston. The comparative effects of clonidine hydrochloride and nifedipine in the treatment of hypertensive crises. *Am Heart J* 1988;115:152.
42. Houston. Treatment of hypertensive emergencies and urgencies with oral clonidine loading and titration. *Arch Intern Med* 1986;146:586.
43. Houston. Treatment of hypertensive urgencies and emergencies with nifedipine. *Am Heart J* 1986;111:963.
44. Isles. Excess smoking in malignant phase hypertension. *Br Med J* 1979;1:579.
45. Jaker. Oral nifedipine vs. oral clonidine in the treatment of urgent hypertension. *Arch Intern Med* 1989;149:260.
46. Kaplan. Hypertensive crises. In Norman Kaplan (Ed.). *Clinical Hypertension*, 6th edition. Williams & Wilkins, Baltimore, 1994;8:281. Review.
47. Kawazoe. Long-term prognosis of malignant hypertension; difference between underlying diseases such as essential hypertension and chronic glomerulonephritis. *Clin Nephrol* 1988;29:53.
48. Keith. Some different types of hypertension: their course and prognosis. *Am J Med Sci* 1939, 197:332.
49. Kincaid-Smith. The clinical course and pathology of hypertension with papilledema (malignant hypertension). *Q J Med* 1958;27:117.

50. Koch-Weser. Medical intelligence: diazoxide. *N Engl J Med* 1976;294:1271.
51. Kumar. Side effects of diazoxide. *JAMA* 1976;235:275.
52. Lake. Adverse drug effects attributed to phenylpropanolamine: a review of 142 case reports. *Am J Med* 1990;89:195.
53. Lavin. Management of hypertension in patients with acute stroke. *Arch Intern Med* 1986;146:66.
54. Lebel. Labetalol infusion in hypertensive emergencies. *Clin Pharmacol* 1985;37: 615.
55. Ledingham. Cerebral complications in the treatment of accelerated hypertension. *Q J Med* 1979;189:25.
56. Linton. Microangiopathic haemolytic anaemia and the pathogenesis of malignant hypertension. *Lancet* 1969;1:1277.
57. Lopez-Ovejero. Medical intelligence: reversal of vascular and renal crises of scleroderma by oral angiotensin-converting-enzyme blockade. *N Engl J Med* 1979;300: 1417.
58. Lunell. Acute effects of an antihypertensive drug, labetalol, on uteroplacental blood flow. *Br J Obstet Gynaecol* 1982;89:640.
59. Mabie. A comparative trial of labetalol and hydralazine in the acute management of severe hypertension complicating pregnancy. *Obstet Gynaecol* 1987;70:328.
60. Mann. Effect of nitroprusside on regional myocardial blood flow in coronary artery disease. *Circulation* 1978;57:732.
61. Mann. Hypertensive emergencies. In John Laragh & Barry Brenner (Eds). *Hypertension: Pathophysiology, Diagnosis, and Management*, 2nd ed. Raven Press, NY 1995;181:3009. Review.
62. McAlister. Hypertensive crisis after discontinuation of angiotensin-converting enzyme inhibitor. *Lancet* 1994;344:1502.
63. McDonald. Intravenous diazoxide therapy in hypertensive crisis. *Am J Cardiol* 1977; 40:409.
64. McDonald. Oral labetalol versus oral nifedipine in hypertensive urgencies in the ED. *Am J Emerg Med* 1993;11:460.
65. Nolan. Malignant hypertension and other hypertensive crises. In: Schrier, Gottschalk. *Diseases of the Kidney*, 5th ed. Little, Brown, and Co., Boston 1992: 1555. Review.
66. Palmer. Medical intelligence: sodium nitroprusside. *N Engl J Med* 1975;292:294.
67. Pickles. A randomized placebo controlled trial of labetalol in the treatment of mild to moderate pregnancy induced hypertension. *Br J Obstet Gynaecol* 1992;99:964.
68. Powers. Acute hypertension after stroke: the scientific basis for treatment decisions. *Neurology* 1993;43:461.
69. Roberts. Clinical and biochemical evidence of endothelial cell dysfunction in the pregnancy syndrome preeclampsia. *Am J Hypertens* 1991;4:700.
70. Rossi. A renin-secreting tumour with severe hypertension and cardiovascular disease: a diagnostic and therapeutic challenge. *Clin Exp Hypertens* 1993;15:325.
71. Sesoko. Predisposing factors for the development of malignant essential hypertension. *Arch Intern Med* 1987;147:1721.
72. Shea. Predisposing factors for severe, uncontrolled hypertension in an inner-city minority population. *N Engl J Med* 1992;327:776.
73. Silver. Acute hypertensive crisis in pregnancy. *Med Clin North Am* 1989;73:623.
74. Sinclair. Secondary hypertension in a blood pressure clinic. *Arch Intern Med* 1987; 147:1289.
75. Spitalewitz. Use of oral clonidine for rapid titration of blood pressure in severe hypertension. *Chest* 1983;83:S404.
76. Steen. Outcome of renal crisis in systemic sclerosis: relation to availability of angiotensin converting enzyme (ACE) inhibitors. *Ann Intern Med* 1990;113:352.
77. Susin. Essential malignant hypertension. *New York State Journal of Medicine* January 1978:54.
78. Thacker. Managing hypertensive emergencies and urgencies in the geriatric patient. *Geriatrics* 1991;46:26.
79. The Joint National Committee on Detection, Evaluation, and Treatment of High Blood Pressure. The 1984 report of the Joint National Committee of Detection,

Evaluation, and Treatment of High Blood Pressure. *Arch Intern Med* 1984;144: 1045.
80. Traub. Hypertension and renal failure (scleroderma renal crisis) is progressive systemic sclerosis. *Medicine (Baltimore)* 1983;62:335.
81. Tschollar. Sublingual captopril in hypertensive crises. *Lancet* 1985:34.
82. Vidt. Current concepts in treatment of hypertensive emergencies. *Am Heart J* 1986; 111:220. Review.
83. Vidt. Round table discussion: pathophysiology of severe hypertension. *Am Heart J* 1986;111:229. Review.
84. Wallace. Blood pressure after stroke. *JAMA* 1981;246:2177.
85. Webster. Accelerated hypertension: patterns of mortality and clinical factors affecting outcome in treated patients. *Q J Med* 1993;86:485.
86. Weingarten. Acute hypertensive encephalopathy: findings on spin-echo and gradient-echo MR imaging. *AJR Am J Roentgenol* 1994;162:665.
87. Werbel. Pheochromocytoma. *Med Clin North Am* 1995;79:131.
88. Wiener. The cellular pathology of experimental hypertension. *Am J Pathol* 1969; 54:187.
89. Wilson. Intravenous labetalol in the treatment of severe hypertension and hypertensive emergencies. *Am J Med* 1993:95.
90. Yu. Malignant hypertension: aetiology and outcome in 83 patients. *Clin Exp Hypertens* 1986;8:1211.

21 Hypercalcemia

Will P. Schmitt and
Cecil H. Coggins

A. Introduction

1. **Definition**—Hypercalcemia is defined as serum calcium concentration >10.5 mg/dl. Because the active, ionized portion of serum calcium is directly related the serum albumin concentration, the measured calcium concentration should be adjusted for the concentration of albumin. A general rule is to increase the serum calcium concentration by 0.8 mg/dl for each 1.0 mg/dl decrement of albumin below 4.0 mg/dl (4). For example, if the measured calcium and albumin concentrations were 10.0 mg/dl and 2.0 mg/dl, respectively, the corrected serum calcium would be 11.6 mg/dl.
2. Mild, moderate, and severe hypercalcemia may be defined as corrected serum calcium levels of 10.5 to 12.0 mg/dl (2.6 to 3.0 mmol/L), 12.0 to 14.0 mg/dl (3.0 to 3.5 mmol/L), and >14.0 mg/dl (>3.5 mmol/L), respectively (4). Mild hypercalcemia is a frequent outpatient finding affecting 1% to 2% of elderly women. However, these patients are often asymptomatic and may merit only careful, long-term surveillance in many cases (31). On the other hand, severe hypercalcemia (>14.0 mg/dl) is a life-threatening condition requiring prompt treatment. Severe hypercalcemia is usually caused by a known malignancy or severe hyperparathyroidism, and it affects up to 0.5% of hospitalized patients (14).
   a. With the routine use of automated screening chemistry panels, asymptomatic mild hypercalcemia is being diagnosed with increasing frequency. At the Mayo Clinic, the diagnosis of hypercalcemia increased almost eightfold, from 8 cases per 100,000 during 1964 to 1974 to 51 cases per 100,000 during 1974 to 1975, the period during which multichannel chemistry panels became routinely available. Most of these "new" cases represent asymptomatic primary hyperparathyroidism, which may constitute more than 80% of all outpatient cases of hypercalcemia (10,18,31).
   b. In a survey of a representative population of 18,000 persons from Sweden, 1.1% of all adults (age >25 years) and 3% of women >60 years old had persistent hypercalcemia. The mean age of these patients was 59 years and 75% were 50 years or older (30,39).
3. More than 90% of all patients with hypercalcemia have either primary hyperparathyroidism or cancer.
   a. For hospitalized patients, the most important cause of hypercalcemia is malignancy. In Fisken's study of 469 hospitalized patients with hypercalcemia (2.7 to 3.0 mmol/L, 66%; 3.0 to 3.5 mmol/L, 23%; 3.5 to 4.0 mmol/L, 7%; >4.0 mmol/L, 4%) the causes of hypercalcemia among nondialysis patients were as shown in Table 21–1 (14).
   b. Among outpatients, the most important cause of hypercalcemia is hyperparathyroidism. In Mundy's study from a period before routine use of automated screening chemistry panels, 207 of the estimated 1 million residents near Birmingham, England, were diagnosed with hypercalcemia. Among these 207 patients, 63% had definite or probable primary hyperparathyroidism and 35% had cancer. Sarcoidosis, thyrotoxicosis, vitamin D excess, and immobilization were the causes of hypercalcemia in the remaining 2% (31).
   c. The incidence of hyperparathyroidism increases with age, and most of these patients are women >70 years old. For example, in Mundy's study,

Table 21-1 Causes of hypercalcemia among hospitalized patients (14)

Cause	%
Malignancy	55%
Primary hyperparathyroidism	15%
Excessive vitamin D	2.5%
Thyrotoxicosis	1%
Recovery phase of acute renal failure	<1%
Malignancy and vitamin D excess	<1%
Sarcoidosis	<1%
Primary hyperparathyroidism and vitamin D excess	<1%
Malignancy and primary hyperparathyroidism	<1%
No apparent cause (most probably primary hyperparathyroidism)	25%

63% of the patients were >70 years old. For patients undergoing parathyroid exploration for hyperparathyroidism, the ratio of women to men was 2:1. Furthermore, the ratio of women to men increased with age, reaching 7:1 among those >70 years old (50). For patients with hyperparathyroidism who undergo neck exploration, 85% are found to have a primary adenoma, 10% have multiglandular hyperplasia, and 5% to 10% have no apparent abnormality. Parathyroid carcinoma is a rare cause of hypercalcemia (50).

d. Multiple endocrine neoplasia (MEN) syndromes are rare causes of hyperparathyroidism. An estimated 30% of patients with multiglandular hyperplasia are found to have MEN-I or less commonly, MEN-IIA (29). The diagnosis of MEN should be considered in any young patient with hypercalcemia, a family history of hyperparathyroidism, or biopsy showing multiglandular hyperplasia (6).

B. Pathophysiology

1. In most cases, hypercalcemia is caused by increased resorption of bone. Calcium intake and gastrointestinal absorption usually do not play a major role, although increased absorption may contribute to hypercalcemia in states of vitamin D excess, including sarcoid (4,33). In all cases of hyperparathyroidism-induced hypercalcemia and probably in most cases of malignancy-associated hypercalcemia (HM), bone resorption is caused by activation of osteoclasts, the regulation of which is complex and not fully understood. Parathyroid hormone (PTH) increases osteoclast activity indirectly by first binding to osteoblasts and the neighboring fibroblasts. The exact mechanism by which PTH increases osteoclast activity is not known, but it may involve a network of local mediators including growth factors and cytokines (22). In addition, PTH directly affects renal calcium clearance by increasing tubular reabsorption of calcium. PTH also indirectly affects renal calcium clearance by stimulating the 1α-hydroxylase enzyme in the kidney. This enzyme converts 25-hydroxyvitamin D (HVD) to the more biologically active 1,25-dihydroxyvitamin D_3 (DHVD), which increases gastrointestinal absorption of calcium (33).
2. Parathyroid hormone–related peptide (PTHrP) is a peptide produced by some tumors that has an amino acid structure similar to that of PTH. PTHrP probably elevates calcium in a manner identical to PTH (7,8). This peptide has been cloned and has been shown to bind to the PTH receptor (25).
3. Vitamin D is actually a hormone rather than a vitamin. Its effects on calcium homeostasis are complex and are reviewed elsewhere (49). In brief, DHVD increases the rate of gastrointestinal absorption of calcium, apparently by upregulating the transcription of a calcium-binding protein. It also appears to increase the number and the activity of osteoclasts, probably by its effects on osteoclast precursors and perhaps by stimulating osteoblasts to release osteoclast-stimulating cytokines (49). PTH stimulates the renal production of DHVD,

which in turn acts on the parathyroid glands to downregulate the expression of PTH. In patients with sarcoidosis and some other granulomatous diseases, independent production of DHVD, probably by activated macrophages, may produce hypercalcemia and hypercalciuria (49).

4. The kidneys provide the first line of defense against the development of hypercalcemia. As the concentration of serum calcium rises, the kidneys compensate by increasing the rate of calcium excretion. Hypercalcemia occurs when the rate of resorption of calcium from bone (or, more rarely, the rate of absorption of calcium from the gut) exceeds the maximal rate of renal calcium excretion.
   a. High levels of PTH and probably PTHrP promote tubular reabsorption of calcium and thereby diminish the ability of the kidneys to excrete calcium.
   b. Hypercalcemic patients are often asymptomatic and remain compensated until they suffer an acute dehydrating event. Diarrhea, nausea, or fever may cause deterioration in a stable hypercalcemic patient by initiating a vicious cycle in which volume depletion impairs the ability of the kidneys to excrete calcium by decreasing the glomerular filtration rate and promoting proximal reabsorption of calcium. High levels of serum calcium may also have a toxic effect on the distal renal tubules, causing a form of nephrogenic diabetes insipidus and further volume depletion (4,32,33).

C. Clinical Presentation

1. The clinical presentation of hypercalcemia usually reflects the underlying disease process as well as the severity of the hypercalcemia. Most patients with mild hypercalcemia are asymptomatic. Patients with HM are usually first identified by symptoms attributable to their cancer rather than to the hypercalcemia. Dehydration, anorexia, nausea, vomiting, fatigue, lethargy, and cognitive changes are common presenting symptoms (31) (see Table 21–2).
2. Among hypercalcemic patients, those with higher levels of serum calcium are more likely to have cancer. For example, in Fisken's study, 33% of those with serum calcium <3 mmol/dl had a malignancy, compared with 79% of those with serum calcium >4 mmol/dl (14).
3. With the increasing use of multichannel chemistry panels for screening, more asymptomatic hypercalcemic patients are being identified, and symptomatic cases of hyperparathyroidism are becoming less common. For example, of the first 343 cases of primary hyperparathyroidism seen at the Massachusetts General Hospital, 57% had clinically evident kidney stones and 23% had bone disease. However, since the advent of these screening panels, <5% of the patients with hyperparathyroidism have clinically evident bone or kidney disease (21).
4. Mental status changes and cognitive defects are common presenting symptoms in the elderly (33).
5. HM rarely presents with nephrolithiasis (33).
6. Cardiovascular effects of hypercalcemia include shortening of the QT interval and enhanced sensitivity to digoxin (4).

D. Diagnosis

1. The differential diagnosis of hypercalcemia is relatively limited. Hyperparathy-

Table 21-2 Presenting signs & symptoms in hypercalcemia (31)

Presentation	N=111
Asymptomatic patients	57%
Acute hypercalcemic syndrome	14%
Lethargy, polyuria	8%
Kidney stones/nephrolithiasis	7%
Hypertension	5%
Psychiatric disorder	5%
Gastrointestinal symptoms	4%

roidism and malignancy account for >90% of all cases of hypercalcemia. Sarcoidosis, hyperthyroidism, and vitamin D excess together cause <5% of all cases (14,31). Other causes of hypercalcemia include vitamin A intoxication, lithium ingestion, and thiazide use, especially in the setting of immobilization.

2. Differentiation of HM from hyperparathyroidism is usually straightforward.
   a. In Fisken's series, 98% of patients who ultimately were diagnosed with HM had known malignancy at the time of diagnosis. In this study, 75% of the patients with HM had obvious signs of metastases, even without the benefit of computed tomography (CT) or bone scans (14). Correspondingly, their prognosis was poor, and 80% of patients with HM in the series died within 1 year (14). The longer a patient has had hypercalcemia, the less likely it is that the hypercalcemia is caused by HM.
   b. The PTH level should be measured in all patients with hypercalcemia, including those with a known tumor, because up to 12% of these patients have both cancer and primary hyperparathyroidism (14,48). The two-site immunoradiometric assay for PTH is both extremely sensitive and specific for distinguishing hyperparathyroidism from HM (34,35). PTH is predictably high in hyperparathyroidism and suppressed in HM. However, PTH levels can be falsely elevated in the setting of renal failure.
3. For patients with no evidence of malignancy and low PTH levels, thyroid function and vitamin D levels should be measured. Vitamin D excess is confirmed by a finding of elevated HVD and suppressed PTH. Patients with sarcoidosis usually have widely disseminated disease that is recognizable on physical examination or chest radiography. These patients usually have an abnormally high level of DHVD compared with the level of HVD (49). If occult malignancy is suspected, serum assay for PTHrP may be useful (48).

E. Hypercalcemia of Malignancy

1. HM occurs in up to 10% of malignant disorders treated in the hospital (19). Hypercalcemia commonly complicates myeloma (30% to 100% of cases) and breast cancer (5% to 40% of cases). It is less common with lung cancer (5% to 16% of cases). Lung and breast cancers account for >50% of HM. Some authors have suggested that HM caused by breast cancer has become less common since the widespread use of tamoxifen (33). Head and neck cancers, renal cell and genitourinary epithelial cancers, and hematologic malignancies (especially myeloma) each account for 10% of HM. Among patients with lymphoma or leukemia related to the human T-cell lymphotropic virus type I (HTLV-I), 100 percent develop some degree of hypercalcemia (33). Even with extensive bony involvement, gastric, colorectal, and prostate cancers rarely cause hypercalcemia (14).
2. For patients with myeloma or breast cancer, HM is virtually always accompanied by metastases. Similarly, two-thirds of the patients with lung cancer–associated hypercalcemia have clinically evident metastases. However, for renal cell and uroepithelial cancers, HM may precede the development of clinically evident metastases. For example, in Fisken's series, only 34% of patients with renal cell or uroepithelial tumors had metastases on initial evaluation, although bone scans and CT evaluations were not performed (14).
3. HM may be caused by two general mechanisms: humoral HM and local osteolytic hypercalcemia. Most cases of humoral HM are associated with high levels of PTHrP. In Ratcliffe's study, 35 (88%) of 40 patients with hypercalcemia and a solid tumor had elevated levels of PTHrP. Three (33%) of the 9 patients with a hematologic malignancy also had elevated levels of PTHrP. Seven (12%) of the 56 hypercalcemic patients in the study with a known malignancy also had coexisting hyperparathyroidism and a low level of PTHrP. There was only a weak association between the level of PTHrP and the degree of hypercalcemia. For 89% of the patients, the diagnosis of cancer was known or made simultaneously with the discovery of hypercalcemia. However, for 2 patients, a suppressed level of PTH and an elevated level of PTHrP led to the discovery of occult tumors (48). Among those with HM and low levels of PTHrP, hypercalcemia may result from activation of local osteoclasts by a number of tumor-derived cytokines and

growth factors. This mechanism is especially important for hematologic malignancies (33).

4. The extent of bony involvement by a tumor is not a good predictor for the development of hypercalcemia, because only one-third of all patients with malignant bony metastases develop hypercalcemia (44).

F. Treatment

1. Hyperparathyroidism

a. Surgical excision is the treatment of choice for patients with severe or symptomatic hyperparathyroidism. For cases of familial polyglandular hyperplasia, three of the glands in entirety and a portion of the fourth gland are excised. For hyperparathyroidism resulting from an adenoma, the gland that is clearly enlarged or abnormal in appearance is excised. In the hands of an experienced surgeon, these techniques are successful in >90% of cases (50).

(1) To date, various preoperative techniques for localizing the abnormal gland or glands have not been found to be more accurate than careful exploration by an experienced surgeon and a pathologist (41,15).

(2) Although parathyroid exploration is generally safe and associated with very low mortality rates, 1% to 2% of patients suffer vocal cord paralysis or permanent hypoparathyroidism. In 5% of cases, no offending lesion is found and reexploration may be necessary. Another 5% of patients may have recurrence of hyperparathyroidism (28,50).

(3) Surgery is usually recommended for hyperparathyroid patients with high levels of calcium (>12 mg/dl) and for those with nephrolithiasis, osteitis fibrosa cystica, refractory peptic ulcer disease, pancreatitis, or other significant symptoms (29). Surgery is probably also indicated for younger patients (<50 years old), those with low cortical bone mass, and those in whom close follow-up is not feasible (42).

b. However, for most hyperparathyroid patients with mild hypercalcemia, the role of surgery is less clear. More than 70% of patients with primary hyperparathyroidism are asymptomatic. Most of these patients are also elderly. There are some data to suggest that in the short term (4 years), these patients do not develop renal or bone disease (20,47). Furthermore, in a small, long-term (14-year) case-control study, there was no difference in the mortality rate among elderly patients with hyperparathyroidism and mild hypercalcemia and the rate among age- and sex-matched normocalcemic controls. However, patients <70 years old had a higher mortality rate, mostly because of cardiovascular disease. No patient with normal renal function at the beginning of the study developed renal dysfunction subsequently. The number of patients in this study was small, and the results have yet to be duplicated (10,30,39). There are no prospective randomized controlled trials (PRCTs) of parathyroid surgery versus watchful waiting in this group of patients.

c. Given the absence of data from randomized controlled trials, a panel of the National Institutes of Health developed consensus guidelines for management of asymptomatic mild hypercalcemia (see Table 21–3) (43).

d. For patients who are monitored medically, the corrected calcium level should be checked every 6 months at first, along with serial evaluations for kidney and bone disease (43). Patients should avoid dehydration, thiazide diuretics, or excessive vitamin D intake, all of which may worsen hypercalcemia.

e. Postmenopausal women may benefit from estrogen replacement, which can reduce the level of serum calcium by 0.5 to 1 mg/dl and decrease the rate of calciuria. It is thought that estrogen and progestins decrease bone resorption by inhibiting the effects of PTH on bone. However, the level of PTH is not significantly reduced by estrogen treatment (10,13,51).

2. **Medical Treatment of Acute Hypercalcemia**—Most authors recommend that hypercalcemic patients with corrected calcium levels >14 mg/dl (>3.5 mmol/L) be admitted and promptly treated with vigorous hydration and an ap-

Table 21-3 NIH guidelines for management of asymptomatic hypercalcemia (43)

Clear Indications for Surgical Treatment	Surgery Probably Preferable to Surveillance
Corrected calcium >11.5–12.0 mg/dl	Patient requests surgery
An episode of life-threatening hypercalcemia	Consistent follow-up is difficult
Reduced creatinine clearance	Patient is <50 y old
Presence of overt kidney or bone disease	Coexistent illness complicates medical management
24-hour urine calcium excretion >400 mg	
Directly measured bone mass reduced by >2 standard deviations	

propriate dose of pamidronate. For patients with severe life-threatening hypercalcemia, calcitonin may be added as first-line therapy. Patients with corrected calcium levels between 12 and 14 mg/dl should also be admitted if they are symptomatic or at risk of becoming volume depleted (4).

a. **Intravenous and Oral Fluid Replacement**—Hydration is usually the first step in the treatment of severe hypercalcemia. As discussed previously, hypercalcemia predisposes to volume depletion by inducing nausea and vomiting and by direct effects on the distal tubules of the kidney. Volume depletion, in turn, decreases renal blood flow and increases the rate of calcium reabsorption in the proximal tubules, decreasing the rate of renal calcium clearance and exacerbating the degree of hypercalcemia. Normal saline given at a rate of 4 L/day to 16 patients with severe hypercalcemia (mean, 14.7 mg/dl or 3.66 mmol/L) resulted in a mean drop in serum calcium of 2.4 mg/dl in 13 patients who responded to treatment. All of these patients had improvement of symptoms. However, it is rare for hydration alone to completely normalize the level of calcium, and almost all patients need additional therapeutic measures (23).

b. **Diuretics**—In the past, loop diuretics have been used in conjunction with hydration for treatment of severe hypercalcemia. By inhibiting sodium reabsorption in the loop of Henle, furosemide can inhibit proximal reabsorption of calcium and promote calciuresis. The administration of loop diuretics should be reserved for patients who are fully volume repleted. In a small study of 8 patients with severe hypercalcemia, the use of furosemide resulted in a mean decrease in the corrected level of serum calcium of 3.1 mg/dl. However, >1000 mg/day of furosemide was administered on the average, and the patients required intensive monitoring because of the potential for electrolyte disturbance, arrhythmia, and renal dysfunction (52). Because less toxic and more effective agents such as pamidronate are now available, most authors recommend use of loop diuretics only as an adjunct to hydration to prevent volume overload, particularly in patients with coexisting myocardial or renal dysfunction (4,33). There are no well-designed trials comparing hydration alone versus forced diuresis therapy.

c. **Bisphosphonates**—Bisphosphonates are a group of pyrophosphate analog compounds that strongly bind to hydroxyapatite in bone and inhibit osteoclast activity through poorly understood mechanisms (33).

   (1) A number of bisphosphonates have been used for treatment of acute hypercalcemia, including clodronate, etidronate, and pamidronate. Of these agents, pamidronate has become the treatment of choice for HM. In randomized controlled trials of clodronate or etidronate versus pamidronate, pamidronate was significantly more effective in normalizing the level of calcium than the other two agents. Pamidronate also worked more rapidly (16,45). Furthermore, pamidronate has the advantage of single-day dosing, whereas etidronate must be given over 3 successive days (16).

(2) In a randomized controlled trial, pamidronate was more effective than mithramycin for treatment of hypercalcemia. Twelve days after initial treatment, 12 of 14 patients treated with pamidronate became eucalcemic, compared with only 3 of 11 patients treated with mithramycin. In another small randomized study, pamidronate was superior to both mithramycin and the combination of calcitonin plus corticosteroids (38,46).

(3) Because pamidronate can cause renal failure, it should be used with caution in patients with preexisting renal disease (16). However, severe deterioration of renal function is rare in patients without preexisting renal disease who are prehydrated (36,53). There appears to be no difference in response to pamidronate between patients with or without bone metastases (16,36). There is limited evidence that high levels of PTHrP may be associated with either resistance or delayed response to pamidronate (12).

(4) Pamidronate is usually given as a single infusion over 24 hours, but lower doses can be given over a shorter period (2 to 4 hours) (9,17). After this infusion, a reduction in the level of calcium can be detected within 48 hours, with a peak effect at 5 to 6 days (36). Pamidronate should be dosed according to the degree of hypercalcemia. For milder cases of hypercalcemia, 30 to 60 mg may suffice and is less likely to cause posttreatment hypocalcemia. However, for patients with more severe hypercalcemia (corrected calcium >13.5 mg/dl), 90 mg should be used (53). These points are well illustrated by Nussbaum's dose-response study involving 50 patients with HM. The effects of 30, 60, and 90 mg of pamidronate given over a 24-hour period are summarized in Table 21-4 (36).

- **(a)** In general, 90 mg was more effective than 30 or 60 mg. With 90 mg of pamidronate, 100% of patients had a normal level of calcium by day 7, compared with 61% and 40% of patients given 60 mg and 30 mg, respectively. However, for patients whose initial calcium level was <13.5 mg/dl, 60 mg of pamidronate normalized the level of calcium in 75%.
- **(b)** Symptom relief was excellent. Nausea and vomiting resolved in 70% to 100% of patients, anorexia improved in 60%, and 62% had improvement in mental function. A small minority (15%) noticed a dramatic decrease in the severity of bone pain (36).
- **(c)** Low-grade fever developed in 20% of the patients in the study.

Table 21-4 Dose-dependent effect of pamidronate therapy for hypercalcemia (36)

	Pamidronate		
	30 mg (n=15)	60 mg (n=18)	90 mg (n=17)
Initial serum calcium (mg/dl)	13.8	13.8	13.3
Calcium at day 7 (mg/dl)	11.6	10.5	9.4
Number of patients (%) with normalized calcium at day 7	6 (40%)	11 (61%)	17 (100%)
Patients with initial calcium >13.5 mg/dl who normalized with therapy	33%	50%	100%
Patients with initial calcium <13.5 mg/dl who normalized with therapy	50%	75%	100%
Mean survival (mo)	1.0	1.7	1.1
Duration of normalized calcium (d)	9.2	13.3	10.8

This effect was not dose related. Three patients developed local reactions at the infusion site. Two patients in the 90-mg group and 1 in the 30-mg group developed transient hypocalcemia. Mortality was predictably high, although 20% of patients lived more than 6 months (36). Although of little clinical significance, hypophosphatemia and hypomagnesemia occurred frequently (40% and 25%, respectively).

(5) The prophylactic use of bisphosphonates in high-risk cancer patients may decrease the number of subsequent hypercalcemic events and the incidence of pathologic fractures. In a double-blind prospective controlled trial involving 173 patients with breast cancer and known bony metastases, daily use of oral clodronate (1600 mg/day) significantly reduced the number of hypercalcemic episodes (28/85 versus 53/88 patients) and the incidence of morbid skeletal events (219 versus 305 per 100 patient-years), compared with control over a mean follow-up period of 14 months (40). Similar results were reported in a small study in which oral pamidronate was given to patients with bony metastases from breast cancer. Pamidronate decreased the subsequent rate of fractures, the severity of bone pain, and the need for radiation therapy (56).

d. Calcitonin

(1) Calcitonin, a 32-amino-acid peptide produced by the parafollicular C cells of the thyroid gland, inhibits bone resorption by decreasing the number and the activity of osteoclasts and increases calciuresis by blocking tubular reabsorption of calcium (11,24). Because of its fast onset of action, calcitonin is a useful adjunct to pamidronate for patients with severe, life-threatening hypercalcemia. Typically, its effects are observed within hours of administration and peak at 12 to 24 hours (11). However, the effects of calcitonin alone are usually short-lived, and rebound hypercalcemia may be observed by 48 hours (5). Salmon calcitonin (4 U/kg) is usually administered subcutaneously or intramuscularly every 12 hours (11). Side effects are rare. Recombinant human calcitonin is also available but is less potent than salmon calcitonin.

(2) The ideal use of calcitonin is as an adjunct to pamidronate for patients who require rapid reduction in the level of serum calcium. Given its low toxicity, it is recommended for patients with severe hypercalcemia (>14 mg/dl) and for those with severe symptoms. However, there are no PRCTs to date that have tested this strategy. In a nonrandomized trial of 34 hypercalcemic patients (mean initial serum calcium, 13 mg/dl) given either pamidronate alone (45 to 60 mg) or pamidronate plus calcitonin suppositories, those treated with the combination had a more rapid decline in calcium (by 2 mg/dl) at 48 hours and an earlier resolution of symptoms (by 2 days), compared with the group treated with pamidronate (54).

e. Gallium—Gallium nitrate is a potent antiresorptive agent in the treatment of HM. Gallium is a group IIIa transition metal that concentrates in bone, binds to hydroxyapatite, and directly inhibits the activity of osteoclasts without affecting their number or the maturation process (55). Gallium nitrate must be given intravenously in a continuous infusion over 5 days.

(1) In a double-blind PRCT comparing gallium nitrate (200 mg/m^2 daily for 5 days) versus etidronate (7.5 mg/kg IV daily for 5 days) in 71 patients with HM, the level of calcium was normalized in 82% of patients treated with gallium, compared with 43% of those treated with etidronate. The median duration of normocalcemia in the group treated with gallium was 8 days. However, the action of gallium was relatively slow, because the calcium level did not normalize until day 5 to day 6 and the nadir was not reached until day 10 (57). There is as yet no randomized trial comparing gallium and pamidronate.

(2) The major problems with gallium are its high cost and the need for a 5-day infusion. Given the proven efficacy and impressive safety record of pamidronate, it is unlikely that gallium will play a major role in the treatment of HM unless it can be administered in a more convenient fashion. In addition, gallium may cause renal insufficiency, particularly in the setting of prior renal disease or concomitant exposure to aminoglycosides (55).

f. **Mithramycin**—Mithramycin is a tumoricidal antibiotic developed initially for the treatment of embryonal cell carcinoma. It interferes with osteoclast activity by blocking RNA synthesis and probably also by inhibiting differentiation of osteoclast precursors. Once used routinely as an antiresorptive agent, it has for the most part been replaced by pamidronate (33). Although mithramycin is potent and relatively fast-acting, it is neither as safe nor as effective as pamidronate. It may cause significant hematologic, renal, and hepatic side effects (27). Furthermore, in two randomized controlled trials, mithramycin was less effective than pamidronate, and those treated with mithramycin tended to have recurrence of hypercalcemia within 4 to 6 days of treatment (38,46).

g. **Corticosteroids**—Corticosteroids have been used to prolong the short-lived effects of calcitonin. The addition of prednisone (30 to 60 mg/day) extends the effects of calcitonin from 24 to 48 hours to 4 to 5 days (5). However, since the introduction of more effective antiresorptive agents such as pamidronate, the role of glucocorticoids is now limited to treatment of the rare cases of hypercalcemia that are caused by sarcoidosis or steroid-responsive lymphoma or myeloma (33). Corticosteroids are thought to suppress abnormal production of DHVD by activated macrophages within granulomatous tissue (1,2).

h. **Ketoconazole**—Ketoconazole is also effective in isolated cases of hypercalcemia caused by granulomatous disease. It may be a reasonable alternative to glucocorticoids for patients with hypercalcemia resulting from sarcoidosis (2,3).

H. Summary

1. More than 90% of all cases of hypercalcemia are caused by hyperparathyroidism or malignancy. Hyperparathyroidism is the most important cause of hypercalcemia among the outpatient population. Because of the routine use of multichannel chemistry screening panels, most patients with hyperparathyroidism are detected early and are asymptomatic at the time of diagnosis. Malignancy is the most important cause of hypercalcemia among the inpatient population. HM is most commonly associated with breast cancer, lung cancer, or myeloma. In >90% of these cases, the diagnosis of cancer has already been established.
2. The PTH level should be checked in all patients with hypercalcemia. An abnormally elevated level of PTH suggests hyperparathyroidism. Malignancy should carefully be excluded in patients with a suppressed level of PTH. The PTH level should be measured even in patients with a known malignancy, because coexisting hyperparathyroidism can occur in up to 12% of these patients. A direct measurement of the PTHrP level may be useful if occult malignancy is suspected. However, renal dysfunction can elevate the levels of PTH and PTHrP. For patients with a suppressed level of PTH but no evidence of malignancy, levels of thyroid-stimulating hormone, HVD, and DHVD should be measured to exclude hyperthyroidism and states of vitamin D excess.
3. Surgical excision is the treatment of choice for symptomatic patients with hyperparathyroidism. There are no data regarding the long-term efficacy of surgery in preventing morbidity or mortality in asymptomatic patients with mild hyperparathyroidism. Therefore, treatment of asymptomatic patients with hyperparathyroidism should be individually tailored.
4. Patients with symptomatic hypercalcemia should be treated with aggressive hydration. Therapy should include pamidronate at a dose adjusted to the severity of hypercalcemia. Fever is a common side effect of pamidronate therapy. In

patients without preexisting renal dysfunction, pamidronate does not cause significant renal dysfunction. Loop diuretics are not recommended as first-line therapy but should be used primarily as an adjunct to hydration to avoid volume overload. Calcitonin should be used as an adjunct to pamidronate in severe cases of hypercalcemia in which a rapid reduction of calcium is desirable. Hypercalcemia caused by granulomatous diseases is best treated with corticosteroids and possibly ketoconazole.

Abbreviations used in Chapter 21

CT = computed tomography
DHVD = 1,25-dihydroxyvitamin D_3
HM = hypercalcemia of malignancy
HTLV-I = human T-cell lymphotropic virus type I
HVD = hydroxyvitamin D
MEN = multiple endocrine neoplasia
P = probability value
PRCT = prospective randomized controlled trial
PTH = parathyroid hormone
PTHrP = parathyroid hormone–related peptide

References

1. Adams. Isolation and structural identification of 1,25 dihydroxyvitamin D_3 produced by cultured alveolar macrophages in sarcoidosis. *J Clin Endocrinol Metab* 1985;60:960.
2. Barbour. Hypercalcemia in an anephric patient with sarcoidosis: evidence of extra renal generation of 1,23 dihydroxyvitamin D. *N Engl J Med* 1981;305:440.
3. Bia. Treatment of sarcoidosis-associated hypercalcemia with ketoconazole. *Am J Kidney Dis* 1991;6:702.
4. Bilezikian. Management of acute hypercalcemia. *N Engl J Med* 1992;326:1196.
5. Binstock. Effect of calcitonin and glucocorticoids in combination on the hypercalcemia of malignancy. *Ann Intern Med* 1980;93:269.
6. Boyd. Neoplastic disorders affecting multiple endocrine organs. In: Isselbacher, ed. *Harrison's Principles of Internal Medicine*, 13th ed. New York: McGraw-Hill, 1994:2052.
7. Broadus. Humoral hypercalcemia of cancer: identification of a novel parathyroid hormone-like peptide. *N Engl J Med* 1988;319:556.
8. Burtis. Immunochemical characterization of circulating parathyroid hormone-related protein in patients with humoral hypercalcemia of cancer. *N Engl J Med* 1990;322:1106.
9. Cantwell. Effect of single high dose infusions of aminohydoxypropylidene diphosphate on hypercalcemia caused by cancer. *Br Med J* 1987;294:467.
10. Davies. Primary hyperparathyroidism: aggressive or conservative treatment? *Clin Endocrinol* 1992;36:325.
11. Deftos. Calcitonin as a drug. *Ann Intern Med* 1981;95:192.
12. Dodwell. Parathyroid hormone-related protein$^{(50\text{-}69)}$ and response to pamidronate therapy for tumour-induced hypercalcemia. *Eur J Cancer* 1991;27:1629.
13. Estrogens and progestins in the management of primary hyperparathyroidism. *J Bone Miner Res* 1991;6(Suppl 2):S125.
14. Fisken. Hypercalcemia: a hospital survey. *Q J Med* 1980;196:405.
15. Gaz. Invited commentary. *World J Surg* 1992;16:661.
16. Gucalp. Comparative study of pamidronate disodium and etidronate disodium in the treatment of cancer-related hypercalcemia. *J Clin Oncol* 1992;10:134.
17. Gucalp. Treatment of cancer-associated hypercalcemia: double-blind comparison

of rapid and slow intravenous infusion regimens of pamidronate disodium and saline alone. *Arch Intern Med* 1994;154:1935.
18. Heath. Primary hyperparathyroidism: incidence, morbidity, and potential economic impact in a community. *N Engl J Med* 1980;302:189.
19. Heath. Parathyroid-hormone-related protein in tumours associated with hypercalcemia. *Lancet* 1990;335:66.
20. Heath. Conservative management of primary hyperparathyroidism. *J Bone Miner Res* 1991;6(Suppl 2):S117.
21. Heath. Clinical spectrum of primary hyperparathyroidism: evolution with changes in medical practice and technology. *J Bone Miner Res* 1991;6(Suppl 2):S63.
22. Holick. Calcium, phosphorus, and bone metabolism: calcium regulating hormones. In: Isselbacher, ed. *Harrison's Principles of Internal Medicine*, 13th ed. New York: McGraw-Hill, 1994:2137.
23. Hosking. Rehydration in the treatment of severe hypercalcemia. *Q J Med* 1981; 200:473.
24. Hosking. Comparison of the renal and skeletal actions of calcitonin in the treatment of severe hypercalcemia of malignancy. *Q J Med* 1984;211:359.
25. Juppner. The PTH-like peptide associated with humoral hypercalcemia of malignancy and parathyroid hormone binds to the same receptor on the plasma membranes of ROS17/2.8 cells. *J Biol Chem* 1988;263:8557.
26. Reserved.
27. Kennedy. Metabolic and toxic effects of mithramycin during tumor therapy. *Am J Med* 1970;49:494.
28. Lafferty. Primary hyperparathyroidism: a review of the long-term surgical and nonsurgical morbidities as a basis for a rational approach to treatment. *Arch Intern Med* 1989;149:789.
29. LiVolsi. Intraoperative assessment of parathyroid gland pathology. *Am J Clin Pathol* 1994;102:365.
30. Ljunghall. Longitudinal studies of mild primary hyperparathyroidism. *J Bone Miner Res* 1991;6(Suppl 2):S111.
31. Mundy. Primary hyperparathyroidism: changes in the pattern of clinical presentation. *Lancet* 1980;1:1317.
32. Mundy. The hypercalcemia of malignancy. *Kidney Int* 1987;31:142.
33. Nussbaum. Pathophysiology and management of severe hypercalcemia. *Endocrinol Metab Clin North Am* 1993;22:343.
34. Nussbaum. Immunoassays for parathyroid hormone 1-84 in the diagnosis of hyperparathyroidism. *J Bone Miner Res* 1991;6(Suppl 2):S43.
35. Nussbaum. Highly sensitive two-site immunoradiometric assay of parathyrin and its clinical utility in evaluating patients with hypercalcemia. *Clin Chemistry* 1987; 33:1364.
36. Nussbaum. Single-dose intravenous therapy with pamidronate for the treatment of hypercalcemia of malignancy: comparison of 30-, 60- and 90-mg doses. *Am J Med* 1993;95:297.
37. Reserved.
38. Ostenstad. Disodium pamidronate versus mithramycin in the management of tumour-associated hypercalcemia. *Acta Oncol* 1992;31:861.
39. Palmer. Survival and renal function in untreated hypercalcemia. *Lancet* 1987;1:59.
40. Paterson. Double-blind trial of oral clodronate in patients with bone metastases from breast cancer. *J Clin Oncol* 1993;11:59.
41. Potts. Diseases of the parathyroid gland and other hyper- and hypocalcemic disorders. In: Isselbacher, ed. *Harrison's Principles of Internal Medicine*, 13th ed. New York: McGraw-Hill, 1994:2151.
42. Potts. Management of asymptomatic hyperparathyroidism. *J Clin Endocrinol Metab* 1990;70:1489.
43. Potts, ed. Consensus development conference statement: Proceedings of the NIH Consensus Development Conference on diagnosis and management of asymptomatic primary hyperparathyroidism, Bethesda, MD, October 29–31, 1990. *J Bone Miner Res* 1991;6(Suppl 2):S9.

44. Ralston. Hypercalcemia and metastatic bone disease: Is there a causal link? *Lancet* 1982;2:903.
45. Ralston. Comparison of three intravenous bisphosphonates in cancer-associated hypercalcemia. *Lancet* 1989;November 18:1180.
46. Ralston. Comparison of aminohydroxypropylidene diphosphate, mithramycin, and corticosteroids/calcitonin in treatment of cancer-associated hypercalcemia. *Lancet* 1985;October 26:907.
47. Rao. Lack of biochemical progression or continuation of accelerated bone loss in mild asymptomatic primary hyperparathyroidism: evidence for biphasic disease course. *J Clin Endocrinol Metab* 1988;67:1294.
48. Ratcliffe. Role of assays for parathyroid-hormone–related protein in investigation of hypercalcemia. *Lancet* 1992;339:164.
49. Reichel. The role of the vitamin D endocrine system in health and disease. *N Engl J Med* 1992;320:980.
50. Satava. Success rate of cervical exploration for hyperparathyroidism. *Arch Surg* 1975;110:626.
51. Selby. Ethinyl estradiol and norethindrone in the treatment of primary hyperparathyroidism in post-menopausal women. *N Engl J Med* 1986;314:1481.
52. Suki. Acute treatment of hypercalcemia with furosemide. *N Engl J Med* 1970;283:836.
53. Thiebauld. Dose-response in the treatment of hypercalcemia of malignancy by a single infusion of bisphosphonate AHPrBP. *J Clin Oncol* 1988;6:762.
54. Thiebauld. Fast and effective treatment of malignant hypercalcemia: combination of suppositories of calcitonin and a single infusion of 3-amino 1-hydroxypropylidene-1-bisphosphonate. *Arch Intern Med* 1990;150:2125.
55. Todd. Gallium nitrate: a review of its pharmacological properties and therapeutic potential in cancer-related hypercalcemia. *Drugs* 1991;42:261.
56. van Holten-Verzantvoort. Reduced morbidity from skeletal metastases in breast cancer patients during long-term bisphosphonate (APD) treatment. *Lancet* 1987;2:983.
57. Warrell. A randomized double-blind study of gallium nitrate compared with etidronate for acute control of cancer-related hypercalcemia. *J Clin Oncol* 1991;9:1467.

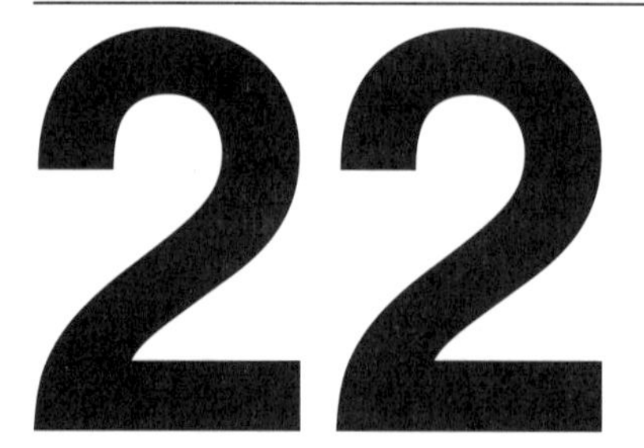

Hyponatremia

Burton W. Lee and
Cecil H. Coggins

A. Physiology

1. **Vascular Compartments**—The estimated total body water is about 60% of the body weight for an average man and 50% of the body weight for an average woman. Roughly, 40% of the total body water is found in the extracellular space and 60% in the intracellular space. The normal intravascular volume (IVV) is about 20% of the extracellular volume (15) (see Table 22–1).
2. **Regulation of Volume and Osmolality**
   a. A normal person typically excretes 500 to 1000 mOsm of solute per day, depending on salt and protein intake. In order to maintain proper fluid and osmotic balance, a healthy kidney regulates the concentration of urine (U_{osm}) at 50 to 1200 mOsm/L. Normal urine output can vary from 400 ml to 10 L or more per day, depending on the concentration of the urine.
   b. The normal osmolality of plasma (P_{osm}) is between 275 and 290 mOsm/kg (15). The major normal contributors to P_{osm} are sodium (P_{Na}), its attendant anions, glucose, and blood urea nitrogen (BUN). P_{osm} can be approximated according to the following equation: $P_{osm}=2(P_{Na}) + \text{Glucose}/18 + \text{BUN}/2.8$.
   c. **Volume Regulation**
      (1) Alterations in volume are sensed by receptors in the atria, the carotid sinuses, the aortic arch, and the afferent arterioles of the kidney. These receptors sense the effective arteriolar volume (EAV) rather than the total body water or the IVV. EAV is a clinically immeasurable part of the IVV that actively participates in tissue perfusion (17).
      (2) The volume receptors in the atria control the release of atrial natriuretic factor. Low atrial pressure decreases the release of atrial natriuretic factor, and high atrial pressure has the opposite effect. Atrial natriuretic factor promotes renal natriuresis (17).
      (3) The volume receptors in the carotid sinuses and the aortic arch influence the sympathetic nervous system. Low EAV stimulates the sympathetic nervous system, and high EAV has the opposite effect. Activation of the sympathetic nervous system causes an increase in the venous tone, the heart rate, and the cardiac output. Furthermore, it enhances renal sodium reabsorption by direct adrenergic effect and by stimulating the renin-angiotensin-aldosterone system (RAAS). In addition to controlling the sympathetic nervous system, these volume receptors also regulate the release of antidiuretic hormone (ADH).

Table 22-1 Estimated total body, extracellular, and intravascular volumes (15)

	Average 70-kg Man	Average 60-kg Woman
Total body water	42 L	30 L
Extracellular volume	17 L	12 L
Intravascular volume	3 L	2.4 L

Low EAV stimulates the release of ADH, and high EAV has the opposite effect. ADH promotes free water conservation and hence volume expansion (17).

(4) The major volume receptors of the kidney are found in the juxtaglomerular apparatus. These receptors regulate the RAAS. Low EAV stimulates the RAAS, and high EAV has the opposite effect. Activation of the RAAS generates angiotensin II, which increases the systemic vascular resistance, stimulates thirst, and enhances renal sodium reabsorption. Angiotensin II also increases the level of aldosterone, which further enhances sodium reabsorption. With low EAV, the kidneys conserve sodium and the concentration of urinary sodium (U_{Na}) usually falls to <10 to 15 mEq/L. With high EAV, sodium is not conserved and U_{Na} usually rises above 20 mEq/L (17).

d. Osmoregulation—The alterations in P_{osm} are detected in the hypothalamus, which modulates the sense of thirst and regulates the secretion of ADH. Thirst stimulates water intake, whereas ADH increases the permeability of the renal collecting tubules to water. ADH relies on an intact osmotic gradient in the renal medulla to promote free water reabsorption. When P_{osm} is <275 mEq/kg, ADH is normally maximally suppressed, free water reabsorption is minimal, and U_{osm} usually falls to <100 mOsm/kg. When P_{osm} is >290 mOsm/kg, ADH secretion increases precipitously, free water is conserved, and U_{osm} typically rises to 600 to 800 mOsm/kg or higher under normal circumstances (16).

e. Volume Regulation Versus Osmoregulation—In addition to P_{osm}, low EAV is also an important stimulus for thirst and ADH release. Either high P_{osm} or low EAV stimulates ADH release, so the presence of one of these stimuli for ADH release overrides the lack of the other. For example, in hypovolemic patients, the stimulatory effect of low EAV on ADH release overrides the inhibitory effect of P_{osm} even when the patients become hyponatremic (15).

B. Differential Diagnosis of Hyponatremia (see Table 22–2).

1. Hyperosmolar Hyponatremia—Although hyperglycemia and mannitol infusion may cause hypernatremia by inducing osmotic diuresis, they are also the most important causes of hyperosmolar hyponatremia. Because glucose and mannitol penetrate the cell membranes poorly, they create an osmotic gradient, causing free water to shift from the intracellular space to the extracellular space. This shift of free water dilutes the P_{Na}. An increase in the concentration

Table 22-2 Differential diagnosis of hyponatremia

Hyperosmolar Hyponatremia	Isoosmolar Hyponatremia	Hypoosmolar Hyponatremia
Mannitol	Hyperlipidemia	Renal failure*
Hyperglycemia†	Hyperproteinemia	Hypoadrenalism
		Hypothyroidism
		Diuretics
		NSAIDS
		SIADH
		Reset osmostat
		Low EAV
		Psychogenic polydipsia

*For patients with high BUN, "effective P_{osm}" rather than P_{osm} should be used for classifying hyponatremia; see section C1b.
†Under certain circumstances, hyperglycemia may be associated with isoosmolar rather than hyperosmolar hyponatremia; see section B2.

of glucose by 60 mg/dl causes a decrease in P_{Na} by about 1 mEq/L. The presence of mannitol (as well as ethanol or ethylene glycol) is suggested by an increased gap between the measured and the calculated P_{osm} (14).

2. **Isoosmolar Hyponatremia**—P_{osm} is determined by measuring the osmotic activity in the plasma water, whereas P_{Na} is determined by measuring the concentration of sodium per liter of whole plasma. Therefore, when the nonwater component of plasma increases because of hyperlipidemia or hyperproteinemia, P_{Na} decreases but P_{osm} remains normal. Because P_{osm} is normal, no therapy is required for these patients. Under certain circumstances, hyperglycemia can also be associated with isoosmolar hyponatremia. For example, if the concentrations of glucose, sodium, and BUN are 300 mg/dl, 131 mEq/L, and 6 mg/dl, respectively, P_{osm} may be 280 mOsm/kg. However, the hyponatremia is mild and of no clinical consequence because the osmolality is normal (14).
3. **Hypoosmolar Hyponatremia**
   a. **Low Effective Arteriolar Volume** (14)
      (1) As described previously, low EAV stimulates renal sodium reabsorption and free water retention. Except under sodium wasting states (*i.e.*, use of diuretics), sodium conservation causes U_{Na} to fall to <10 to 15 mEq/L. Free water retention concentrates the urine, and U_{osm} typically rises to 600 to 800 mOsm/kg or higher in a healthy individual.
      (2) The major causes of hyponatremia associated with low EAV may be divided into edematous and nonedematous states. Edematous causes include congestive heart failure, cirrhosis, and nephrotic syndrome. These patients are typically volume overloaded, but the EAV is low because of decreased cardiac output in the case of congestive heart failure or because of decreased oncotic pressure in the case of cirrhosis or nephrotic syndrome. Nonedematous causes include hypovolemia from GI loss, renal loss, or skin loss. These causes are summarized in Table 22-3.
   b. **Syndrome of Inappropriate Secretion of Antidiuretic Hormone (SIADH) (14)**
      (1) As previously described, patients with low EAV tend to have high levels of ADH. Because this is an adaptive effort to promote volume expansion, these patients are considered to have an appropriate increase in ADH. In patients with SIADH, however, the increased activity of ADH is inappropriate and nonphysiologic. SIADH can result from inappropriate hypothalamic secretion of ADH, ectopic production of ADH, potentiation of ADH effect on the renal collecting tubules, or exogenous administration of ADH or ADH-like drugs. The major causes of SIADH along with its mechanism of action are summarized in Table 22-4 (14).
      (2) In SIADH, hyponatremia is a result of both free water retention and sodium wasting. The former can be attributed to inappropriate ADH activity and the latter to appropriate volume regulation. In contrast to patients with low EAV, renal sodium excretion is not impaired in pa-

Table 22-3 Major causes of hyponatremia associated with low EAV (14)

Edematous States	Nonedematous States		
	GI Loss	Renal Loss	Skin Loss
CHF Cirrhosis Nephrotic syndrome	Vomiting Diarrhea GI bleeding NG Suction	Diuretics Salt Wasting Nephropathy Hypoaldosteronism	Fever Burns Perspiration

Table 22-4 Major causes of SIADH (14)

CNS		Pulmonary		Drugs		Other	
Infection	H	Pneumonia	H	Carbamazepine	H, P	Surgery, trauma	H
Stroke or bleeding	H	Tuberculosis	H, E	Neuroleptics	H	Idiopathic	H
Tumor	H	Respiratory failure	H	Antidepressants	H	Severe nausea	H
Psychosis	H, P	Pneumothorax	H	IV cyclophosphamide	H, P		
Neurosurgery	H	Atelectesis	H	Chlorpropamide	P		
Head trauma	H	Tumor	E	Bromocriptine	H		
				NSAIDs	P		
				Vasopressin/oxytocin	X		

H, Inappropriate hypothalamic secretion of ADH; E, Ectopic production of ADH; P, Potentiation of ADH effect on the renal collecting tubules; X, Exogenous administration of ADH or ADH-like drugs.

tients with SIADH. ADH-mediated free water retention increases EAV, which then stimulates renal sodium excretion. Hence, U_{Na} is typically >20 mEq/L.

(3) The kidneys handle uric acid in a manner similar to sodium. SIADH is associated with a decrease in uric acid reabsorption; consequently, the serum uric acid levels are typically low in patients with SIADH.

c. **Diuretics**

(1) Diuretics induce hypovolemia and renal sodium wasting, both of which may contribute to the development of hyponatremia. For unclear reasons, older women are particularly susceptible to diuretic-induced hyponatremia (2).

(2) Hyponatremia is more often caused by thiazide diuretics than loop diuretics. Loop diuretics destroy the medullary osmotic gradient by blocking sodium reabsorption at the thick ascending limb of the loop of Henle. Consequently, even with maximal ADH activity, the insufficiency of the medullary osmotic gradient limits the ability to conserve free water. In contrast, the ability to conserve free water remains intact in patients treated with thiazide diuretics because these drugs do not interfere with the medullary osmotic gradient. Therefore, hyponatremia is more commonly observed with thiazides than loop diuretics (14).

d. **Hypothyroidism**—The mechanism of development of hyponatremia in hypothyroidism is unknown. However, there is some speculation that thyroxine may counteract the effect of ADH on the kidney. A relative absence of thyroxine would promote an increase in ADH activity. Furthermore, hypothyroidism can cause decreased cardiac output, which may also promote ADH release (14,18).

e. **Hypoadrenalism**—Several mechanisms may be involved in the development of hyponatremia caused by adrenocorticoid deficiency. First, absence of aldosterone causes renal sodium wasting. Second, vomiting, diarrhea, and hypotension cause a volume-mediated increase in ADH secretion. Third, glucocorticoid deficiency can increase ADH activity because cortisol feeds back negatively on ADH release (13,14).

f. **Psychogenic Polydipsia**—Under normal conditions, the kidneys can excrete up to 10 to 15 L of water per day by maximally diluting the urine. For hyponatremia to develop purely from water ingestion, the amount of water intake must exceed the kidneys' ability to excrete free water. This situation is most commonly observed in patients with psychiatric illnesses who use medications with anticholinergic side effects. These drugs often cause dry mouth, which encourages ingestion of free water. In addition to ingesting an enormous amount of free water, these patients typically have a mild stimulus for ADH release, such as the use of diuretics or nausea and vomiting. Patients on IV therapy with hypotonic solutions can also develop an iatrogenic version of this syndrome (14).

g. **Reset Osmostat**—As the name implies, the osmotic threshold for suppression of ADH is altered in patients with reset osmostat. Instead of suppressing ADH when P_{osm} fall to <275 mOsm/kg, these patients suppress at a lower level of P_{osm}. In addition, although these patients are able to sense changes in P_{osm}, most do not have a normal ability to excrete a free water load. Progressive hyponatremia does not usually occur, however, because osmoregulation does function, albeit perhaps imperfectly and at a different threshold. Conditions associated with a reset osmostat include psychosis, pregnancy, malnutrition, and quadriplegia. In addition, some patients with SIADH also have reset osmostat (14).

h. **Acute or Chronic Renal Failure**—In patients with severe renal dysfunction, the ability of the kidney to dilute urine may be impaired. If the kidney is unable to adequately excrete free water, hyponatremia may be observed.

i. **Nonsteroidal Antiinflammatory Drugs (NSAIDs)**—NSAIDs block the synthesis of prostaglandins which counteract the effect of ADH on the kidney. However, they are an uncommon cause of hyponatremia unless the patient is predisposed because of volume depletion, SIADH, or another underlying illness (14).

C. Diagnostic Approach to Hyponatremia

1. Initial blood tests should include P_{osm}, electrolytes, BUN, creatinine, glucose, and uric acid.
   a. P_{osm} can be used to identify patients with hyperosmolar or isoosmolar hyponatremia. This is important because patients with isoosmolar hyponatremia do not need treatment and because management of patients with hyperosmolar hyponatremia is directed not at the hyponatremia but at the underlying cause.
   b. It is important to calculate the effective P_{osm} in patients with renal failure, because BUN is an ineffective osmole. For example, consider a hypothetical patient with P_{Na} of 115 mEq/L, BUN of 112 mg/dl, glucose of 126 mg/dl, and P_{osm} of 280 mOsm/kg. Although P_{osm} appears to be normal, this patient actually has hypoosmolar hyponatremia, because the effective P_{osm} is only 240 mOsm/kg. Effective P_{osm} is approximated by the following formula: Effective P_{osm}=P_{osm} + BUN/2.8=280 + 112/2.8=240 mOsm/kg.
2. Once the diagnosis of hypoosmolar hyponatremia has been confirmed, measurement of U_{osm} should be used to differentiate patients with normal free water excretion from those with impaired free water excretion.
   a. **Conditions With Normal Free Water Excretion** (14)
      (1) If U_{osm} is <100 mOsm/kg, hyponatremia is a result of primary polydipsia or a reset osmostat. Low U_{osm} indicates that the body's ability to excrete free water is intact and that ADH is appropriately suppressed.
      (2) Water restriction can further differentiate primary polydipsia from reset osmostat. In primary polydipsia, water restriction causes U_{osm} to remain low until P_{osm} returns to normal. In reset osmostat, water restriction causes U_{osm} to rise, but P_{osm} does not change because P_{osm} is already at the "reset" level.
   b. **Conditions With Impaired Free Water Excretion**
      (1) If U_{osm} is >100 mOsm/kg, hyponatremia is a result of low EAV, SIADH, diuretics, hypoadrenalism, hypothyroidism, or renal failure. Increased U_{osm} indicates that the ability to excrete free water is limited and that ADH is not maximally suppressed (14).
      (2) Evaluations of thyroid-stimulating hormone, creatinine, and the adrenocorticotropic hormone (ACTH) stimulation test can identify patients with hypothyroidism, renal failure, and hypoadrenalism, respectively. Measurement of U_{Na} can help differentiate among the cases caused by low EAV, use of diuretics, or SIADH. If U_{Na} is <10 to 15 mEq/L, hyponatremia is most likely caused by low EAV (except diuretics). If U_{Na} is >20 mEq/L, use of diuretics or SIADH is the most likely cause. However, hypothyroidism, hypoadrenalism, and low EAV should carefully be excluded before a diagnosis of SIADH is made.
      (3) In equivocal cases, saline infusion or a high-salt diet can help distinguish among patients with true volume depletion, edematous causes of low EAV, or SIADH. In patients with true volume depletion, salt loading helps bring the patient to euvolemia and the ADH level appropriately falls. Because the body no longer retains free water or conserves sodium, U_{osm} decreases and U_{Na} increases. However, because salt loading does not correct the underlying cause of low EAV in patients with congestive heart failure, cirrhosis, or nephrotic syndrome, salt loading may only exacerbate the edema without significantly improving the hyponatremia in these patients. Finally, in patients with SIADH, ADH remains inappropriately high and sodium wasting persists. Therefore, U_{osm} remains high and U_{Na} may increase even further with salt loading in these patients.

(4) In euvolemic patients, SIADH can also be differentiated from other causes by response to free water loading. U_{osm} remains inappropriately high in patients with SIADH despite free water loading (14).

c. **Table 22–5 summarizes the diagnostic clues in patients with hypoosmolar hyponatremia**

D. Clinical Manifestations

1. The retained free water in patients with hypoosmolar hyponatremia causes all tissues to expand, but the brain is the first organ to become physically limited, because of the cranium and the meninges. Therefore, the clinical manifestations of hypoosmolar hyponatremia are primarily neurologic. Early symptoms include nausea, vomiting, malaise, headache, lethargy, and obtundation. Seizures, coma, and death can follow if hyponatremia progresses untreated (14).
2. Both the rapidity of development and the absolute degree of hyponatremia dictate the severity of symptoms. In general, symptoms are rare unless P_{Na} falls to <120 to 125 mEq/L (14). However, the rate of development of hyponatremia is usually more significant than the absolute degree of hyponatremia, because as long as the rate of development does not exceed the capacity of the brain's adaptive mechanism, the central nervous system can protect itself from edema by its ability to extrude excess osmoles when confronted with an hypoosmolar environment (8). In rats with experimentally induced acute hyponatremia, the brain begins to rapidly lose inorganic osmoles (sodium and chloride ions) within 30 minutes and the rate of loss becomes maximal in about 3 hours (12). Similar adaptation takes place during experimentally induced chronic hyponatremia in rats, but the rapid loss of electrolytes accounts for only two-thirds of the observed brain volume regulation; the remaining one-third results from the loss of organic osmolytes (*i.e.*, glutamate, glutamine, taurine, inositol), which also occurs relatively rapidly over a period of 48 hours or less (11,22,23). However, because these adaptations still occur at a finite rate, significant brain edema may develop if hyponatremia develops at a rate that exceeds the ability of the brain to regulate its concentration of osmoles. Consequently, acute hyponatremia is more likely to cause serious neurologic sequelae or death, whereas chronic hyponatremia is usually well tolerated (8).
   a. These points are well illustrated in the following experiment. Arieff studied the effects of artificially induced hyponatremia in four groups of rab-

Table 22-5 Diagnostic clues in patients with hypoosmolar hyponatremia (14)

	U_{osm} (mOsm/kg)	U_{Na} (mEq/L)	Other Clues
Primary polydipsia	<100	Variable	U_{osm} stays low with water restriction
Reset osmostat	<100	>20	U_{osm} increases with water restriction
Low EAV	>100	<10–15	U_{osm} decreases and U_{Na} increases with salt loading*
SIADH	>100	>20	U_{osm} & U_{Na}† remain high with salt loading; U_{osm} remains high with free water loading; serum uric acid level tends to be low.
Diuretics	>100	Usually >20	Hyponatremia improves when the diuretic is stopped
Hypoadrenalism	>100	>20	Abnormal ACTH simulation test; serum potassium level may be high
Renal failure	>100	>20	Elevated BUN and creatine levels

*Since salt loading does not correct the underlying cause of low EAV in patients with CHF, cirrhosis, or nephrotic syndrome, salt loading may only exacerbate the edema without significantly improving the hyponatremia (see text).

†U_{Na} may increase even further with saline loading.

bits. In the first group, acute moderate hyponatremia was induced by decreasing the P_{Na} by 10 mEq/L/hour to 119 mEq/L. In the second group, chronic moderate hyponatremia was induced by decreasing the P_{Na} by 0.21 mEq/L/hour to 122 mEq/L. In the third group, chronic severe hyponatremia was induced by decreasing the P_{Na} by 0.10 mEq/L/hour to 99 mEq/L. The effects of hyponatremia were compared among these three groups and a fourth group of control rabbits (1) (see Table 22–6).

(1) The rate of development of hyponatremia correlated with the degree of cerebral edema, which in turn correlated with the clinical outcome. A rapid (10 mEq/L/hour) reduction in P_{Na} to 119 mEq/L caused marked cerebral edema and death. In contrast, a slower (0.21 mEq/L/hour) reduction of P_{Na} to 122 mEq/L caused less cerebral edema and the rabbits remained asymptomatic.

(2) The absolute degree of hyponatremia also correlated with neurologic symptoms. This is probably a reflection of the importance of sodium for nerve function. A slow (0.10 mEq/L/hour) reduction of P_{Na} to 99 mEq/L caused lethargy, whereas a slow (0.21 mEq/L/hour) reduction of P_{Na} to 122 mEq/L was associated with no clinical manifestations.

b. Similar observations have been made in humans. Cluitmans reviewed all published human cases of hyponatremia with P_{Na} <121 mEq/L. Only those reports in which the rate of development, the rate of correction, and the final outcome were known were included in the analysis. Thirty-eight patients met these criteria (7).

(1) Four patients died and 4 patients suffered serious neurologic sequelae when hyponatremia developed at a rate >0.5 mEq/L/hour.

(2) No deaths or serious neurologic sequelae occurred if hyponatremia developed at a rate <0.5 mEq/L/hour.

c. Based on these observations, the prognosis associated with hyponatremia can be summarized as shown in Table 22-7.

Table 22-6 Effects of artificially induced hyponatremia in rats (1)

	No Reduction in P_{Na}	Rapid Reduction to Moderately Low P_{Na}	Slow Reduction to Moderately Low P_{Na}	Slow Reduction to Very Low P_{Na}
Baseline P_{Na}	139 mEq/L	139 mEq/L	140 mEq/L	139 mEq/L
New P_{Na}	No change	119 mEq/L	122 mEq/L	99 mEq/L
Rate of change	0 mEq/L/hour	10 mEq/L/h	0.21 mEq/L/h	0.10 mEq/L/h
% Gain in brain weight	0%	17%	7%	7%
Outcome	—	88% Mortality	Asymptomatic	Lethargic

Table 22-7 Prognosis of hyponatremia

	Acute Hyponatremia (Rate of Development >0.5 mEq/L/h)	Chronic Hyponatremia (Rate of Development <0.5 mEq/L/h)
Mild hyponatremia (P_{Na} >120 mEq/L)	Good prognosis	Good prognosis
Severe hyponatremia (P_{Na} <110 mEq/L)	Poor prognosis	Good but potentially poor prognosis

E. Therapy

1. Patients with mild hyponatremia usually respond to free water restriction or correction or removal of the offending cause (or both). The management of patients with severe hyponatremia is more controversial.
   a. **Severe Acute Hyponatremia**—In contrast to chronic hyponatremia, acute severe hyponatremia (<110 mEq/L and rate of development >0.5 mEq/L/hour) can be associated with significant morbidity and mortality. These patients may experience the consequences of cerebral edema because a rapid decrease in P_{osm} can overwhelm the brain's ability to extrude the excess osmoles. Therefore, rapid correction may be indicated for severely symptomatic patients with acute hyponatremia, because cerebral edema can be minimized by quickly raising the P_{osm} (18). A study by Cheng supports this observation. This retrospective study involved 13 patients with 27 episodes of seizures caused by acute severe hyponatremia (average P_{Na}, 111 mEq/L) from psychogenic polydipsia. These cases were assumed to be "acute" because all patients were institutionalized and the routine laboratory values were monitored regularly. However, the exact rate of development of the hyponatremia was not known. Hyponatremia was corrected rapidly until P_{Na} rose to 120 to 130 mEq/L. On the average, there was an absolute increase of 15 mEq/L in the first twelve hours. Then the rate of correction was slowed so that an absolute increase of 26 mEq/L was achieved in forty-eight hours. The patients were monitored clinically, by computed tomography, and by magnetic resonance imaging (MRI). After an average of 6.2 years of follow-up, no patient developed central pontine myelinolysis (CPM) or any other long-term neurologic sequelae despite rapid correction (6).
   b. **Severe Chronic Hyponatremia**—As discussed previously, chronic hyponatremia is usually well tolerated because the brain adapts to the hypoosmolar environment by rapidly extruding inorganic and organic osmoles, hence protecting itself from edema (11,12,22,23). Similarly, when recovering from hyponatremia, the brain adapts to the relatively hyperosmolar environment by reaccumulating the inorganic and organic osmoles, hence protecting itself from dehydration. However, there is an important difference between these two processes. In the process of adaptation to hyponatremia, the brain rapidly loses both inorganic and organic osmoles (8). In the process of recovery from hyponatremia, the inorganic osmoles reaccumulate within 24 hours but the organic osmoles (other than glutamate) reaccumulate at a much slower rate over many days (8,11). Consequently, if chronic hyponatremia is corrected too rapidly, the capacity of the brain to regulate its volume may be overwhelmed and the brain may become dehydrated as free water shifts out of the cells into the relatively hyperosmolar environment. This sudden central nervous system dehydration is thought to cause central pontine and extrapontine myelinolysis (CPM), a syndrome characterized by paraparesis or quadriparesis, mutism, dysphagia, dysarthria, emotional lability, ataxia, coma, and death (9). Diagnosis is usually made on a clinical basis, but it can be confirmed by MRI or at autopsy (5,9). Although some investigators still dispute the association between CPM and rapid correction of hyponatremia, most now believe that slower correction decreases the risk of CPM (3–5,7,9,10,21). Nevertheless, the optimal rate of correction still remains controversial.
      (1) Conservative recommendations are to correct at a rate <0.5 mEq/L/hour or <25 mEq/L in 48 hours (3,7,10,19–21). This point is well illustrated by Cluitmans' retrospective review of 117 published cases of chronic hyponatremia with known rates of correction. Chronic hyponatremia was defined as development of hyponatremia at a rate <0.5 mEq/L/hour (7) (see Table 22–8).
         (a) Only 1 patient (2%) developed CPM or other serious neurologic sequelae when hyponatremia was corrected at a rate slower than 0.5 mEq/L/hour.

Table 22-8 Correction of hyponatremia and the risk of neurologic complications

	Rate of Correction <0.5 mEq/L/h			Rate of Correction >0.5 mEq/L/h		
Initial P_{Na} (mEq/L)	N	Risk of CPM	Risk of Other CNS Sequelae	N	Risk of CPM	Risk of Other CNS Sequelae
<105	10	0%	0%	36	53%	28%
105–110	12	0%	0%	17	24%	12%
110–115	9	0%	0%	12	58%	8%
115–120	15	7%	0%	6	0%	0%
Total	46	2%	0%	71	42%	18%

(b) In contrast, the risk of CPM was 42% and the risk of other serious neurologic sequelae was 18% if hyponatremia was corrected at a rate faster than 0.5mEq/L/hour.

(2) Furthermore, it is common practice to correct hyponatremia in two stages. Initially, hyponatremia is corrected relatively quickly to a level of about 120 mEq/L. Then the rate of correction is substantially slowed until P_{Na} is restored to a normal level over many days (14). This approach may be particularly helpful for those with severe symptoms, who may benefit from a relatively rapid rise in serum tonicity to limit the degree of brain edema. Regardless of the exact style of correction, electrolytes should be monitored carefully to avoid overcorrection, and, whenever possible, correction of sodium should not exceed 25 mEq/L in 48 hours for reasons already discussed. Because patients usually tolerate chronic hyponatremia with minimal or no symptoms, a conservative approach to correction is appropriate for most patients. Nevertheless, in the absence of prospective studies that directly compare various rates of correction, the optimal rate of correction remains unknown.

(3) Slow correction does not guarantee that CPM will not occur. For example, in Karp's retrospective review of 14 patients with CPM, 3 patients developed CPM even though the rate of correction was between 0.42 and 0.56 mEq/L/hour (9).

c. Table 22–9 summarizes the pros and cons of rapid versus slow correction of hyponatremia.

2. Specific Treatments

a. True Hypovolemia—For patients with true hypovolemia, treatment of hyponatremia consists of restoration of circulatory volume, for example by

Table 22-9 Comparison of rapid versus slow correction of hyponatremia

	Acute Hyponatremia* (Rate of Development >0.5 mEq/L/h)	Chronic Hyponatremia* (Rate of Development <0.5 mEq/L/h)
Rapid correction (1–2 mEq/L/h)	Therapy is probably well tolerated and may be indicated if the patient is severely symptomatic	Therapy may not be well tolerated and may cause CPM or other serious neurologic sequelae
Slow correction (<0.5 mEq/L/h)	The therapy itself is generally well tolerated but may be inadequate if the patient is severely symptomatic	Therapy is generally well tolerated

*In practice, it is not always possible to reliably distinguish acute hyponatremia from chronic hyponatremia.

IV administration of isotonic saline and ingestion of foods with high salt content (*e.g.*, chicken soup), and removal or correction of the underlying cause if possible, for example by discontinuation of diuretics and administration of antiemetic medications. If hyponatremia is severe, isotonic or hypertonic saline may be used initially until P_{Na} increases to 120 to 125 mEq/L. Careful monitoring of electrolytes is mandatory to ensure that correction occurs at an appropriate rate (14). Table 22–10 illustrates correction of severe hyponatremia at an appropriate rate using isotonic saline.

b. Edematous Causes of Low EAV—Most patients respond to free water restriction and treatment of the underlying condition. Saline infusion should be avoided in these patients because it may exacerbate the existing edema. However, many patients have difficulty in complying with strict free water restriction. In some cases, mild hyponatremia may be permitted so long as the patient remains minimally symptomatic. In patients with severe or symptomatic hyponatremia who remain refractory to conservative measures, furosemide with hypertonic saline may be helpful. Both sodium and water are excreted with furosemide, whereas hypertonic saline replaces more sodium than water. This regimen causes a net negative free water balance, causing P_{Na} to rise.

c. SIADH

(1) Patients with mild hyponatremia caused by SIADH usually respond to free water restriction and oral salt repletion. For patients with severe symptomatic hyponatremia, treatment may be more complicated. Free water handling and osmoregulation are defective in these patients, but sodium handling and volume regulation are normal. If these patients are given isotonic saline, hyponatremia may actually get worse rather than better. High levels of ADH cause retention of the water component of saline, but most of the electrolytes in the saline are excreted since these patients are usually euvolemic. The result is net free water retention and worsening of the hyponatremia. This problem can be overcome by using furosemide and hypertonic saline. Furosemide destroys the medullary osmotic gradient and con-

Table 22-10 Sample correction of severe hyponatremia with isotonic saline

Patient	Hemodynamically stable, 70-kg woman with chronic hyponatremia (P_{Na}=105 mEq/L) due to diuretic use, low-salt diet, and free water ingestion
Goal	To use normal saline to bring the P_{Na} from 105 to 120 mEq/L at a maximal rate of 0.5 mEq/L/h (normal saline contains about 158 mEq/L of sodium)
Definitions	t = Minimum time of infusion V = Volume of saline NewP_{Na} = New target sodium concentration Rate = Maximal rate of infusion to correct at <0.5 mEq/L/h
Calculations	Sodium Deficit = (TBW)(NewP_{Na} − P_{Na}) = (60%)(70 kg)(120 mEq/L − 105 mEq/L) = 630 mEq V = (Sodium Deficit)/(158 mEq/L) = (630 mEq)/(158 mEq/L) = 3987 ml t = (120 mEq − 105 mEq/L)/(0.5 mEq/L/h) = 30 h Rate = (V)/(t) = (3987 ml)/(30 h) = 133 ml/h
Result	Normal saline can be given at 133 mL/h for 30 h. Since this rate is only an estimate, the electrolytes should be monitored carefully. When P_{Na} rises to 120 mEq/L, saline can be discontinued. Then, foods with high salt content such as chicken soup may be given orally with or without free water restriction to gradually bring the P_{Na} to a normal level over few days.

sequently limits the ability of the kidney to conserve free water. As with isotonic saline, most of the electrolytes in hypertonic saline are excreted. However, because there is about 1026 mOsm of solute per liter of hypertonic saline, much more free water must be excreted with the electrolytes for hypertonic saline than for isotonic saline, which contains only about 316 mOsm/L. The result is net free water excretion and improvement of hyponatremia. A more moderate improvement of hyponatremia can be achieved with the use of furosemide and isotonic saline (14).

(2) Maintenance Therapy for SIADH—Mild hyponatremia can be treated with free water restriction plus adequate dietary salt intake. For patients who remain refractory to free water restriction, therapeutic options include furosemide, demeclocycline, lithium, and increased solute loading. As described previously, furosemide decreases the U_{osm} and thus allows more free water to be excreted in the form of dilute urine. Demeclocycline and lithium work by blocking the effects of ADH on the kidney, but they are seldom necessary. Increased solute loading takes advantage of the fact that U_{osm} is relatively fixed in patients with SIADH. Therefore, the volume of urine is primarily determined by the amount of solute excreted. The solute load can be increased by a high-salt and high-protein diet. Alternatively, daily ingestion of 30 to 60 g of urea can be used for the same purpose (14).

d. Other Causes

(1) Psychogenic Polydipsia—Hyponatremia caused by polydipsia is easily corrected by free water restriction alone. Electrolytes should be monitored carefully to avoid too rapid correction.

(2) Reset Osmostat—Unless the underlying cause can be rectified, hyponatremia cannot be corrected. On the other hand, hyponatremia is usually mild in these patients.

(3) Endocrinopathies—Hyponatremia caused by hypothyroidism or hypoadrenalism responds to replacement of the deficient hormone.

F. Summary

1. Symptoms of hyponatremia are primarily neurologic. Early symptoms include nausea, vomiting, malaise, headache, lethargy, and obtundation. Seizures, coma, and death can occur if hyponatremia progresses without therapy. Both the rapidity and the absolute degree of hyponatremia dictate the severity of symptoms. Acute hyponatremia is more likely to cause serious neurologic sequelae or death, whereas chronic hyponatremia is better tolerated. Symptoms do not usually occur unless P_{Na} falls to <120 mEq/L.

2. Diagnostic Approach

a. P_{osm} should be used to identify patients with hyperosmolar or isoosmolar hyponatremia. Patients with isoosmolar hyponatremia do not need treatment, and management of patients with hyperosmolar hyponatremia is directed not at the hyponatremia but at the underlying cause. For patients with renal failure, it is important to calculate the effective P_{osm} because BUN is an ineffective osmole.

b. Once the patient has been confirmed to have hypoosmolar hyponatremia, U_{osm} should be used to differentiate patients with relatively normal free water excretion from those with impaired free water excretion. If U_{osm} is <100 mOsm/kg, free water excretion is normal and the patient has primary polydipsia or a reset osmostat. If U_{osm} is >100 mOsm/kg, free water excretion is impaired and the hyponatremia is caused by low EAV, SIADH, diuretics, hypoadrenalism, hypothyroidism, or renal failure.

c. Evaluations of thyroid-stimulating hormone, creatinine, and ACTH stimulation test can identify those patients with hypothyroidism, renal failure, and hypoadrenalism, respectively. U_{Na} is <10 to 15 mEq/L if hyponatremia is caused by low EAV (except diuretics), but U_{Na} is >20 mEq/L if use of diuretics or SIADH is the cause. Low EAV, hypothyroidism, and hypoadrenalism should carefully be excluded before SIADH is finally diagnosed.

3. Mild hyponatremia usually has a good prognosis. The prognosis of severe hyponatremia depends on whether the hypoosmolar state has developed rapidly or slowly. Chronic severe hyponatremia (<110 mEq/L and rate of development <0.5 mEq/L/hour) is usually well tolerated because the brain has had the time to adapt to the hypoosmolar environment by extruding excess osmoles. In contrast, acute severe hyponatremia (<110 mEq/L and rate of development <0.5 mEq/L/hour) may be associated with high morbidity and mortality.
4. Patients with mild hyponatremia usually respond to free water restriction and/or correction or removal of the offending cause. Rapid correction of patients with chronic severe hyponatremia should be avoided, because it may cause CPM or other serious neurologic sequelae. Although some investigators still dispute the association between CPM and rapid correction of hyponatremia, most now believe that a slower rate of correction decreases the risk of CPM. CPM is characterized by paraparesis or quadriparesis, mutism, dysphagia, dysarthria, emotional lability, ataxia, coma, and death. The diagnosis is usually made on a clinical basis, but it can be confirmed by MRI or at autopsy.
5. The optimal rate of correction for chronic severe hyponatremia is still controversial. Conservative recommendations are to correct no faster than 0.5 mEq/L/hour or 25 mEq/L in 48 hours. However, slow correction does not guarantee that CPM will not occur, and many patients do not develop CPM despite rapid correction. In acute severe hyponatremia, rapid partial correction (1 to 2 mEq/L/hour) is believed to be safe. In patients who are severely symptomatic from acute hyponatremia, rapid correction with furosemide and hypertonic saline may be justified. However, differentiation of acute from chronic hyponatremia is not always possible.

Abbreviations used in Chapter 22

ACTH = adrenocorticotrophic hormone
ADH = antidiuretic hormone
BUN = blood urea nitrogen
CHF = congestive heart failure
CNS = central nervous system
CPM = central pontine myelinolysis
EAV = effective arteriolar volume
GI = gastrointestinal
IV = intravenous
IVV = intravascular volume
MRI = magnetic resonance imaging
NG = nasogastric
NSAIDs = nonsteroidal antiinflammatory drugs
P = probability value
P_{Na} = plasma concentration of sodium
P_{osm} = plasma osmolality
RAAS = renin-angiotensin-aldosterone system
SIADH = syndrome of inappropriate secretion of antidiuretic hormone
TBW = total body water
U_{Na} = urinary sodium concentration
U_{osm} = urinary osmolality
vs = versus

References

1. Arieff. Neurologic manifestations and morbidity of hyponatremia. *Medicine (Baltimore)* 1976;55:121.

2. Ashouri. Severe diuretic-induced hyponatremia in the elderly. *Arch Intern Med* 1986;146:1355.
3. Ayus. Treatment of symptomatic hyponatremia and its relation to brain damage: a prospective study. *N Engl J Med* 1987;317:1190.
4. Berl. Treating hyponatremia: what is all the controversy about. *Ann Intern Med* 1990;113:417.
5. Brunner. Central pontine myelinolysis and pontine lesions after rapid correction of hyponatremia: a prospective magnetic resonance imaging study. *Ann Neurol* 1990;27:61.
6. Cheng. Long-term neurologic outcome in psychogenic water drinkers with severe symptomatic hyponatremia: the effect of rapid correction. *Am J Med* 1990;88:561.
7. Cluitmans. Management of severe hyponatremia: rapid or slow correction. *Am J Med* 1990;88:161.
8. Gullans. Control of brain volume during hyperosmolar and hypoosmolar conditions. *Annu Rev Med* 1993;44:289.
9. Karp. Pontine and extrapontine myelinolysis: a neurologic disorder following rapid correction of hyponatremia. *Medicine (Baltimore)* 1993;72:359.
10. Laureno. Pontine and extrapontine myelinolysis following rapid correction of hyponatremia. *Lancet* 1988;1:1439.
11. Lien. Study of brain electrolytes and organic osmolytes during correction of chronic hyponatremia. *J Clin Invest* 1991;88:303.
12. Melton. Volume regulatory loss of Na, Cl, K from rat brain during acute hyponatremia. *Am J Physiol* 1987;252:F661.
13. Raff. Glucocorticoid inhibition of neurohypophyseal vasopressin secretion. *Am J Physiol* 1987;252:R635.
14. Rose. Hypoosmolal states: hyponatremia. In: Rose. *Clinical Physiology of Acid-Base and Electrolyte Disorders*. New York: McGraw-Hill, 1989:601.
15. Rose. Introduction to disorders of osmolality. In: Rose. *Clinical Physiology of Acid-Base and Electrolyte Disorders*. New York: McGraw-Hill, 1989:589.
16. Rose. Regulation of plasma osmolality. In: Rose. *Clinical Physiology of Acid-Base and Electrolyte Disorders*. New York: McGraw-Hill, 1989:248.
17. Rose. Regulation of the effective circulating volume. In: Rose. *Clinical Physiology of Acid-Base and Electrolyte Disorders*. New York: McGraw-Hill, 1989:225.
18. Skowsky. The role of vasopressin in the impaired water excretion of myxedema. *Am J Med* 1978;64:613.
19. Stern. Osmotic demyelination syndrome following correction of hyponatremia. *N Engl J Med* 1986;314:1535.
20. Sterns. Severe symptomatic hyponatremia: treatment and outcome. A study of 64 cases. *Ann Intern Med* 1987;107:656.
21. Sterns. The treatment of hyponatremia: first do no harm. *Am J Med* 1990;88:557.
22. Verbalis. Adaptation to chronic hypoosmolality in rats. *Kidney Int* 1988;34:351.
23. Verbalis. Hyponatremia causes large sustained reductions in brain content of multiple organic osmolytes in rats. *Brain Res* 1991;567:27

23 Diabetic Ketoacidosis

Jonathan S. Bogan and
Cecil H. Coggins

A. Introduction

1. Diabetic ketoacidosis (DKA) and nonketotic hyperosmolar syndrome (NKHS) represent a continuum of metabolic derangements associated with insulin deficiency. At one extreme, pure DKA without hyperosmolality results from total absence of insulin, with rapid development of acidosis and ketosis accompanied by modest hyperglycemia (typically <300 mg/dl). In contrast, the insulin deficit in pure NKHS is less severe than in DKA. Ketosis does not develop, although profound hyperglycemia (often >1000 mg/dl), volume depletion, and hyperosmolality frequently lead to mental obtundation. DKA is most characteristic of type I (childhood-onset) insulin-dependent diabetes mellitus (DM), but ketosis and acidosis may also occur in type II (non–insulin-dependent) DM with sufficient provocation. Most often, some degree of hyperosmolality is also present in DKA. NKHS most frequently occurs in middle-aged or elderly persons with mild or previously unrecognized type II (adult-onset) DM. Its onset is typically more gradual than that of DKA. The diagnosis of either DKA or NKHS necessitates a search for precipitating factors such as infection, cessation of hypoglycemic therapy, new-onset diabetes, or other metabolic stressors. The focus of this chapter is limited to management of DKA.
2. In a national surveillance study of type I and type II diabetics hospitalized in the United States from 1980 to 1987, DKA was the primary diagnosis for 10.3 to 14.6 per 1000 hospitalized diabetics per year (78). This rate was highest among black males (24.7/1000 in 1987) and lowest among white males (8.7/1000 in 1987, $P<0.001$); the rates for black and white females were similar (12.4/1000 and 12.0/1000, respectively, $P=0.45$). A similar rate of 13.4 episodes of DKA per 1000 patient-years was recorded among 138 type I diabetics in Rochester, Minnesota from 1945 to 1970; the rate among 1398 type II diabetics in that study was 3.3 per 1000 patient-years (41). A higher incidence of DKA was noted among 3250 European type I diabetics participating in the EURODIAB study; 86 per 1000 of these patients reported one or more hospital admissions for DKA in a 12-month time period (72). The incidence of DKA in type I diabetics participating in the Diabetes Control and Complications Trial was similar in the conventional therapy group (18 episodes per 1000 patient-years) and in the intensive therapy group (20 episodes per 1000 patient-years; $P>0.7$) (23).
3. In the United States, the mortality risk attributed to DKA ranged from 0.31 per 1000 diabetics per year in 1980 to 0.25 per 1000 in 1986, or about 2% of those admitted with a primary diagnosis of DKA (78). Other studies from developed countries also report mortality rates of 2% to 5% for patients admitted with DKA (36,70). This mortality risk is lower than the 7% to 12% risk reported in older studies from the 1970s and early 1980s (5,11,20,22,25,27,41).
4. The development of NKHS in middle-aged or older individuals not uncommonly indicates the development of a life-threatening illness in a person with mild or previously unrecognized type II diabetes. Severe dehydration and hyperosmolality may result from delay in seeking medical attention and may contribute to the high mortality risk associated with this condition. Mortality figures for NKHS range from 15% to 70% (7,11,25,36,47).

5. Mortality is increased among elderly persons who present with DKA; one retrospective study observed a 22% mortality rate for patients >65 years of age, compared with 2% for those <65 years (P=0.001) (56). Older age, high serum osmolality, infection (particularly pneumonia and sepsis), myocardial infarction (MI), and renal insufficiency have been associated with a higher risk of death in some but not all studies (13,20,36,41,56). However, an association between mortality and the severity of acidosis has not been described (11,36,66). Although morbidity and mortality in DKA are caused mainly by sepsis or cardiopulmonary complications, patients ≤28 years old are susceptible to fatal cerebral edema, which is estimated to occur during treatment of DKA in 0.7% to 1.0% of episodes (15,37,52).
6. There is no consensus definition for DKA. Although the diagnosis requires the presence of an anion-gap metabolic acidosis (defined as $[Na^+] - ([Cl^-] + [HCO_3^-]) > 16$ mmol/L) and ketonemia, the degree to which these abnormalities are present varies widely. Although most patients with DKA have increased blood glucose, the level may be <200 mg/dl in 1.1% to 7.6% of cases, or it may be in the extreme high range more typical of NKHS (40,59). Ketoacidosis usually denotes an arterial blood pH ≤7.30 or a serum bicarbonate level <10 to 15 mmol/L, or both (33,52). The distinction between ketosis (hyperglycemia and ketosis without overt acidosis) and ketoacidosis is clinically useful, because known diabetics with a pH >7.30 and plasma osmolality <320 mOsm/L can usually be treated on an outpatient basis (17,33,52). Patients with an arterial blood pH ≤7.20 should be hospitalized for intensive management (52).

B. Clinical Presentation of DKA

1. Precipitating Factors

a. **Infection**—About 30% to 50% of the cases of DKA are precipitated by infection (5,25,39,41,44,58,70). Urinary tract infections (including pyelonephritis) and pneumonia are the most common, and septicemia is often present. Other infectious precipitants include occult sinusitis, tooth abscess, axillary furuncle, and perirectal abscess. Rarely, infections such as renal aspergilloma may present with DKA (9). Mucormycosis is a rare infection that is particularly associated with DKA and is rapidly lethal if not treated promptly; it may be suggested by the presence of facial pain, bloody nasal discharge, orbital swelling and proptosis, and blurred vision (11,32). Other precipitants include cholecystitis, pancreatitis, appendicitis, diverticulitis, perforated viscus, or ischemic bowel, particularly if abdominal pain is present. In one series, abdominal disorders accounted for 5% of cases (70).

b. **Insulin**—Omission of insulin or inadequate insulin therapy accounts for 10% to 30% of the cases of DKA (41,58,70). The use of an insulin pump for continuous subcutaneous insulin infusion has been associated with an increased risk of DKA, typically because of dislodgment or obstruction of the catheter or mechanical failure. However, this risk appears to be decreasing as these devices improve (48,70). DKA may develop postoperatively if perioperative insulin dosing is not appropriate; a good rule of thumb is to administer one-third to one-half of the patient's usual total daily dose in the form of long-acting insulin (NPH or Lente) on the morning of surgery, in conjunction with dextrose-containing IV fluid.

c. **New-Onset Diabetes Mellitus**—New-onset or previously undiagnosed DM accounts for 5% to 22% of the cases of DKA (25,58). In the Mayo series, 26% and 15% of the cases of DKA among type I and type II diabetics, respectively, led to a new diagnosis of DM (41). Using less stringent criteria for DKA (HCO_3^- <21 mmol/L), Snorgaard found that 69 (39%) of 175 episodes of DKA coincided with an initial diagnosis of DM (70). Westphal noted that ketosis was the initial presentation of diabetes in 62 (27%) of 226 patients hospitalized with DKA (77).

d. **Myocardial Infarction**—In one study among known diabetics, 6 of the 106 episodes of DKA were precipitated by an MI; 4 of these cases were fatal

(70). In another study, 6 of 92 episodes of DKA were associated with an acute MI, and MI was the single greatest cause of death within 48 hours of hospitalization for patients with DKA (41). These rates are similar to older data in which 11 of 257 patients who presented with DKA had MIs (11).

e. **Drugs**—Numerous drugs can increase the risk of developing DKA or NKHS. Among the most common are the glucocorticoids, which induce a catabolic state, increase peripheral insulin resistance, and perhaps contribute to hepatic ketogenesis (69). β-Adrenergic agonists (*e.g.*, terbutaline), and sympathomimetics (including dobutamine) can also increase insulin resistance. Cocaine use can also precipitate DKA (58). β-Adrenergic antagonists, phenytoin, calcium channel blockers, and alcohol can decrease insulin secretion (69). Pentamidine is toxic to pancreatic β-cells and can cause secondary diabetes and DKA (51). Thiazides may cause hypokalemia and thereby inhibit insulin secretion and increase insulin resistance (69).

f. **Pregnancy**—Insulin requirements are increased in the second half of pregnancy, and failure to appropriately adjust the dose of insulin may lead to poor glycemic control or overt DKA (30). Severe DKA during pregnancy has been associated with a very high (about 65%) fetal mortality rate (11). Starvation ketosis occurs commonly in pregnant or postpartum (lactating) women and results in true ketoacidosis even in the absence of diabetes (21,55)

g. **Noncompliance and Psychological Factors**—Among individuals with multiple hospitalizations for DKA, noncompliance with diet or medication accounted for 43% of the episodes in one series (25). In a 12-year follow-up study involving brittle diabetics, psychological or social factors accounted for up to 80% of the recurrent episodes of DKA (73). The mechanism by which these factors precipitate DKA is not entirely known but may be related to dietary indiscretion or omission of insulin. However, it is also possible that severe emotional stress may itself precipitate DKA among brittle diabetics.

h. **Miscellaneous Conditions**

(1) Stroke can precipitate DKA, and it is the major contributing cause of death in up to 10% of the fatalities associated with DKA or NKHS (13,36).

(2) Pancreatitis has been reported to cause 1% to 8% of the cases of DKA, perhaps varying with the underlying rate of alcoholic pancreatitis in different populations (11,41,70).

(3) There have been case reports of DKA in the context of Cushing's syndrome, acromegaly (with cessation of octreotide therapy), glucagonoma, or somatostatinoma (30).

(4) The precipitating event is unknown in 14% to 25% of the cases (39, 44,70).

2. **Clinical Manifestations**—The symptoms and signs associated with DKA are generally nonspecific. Patients classically present with polyuria, thirst, nausea, vomiting, weakness, air hunger, and altered sensorium. Abdominal pain occurs in about 30% of the cases and can be caused by the DKA itself or by an underlying pathologic process that may have precipitated the DKA (33,69). Tachycardia is usual, but blood pressure is generally maintained; hypotension was present in 9% of the patients in one series (11). Kussmaul respiration may be present and usually indicates a serum pH <7.2 (69). A shallow respiratory pattern may indicate more severe acidosis. The exhaled air may have the characteristic "fruity" scent of acetone. Body temperature is often below normal. Therefore, the lack of a fever does not exclude the presence of an infection. Conversely, if fever is present, there is a very high likelihood of infection (5). Approximately one-fifth of the patients are alert, but 10% are obtunded; the remainder have varying degrees of alertness between these two extremes. Obtundation correlates well with high plasma osmolality (>340 mOsm/L) and carries a poor prognosis (5,11,69). Dehydration may cause poor skin turgor, dry mucous membranes, and orthostasis.

3. **Laboratory Manifestations**—Summarized in Table 23-1 are the average initial laboratory values of patients presenting with DKA in three published series. Beigelman's series includes data from nonfatal cases only (11).

a. **Glucose**

(1) The blood glucose is quite variable and may even be <200 mg/dl, particularly in late pregnancy or in the setting of a prolonged fast before presentation. In one early series of 200 episodes of DKA, 37 were characterized by glucose levels <300 mg/dl and serum bicarbonate <10 mmol/L (59). These episodes were preceded by a reduction in carbohydrate intake because of vomiting, nausea, or, in one case, a dental abscess. In 27 episodes, patients had taken either the usual or an increased dose of insulin. A more recent study of type I diabetics demonstrated that after a 32-hour fast the rate of ketogenesis is accelerated and hepatic glycogenolysis is suppressed, resulting in rapid development of euglycemic ketoacidosis (18). The development of DKA despite frequent, normal capillary blood glucose measurements has been described, and emphasizes the utility of testing urine for ketones (14).

(2) Because glucose is effectively cleared by normally functioning kidneys when moderate hyperglycemia is present, extreme degrees of hyperglycemia suggest profound volume depletion and impaired glomerular filtration. Prospective studies have demonstrated a decrease in blood glucose concentrations attributable to glycosuria after treatment with IV fluid but not insulin (61,75).

b. **Sodium**—The serum sodium concentration may vary substantially, although a total body sodium deficit is invariably present. Often, a transiently low sodium concentration reflects the osmotic activity of the blood glucose, which draws water into the extracellular space and dilutes the serum sodium. The sodium concentration that would be present if the hyperglycemia were corrected may be approximated from the existing sodium concentration (in mmol/L) and serum glucose level (in mg/dl) by the following formula (33): Corrected $[Na^+]=[Na^+] + 1.6\ (\text{Glucose} - 100)/100$. As many as 11% of patients presenting with DKA have triglyceride levels >1000 mg/dl (11.3 mmol/L) (34). Such patients may have artifactually low serum sodium measurements as well as milky plasma and lipemia retinalis (39). The hypertriglyceridemia usually returns to normal after resolution of DKA and 6 to 8 months of improved blood glucose control (34).

c. **Potassium and Phosphate**—The initial serum potassium concentration is typically normal or high because of acidosis, but the total body potas-

Table 23-1 Initial laboratory findings in DKA

	Kitabchi (49) (N=123)	Foster (31) (N=88)	Beigelman (11) (N=308)
Glucose (mg/dl)	606	475	675
Sodium (mmol)	135	132	131
Potassium (mmol)	5.7	4.8	5.3
Bicarbonate (mmol)	6.3	<10	6
Blood urea nitrogen (mg/dl)	29	25	32
Acetoacetate (mmol)	3.1	4.8	—
β-hydroxybutyrate (mmol)	9.8	13.7	—
Lactate (mmol)	2.5	4.6	—
Osmolality (mOsm)	316	310	323
pH	7.11	—	—

Adapted from Foster (31) with permission.

sium is usually depleted (32). Marked hyperkalemia was associated with increased mortality in one retrospective study, perhaps because of circulatory insufficiency and decreased renal perfusion (11). Similarly, the initial phosphate concentration may be normal or high, but total body phosphorus is usually depleted (32,79).

d. **Blood Urea Nitrogen and Creatinine**—Increases in blood urea nitrogen (BUN) and creatinine usually indicate the degree of prerenal azotemia that has resulted from osmotic diuresis or vomiting. In one series of 10 patients, the average initial creatinine clearance was mildly reduced at 82 ml/minute (61). High plasma ketone concentrations cause artifactually high creatinine measurements in most assays and may result in an incorrect diagnosis of renal failure (76).

e. **Ketones and Ketoacids**—Acetoacetate and β-hydroxybutyrate ("ketone") concentrations are usually not precisely measured, but they are the primary reason for the anion-gap acidosis. Lactic acid is also increased and, along with free fatty acids, contributes to the metabolic acidosis. The semiquantitative test strips or tablets commonly used to test for the presence of ketones detect acetone and acetoacetate but not β-hydroxybutyrate. A "large" reading usually corresponds to at least 2 mmol/L acetoacetate (and an equal concentration of acetone) (33). A positive urine test for "large" ketones may be caused by starvation ketosis alone, whereas the presence of large ketones in plasma diluted 1:1 or more usually indicates ketoacidosis (33). Also, a false-positive urine test for acetone may be caused by captopril (reported by the manufacturer).

f. **Bicarbonate**—The acid load in DKA decreases the plasma bicarbonate concentration and increases the anion gap. In a given patient, these changes need not be proportional, and some degree of hyperchloremic acidosis is often present. Adrogué found that a greater degree of prerenal azotemia correlates with more anion-gap acidosis and less hyperchloremic acidosis; conversely, normal renal perfusion correlates with more hyperchloremic acidosis and less of an anion gap (3). Patients with more severe hyperchloremic acidosis recovered more slowly than those with pure ketoacidosis. This is because ketones lost in the urine as salts are no longer available to be metabolically converted to bicarbonate and therefore do not consume excess hydrogen ions. Most of these excess hydrogen ions are excreted by the kidney as ammonium over a longer time period (2). Even if it is not present initially, hyperchloremic acidosis develops in most patients with DKA during the first 4 to 8 hours of treatment (3). This, too, is a result of the excretion of ketones as sodium or potassium salts (rather than as acid), which results in relatively greater renal retention of chloride than of sodium.

g. **Amylase and Lipase**—In one series, the serum amylase concentration was increased in 79% of patients with DKA (74). Pancreatic, salivary, and mixed isoenzyme patterns were all observed, and there was no correlation with abdominal symptoms or hypertriglyceridemia. If the lipase levels are also elevated, the diagnosis of pancreatitis is more likely. However, artifactually high lipase concentrations may also be observed during DKA (33).

h. **Complete Blood Count**—Leukocytosis is characteristic of DKA and does not necessarily indicate that infection is present (5). Hematocrit and erythrocyte mean cell volume may be increased because of osmotic swelling in the setting of increased glucose and normal serum tonicity; this is because glucose (and not sodium) is an osmole that is freely distributed across the erythrocyte membrane (16).

C. **Treatment of DKA**—Prompt diagnosis and therapy are essential for optimal care of the patient with DKA. One retrospective study suggested that the deaths associated with DKA would have been avoidable if complications had been recognized earlier during the hospital course, and that the deaths associated with NKHS would have been avoidable if the symptoms of new-onset DM had been recognized prior to hospitalization (36). Subtle metabolic abnormalities of early DKA may be missed initially if the precipitating illness (*e.g.*, infection, MI, stroke) becomes the main focus of clinical attention (44). In addition, because β-hydroxybutyrate is not detected by the commonly used semiquantitative assays for ketones, ketosis may be underestimated if β-hydroxybutyrate increases out of proportion to the increase in acetate, as may occur in the setting of ethanol ingestion or hypoxia (33). The goals of therapy include rehydration, correction of pH and elimination of ketonemia, normalization of blood glucose, and prevention of complications.

1. Intravenous Fluid

a. IV fluid is important for (a) maintaining cardiac output and renal perfusion, (b) reducing blood glucose concentration and plasma osmolality, and (c) decreasing the concentrations of glucagon, cortisol, and other counter-regulatory hormones implicated in ketogenesis (61,75). Fluid does not, by itself, reverse acidosis or ketonemia. Several uncontrolled studies have evaluated the effects of IV fluid administration in DKA.

(1) In a study involving 8 patients with DKA and 2 with NKHS, administration of hypoosmolal fluid (220 mOsm) without any insulin decreased the mean blood glucose concentration by 32% (range, 17% to 80%) (75). The urine levels of glucose and the plasma levels of lactate, cortisol, epinephrine, norepinephrine, aldosterone, and renin also decreased significantly. Among those with DKA, the serum pH increased from 7.04 to 7.21 ($P<0.005$), but bicarbonate was given to 7 patients whose initial serum pH was <7.20. Patients were later given insulin after the blood glucose concentration ceased to fall any further with IV fluid therapy. On average, patients received 4.4 L of IV fluid.

(2) Similarly, in a study involving 10 patients presenting with DKA, hydration with IV 0.45% saline solution (1/2NS) without any insulin decreased the concentration of blood glucose by 30% over an interval of 3 to 5 hours ($P<0.05$) (61). Based on measurements of urine glucose, the fall in blood glucose concentration appears to have been caused primarily by glycosuria rather than dilution. The mean rise in the measured glomerular filtration rate was not statistically significant. No effect was observed on arterial pH or on plasma concentrations of ketones or bicarbonate.

b. For a typical adult patient presenting with DKA, the average fluid deficit is 3 to 5 L (32). For any individual patient, the fluid deficit (in liters) can be estimated by subtracting the patient's weight on admission (in kilograms) from the last known weight before admission. Even though most patients have a free water deficit as well as a volume deficit, correction of the serum osmolality should be attempted only after volume replacement has been accomplished, especially if clinically significant circulatory insufficiency is present (33,52). An estimation of the serum osmolality (in mOsm/L) may be calculated from the concentrations of sodium and potassium (in mmol/L), the serum glucose level (in mg/dl), and the BUN (in mg/dl) by the following equation: $Osm_{calc} = 2\,[Na^+ + K^+] + Glucose \div 18 + BUN \div 2.8$. BUN contributes to the total osmolality but is often excluded from the calculation because it crosses membranes freely and does not contribute to the free water deficit (30,52). In DKA, hyperosmolality reflects dehydration, and the calculated and measured osmolality are approximately equal. If the measured osmolality is greater than the calculated osmolality, an unmeasured contributor to the osmolality (*e.g.*, ethanol) may be present. As noted previously, patients with DKA and stupor or obtundation often have a measured serum osmolality >340 mOsm/L. These patients are typically quite dehydrated and should receive rapid infusion of isotonic fluids as the initial fluid therapy—either 0.9% saline solution (normal saline, NS) or lactated Ringer's solution (48).

c. For initial treatment of DKA, most authors advocate the use of NS or lactated Ringer's solution rather than 1/2NS (33,42,48,52). Although repletion of the extracellular fluid volume may be the primary reason for this approach, some authors suggest that the use of isotonic fluid may help prevent the development of clinically significant cerebral edema in children. The use of hypotonic fluid may cause a rapid fall in the sodium concentration of the extracellular fluid and thereby promote entry of free water into cells, including the cells of the central nervous system. Others suggest that this same process may also produce mild noncardiogenic pulmonary edema, which may account for the significant increase in the alveolar-arterial oxygen gradient that was prospectively observed during treatment of 18 adults with DKA (26). Although these are theoretical reasons to avoid the use hypoosmolar solutions for treatment of DKA, the results of the retrospective clinical studies on this topic have been mixed.

(1) Duck's retrospective study of 42 cases of brain herniation during treatment of DKA in children noted a weak but significant inverse correlation between the rate of fluid administration and the time to development of neurologic signs, as assessed by linear regression ($r=-0.32$; $P=0.04$) (24). At the time of herniation, the calculated ("corrected") serum sodium values had fallen significantly and were <130 mmol/L in one third of the cases. The authors suggested that excessive vasopressin activity may exacerbate brain edema and that it may be prudent to limit the rate of fluid administration in DKA.

(2) In another retrospective analysis involving 219 children with DKA, 20 cases were complicated by headache, neurologic signs, or death resulting from cerebral edema (37). The calculated plasma osmolality was significantly lower among the complicated cases than among uncomplicated cases. Moreover, the serum sodium concentration remained low during treatment in 54% of uncomplicated episodes and in 95% of complicated episodes ($P<0.01$). Both the rate of infusion and the sodium concentration of the IV fluid correlated with these parameters, leading the authors to conclude that rapid administration of hypotonic fluid may be responsible for the brain edema that can develop during treatment of DKA.

(3) In contrast to the studies just described, Rosenbloom's retrospective analysis of sixty-nine children with DKA did not find any significant relation between the rate or the osmolality of the administered fluid (or the rate of decrease in the blood glucose) and the development of clinically significant cerebral edema (64). Moreover, there were no data to support an association of low corrected sodium concentrations and significant cerebral edema; only 22% of patients for whom data was available reached a corrected sodium concentration of <130 mmol/L.

(4) In a small prospective series, 58 episodes of DKA were managed according to a 48-hour protocol designed to minimize the volume of free water administered, with the goal of increasing sodium by 1 to 2 mmol/L for every 100 mg/dl decline in the glucose concentration (37). Aside from 2 patients with headache, there were no complications in this group; therefore, the rate of complications was lower than the rate observed in the previous retrospective analysis by the same authors. However, this study was too small to arrive at a statistically significant result.

d. The rate of fluid administration (and the type of fluid administered) may also influence the degree of hyperchloremic acidosis that develops during recovery from DKA. However, there is no evidence that hyperchloremic acidosis alone causes any significant adverse effects.

(1) Androgué conducted a prospective, randomized, controlled trial comparing high-rate IV NS infusion (1000 ml/hour for the first 4 hours, then 500 ml/hour) versus low-rate IV NS infusion (500 ml/hour for the first 4 hours, then 250 ml/hour) in adults with DKA (1). After excluding patients with extreme volume deficits, 12 patients were randomly assigned to receive the high-rate infusion and 11 to receive the low-rate infusion. All patients received an IV 10-U bolus of insulin, followed by a constant infusion at 0.1 U/kg/hour. The plasma bicarbonate level normalized more rapidly in the low-rate group and was significantly higher than baseline at 4 hours and at 24 hours. Although both groups developed hyperchloremic acidosis during recovery as expected, the hyperchloremic acidosis was less severe with the lower rate of infusion. The authors suggested that these results resulted from regeneration of bicarbonate from ketone salts, which would have been excreted more rapidly in the group receiving the higher infusion rate.

(2) Foster favors the use of more rapid initial rates of infusion (*i.e.*, 1 L/hour for the first 2 to 3 hours), but suggests that lactated Ringer's solution rather than NS be administered so as to decrease the risk of developing hyperchloremic acidosis (33).

e. In summary, there are no data to support the use of hypotonic fluid in the initial management of DKA. Furthermore, in the absence of circulatory insufficiency, the rate of fluid administration need not be rapid. Some data suggest that recovery may even be faster with less rapid rates of fluid administration. A reasonable goal is to use NS (or lactated Ringer's solution) at rates that will replenish the volume deficit over 12 to 24 hours (48 hours in children) rather than in 8 hours (52). The total fluid deficit is usually 3 to 5 L in adults; urine output and insensible losses also must be replaced. A reasonable replacement schedule would be NS at a rate of 1 L/hour for the initial hour, followed by 500 ml/hour during the next 8 hours (42). On the other hand, if significant circulatory insufficiency is present, aggressive treatment with IV crystalloid solutions is indicated; some authors recommend the use of colloid solutions for rapid intravascular volume expansion, but this point is controversial (8,52).

f. After the initial period of volume replacement, it is reasonable to use 1/2NS rather than NS if the serum sodium concentration exceeds 150 mmol/L (52). Most investigators recommend changing to an IV dextrose solution such as 5% dextrose in 1/2NS once the blood glucose concentration has decreased to 250 to 300 mg/dl in order to avoid hypoglycemia and to replete the free water deficit (33, 42). The rate of IV dextrose administration must be balanced with the amount of insulin administered (see later discussion).

2. Insulin

a. The effects of insulin in DKA are (a) to decrease glucagon production by the pancreas, (b) to counteract the ketogenic and gluconeogenic action of glucagon in the liver, (c) to increase the rate of glucose utilization in fat and muscle, and (d) to inhibit lipolysis in fat, thereby decreasing the availability of substrates for hepatic ketogenesis (33). Because movement of glucose out of the intravascular compartment is accompanied by movement of water, IV fluid should be administered concurrently with insulin to avoid further intravascular volume depletion, hypernatremia, or even circulatory collapse (69).

b. Before the mid-1970s, relatively large doses of insulin (*e.g.*, 50 U/hour given subcutaneously) were used for treatment of DKA, and rehydration was considered less important (48,49). However, a large body of literature in the late 1970s and early 1980s demonstrated the effectiveness of low-dose IM or IV insulin regimens (*e.g.*, 5 U/hour) as well as a reduced incidence of hypoglycemia and hypokalemia with low-dose insulin protocols. These studies established the insulin dosing range that remains the current standard of care.

(1) Alberti's 1973 series was the first to demonstrate that small doses of IM insulin (16 U initially, then 5 to 10 U hourly thereafter) caused a steady and predictable decrease in the blood glucose (90 mg/dl/hour), but that study was retrospective and relied on historical controls (6). Similar findings were reported by other investigators using continuous IV insulin infusions at comparable doses (45,63,67).

(2) In 1976, Kitabchi reported the first prospective, randomized clinical trial comparing high-dose and low-dose insulin protocols in adults with DKA (46). Forty-eight patients were randomly assigned to receive either high-dose insulin (40 to 150 U IM initially, then 15 to 50 U SC hourly) or low-dose insulin (0.1 U/kg IM initially, then 5 U SC hourly). The rate of decrease of glucose and ketones in the blood, the time to normalization of blood pH and bicarbonate, and the improvement in cortisol and glucagon levels were not significantly different between the two groups. Hypokalemia ($[K^+]$ <3.4 mmol/L) was more common in the high-dose group (7 of 24 patients) than in the low-dose group (1 of 24 patients). Development of hypoglycemia (glucose <50 mg/dl) during the first 12 hours of treatment was also more common in the high-dose group (6 of 24 patients) than in the low-dose group (1 of 24 patients). Additional prospective, randomized trials have confirmed the efficacy and the low complication rate of low-dose insulin protocols (6 to 7 U/hour, IM or IV) (29,38,65,68).

(3) The blood levels of insulin attained with low-dose protocols were similar or slightly higher than those observed in normal subjects after a carbohydrate load. In contrast, with the high-dose protocols blood insulin reached supraphysiologic levels without additional therapeutic benefit (4,62). A moderate degree of insulin resistance is present in patients with DKA as compared with normal individuals, but only rarely is this resistance profound enough to require large doses of insulin (10,54). A useful guideline is to increase the insulin dose if the anion gap has not decreased within 4 hours after initiation of therapy (33).

c. As a general rule, the initial insulin should be administered intravenously. Insulin has a half-life of only 5 to 10 minutes, and data from the pediatric population suggest that a loading dose can be omitted if a continuous IV infusion is used (19). However, for patients who are treated with intermittent IM injections of regular (short-acting) insulin, an initial IV insulin bolus should be given. The dose of this bolus is not critical; although most patients respond to 10 U, some authors recommend as much as 50 U (33). Most investigators prefer a continuous IV infusion because of the ease with which the dose can be titrated. Absorption of insulin from an SC depot takes longer than from an IM injection site and is likely to be unreliable if significant dehydration is present. If the tissue perfusion is poor, some authors also warn against IM injection (52).

(1) One randomized, prospective study compared SC, IM, and IV insulin administration in 45 patients presenting with DKA (29). Patients received an initial weight-adjusted dose of regular insulin (0.33 U/kg) by one of the three routes; subsequent doses were 7 U/hour by the respective routes. The group receiving IV insulin had a significantly more rapid reduction in the levels of blood glucose ($P<0.01$) and ketone bodies ($P<0.05$) in the first 2 hours of treatment, compared with the other two groups. In addition, only 1 of 15 patients in the IV group required a repeat loading dose, compared with 3 of 15 in the SC group and 5 of 15 in the IM group (29,65). Thereafter, there were no significant differences in the rates of resolution of hyperglycemia or ketoacidosis among the three groups.

(2) In a follow-up prospective, randomized trial, the same investigators compared the effects of IM versus IV insulin therapy. Patients were divided into two groups and were given an initial bolus of regular insulin, either 0.22 U/kg IV plus 0.22 U/kg IM or 0.44 U/kg IV only; this was followed by administration of 7 U/hour of insulin, intramuscularly in the first group and intravenously in the second group (65). No difference was found in the therapeutic responses of the two groups, establishing that IM therapy can be as effective as IV therapy if one half of the initial loading dose is given as an IV bolus. The same authors demonstrated in yet another prospective, randomized trial that the loading dose is not necessary if continuous IV therapy is used to treat children with DKA, although an initial IV bolus of insulin is still recommended by others (19,33).

d. In summary, the recommended treatment for patients presenting with DKA includes continuous IV infusion of insulin at a rate of 5 to 25 U/hour, with or without an initial bolus of IV insulin (33,48,52). Alternatively, an initial IV bolus of 10 to 50 U may be given, followed by hourly IM injections of 5 to 10 U regular insulin. After the serum glucose level decreases to 250 to 300 mg/dl, it is prudent to start IV administration of 5% dextrose in water or in 1/2NS to avoid hypoglycemia, replete the free water deficit, and maintain the glucose in the range of 200 to 300 mg/dl while ketoacidosis resolves. The end point of treatment is elimination of ketonuria. An empirically derived infusion protocol, based on hourly glucose measurements, such as that shown in Table 23-2, may be useful (33).

e. Regarding when to resume use of regular or intermediate-acting SC insulin, data are few, but various authors suggest starting after the patient is able to eat or when ketoacidosis has resolved. In general, patients should be allowed to eat as soon as they are able. In one study based on chart reviews, the risk of hypoglycemia was significantly associated with restriction of oral intake (nothing by mouth) during hospitalization for DKA (57). In addition, a retrospective study noted a significant inverse correlation between the time to initiation of intermediate- or long-acting insulin and the length of hospital stay (58). If continuous IV insulin is used for the initial treatment, it is important to continue the infusion until the action of the SC dose begins to peak: 1 to 2 hours after the administration of regular insulin or 3 to 4 hours after the administration of intermediate-acting insulin.

3. Potassium

a. Osmotic diuresis results in total body potassium depletion in most patients with DKA. Despite this, the initial serum potassium is often increased because of acidosis and, to some degree, hyperglycemia. As these processes are corrected, redistribution of potassium from the extracellular space into the intracellular space may result in a precipitous decrease in the serum potassium concentration, with the attendant risk of ventricular arrhythmia. Therefore, it is important to anticipate this decrease and administer potassium to nonoliguric patients while serum levels are still within the normal range.

b. Retrospective studies demonstrate that although potassium requirements vary enormously (*e.g.*, from 0 to 620 mEq), the usual total replacement dose is approximately 170 to 240 mEq over 16 hours in patients not receiving large amounts of bicarbonate (12,71). This is consistent with the estimate of other authors, who noted a deficit of 3 to 5 mEq/kg of body weight (32). Androgué's prospective study comparing rates of IV hydration in 23 patients without extreme volume deficit noted a trend toward reduced potas-

Table 23-2 IV infusion protocol for treatment of DKA

Blood Glucose (mg/dl)	Insulin Infusion (U/h)	5% Dextrose in Water (ml/h)
<70	0.5	250
71–100	1	225
101–150	2	200
151–200	3	175
201–250	4	150
251–300	6	100
301–350	8	50
351–400	10	0
401–450	12	0
451–500	16	0
>500	20	0

From Foster (33) with permission.

sium requirements in patients who received a lower rate of IV fluid (124 mEq/24 hours), compared with those who received more aggressive hydration (177 mEq/24 hours) (1).

c. If the initial potassium concentration is normal or low, replacement should be started as soon as adequate urine output is demonstrated. An infusion of 20 to 40 mEq/hour of either potassium chloride or potassium phosphate (see later discussion) is usually appropriate, depending on the serum potassium concentration and the rate of IV fluid administration. For example, 40 mEq/hour can be given for patients with [K^+] <3 mmol/L, 30 mEq/hour for [K^+] <4 mmol/L, and 20 mEq/hour for [K^+] <5 mmol/L, with an IV fluid rate of 500 to 1000 ml/hour (30). Because about half of the administered potassium may be excreted in urine (71), extreme caution must be exercised in oliguric patients to avoid hyperkalemia.

d. If the initial potassium concentration is high, replacement of potassium should be delayed for two to four hours after the fluid and insulin therapies have been initiated (32). Electrocardiographic (ECG) monitoring is important; if only peaked T waves are present, then insulin and fluid are usually sufficient. Rarely, marked hyperkalemia may necessitate emergency infusion of bicarbonate (30). It is important to monitor electrolytes frequently (*e.g.*, every 2 hours) during the initial stage of therapy. Ideally, serum potassium concentrations should be maintained at ≥4 mmol/L (52).

4. Phosphate

a. Like potassium, total body phosphate is typically depleted in DKA because of urinary losses; yet, initial serum concentrations may be normal or high. In addition, treatment of DKA causes a shift of phosphate from the extracellular to the intracellular compartment and may be associated with a marked decrease in the serum phosphate concentration. In contrast to potassium, the development of hypophosphatemia during treatment of DKA is not generally associated with untoward effects. Nevertheless, severe hypophosphatemia can cause weakness, rhabdomyolysis, hemolysis, heart failure, and respiratory depression; none of these are commonly observed in DKA. Depletion of erythrocyte 2,3-diphosphoglycerate (DPG) has been observed in DKA and has been hypothesized to reduce oxygen delivery by shifting the hemoglobin dissociation curve; however, this effect may be counterbalanced by acidemia and does not appear to be clinically significant. Therefore, the consensus among most investigators is that phosphate therapy is not an essential part of treatment in most patients with DKA (30,33,52,69).

(1) Keller studied the effect of 65 mmol sodium phosphate in a prospective, randomized trial including 24 patients with DKA and 16 with NKHS (43). Although this dose was sufficient to prevent hypophosphatemia and to transiently increase the DPG concentration, no benefit was observed for clinical end points such as resolution of hyperglycemia, improvement in mental state, or mortality.

(2) Wilson conducted a prospective, randomized trial of 44 patients with DKA that compared therapy with no phosphate versus 15 mmol sodium phosphate at 4 hours after the initiation of other treatments versus 15 mmol sodium phosphate at 2, 6, and 10 hours after initiation of other treatments (45 mmol total) (79). Only one patient in the last group developed severe hypophosphatemia (phosphate <1.5 mg/dl), and this group had significantly higher phosphate levels than the control group. However, no significant differences were noted in the duration of acidosis or hyperglycemia, muscle enzyme levels, or morbidity and mortality among the three groups.

(3) Fisher randomly assigned 30 patients with DKA to receive either phosphate therapy (8.5 mmol/hour or about 6 g of phosphate in 24 hours) or no phosphate therapy (28). Although a significant difference in serum phosphate levels was achieved, no difference was observed in DPG concentrations, oxyhemoglobin dissociation, or any of a variety of indices designed to assess recovery from DKA. Both groups had some degree of hypocalcemia, but hypocalcemia was significantly more marked in the group treated with phosphate.

b. The preceding studies leave open the possibility that phosphate may have some beneficial effect in certain patients (*e.g.*, if cardiopulmonary compromise is present). Some authorities recommend measurement of the phosphate concentration at 6 hours after the initiation of treatment and consideration of repletion if it is <1 to 2 mg/ml at any time during the course of therapy (48,52,69). Repletion therapy may be given as potassium phosphate, which contains 30 mmol phosphate for each 44 mEq potassium at neutral pH, or as sodium phosphate. It is important to monitor the serum calcium, because hypocalcemia may be induced by phosphate infusion.

5. Bicarbonate

a. The use of bicarbonate in the treatment of DKA has been controversial, and no clear benefit has yet been demonstrated in prospective, randomized trials. Severe acidosis can contribute to hypotension, decreased myocardial contractility, and depression of consciousness (33). On the other hand, potential disadvantages of bicarbonate therapy include worsened hypokalemia and lactic acidosis, paradoxical acidification of cerebrospinal fluid, increased carbon dioxide production, and hypoxia (60).

(1) In a retrospective review of 73 episodes of DKA in which bicarbonate was administered and 22 episodes in which it was not, Lever was unable to find any significant difference in the rate of biochemical or neurologic recovery, or in the incidence of hypoglycemia or hypokalemia (53).

(2) Hale randomly assigned 38 patients with DKA to receive NS, either with or without 150 mEq of sodium bicarbonate added during the second hour of treatment (35). At the end of 2 hours, the increases in pH and serum bicarbonate were significantly greater in the group receiving bicarbonate ($P<0.01$), but this group also had significantly slower clearance of ketones and lactate ($P<0.02$). These findings were thought to be consistent with the effects of worsened tissue hypoxia in the bicarbonate-treated group. No difference was noted in the rate of decline of blood glucose.

(3) Morris studied 21 patients with severe DKA (arterial pH 6.90 to 7.14) in a randomized, prospective protocol in which patients in the treatment group initially received 1 to 3 ampules (44.6 to 133.8 mEq) of sodium bicarbonate, depending on the pH, and the control group was treated with saline alone. Additional bicarbonate was administered to the treatment group every 2 hours until the pH was ≥7.15. No significant difference in the resolution of acidosis, ketosis, or hyperglycemia was noted between the two groups. In addition, cerebrospinal fluid concentrations of glucose, bicarbonate, lactate, ketones, and pH were not significantly different between the two groups.

b. The available data indicate that there is no clear benefit to bicarbonate administration in patients with DKA who have an arterial pH ≥6.9. For patients who are more acidemic, no data are available, although some authors would consider bicarbonate administration for patients with a pH ≤7.0 (33,48,69). Lebovitz suggested that sodium bicarbonate be used only in the case of impending cardiovascular collapse (52), whereas Fleckman noted that lactic acidosis and severe hyperkalemia with life-threatening ECG abnormalities are reasonable indications (30). Each ampule of bicarbonate constitutes a significant sodium load and should therefore be diluted in 250 to 1000 ml of 1/2NS to avoid worsening of hyperosmolarity in patients with DKA. In patients without hyperkalemia, 10 to 20 mEq of potassium chloride should be given with each ampule of sodium bicarbonate.

6. Heparin—Although there are no data from well-controlled studies, one reviewer recommended use of low-dose heparin prophylaxis against thromboembolic complications for older patients presenting with DKA or NKHS (52).

Other investigators suggest that low-dose heparin is best avoided and advocate aggressive rehydration as the best prophylaxis (20,33).

7. **Monitoring of Therapy**
   a. Use of a flow sheet for timed recording of therapeutic interventions, vital signs, urine output, and laboratory data is essential if iatrogenic complications are to be avoided (30,33). Capillary glucose measurements can be made on an hourly basis initially. Because the anion gap and pH usually begin to normalize before the serum bicarbonate increases significantly, resolution of acidosis is best assessed by monitoring the anion gap at 1- to 2-hour intervals. Alternatively, some authors suggest repeated evaluations of venous pH, which can be correlated with arterial pH at the initial measurement and is usually lower by about 0.03 (30,48). Serial determinations of serum ketones are generally not helpful. As recovery progresses, the frequency of monitoring can be decreased.
   b. The initial evaluation is often done in an emergency room, where laboratory studies and therapy can be instituted in a timely manner. There are few data to aid in determining the subsequent disposition. Patients with mental obtundation are best cared for in an intensive care unit, where adequate monitoring is available (48). One retrospective review of 92 cases of DKA found no correlation between length of stay and level of nursing care, degree of acidosis, or disease severity score (58). Length of stay was shorter in patients managed by diabetologists and longer if the patient was admitted in the evening or had a positive bacterial culture.
8. Patient education and the availability of a support team may help prevent future episodes of DKA and are important aspects of management. Identification of precipitating factors and attempts to prevent their recurrence are essential. The utility of urine testing for ketones, in addition to capillary blood glucose testing, may need reemphasis.

D. Complications

1. Cerebral edema is estimated to occur in 1% of the episodes of DKA in children, and it carries a mortality rate of 60% to 80% (64). Subclinical brain swelling is common during therapy for DKA in children, and it is likely that neurologic complications represent an extreme of this phenomenon (50). The onset is acute, with headache and deterioration of consciousness or neurologic deficits usually occurring 6 to 24 hours after initiation of therapy. Papilledema may be present. Computed tomography scanning confirms the diagnosis.
   a. Rosenbloom's review of 69 cases suggested that prompt intervention with mannitol, hyperventilation, and/or dexamethasone may be lifesaving; 13 of 23 patients who were treated early survived with mild or no neurologic deficits. In contrast, only 3 of 46 patients who were treated late or not at all survived without neurologic deficits ($P<0.0001$) (64).
   b. In another series of 11 children, 7 of 8 patients with cerebral edema who were treated within 2 hours of onset with mannitol (0.5 to 1.0 g/kg, repeated as needed up to a total dose of 2.5 g/kg) survived, and 5 of the 7 had normal neurologic function (15). No hyperventilation therapy or glucocorticoids were used.
   c. Subclinical brain swelling has also been documented in adults with DKA. However, clinically significant cerebral edema is rare (52). Neurologic deficits occurring during DKA in adults may be caused by thrombosis in cerebral vessels.
2. Thrombosis may occur in any muscular artery and is most likely caused by the combination of increased viscosity and dehydration leading to slow blood flow; atherosclerosis probably also plays a role (33). In one retrospective study of mortality in DKA and NKHS, mesenteric and iliac thromboses accounted for 5 of 12 deaths in the NKHS group and 1 of 26 deaths in the DKA group (36). Cerebral hemorrhage or thrombosis occurred in 2 patients in the NKHS group and in 1 patient in the DKA group. MI may complicate, as well as precipitate, DKA and NKHS.

3. Other complications of DKA include shock, adult respiratory distress syndrome, acute gastric dilatation or erosive gastritis, and pancreatitis (30,33). Hepatic infarction, pituitary apoplexy, rhabdomyolysis, and arrhythmias resulting from magnesium deficiency have also been described (42).

E. Summary

1. DKA and NKHS represent a continuum of metabolic derangements associated with insulin deficiency. DKA is most characteristic of type I DM, but ketosis and acidosis may also occur in type II DM with sufficient provocation. In the United States, the incidence of DKA requiring hospitalization is 10 to 20 per 1000 diabetics per year. The mortality risk attributed to DKA ranges from 0.25 to 0.3 per year per 1000 diabetics, or about 2% of those admitted with a primary diagnosis of DKA. Other studies from developed countries also report mortality rates of 2% to 5% for patients admitted with DKA. There is no consensus definition for DKA. Although the diagnosis requires the presence of an anion-gap metabolic acidosis and ketonemia, the degree to which these abnormalities are present varies widely.
2. About 30% to 50% of the cases of DKA are precipitated by infection. Urinary tract infections, including pyelonephritis, and pneumonia are the most common. Other common precipitants include omission of insulin or inadequate insulin therapy (10% to 30%) and new-onset or previously undiagnosed DM (5% to 27%). MI, stroke, pancreatitis, drugs, pregnancy, and psychological factors may also play a role in precipitation of DKA. The precipitating event remains unknown in 14% to 25% of cases.
3. Prompt diagnosis and therapy are essential for optimal care of the patient with DKA. Goals of therapy include rehydration, correction of pH and elimination of ketonemia, normalization of blood glucose, and prevention of complications. IV fluid is important for (a) maintaining cardiac output and renal perfusion, (b) reducing blood glucose concentration and plasma osmolality, and (c) decreasing the concentrations of glucagon, cortisol, and other counterregulatory hormones implicated in ketogenesis.
4. There are no data to support the use of hypotonic fluid in the initial management of DKA. In the absence of circulatory insufficiency, the rate of fluid administration need not be rapid. A reasonable replacement schedule for most adults would be NS at a rate of 1 L/hour for the initial hour, followed by 500 ml/hour during the next 8 hours. After the initial period of volume replacement, 1/2NS rather than NS may be used if the serum sodium concentration exceeds 150 mmol/L. Most investigators recommend changing to an IV dextrose solution (*e.g.*, 5% dextrose in 1/2NS) after the blood glucose concentration decreases to 250 to 300 mg/dl in order to avoid hypoglycemia and to replete the free water deficit.
5. The effects of insulin in DKA are (a) to decrease glucagon production by the pancreas, (b) to counteract the ketogenic and gluconeogenic action of glucagon in the liver, (c) to increase the rate of glucose utilization in muscle and fat, and (d) to inhibit lipolysis in fat, thereby decreasing the availability of substrates for hepatic ketogenesis. It is important to administer IV fluid concurrently with insulin to avoid further intravascular volume depletion, hypernatremia, or even circulatory collapse.
6. The recommended treatment for patients presenting with DKA includes continuous IV infusion of insulin at a rate of 5 to 25 U/hour, with or without an initial bolus of IV insulin. Alternatively, an initial IV bolus of 10 to 50 U may be given, followed by intermittent IM injections of regular insulin, 5 to 10 U hourly. After the serum glucose level decreases to 250 to 300 mg/dl, it is necessary to start 5% dextrose in water or in 1/2NS intravenously to avoid hypoglycemia, replete the free water deficit, and maintain the glucose in the range of 200 to 300 mg/dl while ketoacidosis resolves. In general, regular- and intermediate-acting SC insulin can be started after the patient is able to eat. If continuous IV insulin is used for the initial treatment, it is important to continue the infusion until the action of the subcutaneous dose begins to peak.

7. During the course of treatment of DKA, serum levels of potassium must be monitored closely. If the initial potassium concentration is normal or low, replacement should be started as soon as adequate urine output is demonstrated. Extreme caution must be exercised in oliguric patients in order to avoid hyperkalemia. There is consensus among most investigators that phosphate therapy is not an essential part of treatment in most patients with DKA. However, some authorities recommend measurement of the phosphate concentration at 6 hours after the initiation of treatment and administration of sodium or potassium phosphate if the serum phosphate concentration is <1 to 2 mg/ml at any time during the course of therapy.
8. The available data indicate that there is no clear benefit to bicarbonate administration in patients with DKA who have an arterial pH ≥ 6.9. For patients who are more acidemic, no data are available, although some authors would consider bicarbonate administration for patients with pH ≤ 7.0. Lebovitz suggested that sodium bicarbonate should be used only in the case of impending cardiovascular collapse, whereas Fleckman noted that lactic acidosis and severe hyperkalemia with life-threatening ECG abnormalities are reasonable indications.
9. Use of a flow sheet for timed recording of therapeutic interventions, vital signs, urine output, and laboratory data is essential if iatrogenic complications are to be avoided. Capillary glucose measurements can be made on an hourly basis initially. The anion gap and pH usually begin to normalize before the serum bicarbonate increases significantly, so resolution of acidosis is best assessed by monitoring the anion gap at 1 to 2 hour intervals. Serial determinations of ketonemia are generally not helpful. As recovery progresses, the frequency of monitoring can be decreased. The end point of the acute treatment of DKA is elimination of ketonuria.
10. Patient education and the availability of a support team may help prevent future episodes of DKA and are important aspects of management. Identification of precipitating factors and attempts to prevent their recurrence are essential. The utility of urine testing for ketones, in addition to capillary blood glucose testing, may need reemphasis.

Abbreviations used in Chapter 23

1/2NS = 0.45% saline solution
BUN = blood urea nitrogen
DKA = diabetic ketoacidosis
DM = diabetes mellitus
DPG = 2,3-diphosphoglycerate
ECG = electrocardiographic
IM = intramuscular
IV = intravenous
MI = myocardial infarction
N = number of patients
NKHS = nonketotic hyperosmolar syndrome
NS = normal saline, 0.9% saline solution
SC = subcutaneous
vs. = versus

References

1. Adrogué. Salutary effects of modest fluid replacement in the treatment of adults with diabetic ketoacidosis: use in patients without extreme volume deficit. *JAMA* 1989;262:2108.

2. Adrogué. Diabetic ketoacidosis: role of kidney in the acid-base homeostasis re-evaluated. *Kidney Int* 1984;25:591.
3. Adrogué. Plasma acid-base patterns in diabetic ketoacidosis. *N Engl J Med* 1982; 307:1603.
4. Alberti. Low-dose insulin in the treatment of diabetic ketoacidosis. *Arch Intern Med* 1977;137:1367.
5. Alberti. Diabetic coma: a reappraisal after five years. *Clin Endocrinol Metab* 1977; 6:421.
6. Alberti. Small doses of intramuscular insulin in the treatment of diabetic "coma." *Lancet* 1973;2:515.
7. Arieff. Cerebral edema and depression of sensorium in nonketotic hyperosmolar coma. *Diabetes* 1974;23:525.
8. Axelrod. Diabetic emergencies and the Loch Ness monster. *Intensive Care Med* 1987; 13:1.
9. Baird. Diabetic ketoacidosis as the presentation of renal aspergilloma. *Am J Med* 1988;85:453.
10. Barrett. Insulin resistance in diabetic ketoacidosis. *Diabetes* 1982;31:923.
11. Beigelman. Severe diabetic ketoacidosis (diabetic "coma"). *Diabetes* 1971;20:490.
12. Beigelman. Potassium in severe diabetic ketoacidosis. *Am J Med* 1973;54:419.
13. Beigelman. Thirty-two fatal cases of severe diabetic ketoacidosis, including a case of mucormycosis. *Diabetes* 1973;22:847.
14. Bell. Ketoacidosis without hyperglycemia during self-monitoring of diabetes. *Diabetes Care* 1983;6:622.
15. Bello. Cerebral edema in diabetic ketoacidosis in children. *Lancet* 1990;336:64.
16. Bock. Real and artifactual erythrocyte swelling in hyperglycemia. *Diabetologia* 1985; 28:335.
17. Bonadio. Outpatient management of diabetic ketoacidosis. *Am J Dis Child* 1988; 142:448.
18. Burge. Short-term fasting is a mechanism for the development of euglycemic ketoacidosis during periods of insulin deficiency. J Clin Endocrinol Metab 1993;76: 1192.
19. Burghen. Comparison of high dose and low dose insulin by continuous infusion in the treatment of diabetic ketoacidosis in children. *Diabetes Care* 1980;3:15.
20. Carroll. Uncontrolled diabetes mellitus in adults: experience in treating diabetic ketoacidosis and hyperosmolar nonketotic coma with low-dose insulin and a uniform treatment regimen. *Diabetes Care* 1983;6:579.
21. Chernow. "Bovine ketosis" in a nondiabetic postpartum woman. *Diabetes Care* 1982;5:47.
22. Clements. Fatal diabetic ketoacidosis: major causes and approaches to their prevention. *Diabetes Care* 1978;1:314.
23. DCCT Research Group. The effect of intensive treatment of diabetes on the development and progression of long term complications in insulin-dependent diabetes mellitus. *N Engl J Med* 1993;329:977.
24. Duck. Factors associated with brain herniation in the treatment of diabetic ketoacidosis. *J Pediatr* 1988;113:10.
25. Faich. The epidemiology of diabetic acidosis: a population-based study. *Am J Epidemiol* 1983;117:551.
26. Fein. Relation of colloid osmotic pressure to arterial hypoxemia and cerebral edema during crystalloid volume loading of patients with diabetic ketoacidosis. *Ann Intern Med* 1982;96:570.
27. Fishbein. Diabetic ketoacidosis, hyperosmolar nonketotic coma, lactic acidosis and hypoglycemia. In: Harris, ed. *Diabetes in America.* National Diabetes Group. Washington, DC: US Department of Health and Human Services, 1985:1.
28. Fisher. A randomized study of phosphate therapy in the treatment of diabetic ketoacidosis. *J Clin Endocrinol Metab* 1983;57:117.
29. Fisher. Diabetic ketoacidosis: low dose insulin therapy by various routes. *N Engl J Med* 1977;297:238.
30. Fleckman. Diabetic ketoacidosis. *Endocrinol Metab Clin North Am* 1993;22:181.

31. Foster. Diabetes mellitus. In: Isselbacher, ed. *Harrison's Principles of Internal Medicine*, ed 13. New York: McGraw-Hill, 1994:1979.
32. Foster. The metabolic derangements and treatment of diabetic ketoacidosis. *N Engl J Med* 1983;309:159.
33. Foster. Diabetes mellitus: acute complications, ketoacidosis, hyperosmolar coma, lactic acidosis. In: DeGroot, ed. *Endocrinology*, ed 3. Philadelphia: WB Saunders, 1985:1506.
34. Fulop. Severe hypertriglyceridemia in diabetic ketosis. *Am J Med Sci* 1990;300:361.
35. Hale. Metabolic effects of bicarbonate in the treatment of diabetic ketoacidosis. *Br Med J* 1984;289:1035.
36. Hamblin. Deaths associated with diabetic ketoacidosis and hyperosmolar coma, 1973–1988. *Med J Aust* 1989;151:439.
37. Harris. Minimizing the risk of brain herniation during treatment of diabetic ketoacidemia: a retrospective and prospective study. *J Pediatrics* 1990;117:22.
38. Heber. Low-dose continuous insulin therapy for diabetic ketoacidosis. *Arch Intern Med* 1977;137:1377.
39. Hockaday. Diabetic coma. *Clin Endocrinol Metab* 1972;1:751.
40. Jenkins. Euglycemic diabetic ketoacidosis: does it exist? *Acta Diabetol* 1993;30:251.
41. Johnson. Diabetic ketoacidosis in a community-based population. *Mayo Clin Proc* 1980;55:83.
42. Keller. Diabetic ketoacidosis: current views on pathogenesis and treatment. *Diabetologia* 1986;29:71.
43. Keller. Prevention of hypophosphatemia by phosphate infusion during treatment of diabetic ketoacidosis and hyperosmolar coma. *Diabetes* 1980;29:87.
44. Keller. Course and prognosis of 86 episodes of diabetic coma: a five year experience with a uniform schedule of treatment. *Diabetologia* 1975;11:93.
45. Kidson. Treatment of severe diabetes mellitus by insulin infusion. *Br Med J* 1974;2:691.
46. Kitabchi. The efficacy of low dose versus conventional therapy of insulin for treatment of diabetic ketoacidosis. *Ann Intern Med* 1976;84:633.
47. Kitabchi. Diabetic ketoacidosis and hyperosmolar hyperglycemic nonketotic coma. *Med Clin North Am* 1988;72:1545.
48. Kitabchi. Diabetic ketoacidosis. *Med Clin North Am* 1995;79:9.
49. Kitabchi. Diabetic ketoacidosis: reappraisal of therapeutic approach. *Annu Rev Med* 1979;30:339.
50. Krane. Subclinical brain swelling in children during treatment of diabetic ketoacidosis. *N Engl J Med* 1985;312:1147.
51. Lambertus. Diabetic ketoacidosis following pentamidine therapy in a patient with the acquired immunodeficiency syndrome. *West J Med* 1988;149:602.
52. Lebovitz. Diabetic ketoacidosis. *Lancet* 1995;345:767.
53. Lever. Sodium bicarbonate therapy in severe diabetic ketoacidosis. *Am J Med* 1983;75:263.
54. Luzi. Metabolic effects of low-dose insulin therapy on glucose metabolism in diabetic ketoacidosis. *Diabetes* 1988;37:1470.
55. Mahoney. Extreme gestational starvation ketoacidosis: case report and review of pathophysiology. *Am J Kidney Dis* 1992;20:276.
56. Malone. Characteristics of diabetic ketoacidosis in older versus younger adults. *J Am Geriatr Soc* 1992;40:1100.
57. Malone. Frequent hypoglycemic episodes in the treatment of patients with diabetic ketoacidosis. *Arch Intern Med* 1992;152:2472.
58. May. Resource utilization in the treatment of diabetic ketoacidosis in adults. *Am J Med Sci* 1983;306:287.
59. Munro. Euglycemic diabetic ketoacidosis. *Br Med J* 1973;2:578.
60. Narins. Bicarbonate therapy for organic acidosis: the case for its continued use. *Ann Intern Med* 1987;106:615.
61. Owen. Renal function and effects of partial rehydration during diabetic ketoacidosis. *Diabetes* 1981;30:510.

62. Padilla. "Low-dose" versus "high-dose" insulin regimens in the treatment of uncontrolled diabetes: a survey. *Am J Med* 1977;63:843.
63. Page. Treatment of diabetic coma with continuous low-dose infusion of insulin. *Br Med J* 1974;2:687.
64. Rosenbloom. Intracerebral crises during treatment of diabetic ketoacidosis. *Diabetes Care* 1990;13:22.
65. Sacks. Similar responsiveness of diabetic ketoacidosis to low-dose insulin by intramuscular injection and albumin-free infusion. *Ann Intern Med* 1979;90:36.
66. Schade. Diabetic ketoacidosis: pathogenesis, prevention and therapy. *Clin Endocrinol Metab* 1983;12:321.
67. Semple. Continuous intravenous infusion of small doses of insulin in the treatment of diabetic ketoacidosis. *Br Med J* 1974;2:694.
68. Sheppard. The effect on mortality of low-dose insulin therapy for diabetic ketoacidosis. *Diabetes Care* 1982;5:111.
69. Siperstein. Diabetic ketoacidosis and hyperosmolar coma. *Endocrinol Metab Clin North Am* 1992;21:415.
70. Snorgaard. Diabetic ketoacidosis in Denmark: epidemiology, incidence rates, precipitating factors and mortality rates. *J Intern Med* 1989;226:223.
71. Soler. Potassium balance during treatment of diabetic ketoacidosis, with special reference to the use of bicarbonate. *Lancet* 1972;2:665.
72. Stephenson. Microvascular and acute complications in IDDM patients: the EURODIAB IDDM complications study. *Diabetologia* 1994;37:278.
73. Tattersall. Course of brittle diabetes: 12 year follow up. *Br Med J* 1991;302:1240.
74. Vinicor. Hyperamylasemia in diabetic ketoacidosis: sources and significance. *Ann Intern Med* 1979;91:200.
75. Waldhäusl. Severe hyperglycemia: effects of rehydration on endocrine derangements and blood glucose concentration. *Diabetes* 1979;28:577.
76. Watkins. The effect of ketone bodies in the determination of creatinine. *Clin Chim Acta* 1967;18:191.
77. Westphal. The occurrence of diabetic ketoacidosis in non-insulin-dependent diabetes and newly diagnosed diabetic adults. *Am J Med* 1996;101:19
78. Wetterhall. Trends in diabetes and diabetic complications, 1980–1987. *Diabetes Care* 1992;15:960.
79. Wilson. Phosphate therapy in diabetic ketoacidosis. *Arch Intern Med* 1982;142:517.

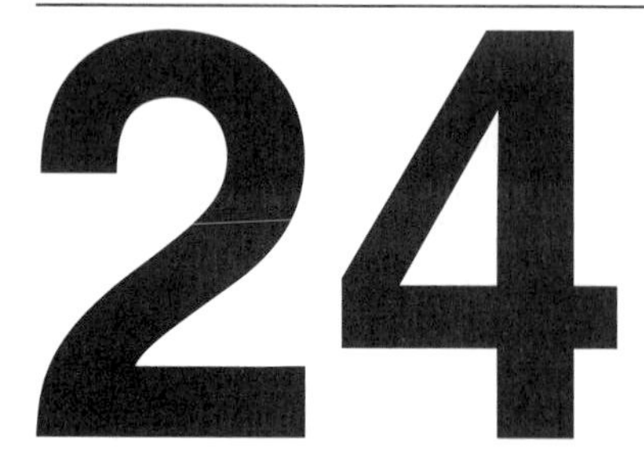

HIV Antiretroviral Therapy

Albert C. Shaw and
Morton N. Swartz

A. Introduction

1. Epidemiology

a. In 1981, the reports of Kaposi's sarcoma and *Pneumocystis carinii* pneumonia (PCP) among homosexual men from New York City, Los Angeles, and San Francisco signaled the clinical appearance in the United States of the human immunodeficiency virus type 1 (HIV-1) (10,11). Transmission of HIV was subsequently found to occur by perinatal, sexual, or parenteral routes (blood products or IV drug use). Since that time, the scope of the HIV pandemic has continued to expand. More than 1 million people in the United States have been infected with HIV, and by 1995 there were >500,000 cases of acquired immunodeficiency syndrome (AIDS) and >300,000 deaths from AIDS (14).

b. Although transmission by male same-sex contact represented 43% of the cases in 1994, this proportion was less than the 1985 figure of 66% (13). However, HIV infection acquired through IV drug use (27% of the cases in 1994) and heterosexual contact (10% of the cases in 1994) has increased in importance (13,15). Furthermore, the incidence of AIDS among women continues to rise dramatically; only 7% of AIDS patients were female in 1985, compared with 18% in 1994 (16). Correspondingly, increasing numbers of children are being affected by HIV; 1017 infants were born infected with HIV in the United States in 1994, compared with 8% in 1993 (15).

c. Worldwide, the most common route of transmission is by heterosexual contact. Estimates for 1995 indicate that 24 million adults and 1.5 million children in the world have been infected with HIV; 5 million have died from AIDS (78). Seventy percent of the adults and 90% of the children infected with HIV are from sub-Saharan Africa, where the epidemic has been particularly devastating. For example, urban areas in Rwanda report an HIV-positive seroprevalence rate of 18% among the general population but as high as 30% among persons between the ages of 26 and 40 years (44). Recent estimates suggest seroprevalence rates of >40% in high-risk urban areas of East Africa (88). HIV has taken a heavy toll even in rural areas; in a group of Ugandan villages, where the seroprevalence rates are <10%, HIV disease accounts for >50% of the mortality among adults and >80% of the deaths among adolescents and young adults between the ages of 13 and 44 years (67).

d. However, epidemiologic data indicate that HIV is currently spreading most rapidly in Southeast Asia. For example, Thailand and India have reported alarming rates of HIV infection among female sex workers and IV drug users, with seroconversion rates of 3% to 5% per month for both groups (51,81). Up to 40% and 65% of the female sex workers in India and Thailand, respectively, are infected with HIV (5,17). Furthermore, of 2417 Thai military recruits studied in one report from 1993, 12% were found to be HIV-positive (69). With the institution of aggressive public education programs, including the promotion of universal condom usage among commercial sex workers, the HIV seroprevalence rate decreased to 6.7% among military draftees surveyed in 1995 (68). Nevertheless, projections of the World

Health Organization suggest that Southeast Asia may surpass sub-Saharan Africa in the incidence of HIV infection by the year 2000 (77). The cumulative global estimate of the number of cases of HIV infection by the year 2000 is 40 million, with >90% of these from developing nations (78).

2. Pathogenesis

a. HIV-1 is a member of the lentivirus family of retroviruses. The structure of the HIV-1 genome is described in this section (56,73).

(1) The *gag* genes encode the capsid proteins including p24, which can be detected in the serum of infected patients.

(2) The *pol* gene encodes the HIV-1 reverse transcriptase which transcribes viral genomic RNA into DNA, the integrase protein which mediates the integration of the viral DNA into the host genome, and the HIV-1 protease which cleaves a fusion protein containing the juxtaposed gag and pol polypeptides into functional gag and pol. The HIV-1 reverse transcriptase is the major target of the currently available antiretroviral agents such as azidothymidine (AZT). The HIV-1 integrase and the protease are the targets for newer antiretroviral agents. The significant error rate of the HIV-1 reverse transcriptase is responsible for the frequent mutations in the sequence of the viral proteins and has frustrated many attempts to develop effective antiretroviral agents.

(3) The *env* gene encodes viral envelope proteins such as gp120 (for glycoprotein of 120,000 Da molecular weight) and gp41, which form the external protein coat of the virion. It appears that the gp120 protein interacts with the CD4 protein on the surface of human helper T lymphocytes and, together with gp41, facilitates entry of the virus into T cells. The env proteins have formed the basis for prototype HIV-1 vaccines.

(4) However, the CD4 molecule alone is not sufficient for HIV infection, since nonhuman cells expressing human CD4 cannot be infected; recent experiments from several groups have implicated proteins in the α- and β-chemokine receptor families as HIV-1 coreceptors that act in concert with CD4 to facilitate viral infection (18,31,33,34,38). The coreceptor function may be fulfilled by different receptor family members in different cell types and in different viral strains. These findings suggest new avenues for the development of animal models of HIV infection as well as potential targets for new classes of therapeutic agents.

(5) The *tat* gene encodes an essential protein that augments transcription of the HIV-1 genes. This protein is also a target for experimental antiretroviral agents.

(6) The *rev* gene encodes an essential protein that regulates splicing of viral RNA species and promotes the export of viral RNAs from the host nucleus; these viral RNAs facilitate the generation of new viral particles in productive, as opposed to latent, infection.

(7) At least four additional proteins, whose functions remain unclear, are also encoded by the HIV-1 genome. One of these proteins, encoded by the *nef* gene, has recently been of particular interest. A single American hemophiliac (50) and a cohort of 7 Australian patients (30) were reported to be infected with HIV for >10 years without any clinical manifestations of immunodeficiency. The Australian patients had all received blood transfusions from an HIV-positive donor carrying a virus whose *nef* gene was inactivated by mutation; similar *nef* mutations were found in virus isolated from the hemophiliac, leading to the intriguing possibility that a defective *nef* gene can disarm the pathogenic potential of HIV-1.

(8) It is evident that HIV-1 contains a sophisticated genetic regulatory system which potentially allows it to react to conditions within the host cell (*e.g.*, using the rev protein to control the types of RNA available for protein translation and optimize the conditions for viral reproduction).

b. A full discussion of the pathogenesis of HIV-1 infection is beyond the scope of this chapter. However, two recent developments have yielded important insights.

(1) A nagging paradox has been the difficulty in detecting HIV-1–infected T cells in the circulation during the clinical latency period—that is, when the patient is asymptomatic but the number of CD4-positive T lymphocytes (CD4 count) is decreasing. This paradox has been the basis for the opinions that have gone so far as to claim that HIV-1 is actually not the cause of AIDS. Such arguments have been convincingly repudiated by those experiments demonstrating that HIV-1 is sequestered in lymphoid tissue during early infection; viral DNA and RNA were found in increased amounts in lymph nodes compared with the much lower levels of DNA and RNA isolatable from peripheral blood lymphocytes. In late stages of AIDS, lymphoid architecture is destroyed, presumably releasing sequestered virus and resulting in high-grade viremia detectable in peripheral blood (35,72). Consequently, a clinical but not a microbiologic latency is present in HIV-1 infection.

(2) Recent studies employing mathematical modeling to examine the kinetics of CD4-positive T cells and HIV-1 in the setting of antiretroviral therapy have revealed extraordinary turnover rates for both T lymphocytes and virions. The mean half-life of HIV in plasma was calculated at 6 hours; the immune system appears to clear 10^8 to $>10^{10}$ viral particles per day, or approximately one-third of the average total virus load in a patient. Moreover, 2×10^9 CD4-positive T lymphocytes are lost per day (with an average lifespan of 2.2 days), presumably killed by the cytotoxic T lymphocytes that recognize and destroy the virus-infected cells. In early HIV disease, this clearance of viruses and infected cells may keep clinical progression in abeyance. Even in those patients with late-stage AIDS, it appears that the battle continues to wage between the rapidly mutating viruses and the immune system. Ultimately, however, the ability to replenish infected T lymphocytes is overwhelmed, resulting in irreparable immune system injury and clinical immunodeficiency (47,74,92). The finding of vigorous viral replication at early stages of HIV disease argues strongly for early therapeutic intervention.

3. Clinical Classification

a. The diagnostic criteria for AIDS were revised by the Centers for Disease Control (CDC) in 1993. Added to the list of AIDS-defining illnesses were recurrent pneumonia, pulmonary tuberculosis, and invasive cervical cancer. In addition, HIV-positive patients with CD4 counts <200 cells/ml and those with a ratio of $CD4^+$ to total lymphocytes $<14\%$ were also included. These changes had the effect of increasing the number of AIDS cases on the basis of definition alone.

b. The current CDC listing of AIDS-defining illnesses includes the following (12): candidiasis of the bronchi, trachea, lungs, or esophagus; invasive cervical carcinoma; coccidioidomycosis (disseminated or extrapulmonary); extrapulmonary cryptococcosis; cytomegalovirus (CMV) infection (except liver, spleen, and nodes); CMV retinitis; HIV encephalopathy; herpes simplex virus (chronic ulcers >1 month duration, bronchitis, pneumonitis, or esophagitis); histoplasmosis (disseminated or extrapulmonary); isosporiasis; Kaposi's sarcoma; immunoblastic or Burkitt's lymphoma; primary central nervous system lymphoma; infection with *Mycobacterium avium* complex, *Mycobacterium kansasii*, or other *Mycobacterium* species (disseminated or extrapulmonary); pulmonary or extrapulmonary tuberculosis; PCP; recurrent pneumonia; progressive multifocal leukoencephalopathy; recurrent *Salmonella* septicemia; central nervous system toxoplasmosis; and HIV wasting syndrome.

c. The CDC clinical classification of HIV disease has frequently been used to stratify patients in clinical trials. For example, several studies of antiretroviral therapy employ progression to CDC group IV disease as an end point. Based on the 1987 definitions of HIV disease, group IV describes symptomatic patients with constitutional disease (*i.e.*, HIV wasting syndrome; group IV-A); neurologic disorders including HIV encephalopathy (group IV-B); secondary infectious diseases including AIDS-defining illnesses (group IV-C1) and others such as oral thrush, oral hairy leukoplakia, and herpes zoster (group IV-C2); and secondary malignancies (IV-D). In practice, these classifications are not clinically useful (despite significant simplification in the revised 1993 system). Clinically useful manifestations of worsening immunosuppression that correlate with the risk of progression to AIDS include oral candidiasis and oral hairy leukoplakia (8,43,52,65).

d. The CD4 count is the most commonly employed laboratory test for assessing HIV disease progression, although other immunologic markers such as β_2-microglobulin are also predictive (37). In one cohort from the San Francisco General Hospital, the 3-year risk of progression to AIDS was 87% for subjects with CD4 counts <200/μl, 46% for 200 to 400/μl, and 16% for >400/μl (65). Similar results have been reported in other studies (42,76).

(1) The CD4 count demonstrates diurnal variation, so that mean differences of 59/μl have been observed during a 24-hour period in HIV-positive subjects (58). In addition, laboratory variation in CD4 count determinations may also be significant (82). These factors should be considered to correctly use the CD4 count for prognostic purposes.

(2) At present, the CD4 count remains a useful parameter in helping to decide when to initiate antiretroviral therapy or prophylactic therapy against opportunistic infections. However, recent evidence suggests that the CD4 count is an imperfect indicator for HIV disease progression, particularly in the setting of antiretroviral therapy with AZT (19,29) or coinfection with human T-cell lymphotropic virus type I (84). As additional information on the course of HIV disease is elucidated, other biologic markers (*e.g.*, syncytium-forming viral phenotype) may prove to be informative (53).

e. Recent studies suggest that HIV RNA, detected and quantitated by amplification of RNA from plasma, is an independent predictor of clinical course, even in patients with unchanged CD4 counts. This important topic is addressed in section F.

4. To date, almost all of the prospective randomized controlled trials (PRCTs) of antiretroviral therapy have focused on the effects of nucleoside analogs on the rate of progression of HIV-1 disease. These drugs inhibit the activity of the viral reverse transcriptase with the goal of blocking the conversion of viral RNA to DNA, a step that is essential for viral integration and replication within the host cell.

a. Because of patient demographics at the beginning of the AIDS epidemic, the overwhelming majority of subjects in these trials were white men. At present, these data must be extrapolated to reach conclusions for other racial groups and for women.

b. In several studies, changes in clinical practice driven by newly published information mandated modification of the study protocol during the course of a trial (*e.g.*, offering open-label drug to patients). Although these changes were necessary for ethical reasons, they sometimes complicated the analysis of the data and may have weakened the conclusions of some trials.

B. Azidothymidine (Zidovudine)

1. AZT Versus Placebo in Patients With AIDS or AIDS-Related Complex— The first study to demonstrate a beneficial effect of AZT in patients with AIDS or AIDS-related complex (ARC) was published by Fischl in 1987 (39). This double-blind PRCT randomly assigned 282 patients (269 males) with AIDS or ARC and CD4 counts of <500/μl to receive either AZT (250 mg PO q 4 hours) or placebo. AIDS was defined as occurrence of a first episode of PCP within 4 months before randomization. Patients with recurrent PCP, malignancy, or other opportunistic infections were excluded. ARC was defined as the presence of either unexplained weight loss (>6.8 kg or 10% of body weight within 3 months of randomization) or oral thrush and one of the following features: unexplained fever, night sweats or diarrhea, herpes zoster, oral hairy leukoplakia, or extrainguinal lymphadenopathy. Clinical end points were survival, rate of opportunistic infections, AIDS-related malignancies, Karnofsky score, body weight, and the severity of HIV-related symptoms. Twenty-one patients receiving AZT and 40 receiving placebo dropped out of the study before completion. Although the trial was designed to continue for 6 months, it was stopped after a mean follow-up of 4 months.

a. **Survival**—Nineteen patients in the placebo group but only 1 in the AZT group died during the trial ($P<0.001$). The 24-week survival rate was 98% for the AZT group and 78% for the placebo group ($P<0.001$). A similar survival benefit was observed for the subgroups of patients with AIDS (96% with AZT versus 76% placebo, $P<0.001$), ARC (100% versus 81%, $P<0.016$), CD4 count <100/μl (96% versus 70%, $P<0.001$), and CD4 count <100/μl (100% versus 91%, $P=0.028$). Subsequent follow-up at 36 weeks revealed a mortality rate of 6.2% for the AZT group and 39.3% for the placebo group.
b. **Risk of Opportunistic Infections**—Forty-five and 24 opportunistic infections occurred in the placebo and AZT groups, respectively. The probability of developing an opportunistic infection was 0.23 with AZT and 0.43 with placebo ($P<0.001$).
c. **CD4 Count**—AZT therapy was associated with a significant increase in the CD4 count. For patients with AIDS, the mean baseline count of 66/μl rose to 152/μl after 4 weeks of therapy. In contrast, subjects taking placebo demonstrated a progressive decrease in the CD4 count during the study. The AZT-induced increase in the CD4 count appeared to wane after 12 weeks, so that the mean count was at baseline by week 20.
d. **Miscellaneous Effects**—No statistically significant difference was observed in the incidence of Kaposi's sarcoma. Statistically significant improvements in Karnofsky score and body weight were noted with AZT.
e. Conducted nearly a decade ago, this trial in a patient population with advanced immunosuppression (as indicated by mean CD4 count) predated the general use of PCP prophylaxis. In addition, the mean duration of follow-up was only 6 months, and the trial's limited definition of AIDS (first-episode PCP) would not be used today. However, its importance is clear as the first trial to demonstrate clinical efficacy of an agent against HIV; in addition, these results still have practical value in indicating a benefit for AZT monotherapy in previously untreated advanced HIV disease.

2. **AZT Versus Placebo in Patients With Early HIV Infection**—AIDS Clinical Trials Group (ACTG) protocol 016 was the first trial to demonstrate a benefit of AZT therapy for patients with ARC and CD4 counts <500/μl (40). This double-blind PRCT examined the efficacy of AZT (200 mg q 4 hours) versus placebo among 711 HIV-positive patients (672 male) with mildly symptomatic early HIV infection. These patients had CD4 counts between 200 and 800/μl and up to two of the following: oral thrush, oral hairy leukoplakia, single dermatomal herpes zoster, or weight loss (>4.5 kg or 10% of body weight), all documented up to 3 years before enrollment; recurrent seborrheic dermatitis or folliculitis, intermittent diarrhea (within 4 months before enrollment, for ≥14 days); or chronic fatigue within 6 months before enrollment. Patients with AIDS were excluded. Clinical end points were progression to AIDS or advanced ARC; ARC was defined as a CD4 count <200 cells/ml on two consecutive measurements plus two of the following: recurrent oral thrush, oral hairy leukoplakia, multidermatomal herpes zoster, weight loss (as defined previously), recurrent fever (>38.5° C for at least 2 weeks or for 15 days out of 30), or severe diarrhea (more than three stools per day for 1 month or longer). Almost one-third of the

enrolled subjects (224 patients) withdrew from the trial; 41 did so when they reached a clinical end point, 16 because of toxicity, 2 because of death, and 164 (93 receiving placebo, 71 receiving AZT) because of noncompliance or individual request. An additional 38 patients were lost to follow-up. The data were analyzed on an intention-to-treat basis. Twenty months into the study, the protocol was revised to allow PCP prophylaxis with aerosolized pentamidine. The study was terminated early after a mean follow-up of 11 months.

a. **Progression to AIDS or Advanced ARC**—Clinical end points were reached in 36 of the placebo group and 15 of the AZT group, (P=0.0013; RR, 2.68 for placebo; 95% CI, 1.47 to 4.92). The 18-month event-free survival rates were 81% (95% CI, 74% to 88%) for the placebo group and 91% (95% CI, 87% to 96%) for the AZT group.
   (1) The benefit of AZT was most evident for patients with CD4 counts between 200 and 500/μl. Among these subjects, 34 reached clinical end points in the placebo group and only 12 in the AZT group; the 18-month event-free survival rates were 76% (95% CI, 68% to 85%) for the placebo group and 90% (95% CI, 84% to 96%) for the AZT group (P=0.0002; RR, 3.23 for placebo; 95% CI, 1.67 to 6.24).
   (2) For patients with CD4 counts between 500 and 800/μl, there was no significant difference in the rate of disease progression (two events among 96 patients receiving placebo, three events among 98 patients receiving AZT; P=0.63).
   (3) No mortality data were reported.
b. **CD4 Count**—CD4 counts improved significantly for patients with baseline values between 200 and 500/μl as well as for those with values between 500 and 800/μl. However, the improvement was transient in both cases, with a subsequent decrease in CD4 counts to baseline after 40 weeks in the former group and after 8 weeks in the latter.
c. **Adverse Effects**—Neutropenia (absolute neutrophil count [ANC] <750/μl) was more common with AZT than with placebo (4% versus 1%, respectively; P=0.03). Anemia (hemoglobin <8.0 g/dl) occurred in 5% of those receiving AZT but in no patients in the placebo group. Nonspecific symptoms such as malaise, nausea, vomiting, bloating, and dyspepsia were also more common with AZT.

3. **AZT Versus Placebo in Asymptomatic HIV-Positive Patients**—ACTG protocol 019 specifically evaluated the benefit of antiretroviral therapy for asymptomatic HIV-positive patients (91). The study also tested the relative efficacy of 500 versus 1500 mg per day of AZT. The 1338 HIV-positive patients (92% male, 91% Caucasian) with CD4 counts <500/μl and no prior diagnosis of AIDS or ARC were randomly assigned to receive either placebo, 500 mg/day of AZT (100 mg q 4 hours while awake), or 1500 mg/day of AZT (300 mg q 4 hours while awake). Clinical end points were onset of AIDS, advanced ARC (defined as in the ACTG 016 study), or severe side effects. In general, patients did not receive PCP prophylaxis. Revision of the protocol 1 month before its termination did allow aerosolized pentamidine to be given to patients with CD4 counts <200/μl, but these patients were evenly distributed among the three groups. The code for the trial was broken after a mean follow-up of 55 weeks. A total of 265 patients withdrew from the trial, including 111 from the placebo group, 73 from the low-dose group, and 81 from the higher-dose group. An additional 87 patients were lost to follow-up, including 41 from the placebo group (P=0.05), 19 from the low-dose group, and 27 from the higher-dose group.

a. **Progression of Disease**—Thirty-three of those patients receiving placebo developed AIDS. In contrast, 11 patients receiving 500 mg/day of AZT developed AIDS (RR, 2.8 for placebo; 95% CI, 1.4 to 5.6), as did 14 of those receiving 1500 mg/day (RR, 1.9 for placebo; 95% CI, 1.0 to 3.5). Similarly, 38 patients receiving placebo developed AIDS or advanced ARC, compared with 17 in the low-dose AZT group (RR, 2.1 for placebo; 95% CI, 1.2 to 3.7) and 19 in the higher-dose AZT group (RR, 1.6 for placebo; 95% CI, 0.9 to 2.7).

b. **CD4 Counts**—Compared with placebo therapy, the CD4 counts significantly improved with either dose of AZT. On an annual basis, the CD4 counts increased by a median of 39/μl in the low-dose AZT group and 26/μl in the high-dose AZT group, whereas they decreased by 16/μl in the placebo group.

c. **Adverse Effects**—The 500 mg/day AZT regimen was well tolerated; the incidence of anemia (hemoglobin <8 g/dl) or neutropenia (ANC <750 cells/μl) was higher for patients receiving low-dose AZT compared with placebo, but the difference was not statistically significant. Five patients receiving low-dose AZT developed anemia, compared with 1 patient receiving placebo (P=0.10), and there were 8 cases of neutropenia with low-dose AZT, compared with 7 cases with placebo (P=0.78). In contrast, the risk of developing anemia or neutropenia was significantly higher with the 1500 mg/day regimen. Twenty-nine patients receiving high-dose AZT developed anemia (P<0.0001 compared with placebo), and 29 became neutropenic (P<0.0001 compared with placebo).

d. Compliance was assessed by measuring serum AZT levels. Of the 371 representative assays, AZT was detected in 84% of the patients receiving 500 mg/day, 79% of those receiving 1500 mg/day, and 9% of those receiving placebo.

e. Together with the ACTG 016 study (40), the ACTG 019 protocol confirmed the benefit of AZT for slowing the rate of progression to AIDS in symptomatic and asymptomatic patients with CD4 counts <500 cells/μl. In addition, the regimen of 500 mg/day AZT was shown to be as effective and less toxic than the 1500 mg/day regimen used in previous trials. Despite these benefits, however, no improvement in the rate of survival was demonstrated except for those patients already diagnosed with AIDS or advanced ARC. For HIV-positive patients without AIDS or advanced ARC, the optimal time to initiate antiretroviral therapy remained unresolved.

4. **Early Versus Late Initiation of AZT**

a. **Veterans Affairs Cooperative Study**—In a double-blind PRCT, the Veterans Affairs Cooperative Study compared early versus late initiation of AZT therapy among 338 patients (99% male) with ARC and CD4 counts of 200 to 500/μl (46). Patients with AIDS or prior antiretroviral therapy were excluded. The patients were stratified by CD4 count (200 to 299 versus 300 to 500/μl) and then randomly assigned to receive either immediate (early) AZT therapy (250 mg q4) or placebo (late therapy). The 168 patients assigned to placebo received AZT when the CD4 count decreased below 200 cells/μl. The clinical end points were death or progression to AIDS. Patients reaching an end point began taking open-label AZT (250 mg q 4 hours). Almost all patients received PCP prophylaxis (98% of those eligible in the early group and 90% of those eligible in the late group; P=NS). The mean duration of follow-up was 27 months for the early group and 28 months for the late group; 15 patients were lost to follow-up. Both groups appeared compliant on the basis of clinic attendance, pill counts (94% to 95% of expected), plasma AZT levels (90% to 92% of levels within range), and measurements of mean corpuscular volume (MCV).

(1) **Survival**—No difference in the mortality rate was observed. The 3-year survival rate was 77% for the early group and 83% for the late group.

(2) **Progression of Disease**—Early therapy appeared to decrease the rate of progression to AIDS. Twenty-eight patients developed AIDS in the early group, compared with 48 in the late group (RR, 1.75 for late therapy; 95% CI, 1.1 to 2.8; P=0.02). At 3 years, 82% of the patients in the early group had not progressed to AIDS, compared with 65% of the patients in the late group.

(3) **CD4 Counts**—Early therapy increased CD4 counts by an average of 11.5/μl over baseline at 4 months. However, at 12 months, the average CD4 count was only 0.3/μl above baseline, and at 20 months, the average CD4 count had decreased to 35.5/μl below baseline. In the late

group, the average CD4 count decreased progressively to 8.6/µl below baseline at 4 months and 83.6/µl below baseline at 20 months.

(4) **Adverse Effects**—With the relatively high dose of AZT used in the trial, leukopenia and anemia were common. Neutropenia (ANC <1000 cells/µl) developed in 14% of the early group and 10% of the late group. Severe anemia requiring a transfusion (criteria not defined) developed in 5% of the early group and 2% of the late group. In addition, nausea, vomiting and diarrhea occurred more frequently in the early group (40% versus 23%, $P<0.01$).

(5) In the late group, 39 of the 168 patients began taking open-label AZT before reaching a clinical end point defined in the protocol. Therefore, a potential survival benefit for early use of AZT may have been underestimated. In addition, the use of open-label AZT in all patients reaching a clinical end point may have blurred the distinction between the two groups.

(6) As in the earlier trials, the Veterans Affairs study demonstrated that initiation of AZT in patients with CD4 counts <500/µl slowed the rate of progression to AIDS. However, no mortality difference was observed.

b. **European-Australian Collaborative Group Study**—The benefit of AZT in HIV-positive patients with CD4 counts >500/µl was evaluated by the European-Australian Collaborative Group (24). This double-blind PRCT enrolled 984 asymptomatic patients (86% male, 96% white) with CD4 counts >400/µl (mean, 650/µl) to receive either AZT (500 mg q 12 hours) or placebo. The end points were AIDS, severe ARC, CDC group IV-C2 disease, or CD4 count <350/µl. As new information from other studies became available, the criteria for the use of open-label AZT evolved during the trial. Ultimately, open-label therapy was offered to patients developing CDC group IV disease and those with CD4 counts <350 cells/µl. Intention-to-treat analysis was employed, but data were censored beginning 3 months after the initiation of open-label therapy. The median duration of follow-up was 93 weeks.

(1) **Progression of Disease**—A total of 129 of the patients receiving placebo but only 76 of those receiving AZT ($P<0.001$) reached one of the four end points. However, no difference between the two treatment arms was observed when the "hard" clinical end points of progression to AIDS or severe ARC were used; 10 patients in the placebo group and 6 in the AZT group reached these end points (P=NS). The development of CDC group IV disease was decreased by AZT (22 in the placebo group versus 11 in the AZT group; $P=0.049$), and the development of a CD4 count <350/µl was also significantly diminished by AZT (113 in the placebo group versus 70 in the AZT group; $P<0.001$).

(2) **Adverse Effects**—Despite the use of a relatively high dose of AZT in this trial, <1% of the AZT-assigned subjects developed severe anemia (hemoglobin <8 g/dl), and 2% in each group developed neutropenia (ANC <750/µl). Nausea, headache, and anorexia were more common in the AZT group. Seventy-eight percent of the patients in the AZT group and 88% of those in the placebo group did not require an alteration of the dosage of the study medication for at least 90% of the trial period.

(3) This trial, which had a significantly longer follow-up period than in others, suggested a potential advantage of early AZT therapy even for patients with CD4 counts >400/µl. However, a survival benefit was not demonstrated. In addition, although a significant benefit of AZT was demonstrated for a broader range of end points, AZT did not significantly slow the rate of progression to the clinical end points of AIDS or ARC. This discrepancy may be attributed to censorship of the data beginning 3 months after blinded therapy was discontinued,

which resulted in a smaller number of events. Furthermore, there was a high rate of patient withdrawal from the protocol (135 from the placebo group and 173 from the AZT group), which potentially complicated the interpretation of these results.

c. **European Concorde Trial**—The publication of the European Concorde trial in 1994 renewed the controversy over the role of AZT (21). In a double-blind PRCT, 1749 (85% male) asymptomatic HIV-positive patients (regardless of CD4 count) were randomly assigned to receive either immediate therapy with AZT (250 mg q 4 hours) or placebo (deferred therapy). Patients assigned to placebo were crossed over to AZT when they developed AIDS or ARC. However, after the results of the ACTG 019 trial became available, the protocol was modified at 1 year into the enrollment period to offer open-label AZT to all patients with CD4 counts <500/μl at the clinician's discretion (65% of subjects had already been randomly assigned to treatment by this point). The study design was also modified at that time to allow for PCP prophylaxis. Ninety-four percent of patients had CD4 counts >200/μl, and 42% had counts >500/μl. Clinical end points were survival, serious adverse events, and progression to AIDS or CDC group IV disease. The median duration of follow-up was 3.3 years.

(1) **Survival**—No significant difference in survival rate was observed between the immediate and the deferred therapy groups (96 versus 76 deaths, respectively). The probability of death at 3 years was 8% for the immediate therapy group and 6% for the deferred therapy group.

(2) **Progression of Disease**—No difference in the rate of progression to AIDS, ARC, or death was observed (267 with immediate therapy versus 284 with deferred therapy; *P*=NS). There was an initial advantage of immediate therapy regarding disease progression at 1 year (RR, 0.77; 95% CI, 0.62 to 0.96; *P*=0.003), but this benefit disappeared by year 3. Most of the initial benefit of early AZT resulted from delay of the onset of ARC.

(3) **CD4 Counts**—Immediate therapy was associated with higher CD4 counts. There was a median increase of 20/μl over baseline at 3 months in the immediate therapy group and a median decrease of 9/μl at 3 months in the deferred therapy group (*P*<0.0001). After 6 months, the CD4 counts fell in both groups, but a difference of 30/μl (higher in the immediate therapy group) persisted for the duration of the trial.

(4) **Adverse Effects**—Ninety-nine subjects in the immediate therapy group and 38 in the deferred therapy group discontinued the study drug because of toxicity. Malaise, gastrointestinal symptoms, and neurologic symptoms (*e.g.*, headache) were common. Anemia (hemoglobin <10 g/dl) affected 8% of the immediate therapy group and 2% of the deferred therapy group at 3 years. During the same time period, neutropenia (ANC <800/μl) was observed in 9% and 3% of the immediate and deferred therapy groups, respectively.

(5) **Compliance**—Measurements of MCV and serum AZT concentrations were used to monitor compliance in a cross-sectional sample of patients from each group. At 132 weeks of follow-up, the MCV was >3 standard deviations above baseline in 87% and 1.4% of the immediate and deferred therapy groups, respectively. Serum AZT concentrations were detectable in 81% of the immediate therapy group; however, in 32 of the 46 immediate therapy patients with undetectable AZT concentrations, proper timing of sample collection (within 6 hours of dosing) could not be verified. Only 3% of the samples in the deferred therapy group had detectable levels of AZT; half of these were thought to be spurious for technical reasons, and none showed elevated levels of MCV.

(6) Among the patients in the deferred therapy group, 48% eventually received AZT during the trial; 15% began taking open-label drug after progression to ARC or AIDS, and an additional 27% began taking AZT

because of low CD4 counts (after protocol modification to accommodate the findings of the ACTG 019 trial). However, the percentage of trial time during which AZT was taken differed sharply between the immediate and deferred therapy groups (80% versus 23%, respectively). Consequently, the authors of the study argued that the confounding effect of open-label AZT therapy was not likely to have been significant.

(7) With its large patient population, exceptionally long period of follow-up, and high number of patient outcomes, the Concorde study is a compelling trial whose results must be carefully considered, albeit with some reservations concerning the influence of open-label AZT usage. These results may be viewed as an extension of the previous trials (*e.g.*, ACTG 019), in which the observed delay in disease progression did not translate into extended survival. The Concorde study confirmed this lack of survival benefit with early AZT therapy and further demonstrated that the delay in progression to ARC or AIDS was transient when patients were compared at extended follow-up. In addition, by dissociating an increase in the CD4 count from improved prognosis, this trial called into question the common practice of using the CD4 count as a surrogate marker for disease progression as well as the use of the CD4 count as a valid clinical end point in previous clinical trials.

d. ACTG 019 Trial—Long-term follow-up of the patients in the ACTG 019 Trial has corroborated many of the findings from the Concorde study (90). After the initial analysis (91) had demonstrated a twofold to threefold decrease in the rate of progression to AIDS with AZT (500 or 1500 mg/day), all patients were offered open-label AZT (500 mg/day). From the original cohort of 1338, with 227 additional subjects, 1030 patients began open-label therapy when the trial was unblinded. Clinical end points were death or development of AIDS. An intention-to-treat analysis was used to compare the clinical outcome among those given immediate AZT therapy (early AZT) versus those given AZT later as part of open-label therapy (delayed AZT).

(1) No difference in mortality was observed.

(2) Compared with patients in the delayed AZT group, the rate of progression to AIDS or death (232 subjects) was significantly delayed with early AZT therapy (pooled low-dose and high-dose AZT groups, $P=0.008$; low-dose group alone, $P=0.004$). The benefit of early AZT therapy appeared to be most prominent in patients with CD4 counts >300/µl. However, the advantage of early AZT therapy waned with time, so that the RR of disease progression or death (placebo versus AZT) was 1.0 after 2.1 years.

e. An additional arm of ACTG protocol 019 specifically examined the effect of AZT in asymptomatic patients with CD4 counts >500/µl (89). Subjects were randomly assigned to receive either placebo, AZT at 500 mg/day, or AZT at 1500 mg/day. When initial results from ACTG 019 demonstrated some clinical benefit for patients with CD4 counts <500/µl, the protocol was modified in 1989 to offer open-label AZT at 500 mg/day to enrolled subjects whose CD4 counts had dropped to <500/µl. Consequently, this study was able to examine the clinical benefit of immediate versus deferred AZT therapy. A total of 1637 patients were randomly assigned to treatment (90% white male, 69% homosexual); the median CD4 count was 655/µl. The median follow-up was 4.8 to 4.9 years. Clinical end points were death or progression to AIDS. Of the 1609 subjects who actually began receiving therapy, 591 (37%) withdrew voluntarily while receiving blinded therapy and an additional 353 (22%) left the study while receiving open-label AZT; the patients who withdrew appeared to be evenly distributed among the three groups. The 569 patients (35%) who were lost to follow-up were also distributed evenly among the three groups. These data were examined using an intention-to-treat analysis.

(1) **Clinical End Points**—There was no difference in mortality among the three groups (about 8% of the patients in each group died during the study) and no difference in the progression to AIDS or death.

(2) The decline in CD4 count was slowed in patients receiving immediate AZT, with the median time to a CD4 count <500/μl being 1.5 years in the 500 mg/day and 1500 mg/day AZT groups, compared with 1 year in the placebo (deferred therapy) group ($P<0.001$). This difference was accentuated in patients with starting CD4 counts >650/μl.

(3) Adverse effects occurred at a similar rate in the deferred AZT and 500 mg/day AZT groups. The 1500 mg/day AZT group had statistically significant increased occurrences of anemia (4%) and thrombocytopenia (5.6%).

(4) Therefore, no additional benefit to institution of AZT therapy at CD4 counts >500/μl could be demonstrated in this study. However, the high rate (>50%) of patient withdrawal could have obscured a modest clinical effect.

5. An attractive explanation for the transient effect of AZT is the development of resistant strains of HIV-1 with prolonged therapy. In a prospective study involving 50 patients receiving long-term AZT therapy (all of whom had received no antiretroviral therapy for at least 3 months before the study), the incidence of AZT resistance was 64% at 180 weeks, and the median time to isolation of a resistant strain was 120 weeks (64). Development of resistance was assessed with the use of viral cultures and susceptibility testing every 12 weeks. In a multivariate analysis, a decreased CD4:CD8 ratio was found to be associated with an increased risk for resistance, but this observation did not achieve statistical significance ($P=0.10$). The RR for progression of disease with the development of AZT resistance was 1.98 (95% CI, 1.36 to 2.89). Although this association does not prove causality, it seems plausible that long-term use of AZT may lead to eventual treatment failure because it selects for resistant strains of HIV-1, especially in view of the high mutation rate of the *pol* gene, where the mutations causing resistance usually are found.

6. **AZT Versus Placebo to Decrease the Risk of Maternal-Fetal Transmission**—Perhaps the most compelling evidence for the benefit of AZT comes from a trial examining its effect on the rate of maternal-fetal transmission of HIV-1 (23). AZT (100 mg five times daily) was compared with placebo in a double-blind PRCT (ACTG protocol 076) involving 409 HIV-positive, pregnant women (14 to 34 weeks' gestation at the time of enrollment) with CD4 counts >200/μl (median, 550/μl). Those in the AZT group were also treated during labor (2 mg/kg IV AZT over 1 hour, then 1 mg/kg/hr AZT until delivery), and the infants were subsequently given AZT (2 mg/kg PO q 6 hours for 6 weeks), commencing at 8 to 12 hours of life. Women given prior antiretroviral therapy during pregnancy and those who had life-threatening fetal anomalies, oligohydramnios in the second trimester or polyhydramnios in the third trimester, fetal hydrops, and mothers with anemia, or ascites were excluded. The children were monitored with HIV cultures at birth, 12, 24, and 78 weeks; HIV enzyme-linked immunosorbent assays and Western blot analyses were obtained at 72 and 78 weeks. Maternal-fetal transmission of HIV was the primary clinical end point. The median gestational age at trial entry was 26 weeks, and the 409 subjects gave birth to 415 children. Median gestational age, birth weight, incidence of prematurity, and mode of delivery were comparable between the two groups.

   a. **Survival**—No women died during the study in either group. Five infants from the AZT group died, as did 3 in the placebo group, but none of the deaths was thought to have been related to HIV infection.

   b. **Maternal-Fetal Transmission**—HIV culture results were unavailable for 46 children (25 in the AZT group, 21 in the placebo group), who were excluded from the analysis. Of the remaining 363 infants, 13 of 180 in the AZT group and 40 of 183 in the placebo group were infected. The estimated incidence of infection at 18 months was 8% with AZT (95% CI, 3.9% to 12.8%)

and 25% with placebo (95% CI, 18.4% to 32.5%), a 67% reduction (*P*= 0.00005).

c. **Adverse Effects**—AZT was well tolerated; only 3 subjects in each group stopped therapy because of adverse effects. Nearly equal numbers of women in the AZT and placebo groups had anemia, thrombocytopenia, neutropenia, electrolyte abnormalities, or elevated liver function tests; many of these findings were thought to be related to labor and delivery. Aside from a decreased level of hemoglobin among the infants born to mothers assigned to AZT (which resolved by 12 weeks), no other adverse effects were observed. The incidence of congenital anomalies was equivalent in the two groups.

d. Therefore, for women with early HIV disease and limited prior exposure to antiretroviral agents, AZT significantly decreased the risk of maternal-fetal transmission of HIV. However, many questions still remain. For example, is it essential to treat the mother during pregnancy, labor, and delivery and the infant for the first 6 weeks (a question which is particularly relevant for optimizing the use of AZT in developing nations)? What is the effect of AZT on mothers with more advanced disease and/or prior exposure to antiretroviral therapy? Is there a threshold level of maternal HIV viremia that predicts fetal transmission, and if so, can it be used to select mothers and neonates who would benefit from antiretroviral therapy during pregnancy to prevent transmission? Finally, are there any long-term consequences of AZT therapy on treated infants (*e.g.*, a delay in cognitive development)?

C. **Didanosine and Zalcitabine**—The family of HIV reverse transcriptase inhibitors was extended with the development of didanosine (ddI) and zalcitabine (ddC). Unpublished trials had indicated that both of these agents were inferior to AZT when used for primary therapy against HIV. However, with persistent questions regarding the duration of benefit of AZT, ddI and ddC were examined as therapeutic alternatives.

1. **AZT Versus ddI**—ACTG protocol 116B/117 enrolled patients with ARC or AIDS and CD4 counts <300/μl and those with asymptomatic HIV infection and CD4 counts <200/μl (who would meet current criteria for AIDS), all of whom had been treated with AZT for at least 16 weeks before enrollment (49). In a double-blind PRCT, 913 patients (96% male, 82% white) were randomly assigned to continue oral AZT (600 mg/day), to begin low-dose oral ddI (500 mg/day), or to begin high-dose oral ddI (750 mg/day). Ninety-three percent of the subjects received aerosolized pentamidine monthly for PCP prophylaxis. The median duration of prior AZT therapy was 13.9 months, and the median CD4 count was 95/μl. For asymptomatic patients and for those with ARC, the clinical end points were death or development of any AIDS-defining illness (using 1987 CDC criteria). For patients with AIDS, the end points were death or a new AIDS-defining illness. In addition, the total number of AIDS-associated events (*i.e.*, both recurrent and new AIDS-defining illnesses) was also monitored for each group. Mean duration of follow-up was 55 weeks. Overall, 57% of the subjects withdrew from the study before completion. However, significantly more patients in the AZT group stopped the assigned drug than in either of the two ddI groups. Most who withdrew desired to take a different antiretroviral agent, and it is possible that these patients may have had more advanced HIV disease. An additional 5% of subjects, equally distributed among the three groups, were lost to follow-up. An intention-to-treat analysis was used.

a. **Progression to Death or Disease**—No difference in survival was observed. However, death or development of a new AIDS-defining illness occurred in 41% of the patients receiving continued AZT, 32% of those in the low-dose ddI group (500 mg/day), and 37% of those in the high-dose ddI group (750 mg/day). Compared with patients assigned to AZT, the combined risk of death or development of a new AIDS-associated event was significantly lower for those assigned to low-dose ddI (*P*=0.015; RR, 1.39 for AZT, 95% CI, 1.06 to 1.82). There was a similar trend for those assigned to the high-dose ddI group, but the difference did not achieve statistical significance.

(1) The decrease in the combined risk of death or development of an AIDS-related event was observed primarily among asymptomatic patients and those with ARC.

(2) For patients with AIDS, there was no significant difference in the risk of death or development of an AIDS-related event among the three treatment arms. However, the power of the study was insufficient to adequately evaluate this subgroup.

(3) No correlation was observed between patient outcome and the duration of prior AZT use.

b. **CD4 Count**—CD4 counts increased slightly in the two ddI groups (mean increase, 2 to 5 cells/μl) but subsequently returned to baseline by week 12. CD4 counts declined steadily in the AZT group.

c. **Risk of Progression and AZT Resistance**—In a retrospective review of a sample of 187 patients from this trial who had baseline HIV-1 viral isolates, high-level AZT resistance was an independent risk factor for a new AIDS-defining illness or death (RR, 1.74; 95% CI, 1.00 to 2.03) and for death alone (RR, 2.78; 95% CI, 1.21 to 6.39), after controlling for baseline CD4 count, disease stage, presence of syncytium-inducing strains of HIV, and therapy arm (26).

d. **Adverse Effects**—Patients assigned to ddI had an increased incidence of pancreatitis, compared with those assigned to AZT. However, this difference was statistically significant only for those assigned to high-dose ddI (13% in the group receiving 750 mg/day ddI versus 3% in the group receiving AZT; $P=0.001$). In both ddI groups, the incidence of hyperamylasemia (>1.3 times baseline) was significantly higher than in the AZT group (20% in the low-dose ddI group and 30% in the high-dose ddI group, versus 6% in the AZT group; $P=0.001$ and $P<0.001$ respectively). Patients receiving AZT had an increased incidence of anemia, leukopenia, and neutropenia, compared with those receiving ddI.

e. These results suggest that ddI may decrease the combined risk of death or development of an AIDS-related event in patients with relatively advanced HIV infection and prolonged prior exposure to AZT monotherapy (mean, 13.9 months). However, the high rate of voluntary patient withdrawal from the trial, especially among those in the AZT group, could have obscured even a larger difference between AZT and ddI therapy.

2. **Continuing AZT Versus Switching to ddI for Patients Failing AZT**—In a double-blind PRCT, Spruance examined the role of ddI among 312 HIV-positive patients (96% male, 67% white) with CD4 counts <300/μl (60% with counts <100/μl) and evidence of disease progression despite at least 6 months of AZT therapy (85). All subjects had evidence of clinical deterioration within 12 weeks before randomization. Clinical deterioration was defined as a new or recurrent AIDS-defining illness; involuntary weight loss of more than 5% of body weight; a decrease in Karnofsky score of 20 points or more; unexplained fever >38° C for >1 week; new or recurrent oral thrush, oral hairy leukoplakia, or herpes zoster; chronic herpes simplex ulcers unresponsive to acyclovir (ACV); new or recurrent HIV-associated dermatologic disorders (*e.g.*, psoriasis, molluscum contagiosum); or a 50% decrease in the CD4 count from the beginning of AZT therapy. Patients were randomly assigned to receive either AZT (100 mg six times per day) plus placebo or ddI (375 mg BID) plus placebo. Clinical end points were death, a new AIDS-defining illness, or two new opportunistic infections together with a 50% decrease in the CD4 count. Patients who reached an end point or experienced drug toxicity at least 12 weeks after beginning the study drugs were crossed over to the other group. The median duration of follow-up was 47 weeks. The median duration of prior AZT therapy was 18 months, and 85% of patients received PCP prophylaxis. Fewer than 20% of the subjects had taken AZT for <12 months.

a. **Survival**—There was no significant difference in the rate of death between the two groups.

b. **Disease Progression**—Disease progression was significantly less common among patients receiving ddI than among those receiving AZT; 67 of 160 patients in the ddI group progressed, compared with 82 of 152 patients in the AZT group (RR, 1.5 for AZT; 95% CI, 1.1 to 2.0). The combined risk of dying or developing a new AIDS-defining illness was also lower with ddI, but this difference did not achieve statistical significance (P=0.09; RR, 1.3; 95% CI, 1.0 to 1.9).
   (1) According to subgroup analysis, patients with higher CD4 counts were more likely to benefit from the switch to ddI. For example, among those with CD4 counts >100/μl, 12 patients in the ddI group progressed to an end point, compared with 24 in the AZT group (P=0.03; RR, 2.2; 95% CI, 1.1 to 4.4). In contrast, among those with CD4 counts <100/μl, 55 and 57 progressed in the ddI and AZT groups, respectively (P=0.22).
   (2) In similar subgroup analysis, patients who had been treated with AZT for >1 year appeared to benefit more from the switch to ddI. For example, among those who had been receiving AZT for >12 months before enrollment, 49 and 62 patients progressed in the ddI and AZT groups, respectively (P=0.02; RR, 1.5; 95% CI, 1.1 to 2.3). In comparison, among those who had been receiving AZT for <12 months before enrollment, 18 and 20 patients progressed, respectively (P>0.2).

c. **CD4 Counts**—CD4 counts initially increased in the ddI group but returned to baseline by about 12 to 16 weeks; CD4 counts decreased steadily in the AZT group.

d. **Adverse Effects**—Aside from an increased incidence of granulocytopenia (ANC <750/μl) in the AZT arm (33 patients, versus 15 in the ddI arm; P= 0.005), the occurrences of pancreatitis, hyperamylasemia, anemia, and neuropathy were equivalent between the two groups.

e. There was a high rate of patient attrition from the trial; 60% of the ddI group and 70% of the AZT group did not complete the course of intended therapy. Included among these subjects were 10% of the AZT group and 27% of the ddI group, who crossed over to the other treatment arm. Overall, almost 50% of the patients in the trial discontinued all study medications.

f. Although the high rate of patient withdrawal is of concern, this trial indicates that patients who experience clinical deterioration despite long-term AZT monotherapy may slow disease progression by changing to ddI.

3. **Changing From AZT to ddI in Clinically Stable Patients**—In a multicenter, double-blind, randomized controlled trial from the Canadian HIV Trials Network (63), entry criteria included a CD4 count between 200 and 500/μl and a prior history of at least 6 months of AZT therapy at 500 mg or more per day. Subjects were randomly assigned either to receive continued AZT (at 600 mg/day) or to begin ddI monotherapy (for patients weighing at least 60 kg, 250 mg BID for ddI sachets, changed to 200 mg BID when ddI tablets became available). The primary clinical end points were death or a new AIDS-defining illness. A total of 245 patients were enrolled, 127 in the AZT arm and 118 in the ddI arm; 94% were white, 95% male, and 84% homosexual or bisexual. Only 4% carried a diagnosis of AIDS on enrollment; 66% were asymptomatic. The median CD4 count was 320/μl, and the median duration of prior AZT therapy was 471 days. The protocol specified formal follow-up of 48 weeks; the median long-term follow-up period was 764 days for the AZT group and 737 days for the ddI group. Only 74% of the ddI group and 60% of the AZT group (a statistically significant difference) completed the full 48 weeks of randomized therapy. More patients in the AZT group stopped randomized therapy because of a drug reaction (26 versus 13 patients; P=0.06) or because of clinical deterioration (14 versus 2 patients; P=0.007). Intention-to-treat analysis was employed.

   a. **Clinical End Points**—No significant difference in mortality was observed; there were nine deaths during long-term follow-up in the ddI group and eight in the AZT group. However, of the nine new AIDS-defining illnesses reported during the first 48 weeks of follow-up, eight were in the AZT group (RR, 7.9; 95% CI, 1.0 to 63.3; P=0.02). In addition, a statistically significant difference in the number of clinical end points (*i.e.*, AIDS-defining illness or death) was observed, with 28 events in the AZT group and 14 in the ddI group during long-term follow-up (RR, 1.9 for AZT; 95% CI, 1.0 to 3.6; P=0.05).

b. **CD4 Count**—An increase in CD4 count by approximately 50 to 60/μl was associated with ddI use, and significantly higher CD4 counts were maintained in the ddI group throughout the 48 weeks of formal follow-up.

c. **Viral Susceptibility**—*In vitro* susceptibility assays were carried out on isolates from 53 unselected AZT group subjects and 49 patients in the ddI group. A substantial proportion of both groups (28% of the AZT group and 21% of the ddI group) had high-level AZT resistance at the beginning of the trial. Continued AZT monotherapy was associated with a 59% 1-year probability of acquiring high-grade AZT resistance, whereas a much lower probability (approximately 15%) was associated with ddI therapy. This correlated with progressively increasing mean 50% inhibitory concentrations for AZT observed in the AZT group; in contrast, the mean 50% inhibitory concentrations for AZT decreased in patients receiving ddI. Resistance to ddI was rarely seen during the protocol.

d. **Adverse Effects**—Both agents appeared to be well tolerated. AZT was associated with significantly higher rates of abdominal pain, leukopenia, and neutropenia, whereas ddI users had a significantly higher incidence of hyperuricemia and a trend toward more frequent hyperamylasemia. Thrombocytopenia and neuropathy were observed at equivalent rates in the two groups.

e. By extending the use of ddI in AZT-experienced patients to individuals in earlier-stage HIV disease, and by combining clinical end points with viral susceptibility data, this study suggested a role for initiation of ddI monotherapy even in the absence of evident clinical deterioration in those receiving AZT.

4. **AZT Versus ddI in Patients With Minimal Prior AZT Experience and Advanced HIV Disease**—The ACTG 116A protocol (32) was a double-blind PRCT that enrolled asymptomatic HIV-positive patients who had CD4 counts <200 cells/μl (again meeting current criteria for AIDS) and patients with AIDS or ARC who had CD4 counts <300 cells/μl. However, unlike the population of ACTG protocol 116B/117, which consisted of many subjects with prolonged prior AZT use, participants in ACTG 116A had either no prior AZT therapy or no more than 16 weeks of AZT. Subjects were randomly assigned to receive either AZT, high-dose ddI (750 mg/day, or 500 mg/day for patients weighing <60 kg), or low-dose ddI (500 mg/day, or 334 mg/day for patients weighing <60 kg). The AZT group received 1200 mg/day in 1989 and 1990, and subsequently 600 mg/day (all q 4 hours). The protocol specified dose reductions for severe toxicity. Endpoints were the onset of a new AIDS-defining illness or death, and patients with a new AIDS-related event or severe drug toxicity could cross over to the alternate therapeutic arm. A total of 617 patients were enrolled, with 212 in the AZT group, 197 in the low-dose ddI group, and 208 in the high-dose ddI group. The median CD4 count was 130/μl, and 39% of patients had CD4 counts <100/μl. Sixty-two percent of the subjects in the protocol had no prior AZT experience, 19% had received AZT for <8 weeks, and another 19% had received AZT for 8 to 16 weeks. Of the >80% of subjects receiving PCP prophylaxis, 62% used aerosolized pentamidine and 31% used trimethoprim-sulfamethoxazole. Compliance was assessed with serum ddI measurements and MCV determinations. The median follow-up was 85 weeks; 46% of the subjects stopped randomized therapy before the end of the trial. Intention-to-treat analysis was used.

a. **Clinical Endpoints**—The advanced stage of HIV disease in the study population was reflected in a high number of clinical end points, which occurred in 249 (40%) of the patients.

(1) No overall difference in the number of clinical endpoints was observed among the three treatment arms.

(2) Among patients who were AZT-naive, AZT therapy was associated with a significant decrease in the number of clinical end points, compared with high-dose ddI (RR, 1.43 for ddI; 90% CI, 1.02 to 2.00). A similar trend that did not reach statistical significance favored AZT over low-dose ddI (RR, 1.21; 90% CI, 0.86 to 1.71). For subjects with not more than 8 weeks of prior AZT therapy, no difference among the treatment arms was noted.

(3) Patients with 8 to 16 weeks of prior AZT therapy appeared to benefit more from low-dose ddI than from AZT (RR, 0.48 for ddI; 90% CI, 0.27 to 0.86). A similar trend was seen for high-dose ddI (RR, 0.61; 90% CI, 0.36 to 1.03) but was not statistically significant.

(4) No differences were observed between the two ddI groups.

b. Survival

(1) In AZT-naive patients, significantly longer survival was associated with AZT than with low-dose ddI (RR, 1.88: 90% CI, 1.1 to 2.27); the RR for high-dose ddI compared with AZT was 1.51, although this comparison did not reach statistical significance.

(2) No difference in survival was found for patients with <8 weeks of prior AZT; however, subjects with 8 to 16 weeks of prior AZT experience demonstrated significantly improved survival with high-dose ddI (750 mg/day) compared with AZT therapy (RR, 0.39; 90% CI, 0.19 to 0.80). The RR for survival in the low-dose ddI group (500 mg/day) compared with the AZT group was 0.51 (again, not statistically significant).

(3) No survival differences were reported when the two ddI arms were compared with each other.

c. CD4 Count—No significant differences were observed in the decline in CD4 count among the three treatment arms for patients with no more than 16 weeks of prior AZT therapy. In patients who were AZT-naive, there was a significant increase in CD4 count with AZT therapy and a slowed decline with low-dose ddI therapy; however, these differences were observed only in the first 2 weeks of therapy.

d. Adverse Effects—Neutropenia occurred in 18% of the AZT group, which was significantly more often than in the low-dose ddI group (6%; $P=0.001$) or in the high-dose ddI group (7%; $P=0.0001$). Pancreatitis was significantly more common in the high-dose ddI group (9%) than in the AZT group (4%; $P=0.03$). In the low-dose ddI group, there was a trend toward increased pancreatitis (7%) that did not reach statistical significance. There was an increased incidence of hyperamylasemia (>1.4 times the upper limit of normal) in both the low-dose ddI group (18%, $P=0.01$) and the high-dose ddI group (19%, $P=0.02$) compared with the AZT group (10%). No significant differences were observed in the incidence of hepatotoxicity or peripheral neuropathy.

e. These results may have been influenced by the high (46%) withdrawal rate from the protocol despite intention-to-treat analysis; however, it is reassuring that 81% of the reported clinical end points occurred either while the patient was receiving the study therapy or within 30 days of stopping treatment. The significant occurrence of PCP probably reflected the predominant use of aerosolized pentamidine for prophylaxis rather than trimethoprim-sulfamethoxazole; however, it is unclear whether any of the treatment arms were preferentially influenced.

f. The ACTG 116A protocol demonstrated that for patients with advanced HIV disease, AZT is superior to ddI in patients without prior AZT therapy. However, for subjects with less than 16 weeks of AZT experience, ddI was more beneficial. In each case, a decreased number of clinical end points and a clear improvement in survival were demonstrated. The implication of these results is that a change to ddI monotherapy after a short course of AZT may be beneficial for this patient population. However, the authors pointed out that this study was not designed to prospectively evaluate this specific hypothesis and that additional trials are needed to address this question.

5. **ddI Versus ddC in Advanced HIV Disease**—Abrams conducted a multicenter, randomized, open-label trial examining either ddI or ddC as an alternative to AZT (2). This study randomly assigned 467 HIV-positive patients (90% male, 65% white) who had previously been treated with AZT to receive either ddI (250 mg BID) or ddC (750 mg TID). All patients either had AIDS or had CD4 counts <300/μl; all had previously been treated with AZT (mean duration, 17 months) and had either drug intolerance (approximately two thirds of the patients) or disease progression despite AZT therapy. Disease progression was defined as occurrence of one or more of the following during therapy: a new or recurrent opportunistic infection or neoplasm (excluding Kaposi's sarcoma); AIDS dementia complex; or failure to thrive resulting in loss of more than 10% of body weight with either unexplained diarrhea or fever and chronic weakness for >1 month. The median baseline CD4 counts were 40 and 34/μl in the DDI and ddC groups, respectively. Patients were allowed to cross over to the alternate treatment arm for drug toxicity or clinical progression occurring after 12 weeks of study therapy; one such crossover was permitted during the trial. Clinical endpoints were survival and disease progression. An intention-to-treat analysis was used. The median duration of follow-up was 16 months.
   a. **Survival**—There was no significant difference in the number of deaths between the two groups (100 with ddI versus 88 with ddC; $P=0.09$; RR, 0.78; 95% CI, 0.58 to 1.04). With either therapy, the mortality rate was high despite antiretroviral therapy. At 16 months, 45.8% of those in the ddI group and 36% of those in the ddC group had died.
   b. The combined risk of death or clinical progression was similar between the two groups.
   c. **CD4 Counts**—For the first 2 months of treatment, CD4 counts increased in about half of the patients in both groups. However, after the second month, the CD4 counts decreased at a rate of about 3/μl per month in both groups.
   d. **Adverse Effects**—Peripheral neuropathy was more common in the ddC group than in the ddI group (69 versus 33 patients, respectively; $P=0.002$). However, diarrhea (48 versus 9 patients; $P<0.001$) and abdominal pain (16 versus 7 patients; $P=0.03$) were more common in the ddI group. Four patients developed pancreatitis, all in the ddI group, and 8 developed stomatitis, all in the ddC group.
   e. By 1 year after randomization, 62% and 55% of the patients in the ddI and ddC groups, respectively, had stopped their study drug. In addition, 12% and 19% of the patients in the ddI and ddC groups, respectively, had resumed AZT at 1 year.
   f. It appears that ddC and ddI are equally effective for HIV-positive patients with advanced disease who have clinical deterioration despite treatment with AZT and for those who are intolerant of AZT because of drug-related adverse effects. However, the high mortality rates in this study suggest that these antiretroviral agents do not significantly alter the course of advanced HIV disease.
6. **Monotherapy Versus Combined** AZT and ddC—A large double-blind PRCT was undertaken to examine the efficacies of AZT or ddC monotherapy and AZT plus ddC combination therapy in patients with advanced HIV disease (41). The study enrolled 1001 subjects (90% male, 82% white; median baseline CD4 count, 119/μl) with symptomatic HIV infection and CD4 counts <300/μl or asymptomatic HIV infection and CD4 counts <200/μl. All patients had been treated with AZT for at least 6 months before enrollment (median, 8 months). Patients were randomly assigned to receive either continued oral AZT monotherapy (200 mg q 8 hours), oral ddC (750 mg q 8 hours), or the combination of oral AZT and ddC. The clinical endpoints of the study were death or development of an AIDS-defining illness. The median length of follow-up was 18 months. All study drugs were discontinued for patients who developed significant drug toxicity; after a period of recovery, blinded therapy was resumed at half the previous dose. Treatment

was interrupted significantly more often in patients whose CD4 counts were <50/μl (90%) than in those whose counts were >150/μl (66%; *P*<0.001). However, all treatment drugs appeared to be well tolerated in general; the time to interrupted therapy was equivalent among the three groups. The proportion of follow-up sessions when full-dose study drugs were given was 73% in the combination group and 78% in each of the AZT and ddC groups.

a. **Survival**—There were no significant differences in mortality rates among the three groups (15%, 18%, and 18% in the AZT, ddC, and combination groups, respectively). Stratification of patients according to baseline CD4 count did not alter this finding.
b. **Disease Progression**—There were no significant differences in the overall rate of disease progression among the three groups (42%, 43%, and 39% in the AZT, ddC, and combination groups, respectively).
c. **Subgroup Analysis**—Patients with CD4 counts >150/μl had fewer clinical end points with combination therapy than with AZT (RR, 0.51; 95% CI, 0.28 to 0.93; *P*=0.029); this benefit was not observed for patients with CD4 counts between 50 and 150/μl or <50/μl. (These CD4 subgroups were specified before the initial data review). No differences were observed between ddC and AZT or between combination therapy and AZT in any CD4 subgroup.
d. **CD4 Count**—There was a higher initial increase (about 20% to 25% over baseline) and a slower subsequent decline in the CD4 count with combination therapy than with AZT, but there was no significant difference in CD4 counts between combination therapy and ddC monotherapy. This effect was most striking for patients with CD4 counts >150/μl. For patients with CD4 counts <50/μl, none of the three antiretroviral regimens significantly increased the CD4 count.
e. **Adverse Effects**—Neutropenia was more commonly associated with AZT, and peripheral neuropathy with ddC. The incidence of pancreatitis was equivalent among the three treatment arms. Severe drug toxicity occurred more often in patients with CD4 counts <50/μl.
f. Overall, there were no significant differences in the rates of death or disease progression among the three groups. However, for patients with CD4 counts >150 cells/μl who have had prolonged exposure to AZT, this study did provide some support for switching from AZT monotherapy to the combination of AZT and ddC. The authors pointed out that the rigorous management of drug toxicity (*i.e.*, stopping all study medications and resuming later at a lower dose after recovery) could have obscured an advantage of combination treatment. In practice, moreover, most clinicians would probably stop the agent believed to be responsible for the adverse effect rather than discontinue all medications.

7. **AZT or ddI Monotherapy Versus Combination Therapy**—The ACTG 175 protocol was a double-blind PRCT that sought to elucidate the roles of monotherapy and combination therapy in antiretroviral-naive and AZT-experienced patients (1,46a). Enrollment requirements were a CD4 count between 200 and 500/μl without prior AIDS-defining illnesses (minimal Kaposi's sarcoma was permitted).
   a. A total of 2467 patients were randomly assigned to one of four study arms: (a) AZT at 600 mg/day with ddI and ddC placebos (AZT group), (b) ddI at 400 mg/day (250 mg/day for patients weighing <60 kg) with AZT and ddC placebos (ddI group), (c) AZT at 600 mg/day plus ddI at 400 mg/day with a ddC placebo (AZT/ddI group), and (d) AZT at 600 mg/day plus ddC at 2.25 mg/day (1.5 mg/day for patients with creatinine clearance <40 ml/minute) with a ddI placebo (AZT/ddC group).
      (1) Of the 2467 subjects, 1400 had previously taken antiretroviral medications (99% had used AZT, 4% had used other agents), and 1067 were antiretroviral-naive. The AZT-experienced subjects generally had extensive prior AZT exposure (80% >6 months, 66% >1 year, 42% >2 years). The mean starting CD4 count was 338/μl in the antiretroviral-

experienced group and 372/μl among antiretroviral-naive subjects. Reflecting these higher CD4 counts, 82% of all patients in the trial were asymptomatic, with the remaining 18% consisting of patients with candidiasis, oral hairy leukoplakia, or herpes zoster within the month before randomization. As in previous ACTG protocols, most enrolled subjects were white (70%) and male (82%); however, increased numbers of women (18%) as well as black (17%) and Hispanic (12%) patients participated.

(2) Clinical endpoints were decreased CD4 count to 50% of baseline, development of an AIDS-defining illness, and death. Patients reaching one of the first two end points changed therapies; those in the AZT or ddI monotherapy groups were randomly assigned in a blinded fashion to begin either AZT/ddI or AZT/ddC, whereas those initially receiving combination therapy were switched to the other combination therapy group in a blinded fashion. Consequently, the effect of immediate versus delayed combination therapy could be assessed; patients beginning in the AZT/ddI or AZT/ddC groups formed the immediate combination therapy arm, and those initially assigned to AZT or ddI monotherapy who began combination therapy after reaching a clinical end point made up the delayed group. Overall, 332 patients (13%) switched therapy arms during the trial; 91% of these changes were provoked by a 50% decrease in CD4 count.

(3) The median length of follow-up was 143 weeks. Fifth-three percent of the enrolled patients (>1300 subjects) stopped their randomized treatment before the end of the trial. These patients were evenly distributed between the antiretroviral-naive and -experienced groups; however, among antiretroviral-naive subjects, significantly fewer patients dropped out of the ddI monotherapy stratum compared with the other three arms. For antiretroviral-experienced subjects, a statistically significant decrease in trial withdrawal was seen in the AZT/ddI group compared with the AZT monotherapy arm. A total of 474 patients (19%) were lost to follow-up, including 25% of the antiretroviral-naive group and 15% of the antiretroviral-experienced group. Within the antiretroviral-naive group, significantly fewer patients receiving ddI monotherapy were lost to follow-up than in each of the other three treatment groups. Intention-to-treat analysis was employed. Although the protocol was powered only to examine the overall patient population, the subgroup analysis of antiretroviral-naive and -experienced subjects, as well as comparisons among the four treatment arms, was preplanned.

b. Clinical endpoints were observed in 565 patients; 69% of these subjects were in the antiretroviral-experienced group. For most of these patients (71%), a 50% drop in CD4 count was the first clinical end point reached.

c. Treatment arms were compared in a pairwise fashion (*i.e.*, AZT/ddI or AZT/ddC versus AZT, ddI versus AZT, AZT/ddI or AZT/ddC versus ddI, and AZT/ddI versus AZT/ddC). The ratio of events for two treatment groups, normalized for patient number, was expressed as a hazard ratio; a ratio of 1 indicated equivalence of the two arms in question, and a ratio of 0.5 denoted a 50% decrease in risk.

(1) There were significantly fewer clinical endpoints in the AZT/ddI group (hazard ratio, 0.50; 95% CI, 0.39 to 0.63; $P<0.001$), the AZT/ddC group (hazard ratio, 0.54; 95% CI, 0.43 to 0.68; $P<0.001$), and the ddI monotherapy group (hazard ratio, 0.61; 95% CI, 0.49 to 0.76; $P<0.001$) than in the AZT monotherapy group.

(a) These differences persisted in subgroup analysis of antiretroviral-naive and -experienced subjects.

(b) Among antiretroviral-naive patients only, fewer clinical end points were seen in the AZT/ddC group compared with the ddI group (hazard ratio, 0.62; 95% CI, 0.38 to 0.99; $P=0.04$); this effect was not observed in the overall patient group.

(c) No significant differences were reported in comparisons of the AZT/ddI and ddI groups or the AZT/ddI and AZT/ddC regimens.

(2) When only the clinical endpoints of AIDS-defining illness or death were examined, both AZT/ddI combination therapy (hazard ratio, 0.64; 95% CI, 0.46 to 0.87; $P=0.005$) and ddI monotherapy (hazard ratio, 0.69; 95% CI, 0.51 to 0.94; $P=0.019$) were superior to AZT alone in the study population overall.

(a) For antiretroviral-naive subjects, AZT/ddC combination therapy was associated with a significantly lowered incidence of AIDS or death than AZT monotherapy (hazard ratio, 0.49; 95% CI, 0.27 to 0.89; $P=0.016$). There were trends toward a potential benefit with AZT/ddI (hazard ratio, 0.61; 95% CI, 0.35 to 1.07; $P=0.08$) and ddI (hazard ratio, 0.65; 95% CI, 0.38 to 1.11; $P=0.11$) which did not reach statistical significance.

(b) Within the antiretroviral-experienced group, AZT/ddI was more effective than AZT alone (hazard ratio, 0.65; 95% CI, 0.44 to 0.95; $P=0.025$), and there was a trend favoring ddI over AZT (hazard ratio, 0.72; 95% CI, 0.49 to 1.04; $P=0.08$). In contrast to the situation with antiretroviral-naive patients, AZT/ddC in antiretroviral-experienced subjects appeared to be equivalent to AZT alone (hazard ratio, 0.91; 95% CI, 0.64 to 1.29; $P=0.60$).

(3) A statistically significant mortality benefit was observed for AZT/ddI (hazard ratio, 0.55; 95% CI, 0.36 to 0.86; $P=0.008$) and for ddI (hazard ratio, 0.51; 95% CI, 0.32 to 0.80; $P=0.003$) compared with AZT alone, both in the cohort as a whole and in the antiretroviral-experienced subgroup. However, no significant difference in survival among the therapeutic groups was observed for antiretroviral-naive subjects.

(4) No significant difference in progression to AIDS or death, or in progression to death alone, was evident when immediate and delayed combination antiretroviral therapies were compared.

d. Surrogate Markers of HIV Infection—CD4 counts were lowest among subjects receiving AZT monotherapy; there was no significant difference in mean CD4 count among the ddI, AZT/ddI, and AZT/ddC arms and in an analysis of a subgroup of 391 subjects, CD4 counts were not correlated with the risk for disease progression or death. In contrast, plasma HIV RNA level, as well as presence of the syncytium-inducing viral phenotype, were significantly associated with death or progression to AIDS. Specifically, a 10-fold reduction in plasma HIV RNA at 56 weeks of randomized therapy led to a 90% decrease in this risk of progression or death (49b). Of note, the mean decreases in plasma HIV RNA after 8 weeks of randomized therapy were significantly greater for the AZT/ddI and AZT/ddC groups (0.93 and 0.89 log, respectively) than for the ddI monotherapy group (0.65 log). Similarly, preliminary analysis of HIV RNA levels indicated significantly higher levels in the AZT group compared with the other three arms.

e. Adverse Effects

(1) A total of 461 subjects (19%) experienced treatment-associated signs or symptoms during the trial. These patients were evenly distributed among the four strata of the protocol, and no specific organ system was preferentially affected in any group. Similar results were found in subgroup analysis of antiretroviral-experienced patients; however, antiretroviral-naive subjects had more signs or symptoms associated with AZT monotherapy.

(2) A total of 506 patients (21%) developed laboratory abnormalities during the study. Although the rate of these abnormalities was similar among the four treatment arms, a significantly higher percentage of subjects taking AZT/ddI had abnormal hepatic enzyme values, compared with those receiving AZT ($P=0.033$) or ddI ($P=0.045$) monotherapy. Hematologic parameters were aberrant significantly more often in the AZT/ddC group than in the other three arms. Pancreatitis was uncommon in this patient population (0.6% incidence), and no difference was observed among the treatment subgroups.

f. This complex and provocative trial advances the present management of early HIV infection beyond AZT monotherapy by demonstrating both clinical and survival benefits associated with ddI monotherapy and AZT combination therapy. The results can be summarized as follows.

(1) For antiretroviral-naive patients, ddI, AZT/ddI, and AZT/ddC were all found to decrease the incidence of clinical endpoints (CD4 count decreased by 50%, AIDS, or death) in comparison with AZT monotherapy. For the hard clinical endpoints of AIDS or death, AZT/ddC was superior to AZT, with trends not attaining statistical significance for ddI and AZT/ddI. No treatment arm clearly affected survival.

(2) For antiretroviral-experienced patients (almost all of whom previously received AZT), AZT/ddI or ddI alone significantly improved survival, compared with AZT alone. Although AZT/ddC decreased the occurrence of clinical end points compared with AZT, no survival benefit or protection from progression to AIDS or death was observed.

(3) No statistically significant difference was observed for the institution of immediate versus delayed combination antiretroviral therapy.

g. Clearly, the high rate of patient withdrawal from the trial (53%) could have influenced these results. Most (76%) of the study end points occurred while participants were receiving randomized therapy or within 3 months after stopping therapy; however, only 51% of the hard end points of AIDS or death occurred within this time, and 25% of these events took place >1 year after the study medication was discontinued. It seems likely that more subtle differences between the treatment arms could have been obscured by patient attrition; whether the main conclusions were influenced by these factors awaits further analysis of the patients who withdrew from the protocol.

h. In addition, the authors pointed out that the magnitude of the response to AZT in the trial, as manifested by the mean increase in CD4 count, was 14 cells/μl, whereas the more typical increase in other trials was 30 to 40 cells/μl in other trials. Although this may suggest an unexplained diminished effect of AZT, it is difficult to draw conclusions by comparing such data across differing trials. Moreover, there was no clear evidence of noncompliance from MCV measurements (although no AZT levels were obtained) or of undocumented prior AZT use that could have selected for viral resistance and a more modest CD4 response.

i. The results of this trial appear to contrast with those of ACTG 116A (32), in which AZT appeared to confer a survival benefit over ddI in AZT-naive patients. However, the patient populations studied in these two protocols were distinct. That of ACTG 116A consisted of patients with more advanced HIV disease (median CD4 count, 120/μl), and asymptomatic subjects comprised only 7% of the study group; in contrast, the mean CD4 count in ACTG 175 was 352/μl, and 82% of patients were asymptomatic. It is conceivable that antiretroviral agents may exert distinct effects at different stages of HIV disease; for example, at later stages, when more rapid onset of AIDS-related events may be expected, a more dramatic benefit of a drug may be observed than in early disease.

j. Complementary results were obtained in the European Delta trial (30a), which evaluated 3207 antiretroviral-naive and antiretroviral-experienced (median prior AZT 17.2 months) individuals with CD4 counts <350/μl. These patients had generally more advanced immunodeficiency than those in ACTG 175, with a mean CD4 count of 205/μl; they were randomized to receive either AZT monotherapy (600 mg/day), AZT plus ddI (400 mg/day), or AZT plus ddC (2.25 gm/day). After a median follow-up time of 30 months, statistically significant decreases in mortality by 32% and 42% were observed for antiretroviral-naive patients in the AZT/ddC and AZT/ddI groups, respectively, compared to AZT alone. For antiretroviral-experienced individuals, a significant mortality benefit was only seen for AZT/ddI (23% decrease). Protection from disease progression was associated with AZT/ddI therapy in both antiretroviral-naive (54% relative reduction, p=0.0008) and experienced patients (40% relative reduction, p=0.04); as in ACTG 175, significant decrease in progression with AZT/ddC was seen only for antiretroviral-naive individuals (44% decrease, p=0.006).

k. Interestingly, Saravolatz recently reported results from a trial enrolling 1102 patients (80a) whose design closely resembled that of the Delta trial, but examined individuals with advanced HIV disease (mean CD4 count 119/μl). Using the same three treatment arms of AZT alone, AZT/ddI, and AZT/ddC, participants were followed for a median time of 35 months. No statistically significant difference in the frequency of disease progression or death (ranging fom 62–66%) was observed for any of the treatment groups. In subgroup analysis, a decrease in progression or death was found for AZT/ddI in antiretroviral-naive patients (RR 0.57, 95% CI, 0.36–0.90), and for AZT/ddC in those with 12 months or less or prior AZT therapy (RR 0.72, 95% CI, 0.54–0.96).

l. The results from these three trials mark the beginning of the next generation of antiretroviral therapy; by evaluating patients in early and late stages of immunodeficiency, they convincingly establish the decrease in disease progression and mortality associated with AZT/ddI and AZT/ddC for antiretroviral-naive patients; for AZT-experienced individuals, the addition of ddI but not ddC was beneficial. Consequently, AZT monotherapy can no longer be considered the initial regimen of choice in HIV antiretroviral therapy.

D. Impact of Antiretroviral Therapy on Quality of Life

1. In a retrospective review (55) of the data from the ACTG 019 study (91), the quality of life for patients receiving antiretroviral therapy was examined. For asymptomatic patients with CD4 counts <500 cells/μl, AZT (500 mg/day) decreased the rate of clinical progression in this trial. However, because the benefit of AZT was subsequently shown to be transient, the advantage of slower disease progression was compared with the impact of therapy on the patient's quality of life, which was inferred from the quality-of-life–adjusted time without symptoms of disease or toxicity (Q-TWiST). Calculation of Q-TWiST uses coefficients that weigh the benefit of decreased progression in relation to the adverse effects of toxicity; these coefficients presumably differ from patient to patient. Only severe or life-threatening events were counted.

a. The average time without adverse events or disease progression was 15.7 months in the placebo group, 15.6 months in the 500 mg/day AZT group, and 14.8 months in the 1500 mg/day AZT group.

b. When patients in the 500 mg/day AZT group were compared with those in the placebo group, the former group were free of clinical progression for an average of 0.5 months longer. However, the patients in the placebo group were free of drug toxicity for an average of 0.6 months longer than those in the AZT group.

c. In this study, adverse events were equally weighted in terms of their impact on the quality of life. Although only severe or life-threatening events were recorded, it seems likely that some drug-related toxicities would have more significant impact on the quality of life than others. Nevertheless, this study underscores the importance of assessment of quality of life in planning and monitoring antiretroviral therapy in future studies. Similarly, quality of life issues should be considered by the physician and the patient before an antiretroviral regimen is chosen.

E. Acyclovir and Antiretroviral Therapy

1. The routine use of ACV for HIV-positive patients is controversial. As a single agent, ACV does not possess significant intrinsic activity against HIV-1. However, limited evidence suggests that there may be synergistic antiviral activity when ACV is combined with AZT *in vitro* (62). In addition, three clinical studies have suggested a survival benefit when ACV is used in HIV disease; these studies are summarized in the following sections.

a. Youle (94) undertook a double-blind PRCT that enrolled 302 HIV- and CMV-seropositive patients (97% male, 96% white) with CD4 counts <150/μl and advanced disease (CDC stage IV, and meeting current criteria for AIDS) but no prior history of AIDS-defining illnesses caused by a herpesvirus (*e.g.*, CMV retinitis, herpes zoster). The subjects were randomly assigned to receive either oral ACV (800 mg QID) or placebo. Antiretroviral therapy and PCP prophylaxis were continued on an open-label basis; 81% of the patients in the placebo arm and 84% of those in the ACV arm received AZT. The original end point of the trial was CMV disease, but the protocol was amended to examine survival as well. The study protocol called for 48 weeks of randomized therapy; patients who reached a clinical end point were monitored for four additional weeks. The mean duration of follow-up was 259 days in the placebo group and 274 days in the ACV group. A total of 102 patients withdrew from the trial. Overall, 64 of 149 patients in the placebo group and 69 of 153 in the ACV group completed 48 weeks of randomized therapy or reached a clinical end point. An intention-to-treat analysis was used.

(1) Survival—ACV significantly improved survival; 43 patients died in the placebo group, compared with 27 in the ACV group (P=0.018). Correcting for antiretroviral therapy, the RR of death for those receiving ACV (versus placebo) at 1 year was 0.54 (95% CI, 0.33 to 0.89; P=0.013). The use of PCP prophylaxis did not alter this apparent protective effect of ACV.

(2) Herpetic Infections—However, there was no significant difference in the risk of CMV infection between the two groups. The average time to development of a herpes simplex infection was significantly decreased in the ACV group, compared with the placebo group (P=0.00001).

(3) CD4 Count—ACV did not significantly change the CD4 count.

(4) Adverse Effects—ACV was well tolerated, and adverse events specifically attributable to ACV were rare.

(5) Although a survival benefit of ACV is evident from these results, the duration of this protective effect is unknown given the relatively short period of follow-up in this trial (only 4 weeks after cessation of randomized therapy).

b. An earlier trial (25) randomly assigned patients with AIDS or ARC to receive either oral AZT (250 mg QID) plus oral ACV (800 mg QID) or AZT plus placebo. An initial 1-year survival benefit favoring ACV disappeared when the data were adjusted for baseline CD4 counts and HIV-associated symptoms.

c. Results from an observational study from the Multicenter AIDS Cohort Study gave support for the use of combination therapy with ACV and AZT (87). From this database of >2600 homosexual or bisexual men, 786 patients who had begun AZT before being diagnosed with AIDS were asked if they had used any other medication for HIV infection or another health reason; 242 reported taking ACV for HIV or AIDS, and 488 had used ACV for non-HIV–related purposes. An intention-to-treat analysis was used.

(1) Survival

(a) For patients who had been using ACV together with AZT for any reason, the risk of death was decreased by 26% (P=NS; relative hazard, 0.74; 95% CI, 0.53 to 1.03), and by 36% (P=0.01; relative hazard, 0.64; 95% CI, 0.45 to 0.91) for those taking ACV specifically for AIDS. This survival advantage was most evident for subjects who began taking ACV after a clinical diagnosis of AIDS; the relative hazard was 0.56 (95% CI, 0.37 to 0.86; P=0.007) for ACV used for any indication and 0.57 (95% CI, 0.38 to 0.84; P=0.005) for ACV used for HIV treatment.

(b) No survival benefit was observed when ACV was begun before AIDS was diagnosed; the authors suggested that higher mortality in patients with advanced AIDS may have accentuated an ACV-associated difference in death rates. The CD4 count, the presence of HIV-related symptoms, and the baseline hemoglobin concentration correlated positively with the probability of survival. Overall, ACV appeared to prolong survival by approximately 1 year.

(c) Survival times associated with the use of ACV were calculated through multivariate analysis employing landmark time points. Two landmarks were chosen: the point 1 year after commencement of AZT, and late indicators of CD4 count <50/μl or diagnosis of AIDS. At the first landmark (1 year after AZT), the 90% survival times were 1325 days for patients who were taking ACV before or at the landmark, and 982 days for those who did not receive ACV (P=0.009). At the second landmark (CD4 count <50/μl or AIDS diagnosis), the 90% survival times were 398 days and 176 days (P= 0.004), respectively.

(2) Disease Progression—In a multivariate analysis, there was no significant difference in mean time to development of CMV infection or progression to AIDS.

(3) There was no dose-dependent effect of ACV. The median dosage was 600 to 800 mg/day, much lower than the dose used in the previously discussed randomized trials.

(4) As with any observational study, potentially confounding, uncontrolled variables may have influenced the data (*e.g.*, an unknown factor that prolonged survival but also correlated with the use of ACV). Another puzzling finding is the decrease in mortality without a corresponding decrease in the rate of disease progression.

d. The potential advantage of combining AZT with ACV is intriguing but remains unproven. Double-blind PRCTs specifically designed to address this issue are in progress and should provide clarification. In the absence of definitive trials, the decision to combine ACV with AZT should be made only after careful consideration of the potential risks (*e.g.*, selecting for resistant herpesvirus strains) and benefits.

F. Utility of HIV Viral Load in the Management of Antiretroviral Therapy

1. HIV viral load can be estimated by measuring plasma concentrations of HIV-specific RNA. Three techniques are currently available to quantitate plasma HIV RNA (6).

a. In the polymerase chain reaction (PCR), template DNA is first synthesized from sample RNA using reverse transcriptase and is then amplified with successive rounds of heat denaturation of DNA to single strands, annealing of HIV-specific primers, and DNA synthesis using a heat-stable polymerase.

b. In nucleic acid sequence-based amplification, sample RNA is directly amplified with the use of reverse transcriptase to generate double-stranded DNA copies of the RNA; this is followed by transcription of the DNA by an RNA polymerase to yield large amounts of RNA copies.

c. The branched chain DNA assays employ branched DNA amplifier molecules which hybridize to sample RNA and detection probes linked to the enzyme alkaline phosphatase, thus allowing chemiluminescent quantitation.

d. For PCR and nucleic acid sequence-based amplification, quantitation is achieved through the coamplification of internal standard RNA in each reaction; branched DNA assays rely on a standard curve generated with each analysis. The PCR and branched DNA assays are more commonly employed at present.

2. The PCR and branched DNA assay results are highly correlated, with a rank correlation coefficient of 0.89; values from the two tests were similar over a three-log range (10^4 to 10^7 copies per milliliter) (7). In general, however, caution should be used in comparing HIV RNA levels derived from different methodologies or even from different manufacturers. Even with the same technique (*e.g.*, PCR), significant interassay variability (as much as two orders of magnitude) may be observed (57).

3. Intra-assay variability is much more limited, and for PCR is on the order of 0.2 log. Serial testing of clinically stable patients demonstrated RNA levels that varied by an average of 0.3 log (93). Therefore, it has been suggested that changes of >0.5 log (about threefold) in HIV plasma RNA should be considered significant (79). Recent studies have shown that influenza vaccination is associated with a marked but transient increase in HIV plasma RNA that peaks at 1 to 2 weeks after vaccination and appears to return to baseline by 4 weeks (70,86). The basis for this effect is unclear, but it is conceivable that generation of a host immune response to the vaccine antigen, with cytokine release, may also activate replication of HIV-1. Certainly this phenomenon may affect HIV plasma RNA quantitation when tested near the time of vaccination. The long-term consequences of this increase in replication are unknown; at present, in the absence of additional data, many practitioners offer vaccinations for HIV-positive patients, given the transient nature of the increase weighed against the significant risk for morbidity and mortality caused by influenza, pneumococcal, and other diseases for which effective prophylaxis is available.
4. HIV plasma RNA is detectable at all stages of infection (48,75) and several studies have implicated it as a more powerful independent predictor of disease progression than the CD4 count.
   a. The most compelling evidence for the correlation between HIV RNA level and disease progression comes from a study of 180 men enrolled in the Multicenter AIDS Cohort Study from whom plasma samples were obtained at study entry and at 6-month intervals (61). Plasma HIV RNA was quantitated using a branched DNA assay. Median follow-up was 5.6 years for patients who progressed to AIDS and 10.6 years for those seropositive subjects who did not develop AIDS.
      (1) A single baseline measurement of plasma HIV RNA level was predictive of disease progression and death (Table 24–1). The prognostic value of plasma HIV RNA was enhanced if the mean of the baseline and 6-month follow-up levels was used in these calculations. In contrast, baseline CD4 counts were less predictive; only those counts <321/μl (the lowest stratified group) were significantly associated with earlier disease progression or death, and use of the mean of two CD4 measurements did not improve outcome stratification.
      (2) Among patients with CD4 counts >500/μl, the median survival rate was significantly greater for those with baseline HIV RNA levels lower than the median value of 10,190 copies per milliliter ($P<0.001$).
      (3) The relative hazard of death was 1.55 for each threefold increase in plasma HIV RNA level ($P<0.001$), based solely on the single RNA measurement obtained at study entry. A decrease of 100 cells/μl in baseline CD4 count was associated with a nonsignificant 1.03 relative hazard of death. Use of the mean of a baseline and 6-month follow-up measurement resulted in statistically significant hazards of 1.57 for a

Table 24-1 Plasma HIV RNA correlates with prognosis (61)

Range of Plasma HIV RNA (copies/ml)	% of Patients Progressing to AIDS at 5 Y	Median Time to Development of AIDS (y)	% Mortality at 5Y	Median Survival (y)
≤4,530	8	>10	5	>10
4,531–13,020	26	7.7	10	9.5
13,021—36,270	49	5.3	25	7.4
>36,270	62	3.5	49	5.1

threefold RNA increase and 1.33 for a decrease in CD4 count of 100/μl.

b. The utility of measurement of the plasma HIV RNA level in monitoring antiretroviral therapy was well illustrated by subgroup analysis of the ACTG175 trial group (49b), and also by a report derived from the Veterans Affairs Cooperative Study (46), which randomly assigned patients with CD4 counts of 200 to 500/μl to receive either immediate or deferred AZT therapy. Plasma samples were available for 270 of the 338 enrolled subjects (129 of those receiving immediate therapy and 141 of those receiving deferred AZT) and were analyzed for viral load, CD4 count, and level of β_2-microglobulin (71).

(1) The baseline plasma viral RNA was significantly associated with progression to AIDS (RR, 1.27 for each 0.5-log increase; $P<0.001$), as was the CD4 count (RR, 0.85 for each increase of 35/μl; $P=0.001$), but not the level of β_2-microglobulin. With the use of serial measurements after randomization to immediate or deferred therapy, the RR for progression to AIDS was 1.5 per 0.5 log increase in plasma HIV RNA level (95% CI, 1.23 to 1.83) and 0.83 for the increase in CD4 count (95% CI, 0.76 to 0.91).

(2) In multivariate analyses, a 75% decrease in plasma HIV RNA level (about 0.6 log) was associated with an RR for progression of 0.44 (95% CI, 0.23 to 0.81, $P=0.009$); the RR for a 10% increase in CD4 count was 0.48 (95% CI, 0.28 to 0.82; $P=0.007$).

(3) Calculations based on Cox proportional hazard models revealed that a 75% decrease in plasma HIV RNA level explained 59% of the decreased risk for progression to AIDS, whereas a 10% increase in CD4 count explained only a 31% decreased risk for progression to AIDS; this suggests that plasma HIV RNA level is a better predictor of clinical course. However, the CD4 count does provide additional prognostic information; the combination of a 75% decrease in RNA and a 10% increase in CD4-positive cells explained 79% of the influence of antiretroviral therapy.

(4) This study confirms the utility of measurements of HIV RNA levels in providing a risk assessment for progression to AIDS in patients receiving antiretroviral therapy, and it also supports the use of a 0.5-log threshold for significant change in viral load.

c. For these reasons, plasma HIV RNA has gained acceptance as an effective marker to assess antiretroviral treatment and disease progression. It should be noted, however, that plasma viral RNA is only a representation of true viral load, given the significant sequestration of HIV within lymphoid tissue and other sites, particularly in early stages of disease. HIV replication within lymphoid tissues may be independent of those processes that control replication of circulating virus. Toward this end, measurement of HIV RNA level within peripheral blood mononuclear cells (80) and studies attempting to quantitate extravascular reservoirs of HIV may provide additional clinical information.

G. New Antiretroviral Agents

1. Nonnucleoside reverse transcriptase inhibitors are presently in clinical trials. One member of this family, nevirapine, was recently evaluated in a PRCT enrolling 398 patients with CD4 counts <350/μl and >6 months of prior nucleoside therapy (27). Patients received unblinded AZT (600 mg/day), ddI (400 mg/day), and either nevirapine (200 mg/day for the first 2 weeks, then 400 mg/day) or placebo. The study was 48 weeks in duration.

a. No difference in disease progression was observed, although the study had only moderate power to detect a 2.5-fold increase in time to disease progression.

b. Modest but statistically significant improvements in surrogate markers of infection were observed (mean CD4 count 18% higher and mean plasma HIV RNA level 0.25 log lower).

c. Severe rashes were significantly more common in the nevirapine group (9%, versus 2% in the placebo group; $P=0.002$).

d. Because clinical progression was not obviously affected in this trial, the role of nevirapine in antiretroviral therapy requires additional clarification.

2. New Nucleoside Analogs

a. Lamivudine (3TC) appears to be a particularly promising drug, especially when combined with AZT (the rapid development of drug resistance precludes 3TC monotherapy). *In vitro* analysis has revealed that the mutation in the viral reverse transcriptase associated with the use of 3TC causes HIV to remain AZT-sensitive, even in the presence of mutations linked to AZT resistance; this presumably occurs through effects on the protein structure of reverse transcriptase that antagonize the effect of AZT-neutralizing mutations (54). Prospective trials examining outcomes have not yet been published; however, encouraging results have been reported with the use of surrogate markers of disease progression.

(1) A recent PRCT enrolled 366 patients with CD4 counts of 200 to 500/μl and <4 weeks of prior AZT use (36). The patients were randomly assigned to one of four arms: AZT monotherapy (200 mg PO TID), 3TC monotherapy (300 mg PO BID), AZT plus low-dose 3TC (150 mg BID), or AZT plus high-dose 3TC (300 mg BID). The differences in CD4 count and plasma HIV RNA level for the AZT/3TC arms were statistically significant when compared with AZT monotherapy (Table 24–2). In a subgroup of patients with baseline HIV RNA values >20,000 copies per milliliter, maximal median decreases of 2 logs (100-fold) were observed in the combination therapy arms. Adverse effects were largely those associated with AZT use; 3TC was in general well tolerated. However, 25% of patients, equally distributed among the four treatment arms, had withdrawn from the study by 24 weeks. Similar results were reported in a European trial which compared AZT monotherapy and AZT/3TC (49a).

(2) A second PRCT compared AZT/3TC combination therapy (with low-dose and high-dose 3TC arms in the same doses as before) with AZT/ddC (the latter at 750 mg TID) (4). A total of 254 patients with CD4 counts between 100 and 300 cells/μl and extensive prior AZT exposure (median duration, 20 months) were enrolled; 22% stopped the study medication before 24 weeks, and 37% by 52 weeks. Both AZT/3TC arms were associated with increases in CD4 count at 52 weeks that were significantly higher than those in the AZT/ddC group. Decreases in plasma HIV RNA level were comparable among the three arms (0.48 and 0.51 log copies per milliliter for the low-dose and high-dose AZT/3TC arms, respectively, and 0.39 log for the AZT/ddC group).

(3) Therefore, AZT and 150 mg BID of 3TC induce impressive and apparently durable improvements in HIV RNA level and CD4 count. Ongo-

Table 24-2 CD4 count and plasma HIV RNA during AZT, 3TC, and AZT/3TC therapy (36)

Regimen	Median Change in CD4 Count at 24 Wk (cells/μl)	Median Change in CD4 Count at 52 Wk (cells/μl)	Median Change in Log HIV RNA at 24 Wk (copies/ml)	Median Change in Log HIV RNA at 52 Wk (copies/ml)
AZT alone	+11.9	−26.5	−0.31	−0.20
3TC alone	+24	+5.8	−0.60	−0.29
AZT/low-dose 3TC	+66.3	+69.4	−1.20	−0.81
AZT/high-dose 3TC	+41.3	+66	−1.10	−1.00

ing studies are addressing whether these changes in surrogate markers of infection correlate with improved clinical outcome.

b. Stavudine (d4T) has recently gained approval from the US Food and Drug Administration. Limited data suggest that d4T monotherapy may improve clinical outcome in patients with >6 months of prior AZT experience and CD4 counts between 50 and 500 cells/µl (3). Combination therapy with d4T is under investigation; d4T/3TC is well tolerated, whereas d4T/ddI can be complicated by the additive effects of peripheral neuropathy, which can be induced by either agent. No outcomes data on these combinations have yet emerged.

3. Protease Inhibitors—These agents, which block the action of the HIV-encoded protease and prevent the post-translational cleavage of a viral polypeptide chain into functional components, have potent effects against HIV and represent a particularly promising new class of antiretroviral drugs. Because of the rapid development of resistance when they are used as monotherapy, including cross-resistance to other protease inhibitors (22), these agents must be used in combination regimens. Three members of this class of drugs are currently available.

a. Saquinavir was the first protease inhibitor to receive approval from the US Food and Drug Administration. Although it has potent in vitro activity, its clinical use is hampered by a poor oral bioavailability (about 4%), although 90% inhibitory concentrations can be achieved in plasma with a 600-mg dose. The drug must be taken with food (optimally with a high fat content) to enhance absorption (66). Saquinavir is generally well tolerated, although associated nausea, vomiting, abdominal pain, and diarrhea have been reported. Concomitant rifampin or rifabutin use may significantly lower plasma saquinavir levels, as may corticosteroids or anticonvulsants. In addition, saquinavir metabolism may increase concentrations of other drugs, such as the antihistamines terfenadine and astemizole (associated with cardiac arrhythmias when present at high levels) (3).

(1) ACTG protocol 229 was a double-blind PRCT enrolling 297 patients with CD4 counts between 50 and 300 cells/µl and >4 months of prior AZT treatment (20). Patients were randomly assigned to one of three treatment arms: open-label AZT (600 mg/day) plus ddC (2.25 mg/day), AZT plus saquinavir (600 mg TID), or AZT combined with ddC and saquinavir.

(a) At 24 weeks of treatment, the number of patients with CD4 counts above baseline was significantly greater in the AZT/ddC/saquinavir group than in the AZT/ddC group ($P<0.001$). Although the AZT/saquinavir group appeared equivalent to the three-drug arm by this measure, follow-up at 48 weeks favored the three-drug regimen over the other two groups.

(b) The decrease in median plasma HIV RNA level was significantly greater in the AZT/ddC/saquinavir group than in the AZT/saquinavir or AZT/ddC arms; the maximal difference from baseline plasma RNA at 24 weeks was about 0.5 log. Direct determination of HIV titer using culture of peripheral blood mononuclear cells revealed a mean decrease in titer of 0.8 log in the three-drug group, a mean decrease of <0.4 log in the AZT/ddC group, and no change in the AZT/saquinavir group.

(2) Additional studies with saquinavir, with outcomes correlations, are needed to draw firmer conclusions regarding its efficacy. In addition, recent evidence suggests that higher doses of saquinavir (3600 to 7200 mg/day) are well tolerated and yield greater improvements in HIV RNA level and CD4 count than the standard regimen of 1800 mg/day (although the two doses were not directly compared) (83); these findings deserve further study in clinical trials.

b. Ritonavir is a protease inhibitor with excellent oral bioavailability. In short-term studies (28,59), ritonavir, at a dose of 600 mg BID, was associated with significant increases in CD4 count and decreases (on the order of

10-fold) in plasma HIV RNA level. Adverse reactions were almost universal; the most common were nausea, vomiting, diarrhea, headache, circumoral paresthesias, alterations in taste, and elevated serum triglycerides and transaminases. In addition to corticosteroids, rifampin, rifabutin, and antihistamines, ritonavir interacts with numerous additional classes of drugs; a partial list includes narcotics, nonsteroidal antiinflammatory drugs, anticonvulsants, antifungal agents, macrolide antibiotics, antidepressants, antiemetics, antihypertensive agents, β-blockers, calcium channel blockers, antiulcer agents, oral hypoglycemics, neuroleptic agents, and benzodiazepines.

(1) Results from an unpublished trial suggest a clinical benefit for ritonavir (3). When added to antiretroviral regimens in >1000 patients with advanced HIV disease and heavy prior antiretroviral drug exposure, ritonavir but not placebo decreased the rate of disease progression or death. An ongoing trial of 12 patients newly diagnosed with HIV-1 infection examined the effect of triple therapy with AZT/3TC/ritonavir (60). All 12 subjects had plasma HIV RNA levels below the limit of detection (<500 copies per milliliter) by a branched DNA assay, at follow-up times ranging from 28 to 240 days.

c. Indinavir (IDV) is another newer-generation protease inhibitor with good oral bioavailability, but fewer drug interactions than ritonavir (rifampin, rifabutin, ketoconazole, and possibly antihistamines, certain benzodiazepines, and cisapride). Decreased absorption of ddI may occur if IDV is taken simultaneously. IDV is generally better tolerated than ritonavir, with nephrolithiasis (2% to 3% incidence) and indirect hyperbilirubinemia among the most common adverse effects (3).

(1) As with the protease inhibitors in general, few data on outcomes are available at present for IDV. However, an ongoing clinical trial contains encouraging information using surrogate markers of infection (45). Ninety-seven patients with CD4 counts between 50 and 400/μl (median, 142/μl), ≥6months of prior AZT therapy (median, 31 months), and ≥20,000 copies per milliliter of plasma viral RNA (median, 41,130) were randomly assigned to one of three arms: IDV alone (800 mg q 8 hours), AZT (200 mg q 8 hours) plus 3TC (150 mg q 12 hours), or triple therapy with AZT/3TC/indinavir. After 24 weeks of therapy, 22 (92%) of 24 patients receiving the triple therapy had plasma viral RNA levels <500 copies per milliliter (*i.e.*, below the level of assay detection). In contrast, 9 (38%) of 24 patients in the IDV group and 0 of 22 in the AZT/ 3TC group had undetectable levels. These findings appeared to be sustained at 44 weeks, although numbers of reportable patients were small (Table 24–3).

d. These remarkable results have stimulated the hope that combinations of nucleoside analogs and protease inhibitors may induce durable remissions from the progressive immunosuppression of HIV infection. However, no data correlating these promising findings with hard clinical end points of disease progression or survival are yet available. In particular, the key question at present is whether resistant viral strains selected by these com-

Table 24-3 CD4 count and plasma HIV RNA in AZT, IDV, and AZT/3TC/IDV therapy (45)

Regimen	Median Change in CD4 Count at 24 Wk (cells/μl)	Median Change in CD4 Count at 44 Wk (cells/μl)	Median Change in Log Plasma HIV RNA at 24 Wk	Median Change in Log Plasma HIV RNA at 44 Wk
AZT/3TC/IDV	+126	+218	−2.2	−2.2
IDV	+105	+158	−0.7	−0.9
AZT/3TC	+14	+14	−0.6	−0.2

bination drug regimens will be pathogenic and eventually cause therapeutic failure, or whether specific combinations of antiretroviral agents will result in prolonged suppression of viral replication.

H. Conclusions

1. Therapy with the first generation of HIV antiretroviral agents was established by the ACTG 016 study with symptomatic patients (40) and the ACTG 019 protocol with asymptomatic patients (91).
   a. AZT therapy significantly slowed the rate of disease progression for HIV-positive patients with CD4 counts <500/μl.
   b. In comparing immediate AZT versus AZT therapy delayed until the onset of symptoms among patients with CD4 counts of 200 to 500/μl, the Veterans Affairs study demonstrated a decrease in the rate of disease progression but no difference in mortality associated with the immediate use of AZT (46).
2. However, it appears that the benefit of AZT is transient and that selection for resistant virus limits its efficacy (26,64).
   a. On the basis of long-term analysis of the ACTG 019 cohort (90), the duration of the protective effect of AZT appears to be at most 2 years.
   b. In the Concorde study (21), a large trial with a particularly long average follow-up period (3.3 years), there was no improvement in the overall rate of progression or survival associated with immediate AZT therapy.
   c. Consequently, in the asymptomatic patient a with CD4 count of 200 to 500/μl, immediate initiation of AZT and deferral of AZT until the onset of symptoms appear to be equivalent therapies. Currently, plasma HIV RNA levels would also be measured to identify individuals with high viral loads who would be at high risk for disease progression.
3. At present, the evidence does not support additional clinical benefit from beginning AZT when CD4 counts are >500/μl. Again, plasma viral load can be employed for risk stratification.
   a. Although a decrease in the rate of disease progression was found with AZT in the European-Australian trial of patients with CD4 counts >400/μl (24), the use of the CD4 count itself as a clinical end point in the study may have biased the interpretation of the data. For example, had progression to a lower CD4 count been included as an end point in the Concorde trial, a clear benefit for early AZT treatment would have been shown.
   b. An arm of ACTG 019 specifically examining the role of AZT for patients with CD4 counts >500/μl did not demonstrate a significant clinical impact, although in this HIV therapeutic trials, like many others, a high rate of patient withdrawal (50%) may have obscured a modest effect (89).
4. Several studies support the use of ddI in patients with prior AZT experience.
   a. For patients with AIDS or ARC who had been previously exposed to prolonged courses (median duration, >1 year) of AZT, ACTG 116B/117 (49) showed that changing to ddI (500 mg/day) was associated with less frequent disease progression compared with continuing AZT therapy, although there was no difference in survival rate.
   b. The ACTG 116A study examined a patient population similar in disease stage to that of ACTG 116B/117 but with <16 weeks of AZT experience; in this population, ddI (500 mg/day) also appeared to be more effective than AZT in decreasing progression and prolonging survival, but only in subjects with 8 to 16 weeks of prior AZT therapy. However, there was a benefit for AZT monotherapy over ddI in patients with ARC or early AIDS (median CD4 count, 130 cells/μl) and no prior antiretroviral experience (32).
   c. Spruance (85) demonstrated that patients with advanced disease and signs of clinical deterioration on AZT had decreased progression when switched to 750 mg/day ddI, with no demonstrable survival advantage.
   d. The Canadian trial (63) of clinically stable patients with CD4 counts of 200 to 500/μl and prolonged previous AZT exposure showed that 400 to 500 mg/day of ddI was more effective than AZT in decreasing incidence of clinical progression or death.

e. For patients with AZT toxicity or treatment failure with advanced AIDS (median CD4 count, <50/μl), ddI (500 mg/day) and ddC (2.25 mg/day) monotherapy were equivalent (2). However, the high mortality rates in this patient population suggest that antiretroviral therapy may not have significantly influenced the clinical course.

5. The results of the ACTG 175 protocol (1,46a) provided the clearest evidence that in antiretroviral-naive patients ddI, AZT/ddI, and AZT/ddC all were more effective than AZT alone in decreasing clinical progression. For subjects with (usually heavy) prior AZT therapy, ddI and AZT/ddI were more beneficial than AZT in slowing clinical progression and in prolonging survival. No difference between immediate versus delayed combination antiretroviral therapy could be elucidated. Similar results were found for AZT/ddI in AZT-naive and experienced patients, and for AZT/ddC in AZT experienced individuals, in two other PCRT's which enrolled subjects with more advanced HIV disease (30a,80a). Based on these findings, AZT monotherapy, previously the initial regimen of choice, should no longer be considered as the standard of care.

6. The use of ACV in antiretroviral regimens remains controversial. Limited data suggest a survival benefit for high-dose ACV (800 mg QID) in patients who are also receiving conventional antiretroviral agents (usually AZT). However, the mechanism for this possible benefit is unclear, and prospective trials specifically addressing the question of ACV-associated improvement in clinical progression remain to be completed.

7. Viral load, as measured by plasma HIV RNA levels, can provide prognostic information as well as an assessment of therapeutic response and appears to be more sensitive than the CD4 count.
   a. A single baseline determination of plasma HIV RNA level can stratify patients by risk for clinical progression and death, and serial measurements appear to improve predictive ability. Patients at lowest risk for clinical progression of HIV disease have viral loads of <5000 to 10,000 copies per milliliter
   b. The intraassay variability of plasma HIV RNA determination is about 0.2 log. Immunization can induce a transient but significant increase in plasma HIV RNA, which returns to baseline within about 4 weeks. In a clinically stable patient, viral load may vary by as much as 0.3 log. Hence, changes in plasma RNA of >0.5 log are considered significant.

8. A new generation of antiretroviral agents has demonstrated considerable potency in short-term studies using surrogate markers of HIV infection (CD4 count and plasma viral RNA level).
   a. 3TC, by inducing HIV reverse transcriptase mutations that preserve AZT susceptibility, provides synergistic activity when combined with AZT.
   b. The protease inhibitors saquinavir, ritonavir, and indinavir represent a particularly promising new class of antiretroviral agents which significantly enhance the potency of combination regimens.
      (1) Saquinavir, the oldest protease inhibitor, at present appears to be the least potent, although it is well tolerated. Additional studies investigating doses higher than the currently approved 1800 mg/day and newly developed formulations with enhanced bioavailability may provide evidence of improved efficacy.
      (2) The recently approved drugs ritonavir and indinavir are both potent protease inhibitors. Indinavir appears to be better tolerated than ritonavir, which has a high incidence of adverse effects and potential drug interactions.
   c. d4T also appears to have utility, especially in combination with other agents. No clear role for the nonnucleoside analog nevirapine has yet been established.
   d. There is encouraging preliminary evidence of significant decreases in plasma viral load associated with combination therapy with two nucleoside analogs and a protease inhibitor, offering the hope for a durable remission of HIV disease. Ongoing trials should provide long-term data on survival and indices of clinical progression. Crucial questions concerning the

frequency of treatment failure and the optimal timing for initiation of these combination regimens remain to be resolved. In addition, the intriguing possibility that aggressive antiretroviral therapy early in the course of HIV infection may severely diminish or even eradicate the viral burden is currently under investigation.

9. Other factors may also influence the choice of an antiretroviral agent in addition to clinical efficacy data and toxicity (75a), including the following examples.

a. Drug interactions may augment toxicity; for example, ddC or ddI can potentially increase the risk for pancreatitis when given with IV pentamidine, can AZT worsen ganciclovir-associated leukopenia).

b. Interactions may interfere with the absorption or metabolism of an antiretroviral agent or other drug. For example, ddI decreases absorption of dapsone, itraconazole, and ketoconazole; and AZT affects the metabolism of phenytoin; and decreased levels of protease inhibitors are associated with rifampin or rifabutin.

c. The patient may lack the ability to follow an increasingly complex medical regimen; for example, the ddI dose should be timed for at least 2 hours after intake of dapsone, itraconazole, or ketoconazole.

d. Quality of life issues associated with drug toxicities are particularly relevant when choosing HIV therapy and should be individually considered for each patient.

10. Given the pathophysiologic evidence for active viral replication even at the earliest stages of HIV disease, it seems likely that early intervention with combination antiretroviral therapy will become the state of the art. Developing and optimizing drug therapies for intervention at early and late phases of the natural history of HIV disease remains a pressing challenge, and recent advances offer hope for further improvements in treatment.

I. Current Recommendations (9)

1. The 1996 Consensus Statement on antiretroviral therapy employs both viral load and CD4 count in criteria for the institution of antiretroviral agents.

a. Symptomatic HIV disease (*i.e.*, oral candidiasis, oral hairy leukoplakia, chronic unexplained fever, sweats, weight loss) and AIDS (defined either by CD4 count <200/μl or by an AIDS-defining illness) require therapy.

b. Antiretroviral agents were also recommended for asymptomatic patients with CD4 counts <500/μl; an alternative approach would be to delay therapy for patients with CD4 counts of 350 to 500/μl if plasma viral RNA levels are <5000 to 10,000 copies per milliliter, placing such individuals at low risk for impending disease progression.

c. At present, clinical benefit from beginning antiretroviral therapy at CD4 counts >500/μl has not been established. However, patients at high risk for progression, as defined by a rapid decline in CD4 count or high plasma viral RNA levels (>30,000 copies per milliliter) should be treated, pending further clinical data.

2. There is no single regimen of choice for the antiretroviral-naive patient. The controversy over whether all HIV-infected patients should be placed on the most powerful regimen available, currently consisting of two nucleoside analogs and a protease inhibitor, has not been resolved. Crucial information on improvements in clinical end points, the duration of these improvements, and the pathogenic potential of resistant viral strains remains to be elucidated. Although a regimen containing a protease inhibitor may be indicated in a patient whose CD4 counts and HIV RNA levels portend clinical progression, current recommendations support the use of nucleoside analogs as an initial choice.

a. AZT/ddI, AZT/ddC, or ddI monotherapy is recommended for initial treatment; the Consensus Statement appears to favor combination therapy over monotherapy, given the larger decreases in viral load observed at 8 weeks in the combination therapy arms of ACT6175 (49b).

b. The combination of AZT/3TC is well tolerated and has at least comparable efficacy, as manifested by improvements in CD4 counts and plasma HIV RNA levels. AZT/3TC may also be a useful initial regimen, although data with clinical end points are not yet available.

c. Therapy with d4T, as monotherapy or in combination with ddI, 3TC, or other agents, has shown promise in preliminary studies but has not yet been extensively evaluated by clinical end point criteria.

3. Both CD4 count and plasma viral RNA can be used to monitor therapeutic response.

   a. The effect of antiretroviral therapy should be reflected in plasma HIV RNA within 3 to 4 weeks; increases to within 0.3 to 0.5 log of baseline may reflect loss of efficacy.

   b. Changes in CD4 count are more difficult to employ in assessing therapy, although a decrease to the baseline CD4 count or a rapidly declining count may indicate therapeutic failure.

   c. The CD4 count and especially the plasma HIV RNA level may provide early information on response to treatment so that opportunistic infections, as late manifestations of clinical failure, may be prevented.

4. In patients previously treated with antiretroviral agents who require a change in treatment because of toxicity, clinical progression, or a less efficacious prior regimen, several options again exist.

   a. Patients on AZT monotherapy may benefit from the addition of ddI, ddC, or 3TC (although, again, outcomes data are lacking for AZT/3TC). Alternatively, ddI monotherapy may be used, especially for those with intolerance to AZT. For patients with advanced HIV disease or with significant risk for clinical progression (by clinical history, CD4 counts, or plasma HIV RNA levels), a more aggressive regimen consisting of AZT/3TC or the addition of a protease inhibitor to two nucleoside analogs may significantly decrease HIV replication and improve clinical outcome.

   b. Patients already receiving combinations of two nucleoside analogs, as well as those treated with two nucleoside analogs plus a protease inhibitor, should begin new regimens containing at least two new agents.

   c. Cross-resistance to other antiretroviral agents may be induced by prior therapy and may limit the choice of alternate regimens or diminish clinical efficacy. Such cross-resistance appears to occur for protease inhibitors

Table 24-4 Alternative antiretroviral regimens for primary treatment failure

Initial Regimen	Alternative Regimens
AZT	AZT/DDI ±protease inhibitor AZT/3TC ±protease inhibitor DDI ±protease inhibitor d4T/DDI ±protease inhibitor
DDI	AZT/3TC ±protease inhibitor AZT/DDI/protease inhibitor d4T/protease inhibitor
AZT/DDI	AZT/3TC ±protease inhibitor d4T/protease inhibitor
AZT/DDC	AZT/3TC ±protease inhibitor d4T/protease inhibitor DDI/protease inhibitor
AZT/3TC	DDI/protease inhibitor d4T/protease inhibitor d4T/DDI d4T/3TC

Adapted from (9).

Table 24-5 Alternative antiretroviral regimens for drug toxicity

Initial Regimen	Alternative Regimens
AZT	DDI
	DDI/d4T
	d4T
	d4T/3TC
DDI	AZT/3TC
	d4T/3TC
	d4T/protease inhibitor
AZT/DDC, with AZT toxicity	DDI
	DDI protease inhibitor
	DDI/d4T
	3TC/protease inhibitor
AZT/DDC, with DDC toxicity	AZT/3TC ±protease inhibitor
AZT/3TC	DDI/protease inhibitor
	d4T/protease inhibitor
	DDI/d4T

Adapted from (9).

and may occur for nucleoside analogs as well, but definitive guidelines are incomplete.

d. Examples of alternate treatment options for clinical failure or drug toxicity are illustrated in Tables 24-4 and 24-5, respectively. Note that not all regimens have demonstrated clinical efficacy as assessed by decreased clinical progression or death.

Abbreviations used in Chapter 24

ACTG = AIDS Clinical Trials Group
ACV = acyclovir
AIDS = acquired immunodeficiency syndrome
ANC = absolute neutrophil count
ARC = AIDS-related complex
AZT = azidothymidine (zidovudine)
BID = twice daily
CDC = Centers for Disease Control
CI = confidence interval
CMV = cytomegalovirus
d4T = stavudine
ddC = dideoxycytidine
ddI = didanosine
DNA = deoxyribonucleic acid
HIV = human immunodeficiency virus
IDV = indinavir
MCV = mean corpuscular volume
NS = not statistically significant
P = probability value
PCP = *Pneumocystis carinii* pneumonia
PCR = polymerase chain reaction
PO = per os
PRCT = prospective randomized controlled trial
q = every
QID = four times daily
Q-TWiST = quality of life–adjusted time without symptoms of disease or toxicity
RNA = ribonucleic acid
RR = relative risk
3TC = lamivudine
TID = three times daily
vs. = versus

References

1. AIDS Clinical Trials Group 175. Executive summary. 1995.

2. Abrams. A comparative trial of didanosine or zalcitabine after treatment with zidovudine in patients with human immunodeficiency virus infection. *New Engl J Med* 1994;330:657.
3. Anonymous. New drugs for HIV infection. *Med Lett Drugs Ther* 1996;38:35.
4. Bartlett. Lamivudine plus zidovudine compared with zalcitabine plus zidovudine in patients with HIV infection: a randomized, double-blind, placebo-controlled trial. *Ann Intern Med* 1996;125:161.
5. Bollinger. The human immunodeficiency virus epidemic in India: current magnitude and future projections. *Medicine (Baltimore)* 1995;74:97.
6. Caliendo. Laboratory methods for quantitating HIV RNA. *AIDS Clin Care* 1995; 7:89.
7. Cao. Clinical evaluation of branched DNA signal amplification for quantifying HIV type 1 in human plasma. *AIDS Res Hum Retroviruses* 1995;11:353.
8. Carne. From persistent generalised lymphadenopathy to AIDS: who will progress? *Br Med J* 1987;294:868.
9. Carpenter. Antiretroviral therapy for HIV infection in 1996: recommendations of an international panel. *JAMA* 1996;276:146.
10. Centers for Disease Control. Kaposi's sarcoma and *Pneumocystis* pneumonia among homosexual men. *MMWR Morb Mortal Wkly Rep* 1981;30:305.
11. Centers for Disease Control. *Pneumocystis* pneumonia Los Angeles. *MMWR Morb Mortal Wkly Rep* 1981;30:250.
12. Centers for Disease Control. 1993 revised classification system for HIV infection and expanded surveillance case definition for AIDS among adolescents and adults. *MMWR Morb Mortal Wkly Rep* 1992;41 (RR-17):1.
13. Centers for Disease Control. Heterosexually acquired AIDS—United States, 1993. *MMWR Morb Mortal Wkly Rep* 1994;43:155.
14. Centers for Disease Control. HIV/AIDS surveillance report 1995. 1995;7:1.
15. Centers for Disease Control. Update: acquired immunodeficiency syndrome—United States, 1994. *MMWR Morb Mortal Wkly Rep* 1995;44:64.
16. Centers for Disease Control. Update: AIDS among women—United States, 1994. *MMWR Morb Mortal Wkly Rep* 1995;44:81.
17. Celentano. HIV-1 infection among lower class commercial sex workers in Chiang Mai, Thailand. *AIDS* 1994;8:533.
18. Choe. The β-chemokine receptors CCR3 and CCR5 facilitate infection by primary HIV-1 isolates. *Cell* 1996;85:1135.
19. Choi. CD4+ lymphocytes are an incomplete surrogate marker for clinical progression in persons with asymptomatic HIV infection taking zidovudine. *Ann Intern Med* 1993;118:674.
20. Collier. Treatment of human immunodeficiency virus infection with saquinavir, zidovudine, and zalcitabine. *New Engl J Med* 1996;334:1011.
21. Concorde Coordinating Committee. Concorde: MRC/ANRS randomised double-blind controlled trial of immediate and deferred zidovudine in symptom-free HIV infection. *Lancet* 1994;343:871.
22. Condra. In vivo emergence of HIV-1 variants resistant to multiple protease inhibitors. *Nature* 1995;374:569.
23. Connor. Reduction of maternal-infant transmission of human immunodeficiency virus type 1 with zidovudine treatment. *New Engl J Med* 1994;331:1173.
24. Cooper. Zidovudine in persons with asymptomatic HIV infection and CD4+ cell counts greater than 400 per cubic millimeter. *New Engl J Med* 1993;329:297.
25. Cooper. The efficacy and safety of zidovudine alone or as cotherapy with acyclovir for the treatment of patients with AIDS and AIDS-related complex: a double-blind, randomized trial. *AIDS* 1993;7:197.
26. D'Aquila. Zidovudine resistance and HIV-1 disease progression during antiretroviral therapy. *Ann Intern Med* 1995;122:401.
27. D'Aquila. Nevirapine, zidovudine, and didanosine compared with zidovudine and didanosine in patients with HIV-1 infection: a randomized, double-blind, placebo-controlled trial. *Ann Intern Med* 1996;124:1019.
28. Danner. A short-term study of the safety, pharmacokinetics, and efficacy of ritonavir, an inhibitor of HIV-1 protease. *New Engl J Med* 1995;333:1528.

29. De Gruttola. Modeling the relationship between survival and CD4 lymphocytes in patients with AIDS and AIDS-related complex. *J Acquir Immune Defic Syndr* 1993;6:359.
30. Deacon. Genomic structure of an attentuated quasi species of HIV-1 from a blood transfusion donor and recipients. *Science* 1995;270:988.
30a. Delta Coordinating Committee. Delta: a randomised double-blind controlled trial comparing combinations of zidovudine plus didanosine or zalcitabine with zidovudine alone in HIV-infected individuals. *Lancet* 1996;348:283.
31. Deng. Identification of a major co-receptor for primary isolates of HIV-1. *Nature* 1996;381:661.
32. Dolin. Zidovudine compared with didanosine in patients with advanced HIV type I infection and little or no previous experience with zidovudine. *Arch Intern Med* 1995;155:961.
33. Doranz. A dual-tropic primary HIV-1 isolate that uses fusin and the β-chemokine receptors CKR-5, CKR-3, and CKR-2b as fusion cofactors. *Cell* 1996;85:1149.
34. Dragic. HIV-1 entry into CD4+ cells is mediated by the chemokine receptor CC-CKR-5. *Nature* 1996;381:667.
35. Embretson. Massive covert infection of helper T lymphocytes and macrophages by HIV during the incubation period of AIDS. *Nature* 1993;362:359.
36. Eron. Treatment with lamivudine, zidovudine, or both in HIV-positive patients with 200 to 500 CD4+ cells per cubic millimeter. *New Engl J Med* 1995;333:1662.
37. Fahey. The prognostic value of cellular and serologic markers in infection with human immunodeficiency virus type 1. *New Engl J Med* 1990;322:166.
38. Feng. HIV-1 entry cofactor: functional cDNA cloning of a seven-transmembrane, G protein–coupled receptor. *Science* 1996;272:872.
39. Fischl. The efficacy of azidothymidine (AZT) in the treatment of patients with AIDS and AIDS-related complex. *N Engl J Med* 1987;317:185.
40. Fischl. The safety and efficacy of zidovudine (AZT) in the treatment of subjects with mildly symptomatic human immunodeficiency virus type 1 (HIV) infection. *Ann Intern Med* 1990;112:727.
41. Fischl. Combination and monotherapy with zidovudine and zalcitabine in patients with advanced HIV disease. *Ann Intern Med* 1995;122:24.
42. Goedert. Effect of T4 count and cofactors on the incidence of AIDS in homosexual men infected with human immunodeficiency virus. *JAMA* 1987;257:331.
43. Greenspan. Relation of oral hairy leukoplakia to infection with the human immunodeficiency virus and the risk of developing AIDS. *J Infect Dis* 1987;155: 475.
44. Rwandan HIV Seroprevalence Study Group. Nationwide community-based serological survey of HIV-1 and other human retrovirus infections in a central African country. *Lancet* 1989;1:941.
45. Gulick. Potent and sustained antiretroviral activity of indinavir (IDV), zidovudine (ZDV) and lamivudine (3TC). Presented at the Eleventh International Conference on AIDS, Vancouver, BC, Canada, 1996.
46. Hamilton. A controlled trial of early versus late treatment with zidovudine in symptomatic human immunodeficiency virus infection: results of the Veterans Affairs Cooperative Study. *New Engl J Med* 1992;326:437.
46a. Hammer. A trial comparing nucleoside monotherapy with combination therapy in HIV-infected adults with CD4 cell counts from 200 to 500 per cubic millimeter. *New Engl J Med* 1996;335:1081.
47. Ho. Rapid turnover of plasma virions and CD4 lymphocytes in HIV-1 infection. *Nature* 1995;373:123.
48. Holodniy. Detection and quantitation of human immunodeficiency virus RNA in patient serum by use of the polymerase chain reaction. *J Infect Dis* 1991;163: 862.
49. Kahn. A controlled trial comparing continued zidovudine with didanosine in human immunodeficiency virus infection. *New Engl J Med* 1992;327:581.
49a. Katlama. Safety and efficacy of lamivudine-zidovudine combination therapy in antiretroviral-naive patients. A randomized controlled comparison with zidovudine monotherapy. *JAMA* 1996;276:118

49b. Katzenstein. The relation of virologic and immunologic markers to clinical outcomes after nucleoside therapy in HIV-infected adults with 200 to 500 CD4 cells per cubic millimeter. *New Engl J Med* 1996;335:1091.
50. Kirchhoff. Brief report: absence of intact *nef* sequences in a long-term survivor with nonprogressive HIV-1 infection. *New Engl J Med* 1995;332:228.
51. Kitayaporn. HIV-1 incidence determined retrospectively among drug users in Bangkok, Thailand. *AIDS* 1994;8:1443.
52. Klein. Oral candidiasis in high-risk patients as the initial manifestation of the acquired immunodeficiency syndrome. *New Engl J Med* 1984;311:354.
53. Koot. Prognostic value of HIV-1 syncytium-inducing phenotype for rate of CD4+ cell depletion and progression to AIDS. *Ann Intern Med* 1993;118:681.
54. Larder. Potential mechanism for sustained antiretroviral efficacy of AZT-3TC combination therapy. *Science* 1995;269:696.
55. Lenderking. Evaluation of the quality of life associated with zidovudine treatment in asymptomatic human immunodeficiency virus infection. *New Engl J Med* 1994;330:738.
56. Levy. Pathogenesis of human immunodeficiency virus infection. *Microbiol Rev* 1993;57:183.
57. Lin. Multicenter evaluation of quantification methods for plasma human immunodeficiency virus type 1 RNA. *J Infect Dis* 1994;170:553.
58. Malone. Sources of variability in repeated T-helper lymphocyte counts from human immunodeficiency virus type 1–infected patients: total lymphocyte count fluctuations and diurnal cycle are important. *J Acquir Immune Defic Syndr* 1990;3:144.
59. Markowitz. A preliminary study of ritonavir, an inhibitor of HIV-1 protease, to treat HIV-1 infection. *New Engl J Med* 1995;333:1534.
60. Markowitz. Triple therapy with AZT, 3TC, and ritonavir in 12 subjects newly infected with HIV-1. Presented at the Eleventh International Conference on AIDS, Vancouver, BC, Canada, 1996.
61. Mellors. Prognosis in HIV-1 infection predicted by the quantity of virus in plasma. *Science* 1996;272:1167.
62. Mitsuya. Strategies for antiviral therapy in AIDS. *Nature* 1987;325:773.
63. Montaner. Didanosine compared to continued zidovudine therapy for HIV-infected patients with 200–500 CD4 cells/mm^3. A double-blind, randomized, controlled trial. *Ann Intern Med* 1995;123:561.
64. Montaner. Clinical correlates of in vitro HIV-1 resistance to zidovudine: results of the Multicentre Canadian AZT Trial. *AIDS* 1993;7:189.
65. Moss. Seropositivity for HIV and the development of AIDS or AIDS-related condition: three year follow up of the San Francisco General Hospital cohort. *Br Med J* 1988;296:745.
66. Muirhead. Pharmacokinetics of the HIV-proteinase inhibitor, Ro 318959, after single and multiple oral doses in healthy volunteers. *Br J Clin Pharmacol* 1992;34:170.
67. Mulder. Two-year HIV-1–associated mortality in a Ugandan rural population. *Lancet* 1994;343:1021.
68. Nelson. Changes in sexual behavior and a decline in HIV infection among young men in Thailand. *New Engl J Med* 1996;335:297.
69. Nelson. Risk factors for HIV infection among young adult men in Northern Thailand. *JAMA* 1993;270:955.
70. O'Brien. Human immunodeficiency virus-type 1 replication can be increased in peripheral blood of seropositive patients after influenza vaccination. *Blood* 1995;86:1082.
71. O'Brien. Changes in plasma HIV-1 RNA and CD4+ lymphocyte counts and the risk of progression to AIDS. *New Engl J Med* 1996;334:426.
72. Pantaleo. HIV infection is active and progressive in lymphoid tissue during the clinically latent stage of disease. *Nature* 1993;362:355.
73. Pantaleo. The immunopathogenesis of human immunodeficiency virus infection. *New Engl J Med* 1993;328:327.

74. Perelson. HIV-1 dynamics in vivo: virion clearance rate, infected c
viral generation time. *Science* 1996;271:1582.
75. Piatak. High levels of HIV-1 in plasma during all stages of infection deter
competitive PCR. *Science* 1993;259:1749.
75a. Piscitelli. Drug interactions in patients infected with human immunodeficienc
virus. *Clin Infect Dis* 1996;23:685.
76. Polk. Predictors of the acquired immunodeficiency syndrome developing in a cohort of seropositive homosexual men. *New Engl J Med* 1987;316:61.
77. Quinn. The epidemiology of the acquired immunodeficiency syndrome in the 1990s. *Emerg Med Clin North Am* 1995;13:1.
78. Quinn. Global burden of the HIV pandemic. *Lancet* 1996;348:99.
79. Saag. HIV viral load markers in clinical practice. *Nature Med* 1996;2:625.
80. Saksela. HIV-1 messenger RNA in peripheral blood mononuclear cells as an early marker of risk for progression to AIDS. *Ann Intern Med* 1995;123:641.
80a. Saravolatz. Zidovudine alone or in combination with didanosine or zalcitabine in HIV-infected patients with the acquired immunodeficiency syndrome or fewer than 200 CD4 cells per cubic millimeter. *New Engl J Med* 1996;335:1099.
81. Sawanpanyalert. HIV-1 seroconversion rates among female commercial sex workers, Chiang Mai, Thailand: a multi cross-sectional study. *AIDS* 1994;8:825.
82. Sax. Potential clinical implications of interlaboratory variability in CD4+ T-lymphocyte counts of patients infected with human immunodeficiency virus. *Clin Infect Dis* 1995;21:1121.
83. Schapiro. The effect of high-dose saquinavir on viral load and CD4+ T-cell counts in HIV-infected patients. *Ann Intern Med* 1996;124:1039.
84. Schechter. Coinfection with human T-cell lymphotropic virus type I and HIV in Brazil: impact on markers of HIV disease progression. *JAMA* 1994;271:353.
85. Spruance. Didanosine compared with continuation of zidovudine in HIV-infected patients with signs of clinical deterioration while receiving zidovudine: a randomized, double-blind clinical trial. *Ann Intern Med* 1994;120:360.
86. Staprans. Activation of virus replication after vaccination of HIV-1–infected individuals. *J Exp Med* 1995;182:1727.
87. Stein. The effect of the interaction of acyclovir with zidovudine on progression to AIDS and survival: analysis of data in the Multicenter AIDS Cohort Study. *Ann Intern Med* 1994;121:100.
88. Van de Perre. The epidemiology of HIV infection and AIDS in Africa. *Trends Microbiol* 1995;3:217.
89. Volberding. A comparison of immediate with deferred zidovudine therapy for asymptomatic HIV-infected adults with CD4 cell counts of 500 or more per cubic millimeter. *New Engl J Med* 1995;333:401.
90. Volberding. The duration of zidovudine benefit in persons with asymptomatic HIV infection: prolonged evaluation of protocol 019 of the AIDS Clinical Trials Group. *JAMA* 1994;272:437.
91. Volberding. Zidovudine in asymptomatic human immunodeficiency virus infection: a controlled trial in persons with fewer than 500 CD4-positive cells per cubic millimeter. *New Engl J Med* 1990;322:941.
92. Wei. Viral dynamics in human immunodeficiency virus type 1 infection. *Nature* 1995;373:117.
93. Winters. Biological variation and quality control of plasma human immunodeficiency virus type 1 RNA quantitation by reverse transcriptase polymerase chain reaction. *J Clin Microbiol* 1993;31:2960.
94. Youle. Effects of high-dose acyclovir on herpesvirus disease and survival in patients with advanced HIV disease: a double-blind, placebo-controlled study. *AIDS* 1994;8:641.

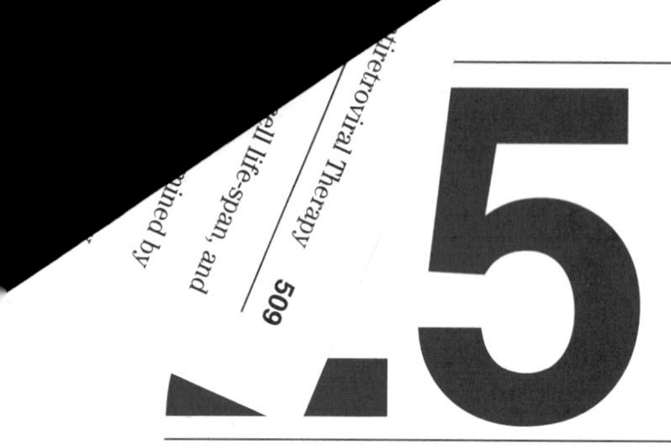

Pneumocystis carinii Pneumonia in HIV Infection

Albert C. Shaw and
Morton N. Swartz

A. Introduction

1. Epidemiology

a. In 1981, reports of *Pneumocystis carinii* pneumonia (PCP) in 15 previously well individuals signalled the beginning of the acquired immunodeficiency syndrome (AIDS) epidemic in the United States (36,62). Before the AIDS epidemic, PCP was rare, occurring most often in premature or malnourished infants or in immunocompromised patients who had undergone chemotherapy or organ transplantation (43,108).

b. Early in the epidemic, PCP was particularly devastating, affecting >60% of AIDS patients (15), with a mortality rate >40% (52). The incidence of PCP has now declined substantially owing to advances in diagnostic technique, antiretroviral therapy, and prophylaxis. For example, in the Multicenter AIDS Cohort Study of 2627 homosexual or bisexual men infected with the human immunodeficiency virus (HIV), the incidence of PCP among those with CD4-positive T lymphocyte counts <100/μl was 62% in 1986—1987 (without PCP prophylaxis) but dropped to 10% in 1990—1991 (with PCP prophylaxis) (74). Nonetheless, PCP remains a significant AIDS-defining illness and may be especially important for patients with poor access to health care and for those who are unaware of their HIV infection (71).

c. PCP appears to be less common among HIV-infected patients in the developing world (1,5). In these countries, patients may succumb first to tuberculosis or bacterial infections before PCP has an opportunity to affect morbidity or mortality. Alternatively, there may be differences in host susceptibility or in the ecology of *P. carinii*. Nevertheless, a much higher rate for PCP (33%) has recently been reported in a small cohort of HIV-infected patients from Zimbabwe. More studies are needed to better document the natural history of PCP worldwide (60).

2. Pathogenesis

a. Through ultrastructural microscopy, three stages can be identified in the life cycle of *P. carinii*: the trophozoite (visible with Giemsa stain), the large cyst (stains with methenamine silver), and the intermediate precyst. Both asexual and sexual phases of reproduction occur, but precise details remain unknown (107). Despite a life cycle that is reminiscent of protozoa, taxonomic analysis of *P. carinii* ribosomal RNA and the organization of genes encoding metabolic enzymes reveals homology with fungi (22–24). However, the relative lack of ergosterol in the plasma membrane is not consistent with a typical fungus and explains the inactivity of conventional antifungal agents against PCP (106).

b. The relative contribution of newly acquired infection versus reactivation of latent infection is not known.

(1) Observations Suggesting Newly Acquired Infection—Horizontal transmission of *P. carinii*, presumably by an airborne route, can be demonstrated in primate and rodent models (95,104). Small clusters of PCP have also been reported among hospitalized immunocompromised patients in close proximity to each other (17,38). However, limitations in distinguishing different genetic strains of *P. carinii* hamper definitive proof of nosocomial outbreaks.

(2) **Observations Suggesting Reactivation**—*P. carinii* has a worldwide distribution, and serologic studies indicate the presence of specific *Pneumocystis* antibodies in >85% of children older than 30 months of age (80). However, *P. carinii* cannot be demonstrated in the respiratory tract of asymptomatic immunocompetent hosts, which argues against the widespread colonization that might be predicted by this antibody data (65,81).

3. **CD4 Count and Risk of Acquiring PCP**—HIV-infected patients with CD4 counts <200/μl are at highest risk for development of PCP (20,63,82). Table 25-1 illustrates the relation between the CD4 count and the subsequent risk of developing PCP as found in the Multicenter AIDS Cohort Study, a study which included 1665 homosexual or bisexual HIV-positive men (82). The RR for development of PCP was 4.9 (95% CI, 3.1 to 8.0) for patients with a baseline CD4 count <200 cells/μl. In multivariate analysis, thrush (RR, 1.86; 95% CI, 1.13 to 3.06) and fever >37.8° C for >2 weeks (RR, 2.15; 95% CI, 1.02 to 4.54) were additional independent predictors for development of PCP (82). Nevertheless, PCP can still occur in 6% to 21% of patients whose CD4 counts are >200 cells/μl (20,63,82).

B. Clinical Manifestations of PCP

1. Among 48 HIV-positive patients presenting with PCP in Kovacs' study, the most common symptoms and signs were fever, nonproductive cough, and dyspnea (52). The median duration of symptoms was 28 days emphasizing the frequently indolent course of this disease. These features are summarized in Table 25-2.
2. In the same study by Kovacs, a lower respiratory rate, lower alveolar-arterial oxygen tension gradient ($P(A\text{-}a)O_2$), higher partial pressure of oxygen in arterial blood with room air (PaO_2), higher lymphocyte count, and higher serum albumin level were associated with improved survival (52). In other studies, a $P(A\text{-}a)O_2$ >35 mm Hg or a PaO_2 <70 to 80 mm Hg at presentation predicted poor survival (12,25,30,75).
3. The classic radiographic appearance of PCP consists of bilateral perihilar interstitial infiltrates. However, focal or nodular infiltrates, miliary disease, cyst for-

Table 25-1 CD4 count correlates with incidence of PCP (82)

CD4 Count at Entry	N	% With PCP by 12 M
<200	77	18.4
201–350	217	4.0
351–500	389	1.4
501–700	483	0.4
>700	499	0

Table 25-2 Frequency of signs and symptoms in 48 HIV+ patients with PCP (52)

Symptoms and Signs of PCP	
Fever	81%
Cough	81%
Dyspnea	68%
Rales	30%
Chills	26%
Sputum	23%
Chest pain	23%
Median respiratory rate	24 breaths/min
Median duration of symptoms	28 d

mation, pneumatoceles, and cavitary lesions have also been described (50). For patients on aerosolized pentamidine (AP) prophylaxis, there is an increased incidence of upper lobe disease, presumably from poor distribution of AP to these areas (47); however, upper lobe presentation may also occur in patients not receiving AP (50). About 5% to 10% of patients have a normal chest radiographic film (40).

4. Several studies have demonstrated that serum lactate dehydrogenase (LDH) is usually elevated in AIDS patients with PCP (30,49,113). In fact, in these studies (involving a total of 234 patients with PCP), only 0% to 7% had a normal serum LDH. In the largest of these studies, elevated LDH had a sensitivity of 94% and a specificity of 82% for distinguishing PCP from other lung diseases in AIDS patients (30). In another study, the serum LDH increased by at least 50 IU from the premorbid level (median increase, 140 IU) in 39 (89%) of 44 patients who developed PCP (113). Therefore, serum LDH can be a useful diagnostic test, because a normal LDH is distinctly unusual in patients with PCP. Furthermore, LDH decreases with treatment in most patients who recover (30,113). On the other hand, elevated LDH is not specific for PCP, because it may be elevated in various other disorders, including lymphoma, lymphocytic interstitial pneumonitis, and pulmonary toxoplasmosis. Table 25-3 summarizes these observations.

C. Diagnosis—Before the AIDS epidemic, diagnosis of PCP required histologic demonstration of *P. carinii* in an open or transbronchial lung biopsy specimen. However, less invasive alternatives are now available, including induced sputum (IS) analysis and bronchoalveolar lavage.

1. Induced Sputum Analysis—Several studies have evaluated the utility of IS examination for diagnosis of PCP. The sensitivity of IS for PCP varies from 55% to 95%, and the NPV varies from 39% to 96% (6,56,77,83,114). Table 25-4 summarizes the diagnostic utility of IS examination. The variability in the accuracy of IS probably reflects differences in the induction protocol, operator experience in obtaining the sample, and, in particular, operator experience in staining and interpreting specimens. Centers with a low incidence of PCP and no dedicated personnel for the procedure have reported lower success rates (69).

a. Aerosolized pentamidine prophylaxis may decrease the sensitivity of sputum induction; in one study comparing 44 episodes of PCP in patients on no prophylaxis with 28 episodes in patients receiving pentamidine, the diagnostic yield of IS was 92.3% in those who had received prophylaxis and 64.3% in those who did not (59). However, another study using a different staining method failed to detect such an effect (75a).

2. Immunofluorescent Stain—The indirect immunofluorescence assay using monoclonal antibodies specific to *P. carinii* has facilitated the analysis of specimens obtained by IS or bronchoscopy. This method allows rapid scanning of specimens for specific fluorescence against a dark background. It has the advantage of rapid processing and short turn-around time and has become one

Table 25-3 Serum LDH levels in PCP

	Zaman (113)	Garay (30)	Kagawa (49)
No. with PCP/ no. controls	54/30	150/671	30/11
Control group	Non-PCP lung disease	AIDS and non-PCP lung disease	AIDS/ARC without PCP or pneumococcal disease
% with PCP and normal LDH	7%	5%	0%
Mean LDH (IU)			
PCP	361	465	509
Control	224	211	217
P	<0.05	<0.05	<0.05

Table 25-4 Induced sputum analysis for the diagnosis of PCP

Location of Study (Reference)	N	PCP (no patients).	Sensitivity	Negative Predictive Value	Comments
San Francisco(6)	43	25	56%	39%	Only those with a negative IS underwent bronchoscopy
Miami (83)	43	20	55%	72%	IS preceded all bronchoscopies
Brooklyn (114)	40	28	78%	71%	Mucolytic agent was added to samples. IS preceded all bronchoscopies
Denver (77)	38	38	66%	62%	Nebulized water, rather than saline, was used
London (56)	51	19	95%	96%	Patients brushed buccal mucosa, tongue, and gums prior to sputum induction

of the most commonly employed methods for diagnosis of PCP. In a study using IS samples from patients with PCP, the immunofluorescent stain detected 92% of the cases and appeared to be more sensitive in direct comparisons with methenamine silver and toluidine blue O; moreover, no false-positive results were observed (53).

3. **Bronchoscopy**—Given the significant false-negative rate associated with IS, bronchoscopy remains an important modality for diagnosis of PCP.
   a. In one prospective study, 171 patients who had AIDS or were at risk for AIDS underwent 276 bronchoscopic examinations. The bronchoalveolar lavage (BAL) or transbronchial biopsy samples were processed with methenamine silver or Giemsa stains. Patients with nondiagnostic studies were observed clinically for at least 4 weeks after the procedure to exclude false-negative tests (13). Overall, 173 pathogens were isolated, including *P. carinii* (57%), cytomegalovirus (CMV; 43%), *Mycobacterium avium* complex (10%), *Mycobacterium tuberculosis* (2%), *Cryptococcus* (2%), *Coccidioides* (0.5%), and *Histoplasma*.
      (1) For all pulmonary pathogens excluding CMV, the sensitivities were 86%, 87%, and 96% for BAL alone, transbronchial biopsy alone, and BAL plus biopsy, respectively. For PCP, the sensitivities were 89%, 97%, and 100%, respectively. Similarly, the NPVs for PCP were 62% to 92%, 92% to 97%, and 92% to 100% with BAL alone, biopsy alone, and BAL plus biopsy, respectively, depending on the true outcome of patients lost to follow-up (Table 25–5). Pneumothorax complicated 9% of the procedures, and when it occurred it was invariably associated with transbronchial biopsy; no complications were associated with BAL alone. Similar findings were reported in a smaller study (99).
      (2) There was an absence of alveolar macrophages in many of the false-negative BAL samples, suggesting that these were inadequate specimens. Therefore, the sensitivity of BAL may have been higher if only adequate specimens had been analyzed. Furthermore, methenamine silver or Giemsa stain was used to detect PCP; if indirect immunofluorescence had been used instead, the sensitivity of BAL for PCP would probably have been higher as well.
   b. Other studies report sensitivities of 97% to 98% for subsegmental BAL when clinical follow-up is used to assess the validity of a negative BAL (34,79). In another report, bilateral BAL, compared with subsegmental lavage, further increased the diagnostic yield of bronchoscopy for PCP (68). As with IS examination, AP prophylaxis may also decrease the diagnostic yield of BAL (47).
   c. In summary, properly performed BAL offers very high sensitivity for PCP. The addition of transbronchial biopsy to bronchoalveolar lavage may offer slightly better diagnostic yield than BAL alone for PCP (13). However, for most circumstances, BAL is sufficient because it still has a high sensitivity for the diagnosis of PCP but is without the risks associated with a blind biopsy.
4. **Gallium Scan**—Gallium 67 citrate scintigraphy has been advocated for diagnosis of PCP. Diffuse lung uptake of gallium is the classic appearance of PCP, although focal uptake may also be seen (54). Excellent sensitivities approaching 100% have been reported (54,111), but the specificity has been estimated at only 51% (55). The routine use of gallium scan for diagnosis of PCP is not rec-

Table 25-5 Comparison of BAL, TBB, or both for the diagnosis of PCP

	BAL	TBB	BAL plus TBB
Sensitivity for PCP	89%	97%	100%
NPV for PCP	62–92%	92–97%	92–100%

ommended because of its relatively high cost, the length of time required for imaging (usually 72 hours), low specificity, and lack of microbiologic information compared to IS or BAL.

5. **Current Recommendations for Diagnosis of PCP**
   a. Numerous other pulmonary processes may mimic the presentation of PCP in HIV-infected patients, including infections by bacteria, mycobacteria, fungi, viruses, *Mycoplasma*, *Legionella*, *Chlamydia*, and *Strongyloides* as well as Kaposi's sarcoma, lymphoma, and congestive heart failure. Consequently, appropriate evaluation of specimens obtained by IS analysis or BAL is essential for proper management of HIV-infected patients who present with clinical features compatible with PCP.
   b. IS examination should be the initial diagnostic step in evaluation for PCP. Provided the sample is acquired and analyzed by experienced personnel, it is a highly effective test for PCP. For patients with a negative IS analysis in whom a suspicion of PCP remains, BAL should be the next diagnostic step. Transbronchial biopsy does not appear to be routinely needed, because the sensitivity of BAL for PCP approaches 97% to 98% and biopsy is associated with a small but significant risk of pneumothorax.
   c. Alternatively, for cases that are highly suspicious for PCP, some practitioners would empirically treat for PCP even if the IS examination is negative, reserving bronchoscopy for those who do not tolerate empiric therapy and those who fail to respond to treatment. Some even support empiric therapy for PCP without any IS examination for selected, clinically stable outpatients with CD4 counts <200/μl who present with pneumonia (64). However, no prospective studies have yet been reported.
   d. A decision analysis model reported by Tu favored empiric therapy over early bronchoscopy if the probability of PCP by BAL was estimated at 72% in the setting of a negative IS examination (103). However, at centers with more experience with IS analysis, the probability of a positive BAL in the setting of a negative IS examination may be only 32% (41). If this value were used in the same decision analysis model, there would be a slight advantage for early bronchoscopy over empiric therapy.

E. **Treatment**—The current treatment of choice for PCP is trimethoprim-sulfamethoxazole (TMP-SMX). Alternative treatment options include pentamidine, trimethoprim-dapsone (TMP-DAP), clindamycin-primaquine, atovaquone, and trimetrexate-leucovorin. For selected patients with severe PCP infection, prednisone has an important adjunctive therapeutic role.

1. **Trimethoprim-Sulfamethoxazole Versus Pentamidine**—Three studies have directly compared TMP-SMX with pentamidine for treatment of PCP (51,91, 109). Two of these studies found no statistically significant difference in survival between these two treatment strategies (51,109). However, in these studies, 60% to 80% of the patients did not complete their initially assigned therapy because of clinical deterioration or adverse drug effects, and crossed over to the alternate arm; this may have diluted any potential difference in outcome between the two groups. In the third study, which did not allow crossover to the alternate arm, TMP-SMX was clearly superior to pentamidine (Table 25–6) (91). This study by Sattler was a prospective, randomized, non-blinded comparison of TMP-SMX versus pentamidine for treatment of PCP. Of the 69 patients with PCP in the study (86% with their first episode of PCP), 36 were randomly as-

Table 25-6 TMP-SMX compared with pentamidine for PCP (91)

	Pentamidine (N=33)	TMP-SMX (N=36)	*P*
Mean baseline $D(A\text{-}a)O_2$	41 mm Hg	44 mm Hg	NS
Survival without ventilatory support	61%	86%	0.03

signed to TMP-SMX (15 to 20 mg/kg/day trimethoprim and 75 to 100 mg/kg/day SMX, IV in three divided doses), and 33 to pentamidine (4 mg/kg/day IV over 90 minutes). Patients were treated for 17 to 21 days. For those assigned to TMP-SMX, the dose was adjusted to maintain a serum trimethoprim concentration of 5 to 8 μg/ml. Pentamidine dosage was adjusted empirically if serum creatinine increased by >1 mg/dl during therapy. Acetaminophen and diphenhydramine were used to minimize febrile and pruritic symptoms, respectively. Crossover to the alternate arm was permitted only for life-threatening toxicity.

a. Survival was significantly improved with TMP-SMX; 86% of patients treated with TMP-SMX were alive without ventilatory assistance at the end of treatment, compared with 61% of those treated with pentamidine (P=0.03). All deaths were caused by respiratory failure except for 1 patient who died of pentamidine-associated hypoglycemia. The number of days to a 10 mm Hg decrease in $P(A - a)O_2$ was significantly decreased in the TMP-SMX group (7 ± 1 vs. 15 ± 26 days, P = 0.04) as well.

b. A dose reduction of the assigned drug was required in 25 of 36 patients receiving TMP-SMX, but only 8 of 33 patients receiving pentamidine. Rash (44% versus 5%; P=0.001) and anemia (39% versus 24%; P=0.03) were more common in the TMP-SMX group. No episodes of Stevens-Johnson syndrome or exfoliative dermatitis were reported. In contrast, azotemia (64% versus 14%; P<0.0001), hypoglycemia (21% versus 0%; P=0.01), and hypotension (27% versus 0%; P=0.002) were more common in the pentamidine group.

c. All three of these trials were conducted before the widespread use of antiretroviral therapy, PCP prophylaxis, or adjunctive corticosteroid therapy. Therefore, the results may or may not be applicable to the present-day patients at risk for PCP.

2. Trimethoprim-Dapsone—Given the significant incidence of adverse effects associated with both TMP-SMX and pentamidine, better tolerated regimens have been sought. Among the first to be investigated was the combination TMP-DAP. After a preliminary report demonstrated efficacy in 15 patients (58), Medina conducted a double-blind, prospective randomized trial enrolling 60 AIDS patients with their first episode of PCP (67). Participants all had mild to moderate PCP; those with a room air PaO_2 <60 mm Hg and those with glucose-6-phosphate dehydrogenase (G6PD) deficiency were excluded. Thirty subjects each were randomly assigned to receive either TMP-DAP (20 mg/kg/day of oral TMP in four divided doses and 100 mg/day of oral DAP for 21 days) or TMP-SMX (20 mg/kg/day of oral TMP and 100 mg/kg/day of oral SMX in four divided doses for 21 days). Pills were counted to assess compliance with the randomized therapy. At the discretion of study investigators, patients with clinical deterioration or significant adverse effects were switched to IV pentamidine (4 mg/kg/day).

a. The overall response rate was 92% for all patients. The rates of survival, relapse, and treatment failure were not significantly different between the two groups. Other measures of disease severity (*e.g.*, PaO_2, carbon monoxide diffusion capacity of the lung, degree of dyspnea, LDH, respiratory rate) were similar between the two treatment arms both before and after therapy. Chest radiographs appeared to worsen during the first six days of therapy in 57 of 60 patients; this observation has also been reported by Wharton (109).

b. Major adverse effects requiring discontinuation of randomized therapy occurred in 17 patients in the TMP-SMX group but in only 9 patients in the TMP-DAP group (P=0.025). Significant elevation of alanine aminotransferase or aspartate aminotransferase (more than five times normal) occurred in 6 patients in the TMP-SMX group but in only 1 patient in the TMP-DAP group (P=0.05). Minor adverse reactions occurred in almost all patients. Rash occurred in 30% and 37% of the TMP-DAP and TMP-SMX groups, respectively; nausea was reported in >90% of patients in both groups; neutropenia (<50% of baseline value) was more common with

TMP-SMX (17 versus 9 patients; $P=0.03$); hyperkalemia was more common with TMP-DAP (53% versus 20%; $P<0.001$); and asymptomatic methemoglobinemia was observed in a third of the patients assigned to TMP-DAP.

c. For patients with mild to moderate PCP, TMP-DAP and TMP-SMX appear to be equally effective, and both may be suitable for outpatient treatment of mild PCP. Further studies are needed to assess its efficacy for more severe cases. However, because the study was small in size, a small but significant difference in efficacy between the two regimens may have been missed.

3. Clindamycin-Primaquine

a. The AIDS Clinical Trials Group (ACTG) protocol 044 evaluated the efficacy of a clindamycin-primaquine combination for treatment of PCP in an uncontrolled study (7). All patients had a P(A-a)O_2 <40 mm Hg with room air. In the first part of this study, 22 patients (the IV/PO group) received 21 days of primaquine base (30 mg PO QD) plus 10 days of IV clindamycin (900 mg q 8 hours), followed by 11 days of oral clindamycin (450 mg q 6 hours). In the second part of the study, 38 additional subjects (the PO group) received 21 days of primaquine base (30 mg/day) plus 21 days of oral clindamycin (600 mg q 8 hours). The mean PaO_2 and the mean P(A-a)O_2 were 80.3 and 24.7 mm Hg, respectively, for the PO group and 83.9 and 23.1 mm Hg, respectively, for the IV/PO group.

(1) Sustained clinical improvement was observed in 91% of the IV/PO patients and 92% of the PO patients. The 90-day survival rate was also similar between the two groups (96% for IV/PO; 100% for PO).

(2) Both regimens were generally well tolerated, and 77% of the patients finished all 3 weeks of therapy. Most drug-related side effects were mild. A maculopapular rash occurred in 62% of all patients and usually resolved without the need for interruption of therapy; 40% developed >10% methemoglobinemia, but no patient was symptomatic or required therapy; 12% developed diarrhea (all *Clostridium difficile* toxin–negative).

(3) Although this study lacked a control group, the clindamycin-primaquine combination appears to be effective for treatment of mild PCP.

b. In an earlier study, the clindamycin-primaquine combination successfully treated 24 of 28 cases of PCP (101). Seventeen of these patients had previously failed or had become intolerant to other therapies. Encouraged by this and other results, 65 AIDS patients with PCP (>90% male; mean CD4 count, 75/μl; baseline PaO_2 >70 mm Hg for about half) were randomly assigned in a double-blind trial to receive either TMP-SMX or clindamycin-primaquine (100). PCP was microbiologically established in only 75% of the cases. Patients with G6PD deficiency or PaO_2 <50 mm Hg were excluded. In the TMP-SMX group, 31 patients were assigned receive to 3 weeks of folinic acid (5 mg/day PO) plus IV TMP-SMX (240 mg TMP and 1200 mg SMX q 6 hours for patients weighing <60 kg, or 320 mg TMP and 1600 mg SMX q 6 hours for those weighing >60 kg). In the clindamycin-primaquine group, 34 patients were assigned to receive primaquine (15 mg/day for 21 days PO) plus IV clindamycin (600 mg q 6 hours for patients weighing > 60 kg, or 450 mg q 6 hours for those weighing <60 kg) for 10 days, followed by 450 mg q 6 hours (for those >60 kg) or 300 mg q 6 hours (for those <60 kg) for 11 days PO. Diphenhydramine was given to both groups beginning on day 5 of therapy.

(1) There was no significant difference in the rate of response to therapy (about 90% overall). Treatment failure occurred in 2 patients assigned to TMP-SMX and 3 patients assigned to clindamycin/primaquine. No patient died while receiving the randomized therapy, and there was no significant difference in the rate of survival with further follow-up.

(2) Both therapies were generally well tolerated; change in therapy was required in 20% and 18% of the TMP-SMX and clindamycin-primaquine groups, respectively. Hyponatremia and nausea were more common in the TMP-SMX group, whereas rash and diarrhea were more common in the clindamycin-primaquine group. No episodes of methemoglobinemia were reported.

(3) This trial compared TMP-SMX with clindamycin-primaquine and found the two regimens to be equally effective for patients with mild to moderate PCP. Further studies are needed to assess the efficacies of these regimens for more severe cases. However, because the study was small in size, a small but significant difference in efficacy between the two regimens may have been missed. Furthermore, the addition of folinic acid to the TMP-SMX arm may have adversely affected the outcome for this group; recent evidence suggests that this combination may increase the risk of therapeutic failure and death (89).

4. ACTG protocol 108 compared oral therapy with TMP-SMX, TMP-DAP, and clindamycin/primaquine for mild to moderate PCP (88). This double-blind prospective randomized controlled trial (PRCT) enrolled 181 patients with AIDS-related PCP and a P(A-a)O_2 ≤45 mm Hg. Sixty-four patients were randomly assigned to receive TMP-SMX dosages based on body weight: two double-strength tablets (320 mg TMP and 1600 mg SMX) TID for patients weighing 51 to 80 kg, or 1.5 double-strength tablets (240 mg TMP and 1200 mg SMX) TID for those weighing 36 to 50 kg, or 2.5 double-strength tablets (400 mg TMP and 2000 mg SMX) for those weighing 81 to 99 kg. Fifty-nine subjects were randomly assigned to receive DAP (100 mg PO QD) plus PO trimethoprim (300 mg TID for patients weighing 51 to 80 kg, or 200 mg TID for those weighing 36 to 50 kg, or 400 mg TID for those weighing 81 to 99 kg). Finally, 58 patients were assigned to receive clindamycin (600 mg PO TID) with primaquine base (30 mg PO QD). Participants with a prior history of TMP-SMX intolerance were randomly assigned to one of the other two treatment arms. Patients with a P(A-a)O_2 of 35 to 45 mm Hg received adjunctive steroid therapy (see later discussion), and all therapies were given for 3 weeks. Eighty-nine percent of the patients were male; only 9.5% had a prior history of PCP. The primary clinical end point was therapeutic failure, defined as any of the following: >20 mm Hg increase in P(A-a)O_2, change in therapy not related to toxicity, intubation, or death.

a. There were no statistically significant differences among the three treatment arms in mortality (follow-up extended to 2 months after therapy), therapeutic failure (9% overall), or completion of a full course of randomized treatment (accomplished by 54% of subjects). However, small but statistically significant differences among the three oral regimens could have escaped detection, because the study had 80% power to delineate differences of >20%.

b. The rates of dose-limiting toxicity were also comparable among the three groups, although again small differences may not have been detected because of the limitations in study power. Rash was the most common adverse event, occurring in 19% of the TMP-SMX group, 10% of the TMP-DAP group, and 21% of the clindamycin/primaquine group (P=0.2). Nausea and vomiting, the second most common type of dose-limiting toxicity, occurred in 9.4%, 8.5%, and 3.4% of the three groups, respectively. Elevations in serum aminotransferase levels greater than fivefold above baseline occurred in 7 patients, 6 of whom were receiving TMP-SMX (P=0.003); hematologic toxicity (anemia, neutropenia, thrombocytopenia, or methemoglobinemia) was significantly more common in the clindamycin-primaquine group. These adverse effect profiles may guide the choice of oral therapeutic regimen.

5. Atovaquone (1,4-hydroxynaphthoquinone)

a. Atovaquone versus Pentamidine—A recent, open-label study randomly assigned 109 TMP-SMX–intolerant patients with AIDS and histologically-confirmed PCP to receive either oral atovaquone (750 mg TID with food) versus IV pentamidine (3 to 4 mg/kg/day) (21). All subjects had P(A-a)O_2 <45 mm Hg; all but 5 patients were male; 68% had mild disease (defined as $P(A\text{-}a)O_2$ <35 mm Hg); and 58% had no prior history of PCP. Intention-to-treat analysis was used.

(1) Therapeutic success rates were statistically similar between the two groups; 29% of patients receiving atovaquone and 17% of those receiving pentamidine did not respond to therapy (P=0.18). Furthermore, no difference in survival was observed at 4 weeks (7 deaths with atovaquone versus 4 with pentamidine, P=0.53) (Table 25–7).

(2) Atovaquone was better tolerated than pentamidine; 4% of the former and 36% of the latter group failed therapy because of severe adverse effects (P<0.001). Hypotension (6%), hypoglycemia (11%), nausea (8%), and vomiting (7%) all occurred exclusively in the pentamidine group. Furthermore, increased creatinine and renal failure were more likely with pentamidine than with atovaquone. However, increased cough was reported more often with atovaquone (14% versus 1%; P=0.009).

(3) This trial tested the hypothesis that atovaquone was not worse than pentamidine for the treatment of mild to moderate PCP, and the results suggest that the two agents are comparable. However, the study's small size means that a small but significant difference in efficacy may have been missed therefore limits the strength of these conclusions. In addition, the unblinded nature of the study may have introduced other forms of bias. Nevertheless, the size of the study was sufficient to examine the rates of treatment-limiting toxicity, and atovaquone was clearly better tolerated than pentamidine.

b. Atovaquone Versus TMP-SMX—In a large prospective, randomized, double-blind trial, 284 patients with AIDS and PCP ($P(A\text{-}a)O_2$ <45 mm Hg and PaO_2 ≥60 mm Hg) were randomly assigned to receive either 21 days of oral TMP-SMX (320 mg TMP and 1600 mg SMX TID) or 21 days of oral atovaquone (750 mg TID) (42). Compliance was monitored by measurement of serum atovaquone and TMP-SMX levels. Steroid therapy was given to patients with $P(A\text{-}a)O_2$ <35 to 45 mm Hg. Criteria for therapeutic failure were (a) for day 3 of therapy, requirement for mechanical ventilation; (b) for day 7 of therapy, any two of the following: $P(A\text{-}a)O_2$ >30 mm Hg with an increase of >20 mm Hg, worsening chest film, or worsening symptoms; (c) for day 10 of therapy, no improvement in the $P(A\text{-}a)O_2$, chest film, or symptoms; or (d) institution of alternative treatment. Intention-to-treat analysis was used.

(1) One month after completion of randomized therapy, therapeutic failure was observed in 20% and 7% of the atovaquone and TMP-SMX patients, respectively (P=0.002). Eleven patients assigned to atovaquone died during the study, compared with 1 patient assigned to TMP-SMX (P=0.003) (Table 25–8).

(2) Atovaquone was better tolerated than TMP-SMX; 20% of the TMP-SMX patients and 7% of the atovaquone patients could not tolerate a full course of therapy (P=0.001). In particular, the rates of nausea (44% versus 20%), vomiting (35% versus 14%), constipation (17% versus 3%), dizziness (8% versus 3%), fever (25% versus 14%) and rash (34% versus

Table 25-7 Atovaquone compared with pentamidine for PCP (21)

	Atovaquone (N=56)	Pentamidine (N=53)	*P*
Therapeutic failure	29%	17%	NS
4-Wk mortality rate	12%	7%	NS
Therapy-limiting toxicity	4%	36%	<0.001

23%) were all significantly higher with TMP-SMX. Diarrhea was more common with atovaquone (20% versus 7%, $P<0.05$).

(3) In logistic regression analysis, the plasma concentration of atovaquone correlated with therapeutic efficacy. In contrast, TMP-SMX concentration did not correlate with successful outcome. In the atovaquone group only, preexisting diarrhea was a predictor of mortality ($P<0.001$), therapeutic failure ($P<0.001$), and plasma atovaquone concentration ($P=0.009$).

c. Atovaquone is a useful alternative drug for patients with mild-to moderate PCP but appears to be less effective than TMP-SMX. The major advantage of atovaquone is its low toxicity profile. However, it is poorly absorbed and must be used with caution, especially in patients with diarrhea or malabsorption. The recently released elixir form of atovaquone has improved oral bioavailability and may have better efficacy against PCP, but this remains to be demonstrated in clinical trials (110).

6. Trimetrexate-Leucovorin—The dihydrofolate reductase inhibitor, trimetrexate, has potent in vitro activity against *P. carinii* (28). Leucovorin rescue, which has no direct effect on *P. carinii*, is required to prevent severe myelosuppression in the human host. After a small pilot study which reported a 63% to 69% response rate to trimetrexate-leucovorin (3), 215 AIDS patients with confirmed PCP ($P(A\text{-}a)O_2 > 30$ mm Hg) were randomly assigned in a double-blind fashion to receive either 21 days of trimetrexate (45 mg per m^2 of body surface area IV once daily) plus leucovorin (20 mg/m^2 q 6 hours) versus 21 days of TMP-SMX (dosed by 5 mg/kg of TMP q 6 hours) (92). The doses of trimetrexate and leucovorin were adjusted with the use of defined algorithms for hematologic toxicity. Steroid therapy, whose efficacy had not yet been demonstrated at the time of this study, was not given. Almost half of the participants had a $P(A\text{-}a)O_2 > 45$ mm Hg. After day 10, patients who were able to leave the hospital continued on assigned therapy of either IV trimetrexate plus oral leucovorin or oral TMP-SMX. The criteria for therapeutic failure at day 10 were any of the following: respiratory rate >50/minute, >20 mm Hg increase in $P(A\text{-}a)O_2$, requirement for new PCP therapy (pentamidine 4 mg/kg/day IV), or death. The criteria for successful treatment at day 21 were all of the following: survival, no increase in $P(A\text{-}a)O_2$ >than 20 mm Hg, no need for supplemental oxygen or mechanical ventilation, no alteration in therapy, and improved pulmonary signs and symptoms.

a. By day 21, treatment failure or death was significantly more likely with trimetrexate than with TMP-SMX (38% versus 20%, respectively; $P=0.008$) (Table 25–9). In addition, 6 patients had relapsed within 1 month of completing assigned therapy; all relapses occurred in the trimetrexate group ($P=0.014$).

b. One month after completion of randomized treatment, 16% of the patients in the TMP-SMX arm had died, compared with 31% of the trimetrexate patients ($P=0.028$).

c. Trimetrexate was better tolerated than TMP-SMX; treatment-limiting toxicity occurred by day 21 in 28% of patients on TMP-SMX, compared with 8% of those on trimetrexate ($P<0.001$).

d. Because many of the patients in this trial would have met the criteria for adjunctive corticosteroid therapy (see later discussion), it is of interest to

Table 25-8 Atovaquone compared with TMP-SMX for PCP (42)

	Atovaquone (N=138)	TMP-SMX (N=146)	*P*
Therapeutic failure	20%	7%	0.002
Mortality rate	8%	0.6%	0.003
Therapy-limiting toxicity	7%	20%	0.001

Table 25-9 Trimetrexate compared with TMP-SMX for PCP (92)

	Trimetrexate	TMP-SMX	*P*
	(N=106)	(N=109)	
Therapeutic failure or death on day 10	27%	16%	NS
Therapeutic failure or death on day 21	38%	20%	0.008
Mortality rate on day 49	31%	16%	0.028
Therapy-limiting toxicity	8%	28%	<0.001

know whether further therapeutic benefit could have been derived from combining trimetrexate with steroids.

e. Trimetrexate is a well-tolerated alternative drug for patients with PCP and may be effective in patients with more severe disease. However, it appears to be less efficacious than TMP-SMX.

7. Adjunctive Corticosteroids—Based on the observation that some patients with PCP initially experience clinical deterioration during the first few days of treatment, it was hypothesized that killing of *P. carinii* may elicit an augmented immunologic response causing release of inflammatory mediators and further lung injury. Consequently, several clinical trials have evaluated the benefit of adjunctive corticosteroid therapy in patients with PCP, with the goal of blunting this inflammatory response and minimizing the extent of lung injury (11,29,73). Based on the results of these randomized studies, the 1990 National Institutes of Health–University of California Expert Panel recommended administration of adjunctive corticosteroids for adult patients with PCP and PaO_2 <70 mm Hg or $P(A\text{-}a)O_2$ >than 35 mm Hg (75). The recommended doses for prednisone were as follows: 40 mg PO BID for days 1 through 5, 40 mg PO QD for days 6 through 10, and 20 mg PO QD for days 11 through 21. Methylprednisolone (at 75% of the prednisone dose) may be substituted if IV delivery is desired (11,75). The original studies by Bozzette (11) and Gagnon (29) are described for illustration.

a. Bozzette described the results of an unblinded, prospective randomized comparison of prednisone (40 mg PO BID for days 1 through 5; 40 mg PO QD for days 6 through 10; 20 mg PO QD for days 11 through 21) versus no prednisone in 251 AIDS patients with PCP (11). Prednisone was started within 36 hours of initiation of antimicrobial therapy; the choice of antimicrobial therapy was made by the responsible physicians. Twenty-five percent had mild disease, defined as a ratio of PaO_2 to fractional concentration of inspired oxygen (FiO_2) ≥350 mm Hg; 48% had moderate PCP (PaO_2/FiO_2 ratio, 250 to 350 mm Hg); and 27% had severe PCP (PaO_2/FiO_2 ratio, 75 to 250 mm Hg). Patients requiring mechanical ventilation and those with a PaO_2/FiO_2 ratio <75 mm Hg were excluded.

(1) The risk of respiratory failure by day 21 (13% versus 28%; *P*=0.004), the risk of death by day 21 (9% versus 18%; *P*=0.024), and the risk of death by day 84 (16% versus 26%; *P*=0.026) were all significantly lower in the prednisone-treated group. The risk of relapse was not different between the two groups (Table 25–10).

(2) When patients were stratified based on the severity of illness at presentation, a statistically significant benefit of adjunctive corticosteroid therapy was observed only for those with moderate or severe PCP. No benefit could be demonstrated for those with mild disease.

(3) More patients in the prednisone group were able to complete at least 14 days of therapy (70% versus 54%; *P*=0.03). The incidence of dose-limiting toxicity was also lower with prednisone, but the difference did not reach statistical significance.

(4) By day 84 of follow-up, the risk of herpes simplex virus reactivation was significantly higher with prednisone than with control (26% versus 15%; $P=0.04$). There was also a trend toward higher incidence of thrush in the prednisone arm, but this difference did not reach statistical significance.

b. Gagnon reported the results of a double-blind, placebo-controlled, randomized comparison of methylprednisolone (40 mg IV q 6 hours for 1 week) versus placebo in 23 AIDS patients with PCP (29). Patients were enrolled within 72 hours of receiving antimicrobial therapy for PCP. All patients were treated with 21 days of TMP-SMX (based on 15 mg/kg/day of TMP); the mean $P(A\text{-}a)O_2$ was approximately 65 mm Hg with on room air; 22 of 23 patients had no prior history of PCP; and all patients had severe PCP, defined as respiratory rate >30/minutes, $P(A\text{-}a)O_2$ >30 mm Hg with room air, and PaO_2 <75 mm Hg with 35% oxygen but >60 mm Hg with 100% oxygen. Those requiring mechanical ventilation were excluded.

(1) For ethical reasons, the study was terminated early because significant excess mortality was observed in the placebo group (Table 25–11). Nine of 12 patients in the corticosteroid group survived to discharge, compared with only 2 of 11 patients in the placebo group ($P<0.008$).

(2) Patients treated with corticosteroids were less likely to experience respiratory failure (25% versus 82%; $P<0.008$) and more likely to receive the full 21 days of TMP-SMX therapy (83% versus 36%; $P<0.024$). When corticosteroids were discontinued after 7 days, 4 patients had a subsequent clinical deterioration but improved with resumption of adjunctive corticosteroid therapy.

(3) Despite its small size, this trial was noteworthy for demonstrating a significant benefit of adjunctive corticosteroid therapy for patients with severe PCP and AIDS. In addition, this study provided support for longer duration of corticosteroid therapy, since a third of the corticosteroid-treated patients deteriorated when the high dose methylprednisolone was stopped after 7 days. Based on this observation and the experience in Bozzette's trial (11), a tapering course of corticosteroids over 21 days is now recommended (75).

Table 25-10 Adjunctive corticosteroids in 251 patients with mild-to-severe PCP (11)

	Corticosteroids (N=128)	No Corticosteroids (N=123)	*P*
Respiratory failure by day 21	13%	28%	0.004
Risk of death by day 21	9%	18%	0.024
Risk of death by day 84	16%	26%	0.026
Dose-limiting toxicity by day 21	22%	31%	NS
Completed >14 days of therapy	70%	54%	0.03
HSV reactivation	26%	15%	0.04
Risk of relapse by day 84	9%	8%	NS

Table 25-11 Adjunctive corticosteroids in 23 patients with severe PCP (29)

	Corticosteroids (N=12)	No Corticosteroids (N=11)	*P*
Survival to discharge	75%	18%	<0.008
Respiratory failure	25%	82%	<0.008
Length of stay in intensive care unit	1.2 d	6.3 d	<0.001

c. In contrast to these trials, Walmsley reported the results of another double-blind PRCT which calls attention to the limitations of adjunctive corticosteroid therapy (105). 78 patients with moderate to severe PCP (PaO_2 <70 mm Hg with room air or $P(A\text{-}a)O_2$ >40 mm Hg) were enrolled within 24 hours of beginning antimicrobial therapy and randomly assigned to receive either methylprednisolone (40 mg IV q 12 hours for 10 days) or placebo. The choice of antimicrobial therapy was determined by the primary physicians. The mean baseline PaO_2 was 56 mm Hg, and the mean $P(A\text{-}a)O_2$ was 76 and 85 mm Hg in the corticosteroid and placebo arms, respectively. The primary clinical end points were any of the following: death before discharge, need for mechanical ventilation for >6 days, or PaO_2 < 70 mm Hg on day 10 of therapy.

- **(1)** In contrast to the studies previously described (11,29), there were no statistically significant differences between the two groups in terms of the risk of death (overall death rate, 13%), the need for mechanical ventilation, or the percentage of patients with PaO_2 <70 mm Hg on day 10. A subgroup analysis of 27 patients with baseline PaO_2 <50 mm Hg also failed to demonstrate any significant benefit of corticosteroid therapy.
- **(2)** However, the mean $P(A\text{-}a)O_2$ was significantly lower with corticosteroid therapy than with placebo (P=0.04). In addition, among the 64 patients treated with TMP-SMX, rash and fever were less likely to occur in those randomly assigned to receive to corticosteroids (4 versus 11 patients, P=0.039).
- **(3)** Different corticosteroid dosing regimens may have been responsible for the conflicting findings in these trials. In addition, the severity of illness may have been different among these trials, as reflected by an overall mortality rate of only 14% in Walmsley's study but 82% in Gagnon's study (29). Potentially, a much larger study population would have been required in Walmsley's study to demonstrate a mortality benefit.
- **(4)** The study by Walmsley (105) evaluated different clinical end points than those evaluated in the three earlier studies (11,29,73). In addition to the mortality rate, the three earlier studies examined end points that were indicators of early deterioration, such as the risk of respiratory failure or a decrease in the oxygen saturation. In contrast, Walmsley evaluated end points more reflective of the potential for recovery, such as the need for prolonged mechanical ventilation or sustained hypoxemia at day 10 (10). The results of these studies are consistent with the hypothesis that the benefit of adjunctive corticosteroid therapy is in blunting the early paradoxical increase in inflammatory response associated with treatment of PCP.

F. Prophylaxis—In the absence of prophylaxis, patients who recover from an episode of PCP have a significant risk of relapse, as high as 50% at 7 months in one study (16,72). Even among those without a prior history of PCP, HIV-infected patients (in the Multicenter AIDS Cohort Study) with CD4 counts <200/µl had an 18.4% incidence of PCP by 12 months (82). Thrush (RR, 1.86; 95% CI, 1.13 to 3.06) and fever >37.8° C for >2 weeks (RR, 2.15; 95% CI, 1.02 to 4.54) are additional independent risk factors (82). An early prospective, randomized, blinded trial demonstrated the effectiveness of PCP prophylaxis in non-HIV–infected children with cancer (44), and numerous studies since have confirmed its benefit among selected HIV-infected patients. PCP prophylaxis should be administered to patients with a CD4 count <200/µl but no prior history of PCP (primary prophylaxis) and to those with a prior history of PCP regardless of the CD4 count (secondary prophylaxis). The current options for PCP prophylaxis include AP, TMP/SMX, and DAP.

1. Aerosolized Pentamidine—Numerous studies have demonstrated the efficacy of AP for primary (39,85) and secondary (31,57,72) prophylaxis against PCP. Representative studies are described here.

a. Primary Prophylaxis With AP—In a PRCT involving 223 HIV-infected patients with no prior history of PCP, AP (300 mg q 28 days) significantly decreased the risk of developing PCP but did not lower the risk of death (39). All patients had at least 5 points in a following scoring system: CD4 <200/μl, 5 points; AIDS-defining illness, 5 points; oral thrush, 3 points; weight loss, 3 points; Kaposi's sarcoma, 2 points; positive p24 antigenemia, 2 points.

(1) The risk of developing PCP was significantly lower with AP (8.6% versus 27.1% per patient-year; $P=0.0021$). There was no significant difference in survival (Table 25–12).

(2) The most common adverse effect of AP was cough, which affected 33% of patients, but only 4 patients had to withdraw because of side effects.

b. **Secondary Prophylaxis With AP**—In a PRCT involving 162 HIV-infected patients who had their first episode of PCP within 2 to 4 weeks of the time of enrollment, AP (60 mg given five times over the first 2 weeks then q 2 weeks) significantly decreased the risk of PCP but did not lower the risk of death (72). The mean follow-up was 15 weeks.

(1) The risk of developing PCP was significantly lower with AP (9% versus 50% over 24 weeks; $P<0.001$), but there was no significant difference in survival (Table 25–13).

(2) Adverse effects were more common with AP (33% versus 19%; $P=0.04$), but none required discontinuation of therapy.

c. As demonstrated by these studies, AP appears to be effective for both primary and secondary prophylaxis against PCP. A monthly administration of AP (300 mg) is the most common regimen. In a prospective, randomized, non-blinded comparison of various dosing regimens of AP, 300 mg q month or 150 mg q 2 weeks was found to be superior to 30 mg q 2 weeks (57). In this study (median follow-up, 212 days), the risks of developing PCP were 26%, 31%, and 42% for the three dosages, respectively ($P=0.02$ for 300 mg q month versus 30 mg q 2 weeks). There were no differences in survival among the three groups. Although some studies have used other devices with success (72), only the Respirgard II nebulizer system is approved for AP prophylaxis in the United States.

d. However, several important disadvantages limit the use of AP.

(1) Because AP is poorly absorbed systemically, it does not provide effective prophylaxis against extrapulmonary pneumocystosis, a rare (1% to 3%) complication of HIV infection. Although almost any tissue may be affected, common sites of extrapulmonary infection include the lymph nodes, spleen, liver, and bone marrow. *P. carinii* may also infect the eye, thyroid, gastrointestinal tract, adrenals, and vasculature (19,76,86). In retrospective studies, monthly administration of IV or IM pentamidine appeared to be an effective prophylaxis for both pul-

Table 25-12 Aerosolized pentamidine for primary PCP prophylaxis (39)

	AP (N=114)	Placebo (N=109)	*P*
Withdrew from study	32	37	NS
Risk of PCP per patient-year	8.6%	27.1%	<0.0021
Mortality rate	4.4%	4.6%	NS

Table 25-13 Aerosolized pentamidine for secondary PCP prophylaxis (72)

	AP (N=114)	Placebo (N=109)	*P*
Withdrew from study	32	37	NS
Risk of PCP per patient-year	8.6%	27.1%	<0.0021
Mortality rate	4.4%	4.6%	NS

monary and extrapulmonary pneumocystosis, but prospective data are lacking (18,26). On the other hand, the risk of adverse effects appear to be higher with systemic administration than with aerosolization.

(2) Furthermore, experienced personnel are required for proper administration of AP. Use of effective nebulizer equipment is mandatory, and the position of the patient must be altered periodically during the procedure in order to achieve even distribution of the drug throughout the lungs. Inadequate or unequal drug delivery may be responsible for some therapeutic failures, especially in the lung apices (59). There is also some risk of transmission of respiratory pathogens (*e.g.*, mycobacteria) during treatment.

(3) Most importantly, AP appears to be less effective than TMP-SMX, as discussed in the following section.

2. TMP-SMX is currently the most effective prophylactic regimen against PCP, although a high incidence of adverse effects limits its applicability for some patients. Representative studies that compared TMP-SMX to various other regimens are discussed here (27,37,66,93).

a. TMP-SMX Versus Control—Fischl in 1988 demonstrated that primary prophylaxis with TMP-SMX clearly lowers the risk for development of PCP as well as the overall mortality rate (27). In a prospective, randomized study, 60 HIV-positive men with Kaposi's sarcoma but no prior history of opportunistic infections were enrolled. Patients receiving antiretroviral therapy, those with a known sulfa allergy, and those receiving other drugs with known anti-PCP activity were excluded. Thirty patients were randomly assigned to receive TMP-SMX (160 mg TMP and 800 mg SMX PO BID) plus calcium leucovorin (5 mg PO QD), and 30 patients were randomly assigned to no therapy. The minimum duration of follow-up was 2 years.

(1) Patients assigned to TMP-SMX were less likely to develop PCP (13% versus 53%) and more likely to survive (60% versus 93% mortality, $P<0.002$) (Table 25–14). If the analysis is limited to those who actually took the assigned drug, no cases of PCP occurred among patients taking TMP-SMX.

(2) However, 50% of the patients in the TMP-SMX group experienced a drug-related adverse effect, and 17% had to discontinue therapy because of the adverse effect. Erythroderma, without mucous membrane involvement or exfoliation, was the most frequent side effect; 4 patients had to discontinue therapy because of severe rash involving mucous membranes and fever. One patient had to discontinue therapy because of neutropenia. The high incidence of side effects may have been a reflection of the relatively high doses of TMP-SMX used.

(3) It should also be noted that this study was conducted before the general use of antiretroviral therapy became standard.

b. TMP-SMX Versus AP for Primary Prophylaxis—Two major studies directly compared TMP-SMX versus AP for primary prophylaxis against PCP (66,93). A prospective, non-blinded French trial randomly assigned 214 patients to receive either AP (300 mg q month) or TMP-SMX (80 mg of TMP and 400 mg of SMX QD) (66). In an intention-to-treat analysis, the risk of PCP was comparable between the two groups (3.1% per year with AP ver-

Table 25-14 TMP-SMX for primary PCP prophylaxis (27)

	TMP-SMX (N=30)	Control (N=30)	*P*
Risk of PCP	13%	53%	—
Mortality rate	60%	93%	<0.002
Mean survival	23 mo	13 mo	<0.002

sus 1.3% per year with TMP-SMX). However, both patients who developed PCP in the TMP-SMX group had switched to AP 7–8 months earlier because of treatment-limiting toxicity. Furthermore, 45% of the subjects withdrew from this trial, complicating interpretation of these results. In contrast, in another randomized study, TMP-SMX was significantly better than AP for primary prophylaxis against PCP (93). This study was a prospective, randomized, non-blinded comparison involving 213 HIV-infected patients with CD4 counts <200/μl but no prior history of PCP. Three treatment arms were compared: AP (300 mg q month, with albuterol premedication), single-strength TMP-SMX (80 mg TMP and 400mg SMX QD), and double-strength TMP-SMX (160 mg TMP and 800 mg SMX QD). The length of follow-up was 264 to 288 days in the treatment groups. The three groups were comparable in age, sex, CD4 count, and risk factors; however, use of zidovudine (AZT) was more common in the AP arm (65%) than in either of the TMP-SMX groups (44% to 55%; *P*=0.04). Seventeen subjects withdrew from the study, in equal proportions among the three arms. An intention-to-treat analysis was used.

(1) No case of PCP occurred in either of the TMP-SMX groups, but the annual risk of PCP was 11% for the group treated with AP (*P*=0.002). In addition, no case of toxoplasmosis occurred in either of the TMP-SMX groups, but 3 such cases occurred among those treated with AP (*P*=0.03). However, no difference in mortality was observed; none of the deaths appeared to be PCP-related.

(2) AP was significantly better tolerated than TMP-SMX. Treatment-limiting toxicity occurred in only 2 patients receiving AP but in 17 and 18 patients receiving the low-dose and high-dose TMP-SMX regimens, respectively. Cough and bronchospasm were the major treatment-limiting side effects of AP. Fever, rash, nausea, and vomiting were the most common adverse reactions associated with TMP-SMX. The mean number of days to an adverse event was 16 in the high-dose TMP-SMX group and 57 in the low-dose TMP-SMX group (*P*=0.02).

(3) Based on these studies, TMP-SMX appears to be superior to AP for primary prophylaxis against PCP. The low-dose and high-dose regimens of TMP-SMX appear to be equally effective. A subsequent report confirmed that the two doses of TMP-SMX were equal in efficacy even after median follow-up of 376 days (94). However, toxicity was significantly more common and occurred earlier with the high-dose regimen.

c. TMP-SMX Versus AP for Secondary Prophylaxis—In a prospective, randomized, non-blinded comparison involving 310 HIV-infected patients (mean CD4 count, 56 cells/μl) recovering from their first episode of PCP, TMP-SMX was once again superior to AP for prophylaxis against PCP (37). The study compared AP (300 mg q month) versus TMP-SMX (160 mg TMP and 800 mg

Table 25-15 TMP-SMX compared with AP for primary PCP prophylaxis (93)

	Low-Dose TMP-SMX (N=72)	High-Dose TMP-SMX (N=71)	AP (N=72)	*P*
Risk of PCP per y	0%	0%	11%	0.002
Number of cases of toxoplasmosis	0	0	3	0.03
Number of deaths	5	5	8	NS
Treatment-limiting adverse effects	24%	25%	2.8%	<0.001
Mean number of days until onset of adverse effects	57 d	16 d	—	0.02

SMX QD). All patients were treated with AZT or another antiretroviral agent after enrollment. The median length of follow-up was 17.4 months; 31 subjects were lost to follow-up. An intention-to-treat analysis was used.

(1) The 18-month relapse rate for PCP was significantly lower with TMP-SMX (11.4% and 27.6% for TMP-SMX and AP groups, respectively, *P*<0.001) (Table 25–16). One episode of extrapulmonary pneumocystosis occurred in a patient assigned to AP. Furthermore, 7 of the 14 cases of PCP in the TMP-SMX group occurred among those who had switched to AP. Three other patients in the TMP-SMX group developed PCP within 3 weeks of beginning the randomized therapy, which suggests that they may have had incompletely treated primary disease rather than true relapse.

(2) There was no difference in the risk of developing toxoplasmosis, but the risk of bacterial infection was significantly lower with TMP-SMX (19 versus 38 cases, *P*=0.017). However, there was no difference in mortality between the two groups (25.8 versus 22.8 months median survival time for TMP-SMX versus AP, respectively).

(3) Treatment-limiting toxicity occurred in 27% of the patients assigned to TMP-SMX, compared with 4% of the patients assigned to AP. However, the rates of hematologic and hepatic toxicities were comparable in the two treatment groups, as were the incidences of fever and rash. Only severe asthenia and abdominal pain were significantly more common among those receiving TMP-SMX.

d. Low-Dose Regimens of TMP-SMX—Because of the significant incidence of drug-related adverse reactions, several studies have examined whether successful PCP prophylaxis can be achieved with lower doses of TMP-SMX (14,87,98,112) (Table 25–17). In one retrospective study, there were no reported cases of PCP with an intermittent TMP-SMX dosing regimen (160 mg TMP and 800mg SMX on Mondays, Wednesdays, and Fridays only). Forty-five patients were treated for primary prophylaxis (mean follow-up, 18.5 months), and 71 patients were treated for secondary prophylaxis (mean follow-up, 24.2 months) (87). Treatment-limiting toxicity occurred in 13% of the patients in the study. A prospective uncontrolled study also confirmed the efficacy of this intermittent regimen and reported a treatment-limiting toxicity risk of 6.8% for primary prophylaxis patients and 13.3% for secondary prophylaxis patients (98). In another retrospective study involving all secondary prophylaxis patients (median follow-up, 11 months), only one relapse of PCP was reported among 60 patients treated with TMP-SMX (160 mg TMP and 800 mg SMX BID for 2 days per week) (14). Treatment-limiting toxicity occurred in only 3 patients with this lower-dose regimen. Similar efficacy was reported for an every-other-day regimen of TMP-SMX (160 mg TMP and 800 mg SMX) (112). Finally, a recent metaanalysis did not demonstrate a loss of efficacy associated with reduced-dose regimens of TMP-SMX (45). Therefore, although prospective data are sparse, there is support for the the use of intermittent TMP-SMX

Table 25-16 TMP-SMX compared with AP for secondary PCP prophylaxis (37)

	TMP-SMX (N=154)	AP (N=156)	*P*
18-month relapse rate	11.4%	27.6%	<0.001
Number of cases of toxoplasmosis	4	6	NS
Number of cases of bacterial infections	19	38	0.017
Median survival	25.8 mo	22.8 mo	NS
Treatment-limiting adverse effects	27%	4%	—

dosing, especially for those patients who experience treatment-limiting toxicity at conventional doses. Various alternative low-dose regimens are summarized in Table 25-17.

e. Although TMP-SMX is highly effective for prophylaxis against PCP, there is a high incidence of drug-related toxicity among HIV-infected patients, as high as 78% in some studies (35,46,70). The reported adverse reactions include fever, anemia, leukopenia, thrombocytopenia, nausea, vomiting, increased level of transaminases, hyperkalemia, hyponatremia, renal failure, taste disturbance, tremor, toxic epidermal necrolysis, and a sepsis-like syndrome (48).

(1) "Treating Through" Approach—For patients who experience a minor adverse reaction to TMP-SMX (*e.g.*, fever and rash without bullae or mucous membrane involvement), limited data indicate that "treating through" the adverse reaction can be successful, particularly if antihistamines and antipyretics are used judiciously (27,91,96).

(2) Rechallenge Approach—Similarly, many patients with a prior history of non–life-threatening reactions to TMP-SMX appear to tolerate a rechallenge with the drug. For example, in the secondary prophylaxis study by Hardy, 68% of the patients in the TMP-SMX group who had a prior history of non–treatment-limiting toxicity to the drug actually tolerated the therapy (37). Similarly, of 21 patients with a history of febrile or cutaneous reactions to TMP-SMX in treatment doses for PCP, 17 tolerated subsequent prophylactic therapy with TMP-SMX (96). However, these "treating through" or rechallenge approaches should be used with caution, as severe hypersensitivity reactions have been reported with these strategies (48,97).

(3) Desensitization—Some success has been reported with desensitization of patients with a prior history of adverse reactions to TMP-SMX. Representative studies are discussed here. In one prospective study, 28 patients with a prior history of adverse reaction to TMP-SMX (fever or rash) underwent oral desensitization (2). The starting doses were 0.4 mg of TMP and 2 mg of SMX; the doses were gradually increased over 10 days to 160 mg of TMP and 800 mg of SMX. Of the 28 patients in the study, 23 completed this protocol, 6 were lost to follow-up, and 10 were still receiving TMP-SMX prophylaxis at a mean follow-up of 19 weeks. In another prospective study, a similar rate of success was reported with use of a rapid oral desensitization schedule beginning with 0.004 mg of TMP and 0.02 mg of SMX and reaching 160 mg of TMP and 800 mg of SMX over a 5-hour period. Of the 22 patients in the study, 19 completed this protocol, and 15 were still receiving TMP-SMX prophylaxis at a mean follow-up of 14 months (33). No episodes of anaphylaxis were observed with these regimens.

3. Dapsone—DAP, given either alone or in combination with pyrimethamine, is also effective for PCP prophylaxis. Several PRCTs have examined the efficacy of DAP (8,9,90,102) or the DAP-pyrimethamine combination (4,32,61,78,84) for prophylaxis against PCP (Table 25–18). Based on these studies, it appears that DAP (a minimum of 100 mg/day) or the DAP-pyrimethamine combination (a minimum of 200 mg/week of DAP with 50 to 75 mg pyrimethamine) is as effective as AP for PCP prophylaxis. However, in one study, DAP was associated with an increased

Table 25-17 Low-dose TMP-SMX regimens for PCP prophylaxis

Alternative Low-Dose Regimens	Reference
160 mg TMP/800 mg SMX on Monday, Wednesday, Friday only	(87, 98)
160 mg TMP/800 mg SMX bid for 2 d/wk	(14)
160 mg TMP/800 mg SMX every other day	(112)

risk of death compared with AP when used for secondary prophylaxis in patients with advanced AIDS (90). Furthermore, these DAP-based regimens appear to be less effective than TMP-SMX. Nevertheless, they offer a low-cost alternative for those who are intolerant to TMP-SMX, and, because both daily and weekly regimens appear to be efficacious, they allow flexible dosing schedules. Finally, like the TMP-SMX combination, the DAP-based regimens are associated with a significant risk of adverse reactions, especially when compared to AP. In particular, patients with G6PD deficiency should not receive DAP because of the risk of DAP-associated hemolysis.

a. **Dapsone Alone**—Numerous studies that have compared the efficacy of DAP versus other regimens for PCP prophylaxis are summarized in Table 25-18.

Table 25-18 Summary of trials of dapsone for PCP prophylaxis

Reference	Design of the Study	Findings
(8)	1. Prospective, randomized, nonblinded study involving 86 patients with a median follow-up of 341 to 352 d. The mean CD4 counts were 111/μl for DAP and 118/μl for TMP-SMX. 2. Compared DAP (100 mg/d) vs. TMP-SMX (160 mg of TMP plus 800 mg of SMX QD) for primary prophylaxis against PCP.	1. There was only one episode of PCP in each group. For the DAP group, 1 compliant patient developed PCP; for the TMP-SMX group, 1 noncompliant patient developed PCP only 11 d after enrollment. 2. Treatment-limiting toxicity occurred in 70% of patients in the DAP group and 64% of patients in the TMP-SMX group. Eleven patients assigned to TMP-SMX crossed over to DAP because of toxicity; 6 of the 11 tolerated DAP. Ten patients assigned to DAP crossed over to TMP-SMX; 4 of the 10 tolerated TMP-SMX.
(102)	1. Prospective, randomized, nonblinded study involving 190 evaluable patients with mean follow-up of 42 to 44 weeks. All patients had CD4 count <250 cells/ml (mean, 163 to192 cells/μl) 2. Compared DAP (100 mg twice per wk) vs. AP (100 mg twice per wk for 1 wk; 100 mg q wk for 4 wk; then 100 mg twice per mo). About 40% were for secondary prophylaxis; rest were for primary prophylaxis.	1. There was no significant difference in the rate of PCP between the two groups (17% for DAP and 14% for AP, *P*=NS). There was still no difference when primary and secondary prophylaxis patients were analyzed separately. 2. There was no difference in survival between the two groups. 3. Treatment-limiting toxicity occurred in 15 patients given DAP (11 rash, 2 hepatitis, 1 hemolysis) and 3 patients given AP (bronchospasm).
(9)	1. Prospective, randomized, nonblinded study involving 842 HIV-infected patients with CD4 counts <200/μl with a median follow-up of 3.25 y. 2. Compared DAP (50 mg BID) vs. AP (300 mg q mo) vs. TMP-SMX (160 mg of TMP plus 800 mg of SMX BID) for primary prophylaxis against PCP.	1. Using intention-to-treat analysis, there was no significant difference in the 3-y cumulative risk of PCP among the three groups (18% for TMP-SMX, 17% for DAP, and 21% for AP). Nevertheless, only 4 of 34 confirmed cases of PCP in the TMP-SMX group occurred in patients actually taking the drug, compared with 21 of 33 in the DAP group and 37 of 38 in the AP group.

Table 25-18 (continued)

Reference	Design of the Study	Findings
		2. There was no significant difference in survival among the three groups. 3. AP was the best-tolerated drug; 88% of the patients in the AP group continued on the assigned drug, compared with 21% and 25% of the patients assigned to TMP-SMX and DAP, respectively.
(90)	1. Prospective, randomized, non-blinded study involving 196 HIV-infected patients with mean follow-up of about 1 y. 2. Compared DAP (50 mg QD) vs. AP (300 mg q mo) for secondary prophylaxis against PCP. 3. Mean CD4 counts were lower in the DAP group (49/μl) compared to the AP group (82/μl; $P<0.002$)	1. Patients in the AP group were more likely to experience a relapse of PCP, but the difference was not statistically significant (11.7% with AP vs. 5.7% with DAP, P=NS). 2. However, patients in the DAP group had a higher 18-mo mortality rate compared with those in the AP group (53.1% with DAP vs. 24.6% with AP). 3. The rate of crossover to alternate therapy was 34% for the DAP group and 19% for the AP group ($P<0.03$). The reason for crossing over was primarily because of toxicity in the DAP group but because of prophylaxis failure in the AP group.

b. Dapsone Plus Pyrimethamine—Numerous studies that have compared the efficacy of the DAP-pyrimethamine combination versus other regimens are summarized in Table 25-19.

c. Representative studies that have evaluated the efficacy of DAP for primary or secondary prophylaxis against PCP are described here for illustration.

(1) Dapsone for Primary Prophylaxis—ACTG protocol 081 was the largest trial to prospectively compare DAP, TMP-SMX, and AP for primary prophylaxis against PCP and had a median follow-up of 3.25 years (9). This randomized, non-blinded study enrolled 842 HIV-infected subjects with CD4 counts <200/μl (mean count, 150 cells/μl); 276 patients were randomly assigned to receive TMP-SMX (160 mg of TMP and 800 mg SMX BID), 288 to DAP (50 mg BID), and 278 to AP (300 mg q month). To minimize crossover, patients in the TMP-SMX and DAP groups who developed significant toxicity were first treated with a lowered dose of the originally assigned drug. Patients receiving TMP-SMX or DAP who could not tolerate the lowered dose were assigned to the alternate drug; finally, those who were intolerant of the alternate systemic therapy were assigned to AP. Patients in the AP group who developed treatment-limiting toxicity were crossed over to TMP-SMX, followed by dose reduction and change to DAP as needed.

(a) By intention-to-treat analysis, there was no significant difference in the 3-year cumulative risk of PCP among the three groups (18% for TMP-SMX, 17% for DAP, and 21% for AP). There was no significant difference in survival among the three groups; the median survival time ranged from 39 to 42 months.

(b) Nevertheless, TMP-SMX is probably still more effective than the other agents, since only 4 of 34 confirmed cases of PCP in the TMP-

Table 25-19 Summary of trials of dapsone-pyrimethamine for PCP prophylaxis

Reference	Design of the Study	Findings
(32)	1. Prospective, randomized, non-blinded study involving 349 HIV-infected patients with a median follow-up of 539 d. 2. Compared DAP (50 mg QD plus pyrimethamine (50 mg q wk) plus folinic acid (25 mg q wk) vs. AP (300 mg q mo) for primary prophylaxis against PCP.	1. No difference in risk of PCP (5.8% with DAP-pyrimethamine vs. 5.7% with AP). 2. No difference in mortality (45 deaths with DAP-pyrimethamine vs. 41 deaths with AP). 3. More patients in the DAP-pyrimethamine group required interruption of therapy because of toxicity (24% with DAP-pyrimethamine vs. 1.7% with AP, $P<0.001$). 4. Study is weakened by the fact that 130 of the 349 patients dropped out of the study.
(61)	1. Prospective, randomized, non-blinded study involving 331 HIV-infected patients with a mean follow-up of 314 d; 45 patients were lost to follow-up 2. Compared DAP (100 mg q wk) plus pyrimethamine (25 mg q wk) vs. TMP-SMX (160 mg of TMP plus 800 mg of SMX 3 d/wk) vs. AP (300 mg q mo) for primary prophylaxis against PCP.	1. No statistically significant difference in the annual risk of PCP according to intention-to-treat analysis (8.3% with DAP-pyrimethamine vs. 3% for TMP-SMX vs. 5.6% for AP). 2. However, only 1 of the 3 failures in the TMP-SMX group occurred while on assigned therapy. In contrast, all of the failures in the AP group and 7 of the 8 failures in the DAP-pyrimethamine group occurred while on assigned therapy. 3. No difference in mortality (20, 18, and 17 deaths in the DAP-pyrimethamine, TMP-SMX, and AP arms, respectively). 4. Incidence of treatment-limiting toxicity was highest for TMP-SMX (9.4%), intermediate for DAP-pyrimethamine (5.2%), and lowest for AP (0%).
(4)	1. Prospective, randomized, non-blinded study involving 197 HIV-infected patients with a mean follow-up of 216 d; 16 patients were lost to follow-up. 2. Compared DAP (100 mg q wk) plus pyrimethamine (25 mg twice per wk) vs. TMP-SMX (160 mg of TMP plus 800 mg of SMX every other d) vs. AP (300 mg q mo) for primary prophylaxis against PCP.	1. Risk of developing PCP was highest for DAP- pyrimethamine (32.1 per 100 patient-years), intermediate for AP (10.2 per 100 patient-years), and lowest for TMP-SMX (2 per 100 patient-years). Only the difference between the DAP-pyrimethamine and the TMP-SMX groups was statistically significant ($P=0.007$). 2. Relative risk of death while taking DAP-pyrimethamine compared with TMP-SMX was 2.8 (95% CI, 1.1–7.3; $P=0.037$). 3. No difference in the incidence of treatment-limiting toxicity among the three groups.

Table 25-19 (continued)

Reference	Design of the Study	Findings
(84)	1. Prospective, randomized, non-blinded study involving 200 HIV-infected patients with a median follow-up of 430 d. 2. Compared DAP (100 mg twice per wk) plus pyrimethamine (50 mg twice per wk) vs. TMP-SMX (160 mg of TMP plus 800 mg of SMX BID twice per wk) for primary prophylaxis against PCP.	1. Risk of PCP was significantly lower with TMP-SMX (0%) than with DAP-pyrimethamine (6.3%, $P<0.0001$). No difference in the risk of bacterial infections. Using intention-to-treat analysis, the 2-year risk of developing PCP was 0% for TMP-SMX and 11% for DAP-pyrimethamine ($P=0.014$). 2. No difference in mortality (14 deaths with DAP-pyrimethamine vs. 15 with TMP-SMX). 3. Treatment-limiting toxicity occurred in (9) patients assigned to DAP-pyrimethamine and 10 patients assigned to TMP-SMX.
(78)	1. Prospective, randomized, non-blinded study involving 533 HIV-infected patients with a median follow-up of 483 days. 2. Compared DAP (200 mg q wk) plus pyrimethamine (75 mg q wk) vs. AP (300 mg q mo) for primary (81%) or secondary (19%) prophylaxis against PCP	1. In an intention-to-treat analysis, there was no significant difference in the risk of PCP (12 cases for DAP-pyrimethamine vs. 13 cases for AP). 2. No difference in mortality (77 deaths with DAP-pyrimethamine vs. 73 deaths with AP). 3. Because of drug-associated toxicity, 30% of the patients in the DAP-pyrimethamine arm and 4% of the patients in the AP arm crossed over to be treated with the other regimen. The high rate of crossover may have diluted small but significant differences in efficacy between the two groups.

SMX group occurred among patients actually taking the drug (either full or reduced dose), compared with 21 of 33 in the DAP group and 37 of 38 in the AP group.

(c) Incidentally, the risk of PCP increased when the 50-mg BID dose of DAP was reduced to once a day.

(d) In a subgroup analysis of patients with CD4 counts <100/μl, there was a trend toward a lower 3-year risk of PCP with TMP-SMX or DAP, but this difference did not reach statistical significance (19% with TMP-SMX versus 22% with DAP versus 33% with AP; $P=0.06$ for comparison of the combined TMP-SMX and DAP groups with AP). No such trend was apparent for those with CD4 counts >100/μl.

(e) AP was the best-tolerated drug; 88% of the patients in the AP group continued on the assigned drug at full dose, compared with 21% and 25% of those in the TMP-SMX and DAP groups, respectively.

(f) Although there was no significant difference in efficacy among the three regimens according to intention-to-treat analysis, an "as-treated" analysis suggested that treatment failures were fewest with TMP-SMX. Furthermore, 100 mg/day of DAP appeared to be more effective than 50 mg/day (in the absence of pyrimethamine). However, this study also illustrates the difficulty in maintaining progressively immunosuppressed patients on prophylactic regimens with significant associated toxicities.

(2) Dapsone for Secondary Prophylaxis—A recent prospective, randomized, non-blinded trial compared DAP (50 mg QD) versus AP (300 mg q month) among 196 HIV-infected patients who had recovered from PCP within 2 months of enrollment (90). Half of the participants had CD4 counts <50/μl; mean follow-up was approximately 1 year. Intention-to-treat analysis was used.

(a) Patients in the AP group were more likely to experience a relapse of PCP, but the difference was not statistically significant (11.7% with AP versus 5.7% with DAP; *P*=NS).

(b) However, patients in the DAP group had a significantly higher 18-month mortality rate than those in the AP group (53.1% versus 24.6%). Adjusting for age, CD4 count, and duration of AIDS diagnosis, the RR of death for patients assigned to DAP was 2.18 (95% CI, 1.27 to 3.14).

(c) The rate of crossover to alternate therapy was 34% for the DAP group and 19% for the AP group (*P*<0.03). The reason for crossing over was primarily toxicity in the DAP group but prophylaxis failure in the AP group.

(d) The baseline CD4 counts were comparable at the beginning of the trial; however, during the study, the mean CD4 counts were significantly lower with DAP than with AP (49 versus 83 cells/μl, *P*<0.002).

(e) The reason for the excess mortality in the DAP group is unclear, and additional studies are needed to verify this observation. The authors' speculations include an unspecified oxidant effect or a toxicity associated with an iron salt in the DAP preparation. For now, it may be prudent to avoid the use of DAP for secondary prophylaxis against PCP in patients with advanced HIV disease.

G. Summary

1. The most common symptoms and signs of PCP are fever, nonproductive cough, and dyspnea. The classic radiographic appearance of PCP is bilateral perihilar interstitial infiltrates but focal or nodular infiltrates, miliary disease, cyst formation, pneumatoceles, cavitary lesions, and a normal chest film have all been described. Serum LDH is usually elevated in AIDS patients with PCP. For patients on AP prophylaxis, there is an increased incidence of upper lobe disease as well as an increased risk of extrapulmonary pneumocystosis.
2. HIV-infected patients with CD4 counts <200/μl are at highest risk for developing PCP. Thrush, fever >37.8° C for >2 weeks, and prior history of PCP are additional independent predictors for development of PCP.
3. IS examination should be the initial diagnostic step for evaluation of PCP. For patients with a negative IS sample in whom clinical suspicion remains high, bronchoscopy with BAL should be the next step. Transbronchial biopsy is not routinely needed, because the sensitivity of BAL for PCP approaches 97% to 98% and transbronchial biopsy is associated with a small but significant risk of pneumothorax. Alternatively, for patients whose clinical presentation is highly suspicious for PCP, some practitioners empirically treat for PCP even if the IS examination is negative, reserving bronchoscopy for those who do not tolerate empiric therapy or who fail to respond to treatment.
4. The current treatment of choice for PCP is 21 days of IV TMP-SMX (15 to 20 mg/kg/day of TMP and 75 to 100 mg/kg/day for SMX in three to four divided doses). Alternative treatment options include pentamidine (4 mg/kg/day IV for 21 days), TMP-DAP, clindamycin-primaquine, atovaquone, and trimetrexate-leucovorin. Adjunctive corticosteroids should be administered for patients with PCP and PaO_2 <70 mm Hg or $P(A\text{-}a)O_2$ >35 mm Hg. The recommended doses are as follows: prednisone 40 mg PO BID for days 1 through 5, then 40 mg PO QD for

days 6 through 10, then 20 mg PO QD for days 11 through 21. Methylprednisolone (at 75% of the prednisone dose) may be substituted if IV delivery is desired.

5. Prophylactic therapy against PCP should be administered to HIV-infected patients with CD4 counts <200/μl but no prior history of PCP (primary prophylaxis) and to those with a prior history of PCP regardless of CD4 count (secondary prophylaxis). TMP-SMX is currently the prophylactic therapy of choice against PCP; a high incidence of adverse effects may limit its applicability for some patients, but lowered prophylactic doses are better tolerated and appear to remain efficacious. AP is the best tolerated prophylactic regimen against PCP, but it is less effective than TMP-SMX. Oral DAP (a minimum of 100 mg/day) or the oral DAP-pyrimethamine combination (a minimum of 200 mg/week of DAP with 50 to 75 mg pyrimethamine) is comparable to AP but is probably less effective than TMP-SMX. However, one study has suggested that DAP may increase the risk of death when it is used for secondary prophylaxis in patients with advanced AIDS.

Abbreviations used in Chapter 25

ACTG = AIDS Clinical Trials Group
AIDS = acquired immunodeficiency syndrome
AP = aerosolized pentamidine
ARC = AIDS-related complex
AZT = zidovudine
BAL = bronchoalveolar lavage
BID = twice daily
CI = confidence interval
CMV = cytomegalovirus
DAP = dapsone
FiO_2 = fraction of inspired oxygen
G6PD = glucose-6-phosphate dehydrogenase
HIV = human immunodeficiency virus
HSV = herpes simplex virus
IM = intramuscular
IS = induced sputum
IV = intravenous
LDH = lactate dehydrogenase
N = number of patients
NPV = negative predictive value
NS = not significant
P = probability value
$P(A\text{-}a)O_2$ gradient = alveolar-arterial difference in partial pressure of oxygen
PaO_2 = arterial partial pressure of oxygen
PCP = *Pneumocystis carinii* pneumonia
PO = per os
PRCT = prospective randomized controlled trial
q = every
QD = once daily
QID = four times daily
RNA = ribonucleic acid
RR = relative risk
SMX = sulfamethoxazole
TBB = transbronchial biopsy
TMP = trimethoprim
TID = three times per day

TMP-DAP = trimethoprim-dapsone
TMP-SMX = trimethoprim-sulfamethoxazole
vs. = versus

References

1. Abouya. *Pneumocystis carinii* pneumonia: an uncommon cause of death in African patients with acquired immunodeficiency syndrome. *Am Rev Respir Dis* 1992;145:617.
2. Absar. Desensitization to trimethoprim/sulfamethoxazole in HIV-infected patients. *J Allergy Clin Immunol* 1994;93:1001.
3. Allegra. Trimetrexate for the treatment of *Pneumocystis carinii* pneumonia in patients with the acquired immunodeficiency syndrome. *N Engl J Med* 1987; 317:978.
4. Antinori. Aerosolized pentamidine, cotrimoxazole and dapsone-pyrimethamine for primary prophylaxis of *Pneumocystis carinii* pneumonia and toxoplasmic encephalitis. *AIDS* 1995;9:1343.
5. Batungwanayo. Pulmonary disease associated with the human immunodeficiency virus in Kigali, Rwanda: a fiberoptic bronchoscopic study of 111 cases of undetermined etiology. *Am J Respir Crit Care Med* 1994;149:1591.
6. Bigby. The usefulness of induced sputum in the diagnosis of *Pneumocystis carinii* pneumonia in patients with the acquired immunodeficiency syndrome. *Am Rev Respir Dis* 1986;133:515.
7. Black. Clindamycin and primaquine therapy for mild-to-moderate episodes of *Pneumocystis carinii* pneumonia in patients with AIDS: AIDS Clinical Trials Group 044. *Clin Infect Dis* 1994;18:905.
8. Blum. Comparative trial of dapsone versus trimethoprim/sulfamethoxazole for primary prophylaxis of *Pneumocystis carinii* pneumonia. *J Acquir Immune Defic Syndr* 1992;5:341.
9. Bozzette. A randomized trial of three antipneumocystis agents in patients with advanced human immunodeficiency virus infection. *N Engl J Med* 1995;332:693.
10. Bozzette. Reconsidering the use of adjunctive corticosteroids in *Pneumocystis* pneumonia? *J Acquir Immune Defic Syndr Hum Retrovirol* 1995;8:345.
11. Bozzette. A controlled trial of early adjunctive treatment with corticosteroids for *Pneumocystis carinii* pneumonia in the acquired immunodeficiency syndrome. *N Engl J Med* 1990;323:1451.
12. Brenner. Prognostic factors and life expectancy of patients with acquired immunodeficiency syndrome and *Pneumocystis carinii* pneumonia. *Am Rev Respir Dis* 1987;136:1199.
13. Broaddus. Bronchoalveolar lavage and transbronchial biopsy for the diagnosis of pulmonary infections in the acquired immunodeficiency syndrome. *Ann Intern Med* 1985;102:747.
14. Carr. Trimethoprim-sulfamethoxazole appears more effective than aerosolized pentamidine as secondary prophylaxis against *Pneumocystis carinii* pneumonia in patients with AIDS. *AIDS* 1992;6:165.
15. Centers for Disease Control. Update: acquired immunodeficiency syndrome—United States. *MMWR Morb Mortal Wkly Rep* 1986;35:757.
16. Centers for Disease Control. Guidelines for prophylaxis against *Pneumocystis carinii* pneumonia for persons infected with human immunodeficiency virus. *MMWR Morb Mortal Wkly Rep* 1989;38(S-5):1.
17. Chave. Transmission of *Pneumocystis carinii* from AIDS patients to other immunosuppressed patients: a cluster of *Pneumocystis carinii* pneumonia in renal transplant recipients. *AIDS* 1991;5:927.
18. Cheung. Intramuscular pentamidine for the prevention of *Pneumocystis carinii* pneumonia in patients infected with human immunodeficiency virus. *Clin Infect Dis* 1993;16:22.

19. Cohen. Extrapulmonary *Pneumocystis carinii* infections in the acquired immunodeficiency syndrome. *Arch Intern Med* 1991;151:1205.
20. Crowe. Predictive value of CD4 lymphocyte numbers for the development of opportunistic infections and malignancies in HIV-infected persons. *J Acquir Immune Defic Syndr* 1991;4:770.
21. Dohn. Oral atovaquone compared with intravenous pentamidine for *Pneumocystis carinii* pneumonia in patients with AIDS. *Ann Intern Med* 1994;121:174.
22. Edman. Isolation and expression of the *Pneumocystis carinii* dihydrofolate reductase gene. *Proc Natl Acad Sci USA* 1989;86:8625.
23. Edman. Ribosomal RNA sequences show *Pneumocystis carinii* to be member of the fungi. *Nature* 1988;334:519.
24. Edman. Isolation and expression of *Pneumocystis carinii* thymidylate synthase gene. *Proc Natl Acad Sci USA* 1989;86:6503.
25. El-Sadr. Survival and prognostic factors in severe *Pneumocystis carinii* pneumonia requiring mechanical ventilation. *Am Rev Respir Dis* 1988;137:1264.
26. Ena. Once-a-month administration of intravenous pentamidine to patients infected with human immunodeficiency virus as prophylaxis for *Pneumocystis carinii* pneumonia. *Clin Infect Dis* 1994;18:901.
27. Fischl. Safety and efficacy of sulfamethoxazole and trimethoprim chemoprophylaxis for *Pneumocystis carinii* pneumonia in AIDS. *JAMA* 1988;259:1185.
28. Fulton. Trimetrexate: a review of its pharmacodynamic and pharmacokinetic properties and therapeutic potential in the treatment of *Pneumocystis carinii* pneumonia. *Drugs* 1995;49:563.
29. Gagnon. Corticosteroids as adjunctive therapy for severe *Pneumocystis carinii* pneumonia in the acquired immunodeficiency syndrome: a double-blind, placebo-controlled trial. *N Engl J Med* 1990;323:1444.
30. Garay. Prognostic indicators in the initial presentation of *Pneumocystis carinii* pneumonia. *Chest* 1989;95:769.
31. Girard. Prevention of *Pneumocystis carinii* pneumonia relapse by pentamidine aerosol in zidovudine-treated AIDS patients. *Lancet* 1989;1:1348.
32. Girard. Dapsone-pyrimethamine compared with aerosolized pentamidine as primary prophylaxis against *Pneumocystis carinii* pneumonia and toxoplasmosis in HIV infection. *N Engl J Med* 1993;328:1514.
33. Gluckstein. Rapid oral desensitization to trimethoprim-sulfamethoxazole (TMP-SMX): use in prophylaxis for *Pneumocystis carinii* pneumonia in patients with AIDS who were previously intolerant to TMP-SMX. *Clin Infect Dis* 1995;20:849.
34. Golden. Bronchoalveolar lavage as the exclusive diagnostic modality for *Pneumocystis carinii* pneumonia: a prospective study among patients with acquired immunodeficiency syndrome. *Chest* 1986;90:18.
35. Gordin. Adverse reactions to trimethoprim-sulfamethoxazole in patients with the acquired immunodeficiency syndrome. *Ann Intern Med* 1984;100:495.
36. Gottlieb. *Pneumocystis carinii* pneumonia and mucosal candidiasis in previously healthy homosexual men. *N Engl J Med* 1981;305:1425.
37. Hardy. A controlled trial of trimethoprim-sulfamethoxazole or aerosolized pentamidine for secondary prophylaxis of *Pneumocystis carinii* pneumonia in patients with the acquired immunodeficiency syndrome. AIDS Clinical Trials Group Protocol 021. *N Engl J Med* 1992;327:1842.
38. Haron. Has the incidence of *Pneumocystis carinii* pneumonia in cancer patients increased with the AIDS epidemic? *Lancet* 1988;2:904.
39. Hirschel. A controlled study of inhaled pentamidine for primary prophylaxis of *Pneumocystis carinii* pneumonia. *N Engl J Med* 1991;324:1079.
40. Hopewell. *Pneumocystis carinii* pneumonia: diagnosis. *J Infect Dis* 1988;157:1115.
41. Huang. Suspected *Pneumocystis carinii* pneumonia with a negative induced sputum examination: Is early bronchoscopy useful? *Am J Respir Crit Care Med* 1995;151:1866.
42. Hughes. Comparison of atovaquone (566C80) with trimethoprim-sulfamethoxazole to treat *Pneumocystis carinii* pneumonia in patients with AIDS. *N Engl J Med* 1993;328:1521.

43. Hughes. *Pneumocystis carinii* pneumonia. *N Engl J Med* 1977;297:1381.
44. Hughes. Successful chemoprophylaxis for *Pneumocystis carinii* pneumonitis. *N Engl J Med* 1977;297:1419.
45. Ioannidis. A meta-analysis of the relative efficacy and toxicity of *Pneumocystis carinii* prophylactic regimens. *Arch Intern Med* 1996;156:177.
46. Jaffe. Complications of co-trimoxazole in treatment of AIDS-associated *Pneumocystis carinii* pneumonia in homosexual men. *Lancet* 1983;2:1109.
47. Jules-Elysee. Aerosolized pentamidine: effect on diagnosis and presentation of *Pneumocystis carinii* pneumonia. *Ann Intern Med* 1990;112:750.
48. Jung. Management of adverse reactions to trimethoprim-sulfamethoxazole in human immunodeficiency virus-infected patients. *Arch Intern Med* 1994;154:2402.
49. Kagawa. Serum lactate dehydrogenase activity in patients with AIDS and *Pneumocystis carinii* pneumonia: an adjunct to diagnosis. *Chest* 1988;94:1031.
50. Kennedy. Atypical roentgenographic manifestations of *Pneumocystis carinii* pneumonia. *Arch Intern Med* 1992;152:1390.
51. Klein. Trimethoprim-sulfamethoxazole versus pentamidine for *Pneumocystis carinii* pneumonia in AIDS patients: results of a large prospective randomized treatment trial. *AIDS* 1992;6:301.
52. Kovacs. *Pneumocystis carinii* pneumonia: a comparison between patients with the acquired immunodeficiency syndrome and patients with other immunodeficiencies. *Ann Intern Med* 1984;100:663.
53. Kovacs. Diagnosis of *Pneumocystis carinii* pneumonia: improved detection in sputum with use of monoclonal antibodies. *N Engl J Med* 1988;318:589.
54. Kramer. Diagnostic implications of Ga-67 chest-scan patterns in human immunodeficiency virus–seropositive patients. *Radiology* 1989;170:671.
55. Kramer. Gallium-67 scans of the chest in patients with acquired immunodeficiency syndrome. *J Nucl Med* 1987;28:1107.
56. Leigh. Sputum induction for diagnosis of *Pneumocystis carinii* pneumonia. *Lancet* 1989;2:205.
57. Leoung. Aerosolized pentamidine for prophylaxis against *Pneumocystis carinii* pneumonia: The San Francisco Community Prophylaxis Trial. *N Engl J Med* 1990; 323:769.
58. Leoung. Dapsone-trimethoprim for *Pneumocystis carinii* pneumonia in the acquired immunodeficiency syndrome. *Ann Intern Med* 1986;105:45.
59. Levine. Effect of aerosolized pentamidine prophylaxis on the diagnosis of *Pneumocystis carinii* pneumonia by induced sputum examination in patients infected with the human immunodeficiency virus. *Am Rev Respir Dis* 1991;144:760.
60. Malin. *Pneumocystis carinii* pneumonia in Zimbabwe. *Lancet* 1995;346:1258.
61. Mallolas. Primary prophylaxis for *Pneumocystis carinii* pneumonia: a randomized trial comparing cotrimoxazole, aerosolized pentamidine and dapsone plus pyrimethamine. *AIDS* 1993;7:59.
62. Masur. An outbreak of community-acquired *Pneumocystis carinii* pneumonia: initial manifestation of cellular immune dysfunction. *N Engl J Med* 1981;305:1431.
63. Masur. CD4 counts as predictors of opportunistic pneumonias in human immunodeficiency virus (HIV) infection. *Ann Intern Med* 1989;111:223.
64. Masur. Empiric outpatient management of HIV-related pneumonia: economical or unwise? *Ann Intern Med* 1996;124:451.
65. Matusiewicz. *Pneumocystis carinii* in bronchoalveolar lavage fluid and bronchial washings. *BMJ* 1994;308:1206.
66. May. Trimethoprim-sulfamethoxazole versus aerosolized pentamidine for primary prophylaxis of *Pneumocystis carinii* pneumonia: a prospective, randomized, controlled clinical trial. *J Acquir Immune Defic Syndr* 1994;7:457.
67. Medina. Oral therapy for *Pneumocystis carinii* pneumonia in the acquired immunodeficiency syndrome: a controlled trial of trimethoprim-sulfamethoxazole versus trimethoprim-dapsone. *N Engl J Med* 1990;323:776.
68. Meduri. Bilateral bronchoalveolar lavage in the diagnosis of opportunistic pulmonary infections. *Chest* 1991;100:1272.
69. Miller. Difficulties with sputum induction for diagnosis of *Pneumocystis carinii* pneumonia. *Lancet* 1990;335:112.

70. Mitsuyasu. Cutaneous reaction to trimethoprim-sulfamethoxazole in patients with AIDS and Kaposi's sarcoma. *N Engl J Med* 1983;308:1535.
71. Moe. *Pneumocystis carinii* infection in the HIV-seropositive patient. *Infect Dis Clin North Am* 1994;8:331.
72. Montaner. Aerosol pentamidine for secondary prophylaxis of AIDS-related *Pneumocystis carinii* pneumonia. *Ann Intern Med* 1991;114:948.
73. Montaner. Corticosteroids prevent early deterioration in patients with moderately severe *Pneumocystis carinii* pneumonia and the acquired immunodeficiency syndrome (AIDS). *Ann Intern Med* 1990;113:14.
74. Munoz. Trends in the incidence of outcomes defining acquired immunodeficiency syndrome (AIDS) in the Multicenter AIDS Cohort Study: 1985–1991. *Am J Epidemiol* 1993;137:423.
75. National Institutes of Health–University of California Expert Panel for Corticosteroids as Adjunctive Therapy for Pneumocystis Pneumonia. Consensus statement on the use of corticosteroids as adjunctive therapy for pneumocystis pneumonia in the acquired immunodeficiency syndrome. *N Engl J Med* 1990;323:1500.
75a. Ng. Lack of effect of prophylactic aerosolized pentamidine on the detection of *Pneumocystis carinii* in induced sputum or bronchoalveolar lavage specimens *Arch Path Lab Med* 1993;117:493.
76. Northfelt. Extrapulmonary pneumocystosis: clinical features in human immunodeficiency virus infection. *Medicine (Baltimore)* 1990;69:392.
77. O'Brien. Diagnosis of *Pneumocystis carinii* pneumonia by induced sputum in a city with moderate incidence of AIDS. *Chest* 1989;95:136.
78. Opravil. Once-weekly administration of dapsone/pyrimethamine vs. aerosolized pentamidine as combined prophylaxis for *Pneumocystis carinii* pneumonia and toxoplasmic encephalitis in human immunodeficiency virus-infected patients. *Clin Infect Dis* 1995;20:531.
79. Orenstein. Value of bronchoalveolar lavage in the diagnosis of pulmonary infection in acquired immune deficiency syndrome. *Thorax* 1986;41:345.
80. Peglow. Serologic responses to *Pneumocystis carinii* antigens in health and disease. *J Infect Dis* 1990;161:296.
81. Peters. A search for latent *Pneumocystis carinii* infection in post-mortem lungs by DNA amplification. *J Pathol* 1991;166:195.
82. Phair. The risk of *Pneumocystis carinii* pneumonia among men infected with human immunodeficiency virus type I. *N Engl J Med* 1990;322:161.
83. Pitchenik. Sputum examination for the diagnosis of *Pneumocystis carinii* pneumonia in the acquired immunodeficiency syndrome. *Am Rev Respir Dis* 1986; 133:226.
84. Podzamczer. Intermittent trimethoprim-sulfamethoxazole compared with dapsone-pyrimethamine for the simultaneous primary prophylaxis of *Pneumocystis* pneumonia and toxoplasmosis in patients infected with HIV. *Ann Intern Med* 1995;122:755.
85. Pretet. Long-term results of monthly inhaled pentamidine as primary prophylaxis of *Pneumocystis carinii* pneumonia in HIV-infected patients. *Am J Medicine* 1993;94:35.
86. Raviglione. Extrapulmonary pneumocystosis: the first 50 cases. *Rev Infect Dis* 1990;12:1127.
87. Ruskin. Low-dose co-trimoxazole for prevention of *Pneumocystis carinii* pneumonia in human immunodeficiency virus disease. *Lancet* 1991;337:468.
88. Safrin. Comparison of three regimens for treatment of mild to moderate *Pneumocystis carinii* pneumonia in patients with AIDS: a double-blind, randomized trial of oral trimethoprim-sulfamethoxazole, dapsone-trimethoprim, and clindamycin-primaquine. *Ann Intern Med* 1996;124:792.
89. Safrin. Adjunctive folinic acid with trimethoprim-sulfamethoxazole for *Pneumocystis carinii* pneumonia in AIDS is associated with an increased risk of therapeutic failure and death. *J Infect Dis* 1994;170:912.
90. Salmon-Ceron. Lower survival in AIDS patients receiving dapsone compared with aerosolized pentamidine for secondary prophylaxis of *Pneumocystis carinii* pneumonia. *J Infect Dis* 1995;172:656.

91. Sattler. Trimethoprim-sulfamethoxazole compared with pentamidine for treatment of *Pneumocystis carinii* pneumonia in the acquired immunodeficiency syndrome: a prospective, noncrossover study. *Ann Intern Med* 1988;109:280.
92. Sattler. Trimetrexate with leucovorin versus trimethoprim-sulfamethoxazole for moderate to severe episodes of *Pneumocystis carinii* pneumonia in patients with AIDS: a prospective, controlled multicenter investigation of the AIDS Clinical Trials Group Protocol 029/031. *J Infect Dis* 1994;170:165.
93. Schneider. A controlled trial of aerosolized pentamidine or trimethoprim-sulfamethoxazole as primary prophylaxis against *Pneumocystis carinii* pneumonia in patients with human immunodeficiency virus infection. *N Engl J Med* 1992; 327:1836.
94. Schneider. Efficacy and toxicity of two doses of trimethoprim-sulfamethoxazole as primary prophylaxis against *Pneumocystis carinii* pneumonia in patients with human immunodeficiency virus. *J Infect Dis* 1995;171:1632.
95. Sepkowitz. DNA amplification in experimental pneumocystosis: characterization of serum *Pneumocystis carinii* DNA and potential *P. carinii* carrier states. *J Infect Dis* 1993;168:421.
96. Shafer. Successful prophylaxis of *Pneumocystis carinii* pneumonia with trimethoprim-sulfamethoxazole in AIDS patients with previous allergic reactions. *J Acquir Immune Defic Syndr* 1989;2:389.
97. Silvestri. Pulmonary infiltrates and hypoxemia in patients with the acquired immunodeficiency syndrome re-exposed to trimethoprim-sulfamethoxazole. *Am Rev Respir Dis* 1987;136:1003.
98. Stein. Use of low-dose trimethoprim-sulfamethoxazole thrice weekly for primary and secondary prophylaxis of *Pneumocystis carinii* pneumonia in human immunodeficiency virus-infected patients. *Antimicrob Agents Chemother* 1991;35: 1705.
99. Stover. Diagnosis of pulmonary disease in acquired immune deficiency syndrome (AIDS): role of bronchoscopy and bronchoalveolar lavage. *Am Rev Respir Dis* 1984;130:659.
100. Toma. Clindamycin/primaquine versus trimethoprim-sulfamethoxazole as primary therapy for *Pneumocystis carinii* pneumonia in AIDS: a randomized, double-blind pilot trial. *Clin Infect Dis* 1993;17:178.
101. Toma. Clindamycin with primaquine for *Pneumocystis carinii* pneumonia. *Lancet* 1989;1:1046.
102. Torres. Randomized trial of dapsone and aerosolized pentamidine for the prophylaxis of *Pneumocystis carinii* pneumonia and toxoplasmic encephalitis. *Am J Medicine* 1993;95:573.
103. Tu. Bronchoscopy versus empirical therapy in HIV-infected patients with presumptive *Pneumocystis carinii* pneumonia: a decision analysis. *Am Rev Respir Dis* 1993;148:370.
104. Vogel. Evidence of horizontal transmission of *Pneumocystis carinii* pneumonia in simian immunodeficiency virus-infected rhesus macaques. *J Infect Dis* 1993; 168:836.
105. Walmsley. A multicenter randomized double-blind placebo-controlled trial of adjunctive corticosteroids in the treatment of *Pneumocystis carinii* pneumonia complicating the acquired immune deficiency syndrome. *J Acquir Immune Defic Syndr Hum Retrovirol* 1995;8:348.
106. Walzer. *Pneumocystis carinii*: recent advances in basic biology and their clinical application. *AIDS* 1993;7:1293.
107. Walzer. *Pneumocystis carinii*. In: Mandell, Bennett, Dolin, eds. *Principles and Practice of Infectious Diseases*. New York: Churchill Livingstone, 1995:2475.
108. Walzer. *Pneumocystis carinii* pneumonia in the United States: epidemiologic, diagnostic, and clinical features. *Ann Intern Med* 1974;80:83.
109. Wharton. Trimethoprim-sulfamethoxazole or pentamidine for *Pneumocystis carinii* pneumonia in the acquired immunodeficiency syndrome: a prospective randomized trial. *Ann Intern Med* 1986;105:37.
110. White. Clinical experience with atovaquone on a treatment investigational new drug

protocol for *Pneumocystis carinii* pneumonia. *J Acquir Immune Defic Syndr Hum Retrovirol* 1995;9:280.

111. Woolfenden. Acquired immunodeficiency syndrome: Ga-67 citrate imaging. *Radiology* 1987;162:383.
112. Wormser. Low-dose intermittent trimethoprim-sulfamethoxazole for prevention of *Pneumocystis carinii* pneumonia in patients with human immunodeficiency virus infection. *Arch Intern Med* 1991;151:688.
113. Zaman. Serum lactate dehydrogenase levels and *Pneumocystis carinii* pneumonia: diagnostic and prognostic significance. *Am Rev Respir Dis* 1988;137:796.
114. Zaman. Rapid noninvasive diagnosis of *Pneumocystis carinii* from induced liquified sputum. *Ann Intern Med* 1988;109:7.

26 Acute Meningitis

Will P. Schmitt, Burton W. Lee, and Morton N. Swartz

A. Epidemiology of Acute Meningitis

1. Aseptic Meningitis (Clinical Features of Meningitis with a Lymphocytic Pleocytosis)

a. By far, viruses are the most common causes of aseptic meningitis. Enteroviruses, such as the coxsackieviruses or the echoviruses, are most often implicated (11). Other viral causes include arboviruses, lymphocytic choriomeningitis virus, mumps virus, Epstein-Barr virus, cytomegalovirus, herpes simplex (primarily type 2), herpes zoster, and human immunodeficiency virus (HIV). Poliomyelitis is now rare in Western nations and appears to have been eliminated from North America except for very rare instances of vaccine-associated infection.

b. Less common infectious causes of aseptic meningitis include *Mycobacterium tuberculosis*, fungi, *Treponema pallidum*, *Leptospira*, and *Borrelia burgdorferi*, the agent responsible for Lyme disease. Other uncommon causes include carcinomatous meningitis, hypersensitivity reactions to vaccinations or drugs (*e.g.*, sulfonamides, nonsteroidal antiinflammatory agents), and rare involvement in Behçet's syndrome or systemic lupus erythematosus.

c. Parameningeal infections (*e.g.*, brain abscess, epidural abscess, or subdural empyema) may also elicit a sympathetic, predominantly lymphocytic pleocytosis. Neurosurgical drainage along with antimicrobial therapy is usually required for these conditions.

2. Acute Bacterial Meningitis

2. Acute Bacterial Meningitis—The following data are from Durand's retrospective observational review of 445 patients with 493 episodes of acute bacterial meningitis. All patients were at least 16 years of age. Cases represent all admissions for acute bacterial meningitis between 1962 and 1988 to the Massachusetts General Hospital, a large urban tertiary care hospital (3)

a. Causes of Bacterial Meningitis in Adults (3) (see Table 21–1)

(1) Community-Acquired Meningitis

(a) The pneumococcus was the predominant cause of community-acquired meningitis (38%), followed in frequency by the meningococcus (14%), *Listeria* (11%), and various streptococci (7%). Culture-negative bacterial meningitis accounted for 13% of the community-acquired cases.

(b) Gram-negative bacilli, *Staphylococcus aureus*, and *Haemophilus influenzae* were relatively uncommon, each accounting for ≤5% of the cases.

(2) Nosocomial Meningitis

(a) Gram-negative bacilli were the predominant cause (38%) of hospital-acquired meningitis. Other common causes included streptococci (9%), *S aureus* (9%), and coagulase-negative staphylococci (9%). Culture-negative meningitis accounted for 11% of the nosocomial cases.

(b) The pneumococcus, the meningococcus, *Listeria*, and *H influenzae* were relatively uncommon, each accounting for <5% of cases.

Table 26-1 Causes of acute bacterial meningitis (3)

	Community-Acquired Meningitis (N=253)	Hospital-Acquired Meningitis (N=151)
Pneumococcus	38%	5%
Gram-negative bacilli	4%	38%
Meningococcus	14%	1%
Streptococcus	7%	9%
Enterococcus	0%	3%
Staphylococcus aureus	5%	9%
Listeria monocytogenes	11%	3%
Haemophilus influenzae	4%	4%
Mixed bacterial species	2%	7%
Coagulase-negative staphylococci	0%	9%
Other organisms	2%	3%
Culture-negative cases	13%	11%

(3) The overall incidence of pneumococcal meningitis (community-acquired plus nosocomial cases) decreased from 35% of the total in the 1960s to 20% in the 1980s. The incidence of meningococcal meningitis also decreased over the same period. Meanwhile, the incidence of gram-negative bacillary meningitis increased from 11% in the 1960s to 24% in the 1980s. The latter trend parallels a rise in the frequency of neurosurgical procedures in a large urban tertiary care hospital.

b. **Risk Factors for Bacterial Meningitis in Adults**—Most patients with bacterial meningitis had one or more identifiable risk factors. Seventy-five percent of community-acquired cases and 92% of hospital-acquired cases involved at least one risk factor for meningitis (3).

(1) Among community-acquired cases, many patients had concurrent infections such as otitis media (26%), sinusitis (12%), pneumonia (15%), or endocarditis (7%). Altered immune state (19%), diabetes mellitus (10%), alcoholism (18%), recent or remote history of head injury (9%), and cerebrospinal fluid (CSF) leak (8%) were other major risk factors.

(2) Most of the community-acquired cases of staphylococcal meningitis in another study were associated with endocarditis, IV drug abuse, abscess, cellulitis, or osteomyelitis (18).

(3) Among nosocomial cases, major risk factors included recent neurosurgery (68%), presence of an indwelling neurosurgical device (32%), altered immune state (31%), a history of recent head injury (13%), and CSF leak (13%).

(4) Cases of recurrent meningitis were relatively common in adults. More than one episode of meningitis occurred in 8% and 14% of patients with community-acquired and nosocomial infections, respectively. Among those with recurrent community-acquired cases, 47% had a prior history of neurosurgery or head trauma and 76% had leakage of CSF. All of the patients with recurrent nosocomial cases had a prior history of a neurosurgical procedure, and 47% had leakage of CSF. Sixty-eight percent of the recurrent nosocomial cases were caused by staphylococcal species or gram-negative bacilli. (3)

(5) Seventy-nine percent of the cases of *H influenzae* meningitis in this series were associated with either recent neurosurgery or leakage of CSF. Therefore, the diagnosis of *H influenzae* meningitis in an adult patient should alert the clinician to the probable presence of a CSF leak (3,20).

B. Clinical Presentation of Meningitis

1. **Clinical Features of Aseptic Meningitis**—The following data are from Lepow's retrospective observational review of 407 patients at the Cleveland Metropolitan General Hospital between 1955 and 1958. Both adults and children were included in the study. Analysis excluded patients shown to have a bacterial cause, flaccid paralysis, acute demyelinating encephalomyelitis, meningoencephalitis, or parotitis. Successful long-term follow-up was achieved in 301 of the 407 patients (11,12).
   - **a.** Typical clinical features of aseptic meningitis included headache, fever, neck stiffness, and vomiting. Less common features included chest or abdominal pain (11.8%), upper respiratory symptoms (14.0%), and rash (1.7%). Photophobia, although a common finding, was not listed as a feature in this particular series. Coxsackievirus B was associated with chest or abdominal pain in a third of the cases. Echovirus type 9 or coxsackievirus A type 9 was isolated in 42% of patients with a rash.
   - **b.** Most of the patients in the study had a benign course, and the total duration of illness was <2 weeks in most cases. However, 11% had serious complications such as seizures, coma, severe lethargy, transient sensory deficits, or significant muscle weakness. On the other hand, some of these patients may have had meningoencephalitis rather than meningitis (see Table 26–2).
   - **c.** Furthermore, approximately half of the patients who had adequate long-term follow-up suffered from some degree of physical disability even several months after the acute illness. However, 95% fully recovered by 1 year.
   - **d.** Several limitations of the study should be noted. First, a referral bias may have exaggerated the percentage of patients with serious complications or long-term disabilities. Second, poliomyelitis and mumps were the third and the fourth most common causes, respectively, of aseptic meningitis in this 1950s study. Because these causes are rare today, these data may not be relevant to modern practice. Furthermore, the technical capability in the 1950s to exclude nonviral or treatable causes of aseptic meningitis was more limited than it is today. Finally, only 28% of the patients in the series were ≥20 years of age.

Table 26-2 Serious complications of aseptic meningitis (11,12)

	Prevalence
Seizures	3.4%
Coma or severe lethargy	3.7%
Transient sensory deficits	3.7%
Significant muscle weakness	1.0%

Table 26-3 Clinical features of bacterial meningitis (3)

Findings on Presentation	Prevalence
Fever ≥100°F	95%
Neck-stiffness	88%
Abnormal mental status	78%
Confused/lethargic	51%
Responsive to pain only	22%
Unresponsive	6%
Seizures	23%
Focal neurologic findings	29%
Papilledema	4%
Rash	11%

2. Clinical Features of Bacterial Meningitis (3)

a. In Durand's study, only two-thirds of patients with community-acquired bacterial meningitis presented with the full triad of fever, change in mental status, and nuchal rigidity. However, all patients had at least one of these findings (3).

b. Other common findings included seizures (23%), focal neurologic signs (29%), and rash (11%). Seventy-three percent of patients who had presented with rash proved to have meningococcal meningitis. Blurring of the optic discs was present in 4%. In only one-third was the CSF pressure markedly elevated (3). In acute bacterial meningitis, papilledema would not be expected because the patient is usually hospitalized within 24 hours of onset of symptoms, a period too short for the development of this finding. The presence of true papilledema in a patient with ostensible meningitis should raise the possibility of a brain abscess or other parameningeal infection (see Table 26–3).

c. Hemiparesis was relatively common in the course of bacterial meningitis, affecting 13% of patients; more than half of these patients either died or were left with permanent hemiparesis (3).

d. The overall risk of death was 25% for a single episode of community-acquired meningitis and 35% for nosocomial meningitis. Age >60 years, obtunded mental status, and seizures within 24 hours of presentation were risk factors associated with increased mortality in the study (3).

3. Clinical Features of Tuberculous Meningitis

a. Meningitis caused by tuberculosis (TB) is rare, with 200 to 400 cases reported annually in United States (15). In Ogawa's retrospective study of 45 consecutive patients with TB meningitis, 33% were immigrants from endemic countries and 16% had a prior history of active TB. Alcoholism (27%), IV drug abuse (16%), recent steroid use (9%), recent head trauma (9%), and pregnancy (9%) were other major risk factors. Only one patient had the acquired immune deficiency syndrome (AIDS) in this study (15).

b. The most common features of TB meningitis in Ogawa's study were fever (80%), neck stiffness (71%), headache (62%), and focal neurologic findings (51%). TB meningitis tended to follow a slower course than bacterial meningitis, with an average prodrome of 14 days. However, focal neurologic findings, weight loss, hyponatremia, and change in mental status were more common with TB meningitis (15). Paresis of the sixth cranial nerve, especially when bilateral, is suggestive of a basilar meningitis, particularly one caused by *M tuberculosis*.

c. Prognosis of TB meningitis is relatively poor. The in-hospital mortality rate was 31% despite combination drug therapy, and 32% of the survivors were left with a significant neurologic deficit (15). If untreated, TB meningitis is usually fatal in 3 to 6 weeks.

4. Clinical Features of Cryptococcal Meningitis

a. Cryptococcal meningitis is relatively common among severely immunocompromised patients. Five percent to 10% of AIDS patients eventually develop cryptococcal meningitis as a complication of their illness (1,2,17). However, it appears to be a late manifestation of HIV disease. In one large trial comparing fluconazole with amphotericin B in HIV-positive patients with cryptococcal meningitis, the mean count of CD4-positive T lymphocytes was 55 cells/μl. Patients with CD4 counts >200 cells/μl were unusual (17).

b. Like TB meningitis, cryptococcal meningitis tends to have a more subtle presentation than bacterial meningitis. In Chuck's retrospective review of 106 AIDS patients with cryptococcal disease, many patients did not have the classic features of meningitis. For example, 44% were afebrile, 73% had no meningeal signs, and 83% had a normal mental status examination on presentation (1). Because the presentation can be subtle, lumbar puncture should be strongly considered for all patients with advanced HIV infection who exhibit headache and fever (see Table 26–4).

C. Diagnosis of Acute Meningitis

1. Bacterial Versus Aseptic Meningitis (19)

Table 26-4 Clinical features of cryptococcal meningitis (1)

Findings on Presentation	Prevalence
Fever >38.4°C	56%
Meningeal signs	27%
Headache	73%
Abnormal mental status	17%
Seizures	4%
Focal neurologic findings	15%

a. Lumbar puncture is the most important procedure for diagnosing meningitis. CSF should be sent for Gram stain, culture, rapid bacterial antigen tests (if available), the VDRL syphilis test, protein, glucose, and complete cell count and differential. Simultaneous serum glucose level should also be obtained. In HIV-infected patients, the cryptococcal antigen test and India ink examination should be performed on CSF, and toxoplasmosis serology should be done on serum. In the appropriate setting, serum Lyme disease antibody titers can be useful. In the setting of a new outbreak of presumed enteroviral aseptic meningitis, the viral agent may be isolated from fecal specimens at a research virology laboratory. Acute and convalescent sera may subsequently demonstrate the presence of neutralizing antibodies.

b. Analysis of CSF and epidemiologic features can usually differentiate bacterial from viral meningitis. The following data are from a retrospective analysis of all immunocompetent patients with acute meningitis who were treated at Duke University between January 1969 and July 1980. Patients with CSF shunts or those with recent neurosurgery were excluded. Patients <1 month of age were also excluded. A positive CSF or blood culture or a positive CSF or urine antigen test was required for the diagnosis of acute bacterial meningitis (19).

(1) Numerous CSF variables correlated with the relative risk of bacterial versus viral meningitis (19) (see Table 26–5).

(a) Gram stain of the CSF was positive in 71% of patients with bacterial meningitis. However, misidentification of the organism occurred in 7% of cases (19). *Listeria* and *H influenzae* were the most frequently misidentified pathogens in Durand's study (3). Furthermore, the Gram stain was falsely positive in 1% of patients with viral meningitis (19).

(b) CSF glucose level was significantly lower in bacterial than in viral meningitis ($P<0.001$). In contrast, the serum glucose level was significantly higher in bacterial than in viral meningitis ($P<0.001$). Correspondingly, the CSF-to-serum glucose ratio was more useful

Table 26-5 CSF & serum values in viral vs. bacterial meningitis (19)

	Viral Meningitis (N=205)	Bacterial Meningitis (N=217)	*P*
% positive gram stain of CSF	1	71	<0.001
Median CSF glucose (mg/dl)	70	36	<0.001
Median serum glucose (mg/dl)	115	147	<0.001
CSF to serum glucose ratio	0.61	0.29	—
Median CSF protein (mg/dl)	45	172	<0.001
Median CSF leukocyte count ($\times 10^6$/L)	100	1195	<0.001
Median CSF % PMN	33	86	<0.001

than the absolute CSF glucose level. For example, 29% of patients with a normal CSF glucose level had a CSF-to-serum glucose ratio of <0.4. A normal CSF glucose (>40 mg/dl) is observed in about half of the cases of bacterial meningitis.

(c) CSF protein level was significantly higher in bacterial than in viral meningitis (*P*<0.001). However, 10% of patients with bacterial meningitis had a normal CSF protein level.

(d) CSF leukocyte count was significantly higher in bacterial than in viral meningitis (*P*<0.001). However, 21% of patients with bacterial meningitis had a CSF leukocyte count <250 cells/ml.

(e) The percentage of neutrophils in the initial CSF sample was significantly higher in bacterial meningitis than in viral meningitis (*P*<0.001). However, 15% of patients with bacterial meningitis had a lymphocyte-predominant CSF, whereas 40% of patients with viral meningitis had a neutrophil-predominant CSF in the early stage. Feigin described a study of 31 pediatric patients with suspected viral meningitis but with a preponderance of polymorphonuclear neutrophils (PMNs) on the initial CSF analysis. Patients underwent repeat lumbar puncture 6 to 8 hours after the initial procedure. The prevalence of PMNs in the CSF dropped from 71% to 27.5% on repeat tap. All of these patients subsequently had negative bacterial cultures (4). These findings have been duplicated in a similar study in adults (22).

(f) The total CSF neutrophil count was more useful than the percentage of PMNs for distinguishing bacterial from viral meningitis. For example, a total CSF neutrophil count >1180 cells/μl had a 99% PPV for bacterial meningitis.

(2) Epidemiologic factors also correlated with the relative risk of bacterial versus viral meningitis (19).

(a) Time of Year—The relative risk of bacterial versus viral meningitis was highest during the months of December and January and lowest during the months of July and August.

(b) Age of the Patient—The risk of bacterial meningitis was highest in children <24 months of age and in elderly patients. The risk of bacterial meningitis was lowest at the age of 22 years.

(3) In Spanos' study, the best predictors of bacterial meningitis were a CSF protein level >220 mg/dL, a CSF-to-serum glucose ratio <0.23, a total CSF neutrophil count >1180 cells/μl, and a positive CSF Gram stain. Furthermore, presentation during the winter months and extremes of age (<2 years old or elderly) also favored bacterial meningitis (19). When these features were present, the probability of bacterial meningitis was very high. However, the absence of these parameters could not exclude bacterial meningitis, because there was significant overlap with the values found in viral meningitis. Therefore, the authors of the study proposed a nomogram that combines these CSF and epidemiologic variables to better differentiate viral from bacterial meningitis (Fig. 26-1). The nomogram was also validated in an independent test sample in the same study.

c. Partially Treated Bacterial Meningitis

(1) Patients with partially treated bacterial meningitis tended to have slightly less PMN predominance, lower CSF glucose levels, and lower CSF protein levels. However, these values lack specificity, because there is significant overlap with the findings in viral or untreated bacterial meningitis (19) (see Table 26–6).

(2) Not surprisingly, pretreatment also decreased the yield for identifying the bacterial pathogen. In Spanos' study, 49% of patients with negative results on Gram stain had received antibiotics before the lumbar puncture was performed, compared with 32% of patients with a posi-

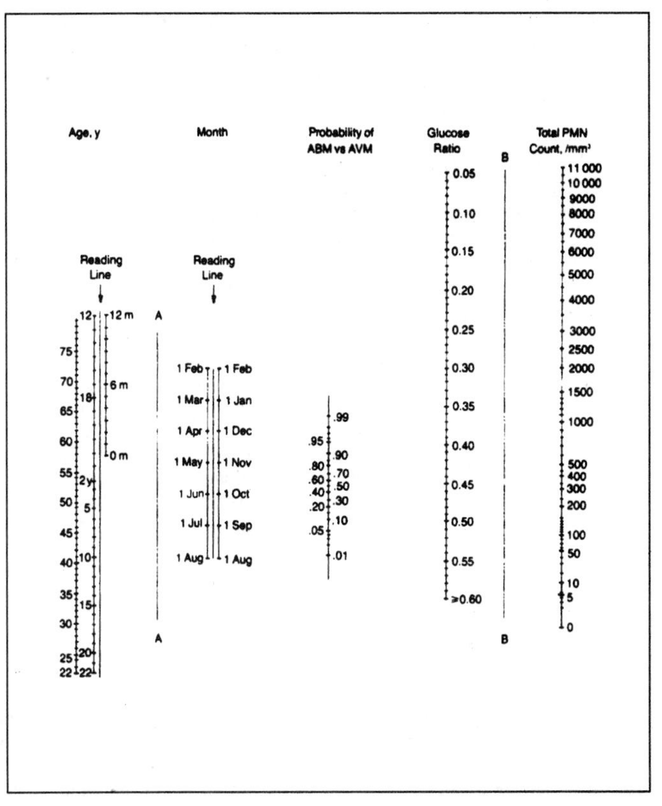

Fig. 26-1. Nomogram for estimating the probability of bacterial (ABM) vs. viral (AVM) meningitis. Step 1, place ruler on reading lines for patient's age and month of presentation and mark intersection with line A. Step 2, place ruler on values for glucose ratio and total polymorphonuclear leukocyte (PMN) count in cerebrospinal fluid and mark intersection with line B. Step 3, use ruler to join marks on lines A and B, then read off the probability of ABM vs. AVM. (Reproduced with permission from (19).)

Table 26-6 CSF profile of untreated vs. pretreated bacterial meningitis (19)

	Untreated Bacterial Meningitis (N=135)	Pretreated Bacterial Meningitis (N=82)	*P*
Median CSF leukocyte count ($\times 10^6$/L)	1350	1090	NS
Median CSF % PMNs	90	82	0.04
Median CSF glucose (mg/dl)	39	25	0.03
Median CSF protein (mg/dl)	200	131	0.009

tive Gram stain ($P=0.04$) (19). Similarly, in Durand's study, 50% of patients with negative bacterial cultures had received antibiotics before lumbar puncture, compared with 38% of patients with positive cultures ($P<0.05$) (3).

2. CSF Findings in TB Meningitis

a. The typical CSF of patients with TB meningitis is characterized by a moderately elevated leukocyte count, lymphocyte predominance, low glucose, and elevated protein. However, these values lack specificity, because there is much overlap with findings in viral or bacterial meningitis. For example, the CSF leukocyte count ranged from 0 to 8600 cells/μl, glucose from 7 to 189 mg/dl, and protein from 35 to 2900 mg/dl. Similarly, there was a neutrophil predominance in 32% of cases (15). However, in 90% to 95% of cases, the CSF leukocyte count is <500 to 600 cells/μl. Therefore, higher CSF cell counts should raise other possible diagnostic considerations. The CSF features of TB meningitis are presented in Table 26-7.

b. In a recent series, the acid-fast stain of CSF was positive in 10%, and only 40% had a positive culture for *M tuberculosis*. A third of the patients had evidence of old or active TB on chest radiographic films. The tuberculin skin test may be misleading, because about 50% of patients are anergic (7,15). In some centers, polymerase chain reaction is being used to improve the diagnostic accuracy. Examination of CSF for tuberculostearic and other organic acids on high-pressure liquid chromatography may be helpful for diagnosis. However, this test is available only in few research laboratories and in the laboratory at the Centers for Disease Control.

3. CSF Findings In Cryptococcal Meningitis

a. CSF findings in patients with cryptococcal meningitis and AIDS can be relatively unimpressive. In Chuck's retrospective analysis of 89 AIDS patients with cryptococcal meningitis, most patients did not have significant abnormalities in CSF glucose, protein, or leukocyte count. In contrast, almost all patients had a positive CSF India ink test, a positive CSF culture, or an elevated CSF cryptococcal antigen titer (1) (see Table 26–8).

b. The analysis of CSF in HIV-infected patients is further complicated by the fact that the CSF is frequently abnormal in these patients even in the absence of a second central nervous system infection. Elevation of CSF protein and pleocytosis are particularly common (6).

Table 26-7 CSF profile of tuberculous meningitis (15)

Median CSF leukocyte count	162 cells/μl
Percent of patients with lymphocyte predominance	68%
Median opening pressure	190 mm H_2O
Median glucose	35 mg/dl
Median protein	151 mg/dl

Table 26-8 CSF profile of cryptococcal meningitis (1)

CSF Features	Prevalence
CSF leukocyte count >20 cells/μl	21%
CSF PMN count >10% of leukocytes	16%
CSF protein >45 mg/dl	55%
CSF glucose <40 mg/dl	24%
Positive CSF India ink test	74%
Positive CSF cryptococcal antigen test	91%

4. Other Useful Tests

a. Brain Imaging Studies

(1) Computed tomography (CT) or magnetic resonance imaging of the head can be useful for patients with suspected meningitis and focal neurologic findings at presentation. If possible, CT scan should be done with a contrast agent to rule out an abscess or other mass lesion, especially in HIV-infected patients. In Durand's study, about half of the patients with a focal neurologic examination had an intracranial abnormality on CT scan (3). If the suspicion for bacterial meningitis is high, antibiotics should not be delayed while the patient waits for the imaging study. In the absence of focal neurologic findings, papilledema, or other suggestions of a parameningeal infection, a CT scan is not mandatory before performance of a lumbar puncture.

(2) The issue of whether lumbar puncture contributes significantly to herniation in patients with meningitis and high CSF pressure has not been resolved. Although herniation has been described after lumbar puncture, there are no well-designed studies that indicate that lumbar puncture actually increases this risk (13). In patients without focal neurologic findings or papilledema, lumbar puncture is safe and should be performed as soon as possible. If markedly increased CSF pressure is found on lumbar puncture, it would be prudent to remove only the small amount of CSF in the manometer, which is usually enough for essential studies. To reduce the CSF pressure, IV infusion of 25 to 50 g of 20% mannitol solution may be used. If the clinical situation requires further efforts to reduce the CSF pressure, IV dexamethasone may be given subsequently.

b. Rapid Bacterial Antigen Tests—Latex agglutination assays for antigens in the CSF (*H influenzae* type b [HIB], meningococcus, group B streptococcus, *Escherichia coli*, and pneumococcus) may be helpful in accelerating diagnosis. It may be particularly useful in patients with culture-negative bacterial meningitis and those who have received antibiotics before presentation. Although these tests are highly accurate, they are not 100% sensitive. False-negative tests may occur if the serotype of the pathogen is not detectable by the assay or if insufficient amounts of antigen are present in the CSF (10,24).

D. Treatment

1. Aseptic Meningitis—The major challenge in the management of patients with suspected aseptic meningitis is to identify those who have treatable causes of meningitis. These causes include TB, cryptococcal infection, syphilis, toxoplasmosis, malignancies, Lyme disease, leptospirosis, herpes simplex, herpes zoster, HIV, and drug hypersensitivity. Care must be given to exclude the possibility of parameningeal infections or partially treated bacterial meningitides, which can also mimic viral meningitis. Once those patients with treatable causes have been excluded, therapy for aseptic meningitis is usually supportive.

2. Acute Bacterial Meningitis

a. Patients with suspected bacterial meningitis should be treated with antibiotics as soon as possible. If the suspicion for bacterial meningitis is high, treatment should not be delayed for imaging studies. Therapy should be guided by the results of the Gram stain of CSF. If the Gram stain is negative, the patient's age and other clinical and epidemiologic factors should guide the choice of empiric antibiotics.

(1) Most cases of community-acquired meningitis in adults are caused by the pneumococcus, meningococcus, *Listeria*, *H influenzae*, or other streptococcal species. To cover these common pathogens, empiric treatment with a third-generation cephalosporin and ampicillin or a third-generation cephalosporin alone has been recommended by experts. Because *Listeria* is an important pathogen among older patients and immunosuppressed patients of all ages, ampicillin should be included in the empiric regimen. A third-generation cephalosporin alone usually suffices for adolescents and immunocompetent younger adults (20,21).

(2) Adequately controlled studies comparing various empiric antibiotic regimens have been done only in children, and these data cannot be generalized to adults (13,20,21).

b. If the Gram stain is positive, the identified organism along with epidemiologic considerations should guide the choice of antibiotics.

(1) In general, bactericidal antibiotics with good CSF penetration should be administered by intermittent IV boluses. Recommended duration of therapy varies from 7 to 14 days for most organisms and 3 weeks for gram-negative bacilli. For patients highly allergic to penicillin, treatment with chloramphenicol or vancomycin is indicated for treatment of pneumococcal meningitis, and chloramphenicol is the alternative for meningococcal meningitis. The major antibiotics that are used to treat meningitis are summarized in Table 26-9 (20,21).

(2) Antibiotic choices for specific pathogens vary depending on institutional preferences and the local antibiotic resistance patterns (20,21). One possible scheme is summarized in Table 26-10.

c. The initial therapy should be tailored for patients belonging to a particular risk group. Patients with a history of IV drug use should receive coverage for staphylococcal species. An aminoglycoside should be added for patients with a urinary tract infection to cover gram-negative rods. If *Pseudomonas* infection is suspected, ceftazidime should be used in place of ceftriaxone or cefotaxime. Patients with nosocomial infections should be treated initially for gram-negative bacillary infection as well as for staphylococcal meningitis. In patients with CNS shunts, vancomycin should be used to cover infections caused by coagulase-negative staphylococci.

d. Strains of pneumococcus with intermediate or high resistance to penicillin have been reported in United States, and penicillin may no longer be suitable for empiric therapy in many areas. A two-drug combination of penicillin, ampicillin, or vancomycin plus a third-generation cephalosporin is now recommended for initial therapy of pneumococcal meningitis. All isolates of *Streptococcus pneumoniae* should be tested for resistance to β-lactam antibiotics. Penicillin or ampicillin should be used alone only after the isolate is proven to be penicillin susceptible (minimal inhibitory concentration [MIC] <0.1 mg/ml). If the pneumococcus is proven resistant to the drug in vitro, penicillin should be omitted from the combination therapy and the third-generation cephalosporin alone (cefotaxime or ceftriaxone) should be continued. In areas where highly resistant (MIC >1.0 mg/ml) pneumococci are endemic, initial therapy should consist of vancomycin plus a third-generation cephalosporin until susceptibility testing has been performed (23).

Table 26-9 Antibiotic dosages for bacterial meningitis

	Typical IV Dosage
Penicillin G	4×10^6 U q 4 h
Ampicillin	2 g q 4 h
Nafcillin	1.5–2.0 g q 4 h
Chloramphenicol	1.0–1.5 g q 6 h
Ceftriaxone	2 g q 12 h
Cefotaxime	2 g q 4 h
Ceftazidime	2 g q 8 h
Vancomycin	500 mg q 6 h
Gentamicin or tobramycin	1.0–1.5 mg/kg of body weight q 8 h
Amikacin	5 mg/kg of body weight q 8 h

Table 26-10 Suggested therapy for bacterial meningitis

Pathogen	Standard Therapy	Alternative Therapy
Pneumococcus	Penicillin G or ampicillin + a third-generation cephalosporin[*]	Vancomycin or chloramphenicol
Meningococcus	Penicillin G or ampicillin	Ceftriaxone, Cefotaxime, or chloramphenicol
Haemophilus influenzae (β-lactamase–negative)	Ampicillin	Ceftriaxone, cefotaxime, or chloramphenicol
Haemophilus influenzae (β-lactamase–positive)	Ceftriaxone or cefotaxime	Chloramphenicol
Listeria monocytogenes	Ampicillin ±aminoglycoside or penicillin G ±aminoglycoside[†]	Trimethoprim/Sulfamethoxazole[†]
Staphylococcus aureus (methicillin-sensitive)	Nafcillin	Vancomycin
Staphylococeus aureus (methicillin-resistant)	Vancomycin	Trimethoprim/Sulfamethoxazole or quinolones[‡]
Staphylococcus epidermidis	Vancomycin + rifampin	Teicoplanin[‡]
Enteric gram-negative rods	Ceftriaxone + aminoglycoside or Cefotaxime + aminoglycoside	Piperacillin + aminoglycoside, azlocillin + aminoglycoside, aztreonam,[‡] or quinolones[‡]
Pseudomonas aeruginosa	Ceftazidime + aminoglycoside	Piperacillin + aminoglycoside, azlocillin + aminoglycoside, imipenem,[‡] aztreonam,[‡] or quinolones[‡]
Streptococcus agalactiae (group B streptococcus)	Ampicillin ±aminoglycoside or penicillin G ±aminoglycoside	Ceftriaxone, cefotaxime, or vancomycin

[*]Two drugs are now used in initial therapy because of the increasing resistance of pneumococci to penicillin. Penicillin or ampicillin should be used alone only after the isolate is proven to be penicillin susceptible (MIC <0.1 μg/ml). If the pneumococci is proven resistant to the drug in vitro, penicillin is omitted from the combination therapy and the third-generation cephalosporin alone (cefotaxime or ceftriaxone) is continued. In areas where highly resistant (MIC >1.0 μg/ml) pneumococci are endemic, initial therapy should consist of vancomycin plus a third-generation cephalosporin until susceptibility testing has been performed.
[†]If patient is allergic to standard therapy, desensitization should be strongly considered.
[‡]Effectiveness of these drugs has not been fully evaluated.

3. Treatment of Cryptococcal Meningitis

a. The optimal regimen for treatment of cryptococcal meningitis is still being evaluated. Saag randomly assigned 194 HIV-positive patients with cryptococcal meningitis to receive either IV amphotericin B (0.3 mg/kg/day) or oral fluconazole (400 mg loading dose, followed by 200 mg/day). Patients who were comatose or those whose life expectancy was <2 weeks were excluded from the study. Flucytosine was added to amphotericin at the discretion of the investigators (17) (see Table 26–11).

(1) Overall at 10 weeks, there was no significant difference in outcome between patients treated with fluconazole and those treated with amphotericin. However, the mortality rate during the first 2 weeks of the study was lower with amphotericin (*P*=NS). Furthermore, the median number of days to negative CSF culture was 42 with amphotericin and 64 with fluconazole (*P*=NS). On the other hand, amphotericin was much more likely to cause toxic side effects (*P*<0.0001).

(2) Because study-defined treatment success was achieved in only 34% to 40% of patients with either drug, therapy for cryptococcal meningitis requires much improvement. Indeed, Saag's study has been criticized because the doses used in both groups (0.3 mg/kg/day of amphotericin B and 200 mg/day of fluconazole) are now considered suboptimal. It is unknown how the two drugs would compare at higher doses.

(3) Some experts advocate the use of flucytosine with amphotericin, but its added value is also unknown. Results of larger, well-designed controlled trials are needed to answer these important questions (8).

b. HIV-infected patients who survive a bout of cryptococcal meningitis should receive chemoprophylaxis for life, because the risk of relapse without maintenance treatment is 50% to 60%. Fluconazole is the current drug of choice. Powderly randomly assigned 218 AIDS patients who had recovered from cryptococcal meningitis to receive either amphotericin B (1 mg/kg IV q week) or fluconazole (200 mg/day PO). All patients had been treated with IV amphotericin B initially. Average follow-up was 286 days (15a) (see Table 26–12).

(1) Overall, fluconazole was superior to amphotericin. The risk of relapse was significantly lower (*P*<0.001) and secondary bacterial infections were less common (*P*=0.004) with fluconazole.

(2) Furthermore, fluconazole was better tolerated than amphotericin B (*P*<0.001).

4. Role of Steroids in Adult Patients With Bacterial Meningitis

a. Introduction

(1) Interest in adjunctive therapy with steroids stems partly from the fact that bacterial meningitis continues to cause significant morbidity and mortality despite modern advances in antibiotic therapy. Much of the damage to the host is thought to be caused by host-pathogen interactions that activate various inflammatory cascades. The latter cause

Table 26-11 Amphotericin B vs. fluconazole for cryptococcal meningitis (17)

	Amphotericin B (N=63)	Fluconazole (N=131)	*P*
Treatment success	40%	34%	NS
Disease progression	11%	20%	NS
Overall mortality rate	14%	18%	NS
2-wk mortality rate	8%	15%	NS
Time to negative CSF culture	42 d	64 d	NS
Patients with no side effects	36%	73%	<0.0001
Severe toxicity requiring cessation of therapy	8%	2%	NS

Table 26-12 Comparison of maintenance therapy for cryptococcal meningitis (15a)

	Amphotericin B (N=99)	Fluconazole (N=119)	*P*
Probability of being relapse-free at 1 y	78%	97%	<0.001
Patients with no adverse effects	33%	62%	<0.001
Risk of bacterial infections	36%	17%	0.004

breakdown of the blood-brain barrier, thrombosis of vessels, infarction of brain tissue, cerebral edema, and increased intracranial pressure. Furthermore, initiation of antibiotics is thought to cause a paradoxical increase in inflammation, because bacteriolysis activates more inflammatory cascades (16).

(2) As an antiinflammatory drug, corticosteroids can decrease the inflammation initiated by the host-pathogen interaction as well as that caused by antibiotic-induced bacteriolysis. On this basis, corticosteroids have been tested in bacterial meningitis to improve clinical outcome.

b. In children with bacterial meningitis, several randomized controlled trials have shown significant benefit of adjunctive therapy with dexamethasone (5,9,14). A representative study by Odio is described here (14). This double-blind, controlled trial randomly assigned 101 infants and children with bacterial meningitis to receive either cefotaxime (50 mg/kg q 6 hours for 7 to 10 days) plus dexamethasone (0.15 mg/kg q 6 hours for 4 days) or cefotaxime (same dosage) plus placebo. The first dose of dexamethasone was given minutes before antibiotic administration. Patients were 6 weeks to 13 years of age. The average length of follow-up was about 15 months (see Table 26–13).

(1) Patients treated with dexamethasone had a decrease in intracranial pressure at 12 hours, whereas patients treated with placebo had an increase in intracranial pressure. Furthermore, steroid therapy decreased the CSF levels of tumor necrosis factor-α and platelet-activating factor.

(2) More importantly, the risk of long-term neurologic sequelae, primarily sensorineural hearing loss and ataxia, was significantly decreased with dexamethasone ($P=0.008$). However, there was no difference in mortality. One patient died in each group.

(3) These studies were done at a time HIB accounted for most cases of childhood meningitis. The favorable results probably reflect the response, primarily of HIB, to corticosteroid therapy. Since the use of HIB protein-conjugate vaccine in children became widespread in this country, the incidence of neurologic complications of HIB meningitis has declined markedly. The effect of corticosteroid therapy on pneumococcal or meningococcal meningitis has not yet been clearly established.

c. Almost all of the patients in these trials were children. For example, the average age of the patients in Odio's study was 16 months, and 75% of the

Table 26-13 Dexamethasone vs. placebo as adjunctive therapy in children (14)

	Dexamethasone (N=52)	Placebo (N=49)	*P*
Opening pressure at 0/12 h (mm H_2O)	180/166	182/199	0.04
TNF α level at 0/12 h (pg/ml)	1040/170	900/700	0.04
Platelet activating factor at 0/12 h (pg/ml)	3140/941	2415/3242	0.04
Significant neurologic or audiologic sequelae	14%	38%	0.007

cases were caused by *H influenzae*, a pathogen that occurs almost exclusively in young children for meningitis. Whether the results of these trials can be generalized to adult patients with other causes of bacterial meningitis is not clear, and therefore the role of corticosteroids in adult patients is more controversial. In the only large study of corticosteroids involving adult patients with bacterial meningitis, only 30% of the 492 patients were >13 years of age. Although dexamethasone was beneficial, steroids decreased the mortality only in those with pneumococcal meningitis, and the benefit was limited to patients <25 years of age (5). Given the paucity of data among adults, most authors recommend use of steroids only for patients with severe cerebral edema or markedly elevated CSF pressure. More studies are needed to better define the role of steroids in adult patients with bacterial meningitis (21).

E. Summary

1. In adults, most cases of community-acquired bacterial meningitis are caused by the pneumococcus, meningococcus, *Listeria*, or various streptococci. Nosocomial cases are most often caused by gram-negative rods, streptococci, *S aureus*, or coagulase-negative staphylococci. *H influenzae* is an uncommon cause of meningitis in adults and, when present, may indicate the presence of a CSF leak. Aseptic meningitis is most often caused by the enteroviruses, such as the coxsackievirus or echoviruses. However, numerous other viruses as well as *M tuberculosis*, *T pallidum*, *Cryptococcus neoformans*, *Toxoplasma gondii*, *B burgdorferi*, parameningeal infections, drug hypersensitivity, and malignancies should also be considered.
2. The relative prevalence of bacterial versus viral meningitis varies with age and season. Viral meningitis is much more common during the summer months, and bacterial meningitis is relatively more common during the winter months. The risk of bacterial meningitis is highest in children <24 months of age and in elderly patients.
3. The typical CSF profile for various types of meningitides are summarized in Table 26-14. However, because there is so much overlap in these values, accurate distinction among various causes of meningitis is not always possible. Other tests of the CSF, such as the Gram stain, rapid antigen tests, acid-fast bacillus smears, VDRL tests, India ink preparations, cryptococcal antigen tests, and cultures for bacteria, fungi, and mycobacteria can provide additional diagnostic information.
4. Treatment of viral meningitis is usually supportive. Treatment of bacterial meningitis is guided by the findings on the initial Gram stain but should be

Table 26-14 Typical CSF profiles in various meningitides

Type of Meningitis	Bacterial	Viral	Cryptococcal	Tuberculous	Normal Values
Opening pressure (mm H_2O)	200–400	90–200	180–300	180–300	90–180
CSF glucose (mg/dl)	<40	50–75	<40	<40*	50–75
CSF protein (mg/dl)	>100	50–100	50–200	100–200	15–40
CSF leukocyte count (cells/μl)	100–5000	10–300	0–200	0–500	0–5
Predominant cell type	Neutrophils	Lymphocytes†	Lymphocytes	Lymphocytes	Lymphocytes

*The CSF glucose concentration may be normal in early stages with subsequent development of hypoglycorrhachia.
†Early viral meningitis may show neutrophil predominance initially.

tailored according to the local patterns of antibiotic resistance and the patient's risk profile. If the Gram stain is negative, empiric therapy with a third-generation cephalosporin is recommended for younger adults with community-acquired bacterial meningitis. A third-generation cephalosporin plus ampicillin is recommended for older adults and for immunosuppressed patients of all ages, in whom an infection with *Listeria* may be suspected. For nosocomial cases, gram-negative bacilli and staphylococcal species should be targeted. Treatment should continue for 7 to 14 days for most of the common community-acquired organisms causing meningitis, and for 3 weeks for gram-negative bacillary infections.

5. In children with bacterial meningitis, adjunctive therapy with dexamethasone significantly decreases the risk of sensorineural hearing loss or ataxia. However, the use of corticosteroids in adult patients is more controversial because adequate trials have not been done in this population. Until the results of such trials become available, the use of corticosteroids in adults should be considered only for those with evidence of brain swelling.

Abbreviations used in Chapter 26

ABM = bacterial meningitis
AIDS = acquired immunodeficiency syndrome
AVM = viral meningitis
CSF = cerebrospinal fluid
CT = computed tomography
HIB = *Hemophilus influenzae* type B
HIV = human immunodeficiency virus
IV = intravenous
MIC = minimum inhibitory concentration
NS = not significant
P = probability value
PMN = polymorphonuclear neutrophils
PO = per os
PPV = positive predictive value
q = every
TB = tuberculosis
TNF = tumor necrosis factor
VDRL = Venereal Disease Research Laboratory
vs. = versus

References

1. Chuck. Infections with *Cryptococcus neoformans* in the acquired immunodeficiency syndrome. *N Engl J Med* 1989;321:794.
2. Dismukes. Cryptococcal meningitis in patients with AIDS. *J Infect Dis* 1988;157: 624.
3. Durand. Acute bacterial meningitis in adults: a review of 493 episodes. *N Engl J Med* 1993;328:21.
4. Feigin. Value of repeat lumbar puncture in the differential diagnosis of meningitis. *N Engl J Med* 1973;289:571.
5. Girgis. Dexamethasone treatment for bacterial meningitis in children and adults. *Pediatr Infect Dis J* 1989;8:848.
6. Hollander. Diagnostic lumbar puncture in HIV-infected patients: analysis of 128 cases. *Am J Med* 1994;96:223.
7. Karandanis. Recent survey of infectious meningitis in adults: review of laboratory findings in bacterial, tuberculous, and aseptic meningitis. *South Med J* 1976;69: 449.

8. Larsen. Fluconazole compared with amphotericin B plus flucytosine for cryptococcal meningitis in AIDS. *Ann Intern Med* 1990;113:183.
9. Lebel. Dexamethasone therapy for bacterial meningitis: results of two double blind, placebo-controlled trials. *N Engl J Med* 1988;319:964.
10. Leinonen. Comparison of counter-current immunoelectrophoresis, latex agglutination, and radioimmunossay in detection of soluble capsular polysaccharide antigens of *Haemophilus influenzae* type b and *Neisseria meningitides* of groups A or C. *J Clin Pathol* 1978;31:1172.
11. Lepow. A clinical, epidemiologic and laboratory investigation of aseptic meningitis during the four-year period, 1955–1958: I. Observation concerning etiology and epidemiology. *N Engl J Med* 1962;266:1181.
12. Lepow. A clinical, epidemiologic and laboratory investigation of aseptic meningitis during the four-year period, 1955–1958: II. The clinical disease and its sequelae. *N Engl J Med* 1962;266:1188.
13. Martin. The spinal tap: a new look at an old test. *Ann Intern Med* 1986;104:840.
14. Odio. The beneficial effects of early dexamethasone administration in infants and children with bacterial meningitis. *N Engl J Med* 1991;324:1525.
15. Ogawa. Tuberculous meningitis in an urban medical center. *Medicine (Baltimore)* 1987;66:317.

15a. Powderly. A controlled trial of fluconazole or amphotericin B to prevent relapse of cryptococcal meningitis in patients with the acquired immunodeficiency syndrome. *NEJM* 1992;326:793.
16. Quagliarello. Bacterial meningitis: pathogenesis, pathophysiology, and progress. *N Engl J Med* 1992;327:864.
17. Saag. Comparison of amphotericin B with fluconazole in the treatment of acute AIDS-associated cryptococcal meningitis. *N Engl J Med* 1992;326:83.
18. Schlesinger. *Staphylococcus aureus* meningitis: a broad-based epidemiologic study. *Medicine (Baltimore)* 1987;66:148.
19. Spanos. Differential diagnosis of acute meningitis: an analysis of the predictive value of initial observations. *JAMA* 1989;262:2700.
20. Swartz. Bacterial meningitis. Lecture given at the Medical Grand Rounds, Massachusetts General Hospital, February 22, 1993.
21. Tunkel. Bacterial meningitis: recent advances in pathophysiology and treatment. *Ann Intern Med* 1990;112:619.
22. Varki. Value of second lumbar puncture in confirming a diagnosis of aseptic meningitis. *Arch Neurol* 1979;36:581.
23. Viladrich. Characteristics and antibiotic therapy of adult meningitis due to penicillin-resistant pneumococci. *Am J Med* 1988;84:839.
24. Williams. Rapid identification of bacterial antigen in blood cultures and cerebrospinal fluid. *J Clin Pathol* 1988;41:691.

27 Fever and Neutropenia

Will P. Schmitt, Burton W. Lee, and Morton N. Swartz

A. Introduction

1. Since the advent of cytotoxic chemotherapy in the late 1950s, researchers have recognized the relationship between risk of infection and the absolute neutrophil count (ANC). The ANC is calculated by adding the total number of neutrophils, metamyelocytes, and band forms per microliter of blood. Bodey's seminal observational study of 52 patients with leukemia and chemotherapy-induced neutropenia is described here. Patients were between 1 and 77 years of age, and all patients had received chemotherapy for biopsy-proven acute myelogenous or lymphocytic leukemia (4).
   a. **Neutropenia Versus Lymphopenia**—The rate of infection was highest when both neutropenia and lymphopenia were present simultaneously. However, the rate of infection was higher when neutropenia was present alone than when lymphopenia was present alone (4) (see Table 27–1).
   b. **Severity of Neutropenia**—The risk of infection was inversely related to the ANC. When the ANC was <100 cells/μl, 43 severe infections occurred per 1000 days of observation. This corresponded to 53% of the observed patient-days being spent with an identified infection. The risk decreased by about half when the ANC was between 100 to 500 cells/μl and was halved again when the ANC was between 500 and 1000 cells/μl. The risk continued to decrease to <5 infections per 1000 days of observation when the ANC was between 1000 and 1500 cells/μl. However, beyond an ANC of 1500 cells/ml, no further decrease in the risk was observed (4).
   c. **Duration of Neutropenia**—The risk of infection also correlated with the duration of neutropenia. Overall, any patient with an ANC <1000 cells/μl had a 39% chance of developing an identified infection. However, if the ANC was <1000 cells/μl for ≥12 weeks, the risk of infection was 100% (4).
2. Neutropenic patients are more susceptible to infection because of two major reasons. First, neutropenia represents the loss of the primary line of defense against bacterial infections. Second, chemotherapy often damages the integrity of the gastrointestinal mucosa. This may cause leakage of oral or fecal flora into the circulation, resulting in transient bacteremia. Therefore, patients remain at increased risk of infection until the integrity of the gastrointestinal mucosa and the granulocyte count are both restored.
3. In neutropenic patients, the clinical manifestations of infection can often be

Table 27-1 Risk of severe infection with leukopenia (4)

Neutropenia (<1000 cells/μL)	Lymphopenia (<1000 cells/μL)	Episodes of Severe Infection per 1000 Days of Observation
Yes	Yes	28
Yes	No	14
No	Yes	6
No	No	3

subtle because of a limited ability to produce an inflammatory response. Therefore, fever is often the only sign of infection. In Sickles' study of 344 neutropenic patients with documented infections, every patient with a urinary tract infection and an ANC <100 cells/μl was febrile, but only 44% had dysuria and only 11% had pyuria. In contrast, among patients with a urinary tract infection and an ANC >1000 cells/μl, 85% had dysuria and 97% had pyuria. Similarly, 98% of patients with pneumonia and an ANC <100 cells/μl were febrile but only 8% had a purulent sputum. For patients with an ANC >1000 cells/μl, 84% had a purulent sputum (72).

4. The cause of fever is often unidentified in febrile neutropenic patients. Pizzo described a prospective observational study of all cases of fever in pediatric cancer patients (average age, 15.7 years) at the National Cancer Institute from 1975 to 1980 (55) (see Table 27–2).
   a. Among the 793 episodes of neutropenic fever (ANC <500 cells/μl), 48% were unexplained. Microbiologically documented infections accounted for 27%, and 25% were clinical infections without microbiologic confirmation.
   b. Infections of the blood stream and the respiratory system were the most common identifiable causes of fever. Infections of the genitourinary tract were relatively uncommon, probably because bladder catheterization was avoided in the study. The nature of the infections did not differ according to the underlying malignancy.

5. The bacteriology of infection in neutropenic patients appears to be changing.
   a. During the 1960s and 1970s, gram-negative rods were responsible for most of the documented infections among febrile neutropenic patients. For example, in the first EORTC (European Organization for Research and Treatment of Cancer) International Antimicrobial Therapy Trial, published in 1978, gram-negative rods caused 63% of the bacteremia in febrile neutropenic patients and gram-positive organisms accounted for only 25% of the bacteremic episodes (24).
   b. However, since the 1980s, infections caused by gram-positive organisms now outnumber those caused by gram-negative organisms (60). For example, of the 151 episodes of bacteremia among febrile neutropenic patients in the eighth EORTC trial, published in 1993, gram-positive and gram-negative organisms were isolated in 69% and 31% of the cases, respectively (22). Similarly, in Pizzo's study of 550 episodes of neutropenic fever, 56% and 40% of the microbiologically identifiable etiologic agents were gram-positive and gram-negative organisms, respectively. The relative frequencies of the major pathogens isolated in Pizzo's study are summarized in Table 27-3 (58).
   c. The incidence of infections caused by viridans streptococci has been increasing among neutropenic patients (2,3,8,10,11,19,39,44,63,75). Traditionally, these organisms were recognized as pathogens primarily in the context of dental infections or endocarditis. More recently, viridans streptococci have emerged as important pathogens among immunocompro-

Table 27-2 Clinical presentation of patients with neutropenic fever (55)

Characteristics	Percent of Episodes
Unexplained fever	48
Documented infection	
Sepsis	13
Pneumonia	11
Infections of the head, eyes, ears, nose, or throat	9
Cellulitis	5
Gastrointestinal infections	4
Genitourinary infections	4
Other infections	6
Total	52

Table 27-3 Microbiology of proven infections in neutropenic fever (58)

Organism	% of Microbiologically Identified Cases
Gram-positive aerobes	
Staphylococcus aureus	17
Staphylococcus epidermidis	17
Streptococci	15
Other	7
Total	56
Gram-negative aerobes	
Escherichia coli	15
Klebsiella pneumoniae	7
Pseudomonas aeruginosa	13
Other	5
Total	40
Anaerobes	4
Fungi	2

mised hosts, accounting for 39% of the bacteremic episodes among febrile neutropenic patients in one study (63). These organisms have been associated with a number of serious infectious complications in neutropenic patients, including adult respiratory distress syndrome (3,8,10,11,19,39), septic shock (11,19,39,75), endocarditis (3,19), and death (2,3,8,10,11,19,39,44, 63,75).

d. The reason for the growing importance of infections caused by gram-positive organisms in febrile neutropenic patients is not entirely clear. However, the more severe mucositis that results from more intensive chemotherapeutic protocols and the prevalent use of indwelling central venous catheters probably contribute to this changing pattern. The increasing use of oral antimicrobial prophylaxis with agents that do not suppress the growth of gram-positive intestinal microorganisms may be an additional contributor.

B. Initial Management of Patients With Fever and Neutropenia

1. Evaluation of the Febrile Neutropenic Patient

a. A careful history and physical examination should be performed expeditiously. The date of the last course of chemotherapy is important, because the nadir of the granulocyte count occurs approximately 14 days after chemotherapy. The type of cancer or chemotherapy, when controlled for the level of ANC, does not appear to change the type of infection for which the patient is at risk. As discussed previously, symptoms and signs of infection are often subtle in this population. Therefore, history and physical examination must be thorough. Examination of the skin, perirectal area, catheter sites, dentition, oropharynx, ears, and the sinuses should not be overlooked (55).

b. Laboratory evaluation should include complete blood count with differential, chest film, blood urea nitrogen, creatinine, electrolytes, liver function tests, urinalysis, urine culture, and two blood cultures. Further tests should be obtained as indicated by the patient's symptoms and signs. If a patient has an indwelling intravenous catheter, one blood culture should be drawn from each port (34).

2. Empiric Antibiotic Therapy—Antibiotic therapy is recommended for all febrile patients ($\geq 38.3°$ C) with ANC <500 cells/μl. Patients should also receive treatment if the initial ANC is between 500 and 1000 cells/μl but is expected to fall to <500 cells/μl within 48 hours. Because the culture results usually are not available at the time of presentation, administration of empiric broad-spectrum antibiotics is necessary. Historically, the mortality rate among neutropenic patients with septicemia had been as high as 70% to 84% (5,7). However, it has declined to 10% to 30% in the modern era, presumably because of the widespread use of broad-spectrum antibiotics (58,59,68).

a. Since Schimpff's first study in 1971, >100 papers have been published comparing various antibiotic regimens for empiric treatment of neutropenic fever (68). However, on the average, these studies are characterized by small size, mediocre design quality, and lack of statistical power (50). There are few data to suggest that any one antibiotic regimen is clearly superior to another (34,60).

(1) The currently recommended empiric regimens include the following (34,60): (a) an aminoglycoside (gentamicin, tobramycin, or amikacin) plus an antipseudomonal β-lactam antibiotic (ticarcillin, azlocillin, mezlocillin, piperacillin, cefoperazone, or ceftazidime); (b) an antipseudomonal penicillin (ticarcillin, azlocillin, mezlocillin, or piperacillin) plus an antipseudomonal third-generation cephalosporin (cefoperazone or ceftazidime); (c) monotherapy with cefoperazone, ceftazidime, or imipenem-cilastatin; and (d) an antipseudomonal β-lactam (ticarcillin, azlocillin, mezlocillin, piperacillin, cefoperazone, ceftazidime) plus an aminoglycoside (gentamicin, tobramycin, or amikacin) plus vancomycin.

(2) For patients allergic to penicillin, aztreonam is an adequate substitute. However, it must be used in combination with another antibiotic because it lacks efficacy against gram-positive organisms (36). Among older patients with baseline serum creatinine levels >1.1 mg/dl, severe renal dysfunction was observed in 26% of those receiving an aminoglycoside. Therefore, if an aminoglycoside is to be used in this group, serum antibiotic levels should be monitored carefully (24). Use of an aminoglycoside should be avoided if possible when other nephrotoxic drugs (*e.g.*, cisplatin, cyclosporine, amphotericin B) are being used simultaneously for other purposes.

b. Monotherapy Versus Combination Therapy—Among the identified organisms causing bacteremic neutropenic fever in Pizzo's study, 56% were gram-positive cocci and 40% were gram-negative aerobes (58). Traditionally, broad-spectrum coverage has been achieved with combination therapy, usually an antipseudomonal β-lactam with an aminoglycoside or with double β-lactam therapy.

(1) More recently, monotherapy with ceftazidime has been shown to be equivalent to combination therapy as the initial treatment for patients with fever and neutropenia (15,58,65). The study by Pizzo is described as an example (58). Pizzo compared ceftazidime versus the combination of cephalothin, gentamicin, and carbenicillin in 550 episodes of neutropenic fever. Neutropenia was defined as an ANC <500 cells/μl or an initial ANC between 500 and 1000 cells/μl falling to <500 cells/μl within 48 hours. A complete blood count, chest film, urinalysis, and at least two blood cultures were obtained before treatment. Routine and fungal cultures of the nose, throat, urine, and stool were also performed before antimicrobial therapy. Modification of the initial antibiotic regimen was permitted as deemed necessary by the patient's clinical condition or microbiologic data. Aminoglycoside levels were monitored closely, and the dose was adjusted as needed. Patients were considered to have "unexplained fever" if no infection was detected within 72 hours of enrollment and initiation of antibiotic therapy. Others were considered to have a "documented infection." The outcome was considered to be a "success without modification" if the patient fully recovered from neutropenic fever without modification of the initial antibiotic regimen, and it was considered to be a "success with modification" if the patient fully recovered from neutropenic fever but required some modification of the initial regimen. Finally, the outcome was considered to be a "failure" if the patient died from a documented or presumed infection during the neutropenic episode (58).

(a) Overall, there was no significant difference in the rate of success between monotherapy and combination therapy. Despite use of monotherapy, significant antibiotic resistance was not observed. In addition, the risk of organ toxicity was lower with monotherapy than with combination therapy (see Table 27–4).

(b) Among patients with unexplained fever, both strategies were highly successful, usually without the need for modification of the initial regimen.

(c) Among patients with a documented infection, both strategies were also highly successful, but modification of the initial regimen was usually required (see Table 27–5).

(2) De Pauw duplicated these findings among patients with more profound and prolonged neutropenia. The risk of adverse events was also significantly lower ($P<0.001$) with monotherapy (8%) than with combination therapy (20%) in this study (15). Nevertheless, some experts still fear that widespread use of monotherapy may eventually select for resistant organisms (46) or that modification of the single regimen may be required often enough to make combination drug therapy preferable as the initial empiric regimen (20,77).

c. Vancomycin—Because gram-positive organisms account for more than half of the identified bacteremic infections in neutropenic patients, several authors have evaluated the role of vancomycin for empiric therapy (23,37, 64). The study by the EORTC is described as an example. This prospective randomized controlled trial (PRCT) compared the efficacy of empiric antibiotic therapy (ceftazidime plus amikacin) with and without vancomycin in 747 patients with neutropenic fever. Neutropenia was defined as ANC <1000 cells/μl. Therapy was classified as a "success" if the fever and the other clinical signs of infection resolved and if the infecting organism was eradicated without modification of the initial regimen. Therapy was classified as a "failure" if the patient died, if the antibiotic regimen required change, if fever and clinical signs did not resolve, or if the infecting organism could not be eradicated (23).

(1) Vancomycin significantly increased the overall success rate from 63% to 76%. On closer inspection, however, although more patients failed without vancomycin, there were no important differences in the mortality rate, the duration of fever, or any other adverse clinical outcome.

Table 27-4 Combination vs. monotherapy in neutropenic fever (58)

	Combination Therapy (N=204)	Monotherapy (N=190)	*P*
Success without modification	78%	77%	NS
Success with modification	20%	21%	NS
Failure	2%	2%	NS
Overall success rate	98%	98%	NS

Table 27-5 Combination vs. monotherapy in documented infections (58)

	Combination Therapy (N=64)	Monotherapy (N=92)	*P*
Success without modification	31%	30%	NS
Success with modification	60%	59%	NS
Failure	9%	11%	NS
Overall success rate	91%	89%	NS

Vancomycin-treated patients did require fewer modifications of the initial antibiotic regimen, which accounted for most of the difference in the success rate between the two groups (see Table 27–6).

(2) In fact, the mortality from bacteremia caused by gram-positive bacteria was only 2%, and no patient died during the first 3 days of empiric therapy. Therefore, survival was not adversely affected by limiting the initial empiric use of vancomycin for patients with a documented infection caused by gram-positive bacteria. In addition, vancomycin was associated with an increased risk of renal dysfunction ($P<0.02$). Finally, concerns about the emergence of resistant organisms have led most authors to argue against the routine empiric use of vancomycin (23,37,60,64). However, if there is a significant likelihood of infection with methicillin-resistant *Staphylococcus aureus* (*i.e.*, in a hospital with high infection rates with this organism or in patients with potential infection related to indwelling central venous catheters), vancomycin should be included in the initial empiric regimen.

d. Hematopoietic Growth Factors—In an effort to reduce the duration and the nadir of granulocytopenia in patients who present with fever and neutropenia, the benefit of adding granulocyte colony-stimulating factor (G-CSF) or granulocyte-macrophage colony-stimulating factor (GM-CSF) to empiric broad-spectrum antibiotics has been recently evaluated (31,69).

(1) G-CSF (Filgrastim)—In a double-blind PRCT, 218 patients with fever and neutropenia (ANC <1000 cells/μl) were randomly assigned to receive either G-CSF (12 μg/kg SC per day) or placebo within 12 hours of starting piperacillin and tobramycin (42). Patients with leukemia and those treated with bone marrow transplantation were excluded from the study. Compared with placebo, G-CSF shortened the duration of neutropenia and hastened the rate of recovery from the febrile neutropenic episode (each by 1 day). However, there was no difference in the overall duration of fever, the overall length of hospitalization, or the frequency of the need to change the initial antibiotic regimen. Therefore, it is unclear whether shortening the duration of neutropenia by 1 day had clinically important benefits (42). In subgroup analysis, G-CSF was most beneficial for patients whose ANC was <100 cells/μl, and some experts recommend limiting the use of G-CSF to this population (69) (see Table 27–7).

Table 27-6 Empiric therapy with & without vancomycin in neutropenic fever (23)

	Ceftazidime + Amikacin (N=370)	Ceftazidime + Amikacin + Vancomycin (N=377)	*P*
Overall success rate	63%	76%	<0.001
Nephrotoxicity	2%	6%	0.02

Table 27-7 G-CSF vs. placebo for adjunctive therapy in neutropenic fever (42)

	G-CSF (N=109)	Placebo (N=107)	*P*
Median duration of neutropenia (ANC <500 cells/μl)	3.0 d	4.0 d	0.005
Time to resolution of febrile neutropenia	5.0 d	6.0 d	0.01
Median duration of fever	3.0 d	3.0 d	NS
Median length of hospitalization	8.0 d	8.0 d	NS
Need to change initial antibiotic regimen	46%	41%	NS

(2) GM-CSF—In a smaller double-blind PRCT involving children with 58 episodes of neutropenic fever (mean ANC, 32 cells/μl), the addition of GM-CSF (5 μg/kg IV over 4 hours daily) to imipenem-cilastatin shortened the duration of neutropenia (ANC <500 cells/μl) from 6.0 to 4.5 days ($P<0.05$) (31). Patients with myeloid leukemia and those treated with bone marrow transplantation were excluded from the study. In contrast to the G-CSF study described previously (42), GM-CSF also shortened the median length of hospitalization from 10.0 to 9.0 days ($P<0.05$). Adverse effects observed with GM-CSF included rash or urticaria (21%), musculoskeletal pain (14%), and new fever (18%).

3. Subsequent Management—After the first few days, patients can be divided into two categories: those with an identified infection and those with fever of unknown source.

a. Treatment of Documented Infections

(1) Once an infection has been documented, antibiotics should be adjusted to optimally treat the identified pathogen. If a gram-negative bacillus is isolated from the blood stream, many authors recommend double coverage, with an aminoglycoside and a β-lactam (60). However, even if an organism has been isolated, the antibiotic coverage should not be narrowed, because the neutropenic patient is still at risk for other infections. For example, in a retrospective review of 39 patients with prolonged neutropenia and documented infection by gram-positive organisms, none who were maintained on broad-spectrum coverage developed a second infection, whereas a gram-negative rod infection developed in 47% of those whose antibiotic coverage was narrowed to a single drug (53). In another study that used ceftazidime monotherapy, 5% of patients had breakthrough or recurrent bacteremia caused primarily by gram-positive cocci (*Staphylococcus epidermidis* and group D streptococci) and resistant gram-negative bacilli (58).

(2) The ideal length of treatment for a documented infection depends on whether the patient remains neutropenic. If the ANC rises to >500 cells/μl and the patient becomes afebrile with no further evidence of infection, a total of 7 to 10 days of parenteral antibiotics is usually sufficient. For the patient with a documented infection who remains neutropenic, the optimum course of antimicrobial therapy is not known. If the infection resolves and the patient remains afebrile with no signs of mucositis or ulceration at 2 weeks, some authors favor discontinuation of antibiotics with close observation. If the patient remains febrile, antibiotics should be continued until the ANC returns to >500 cells/μl and the patient becomes clinically well. A vigorous search for the possibility of a second infection should also be initiated as well (34,57).

b. Treatment of Fever of Unknown Source

(1) Pizzo described a prospective study of 142 patients with neutropenic fever of unknown source. The patient age varied from 1 to 33 years. Neutropenia was defined as an ANC <500 cells/μl or an initial ANC between 500 and 1000 cells/μl falling to <500 cells/μl within 48 hours. A thorough history, physical examination, and laboratory evaluation failed to reveal a clear source of infection by day 7 of the study. All patients were febrile despite 7 days of treatment with cephalothin plus gentamicin plus carbenicillin. Pizzo was able to divide these patients into low-risk and high-risk groups (52).

(a) Low-Risk Group—Among the 142 patients with neutropenic fever of unknown source, 86 were no longer neutropenic by day 7. Five of these 86 patients were still febrile. After antibiotics were discontinued in these 86 patients, there were no further infectious complications. Therefore, for patients with neutropenic fever of unknown source who recover from neutropenia, antibiotics can safely be discontinued, but subsequent clinical reevaluation is important.

(b) **High-Risk Group**—Among the 142 patients with neutropenic fever of unknown source, 56 were still neutropenic on day 7; 23 of these were still febrile and were not discussed further in the study. The remaining 33 patients, who were afebrile, were randomly assigned to either continuation of antibiotics or discontinuation with observation. The group receiving continued antibiotic therapy had significantly fewer episodes of fever and infectious complications than the group assigned to discontinuation ($P=0.024$). Only one patient in the antibiotic group developed fever, but antibiotics had been discontinued in that patient because of side effects (see Table 27–8).

(2) For patients who remain afebrile but neutropenic after 14 days of treatment, some authors recommend stopping the antibiotics if the patient appears otherwise well, can be closely monitored, and has a controlled tumor. However, there are few data to support this practice (34,59).

4. Treatment of Patients With Persistent Fever

a. If a patient remains neutropenic and febrile despite broad-spectrum antibiotics, a vigorous search for a source of infection should be repeated, including a chest film, *Clostridium difficile* test, and cultures of the urine, sputum, and blood. Fungal isolator blood cultures, abdominal computed tomography scan, abdominal ultrasonography, and assays for uncommon organisms such as *Legionella*, cytomegalovirus (CMV), or cryptococci may also be helpful.

b. Antibiotics should be modified as the clinical situation dictates, but they should not be discontinued, because >50% of patients with persistent neutropenic fever (>7 days) develop infectious complications within 3 days of discontinuation of antibiotics (54). If vancomycin was not part of the original regimen, it may be added then, particularly for patients with central venous catheters. Further, if an antipseudomonal penicillin was part of the initial regimen, consideration may be given to switching to ceftazidime.

c. **Empiric Antifungal Therapy**

(1) In patients with prolonged neutropenia, fungal superinfection becomes a frequent complication. Fungal infections in this population must be treated promptly. For example, in a retrospective review of 155 cases of catheter-associated fungemia at the National Cancer Institute, a delay in treatment was associated with a mortality rate of 69%, compared with 38% in patients who were treated promptly (40).

(2) Pizzo described a study of 50 patients with persistent neutropenic fever despite 7 days of empiric broad-spectrum antibiotic therapy (cephalothin, carbenicillin, and gentamicin) (54). The source of the fever was unknown in all cases. Patients were randomly assigned after day 7 to one of three arms: discontinuation of antibiotics (group 1), continuation of antibiotics (group 2), or continuation of antibiotics with addition of amphotericin B (group 3) (see Table 27–9).

(a) Group 1 did poorly; more than half of these patients developed infectious complications, and 38% developed septic shock.

(b) Group 2 had a lower risk of bacterial infection and septic shock, but the risk of fungal infection was substantial at 31%.

(c) Group 3 had the lowest risk of infectious complications. No pa-

Table 27-8 Continuing vs. discontinuing therapy in afebrile neutropenics (52)

	Continued Antibiotics (N=16)	Discontinued Antibiotics (N=17)	P
Fever or infectious complications	6.3%	41%	0.024

Table 27-9 Comparison of 3 strategies in persistent neutropenic fever (54)

	Antibiotics Discontinued (Group 1) (N=16)	Antibiotics Continued (Group 2) (N=16)	Amphotericin Added (Group 3) (N=18)	*P* Group 1 vs. 2	*P* Group 2 vs. 3	*P* Group 1 vs. 3
All infections	56%	38%	11%	?	NS	0.013
Fungal infections	6%	31%	6%	?	?	?
Bacterial infections	19%	6%	0%	?	?	?
Septic shock	38%	0%	0%	<0.02	NS	<0.02
Time to Defervescence	11 d	8 d	6 d	?	?	?
Overall mortality	31%	31%	17%	NS	NS	NS

tient in this group developed septic shock. Furthermore, there was a trend toward improved survival with amphotericin but the difference was not statistically significant.

(3) In a similar randomized study of 132 patients with persistent neutropenic fever despite 4 days of empiric broad-spectrum antibiotic therapy, amphotericin decreased the overall rate of fungal infections from 9.4% to 1.5% (P=0.10). The study was too small to demonstrate a survival benefit (21).

(4) Although other antifungal drugs are available, amphotericin is still the gold standard. One milligram of amphotericin should be administered as a test dose. If the drug is tolerated, 0.5 to 0.6 mg/kg/day is the usual dose. Some authors recommend premedication with antihistamines, meperidine, and acetaminophen (Tylenol) to decrease the risk of drug-induced fever and rigors. Corticosteroids are also used for this purpose. Prehydration with 1 L of normal saline is also recommended to decrease the risk of nephrotoxicity (73). The optimal length of empiric amphotericin therapy is not known. If the physical examination, chest film, abdominal computed tomography scan, and cultures are all unrevealing, some authors recommend that amphotericin be discontinued.

d. Empiric Antiviral Therapy—Currently, there are no data to support the use of empiric antiviral therapy in neutropenic febrile patients. However, documented viral infections should be treated aggressively (herpes simplex virus and varicella-zoster virus with acyclovir; CMV with ganciclovir), and all suspicious mucosal lesions should be cultured for herpes simplex virus.

C. Prophylactic Treatments—Because most episodes of neutropenia are iatrogenic and therefore predictable, there has been much interest in use of prophylactic antibiotics to decrease the incidence of bacteremia. Similarly, hematopoietic growth factors (CSFs) have been studied as a means to shorten the duration of neutropenia. These are areas of active clinical research and ongoing controversy.

1. Isolation of Neutropenic Patients—In Nauseef's randomized study involving 43 neutropenic patients, food sterilization and patient isolation did not decrease the incidence of fever or infection (48). Therefore, there is no role for hospitalization of an afebrile neutropenic patient for the purpose of isolation. However, strict hand washing and standard neutropenic precautions should be used in the care of these patients. In contrast, isolation rooms with filtered air supplies are recommended for patients undergoing bone marrow transplantation (BMT). BMT patients are at much higher risk for aspergillosis and other infections than standard chemotherapy patients.

2. Prophylactic Antibiotic Therapy—Over the years, numerous antibiotics have been tested for prevention of infection in afebrile neutropenic patients. Initially, most of the studies used orally nonabsorbable antibiotics such as gentamicin, vancomycin, nystatin, and polymyxin for decontamination of the gastrointestinal tract (31). However, because of poor patient tolerance and high cost, these agents have been replaced by trimethoprim-sulfamethoxazole (TMP-SMX) or a fluoroquinolone (80,82). The latter drugs may also be preferred over the nonabsorbable agents because they preserve the endogenous anaerobic gastrointestinal flora, which may be important for colonization resistance against pathogenic organisms. Although TMP-SMX was effective in decreasing the risk of infection in this group, concerns regarding antibiotic resistance, fungal superinfection, and potential myelotoxicity have tempered the enthusiasm for this drug (16, 29,31,43,56,76,78,84). More recently, fluoroquinolones have been shown to be more effective than placebo (9,30,38) or orally nonabsorbable antibiotics (80,82). In addition, they appear to be at least as effective and better tolerated than TMP-SMX (6,14,17,41). In general, these studies targeted patients who were expected to develop severe and prolonged neutropenia (*i.e.*, those receiving induction chemotherapy for acute leukemia or undergoing BMT). The representative studies that investigated the value of fluoroquinolone prophylaxis are described here.

a. Quinolones Versus Placebo—Several studies demonstrated that antibiotic prophylaxis with fluoroquinolones may decrease the risk of infection among afebrile neutropenic patients (9,30,38). For example, Karp compared norfloxacin versus placebo in a PRCT of 68 adult leukemic patients with prolonged neutropenia resulting from chemotherapy. All patients had received intensive chemotherapy that produced severe neutropenia (ANC <100 cells/μl). The average duration of neutropenia was 32 days (38) (see Table 27–10).

(1) All patients eventually became febrile, but the average time to first infectious fever was significantly delayed with norfloxacin ($P<0.005$). The percentage of time spent febrile was also decreased with norfloxacin prophylaxis ($P<0.015$).

(2) The risk of gram-negative bacillary infection was significantly reduced by norfloxacin ($P<0.02$), but there were no differences in the rates of infections caused by gram-positive organisms or fungi. Emergence of drug-resistant organisms was not observed during the study period. Nevertheless, there was no significant difference in survival.

b. Quinolones Versus Trimethoprim-Sulfamethoxazole—Several studies have demonstrated that fluoroquinolones are at least as effective and better tolerated than TMP-SMX (6,14,17,41). For example, in a PRCT involving 56 leukemic patients undergoing induction chemotherapy, Dekker randomly compared ciprofloxacin (500 mg PO BID) versus TMP-SMX (160 mg of TMP and 800 mg of SMX q 8 hours) plus colistin (200 mg q 8 hours) for prophylaxis against bacterial infections (begun 1 to 2 days before initiation of cytotoxic chemotherapy). Both groups were treated with oral amphotericin B (17) (see Table 27–11).

(1) The risk of acquiring a bacteriologically documented infection was significantly lower with ciprofloxacin (5 versus 14 episodes; $P<0.05$). In particular, the risk of acquiring an infection caused by gram-negative bacteria was significantly lower with ciprofloxacin (0 versus 7 episodes; $P<0.02$). However, the overall risk of any infection and the risk of acquiring an infection caused by a gram-positive organism were both similar between the two groups.

(2) Based on the results of periodic microbiologic surveillance cultures (obtained from the oropharynx, feces, and urine), gram-negative organisms resistant to the respective drug were commonly isolated from both groups of patients, but this was less likely with ciprofloxacin than with TMP-SMX (8 versus 15 cultures).

(3) Ciprofloxacin was also associated with better compliance with the drug regimen (82% versus 54% of patients, respectively, took 95% or more of the assigned drug; $P<0.05$) as well as a lower risk of gastrointestinal or allergic side effects.

(4) On the other hand, TMP-SMX provided highly effective prophylaxis against *Pneumocystis carinii*, a feature not found with quinolones (32,33). Although generally not of great importance for patients undergoing standard chemotherapy for solid organ tumors, this advantage should be considered in patients with acute leukemias and those undergoing allogeneic BMT (see section *Pneumocystis carinii* prophylaxis).

Table 27-10 Norfloxacin vs. placebo for prophylactic therapy (38)

	Norfloxacin (N=35)	Placebo (N=33)	*P*
Time to onset of first infectious fever	6.3 days	3.7 days	<0.005
Time spent febrile	28%	40%	<0.015
Risk of gram-negative infection	11%	39%	<0.02
Risk of gram-positive infection	46%	39%	NS
Risk of fungal infection	29%	24%	NS
Mortality rate	23%	15%	NS

Table 27-11 Ciprofloxacin vs. TMP/SMX for prophylactic therapy (17)

	Ciprofloxacin (N=28)	Trimethoprim-Sulfamethoxazole (N=28)	*P*
Days with febrile neutropenia	21	17	NS
Overall number of infections	22	25	NS
Number of microbiologically documented infections	5	14	<0.05
Number of aerobic gram-positive infections	4	7	NS
Number of aerobic gram-negative infections	0	7	<0.02

c. **Quinolone Plus Penicillin Versus Quinolone Alone**—It should also be recalled that gram-positive organisms (including viridans streptococci) are now responsible for an increasing proportion of infections among febrile neutropenic patients (2,3,8,10,11,19,39,44,58,60,63,75). Although fluoroquinolones have good activity against gram-negative organisms, they have relatively poor activity against gram-positive organisms (6,17,26,80,82). Ciprofloxacin and ofloxacin are thought to have better gram-positive activity than norfloxacin. However, in general, none of the fluoroquinolones has provided reliable protection against gram-positive infections in the neutropenic population (6,17,26,80,82). Therefore, a recent EORTC study compared penicillin V (500 mg PO BID) plus pefloxacin (400 mg PO BID, a quinolone) versus placebo plus pefloxacin (400 mg PO BID) in a double-blind PRCT involving 536 afebrile neutropenic patients (35). The study drugs were begun immediately after initiation of cytotoxic chemotherapy, and almost all of the patients in the study had leukemia or had undergone BMT (see Table 27–12).
   (1) Fewer patients receiving the combination therapy became febrile or acquired an infection (71% versus 80%; P=0.03). The risk of bacteremia was also significantly reduced with the combination therapy (14% versus 22%; P=0.03).
   (2) Both regimens protected against gram-negative infections successfully. There was a statistically nonsignificant trend toward lower risk of acquiring a gram-positive infection with the combination therapy (13% versus 18%; P=NS). However, the risk of developing streptococcal bacteremia was reduced by 50% with the combination therapy (5% versus 10%: P=0.05).

d. Despite the apparent efficacy of prophylactic antibiotics, there is concern that widespread use of these agents will simply select out resistant organisms. For example, the prevalence of fluoroquinolone resistance among *Escherichia coli* increased from 0% to 28% during the period 1990 to 1993 in centers where the use of these agents increased from 1.4% to 45% (12). More data are needed in this area, because the modest success gained with prophylaxis may be offset by the steep penalty of widespread resistance and superinfection after routine use (47). Furthermore, an overall mortality benefit has yet to be demonstrated with antimicrobial prophylaxis in this population. If prophylactic antibiotics are to be used, they probably should be limited to patients who become profoundly neutropenic for >7 days, such as those with acute leukemias and those undergoing BMT. Current options include TMP-SMX, a fluoroquinolone such as ciprofloxacin or ofloxacin, or a combination of penicillin plus a fluoroquinolone.

3. **Prophylactic Antifungal Therapy**
   a. Prophylactic treatment of BMT patients with fluconazole (400 mg/day) has

Table 27-12 Pefloxacin with and without penicillin for prophylaxis (35)

	Penicillin and Pefloxacin (N=268)	Placebo and Pefloxacin (N=268)	*P*
Mean duration of neutropenia	22 days	21 days	NS
% with episodes of fever or infection	71	80	0.03
% with bacteremia	14	22	0.03
% with bacteremia due to a gram-positive organism	13	18	NS
% with bacteremia due to a gram-negative organism	1	2	NS
% with streptococcal bacteremia	5	10	0.05

been shown in a large double-blind PRCT to decrease the number of fungal infections as well as the mortality from fungemia. However, as with antibiotic prophylaxis, there was no difference in overall survival (27). Similar results have been reported with fluconazole in a double-blind PRCT of leukemic patients undergoing chemotherapy (79).

b. In a recent PRCT involving 820 acute leukemic patients with neutropenia, fluconazole (150 mg once daily PO) was shown to be as efficacious as amphotericin B (500 mg q 6 hours PO) for fungal prophylaxis. Of the patients assigned to fluconazole, 2.6% developed a definite systemic fungal infection and 16% developed a suspected fungal infection requiring empiric antifungal therapy, compared with 2.5% and 21%, respectively, among the patients assigned to amphotericin (*P*=NS in both cases). Side effects were observed in only 1.4% of patients assigned to fluconazole, compared with 7% of those assigned to amphotericin (*P*<0.01). Therefore, fluconazole appears to be better tolerated than and at least as effective as amphotericin suspension for fungal prophylaxis in neutropenic patients (45).

c. As with antibiotic prophylaxis, concern about the emergence of resistant organisms has limited widespread use of antifungal prophylaxis. In a retrospective study of 296 consecutive BMT patients, Wingard found that fluconazole prophylaxis decreased the incidence of fungal infections but increased the number of infections with fluconazole-resistant candidal species such as *Candida kruseii* and *Torulopsis glabrata*. More than 40% of patients receiving fluconazole became colonized with resistant candidal species (79). As with prophylactic antibacterial agents, if prophylactic antifungal drugs are to be used, they should probably be limited to high-risk patients such as those with acute leukemias and those undergoing BMT. Further studies are needed to clarify this controversial issue.

4. Antiviral prophylaxis—In general, antiviral prophylaxis has been limited to BMT patients and those receiving intensive chemotherapy.

a. Several studies demonstrated that ganciclovir can decrease the risk of CMV infection in BMT patients. However, the enthusiasm for ganciclovir prophylaxis has been tempered by the risk of neutropenia (28,70,83). The study by Goodrich is described as an example (28). In a double-blind PRCT, 64 CMV-seropositive allogeneic BMT patients were randomly assigned to receive either ganciclovir (5 mg/kg IV BID for 5 days, then 5 mg/kg QD until day 100) or placebo. Ganciclovir significantly decreased the risk of CMV infection (*P*=0.015) but increased the risk of neutropenia. There was no difference in survival (see Table 27–13).

Table 27-13 Ganciclovir vs. placebo for prophylaxis in BMT (28)

	Placebo (N=31)	Ganciclovir (N=33)	*P*
Risk of CMV disease by day 180	31%	9%	0.015
Risk of neutropenia	0%	30%	0.001
Risk of death	26%	30%	NS

b. Anti-CMV immunoglobulin G (IgG) has also been shown to decrease the risk of CMV infection in patients undergoing BMT or solid organ transplantation. Winston compared anti-CMV IgG versus control in a PRCT of 75 CMV-seropositive BMT patients (81). High-dose IV anti-CMV IgG decreased the risk of clinically significant CMV disease from 46% in the control group to 21% in the treated group (P=0.03). There were fewer CMV-related deaths with anti-CMV IgG, but this trend was not statistically significant. Anti-CMV IgG also decreased the risk of graft-versus-host disease (GVHD). Because of the risk of neutropenia, prophylactic ganciclovir is not commonly used. On the other hand, anti-CMV IgG is given routinely to CMV-seropositive patients undergoing BMT (51).

c. Intravenous acyclovir has been shown in small double-blind PRCTs to decrease the incidence of local herpes reactivations in patients undergoing BMT and intensive chemotherapy for leukemia (66,67).

5. *Pneumocystis carinii* Prophylaxis—In a subgroup of neutropenic patients (*i.e.*, children with leukemia, patients undergoing allogeneic BMT, and other patients receiving immunosuppression for organ transplantation), prophylaxis with TMP-SMX clearly decreases the risk of pneumonia caused by *P carinii*. Three-times-per-week dosing is equivalent to daily dosing in this population (32,33). Prophylaxis is usually not necessary for patients undergoing standard chemotherapy for solid tumors.

6. Use of Colony-Stimulating Factors—Since their introduction in the late 1980s, G-CSF and GM-CSF have been shown to decrease morbidity in patients undergoing intensive chemotherapy or BMT.

a. G-CSF (Filgrastim)

(1) Prophylactic Use for Standard-Dose Chemotherapy—In a double-blind PRCT, the prophylactic use of G-CSF (230 μg/m² SC for days 4 to 17 after each cycle for chemotherapy) for small cell lung cancer significantly reduced the duration of neutropenia, the risk of neutropenic fever, the length of hospital stay, and the overall rate of infection. The use of G-CSF over multiple cycles of chemotherapy reduced the number of hospital days by 50%. However, there was no difference in short- or long-term survival (13) (see Table 27–14).

(2) Bone Marrow Transplantation—Small, uncontrolled studies showed that G-CSF shortened the duration of neutropenia compared with historical controls in patients undergoing autologous BMT for solid tumors and Hodgkin's disease. There are no well-designed, controlled studies of G-CSF in BMT patients (71,74).

Table 27-14 G-CSF vs. placebo for prophylaxis in standard-dose chemotherapy (13)

	Placebo (N=104)	G-CSF (N=95)	*P*
Median no. of days with ANC <500	6.0	3.0	<0.001
Risk of neutropenic fever for cycle 1	57%	28%	<0.001
Median no. of days with neutropenic fever	5.0	4.0	NS
Risk of culture-confirmed infection	13.3%	6.5%	?

b. GM-CSF

(1) Standard-Dose Chemotherapy—There is one relatively large (137 evaluable patients) double-blind PRCT of GM-CSF versus placebo as adjunctive treatment in high grade non-Hodgkin's lymphoma. As with G-CSF, GM-CSF significantly decreased the duration of fever (2.1 versus 4.0 days), infection (28 versus 69 days), and hospital stay (3.5 versus 8.0 days). However, survival was not improved (25).

(2) Bone Marrow Transplantation

(a) Autologous BMT—Data from a double-blind PRCT showed that the use of GM-CSF in autologous BMT can shorten the duration of neutropenia after engraftment by 7 days (19 versus 26 days; $P<0.001$). These patients also required fewer days of antibiotics (24 versus 27 days) and had shorter hospital stays (27 versus 33 days; $P=0.01$) (49). Subsequent studies have since confirmed these findings. The optimal dose of GM-CSF in these patients has not been determined (1). Thus far, GM-CSF does not appear to increase the risk of tumor recurrence (62).

(b) Allogeneic BMT—The use of CSFs in allogeneic BMT has been approached with caution because of fears of exacerbating GVHD. In one small, double-blind PRCT, GM-CSF was used in allogeneic BMT patients. There was a small, nonsignificant decrease in the duration of neutropenia (16 days with placebo versus 13 days with GM-CSF) and no difference in the duration of hospitalization, the risk of infection, or the rate of survival. The risk of GVHD or graft rejection was not increased (61). In a second, slightly larger study of GM-CSF in allogeneic BMT patients, GM-CSF decreased the duration of neutropenia (ANC <500) from 15.6 to 13.2 days ($P<.05$). Furthermore, fewer cases of pneumonia were observed with GM-CSF. Again, the risk of GVHD or graft rejection was not increased (18).

D. Summary

1. The risk of infection is inversely related to the ANC and positively correlated with the duration of neutropenia. About half of the episodes of neutropenic fever are unexplained despite a vigorous search for an organism. Among the identifiable causes, both gram-positive and gram-negative organisms are common. The clinical manifestations of infection are often subtle in neutropenic patients.
2. Prompt initiation of empiric broad-spectrum antibiotics for any neutropenic patient with fever is the cornerstone of therapy. There are few data to suggest that one antibiotic regimen is clearly superior to another. However, cognizance should be taken of the patterns of antimicrobial resistance at a given institution in selecting appropriate antibiotics. The typical doses of the currently recommended drugs are listed in Table 27-15. The dosage should be modified depending on the patient's renal and hepatic condition. The currently recommended empiric regimens are (a) an aminoglycoside plus an antipseudomonal β-lactam; (b) an antipseudomonal penicillin plus an antipseudomonal cephalosporin; (c) monotherapy with ceftazidime, cefoperazone, or imipenem-cilastatin; and (d) an antipseudomonal β-lactam plus an aminoglycoside plus vancomycin.
3. For patients with an identified pathogen, the antibiotic regimen should adjusted to optimally treat the infection but the coverage should not be narrowed. In general, broad-spectrum antibiotics should be continued until the ANC rises to >500 cells/μl. For patients with fever of unknown origin, the antibiotics may be discontinued if the patient is no longer neutropenic; otherwise, antibiotics should be continued until the ANC rises to >500 cells/μl.
4. For patients with persistent neutropenic fever, antibiotics should be modified as needed, but they should not be discontinued. Vancomycin can be added if it was not part of the initial regimen. If an antipseudomonal penicillin was used initially, it can be changed to ceftazidime. Empiric antifungal therapy is recommended for patients with persistent neutropenic fever despite 4 to 7 days of broad-spectrum antibiotic therapy.
5. The role of prophylactic antibiotics or antifungals is controversial at this time.

These agents decrease the number of febrile events and infections but at the possible cost of resistant organisms in the future. Furthermore, they have not been shown to lower mortality. Prophylactic antimicrobial therapy should probably be limited to patients who are expected to become profoundly neutropenic for >7 days (*i.e.*, those with acute leukemias and those undergoing BMT). CSFs consistently shorten the duration of neutropenia, the risk of infection, and the duration of hospitalization. However, they have not been shown to improve survival.

6. Many issues still remain to be answered. Will the use of monotherapy for empiric treatment of neutropenic fever cause emergence of resistant organisms? Will the widespread use of prophylactic antibiotics and antifungals cause emergence of resistant organisms and limit their eventual effectiveness? What are the optimal doses of G-CSF and GM-CSF? Are they cost-effective? Which works better? Are there febrile neutropenic patients who could be treated with oral antibiotics as outpatients?

Table 27-15 Commonly used empiric antibiotics in neutropenic fever

	Usual IV Doses
Aminoglycosides	
Gentamicin	1.0–1.5 mg/kg q 8 h
Tobramycin	1.0–1.5 mg/kg q 8 h
Amikacin	5 mg/kg q 8 h
Antipseudomonal penicillins	
Ticarcillin	3 g q 3–6 h
Azlocillin	2–3 g q 4–6 h
Mezlocillin	3 g q 4 h
Piperacillin	3–4 g q 4–6 h
Antipseudomonal cephalosporins	
Cefoperazone	2–3 g q 6–8 h
Ceftazidime	1–2 g q 8–12 h
Antistaphylococcal agent	
Vancomycin	500 mg q 6 h or 1 g q 12 h

Abbreviations used in Chapter 27

ANC = absolute neutrophil count
BID = twice daily
BMT = bone marrow transplantation
CMV = cytomegalovirus
EORTC = European Organization for Research and Treatment of Cancer
G-CSF = granulocyte colony-stimulating factor
GM-CSF = granulocyte-macrophage colony-stimulating factor
GVHD = graft-versus-host disease
HIV = human immunodeficiency virus
IgG = immunoglobulin G
IV = intravenous
N = number of patients
NS = not statistically significant
P = probability value
PO = per os
PRCT = prospective randomized controlled trial
q = every

SC = subcutaneous
TMP-SMX = trimethoprim-sulfamethoxazole
vs. = versus

References

1. Applebaum. The use of colony stimulating factors in marrow transplantation. *Cancer* 1993;72:3387.
2. Bochud. Bacteremia due to viridans streptococci in neutropenic patients: a review. *Am J Med* 1994;97:256.
3. Bochud. Bacteremia due to viridans streptococcus in neutropenic patients with cancer: clinical spectrum and risk factors. *Clin Infect Dis* 1994;18:25.
4. Bodey. Quantitative relationship between circulating leukocytes and infection in patients with acute leukemia. *Ann Intern Med* 1966;64:328.
5. Bodey. Fever and infection in leukemic patients: a study of 494 consecutive patients. *Cancer* 1978;41:1610.
6. Bow. Comparison of norfloxacin with cotrimoxazole for infection prophylaxis in acute leukemia: the trade-off for reduced gram-negative sepsis. *Am J Med* 1988; 84:847.
7. Bryant. Factors affecting mortality of gram-negative bacteremia. *Arch Intern Med* 1971;127:120.
8. Burden. Viridans streptococcal bacteremia in patients with hematological and solid malignancy. *Eur J Cancer* 1991;27:409.
9. Cassali. Chemoprophylaxis of bacterial infections in granulocytopenic cancer patients using norfloxacin. *Chemioterapia* 1988;7:327.
10. Classen. *Streptococcus mitis* sepsis in bone marrow transplant patients receiving oral antimicrobial prophylaxis. *Am J Med* 1990;89:441.
11. Cohen. Septicemia caused by viridans streptococci in neutropenic patients with leukemia. *Lancet* 1983;2:1452.
12. Cometta. *Escherichia coli* resistant to fluoroquinolones in patients with cancer and neutropenia. *N Engl J Med* 1994;330:1179.
13. Crawford. Reduction by granulocyte colony-stimulating factor of fever and neutropenia induced by chemotherapy in patients with small-cell lung cancer. *N Engl J Med* 1991;325:164.
14. Cruciani. Prophylactic cotrimoxazole versus norfloxacin in neutropenic children: prospective randomized study. *Infection* 1989;17:65.
15. De Pauw. Ceftazidime compared with piperacillin and tobramycin for the empiric treatment of fever in neutropenic patients with cancer. *Ann Intern Med* 1994;120:834.
16. Dekker. Prevention of infection by trimethoprim-sulfamethoxazole plus amphotericin B in patients with acute nonlymphocytic leukemia. *Ann Intern Med* 1981; 95:555.
17. Dekker. Infection prophylaxis in acute leukemia: a comparison of ciprofloxacin with trimethoprim-sulfamethoxazole and colistin. *Ann Intern Med* 1987;106:7.
18. DeWitte. Recombinant human granulocyte-macrophage colony-stimulating factor accelerates neutrophil and monocyte recovery after allogeneic T-cell depleted bone marrow transplantation. *Blood* 1992;79:1359.
19. Elting. Septicemia and shock syndrome due to viridans streptococci: a case-control study of predisposing factors. *Clin Infect Dis* 1992;14:1201.
20. EORTC International Antimicrobial Therapy Cooperative Group. Ceftazidime combined with a short or long course of amikacin for empirical therapy of gram-negative bacteremia in cancer patients with granulocytopenia. *N Engl J Med* 1987; 317:1692.
21. EORTC International Antimicrobial Therapy Cooperative Group. Empiric antifungal therapy in febrile granulocytopenic patients. *Am J Med* 1989;86:668.
22. EORTC International Antimicrobial Therapy Cooperative Group. Single daily dosing of amikacin and ceftriaxone is as efficacious and no more toxic than multiple daily dosing of amikacin and ceftazidime. *Ann Intern Med* 1993;119:584.

23. EORTC International Antimicrobial Therapy Cooperative Group and the National Cancer Institute of Canada–Clinical Trials Group. Vancomycin added to empirical combination antibiotic therapy for fever in granulocytopenic cancer patients. *J Infect Dis* 1991;163:951.
24. EORTC International Antimicrobial Therapy Project Group. Three antibiotic regimens in the treatment of infection in febrile granulocytopenic patients with cancer. *J Infect Dis* 1978;137:14.
25. Gerhartz. Randomized double-blind placebo-controlled phase III study of recombinant human granulocyte-macrophage colony stimulating factor as adjunct to induction treatment of high-grade non-Hodgkin's lymphomas. *Blood* 1994;82:2329.
26. GIMEMA Infection Program. Prevention of bacterial infection in neutropenic patients with hematologic malignancies: a randomized, multicenter trial comparing norfloxacin with ciprofloxacin. *Ann Intern Med* 1991;115:7.
27. Goodman. A controlled trial of fluconazole to prevent fungal infections in patients undergoing bone marrow transplantation. *N Engl J Med* 1992;326:845.
28. Goodrich. Ganciclovir prophylaxis to prevent cytomegalovirus disease after allogeneic marrow transplantation. *Ann Intern Med* 1993;118:173.
29. Gualtier. Double-blind randomized study of prophylactic trimethoprim-sulfamethoxazole in granulocytopenic patients with hematologic malignancies. *Am J Med* 1983; 74:934.
30. Hartlapp. Antimicrobial prophylaxis in immunocompromised patients. *Drugs* 1987; 34(Suppl 1):131.
31. Henry. Symposium on infectious complications of neoplastic disease: Part II. Chemoprophylaxis of bacterial infections in granulocytopenic patients. *Am J Med* 1984;76:645.
32. Hughes. Successful chemoprophylaxis for *Pneumocystis carinii* pneumonitis. *N Engl J Med* 1977;297:1419.
33. Hughes. Successful intermittent chemoprophylaxis for *Pneumocystis carinii* pneumonitis. *N Engl J Med* 1987;316:1627.
34. Hughes. Guidelines for the use of antimicrobial agents in neutropenic patients with unexplained fever. *J Infect Dis* 1990;161:381.
35. International Antimicrobial Therapy Cooperative Group of the European Organization for Research and Treatment of Cancer. Reduction of fever and streptococcal bacteremia in granulocytopenic patients with cancer. *JAMA* 1994;272:1183.
36. Jones. Aztreonam therapy in neutropenic patients with cancer. *Am J Med* 1986; 81:243.
37. Karp. Empiric use of vancomycin during prolonged treatment-induced granulocytopenia. *Am J Med* 1986;81:237.
38. Karp. Oral norfloxacin for prevention of gram-negative bacterial infections in patients with acute leukemia and granulocytopenia. *Ann Intern Med* 1987;106:1.
39. Kern. Streptococcal bacteremia in adult patients with leukemia undergoing aggressive chemotherapy: a review of 55 cases. *Infection* 1990;18:138.
40. Lecciones. Catheter associated fungemia in cancer patients: characteristics and clinical outcome. Program and abstracts of the 29th Interscience Conference on Antimicrobial Agents and Chemotherapy, 1991:112.
41. Liang. Ofloxacin versus cotrimoxazole for prevention of infection in neutropenic patients following cytotoxic chemotherapy. *Antimicrob Agents Chemother* 1990; 34:215.
42. Maher. Filgrastim in patients with chemotherapy-induced febrile neutropenia: a double-blind, placebo-controlled trial. *Ann Intern Med* 1994;121:492.
43. Martino. Cotrimoxazole prophylaxis in patients with leukemia and prolonged granulocytopenia. *Am J Med Sci* 1984;287:7.
44. Menichetti. Viridans streptococci septicemia in cancer patients: a clinical study. *Eur J Epidemiol* 1987;3:316.
45. Menichetti. Preventing fungal infection in neutropenic patients with acute leukemia: fluconazole compared with oral amphotericin B. *Ann Intern Med* 1994; 120:913.
46. Meyer. Nosocomial outbreak of *Klebsiella* infection resistant to late-generation cephalosporins. *Ann Intern Med* 1993;119:353.

47. Murray. Can antibiotic resistance be controlled. *N Engl J Med* 1994;330:1229.
48. Nauseef. A study of simple protective isolation in patients with granulocytopenia. *N Engl J Med* 1981;304:448.
49. Nemunaitis. Recombinant granulocyte-macrophage-colony stimulating factor after autologous marrow transplantation for lymphoid cancer. *N Engl J Med* 1991; 324:1773.
50. Pater. Reporting the results of randomized trials of empiric antibiotic in febrile neutropenic patients: a critical survey. *J Clin Oncol* 1986;4:346.
51. Personal communication. Dr. Tom Spitzer, Bone Marrow Transplant Unit, Massachusetts General Hospital, June 1994.
52. Pizzo. Duration of empiric antibiotic therapy in granulocytic patients with cancer. *Am J Med* 1979;67:194.
53. Pizzo. Treatment of gram-positive septicemia in cancer patients. *Cancer* 1980;45: 206.
54. Pizzo. Empiric antibiotic and antifungal therapy for cancer patients with prolonged fever and granulocytopenia. *Am J Med* 1982;72:101.
55. Pizzo. Fever in the pediatric and young adult patient with cancer: a prospective study of 1001 episodes. *Medicine (Baltimore)* 1982;61:153.
56. Pizzo. Oral antibiotic prophylaxis in patients with cancer: a double-blind randomized placebo-controlled trial. *J Pediatr* 1983;102:125.
57. Pizzo. Approaching the controversies in antibacterial management of cancer patients. *Am J Med* 1984;76:436.
58. Pizzo. A randomized trial comparing ceftazidime alone with combination antibiotic therapy in cancer patients with fever and neutropenia. *N Engl J Med* 1986; 315:552.
59. Pizzo, Preventing infections in cancer patients. In: De Vita VT, ed. *Cancer Principles and Practice of Oncology*, ed 3. Philadelphia: Lippincott, 1989:2092.
60. Pizzo. Management of fever in patients with cancer and treatment induced neutropenia. *N Engl J Med* 1993;328:1323.
61. Polwes. Human recombinant GM-CSF in allogeneic bone-marrow transplantation for leukemia: a double-blind, placebo-controlled trial. *Lancet* 1990;ii:1417.
62. Rabinowe. Long term follow-up of a phase III study of GM-CSF after autologous bone marrow transplantation for lymphoid malignancies. *Blood* 1993;81:1903.
63. Reed. Characteristics of gram-positive septicemia in patients with neutropenic fever. Proceedings of the Fifth International Symposium on Autologous Bone Marrow Transplantation, 1991:267.
64. Rubin. Gram-positive infections and the use of vancomycin in 550 episodes of fever and neutropenia. *Ann Intern Med* 1988;108:30.
65. Sanders. Ceftazidime monotherapy for empiric treatment of febrile neutropenic patients: a meta-analysis. *J Infect Dis* 1991;164:907.
66. Saral. Acyclovir prophylaxis of herpes simplex virus infections: a randomized, double-blind, controlled trial in bone marrow transplant recipients. *N Engl J Med* 1981;305:63.
67. Saral. Acyclovir prophylaxis against herpes simplex virus infection in patients with leukemia. *Ann Intern Med* 1983;99:773.
68. Schimpff. Empiric therapy with carbenicillin and gentamicin for febrile patients with cancer and granulocytopenia. *N Engl J Med* 1971;284:1061.
69. Schimpff. Growth factors and empiric therapy with antibiotics: should they be used concurrently. *Ann Intern Med* 1994;121:538.
70. Schmidt. A randomized, controlled trial of prophylactic ganciclovir for cytomegalovirus pulmonary infection in recipients of allogeneic bone marrow transplants. *N Engl J Med* 1991;324:1005.
71. Sheriden. Granulocyte colony-stimulating factor and neutrophil recovery after high-dose chemotherapy and autologous bone marrow transplantation. *Lancet* 1989;ii: 891.
72. Sickles. Clinical presentation of infection in granulocytopenic patients. *Arch Intern Med* 1975;135:715.
73. Sugar. Empiric treatment of fungal infections in the neutropenic host: review of the literature and guidelines for use. *Arch Intern Med* 1990;150:2258.

74. Taylor. Recombinant human granulocyte colony-stimulating factor hastens granulocyte recovery after high-dose chemotherapy and autologous bone marrow transplantation in Hodgkin s disease. *J Clin Oncol* 1989;7:1791.
75. Villablanca. The clinical spectrum of infections with viridans streptococci in bone marrow transplant. *Bone Marrow Transplant* 1990;6:387.
76. Wade. Selective antimicrobial modulation as prophylaxis against infection during granulocytopenia: trimethoprim-sulfamethoxazole vs. nalidixic acid. *J Infect Dis* 1983;147:624.
77. Wade. Monotherapy for empiric treatment of fever in granulocytopenic cancer patients. *Am J Med* 1986;80(Suppl 5C):85.
78. Wilson. Failure of oral trimethoprim-sulfamethoxazole prophylaxis in acute leukemia: isolation of resistant plasmids from strains of Enterobacteriaceae causing bacteremia. *N Engl J Med* 1982;306:16.
79. Wingard. Increase in *Candida kruseii* infection among patients with bone marrow transplantation and neutropenia treated prophylactically with fluconazole. *N Engl J Med* 1991;325:1274.
80. Winston. Norfloxacin versus vancomycin/polymyxin for prevention of infections in granulocytopenic patients. *Am J Med* 1986;80:884.
81. Winston. Intravenous immune globulin for prevention of cytomegalovirus infection and interstitial pneumonia after bone marrow transplantation. *Ann Intern Med* 1987;106:12.
82. Winston. Ofloxacin versus vancomycin/polymyxin for prevention of infections in granulocytopenic patients. *Am J Med* 1990;88:36.
83. Winston. Ganciclovir prophylaxis of cytomegalovirus infection and disease in allogeneic bone marrow transplant recipients: results of a placebo-controlled, double-blind trial. *Ann Intern Med* 1993;118:179.
84. Young. Antimicrobial prophylaxis in the neutropenic host: lessons of the past and perspective for the future. *Eur J Clin Microbiol Infect Dis* 1988;7:93.

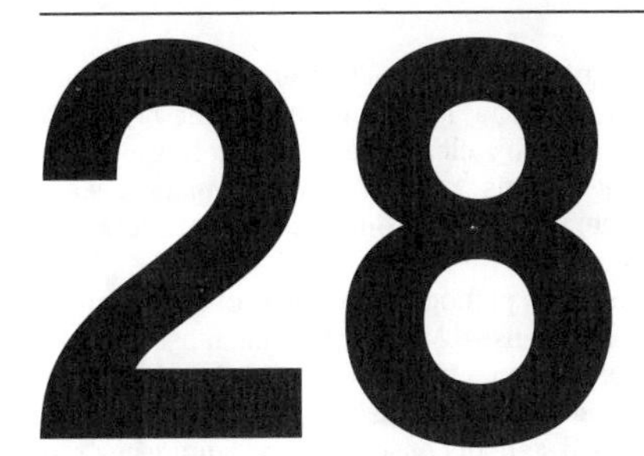

Community-Acquired Pneumonia

Laura A. Napolitano and
Morton N. Swartz

A. Introduction

1. Pneumonia is defined as an inflammatory process within the lung which commonly occurs in response to an uncontrolled proliferation of pathogenic organisms. It is differentiated from bronchitis by its involvement of the most distal portion of the respiratory tract: the respiratory bronchioles and alveoli. Histologically, an inflammatory reaction encompasses the alveolar interstitium and leads to exudative consolidation of the alveoli and impaired gas exchange across the alveolar membrane. In most cases, prompt and appropriate treatment leads to complete resolution of the disease.
2. Community-acquired pneumonia (CAP) is pneumonia that is acquired outside the hospital setting. In most cases, the community setting also includes nursing homes and similar chronic care facilities. Hospital-acquired (nosocomial) pneumonia is a separate clinical entity from CAP, with different causes as well as distinct diagnostic and therapeutic approaches. Nosocomial pneumonia is discussed in detail in Chapter 29.
3. The discussion in this chapter is strictly limited to CAP. Excluded is medical literature that loosely combines CAP with bronchitis into a broader category of "lower respiratory tract infections." Most of the data are derived from inpatient studies and, consequently their applicability to outpatient management of pneumonia is limited. Although they are of major importance, discussions of pneumonia caused by *Mycobacterium tuberculosis* and pneumonia in the immunocompromised host are beyond the scope of this chapter.

B. Epidemiology of Community-Acquired Pneumonia

1. Pneumonia is the sixth leading cause of death in the United States, and the cost of this disease is estimated at $23 billion per year (31,50). There are approximately 4 million cases of CAP yearly, with roughly 20% of affected persons requiring hospitalization (31). Mortality among hospitalized patients with CAP is 13% to 24% but may rise to 40% to 50% in selected groups such as nursing home residents or the critically ill (19,51,53,58,72).
2. Over the past two decades, several factors have contributed to major changes in the epidemiology and treatment of CAP. The population at risk for CAP includes increasing numbers of elderly, immunocompromised, and chronically ill persons. Opportunistic pathogens are more commonly seen. Newly described and characterized etiologic agents, such as *Legionella*, *Chlamydia pneumoniae* (TWAR), *Moraxella catarrhalis*, and hantavirus, have been identified. Advances in diagnostic technology provide more rapid and accurate information. Numerous broad-spectrum antibiotics have been developed, accompanied by a worrisome rise in the incidence of antimicrobial resistance.

C. Pathophysiology of Community-Acquired Pneumonia

1. In the normal host, the upper respiratory tract is colonized by *Streptococcus pneumoniae*, *Streptococcus* species, *Haemophilus* species, *Neisseria* species, and many anaerobic bacteria. *Haemophilus influenzae* and *M catarrhalis* frequently colonize the upper respiratory tracts of smokers. Alcoholics, recently hospitalized patients, diabetics, and residents of chronic care facilities are prone to colonization with gram-negative bacilli (GNRs) (66).

2. The lower respiratory tract is normally sterile. This environment is maintained by structural barriers (nasal vibrissae, larynx, branched airways), protective mechanisms (gag reflex, mucociliary clearance, cough reflex), and immune-mediated defenses (immunoglobulins A and G, alveolar macrophages). Host defenses are weakened by age, smoking, chronic illness (particularly lung disease), and immunosuppression (66).
3. Pneumonia results when respiratory pathogens, by virtue of their quantity and/or virulence, overwhelm the host defenses. Microorganisms most often reach the lungs through inhalation or aspiration. Microaspiration has been demonstrated in 45% of normal persons through the use of nasopharyngeal radiolabelling techniques. Patients with a depressed state of consciousness aspirate at a rate of 70% (41). Occasionally, microorganisms may also reach the lung hematogenously, or by local extension.

D. Pathogens in Community-Acquired Pneumonia

1. **Bacteria**—Table 28-1 describes common bacterial agents and their characteristics.
2. **Viruses**
   a. Viral pneumonia is uncommon in the immunocompetent adult, although it is seen more commonly in an epidemic setting. Before the mid-1980's, viruses accounted for approximately 10% of CAP (35); however, the incidence is rising as the population becomes increasingly immunosuppressed, elderly, and chronically ill. In a recent study in which a viral diagnosis was aggressively pursued, viruses accounted for approximately 18% of CAP (51). Immunosuppressed and nursing home patients constituted 31% of the study population. Among the patients with viral pneumonia, influenza A (30%), cytomegalovirus (24%), parainfluenza (14%), influenza B (13%), respiratory syncytial virus (4%), and parainfluenza 1 (2%) were detected (51). Adenovirus and varicella-zoster virus were not reported in this study but have been detected elsewhere (35).
   b. Incidence of viral CAP is highest in the winter. Closed populations, such as those in military barracks or nursing homes, are more susceptible to epidemic spread. Viral pneumonia cannot be reliably differentiated from bacterial pneumonia on the basis of clinical presentation. Bacterial superinfection of the lung may be seen after viral pneumonia (35).
   c. Influenza is the most common cause of viral CAP, and fatalities in the tens of thousands have occurred during epidemic years. Eighty percent of influenza victims are >65 years of age (16). Bacterial superinfection is most commonly caused by *S pneumoniae*, *H influenzae*, and *S aureus* (35).
   d. Respiratory syncytial virus and parainfluenza are seen predominantly in the pediatric population and decrease in incidence with age. In adults, they are most likely to be seen in the immunosuppressed population, as are cytomegalovirus, herpes simplex virus, and varicella-zoster virus. Adenovirus causes pneumonia in young adults or in immunocompromised persons (35).
   e. In 1994, 24 cases of hantavirus pneumonia were reported in the southwestern United States. Scattered cases have occurred elsewhere, including the northeast United States. A different strain of this virus was previously described in Korea and China, where it causes hemorrhagic fever with renal syndrome. The 1994 outbreak in the Southwest arose from a newly identified, especially virulent hantavirus strain that is responsible for hantavirus pulmonary syndrome. This syndrome is frequently followed by adult respiratory distress syndrome (ARDS) and death. The mortality rate is at least 50%. Infection results from direct contact with excreta of a rodent host or inhalation of aerosolized particles (17).
3. **Aspiration Pneumonia and Anaerobic Necrotizing Pneumonia**
   a. The term "aspiration pneumonia" is most commonly used to describe aspiration of gastric contents and/or bacteria-laden upper respiratory secretions into the lungs. Microaspiration occurs routinely in normal individu-

Table 28-1 Common pathogens in community-acquired pneumonia

Organism	Diagnostic Characteristics	Virulence Factors	Reservoir of Infection	Clinical Characteristics	Extrapulmonary Complications	References
Streptococcus pneumoniae	Lancet-shaped gram-positive diplococci; alpha-hemolytic	Polysaccharide capsule	Upper respiratory tract	Classic presentation includes acute onset, single rigor, high fever, rusty sputum, pleuritic chest pain.* Risk of serious infection increases with advanced age, sickle cell anemia, asplenia, diabetes, systemic lupus erythematosus, chronic heart or lung disease, cirrhosis, immunosuppression, renal failure, hematologic malignancy.	Bacteremia with metastatic infection; meningitis; empyema; endocarditis. Local extension to ears, sinuses.	3, 44

Table 28-1 (continued)

Organism	Diagnostic Characteristics	Virulence Factors	Reservoir of Infection	Clinical Characteristics	Extrapulmonary Complications	References
Haemophilus influenzae	Pleomorphic gram-negative coccobacilli	Polysaccharide capsule	Upper respiratory tract	Upper respiratory tract colonization increases with age and chronic lung disease (often nonencapsulated strains). Risk of infection increases with chronic lung disease, immunosuppression.†	Bacteremia; meningitis. Local extension to ears, sinuses.	54
Legionella species	Fastidious gram-negative bacillus; facultative intracellular parasite	Disruption of phagocyte function; toxins; proteases	Natural and manmade freshwater habitats	Classically accompanied by liver function abnormalities, diarrhea, hyponatremia.* Cases may be epidemic or sporadic; 2–10 d incubation period. Risk of infection increases with smoking, aspiration, steroids, chronic renal disease.	Bacteremia	42, 55
Chlamydia pneumoniae	Pear-shaped elementary body; obligate intracellular parasite	Not defined	Endemic in humans	Classic presentation includes viral-like prodrome, dry cough.* Cases may be epidemic or sporadic with primary infection or reinfection; 10–30 d incubation period.	—	70

Table 28-1 (continued)

Mycoplasma pneumoniae	Smallest free-living organism; no cell wall; filterable; filamentous	H_2O_2 and superoxide release; epithelial cell adhesin; induction of autoantibodies	Endemic in humans	Classically, age <40 y, upper respiratory symptoms, low grade fever, headache, dry or mildly productive cough.* Intrafamilial and epidemic spread are more common than sporadic cases; occurs year-round but most common in fall and winter; 1–3 wk incubation period.	Bullous myringitis; hemolytic anemia; erythema multiforme; encephalitis.	1, 46
Staphylococcus aureus	Plump gram-positive cocci in clusters	Peptidoglycan wall; protein A; enterotoxins A through E	Upper respiratory tract and skin	Classically, moderate to severe illness and slow resolution which may be complicated by cavitation, lung abscess, empyema.* Risk of infection increases with advanced age, diabetes, post-influenza, HIV, chronic lung disease, mechanical ventilation, central line, steroid use, hospitalization, nursing home residence, recent neurosurgery.	Bacteremia with metastatic infection; endocarditis; toxic shock syndrome.	40

Table 28-1 (continued)

Organism	Diagnostic Characteristics	Virulence Factors	Reservoir of Infection	Clinical Characteristics	Extrapulmonary Complications	References
Klebsiella pneumoniae *Escherichia coli* *Pseudomonas aeruginosa*	Gram-negative bacilli	Endotoxin	Upper respiratory tract, skin, and intestines	Risk of infection increases with advanced age, diabetes, alcohol abuse, malnutrition, liver disease, congestive heart failure, nursing home residence, hospitalization, debilitation, cystic fibrosis, aspiration, mechanical ventilation, steroids. May be associated with cavitation, abscess, empyema.	Bacteremia; shock.	18
Moraxella catarrhalis	Kidney bean–shaped gram-negative diplococci	Not defined	Upper respiratory tract	Generally causes bronchitis or mild pneumonia. Predominant risk is chronic lung disease; risk of infection also increases with advanced age and underlying chronic disease. Most common in late fall to mid-spring.	Bacteremia is rare.	75

*Classic clinical presentations are not well corroborated by rigorously controlled studies.
†Asplenia increases the risk of bacteremia with *H influenzae* type b.

als (41); however, host defenses usually prevent the development of pneumonia. Macroaspiration is more likely to overcome the defense mechanisms and result in pneumonia. Risk factors for the development of aspiration pneumonia include history of stroke, neuromuscular disease, sedation, obtundation, alcoholism, dysphagia, intubation, and any chronic illness (15).

b. Clinical presentations are varied. Symptoms may be abrupt, or they may be more insidious with chronic aspiration. The dependent areas of the lung are most often involved radiographically.

(1) Chemical pneumonitis may result from aspiration of sterile gastric secretions. Based upon extrapolation from animal data, approximately 25 ml of gastric secretions at a pH of <2.5 is required to produce pneumonitis in humans (15). After aspiration, fever, tachypnea, and severe hypoxemia are seen in almost all patients. Thirty percent have cough, apnea, or wheezing. Rapid clinical and radiographic improvement may be seen in 3 to 6 days (62%). Alternatively, rapid decline and death (12%) or bacterial superinfection (40%) may occur (10). Up to 35% of patients develop ARDS (15). The risk of bacterial superinfection increases with use of antacids or histamine$_2$ blockers. Antibiotics should be withheld unless there are signs of bacterial superinfection such as new fever, leukocytosis, evidence of leukocytes and bacteria on gram-stained sputum examination, and worsening appearance of chest roentgenogram (CXR) (10,15).

(2) Bacterial pneumonitis may result from primary aspiration of oropharyngeal flora or superinfection after sterile aspiration. Pathogens in the normal host are chiefly oral anaerobes (*Bacteroides*, *Fusobacterium*, *Peptostreptococcus*) and aerobic *Streptococcus* species, which together account for 66% to 87% of community-acquired aspiration pneumonias. Commensal *S aureus* and GNRs may be aspirated by chronically ill or institutionalized patients. Eighteen percent of patients develop putrid sputum, which is indicative of infection with anaerobes and suggestive of necrotizing pneumonia or lung abscess. Resolution can take weeks. Cavitation and abscess (20%), necrotizing pneumonia, or empyema may complicate recovery (28).

4. Other Pathogens—The nonbacterial pathogens, *C pneumoniae* and *Mycoplasma pneumoniae* are common causes of CAP (see Table 28-1). Opportunistic organisms including *Pneumocystis carinii* and fungi can also cause CAP, especially in the immunosuppressed host. *Pneumocystis carinii* pneumonia is discussed in more detail in Chapter 25.

E. Etiology of Community-Acquired Pneumonia

1. Despite extensive diagnostic evaluation, the cause of CAP remains unknown in 35% to 60% of cases (19,51,53,58,72). This is a result of a combination of factors: inadequate performance of sputum cultures and Gram stains, treatment with antibiotics before evaluation, lack of sputum production, and limited ability to detect or identify certain pathogens, particularly viral agents, *Chlamydia*, and *Mycoplasma*. Many studies have sought to identify the most common causes of CAP. Older studies were limited by nonuniform criteria and a diagnostic battery that excluded detection of several newly defined pathogens. Current studies are more uniform in their design, yet interpretation and comparison of these studies is confounded by variations in population, endemic pathogens, seasonal bias, and rigor of diagnostic pursuit.

2. Table 28-2 summarizes the recent etiologic data from several representative studies. *S pneumoniae* is the most common cause of CAP; *H influenzae*, *Legionella*, influenza, GNRs, *M pneumoniae*, and TWAR constitute most of the remaining cases.

a. Although the etiologic profile of patients with CAP requiring admission to an intensive care unit (ICU) was not significantly different from that of patients with CAP in general, the distribution of pathogens was slightly differ-

Table 28-2 Etiologic agents of community-acquired pneumonia

Location	Year	Study Type	# Cases	Five Most Common Etiologies (ranked in order of frequency) 1	2	3	4	5	Unknown	Mortality	Reference
Pittsburgh	1986–1987	Prospective multicenter	359+	total pop: *S. pneumo*, 15%	total pop: *H. flu*, 11%	total pop: *Legionella* sp., 7%	total pop: TWAR, 6%	total pop: GNR, 6%	total pop: 33%	total pop: 13.7%	
				NH pop: *S. pneumo*, 19.6%	NH pop: GNR, 10.9%	NH pop: aspiration 10.9%	NH pop: *H. flu*, 8.7%	NH pop: *Legionella* sp., 6.5%	NH pop: 26.1%	NH pop: 19.6%	(19)
Halifax	1981–1987	Prospective single center	719++	total pop: *S. pneumo*, 8.5%	total pop: aspiration 7.2%	total pop: *M. pneumoniae*, 5.6%	total pop: Influenza A, 5.6%	total pop: *S. aureus*, 4.0%	total pop: 47%	total pop: 21%	
				NH pop: aspiration 14.5%	NH pop: Influenza A 8.5%	NH pop: *S. pneumo*, 6.9%	NH pop: GNR 5.3%	NH pop: *S. aureus*, 5.3%	NH pop: 59%	NH pop: 40%	(51)
Barcelona	1984–1987	Prospective single center ICU only	92*	*S. pneumo*, 15.2%	*Legionella* sp., 14.1%	*M. pneumoniae*, 6.5%	*P. aeruginosa*, 5.4%	α-hemolytic *Streptococci*, 3.3%	48%	22%	(72)
France	1987–1989	Prospective multicenter ICU only	132*	*S. pneumo*, 32.6%	*H. flu*, 10.6%	GNR, 10.6%	*Streptococcus* sp., 6.8%	*S. aureus* 3.8%	28%	24%	(53)

+12.8% cases are NHAP.
++18.2% cases are NHAP.
*Immunosuppressed and HIV patients excluded from study.

ent. One study noted an increased incidence of ICU admissions with CAP caused by *Legionella* compared with other pathogens, but this difference did not reach statistical significance (19).

b. The incidence of aspiration pneumonia was significantly higher with nursing home–acquired pneumonia (NHAP) than with CAP occurring in other settings (51).

c. Despite increased colonization of *H influenzae* in patients with chronic obstructive pulmonary disease (COPD), GNR in alcoholic patients, GNR in nursing home patients, and so on, no particular underlying illness or clinical setting was statistically correlated with infection with any of the five most common pathogens (19,51).

d. Although *M pneumoniae* is classically seen in younger patients, some studies reported a significant number of older patients with this infection (6,20).

F. Clinical Presentation of Community-Acquired Pneumonia

1. Signs and Symptoms—Table 28-3 summarizes the common presenting features of CAP found in two representative studies (19,51).

a. Confusion is statistically more common in the elderly. It is seen in 48% of patients >65 years of age (19,51,73).

b. A lower fever is associated with advanced age (19,73). Up to 60% of CAP patients >65 years old may be afebrile (73).

2. Typical Versus Atypical Presentation

a. Historically, the clinical presentation of pneumonia has been classified as typical or atypical. The term "typical pneumonia" was originally used to describe *S pneumoniae* infection and implied an abrupt onset of illness with purulent sputum, high fever, pleuritic chest pain, and lobar consolidation. Subsequently, other bacterial pathogens such as *H influenzae* and *S aureus* were found to cause similar symptoms. The term "atypical pneumonia" was coined to describe pneumonia of more indolent onset, with a dry cough, lower fever, patchy consolidation on CXR, and gastrointestinal symptoms, generally occurring in a younger population. This presentation is attributed to nonbacterial pathogens such as *M pneumoniae, Chlamydia* species, viruses, and the bacterium *Legionella pneumophila.*

b. However, clinical studies have shown that the cause of pneumonia cannot be reliably determined on the basis of the presenting signs and symptoms (19,20,72). For example, in one study that used a computerized multivariate discriminant function analysis of 441 adults with CAP, the clinical features correctly predicted the etiologic organism in only 42% of the cases (20). Nevertheless, a few isolated clinical features of CAP may still be useful for diagnosis. Diarrhea was found to be more common with "atypical" pathogens ($P<0.05$), and fever >40° C was more common with infections caused by *Legionella* ($P=0.02$) (19).

G. Evaluation of Community-Acquired Pneumonia

1. Diagnostic Criteria—The diagnosis of acute CAP requires the presence of a new infiltrate on CXR (not attributable to some other cause) within 24 to 48

Table 28-3 Clinical manifestations of community-acquired pneumonia

	Fang (19)	Marrie (51)
Cough	88%	78%
Sputum production	71%	56%
Fever	69%	79%
Dyspnea	60%	Not described
Chills	48%	44%
Pleuritic chest pain	30%	36%
Confusion	18%	33%

hours after admission. One or more of the following should be present: cough, fever, sputum production, and leukocytosis (19,51). In some cases, particularly in elderly patients, a constellation of less specific symptoms (*e.g.*, pleuritic chest pain, confusion, dyspnea) may be the only presenting features (34,73).

2. **Medical History and Physical Examination**—The history and the physical examination are important tools in refining the differential diagnosis. They should be used to guide the diagnostic evaluation and the selection of empiric antimicrobial therapy.
   a. The following information should be sought in the history: age; place of residence; comorbid diseases with particular attention to history of lung disease, tobacco use, and alcohol use; recent hospitalizations; prior episodes of pneumonia (including cause and treatment, if known); medication history with particular attention to the use of antibiotics, steroids, or other immunosuppressive agents; allergies; risk factors for infection with the human immunodeficiency virus (HIV); presence or absence of spleen; occupational history; travel history; animal or bird exposure; immunization status; contacts with other ill persons; and clinical presentation.
   b. A complete examination should be performed. Fever >37.8° C, pulse >100 bpm, rales, and decreased breath sounds appear to be significant independent and additive predictors of finding a pulmonary infiltrate on CXR (38). The patient's overall clinical condition, with particular attention to general appearance, vital signs, and cardiorespiratory status, is an essential component of triage. Additional etiologic clues may be obtained from the presence of rash, bullous myringitis, sinusitis, poor dentition, diminished gag reflex, or decreased neurologic status (50).
3. **Laboratory Diagnosis**
   a. **Routine Blood Work**—A complete blood count with differential, a complete chemistry panel (including electrolytes, blood urea nitrogen, creatinine, and liver function tests), and a measurement of arterial oxygenation should be performed on all hospitalized patients. These tests are most useful for risk stratification and as a baseline to measure clinical improvement or deterioration. No specific laboratory values are significantly correlated with specific causes (19). *Legionella* infection traditionally has been associated with hyponatremia and liver function abnormalities (42). However, this association has been disputed by a more recent study (19).
   b. **Radiographic Analysis**—A new infiltrate on CXR is the gold standard for the diagnosis of acute pneumonia. Traditional radiographic interpretations describe bacterial pneumonia as a lobar or segmental infiltrate and nonbacterial pneumonia as a reticulonodular process. However, these classic features are not upheld by the literature. Studies demonstrate that without clinical information, radiologists and clinicians are unable to reliably distinguish typical from atypical pneumonia based solely on radiographic appearance (47,69).
   c. **Sputum Gram Stain**
      (1) The sputum Gram stain is a test whose utility has been contested by some, but a high-quality specimen is generally regarded as useful (8, 32,61). Shortcomings of this test include potential contamination with oropharyngeal flora and inability to identify atypical pathogens. To be of satisfactory quality, the Gram stain should reveal <10 epithelial cells and >25 neutrophils per 100× field, with a preponderant flora of >10 organisms per oil-immersion field (19,61). However, an acceptable specimen is obtained in only 35% to 45% of cases (32,51).
      (2) For diagnosis of pneumococcal pneumonia, the sensitivity and the specificity of the Gram stain have been estimated at 62% and 85%, respectively (61). However, the accuracy of these values is uncertain

because they were derived with the use of sputum culture as the diagnostic gold standard. If the Gram stain preparation of sputum in a typical oil-immersion field reveals no epithelial cells, at least 3 to 4 neutrophils, and ≥10 gram-positive lancet-shaped diplococci, it predicts isolation of *S pneumoniae* in about 90% of patients. In a study that used blood cultures as a gold standard to assess the utility of the sputum Gram stain for a variety of pathogens, the sensitivity was 85%, and the specificity was not calculated (32).

d. Sputum Culture

(1) Routine Culture

(a) The utility of the routine sputum culture is more debated than that of the Gram stain. Because many potential respiratory pathogens colonize the upper airways, interpretation of culture results is confounded by possible growth of these colonizers. In addition, pneumococci may undergo autolysis and fail to be isolated if the sputum is not plated when freshly expectorated.

(b) The concordance rate of sputum and blood cultures varies widely, from 45% to 82% (5,20,51). Although some studies show low diagnostic yield and poor specificity for the sputum culture, others claim better results when specimens are carefully screened and cultures are more strictly quantified (5,20,45,51,71).

(c) The results of sputum culture are not worth consideration unless a Gram stain of the same specimen is of acceptable quality. Although some investigators support forgoing the sputum culture altogether, it is valuable in the determination of antibiotic susceptibility and in the detection of pathogens not present in the normal flora.

(d) A reasonable approach to the interpretation of sputum cultures is through the use of "definitive" versus "probable" diagnosis. Current diagnostic standards for CAP are detailed in Table 28-4.

Table 28-4 Current diagnostic standards for community-acquired pneumonia

Definitive Diagnosis	Presumptive Diagnosis
1. Blood culture yielding pathogen	1. Heavy growth of a predominant bacterial pathogen on sputum culture (10^7CFU/ml)
2. Pleural fluid yielding pathogen	2. Any growth of a bacterial pathogen on sputum culture with compatible Gram stain
3. BAL or induced sputum yielding *Pneumocystis carinii*	3. *Chlamydia pneumoniae* IgM titer ≥1:32
4. Open lung biopsy yielding a pathogen (stains or cultures)	4. *Mycoplasma pneumoniae* CFT ≥1:512
5. Sputum culture yielding *Mycoplasma pneumoniae*	
6. Positive sputum culture or urinary antigen for *Legionella* sp	
7. Fourfold or higher rise in antibody titer for *Legionella* sp, *Chlamydia pneumoniae, Mycoplasma pneumoniae,* or routine respiratory viruses (influenza, parainfluenza, adenovirus, RSV)	
8. Serum- or urine-positive CIE	
9. Positive *Legionella* DFA stain and IgG titer ≥1:256	

Adapted from Fang (19), Levy (45), and Marrie (1).

(2) **_Legionella_ Species Culture**—*Legionella* requires culture on selective media, the buffered charcoal-yeast extract agar, which may contain antibiotics to suppress the growth of less fastidious organisms. Growth of *Legionella* typically takes 3 to 5 days. The sensitivity of the sputum culture for *Legionella* species varies from 11% to 70%, depending presumably on the quality of the expectorated specimen. Higher sensitivities of 65% to 90% are seen in lower respiratory tract specimens such as transtracheal aspirates. By definition, the specificity is 100% (43,55,64).

(3) **_Mycoplasma pneumoniae_ Culture**—This organism requires a specialized culture of agar supplemented with horse serum. Growth typically takes 7 to 10 days. In general, *Mycoplasma* culture is an insensitive diagnostic method; a positive sputum culture may be observed in only 26% of the infected patients. By definition, the specificity is 100% (1).

(4) **_Chlamydia pneumoniae_ Culture**—This intracellular pathogen is difficult to culture and requires tissue culture cell lines for isolation. The diagnostic yield is increased by immunofluorescent staining of cultures, a technique that is not widely available. Serology is the diagnostic method of choice (70) (see Table 28-5).

(5) **Viral Culture**—Viral culture is not routinely indicated (56) but may be helpful in selected cases to establish the onset of a viral outbreak such as an influenza A epidemic. Days to weeks are required to make a diagnosis, and the yield is low. Therefore, rapid antigen detection may be more helpful. Serology of specimens from acutely ill and convalescing patients may be helpful for retrospective diagnosis (6,35,68).

(6) **Induced Sputum**—Induced sputum specimens are superior to spontaneously produced specimens in the diagnosis of *P carinii* pneumonia and tuberculosis. However, in the diagnosis of pneumonia caused by routine bacterial pathogens, induced specimens are no better than spontaneously produced sputum. They offer no significant improvement in the quality of the Gram stain or in the bacteriologic yield of culture (29). The role of induced sputum in the determination of atypical pathogens has not been well studied.

e. **Blood Culture**—Two sets of blood cultures are recommended for all hospitalized patients with pneumonia (56). A positive test is diagnostic, excepting skin contaminants. The utility of this test is limited by the low prevalence of bacteremia in CAP (6% to 20%) and the low sensitivity of this test in the detection of transient bacteremia (2,6,45,51,72). Specificity is virtually 100%. Bacteremia is most common in pneumococcal pneumonia and is present in 9% of 46% of those cases (19,45,51,58,73).

f. **Pleural Fluid Culture**—Hospitalized patients with a significant pleural effusion should be considered for diagnostic thoracentesis (56). A positive test is considered diagnostic, excepting skin contaminants. Specificity is virtually 100%. The utility of this test is limited by the low prevalence of pleural effusions amenable to thoracentesis in CAP (7% to 28%) and the low diagnostic (bacteriologic) yield of thoracentesis (12% to 33%) (6,45, 72,73).

g. **Serologic Analysis**

(1) Serology is most often used in the diagnosis of pathogens that grow poorly or slowly in culture, such as *M pneumoniae*, *Legionella* species, *C. pneumoniae*, and respiratory viruses. This test measures the presence of host antibodies directed against a pathogen. The generation of antibodies does not occur until 1 to 6 weeks after exposure to a pathogen. Consequently, serologic analysis is often nondiagnostic at the time of acute infection, and "convalescent" titers drawn 3 to 6 weeks after the onset of illness are required to confirm a diagnosis. A fourfold or higher difference between the acute and convalescent titers is the gold standard of diagnosis for several respiratory pathogens. In some cases,

Table 28-5 Diagnostic serology

Organism (References)	Diagnostic Criteria for Acute Infection	Time Course of Titer Rise After Infection	Persistence of Antibodies	Comments
Mycoplasma pneumoniae (1)	≥Fourfold rise in CFT or CFT ≥1:512*	CFT, 0–3 wk; IgM, immediate†	CFT, months; IgM, unknown	Cold agglutinins are also useful
Chlamydia pneumoniae (70)	IgM titer ≥1:32* or ≥fourfold rise in IgG or IgM	Primary infection: IgM, 2–4 wk; IgG, 6–8 wk Reinfection: IgM may not rise; IgG, 1–3 wk	IgM, 2–6 mo; IgG, months to years	CFT may also be used but is not species specific and may not rise in reinfection
Legionella sp (42, 55, 74)	≥Fourfold rise in IFA or IFA ≥1.256*	0–8 weeks	IgM, months; IgG, years	Antibodies may not be detected in up to 20% of cases; IFA may crossreact with other organisms
Respiratory viruses (35)	≥Fourfold rise in antibody titers	Varied	Varied	Serology is rarely useful

*Presumptive diagnosis only; requires clinical correlation for interpretation.

†*M pneumoniae* IgM titer shows promise as an early diagnostic test: 42/45 (89%) of patients with *M pneumoniae* infection had an IgM titer of 1:4 or higher at time of presentation (1). However, this test has not yet been broadly applied and its diagnostic utility has not been evaluated in large studies.

highly elevated acute titers may be considered diagnostic in the presence of a compatible clinical picture. However, a high titer of a specific antibody (*e.g.*, *Legionella*) may persist for months or years after an infection (56).

(2) Because of the retrospective nature of serologic diagnosis, routine serology is not recommended in the initial evaluation of CAP. It is most appropriate for academic and epidemiologic purposes but may also be helpful in the management of severely ill patients for whom the routine diagnostic methods fail to yield a diagnosis (56). Table 28-5 provides further details of diagnostic serology.

h. Cold Agglutinins

(1) The cold agglutinin test is sometimes useful in the diagnosis of *M pneumoniae* infection. It may be performed quickly at the bedside or sent to the laboratory. For the rapid bedside test, whole blood is collected in a citrated tube and chilled to 4° C for 1 minute. The development of clumped erythrocytes indicates a positive test of at least 1:128 titer of cold agglutinins. Agglutination should disappear after rewarming to 37° C. The sensitivity of the bedside test is 98%; the specificity is 100% for detection of titer ≥1:64 (36).

(2) A positive cold agglutinin test has been seen in *M pneumoniae* infection, viral illness, psittacosis, mononucleosis, listeriosis, and pneumococcal pneumonia, although a titer of ≥1:128 is most suggestive of *M pneumoniae* infection (46,59).

i. Antigen Detection Assays

(1) *Legionella* urinary antigen assay detects the presence of *L pneumophila* serogroup 1 antigen in the urine. Serogroup 1 is responsible for approximately 50% to 80% of the cases of legionnaires' disease. Some cross-reactivity may be seen with other serotypes. The sensitivity is 70% to 90%, and the specificity is virtually 100%. When detectable, the antigen is present in 66% of cases during the first week of symptoms, and in 100% the by second week. The antigen remains present in the urine for up to 10 weeks (43,64).

(2) Countercurrent immunoelectrophoresis is used to detect soluble antigens of pneumococcus or *H influenzae* in urine, sputum, blood, pleural fluid, or cerebrospinal fluid. In general, this assay is not broadly used because of its low sensitivity (45,50). It may be helpful when prior antibiotic administration results in nondiagnostic culture data.

(3) Many advanced rapid diagnostic techniques for antigen detection of viruses, slow-growing pathogens, and bacteria are being investigated (50,68). Their contribution to the diagnosis and treatment of CAP has not yet been determined.

j. Direct Fluorescent Antibody Test—The direct fluorescent antibody (DFA) test is useful for rapid diagnosis of organisms that grow slowly, or not at all, in culture. It is used primarily on sputum or bronchoalveolar lavage (BAL) samples. For the *Legionella* DFA test, the sensitivity and the specificity depend on the type of reagent used. Polyvalent serum is less specific than monovalent serum. Because of cross-reaction with certain *Bacteroides* and *Pseudomonas* strains, the DFA test for *Legionella* is not recommended on sputum specimens. However, it may be helpful in the evaluation of pleural fluid and transbronchial biopsy specimens (43,55,64).

k. Invasive Diagnostic Techniques

(1) Noninvasive testing is nondiagnostic in 40% to 60% of cases (6,19,45, 51,53,58,72). Determination of the exact cause of CAP may lead to less expensive and less toxic therapy, but it does not confer a survival benefit in most cases (45,58,72). In general, the course of CAP is benign and responds well to properly selected empiric therapy. However, in situations such as failure of therapy, immunosuppression, or severe illness, a precise diagnosis is warranted. Invasive diagnostic methods offer higher diagnostic yields at a cost of higher procedural risk. These techniques have been more broadly studied and applied in ventilator-associated pneumonia. Because of the increased risk associated with invasive procedures and the questionable contribution of etiologic diagnosis toward survival, the routine application of these techniques is not appropriate in CAP (6,52,56,57). They should be reserved only for immunocompromised patients or immunocompetent patients with severe or nonresolving disease.

(2) Transtracheal aspiration is a time-honored means of obtaining lower respiratory specimens free from oropharyngeal contamination. The rate of complications is 5% to 10%. Sensitivity for bacterial pneumonia is as high as 80% but specificity is poor, particularly in cases of chronic bronchitis, aspiration, or chronic illness (13,57). Although formerly a favored method of obtaining sterile specimens, especially in patients who are unable to produce a good sputum sample, this technique is declining in popularity. Percutaneous needle aspiration (PNA) and fiberoptic bronchoscopy offer less patient discomfort and higher specificity.

(3) Fiberoptic bronchoscopy with BAL is routinely used in the diagnosis of opportunistic infections in the immunosuppressed host. It is the procedure of choice for detecting *P carinii* pneumonia and suspected tuberculosis. Its use in the diagnosis of bacterial CAP is limited by the low specificity, which results from upper airway contamination of BAL culture specimens in approximately 33% of cases. There is some utility of BAL in the diagnosis of atypical respiratory pathogens such as *Legionella* and *M pneumoniae*, which do not colonize the bronchial tree, but bronchoscopy with protected brush specimens has better overall specificity in the diagnosis of CAP. The most common complication of fiberoptic bronchoscopy is hypoxia (13% to 23%), which is usually responsive to supplementary oxygen. The risk of serious complications is minimal (52).

(4) Fiberoptic bronchoscopy with protected brush specimen offers improved specificity and precise culture quantification. Concordance with blood cultures is 100% (6). In a study of 19 patients with CAP by Ortqvist, the procedure was diagnostic in 50% of the cases and was considered valuable for management in 79%. The sensitivity was higher in patients who had not received any antibiotics before the procedure (80% versus 12%); the specificity was 100%. There were no major complications associated with the procedure (57).

(5) PNA, also referred to as transthoracic needle aspiration, is commonly done under radiologic guidance. The sensitivity is 60% to 90%, and the specificity is almost 100% (49). In Pachon's study of 34 patients with severe CAP who underwent PNA, the diagnostic yield was 53% (58). The complication rate of ultrathin PNA is 1% to 2% (49,76). Its use is not recommended in ventilated patients.

H. Therapeutic Approach to Patients With CAP

1. Supportive Therapy

a. Supplemental oxygen should be administered to maintain adequate arterial oxygenation. The oxygenation goal should be individualized for each patient. A patient with COPD may rest comfortably at an oxygen saturation of 92%, whereas this degree of oxygenation may induce myocardial ischemia in a patient with coronary artery disease. Mechanical ventilation may be necessary for patients who are unable to adequately oxygenate or ventilate on their own.

b. Chest physiotherapy and bronchodilators are often useful to assist with the clearance of secretions and maintenance of airway patency.

c. Hydration restores volume or electrolyte loss from fever, emesis, diarrhea, or malnutrition.
d. Treatment of active comorbid illness should not be overlooked. In the case of pneumococcal pneumonia, the presence of the following complications should specifically be sought: meningitis, empyema, endocarditis, pericarditis, and septic arthritis.

2. **Antimicrobial Therapy**
   a. **Selection of Antibiotic Therapy**
      (1) Numerous classes of antibiotics are available for the treatment of CAP, and new agents are continuously being developed. Selection of a therapeutic agent must take into consideration its absorption, tissue penetration, *in vitro* and *in vivo* activity, interactions, side effects, and cost of the drug. The mean inhibitory concentration for a given pathogen and the tissue concentration of the antibiotic ultimately determine its therapeutic efficacy.
      (2) The tissue concentration of an antibiotic depends on its ability to enter that tissue. The capillary bed of the lung is nonfenestrated and therefore may limit penetration of less lipid-soluble antibiotics. Examples of lipophilic antibiotics include the macrolides, doxycycline, and trimethoprim. Examples of less lipid-soluble antibiotics include the β-lactams and the aminoglycosides. These agents require a higher concentration gradient to penetrate the lung (48).
      (3) The antimicrobial activity of some agents may be affected by the microenvironment of the lung. For example, the endobronchial pH may fall in the setting of pneumonia, which decreases the efficacy of some pH-sensitive antibiotics (*e.g.*, aminoglycosides) (7).
   b. **Interpretation of Efficacy Data**—The rapid expansion of the number of antimicrobial agents has been accompanied by a plethora of efficacy studies. Interpretation of these data is fraught with many problems, including (a) lack of prospective, randomized, double-blind trials; (b) small sample sizes; (c) lack of distinction between CAP and bronchitis, CAP and hospital-acquired pneumonia, or inpatient and outpatient pneumonias; and (d) poorly defined diagnostic criteria. In addition, many studies have been sponsored by pharmaceutical companies and only marginally peer-reviewed (11). For these reasons, specific antibiotic efficacy data are not presented in this chapter. Instead, general treatment guidelines are presented here. These are based on published algorithms and known *in vitro* efficacy.
   c. **Empiric Antimicrobial Therapy**—The cause of CAP is rarely known at the time of presentation and remains unknown in up to 60% of cases (6,19, 45,51,53,58,72). This necessitates empiric selection of antibiotic therapy based on historical and clinical features such as site of acquisition, local epidemiology, age of the patient, presence of comorbid diseases, severity of the illness, and the findings on the sputum Gram stain. In many cases, initial therapy must encompass several possible organisms and is appropriately broad in spectrum. Therapy may later be directed more specifically, in accordance with the results of the cultures and other diagnostic studies. Table 28-6 reviews the recommendations for initial management of patients hospitalized with CAP and is adapted from recent reviews (50,56). These recommendations apply only to patients who are not infected with, and not at high risk for, HIV infection and to patients in whom the gram-stained smear of the sputum is noninformative. Clinical judgment and local epidemiologic patterns may warrant modification of these guidelines. The use of prophylactic amantadine or rimantadine should strongly be considered when an outbreak of nursing home–acquired pneumonia or severe CAP occurs in a setting consistent with an influenza epidemic.
   d. **Directed Antimicrobial Therapy**
      (1) Detailed information concerning the spectrum of activity and dosage

Table 28-6 Initial empiric therapy of CAP in hospitalized patients

Patient Population	Treatment Recommendations
Non-ICU patients	Cephalosporin, preferably second- or third-generation, ±macrolide **OR** Beta-lactam with a beta-lactamase inhibitor ±macrolide If penicillin-allergic, TMP-SMX + macrolide
ICU patients	Third-generation antipseudomonal cephalosporin + macrolide **OR** Imipenem-cilastatin + macrolide **OR** Ciprofloxacin + macrolide
Patients with nursing home-acquired pneumonia	Penicillin + ciprofloxacin ±macrolide if *Legionella* is suspected **OR** Second- or third-generation cephalosporin ±macrolide if *Legionella* is suspected **OR** Beta-lactam with beta-lactamase inhibitor ±macrolide If highly penicillin-allergic, clindamycin + ciprofloxacin

Adapted from Marrie (50) and Niederman (56).

for each antibiotic class is available elsewhere (12,48). Table 28-7 is intended to serve as a guide for directed antibiotic selection in CAP. These guidelines should be modified as indicated by local epidemiologic trends, the susceptibility profile of the causative agent, and clinical judgment.

(2) Duration of treatment has not been well studied. In general, bacterial pneumonia is treated for 7 to 14 days; pneumonia caused by M pneumoniae or TWAR is treated for 14 days; and Legionella pneumonia is treated for 21 days. Conversion of parenteral to oral therapy is usually appropriate after the patient has remained afebrile for 24 hours and tolerates oral feedings and the clinical condition has improved and stabilized (50,56).

I. Outcome of Community-Acquired Pneumonia

1. **Uncomplicated Course**—The course is uncomplicated in approximately 53% of the cases of inpatient CAP (51).
   - **a.** The rate of clinical improvement from CAP depends on the premorbid condition of the patient and the severity of the pneumonia. In general, some improvement in clinical parameters (temperature, hypoxia, dyspnea, cough, or leukocytosis) can be expected within 48 to 72 hours after initiation of therapy. Treatment should not be altered within the first 72 hours unless there is a significant clinical decline or a specific pathogen is identified that is not covered by the initial antimicrobial therapy (56). By day 4 of antibiotic treatment, most patients should be afebrile, and any leukocytosis should have resolved (56).
   - **b.** Abnormal findings on lung examination may be found persistently for >1 week in up to 40% of patients. Cough and malaise may last several weeks (50,56). Radiographic improvement lags behind clinical response. Modest progression of an infiltrate may occur initially but is often insignificant in the setting of mild disease or clinical improvement. Complete radiographic resolution is usually seen in 4 to 6 weeks, although in some cases it may require 3 to 6 months. COPD, any chronic illness, age >50 years, bacteremia, severe pneumonia, and some organisms (*e.g., Legionella)* are particularly associated with slow radiologic resolution (22,47,50,56). It may be important to document a complete radiographic resolution if postobstructive pneumonia is a concern.
2. **Morbidity**—In the following discussion, the percentage of various complications associated with CAP are provided when available. However, there is no single source that fully describes the frequency of these complications, and the figures may have been derived from only one or two studies.

Table 28-7 Directed antimicrobial therapy in community-acquired pneumonia

Drug	General Antimicrobial Spectrum in CAP	Examples	Comments
Beta-lactams: Penicillins			
Natural penicillins	*S pneumoniae* and oral anaerobes	Penicillin G	Drug of choice against non–penicillin-resistant and moderately penicillin-resistant pneumococci.
Aminopenicillins	Adds some *H influenzae* and *M catarrhalis* coverage to penicillin, but not effective against beta-lactamase producing strains. Some activity against enteric GNRs.	Ampicillin	
Penicillinase-resistant penicillins	Streptococci and penicillinase-producing staphylococci. The incidence of MRSA is increasing.	Nafcillin, methicillin, oxacillin	Nearly all hospital-acquired and >80% of the community-acquired strains of *S aureus* produce penicillinase (58). Most coagulase negative staphylococci are resistant to this class of antibiotic.
Antipseudomonal penicillins	Streptococci. GNRs, including *Pseudomonas* sp. Little antistaphylococcal activity.	Ticarcillin, piperacillin	
Penicillins with beta-lactamase inhibitor	Broadens the antibiotic spectrum of parent drug to include staphylococci as well as beta-lactamase producing strains of *H influenzae*, *M catarrhalis*, GNRs, and anaerobes.	Ampicillin-sulbactam, ticarcillin-clavulnate pipercillin-tazobactam	Beta-lactamase inhibitors also inhibit staphylococcal penicillinases.
Beta-lactams: Cephalosporins	In general, gram-positive activity declines and gram-negative activity improves with advancement from first to third generation.		

Table 28-7 (continued)

First generation	Streptococci, penicillinase-producing staphylococci, non–beta-lactamase–producing enteric GNRs, *H influenzae*, and *M catarrhalis*. Most anaerobes, except *Bacteroides*.	Cephalexin, cefazolin	
Second generation	Cefuroxime: Streptococci, penicillinase-producing staphylococci, and beta-lactamase–producing enteric GNRs, *H influenzae*, and *M catarrhalis*. Most anaerobes, except *Bacteroides*. Cefotetan. As above, with added activity against *Bacteroides; B fragilis* may be resistant.	Cefuroxime, cefotetan	
Third-generation	Ceftriaxone and cefotaxime: Streptococci (including penicillin resistant strains). Beta-lactamase–producing strains of *H influenzae* and *M catarrhalis*. Most enteric and many nonenteric GNRs. Limited activity against *Pseudomonas*, staphylococci, and anaerobes. Ceftazidime: Virtually all GNRs, including *P aeruginosa*. Beta-lactamase–producing strains of *H influenzae* and *M catarrhalis*. Poor activity against most gram-positive organisms and anaerobes.	Ceftriaxone, cefotaxime, ceftazidime	Ceftriaxone and cefotaxime: Drug of choice for highly penicillin-resistant pneumococci. Ceftazidime: Poor choice for monotherapy if gram-positive organism is the potential pathogen.
Beta-lactams: Carbapenems	Streptococci (including most penicillin-resistant strains), penicillinase-producing staphylococci, virtually all GNRs, including *P aeruginosa*. Anaerobes.	Imipenem-cilistatin	

Table 28-7 (continued)

Drug	General Antimicrobial Spectrum in CAP	Examples	Comments
Beta-lactams: Monobactams	Virtually all GNRs, including *P aeruginosa*. Poor activity against gram-positive organisms and anaerobes.	Aztreonam	
Macrolides	Erythromycin: Streptococci, *M pneumoniae*, *Legionella*, *C pneumoniae*. Some staphylococci, *M catarrhalis*, and anaerobes. Poor activity against -GNRs. Clarithromycin and azithromycin: As above with enhanced activity against *H influenzae* and *M catarrhalis*.	Erythromycin, clarithromycin, azithromycin	Erythromycin is drug of choice in *Legionella* and penicillin-allergic patient with pneumococcus. Macrolides are choice agents in CAP with *M pneumoniae* and good alternative to doxycycline for treatment of *Chlamydia*. Azithromycin does not yield high serum levels and has limited use in bacteremia.
Aminoglycosides	Most GNRs, including *P aeruginosa*. *Pseudomonas* resistance varies geographically. Synergistic activity with penicillin against some gram-positive cocci (i.e., enterococci).	Gentamicin, tobramycin, amikacin	Efficacy as a sole agent in CAP may be limited by poor tissue levels and local inactivation by. acidic pH.
Fluoroquinolones	Most GNRs, including *P aeruginosa*. Atypicals: *Legionella*, *M pneumoniae* (limited), *C pneumoniae* (limited). Beta-lactamase–producing strains of *H influenzae* and *M catarrhalis*. Some staphylococci, including some MRSA. Poor streptococcus and anaerobe activity.	Ciprofloxacin	Poor choice as monotherapy if *S pneumoniae* is a potential pathogen. Oral therapy provides similar serum levels as intravenous therapy.
Tetracyclines	Atypicals: *Legionella*, *M pneumoniae*, *C pneumoniae*. Some streptococci staphylococci, *H influenzae*, and *M catarrhalis*, but resistance is rising.	Doxycycline, tetracycline	Drug of choice in chlamydial pneumonia.

Table 28-7 (continued)

Drug	General Antimicrobial Spectrum in CAP	Examples	Comments
TMP-SMX	*H influenzae* and *M catarrhalis*. Most streptococci. Many staphylococci, including some MRSA. Most GNRs, but limited against *Pseudomonas*. Excellent coverage against *Pneumocystis carinii*. Poor activity against anaerobic organisms.		Inexpensive, broad-spectrum alternative to beta-lactam agents. In some areas GNRs are becoming increasingly resistant.
Clindamycin	Streptococci, most staphylococci, all anaerobes.		Alternative to penicillin for aspiration pneumonia.
Vancomycin	Virtually all streptococci and staphylococci, including MRSA. Limited anaerobic spectrum.		Drug of choice in CAP due to MRSA. Also indicated for cephalosporin-resistant (third-generation) pneumococci.
Metronidazole	Anaerobes. Not effective against facultative anaerobes.		Good combination drug for anaerobic CAP.

a. **Infectious Complications**—Empyema (8% of ICU patients), lung abscess, secondary infection (12%), and metastatic infection (in up to 10% of bacteremic patients) may complicate CAP (51,56,72).

b. **Noninfectious Complications**—Respiratory failure requiring mechanical ventilation (18% of all cases; 60% of ICU patients), ARDS (25% of ICU patients), renal failure (2.7% of all cases; 39% of ICU patients), septic shock (24% of ICU patients), cardiac dysrhythmias (22% of ICU patients), myocardial infarction, cardiac failure (11.3% of all cases), disseminated intravascular coagulation (9% of ICU patients), multiple organ dysfunction syndrome, or prolonged debilitation (in up to 55% of elderly patients) may result from CAP (34,50,51,56,72).

c. Progression or failure to respond after 72 hours requires reevaluation of the patient with repeat microbiologic studies and possibly invasive diagnostic measures. The following circumstances must be considered and ruled out.

(1) Complication by empyema, abscess, or ARDS may occur.

(2) Concomitant infection or superinfection with one or more additional organisms may occur.

(3) Inappropriate antimicrobial therapy caused by incorrect empiric selection of antibiotics, unusual or unsuspected etiologic agent, or antibiotic resistance may be responsible for the failure to respond.

(4) **Noninfectious Illnesses**—Neoplasm, bronchiolitis obliterans, Hamman–Rich syndrome, hypersensitivity pneumonitis, drug-induced pneumonitis, pulmonary vasculitis, pulmonary fibrosis, pulmonary alveolar proteinosis, pulmonary hemorrhage, pulmonary embolism, and congestive heart failure can mimic CAP (22,37,56).

3. **Mortality**—CAP requiring hospitalization carries an in-hospital mortality rate of 13% to 24%. The mortality rate is higher among ICU and nursing home patients (19,51,53,58,72). Follow-up studies showed that up to 32% of patients with CAP die within 2 years (50). This finding probably reflects a high prevalence of other serious underlying illnesses in this population.

J. Indications for Hospitalization and Prognostic Indicators in CAP

1. **Indications for Hospitalization**—Well-accepted indications for hospitalization include a severe vital sign abnormality, advanced age, comorbid disease, hypoxia, altered mental status, suppurative infection, infectious complications (*e.g.*, empyema), and severe metabolic or hematologic derangement. In addition, independent predictors of morbidity and mortality have been identified to differentiate high-risk from low-risk patients. Ultimately, the decision to hospitalize should be based on clinical judgment and the overall appearance of the patient.

2. **Predictors of Morbidity**—Fine performed a prospective observational study of patients with CAP (hospital inpatients and outpatients) to identify clinical factors predictive of a complicated course. Age >65 years, presence of comorbid illness, fever >38.3° C, immunosuppression, and "high-risk" cause (*i.e.*, CAP associated with GNRs, staphylococci, aspiration, or obstruction) were independent predictors of a complicated course. Presence of two or more of these factors was considered an indication for hospitalization (25).

3. **Predictors of Mortality**—Numerous studies have attempted to define predictors of mortality in patients with CAP. More than 100 parameters have been identified, and these have been summarized elsewhere (21,50,56). The major prognostic factors are described here.

a. Fine developed a mortality prognostic index which has been well validated. This index classifies patients into one of five risk categories based on six predictors of mortality: age >65 years, mental status changes, severe vital sign abnormality, neoplasia, and "high-risk" cause (*i.e.*, CAP associated with GNRs, staphylococci, aspiration, or obstruction). Pleuritic chest pain was found to be a protective prognostic factor (26,27). In another study which corrected for the presence of comorbid illnesses, healthy elderly patients did not have a higher mortality rate than their younger counterparts (9).

b. Farr applied stepwise logistic regression analysis to 42 previously reported prognostic indicators of CAP. Patients with postobstructive CAP were excluded, and the cause of the pneumonia was not considered. When only the data available at presentation were used, respiratory rate >30 breaths per minute, blood urea nitrogen >7 mmol/L, and diastolic blood pressure <60 mm Hg were found to be independent predictors of death (21).

c. For patients with CAP who required admission to an ICU, progression of radiographic infiltrate, advanced age, and presence of septic shock were found to be predictors of death (53,58,72).

d. Compared with other causes, pneumonias caused by *S aureus* or GNR, particularly *P aeruginosa*, were often associated with a higher mortality rate (50% and 35% to 100%, respectively) (19,26,51,53,72). The lowest mortality rates were observed with pneumonias caused by *M pneumoniae* (0%) or TWAR (4.5%) (19). In addition, patients with bacteremia typically had higher mortality rates (50,53,72).

K. Prevention of Community-Acquired Pneumonia

1. Pneumococcal Vaccine (23-Valent Pneumococcal Polysaccharide Vaccine)

a. At present, the Immunization Practice Advisory Committee of the US Public Health Service recommends pneumococcal vaccination for all persons older than 65 years of age; for those with chronic illnesses (including diabetes mellitus, alcoholism, cirrhosis, chronic lung disease, and chronic heart disease) or immunocompromising disorders (including asplenia, chronic renal failure, organ transplantation, lymphoma, hematologic malignancies, and HIV infection); and for those living in special environments, including institutionalized settings (62). Revaccination may be indicated in selected patients. (14).

b. However, despite this recommendation, the efficacy of the pneumococcal vaccination is intensely debated. Although a randomized controlled trial among South African gold miners (for whom the risk of pneumococcal pneumonia is extremely high) demonstrated an 80% to 90% reduction in the frequency of pneumococcal pneumonia caused by vaccine serotypes (67), other prospective randomized trials failed to demonstrate a benefit of the pneumococcal vaccine in populations similar to that targeted by the Immunization Practice Advisory Committee (4,63,65). Therefore, some investigators argue against the use of this vaccine because of its unproven efficacy and the high cost of widespread vaccination (39). However, others favor aggressive immunization of high-risk groups based on the unequivocal safety and relatively low cost of each dose of vaccine.

c. The advocates of the vaccine claim that the uncertain efficacy results from a lack of large prospective trials with adequate statistical power conducted among patients with proven pneumococcal pneumonia. For example, isolation of *S pneumoniae* from the sputum may simply represent colonization and does not necessarily prove *S pneumoniae* to be the cause of the pneumonia. Therefore, many cases of pneumococcal pneumonia defined by sputum culture in randomized trials may have been caused by another organism, which would have diluted any differences in outcome between the vaccinated and the control groups. This problem was overcome by Shapiro's case-control study involving 1054 prospectively identified patients with *S pneumoniae* isolated from any normally sterile site (blood, pleural fluid, cerebrospinal fluid) who had an indication for pneumococcal vaccination (64a). For each of these patients, a control patient was matched for age; for comorbid illnesses, especially the indication for vaccination; and for site of hospitalization. All patients were >18 years of age. Eighteen percent of the case patients were immunocompromised, but those with the acquired immunodeficiency syndrome were excluded. Of the case patients, 82% and 93% were infected by a serotype represented in the 14-valent and the 23-valent vaccines, respectively.

(1) Overall, 13% of the case patients and 20% of the control patients had been vaccinated against pneumococcus (14- or 23-valent). The protective efficacy was estimated at 56% ($P<0.00001$) against the serotypes represented in the vaccine; it was not effective against unrepresented serotypes. For the subgroup whose only indication for vaccination was age, the protective efficacy was 40% (P=NS). There was no significant difference in case fatality rate between the two groups.

(2) The efficacy of the vaccine varied with the age and immune status of the patient (*i.e.*, immunocompromised versus immunocompetent). For example, among immunocompetent patients <55 years of age, the protective efficacy was 93%, compared with 46% for those ≥85 years old. In the immunocompromised subgroup, the protective efficacy was 21% (P=NS), compared with 61% in the immunocompetent subgroup ($P<0.00001$).

d. These issues are well summarized in a recent metaanalysis (24). As in the case-control study by Shapiro (64a), this metaanalysis demonstrated a benefit of the vaccine for prevention of pneumococcal pneumonia in low-risk patients but not in the high-risk population (elderly and chronically ill persons), for whom the vaccination is usually recommended. No mortality benefit was observed with vaccination. The lack of efficacy in the high-risk subgroup may be explained by an impaired immune response to the vaccine in these persons. Conversely, a benefit may not have been detected because the studies simply lacked sufficient statistical power to identify those who would most benefit from the vaccine. Further trials are needed to settle this debate.

2. Influenza Vaccine—The efficacy of the influenza vaccine is undisputed, and annual vaccination is recommended for the following persons: residents of nursing homes and chronic care facilities; patients with chronic pulmonary, cardiac, or systemic disease (*e.g.*, diabetes, renal failure, immunosuppression); those ≥65 years of age; and health care workers. Vaccine administration is contraindicated in persons with an allergy to eggs. Immunization achieves 65% to 80% protection against infection in young adults; 30% to 40% protection is seen in elderly persons, but a larger benefit is conferred by a reduction in the severity of the illness and a decrease in the mortality rate. Placebo-controlled studies have shown that vaccine-related side effects are significantly less common than had been anecdotally reported (33,60). Systemic adverse reaction was no more likely after receipt of vaccine than after placebo (11% versus 9.4%, respectively; P=NS). Local adverse reactions were reported in up to one third of vaccinated patients and did occur more frequently with vaccine than with placebo (17.5% versus 7.3%, respectively; $P<0.001$) (33).

3. Amantadine or rimantadine is effective for prophylaxis and treatment of influenza A, but not against influenza B. Drug-resistant isolates may develop readily (16,23,30).

L. Summary

1. The epidemiology of CAP has changed over the past several decades. The population at risk for CAP includes increasing numbers of elderly, immunocompromised, and chronically ill patients. Newly described or characterized etiologic agents such as *Legionella*, TWAR, *M catarrhalis*, and hantavirus have been identified. Numerous new, broad-spectrum antibiotics have been developed, accompanied by a worrisome rise in the incidence of antimicrobial resistance against many of the pathogens in CAP.

2. Pneumonia most frequently occurs as a result of aspiration or inhalation of pathogenic organisms into a normally sterile lower respiratory tract. Some pathogens, such as *S pneumoniae*, are commensal organisms in the upper respiratory tract of normal individuals. In other instances, underlying illness leads to colonization of the upper respiratory tract with additional pathogens, thereby increasing the risk of pneumonia caused by these organisms.
3. The cause of CAP remains undefined in up to 60% of the cases, despite rigorous microbiologic evaluation. This is most likely a result of several factors, including prior treatment with antibiotics, inadequate sputum specimens, and an inability to detect or identify certain pathogens.
4. *S pneumoniae* is the most common cause of CAP and accounts for approximately 10% to 40% of cases. *H influenzae* (4% to 10%), GNRs (5% to 10%), *Legionella* (0% to 7%), *M pneumoniae* (2% to 7%), *S aureus* (1% to 4%), TWAR (1% to 6%), and viruses (0% to 9%) are the other major pathogens. Aspiration pneumonia is diagnosed in up to 15% of the cases and is most commonly seen in elderly or chronically ill persons.
5. Cough, sputum production, and fever are the most common presenting signs and symptoms of CAP. However, these features may be absent in some patients, particularly elderly patients. Clinical studies have shown that the cause of pneumonia cannot be reliably identified on the bases of "typical" versus "atypical" presenting features.
6. The history and the physical examination are important tools in the generation of a differential diagnosis. They should be used to guide the diagnostic evaluation and the selection of empiric therapy. The laboratory and microbiologic evaluation of the hospitalized patient with CAP should include a complete blood count with differential, a complete chemistry panel, measure of arterial oxygenation, CXR, sputum Gram stain and culture, two sets of blood cultures, and an analysis and culture of the pleural fluid (if present). Additional studies, such as serology or rapid antigen tests, should be performed as warranted by the clinical setting. Cultures of blood, pleural fluid, or tissue obtained by fiberoptic bronchoscopy provide gold-standard microbiologic data. The sputum Gram stain and culture must be interpreted with attention to the quality of the specimen.
7. Treatment of CAP should include supportive measures such as oxygen and chest physiotherapy as well as antimicrobial treatment. If the sputum Gram stain is not informative, the initial antibiotic selection is empiric and should be broad enough to cover the pathogens most likely to cause CAP in the particular patient. Once a causative organism is identified, a more specific antimicrobial regimen should be selected.
8. CAP is associated with an uncomplicated course in approximately 53% of the cases. The potential complications of CAP include sepsis, respiratory failure, empyema, lung abscess, ARDS, congestive heart failure, cardiac arrhythmia, and renal failure. The mortality rate is 13% to 24% and may be as high as 40% to 50% in ICU or nursing home patients.
9. More than 100 predictors of morbidity or mortality have been identified for patients with CAP. In general, age >65 years, presence of chronic disease, imunosuppression, severe vital sign abnormality, severe metabolic abnormality, sepsis, and bacteremia are commonly viewed as poor prognostic factors.

Abbreviations used in Chapter 28

ARDS = adult respiratory distress syndrome
BAL = bronchoalveolar lavage

bpm = beats per minute
CAP = community-acquired pneumonia
COPD = chronic obstructive pulmonary disease
CFT = complement fixation titer
CFU = colony-forming units
CIE = countercurrent immunoelectrophoresis
COPD = chronic obstructive pulmonary disease
CXR = chest roentgenogram
DFA = direct fluorescent antibody
GNR = gram-negative rod
H_2O_2 = hydrogen peroxide
HIV = human immunodeficiency virus
ICU = intensive care unit
IFA = immunofluorescent antibodies
IgG = immunoglobulin G
IgM = immunoglobulin M
MRSA = methicillin-resistant *Staphylococcus aureus*
NHAP = nursing home–acquired pneumonia
NS = not statistically significant
P = probability value
PNA = percutaneous needle aspiration
RSV = respiratory syncytial virus
TMP-SMX = trimethoprim-sulfamethoxazole
TWAR = *Chlamydia pneumoniae*

References

1. Ali. The clinical spectrum and diagnosis of *Mycoplasma pneumoniae* infection. *Q J Med* 1986;58:241.
2. Aronson. Blood cultures. *Ann Intern Med* 1987;106:246.
3. Austrian. Pneumococcal infections. In: Isselbacher, ed. *Harrison's Principles of Internal Medicine.* New York: McGraw-Hill, 1994:607.
4. Austrian. *Surveillance of Pneumococcal Infection for Field Trials of Polyvalent Pneumococcal Vaccines.* Bethesda, MD: National Institutes of Health. 1980 Publication DAB-VDP-12-84.
5. Barrett-Connor. The nonvalue of sputum culture in the diagnosis of pneumococcal pneumonia. *Am Rev Respir Dis* 1971;103:845.
6. Bates. Microbial etiology of acute pneumonia in hospitalized patients. *Chest* 1992; 101:1005.
7. Boden. Endobronchial pH. Relevance to aminoglycoside activity in gram-negative bacillary pneumonia. *Am Rev Respir Dis* 1983;127:39.
8. Boerner. The value of the sputum Gram's stain in community-acquired pneumonia. *JAMA* 1982;247:642.
9. Brancati. Is pneumonia really the old man's friend? Two year prognosis after community-acquired pneumonia. *Lancet* 1993;342:30.
10. Bynum. Pulmonary aspiration of gastric contents. *Am Rev Respir Dis* 1976;114: 1129.
11. Chow. Antibiotic studies in pneumonia: pitfalls in interpretation and suggested solutions. *Chest* 1989;96:453.
12. Craig. Penicillins. In: Gorbach, ed. *Infectious Diseases.* Philadelphia: WB Saunders, 1992:160.
13. Davidson. Bacterial diagnosis of acute pneumonia. Comparison of sputum, transtracheal aspirates, and lung aspirates. *JAMA* 1976;235:158.
14. Davidson. Immunogenicity of pneumococcal revaccination in patients with chronic disease. *Arch Intern Med* 1994;154:2209.

15. DePaso. Aspiration Pneumonia. *Clin Chest Med* 1991;12:269.
16. Douglas. Prophylaxis and treatment of influenza. *N Engl J Med* 1990;322:443.
17. Duchin. Hantavirus pulmonary syndrome: a clinical description of 17 patients with a newly recognized disease. *N Engl J Med* 1994;330:949.
18. Eisenstein. Diseases caused by gram-negative enteric bacilli. In: Isselbacher, ed. *Harrison's Principles of Internal Medicine.* New York: McGraw-Hill, 1994: 661.
19. Fang. New and emerging etiologies for community-acquired pneumonia with implications for therapy. *Medicine (Baltimore)* 1990;69:307.
20. Farr. Prediction of microbiologic aetiology at admission to hospital for pneumonia from the presenting clinical features. *Thorax* 1989;44:1031.
21. Farr. Predicting death in patients hospitalized for community-acquired pneumonia. *Ann Intern Med* 1991;115:428.
22. Fein. "When the pneumonia doesn't get better." *Clin Chest Med* 1987;8:529
23. Fiebach. Prevention of respiratory infections in adults: influenza and pneumococcal vaccines. *Arch Intern Med* 1994;154:2545.
24. Fine. Efficacy of pneumococcal vaccination in adults: a meta-analysis of randomized controlled trials. *Arch Intern Med* 1994;154:2666.
25. Fine. Hospitalization decision in patients with community-acquired pneumonia: a prospective cohort study. *Am J Med* 1990;89:713.
26. Fine. Prognosis of patients hospitalized with community-acquired pneumonia. *Am J Med* 1990;88:5-1N.
27. Fine. Validation of a pneumonia prognostic index using the Medisgroup comparative hospital database. *Am J Med* 1993;94:153.
28. Finegold. Aspiration pneumonia. *Rev Infect Dis* 1991;13(Suppl 9):S737.
29. Fishman. Use of induced sputum specimens for microbiologic diagnosis of infections due to organisms other than *Pneumocystis carinii. J Clin Microbiol* 1994; 32:131.
30. Gardner. Immunization of Adults. *N Engl J Med* 1993;328:1252.
31. Garibaldi. Epidemiology of community-acquired respiratory tract infections in adults: incidence, etiology, and impact. *Am J Med* 1985;78(Suppl 6B):32.
32. Gleckman. Sputum gram stain assessment in community-acquired bacteremic pneumonia. *J Clin Microbiol* 1988;26:846.
33. Govaert. Adverse reactions to influenza vaccine in elderly people: randomised double blind placebo controlled trial. *Br Med J* 1993;307:988.
34. Granton. Community-acquired pneumonia in the elderly patient. *Clin Chest Med* 1993;14:537.
35. Greenberg. Viral pneumonia. *Infect Dis Clin North Am* 1991;5:603.
36. Griffin. Rapid screening for cold agglutinins in pneumonia. *Ann Intern Med* 1969; 70:705.
37. Gross. Noninfectious pulmonary diseases masquerading as community acquired pneumonia. *Clin Chest Med* 1991;12:363.
38. Heckerling. Clinical prediction rule for pulmonary infiltrates. *Ann Intern Med* 1990; 113:664.
39. Hirschmann. The pneumococcal vaccine after 15 years of use. *Arch Intern Med* 1994; 154:373.
40. Hirschtick. *Staphylococcus aureus* pneumonia: when to suspect, how to treat. *Journal of Critical Illness* 1992;7:1576.
41. Huxley. Pharyngeal aspiration in normal adults and patients with depressed consciousness. *Am J Med* 1978;64:564.
42. Kirby. Legionnaires' disease: report of sixty-five nosocomially acquired cases and review of the literature. *Medicine (Baltimore)* 1980;59:188.
43. Kohler. Update on legionnaires' disease: how to make the diagnosis, how best to treat. *Journal of Critical Illness* 1993;8:771.
44. Kramer. Pneumococcal bacteremia: no change in mortality in 30 years. Analysis of 104 cases and review of the literature. *Isr J Med Sci* 1987;23:174.
45. Levy. Community-acquired pneumonia. Importance of initial noninvasive bacteriologic and radiographic investigations. *Chest* 1988;92:43.

46. Luby. Pneumonia caused by *Mycoplasma pneumoniae* infection. *Clin Chest Med* 1991;12:237.
47. MacFarlane. Comparative radiographic features of community acquired legionnaires' disease, pneumococcal pneumonia, mycoplasma pneumonia, and psittacosis. *Thorax* 1984;39:28.
48. Mandell. Antibiotics for pneumonia therapy. *Med Clin North Am* 1994;78:997.
49. Manresa. Needle aspiration techniques in the diagnosis of pneumonia. *Thorax* 1991; 40:661.
50. Marrie. Community-acquired pneumonia. *Clin Infect Dis* 1994;18:501.
51. Marrie. Community-acquired pneumonia requiring hospitalization: 5-year prospective study. *Rev Infect Dis* 1989;2:586.
52. Meduri. The role of bronchoalveolar lavage in diagnosing nonopportunistic bacterial pneumonia. *Chest* 1991;100:179.
53. Moine. Severe community-acquired pneumonia: etiology, epidemiology, and prognosis factors. *Chest* 1994;105:1487.
54. Musher. Pneumonia and acute febrile tracheobronchitis due to *Haemophilus influenzae*. *Ann Intern Med* 1983;99:444.
55. Nguyen. *Legionella* infection. *Clin Chest Med* 1991;12:257.
56. Niederman. American Thoracic Society guidelines for the initial management of adults with community-acquired pneumonia. Diagnosis, assessment of severity, and initial antimicrobial therapy. *Am Rev Respir Dis* 1993;148:1418.
57. Ortqvist. Diagnostic fiberoptic bronchoscopy and protected brush culture in patients with community-acquired pneumonia. *Chest* 1990;97:576.
58. Pachon. Severe community-acquired pneumonia. Etiology, prognosis, and treatment. *Am Rev Respir Dis* 1990;142:369.
59. Pruzanski. Biologic activity of cold-reacting autoantibodies. *N Engl J Med* 1977:297: 583.
60. Quinnan. Serologic responses and systemic reactions in adults after vaccination with monovalent A/USSR/77, and trivalent A/USSR/77, A/Texas/77, B/Hong Kong/ 72 influenza vaccines. *Rev Infect Dis* 1983;5:748.
61. Rein. Accuracy of Gram's stain in identifying pneumococci in sputum. *JAMA* 1978;239:2671.
62. Recommendations of the Immunization Practices Advisory Committee: pneumococcal polysaccharide vaccine. *MMWR Morb Mortal Wkly Rep* 1989;38:64.
63. Ruben. Efficacy of pneumococcal vaccine in severe chronic obstructive pulmon ary disease. *Can Med Assoc J* 1987;136:361.
64. Ruf. Prevalence and diagnosis of *Legionella* pneumonia: a 3-year prospective study with emphasis on application of urinary antigen detection. *J Infect Dis* 1990;162: 1341.
64a. Shapiro. The protective efficacy of polyvalent pneumococcal polysaccharide vaccine. *N Engl J Med* 1991;325:1453.
65. Simberkoff. Efficacy of pneumococcal vaccine in high-risk patients: results of a Veterans Administration Cooperative Study. *N Engl J Med* 1986;315:1318.
66. Skerrett. Host defenses against respiratory infection. *Med Clin North Am* 1994; 78:941.
67. Smit. Protective efficacy of pneumococcal polysaccharide vaccines. *JAMA* 1977; 238:2613.
68. Smith. New developments in the diagnosis of viral diseases. *Infect Dis Clin North Am* 1993;7:183.
69. Tew. Bacterial or nonbacterial pneumonia: accuracy of radiographic diagnosis. *Radiology* 1977;124:607.
70. Thom. Infections with *Chlamydia pneumoniae* strain TWAR. *Clin Chest Med* 1991; 12:245.
71. Thorsteinsson. The diagnostic value of sputum culture in acute pneumonia. *JAMA* 1975;233:894.
72. Torres. Severe community-acquired pneumonia. Epidemiology and prognostic factors. *Am Rev Respir Dis* 1991;144:312.
73. Venkatesan. A hospital study of community acquired pneumonia in the elderly. *Thorax* 1990;45:254.

74. Winn. *Legionella* and the clinical microbiologist. *Infect Dis Clin North Am* 1993; 7:377.
75. Wright. A descriptive study of 42 cases of *Branhamella catarrhalis* pneumonia. *Am J Med* 1990;88:5A-2S.
76. Zavala. Ultrathin needle aspiration of the lung in infectious and malignant disease. *Am Rev Respir Dis* 1981;123:125.

Nosocomial Pneumonia

Laura A. Napolitano,
Les A. Szekely, and
B. Taylor Thompson

A. Introduction

1. Nosocomial pneumonia (NP) refers specifically to a pneumonia acquired in a hospital setting. By definition, a nosocomial infection must not be evident or incubating at the time of hospital admission. Therefore, most studies of NP require that evidence of lung infection be absent within the first 48 to 72 hours of hospitalization.
2. Ventilator-associated pneumonia (VAP) refers more specifically to a subgroup of NP that develops in patients who have been mechanically ventilated for at least 48 hours. Because much of the clinical data regarding NP are based on those with VAP, these two terms are often used interchangeably in the literature.
3. The clinical investigation of NP has been marred by the lack of a readily available gold standard for diagnosis. Inclusion and diagnostic criteria have varied widely from study to study. Consequently, there is great disparity in the data regarding the epidemiology and treatment of NP, and some of the available data may not be reliable. The recent advances in diagnostic technique and the standardization of diagnostic criteria have improved the quality of available information.
4. The discussion of NP in this chapter is limited to immunocompetent adults. NP refers to both VAP and non-VAP unless otherwise specified.

B. Epidemiology of Nosocomial Pneumonia

1. NP occurs in 0.4% to 1.1% of hospitalized patients. It is the most common infection in intensive care units and the second most common cause of nosocomial infection overall (27,44,53). Intensive care unit incidence is regularly cited to be 21% to 26%, although it may be as low as 9% to 11% when more specific diagnostic methods are employed (1,35). NP has been reported to develop in 25% to 58% of mechanically ventilated patients, depending on the method of diagnosis (35,57). The rate of infection is estimated to be 1% to 3% per day of mechanical ventilation (1,35,44,70).
2. NP is the leading cause of death from nosocomial infection and is responsible for 25,000 to 108,000 deaths per year (15,46,102). VAP carries an estimated mortality of 20–50%. The mortality rate is generally lower for nonintubated patients and for those who were previously healthy (24,27,44,102). However, the mortality rate may be as high as 60% to 100% for those with adult respiratory distress syndrome (ARDS) and for those infected with a more virulent pathogen such as *Pseudomonas aeruginosa* (32,80). On the average, each episode of NP results in 6 to 13 additional days of hospitalization (15,34,102).

C. Pathogenesis of Nosocomial Pneumonia

1. Basic Principles

a. The lower respiratory tract (LRT) is normally sterile. This environment is maintained by structural barriers (nasal vibrissae, larynx, branched airways), protective mechanisms (gag reflex, mucociliary clearance, cough reflex), and immune-mediated defenses (immunoglobulins A and G, alveolar macrophages) (104).
b. Although there are numerous means by which bacteria gain access to the LRT, it is the host factors that typically determine whether or not a pneumonia will develop. Healthy individuals are less susceptible to NP because the normal host immune system is able to overcome most microbial chal-

lenges to the LRT. Thus, NP is most likely to occur in a setting of impaired host defenses, such as recent surgery, sepsis, chronic pulmonary disease, neurologic disease, ARDS, trauma, endotracheal intubation, malnutrition, or advanced age.

2. Airway Colonization

a. In the normal host, the upper respiratory tract is colonized by *Streptococcus pneumoniae*, *Streptococcus* species, *Haemophilus* species, *Neisseria* species, and anaerobic bacteria. *Haemophilus influenzae* and *Moraxella catarrhalis* also frequently colonize the upper respiratory tract of smokers. Normally, the presence of these organisms as well as anaerobes decreases the risk of colonization by gram-negative bacilli (GNRs) (1,104). For example, when healthy volunteers gargled a radiolabelled suspension of GNRs, serial oropharyngeal cultures demonstrated that <1% of the initial inoculum remained after 3 hours (68).

b. However, patients who are ill do not resist bacillary colonization as well. Johanson performed oropharyngeal culture analyses on 253 individuals: 82 healthy outpatients, 47 healthy hospital staff, 20 physically well psychiatric inpatients, 81 moderately ill orthopedic inpatients, and 23 critically ill medical inpatients. Fewer than 6% of the outpatients, hospital staff, and psychiatric inpatients were colonized with oropharyngeal GNRs. Conversely, cultures were positive for GNRs in 35% of moderately ill and 73% of critically ill patients (58).

c. In another study, Johanson demonstrated that bacillary colonization of critically ill patients occurs within the first hospital day for 20% of patients and within the first 4 days for 40%. Twenty-three percent of patients colonized with GNRs developed nosocomial respiratory infection, whereas only 3% of noncolonized patients became infected (60). Numerous risk factors are associated with the risk of GNR colonization; these include a history of prior antibiotic use, severe and prolonged illness, intubation, tracheostomy, major surgery, tobacco use, malnutrition, diabetes mellitus, coma, nasoenteric intubation, alcohol abuse, and preexisting pulmonary disease (1,44,60).

d. The increased rate of GNR colonization is a result of enhanced bacillary adherence to oropharyngeal and tracheal epithelium (59). *P aeruginosa* appears to have a predilection for tracheal epithelium and may colonize the LRT without first colonizing the oropharynx (1,32,44). In addition, the endotracheal tube may also provide a foundation for bacterial colonization. Up to 84% of these tubes may be covered with a bacterial biofilm. This site appears to be impervious to antibiotics (24,56).

3. Aspiration into the LRT

a. NP probably develops as a result of overt or subclinical aspiration of colonizing bacteria. Microaspiration has been demonstrated in 45% of normal individuals by nasopharyngeal radiolabelling. Persons with a depressed state of consciousness aspirate at a rate of 70% (54).

b. Despite the use of a tracheal cuff, patients with an endotracheal or tracheostomy tube may still aspirate. Stagnant bacteria-laden secretions often pool above and around the endotracheal cuff (24,44,72). A properly inflated balloon cuff does not adequately protect against aspiration. Aspiration with a low-volume, high-pressure cuff occurs in up to 87% of tracheostomy patients and 56% of patients with an endotracheal tube. The rate of aspiration with high-volume, low-pressure cuffs is lower, at 15% to 20% (33,72,102).

c. Aspiration may also result from aerosolization of bacteria from the endotracheal biofilm. Furthermore, microemboli of bacteria, possibly generated by suction catheters as they pass through the endotracheal tube, may also be aspirated (72).

4. Mechanical Disruption of Host Defenses—The endotracheal and tracheostomy tubes bypass the normal upper respiratory tract defenses and provide direct access to the LRT. Mucociliary transport is also impaired, and the cough and gag reflexes become ineffective. The presence of a nasogastric tube may similarly inhibit the host defenses (44,72). Direct trauma from the placement or the presence of an endotracheal tube, tracheostomy tube, or nasogastric tube may cause denudation of epithelial cells and create a nidus for bacterial colonization. Blind suctioning procedures may also damage the epithelium (44,72).

5. **Colonization of the Gastrointestinal Tract**
   a. Loss of gastric acidity may promote bacterial overgrowth, which can become a potential reservoir of nosocomial pathogens. Antacids, histamine$_2$ (H_2) blockade, and enteral feedings all increase the pH of gastric secretions. In a study of 60 mechanically ventilated patients receiving antacids or H_2 blockade, the mean gastric pH was 5.52. The gastric aspirate of these patients contained an average bacterial concentration of 10^8 colony-forming units (CFUs) per milliliter, mostly GNRs (31). In addition, even when no alkalinizing agents are used, the gastric pH may rise to above 4 in up to 77% of critically ill patients (1).
   b. Nasoenteric intubation causes disruption of the lower esophageal sphincter and may predispose the patient to gastroesophageal reflux and aspiration. When a radiolabelled solution was infused via a nasoenteric tube into the stomach of critically ill patients, reflux and aspiration were demonstrated in 83% of cases (55). Supine positioning and increased gastric volume due to an ileus or enteral feeding may increase the risk of reflux and aspiration (6).
   c. Several investigators have cultured pathogenic organisms simultaneously from the stomach and the upper respiratory tract and have suggested that upper respiratory tract colonization may originate from a gastric reservoir. Some studies using serial cultures with biotype analysis have shown that pathogenic organisms first colonize the stomach and then are aspirated into the respiratory tract, where they may cause NP. However, other studies investigating the precise sequence of colonization have demonstrated conflicting results (10,31,92,105). Furthermore, some studies suggest that bacterial colonization of the stomach or alkalinization of gastric contents may not predispose to NP. Therefore, the role of gastric colonization in NP remains controversial (see Section K).
6. **Hematogenous or Local Spread of Infection**—NP may be seeded hematogenously from other infectious sources such as catheters, wounds, or urinary infections. Sinusitis may extend locally to involve the respiratory tract, particularly in patients who are nasotracheally intubated (47,52).
7. **Contamination of Hospital Equipment and by Personnel**
   a. Outbreaks of NP have been linked to contaminated respiratory equipment, including ventilator circuits, nebulizers, multidose medication vials, ventilation bags, and spirometers (6,25,44). *P aeruginosa*, *Acinetobacter* species, and *Legionella* species are the most common etiologic agents in outbreaks (6,44).
   b. *Staphylococcus aureus* (usually from the skin or nares) or GNRs (usually from respiratory or intestinal secretions) may be transmitted to patients by unsanitary use of shared equipment or by unwashed hands of medical personnel (6).
   c. A wide variety of pathogens, including GNRs, *S aureus*, and fungi, have been cultured from enteral feeding solutions. One study showed 68% of feeding solutions to be contaminated with *Klebsiella pneumoniae* (6). Contaminated enteral solutions may promote gastric colonization with a potential pathogen.

D. **Risk Factors for Nosocomial Pneumonia**—The risk factors for NP can readily be inferred from an understanding of its pathogenesis. Continuous mechanical ventilation is the strongest risk factor for the development of NP (6- to 21-fold increase in risk). The risk of NP increases with the duration of mechanical ventilation. Advanced age is also a major risk factor for NP. Numerous other risk factors have been identified, and the most significant are summarized in Table 29-1.

Table 29-1 Risk factors for nosocomial pneumonia

Risk Factor	Reference
Mechanical ventilation	14, 24, 44, 48
Thoracoabdominal surgery	14, 24, 44, 48, 62
Advanced age	14, 24, 35, 44, 65
Increased duration of intubation	24, 35, 44, 70, 106
Severity of illness	24, 35, 44, 65
Macroaspiration	14, 106
Depressed level of consciousness	14, 24
Chronic pulmonary disease	14, 24, 44, 106
Prior administration of antibiotics	65
Nasogastric tube	24, 62
Use of antacids or H_2 blockade	30, 92
Reintubation	44, 106
Bronchoscopy	62
Head trauma	24, 44
Intracranial pressure monitor	24, 44
Supine head position	65
Malnutrition[*]	49,[†] 79[‡]

[*]No well-conducted studies address the association between malnutrition and the risk of NP in adults.
[†]Hypoalbuminemia (albumin <3.0) found to be independent predictor of NP among elderly patients.
[‡]Review of the relationship between malnutrition and lung infection.

E. Pathogens in Nosocomial Pneumonia

1. More than 90% of cases of NP are caused by bacteria, because NP is largely a consequence of bacterial colonization. The most common bacterial pathogens are listed in Table 29-2.
   a. NP is most often caused by GNRs, including *P aeruginosa, K pneumoniae, Escherichia coli, Acinetobacter* species, *Serratia* species, and *Enterobacter* species, which together account for 25% to 75% of cases. *S aureus* accounts for 15% to 30% of NP; *S pneumoniae, H influenzae,* and *Streptococcus* species make up most of the remaining cases. Thirty percent to 50% of cases of NP are polymicrobial. The pathogenic role of anaerobes is unclear; their presence is probably most significant in the setting of polymicrobial infection and in the setting of macroaspiration (5,27).
   b. NP caused by *S pneumoniae* or *H influenzae* is more often found in nonintubated patients, in those who have not received antibiotics, and in community hospitals. These organisms are associated with a relatively low mortality risk. Conversely, GNRs and *S aureus* are more frequently found in intubated patients and at university hospitals. NP caused by *P aeruginosa, Acinetobacter* species, *S aureus,* and methicillin-resistant *S aureus* (MRSA) should be considered high risk, because these organisms are associated with a mortality rate of 60% to 100% (5,14,24,27,34,35,44,96,97).
   c. Unequivocal determination of etiologic agents is difficult when routine culture of expectorated sputum or endotracheal aspirates are used for pathogen identification. The distinction between colonizing and infecting organisms often is not possible with these samples.
   d. A history of prior antibiotic use is associated with increased mortality, because these cases of NP are often caused by *P aeruginosa, Acinetobacter* species, or MRSA. Alternatively, prior antibiotic use may correlate with the patients' being sicker (53,96,97). In addition, cystic fibrosis, bronchiectasis, malignancy, neutropenia, glucocorticoid use, and use of respiratory

Table 29-2 Bacterial etiology of nosocomial pneumonia

Reference	Fagon (35)	Horan (53)*	Rello (95)	Bartlett (5)†
Patient population	52 cases of VAP at a single center	Multicenter study of 15,499 cases of VAP and non-VAP	67 cases of VAP at a single center	159 cases of VAP & non-VAP at a single center
Diagnostic method	Protected specimen brush	Not specified	Protected specimen brush, autopsy, and blood culture	Transtracheal aspirate, culture of blood or pleural fluid
Total GNR	61	NA	63	46
Total GPC	38	NA	30	NA
Pseudomonas aeruginosa	31	17	22	9
Staphylococcus aureus	33	15	23	26
Acinetobacter species	15	3	3	NA
Haemophilus influenzae	10	6	20	17
Streptococcus pneumoniae	6	3	5	31
Anaerobes	2	NA	4	35
Polymicrobial	40	NA	28	54

*Data is from the National Nosocomial Infections Surveillance System (NNIS) epidemiological data base. NNIS did not employ rigorous diagnostic standards and NP was grouped into a broader category of nosocomial LRT infections (more than 80% were pneumonia).
†52% of the cases were from a chronic or intermediate care facility; 48% were from an acute medical/surgical floor. The percent of ICU patients or ventilated patients is unspecified.

therapy equipment are also associated with an increased risk of colonization or infection with *P aeruginosa* (32). Higher incidence of colonization or infection with *S aureus* is seen in patients with a history of coma, diabetes mellitus, or recent influenza infection (2,98).

2. The etiologic agent of NP can be predicted to some extent by dividing NP into two categories: early-onset and late-onset NP. Early-onset NP occurs within the first 4 days of intubation. Presumably, the pneumonia develops as a result of bacterial inoculation into the LRT in the peri-intubation period. Consequently, *S pneumoniae, H influenzae*, and *S aureus* are the most common pathogens. GNRs constitute <20% of the cases (24,92). Late-onset NP occurs after the first 4 days of intubation. It is probably caused by colonization and aspiration of bacteria and is most commonly caused by GNRs or *S aureus* (24,92).

3. Nonbacterial or atypical causes of NP are uncommon, but *Legionella* species, fungi, and viruses have each been implicated. Their precise incidence is not well known, because microbiologic assays are not routinely performed for these organisms.

a. *Legionella* organisms usually cause NP in association with a contaminated hospital water supply. Numerous epidemics have been reported (24,64).

b. Viral NP is seen most often in pediatric and psychiatric patients, probably because of the difficulty in enforcing respiratory precautions in these patients. Influenza and respiratory syncytial virus are most common and usually are seen in concert with community epidemics (24,51,115).

c. Fungal NP may be caused by *Aspergillus* species or *Candida albicans*. It is rarely observed in an immunocompetent host. However, critically ill patients may be relatively immunosuppressed and are potentially susceptible to these opportunistic infections (24).

F. Clinical Presentation of Nosocomial Pneumonia

1. Fever, leukocytosis, and radiographic infiltrates may be common among critically ill patients who are intubated and/or have significant comorbid illnesses and do not necessarily imply that the patient has NP. Purulent tracheobronchitis, malignancy, congestive heart failure, atelectasis, ARDS, vasculitis, pulmonary embolism, pulmonary infarction, pulmonary hemorrhage, chemical pneumonitis, pancreatitis, and pulmonary contusion may all mimic NP. Consequently, NP may be overdiagnosed if the diagnosis is based solely on clinical characteristics.

a. In a study involving 84 intubated patients, a team of physicians predicted the presence or absence of NP using clinical judgment with 77% accuracy. The sensitivity and specificity of clinical diagnosis were 62% and 84%, respectively. The absence of NP was more successfully predicted (82% NPV) than its presence (64% PPV) (36).

b. In a prospective analysis of 15 clinical variables measured among 147 ventilated patients with suspected NP, no single clinical parameter differentiated patients with NP from those without it NP (37). In another study, the respective sensitivities and specificities of classic clinical features to predict the presence of NP were as follows: 55% and 58%, respectively, for fever >38° C; 83% and 33%, respectively, for purulent secretions; and 78% and 42%, respectively, for new progressive infiltrate on chest radiograph (107). In several studies, despite high clinical suspicion, only 30% to 60% of symptomatic patients were ultimately found to have NP by rigorous standards such as bronchoscopic and histopathologic analysis (18,80,107,117).

c. Several different clinical criteria have been suggested to predict the presence or absence of NP. Pugin suggested the use of a Clinical Pulmonary Infection Score (CPIS) which is described in Table 29-3 (93). Although not rigorously validated, the results of this scoring system are promising. A recent study compared the accuracy of CPIS to a lung culture and histology and found that a CPIS >6 predicted VAP with 72% sensitivity and 85% specificity (88). Some investigators have adapted the CPIS (42). However, in general, clinical criteria remain unreliable predictors of NP.

2. NP is often underdiagnosed in patients with ARDS. This is probably because of the marked, preexisting abnormalities of oxygenation, temperature, hemody-

Table 29-3 CPIS for the diagnosis of ventilator-associated pneumonia

Temperature °C	≥36.5 and ≤38.4	0 point
	≥38.5 and ≤38.9	1 point
	≥39 or ≤36.0	2 points
Blood leukocytes (cells/mm^3)	≥4,000 and ≤11,000	0 point
	<4,000 or ≥11,000	1 point
	Band forms ≥500	1 point
Tracheal secretions	<14 points of tracheal secretions*	0 point
	≥14 points of tracheal secretions*	1 point
	Purulent secretion	1 point
Oxygenation: PaO_2/FiO_2 (mm Hg)	>240 or ARDS	0 point
	≤240 and no evidence of ARDS	2 point
Pulmonary radiography	No infiltrate	0 point
	Diffuse (or patchy) Infiltrate	1 point
	Localized infiltrate	2 points
Culture of tracheal aspirate (semiquantitative: 0, 1+, 2+, or 3+)	Pathogenic bacteria 0 or 1+	0 point
	Pathogenic bacteria cultured >1+	1 point
	Same bacteria or gram stain >1+	1 point

*The quantity of secretions were estimated by nurse on a scale of 0 to 4 and the total sum was recorded per 24 hours.
Permission granted from Pugin (93).

namics, and chest radiography that may accompany ARDS. When autopsy was used as a gold standard in two studies involving patients with ARDS, the use of clinical features for predicting diagnosis had a false-negative rate of 36% to 62% and a false-positive rate of 10% to 20%. The overall rate of misdiagnosis was 29% to 38% (3,7). For illustration, the data derived from one of the two studies is presented in Table 29-4 (3).

G. Diagnosis of Nosocomial Pneumonia

1. The ultimate gold standard for the diagnosis of NP is histologic examination and quantitative culture of lung tissue. This information is not readily obtainable in most cases of suspected NP. Consequently, the diagnosis of NP has traditionally relied on nonspecific clinical criteria supplemented by other laboratory studies, including sputum analysis. However, these specimens are often contaminated by colonizing bacteria, resulting in false-positive results. The recent development of strict clinical criteria and distal airway sampling techniques may significantly improve diagnostic accuracy of NP.
2. **Medical History and Physical Examination**
   a. Although there are no historical features or physical findings that are specific for NP, the history and physical examination are useful in the following

Table 29-4 Clinical and laboratory features for diagnosis of NP in ARDS.

	Sensitivity %	Specificity %	PPV (%)	NPV (%)
Fever >38.3°C	100	25	63	100
WBC >10,000 or <5,000	100	25	63	100
Pathogens in sputum	86	30	63	60
Asymmetric infiltrate on chest radiograph	57	70	73	54

From Andrews (3).

circumstances: exclusion of NP through diagnosis of an alternative condition; determination of the mechanism of infection, such as aspiration or sinusitis; identification of the most likely pathogen through assessment of risk factors.

b. The following information should be included in the history: age; presenting features; history of tobacco and alcohol use; medication history with particular attention to the use of antibiotics, steroids, or other immunosuppressive agents; allergies; risk factors for human immunodeficiency virus infection; presence or absence of spleen; history of cardiac disease, lung disease, malignancy, or autoimmune disease; risk factors for pulmonary embolism; risk of aspiration; and history of recent trauma, recent surgery, or recent blood transfusion.

c. A complete physical examination should be performed with particular attention to general appearance, vital signs, and cardiorespiratory status. Further diagnostic clues may be obtained by assessing for evidence of trauma, skin lesions, indwelling catheters, sinus drainage, poor dentition, jugular venous distention, edema, calf tenderness or swelling, and aspiration risk.

3. Routine Blood Work—A complete blood count with differential, chemistry panel, and measurement of arterial oxygenation should be performed. More specialized studies, such as an evaluation of vasculitis, should be ordered if indicated.

4. Radiographic Analysis—The chest roentgenogram may be technically limited. Patients with suspected NP are often critically ill, preventing optimal positioning. A lateral view is rarely obtained. In a critically ill patient, the presence of a radiographic infiltrate is often a nonspecific finding. For example, among 69 mechanically ventilated patients who subsequently underwent autopsy, a radiographic infiltrate was present in 80% although only 35% had histologic evidence of pneumonia. Other histologic findings included atelectasis (16%), pulmonary infarction (29%), and pulmonary hemorrhage (38%). Progressive infiltrates represented NP in only 32% of cases (117).

5. Sputum Analysis—Gram stain and culture of proximal airway specimens obtained by expectoration or endotracheal aspiration have traditionally been used to guide management of NP. However, the utility of these sputum specimens is frequently limited and may be misleading. For example, bacterial colonization of the oropharynx, trachea, and endotracheal tube in patients at risk for NP makes it difficult to distinguish between a true pathogen and a mere colonizer. Furthermore, the presence of leukocytes in sputum may represent tracheobronchitis or ARDS, and not necessarily pneumonia.

a. Sputum Gram Stain—Gram stain of the proximal airway specimen provides little useful data. In one study, semiquantitative grading of the Gram stain demonstrated a significant difference between the numbers of polymorphonuclear neutrophils and bacteria present in the endotracheal aspirates of colonized versus infected ventilated patients. However, despite the statistical significance, the differences were small and of limited clinical application unless combined with elastin fiber analysis (described later) (101).

b. Sputum Culture

(1) Expectorated sputum cultures have a false-positive rate of approximately 45%; most of these represent colonization with GNRs. Only 49% of expectorated sputum samples correlated with isolates from blood culture (5,80)

(2) Cultures of endotracheal aspirates carry a sensitivity of 100% but a specificity of only 29% when measured against strict clinical criteria and autopsy specimens (108)

(3) Efforts to improve the quality of endotracheal aspirates include the development of protected specimen techniques and the use of quantitative cultures to distinguish between pathogenic and colonizing bacteria. Although some of these methods appear promising, qualitative correlation with a more specific gold standard is lacking (78,80,109).

c. **Elastin Fiber Analysis**
   (1) Elastin fibers are detected by potassium hydroxide preparation of a proximal or distal airway specimen. The presence of elastin fibers within a sputum specimen signifies necrosis of lung tissue. Necrosis is present in necrotizing pneumonia but may also be seen in conditions such as ARDS or malignancy.
   (2) The presence of elastin fibers in endotracheal aspirates from intubated patients is reported to be 52% sensitive and 100% specific for NP (101). Necrotizing pneumonia is more commonly associated with GNRs than gram-positive cocci; therefore, false-negative results are more common in cases of NP caused by gram-positive cocci. False-positive results are often caused by ARDS, and in this subset of patients the PPV of this test falls to 50% (45,80,93).

d. **Antibody-Coated Bacteria**—The detection of antibodies on the surface of bacteria is intended to distinguish pathogenic from colonizing bacteria. The sensitivity and specificity of this test have been inconsistent, and its applicability is very limited currently.

6. **Blood Cultures**—Positive blood cultures are observed in 4% to 38% of patients with NP. On the average, 11% of patients with NP are bacteremic (5,13,44,102, 110). In patients with suspected NP, positive blood cultures must be interpreted cautiously. Although blood cultures are an incontestable gold standard for community-acquired pneumonia, the high incidence of indwelling lines, catheters, wounds, and concomitant infections in patients at risk for NP makes a positive blood culture more difficult to interpret. Up to 64% of positive blood cultures may be attributable to a source other than the lung (13,82,110).
7. **Miscellaneous Microbiologic Studies**—A positive pleural fluid culture is considered diagnostic, excepting skin contaminants. However, fewer than 15% of patients with NP have a pleural effusion or empyema (5,44). Culture of urine, wounds, sinuses, catheter tips, cerebrospinal fluid, or stool should be performed as indicated to diagnose or exclude extrapulmonary infection.
8. **Bronchoscopic and Nonbronchoscopic Distal Airways Analysis**—The unreliability of proximal airway specimens for diagnosis of NP has led to the development of more invasive but more reliable strategies for sampling the distal airways. These include protected specimen brush (PSB), bronchoalveolar lavage (BAL), and transtracheal aspiration. PSB and BAL may be performed either by fiberoptic bronchoscopy or by blind bronchial sampling (BBS).
   a. **Methods of Distal Airways Analysis**
      (1) **Fiberoptic Bronchoscopy**—Bronchoscopic techniques allow for retrieval of distal airway secretions under direct visualization. However, the bronchoscope must first pass through the upper airway and may transport colonizing bacteria into the LRT. The development of protected bronchoscopic techniques and the implementation of quantitative cultures have diminished the impact of upper airway contamination. A standardized procedural protocol has been published for bronchoscopic diagnosis of VAP (81).
         (a) **Fiberoptic Bronchoscopy Brushings**—Distal airway brushings are usually obtained by PSB or telescoping plugged catheter. PSB is the most widely studied invasive diagnostic technique for NP. A double-catheter system with a protected brush is advanced into a subsegmental bronchus of a radiographically affected region. The brush sample area is small; only 0.01 to 0.001 ml of secretions are retrieved for culture analysis, which is not available for 1 to 2 days.
         (b) **Fiberoptic Bronchoscopy with BAL**—BAL is well established in the diagnosis of pneumonia in the immunocompromised host but is not as well studied for NP. An unprotected or protected bronchoscope is advanced into a subsegmental bronchus of a radiographically affected region. Sterile saline is instilled and aspirated from the lung. A large portion of the distal airway, approxi-

mately 1 million alveoli, is sampled. Microscopic fluid analysis is immediately available. Culture results require 1 to 2 days.

(c) The diagnostic accuracies of various bronchoscopic techniques are summarized in Table 29-5.

(2) Blind Bronchial Sampling

(a) BBS is a general term that describes several different methods of nonbronchoscopic distal airways analysis. Brushings, aspirates, and mini-BAL may each be performed by blind insertion of a catheter into the distal airway. These techniques may safely be performed by a technician and are both less invasive and less expensive than with bronchoscopic methods.

(b) BBS preferentially samples dependent lung regions. Because NP is frequently a result of microaspiration, dependent lung segments are most commonly involved (99). The technique may be less useful when the pneumonia is not in a dependent lung segment.

(c) The diagnostic accuracies of various nonbronchoscopic techniques are summarized in Table 29-5.

(3) Miscellaneous Techniques—The utility of transtracheal aspiration is limited by tracheal colonization and by the high risk of complications in mechanically ventilated patients (80,82). Likewise, the use of transthoracic needle biopsy is limited by a high risk of complications in mechanically ventilated patients (80). Open lung biopsy is rarely indicated because of the reliability of distal airways sampling.

b. Diagnostic Analysis of Distal Airways Specimens

(1) Gram stain analysis of distal airways samples is superior to that of endotracheal aspirates or expectorated sputum. The sensitivity and specificity vary with the mode of sampling. Alveolar lavage yields the best results, with a reported PPV of 92% to 95% and an NPV of 57% to 97% (42,83). Findings on BAL Gram stain correlate closely with BAL culture results (110). Gram stain of PSB specimens carries 88% to 100% specificity, but the sensitivity may be as low as 20% (80,89).

(2) Quantitative Culture

(a) Specimen Quality—The presence of >1% squamous epithelial cells in BAL fluid is an indicator of oropharyngeal contamination (63).

(b) Quantitative bacterial culture has emerged as a means of distinguishing true pathogens (high colony count) from colonizing bacteria (low colony count). According to consensus criteria, pneumonia is considered to be present if bacteria are cultured at a concentration $\geq 10^3$ CFU/ml by PSB, or $\geq 10^4$ CFU/ml by BAL. These cutoffs are derived from comparisons with histologic examination and quantitative culture analysis of lung biopsy specimens (81).

(c) Several investigators have questioned the indiscriminate application of quantitative thresholds. The prior use of antibiotics may alter culture yield and invalidate the usual standards (13,85,109, 117). In addition, many cases of NP are polymicrobial, and each competing pathogen may not achieve growth to the diagnostic threshold (4,61).

(3) Rapid Analysis of Lavage Fluid—Microscopic analysis of cytocentrifuged lavage fluid may provide rapid diagnostic information. Examination of alveolar macrophages for intracellular organisms is a reliable indicator of NP; more than 7% of macrophages with intracellular organisms constitutes a positive test. This test carries a sensitivity of 96%, a specificity of 86%, a PPV of 86%, and an NPV of 96%. (19)

(4) Elastin fiber analysis of distal airway specimens may be performed as previously discussed.

Table 29-5 Diagnostic procedures in nosocomial pneumonia

Diagnostic Method	Diagnostic Threshold CFU/ml	Sample Size	Sensitivity %	Specificity %	Positive Predictive Value	Negative Predictive Value	Gold Standard	Advantages	Disadvantages	Reference
EA	NA	25[*]	100	29	78	100	Path, AR	Low risk, low cost, ease of performance	High contamination risk due to upper airways colonization	108
	10^6	27[†]	NA	78	NA	NA	Clinical			109
	10^6	52	82	83	75	68	Clinical, AR			78
PSB	10^3	25[*]	66	100	100	54	Path, AR	Protected specimen with low contamination risk	Invasive, expensive, small sample area, 1–2 day delay results, variable repeatability	108
	10^3	110[‡]	100	95	89	100	Path, AR			37
	10^3	55[§]	65	93	73	86	Path, AR, clinical[‖]			89
	10^3	18[¶]	100	100	100	100	AR, path, blood cx			18
BAL	10^4	21[¶]	80	69	NA	NA	AR, path, blood cx	Large sample area, rapid results	Unprotected specimen, invasive, expensive	18
	10^3	25[**]	72	71	90	26	Path, AR			110
PBAL	10^4	46	92	97	97	92	Clinical, AR, path	Same as BAL, protected specimen	Invasive, expensive	83

Table 29-5 (continued)

Diagnostic Method	Diagnostic Threshold CFU/ml	Sample Size	Sensitivity %	Specificity %	Positive Predictive Value	Negative Predictive Value	Gold Standard	Advantages	Disadvantages	Reference
BBS								Lower cost, ease of performance, lower complication risk	No airways visualization, applicability to management of NP not yet proven	
P-TPC[††]	10^3	25[*]	61	100	100	50	Path, AR			108
P-TPC[‡‡]	10^3	55	100	88	74	100	Clinical, path, AR			89
PM-BAL[§§]	NA	83	70	69	NA	NA	Path			99

[*]16% of samples were obtained from patients receiving antibiotics; 68% of patients had NP; 32% of patients had CAP.
[†]All patients were mechanically ventilated and without pneumonia. The study was designed to determine the incidence of positive cultures in a population without NP.
[‡]Omits 25% of patients in study with "uncertain" diagnosis.
[§]65% of samples were obtained from patients receiving antibiotics.
[‖]Includes blood and pleural fluid cultures.
[¶]Patients received no prior antibiotics.
[**]Excludes 9 patients with CAP.
[††]Telescoping Plugged Catheter with a protected brush, blindly samples major bronchus.
[‡‡]Telescoping Plugged Catheter with protected aspiration device, performed blindly.
[§§]Protected Mini-BAL, performed blindly.

c. Limitations of Distal Airways Sampling

(1) Prior Antibiotic Use—Several studies suggest that quantitative culture analysis may be misleading in the setting of prior antibiotic use. The sensitivity and specificity of distal airways analysis decreases by as much as 64% in the setting of prior antibiotic use. PSB appears to be more susceptible; false-negative results may occur because of sterilization and false-positive results from overgrowth of resistant colonizing bacteria (20,107–109). In one study, 67% of the patients with positive quantitative cultures by PSB had sterile cultures within 3 days of empiric antibiotic therapy (85). In another study, 68% of patients with a prior history of antibiotic use had sterile or subthreshold quantitative cultures despite histologic evidence of pneumonia (99). In addition, analysis of intracellular organisms has limited utility in patients who have recently received antibiotics (28). It is not clear how many days the antibiotics need to be withheld before the diagnostic accuracy of distal airways analysis begins to improve. Subgroup analysis in one study (n=13) suggests that the odds of a true positive culture increase by 47% with each day off of antibiotics (83).

(2) Borderline Quantitative Cultures—Borderline quantitative culture results (10^2 to 10^3 CFU/ml) have been studied primarily with PSB. For patients with a prior history of antibiotic use, a borderline quantitative culture result may represent NP in up to 45% of cases. For patients without a prior history of antibiotic use, NP may be present in up to 35% of cases. A repeat PSB should be performed within 72 hours if there is still clinical suspicion of NP (29).

d. Complications of Distal Airways Sampling

(1) Fiberoptic bronchoscopy carries some procedural risks but is generally considered a safe procedure in experienced hands. Significant hypoxemia (partial pressure of arterial oxygen [PaO_2] <60 mm Hg with a fraction of inspired oxygen [FiO_2] of 80%) complicates the procedure in approximately 12% of mechanically ventilated patients. Fever, pulmonary hemorrhage, pneumothoraces, and hypotension are also observed (18,45,69,80,83,89,108).

(2) BBS carries few procedural risks, which is one of its primary advantages. Minor hemorrhage or oxygen desaturation <90% may occur in up to 9% of patients (66).

(3) The risk of complications is increased with mechanical ventilation, active bronchospasm, ARDS, recent myocardial infarction, hypotension, severe hypoxia, coagulopathy, or small endotracheal tubes (45,80).

e. Selecting a Method of Distal Airways Sampling

(1) The advantages and disadvantages of the various techniques have been outlined in the tables.

(2) The diagnostic yield of PSB is excellent in cases in which no prior antibiotics have been given (18). The reproducibility of this technique is qualitatively good; however, up to 59% of serial samples may vary quantitatively by more than 1 log (78). The 24- to 48-hour delay for culture results is not ideal and may delay optimal treatment.

(3) BAL allows rapid analysis of intracellular organisms and Gram stain to immediately guide therapy. The lavage technique samples a larger area of lung, which may improve sensitivity (61). The diagnostic accuracy of BAL may not be as good as that of PSB, but BAL appears to be less adversely affected by prior antibiotic use (18,107). Overall, PSB and BAL are considered equivalent in diagnostic efficacy, each with its particular strengths and weaknesses (18,110).

(4) Some investigators suggest performing both PSB and BAL to gain the diagnostic advantages of each; however, this is expensive (18,82). Protected BAL is not well studied but is promising and may combine the advantages of PSB and BAL, with fewer disadvantages (83).

(5) BBS is a novel technique. In some studies, the sensitivity and specificity are comparable to those of the more invasive techniques, with fewer costs and complications (88,89,108). It may be performed in hospitals that do not have capabilities for bronchoscopy or quantitative culture. However, some studies show poor qualitative correlation of BBS with lung cultures or PSB (66,99), and further studies are needed before it can be implemented widely.

(6) Papazian assessed the accuracy of cultures obtained with the use of PSB, BAL, BBS, and protected mini-BAL for the diagnosis of VAP, using postmortem histologic examination of the whole lung as the gold standard (88). Sensitivity, specificity, false-positive rate, false-negative rate, PPV, and NPV were calculated and are summarized in Table 29-6, which directly compares the various diagnostic procedures for NP. BBS had an excellent specificity and sensitivity at a threshold of 10^4 CFU/ml. The PSB was more specific, but this advantage may be outweighed by a higher false-negative rate.

H. Diagnostic Criteria for Nosocomial Pneumonia—Several sets of diagnostic criteria have been issued, and the definitions of NP vary. Clinical criteria and microscopic criteria have been suggested by both the Centers for Disease Control and individual investigators (16,42,83,93). More recently, a consensus conference produced in-depth criteria for the definite and probable diagnosis of the presence of NP (90). Table 29-7 provides a condensed set of diagnostic criteria, and the reader is referred to the original documents for more detail.

I. Therapeutic Approach to Nosocomial Pneumonia

1. Supportive Therapy—Supplemental oxygen should be administered to maintain adequate arterial oxygenation. Mechanical ventilation should be considered for patients who are unable to adequately oxygenate, ventilate, or protect the airway. Nasogastric tubes should be converted to orogastric tubes to minimize the risk of sinusitis. Chest physiotherapy, incentive spirometry, and bronchodilators may be useful in helping to clear secretions, maintain airway patency, and prevent atelectasis. The use of central lines should be minimized. Fluid and electrolyte losses from fever, emesis, or diarrhea should be restored, and all active comorbid illnesses should be treated.

2. Antimicrobial Therapy

a. General Principles of Antimicrobial Therapy in NP

(1) Appropriate antimicrobial therapy has been associated with im-

Table 29-6 Comparison of diagnostic procedures for nosocomial pneumonia

	PSB (N=38)	BAL (N=38)	BBS (N=38)	PM-BAL (N=38)
Diagnostic threshold (CFU/ml)	10^3	10^4	10^4	10^3
Sensitivity for definite VAP* (%)	42	58	83	67
Sensitivity for definite or histologic VAP† (%)	33	50	72	56
Specificity % for definite VAP* (%)	95	95	80	80
Specificity % for definite or histologic VAP† (%)	95	95	80	80
PPV for definite VAP* (%)	83	88	71	67
PPV for definite or histologic VAP† (%)	86	90	77	71
NPV for definite VAP* (%)	73	79	89	80
NPV for definite or histologic VAP† (%)	61	68	76	67

*Postmortem lung cultures positive and histologic evidence of bronchopneumonia
†Postmortem histologic evidence of bronchopneumonia +/−positive postmortem lung cultures
From Papazian (88).

Table 29-7 Condensed diagnostic criteria for nosocomial pneumonia (16,83,90)

Presence of Nosocomial Pneumonia	Absence of Nosocomial Pneumonia
Histopathologic analysis of lung tissue consistent with pneumonia Clinical suspicion of nosocomial pneumonia (fever, leukocytosis, purulent sputum, and radiographic infiltrate) and at least one of the following: 1. Significant growth of pathogen on distal airways analysis 2. Positive blood culture unrelated to another source 3. Positive pleural fluid culture 4. Radiographic evidence of pulmonary cavitation in the absence of malignancy 5. Isolation of respiratory virus or *Legionella* from respiratory secretions 6. Serologic or antigen assay confirmation of infection with respiratory virus or *Legionella*	Histopathologic analysis of lung tissue inconsistent with pneumonia Diagnosis of alternative cause plus no growth on distal airways analysis Resolution of infiltrate, fever, and leukocytosis in the absence of antibiotics

proved survival in NP. Mortality in patients on appropriate therapy is approximately 23% to 31%, whereas inappropriate therapy is associated with a 52% to 92% mortality rate (14,106). Therefore, selection of proper antimicrobial agents is vital.

(2) The capillary bed of the lung is nonfenestrated and therefore may limit the penetration of less lipid-soluble antibiotics. The more lipophilic agents include macrolides, doxycycline, and trimethoprim. Less lipid-soluble antibiotics include β-lactams and aminoglycosides (76). Barriers to tissue penetration may be overcome by strategic dosing regimens. A once-daily aminoglycoside dosing regimen has been shown to improve alveolar antibiotic levels (86,114).

(3) The antimicrobial activity of some agents may be affected by the microenvironment of the lung. Endobronchial pH may fall in the setting of pneumonia and thereby decrease the efficacy of some pH-sensitive antibiotics, such as aminoglycosides (9).

(4) Antibiotics should be used only if absolutely necessary and should be narrowly directed whenever possible. Widespread use of broad-spectrum antibiotics has led to the emergence of multidrug-resistant organisms in hospitals across the world (*e.g.*, MRSA, multidrug-resistant *Klebsiella* or *Pseudomonas* species) (38).

b. Early Antimicrobial Therapy Versus Early Bronchoscopy—The optimal management strategy for NP is a subject of much controversy. In a clinically stable patient with suspected NP, some investigators recommend the early use of bronchoscopic sampling and delay of antibiotic therapy until a definitive diagnosis is available. In an unstable patient, these investigators support early bronchoscopy followed by the administration of empiric antibiotics. Antimicrobial selection is guided by rapid BAL analysis and then modified according to culture results (1,21,80,81). Other investigators advocate early use of empiric antibiotics in all patients with suspected NP. Antimicrobial selection is based on clinical presentation and noninvasive studies. These investigators recommend bronchoscopy only in selected cases (87)

(1) Justification for Early Use of Empiric Antibiotics and Delay of Bronchoscopy in Suspected NP

(a) NP occurs most frequently in a critically ill population, and withholding of antibiotics in this population is potentially dangerous.

(b) Invasive procedures carry an increased cost in both dollars and complications. In addition, many hospitals do not have the facilities necessary for bronchoscopy and quantitative cultures.

(c) No prospective, randomized study has demonstrated that early invasive diagnosis leads to improved outcome, compared with empiric clinical management. Therefore, invasive methods should not be accepted as the standard of care.

(d) Although the diagnostic accuracy of invasive tests falls significantly with prior antibiotic use, 16% to 85% of patients at risk for NP are already taking antibiotics for another reason. Therefore, modification of the antibiotic regimen to empirically treat NP does not necessarily further decrease the diagnostic yield of bronchoscopy (20,89,99,109).

(e) Given the high percentage of patients already taking antibiotics, the true sensitivity and specificity of invasive diagnostic methods are probably lower than those cited in studies which excluded patients who were taking antibiotics. On the other hand, clinical judgment had a sensitivity and specificity in one study of 62% and 84%, respectively; this approaches the sensitivity and specificity of invasive diagnostic methods published in the literature (36).

(2) Justification for Routine Use of Early Bronchoscopy in Suspected NP

(a) Early identification of the pathogen facilitates appropriate antibiotic therapy and probably improves mortality (14,106). Even in the study by Fagon, which reported a diagnostic accuracy of 77% for clinical judgment (without invasive diagnostic techniques), 67% of the antimicrobial regimens that were chosen on the basis of noninvasive testing were inappropriate for those who proved to have NP (36).

(b) Clinical criteria may overdiagnose pneumonia in 35% to 60% of cases; therefore, most patients would unnecessarily receive antibiotic therapy (18,36,80,107,117). For uninfected patients, the potential cost of empiric antibiotic therapy is high. Unnecessary antibiotic therapy increases the cost of medical care as well as the likelihood of antibiotic toxicity. In addition, prior antibiotic treatment has been associated with an increased risk of acquiring NP (65,67), dying from NP (97), and being colonized or infected with a high-risk (32,53,67,96,97) or a resistant (35,67,81,85, 117,118) pathogen.

(c) By some estimates, the cost of PSB pays for itself in 6 days (37). Furthermore, early bronchoscopy may successfully rule out NP and allow pursuit of a proper diagnosis.

(d) Prior antibiotic use has a deleterious effect on the sensitivity and specificity of distal airways analysis. The administration of empiric antibiotics before bronchoscopy may render it nondiagnostic.

(3) This debate remains unsettled until further studies are completed. A compromise may evolve through the combined use of rigorous clinical criteria with BBS (42,88,93). BBS shows promise as a low-risk, low-cost means of routine distal airways analysis. However, more data are needed.

c. Selection of Empiric Therapy—Empiric antibiotics are often initiated before receipt of microbiologic data and must be directed at the most likely pathogens. In order to achieve the highest serum level and lung tissue concentration, antibiotics should be administered intravenously. In NP, antimicrobial selection may be simplified by classifying the patient as having either low risk or high risk of infection with *P aeruginosa* (74,75,77,86). These guidelines should be modified according to clinical judgment and local epidemiologic patterns. Furthermore, empiric therapy for immunosuppressed hosts is not included in these recommendations.

(1) **Low Risk of *Pseudomonas aeruginosa* Infection**—These patients are usually only mildly to moderately ill. In general, they are previously healthy, have received no prior antibiotics, and have received <4 days of mechanical ventilation. They should have no other risk factors for *P aeruginosa* colonization (see previous discussion). Patients in this category are most likely to be infected with *S pneumoniae, H influenzae*, methicillin-sensitive *S aureus*, or lactose-fermenting GNRs. Empiric coverage with a single antibiotic agent (monotherapy) is successful in this population. Combination therapy has been employed but usually is not any more effective (74,86). Table 29-8 summarizes the appropriate antibiotic options for this group (adapted from 74,75,77,86).

(2) **High Risk of *Pseudomonas aeruginosa* Infection**—These patients are moderately to critically ill. They often have received prolonged mechanical ventilation or prior antibiotics, or both. They tend to be at increased risk for *P aeruginosa* infection or colonization, as described previously, and for other high-risk organisms such as *Acinetobacter* species or MRSA. Ciprofloxacin, imipenem-cilastatin, and ceftazidime have each been used successfully as empiric monotherapy against severe NP. However, these single agents carry a failure rate as high as 60% against *P aeruginosa* (41,74,86). For patients who are at low risk for *P aeruginosa*, monotherapy with one of these agents may be sufficient, but for patients with known or suspected *P aeruginosa* infection, combination therapy is strongly advised. The antibiotics that are active against *P aeruginosa* are listed in Table 29-9 below (table

Table 29-8 Empiric therapy of NP in patients at low risk for infection with *P. aeruginosa*

Monotherapy	Combination Therapy
Second-generation cephalosporin (cefuroxime)	First-generation cephalosporin + aminoglycoside
Non-pseudomonal third generation cephalosporin (ceftriaxone)	Clindamycin + aztreonam
Betalactam plus Betalactamase inhibitor (ampicillin-sulbactam)	
Fluoroquinolone (ciprofloxacin)*	
Trimethoprim-sulfamethoxazole	

*Poor coverage of streptococci and anaerobes.

Table 29-9 Empiric therapy of NP in patients at high risk for infection with *P. aeruginosa*

Third-generation antipseudomonal cephalosporin (ceftazidime)
Carbapenem (imipenem-cilastatin)
Aminoglycoside (gentamicin)
Fluoroquinolone (ciprofloxacin)
Antipseudomonal penicillin with betalactamase inhibitor (ticarcillin clavulanate)
Monobactam (aztreonam)

*Combine two agents; see text.

adapted from 74,75,77,86).

(a) In general, with the exception of double β-lactam coverage, any combination of two antibiotics listed Table 29-9 provides acceptable antipseudomonal coverage. Combinations that broadly cover other high-risk pathogens may be most appropriate. For example, combinations that include only gentamicin, aztreonam, or ceftazidime do not provide adequate coverage against *S aureus*. These agents are best combined with an antibiotic with good activity against gram-positive organisms (74,75,86).

(b) The combination of a β-lactam with an aminoglycoside is popular. The popularity of this combination is based on *in vitro* studies that demonstrated antibacterial synergy between these drugs. Aminoglycosides should be used cautiously, with close monitoring of renal function. A β-lactam–fluoroquinolone combination is a reasonable alternative if aminoglycosides are contraindicated. Rigorously designed studies that compare the efficacy of various antibiotic combinations have yet to be performed (74,86).

(3) Empiric treatment against *S. aureus*, MRSA, anaerobes, or *Legionella* species should be initiated as indicated by the presence of known risk factors (see Section E). Vancomycin should be reserved for cases in which there is strong suspicion of a resistant pathogen (74,75,86). Amantadine or rimantidine should be considered in the setting of an influenza epidemic. For nosocomial aspiration pneumonia, penicillin or clindamycin, which is the standard empiric therapy for community-acquired aspiration pneumonia, may be inadequate. Because nosocomial aspiration pneumonias are often caused by a combination of gram-negative and gram-positive organisms, empiric coverage should be broadened to include GNRs, gram-positive cocci, and anaerobes (84).

d. Directed Antimicrobial Therapy—If a precise pathogen is identified, antimicrobial therapy may be narrowed based on antibiotic sensitivities of the isolated organism. *P aeruginosa* warrants combination antimicrobial therapy at all times. Up to 40% of NP is polymicrobial, and therapy may need to be directed at more than just the predominant organism.

e. Duration of Antimicrobial Therapy—There are no data that specify optimal duration of treatment for NP. In general, 14 to 21 days of therapy are recommended. A 10-day course may be sufficient in mild to moderate disease with a low-risk organism in a clinically stable patient. A 28-day course may be needed for severe staphylococcal pneumonia with necrosis. A change to oral therapy may be reasonable after several days of defervescence and clinical improvement, assuming that adequate oral absorption can be expected. Transition to monotherapy with oral ciprofloxacin has shown promise (74,86).

f. Alternative Delivery of Antimicrobial Agents—Endotracheal and aerosolized delivery of aminoglycosides have been studied. No role has yet been defined for these modes of delivery in the acute therapy of NP (12,40).

3. Failure to Respond to Antimicrobial Therapy—There is no universally accepted definition of antimicrobial failure (73,118,119). In general, a poor response to therapy is defined as worsening of the clinical condition, including persistent fever or hemodynamic instability, at least 48 to 72 hours after initiation of antimicrobial therapy (73,118). Further details regarding the expected outcome of NP are discussed in the next section. Given the vagaries of diagnosis of NP, ongoing consideration should be given to alternative causes that may mimic NP (see previous discussion). In the setting of unresponsive or progressive disease, the following options should be considered (80, 118).

a. Repeat cultures of the blood, urine, and other indicated sites should be obtained. Central lines should be removed or changed.

b. Alternative diagnosis should be considered. Additional diagnostic tests such as chest computed tomography, ventilation-perfusion, sinus films, serologic tests, or echocardiography should be obtained as clinically indicated. The list of drugs should be reviewed for the possibility of drug-induced fever or pulmonary toxicity. Empyema, abscess, or metastatic infection should be considered.

c. If not done previously, a distal airways specimen should be obtained. If sampling was done, a repeat study should be considered. In addition to routine microbiologic studies, cytologic analysis to rule out malignancy should be considered, as well as specialized studies for *Legionella* species, viral infection, and opportunistic pathogens.

d. The appropriateness of antibiotic selection and dose should be reviewed. Broadening of antibiotic therapy to empirically cover superinfecting organisms, anaerobes, or nonbacterial pathogens should be considered. If possible, antibiotic therapy should not be broadened until repeat distal airways sampling and other cultures have been completed. In many cases, the disease may progress despite appropriate antimicrobial treatment.

e. If definitive diagnosis is necessary, open lung biopsy should be considered.

J. Outcome of Nosocomial Pneumonia—The natural history of NP is not well defined. The high incidence of severe comorbid illnesses in the population at risk for NP makes outcomes analysis complicated and difficult to perform.

1. Resolution of Nosocomial Pneumonia

a. Resolution can be classified as either clinical or microbiologic. Evidence of clinical resolution includes resolution of fever, leukocytosis, hypoxia, and radiographic infiltrate. The average time to clinical resolution of NP is highly variable (days to months). Delayed resolution of NP (persistence of radiographic infiltrate beyond 4 weeks) is seen more commonly in patients with underlying pulmonary disease and in pneumonias associated with GNRs, aspiration, or mechanical ventilation (73).

b. The average time to microbiologic resolution of NP is somewhat more predictable. Invasive studies have demonstrated sterilization of distal airways secretions within 72 hours of initiation of appropriate antimicrobial therapy (73,85). Failure to achieve growth of $<10^2$ CFU/ml within 3 days of starting antibiotic therapy correlates with poor clinical response to therapy.

c. Complications of NP include prolonged hospitalization, debilitation, respiratory failure requiring mechanical ventilation, lung abscess, superinfection by a resistant organism, ARDS, septic shock, renal failure, myocardial infarction, and multiple organ dysfunction syndrome. Currently, there are no reliable data that describe the incidence of these complications.

2. Mortality in Nosocomial Pneumonia

a. **Crude Mortality**—The overall mortality rate associated with NP is reported to be 20% to 50%. It may be as high as 80% in patients with ARDS or pneumonia caused by a high-risk pathogen. Although some studies report a 2.0- to 2.5-fold higher rate of crude mortality for patients with NP, compared with matched controls without NP (62,80), other studies have not demonstrated a significant contribution of NP to the overall mortality risk (26,95). The latter studies have suggested that NP may be predominantly an indicator of severe illness rather than a primary cause of death.

b. **Attributable Mortality**—The crude mortality rate measures the absolute number of patients who die with NP but does not adjust for deaths resulting from a concomitant illness. The attributable mortality rate is an attempt to more precisely define the contribution of NP to the mortality risk. When patients are matched closely for severity of illness and only the presence of NP distinguishes the case from control subjects, the attributable mortality is estimated to be 27% to 33%. For example, for a crude mortality of 45%, an attributable mortality of 33% implies that only 15% of patients died directly from NP. Consequently, NP may be viewed as both a cause and a consequence of critical illness (34,71).

c. **Risk Factors for Increased Mortality**—Several studies have attempted to identify the predictors of mortality in patients with NP. Advanced age, prolonged mechanical ventilation, malignancy, prior exposure to antibiotics, inappropriate antibiotic use, bacteremia, septic shock, ARDS, supine head position, bilateral disease, and infection caused by *Pseudomonas* species, *Acinetobacter* species, or *S aureus* are among the reported risk factors for increased mortality (14,34,65,71,106).

K. **Prevention of Nosocomial Pneumonia**—Strategies for prevention of NP are reviewed in detail elsewhere (6,17). A brief summary is presented here.

1. **Selective digestive decontamination**—This strategy has been widely investigated for prevention of oropharyngeal and gastric colonization in intubated patients. An antibiotic paste which usually contains a combination of polymyxin, an aminoglycoside, and an antifungal is topically applied to the oropharynx and the gastrointestinal tract through a nasogastric tube. In some instances, a broad-spectrum systemic antibiotic is also administered. Most studies have shown that this procedure decreases the risk of colonization or the rate of NP caused by GNRs, or both. However, it does not clearly improve the mortality (6,17,22). Recent meta-analyses and well designed randomized, double-blind, placebo-controlled studies corroborate these findings (17,22,39,43,94,116). There are several explanations for this observation. First, selective digestive decontamination may promote the emergence of resistant, highly pathogenic organisms. This has been reported by some but not by the majority of investigators, leaving its significance unclear. Alternatively, as previously discussed, NP may merely be a marker of severe illness. Consequently, its prevention may not necessarily confer a mortality advantage. Although selective digestive decontamination may still prove useful for selected populations, its benefit has not been proved and its use should be considered investigational at this time.

2. **Maintenance of Gastric Acidity**—Stress ulcer prophylaxis has been associated with an increased risk of NP, apparently through increased gastric alkalinization and bacterial overgrowth (30,92). Although H_2 blockade and antacids increase the gastric pH and may predispose the patient to gastric bacterial overgrowth, sucralfate does not. In addition, sucralfate has inherent bactericidal activity that may inhibit gastric colonization (23).
   a. Some investigators have suggested that sucralfate is the most appropriate form of stress ulcer prophylaxis in critically ill patients (23,30,92,112). When compared with antacids and H_2 blockade, sucralfate use has been associated with a twofold to threefold decrease in NP, presumably secondary to decreased gastric colonization. However, this finding has been debated (8,103). In particular, it is unclear whether H_2 blockade alone leads to a higher rate of NP than sucralfate. No mortality differences have been reported (6,23,30,92).
   b. Bonton evaluated the effects of sucralfate and antacids on intragastric acidity; colonization of the stomach, oropharynx, and trachea; and incidence of NP. The study was a prospective, randomized, double-blind trial involving 112 patients. The study found that antacids and sucralfate had similar effects on intragastric acidity, colonization, and incidence of NP. They did find that those with stomach colonization had higher gastric pH (11).
   c. Antacids appear to be the least desirable form of stress ulcer prophylaxis. By decreasing gastric pH and increasing gastric volume, it may predispose the patient to bacterial overgrowth, reflux, aspiration, and NP. Although current data favor the use of sucralfate over H_2 blockade, further studies are needed before one of these medications emerges as obviously superior for the prevention of NP (6,17,23,112).

3. **Semirecumbent Positioning**—The supine position has been associated with an increased risk of NP, presumably by increasing the incidence of gastroesophageal reflux and aspiration (65). By instillation of radiolabelled solution through a nasogastric tube, Torres demonstrated that maintenance of head position at a 45° angle, when compared with supine positioning, significantly reduced aspiration of gastric contents (111).

4. **Continuous Subglottic Aspiration**—Using a specialized endotracheal tube with a separate dorsal lumen for aspiration, Valles demonstrated a reduction in the incidence of VAP through continuous aspiration of subglottic secretions. NP developed in 32.5% of those receiving routine ventilator care and only 18.4% of patients who underwent continuous aspiration. No difference in mortality was seen (113).
5. **Appropriate Delivery of Enteral Feeding**—The presence of a nasoenteric tube and infusion of enteral feeding disrupts the lower esophageal sphincter, increases gastric pH, and increases the gastric volume, all of which result in increased colonization, reflux, and aspiration.
   a. The following preventive strategies have been proposed but have not proved clearly effective: decreased size of feeding tube; placement of the feeding tube in the jejunum; continuous feeding to minimize gastric distention; bolus feeding to minimize alkalinization and colonization (6,17).
   b. Unstudied but commonly employed preventive measures include minimization of gastric distention through routine inspection for residual aspirates, use of promotility agents when indicated, and placement of a percutaneous tube in stable patients in whom long-term feeding is anticipated.
   c. **Acidification of Enteral Nutrition**—Most enteral supplements have an alkalinizing effect on gastric pH that may predispose to bacterial overgrowth and NP (91). Heyland demonstrated that acidified enteral feeding (pH <3.5) significantly reduced gastric bacterial growth in comparison with nonacidified feeding. The impact of this finding on the incidence of NP has not yet been determined (50).
6. **Prevention of Cross-Contamination**—Rigorous infection control measures, such as education of physicians, nurses, and respiratory personnel, hand washing, glove use, gown use, proper care and sterilization of respiratory equipment, and surveillance for contamination of enteral solutions or water supply, are routinely employed and are described in detail elsewhere (17).
7. **Miscellaneous Preventive Strategies**
   a. **Elimination of Endotracheal Biofilm**—Advances in the development of biomaterials could lead to the development of an endotracheal tube that does not permit bacterial colonization. Currently, there are no data on this form of prevention.
   b. The use of enteral nutrition is associated with a lower incidence of pneumonia when compared with total parenteral nutrition. It is hypothesized that enteral feeding minimizes translocation of bacteria across the gut and potentially to the lung (79).
   c. Postoperative patients, especially those with chronic lung disease or other conditions predisposing to pulmonary infection, should receive chest physiotherapy, bronchodilator treatment, incentive spirometry, and pain control to minimize atelectasis and the risk of NP.
   d. Continuous lateral rotational therapy has been studied in mechanically ventilated patients. This procedure employs a gently rotating bed to assist in mobilization of pulmonary secretions. Preliminary studies suggest that when this technique is initiated early in hospitalization it may be effective in preventing NP. Larger studies and cost-benefit analysis are needed (100).
   e. Vaccination of all health care personnel and appropriate isolation precautions should be carried out to minimize the impact of viral epidemics.

L. Summary

1. NP is the most common infection in the intensive care unit and the second most common cause of nosocomial infection overall. Bacterial colonization of the upper airway, followed by microaspiration or macroaspiration into the pulmonary tree, is considered to be the primary mechanism for development of NP.
2. More than 90% of cases of NP are bacterial in origin. NP is most often caused by GNRs, including *P aeruginosa*, *K pneumoniae*, *E coli*, *Acinetobacter* species, *Serratia* species, and *Enterobacter* species, which account for 25% to 75% of cases. *S aureus* accounts for 15% to 30% of NP. *S pneumoniae*, *H influenzae*, and *Streptococcus* species make up most of the remaining cases. Thirty percent

to 50% of NP is polymicrobial. Nonbacterial or atypical NP is rare and may be caused by *Legionella* species, viruses, or opportunistic organisms.

3. The classic presenting features of pneumonia, such as fever, leukocytosis, and radiographic pulmonary infiltrate, are nonspecific findings in patients at risk for NP. Multiple conditions such as congestive heart failure, ARDS, or pulmonary hemorrhage may mimic NP. Consequently, NP may be overdiagnosed if the diagnosis is based solely on clinical characteristics.
4. Clinical investigation of NP has been marred by the lack of a readily available gold standard for diagnosis. Consequently, the diagnosis of NP has traditionally relied on nonspecific clinical criteria, supplemented by sputum analysis, which carries a high potential for upper airway contamination from colonizing bacteria.
5. The unreliability of clinical criteria, proximal airway specimens, and blood cultures for diagnosis of NP has led to the development of more invasive, more specific methods of distal airways sampling, such as PSB and BAL. Each may be performed by fiberoptic bronchoscopy or BBS. Overall, PSB and BAL are considered equivalent in diagnostic efficacy, each with its particular strengths and weaknesses. BBS may provide an inexpensive alternative to PSB or BAL.
6. Initial antibiotic selection for NP is empiric and should be broad enough to cover all of the most likely pathogens. Once an organism is identified, antibiotic selection should be directed more specifically.
7. Mortality in patients with NP is 20% to 50%. It is generally lower in patients who were previously healthy or nonintubated, but it may rise to 60% to 100% in the setting of ARDS or infection with a highly virulent pathogen. Because NP tends to occur in the setting of severe illness and impaired host defenses, some investigators have suggested that NP is predominantly an indicator of severe illness rather than a primary cause of death.
8. An understanding of the pathogenesis of NP has led to development of multiple preventive strategies. Rigorous infection control measures have been successful in the prevention of NP. Selective digestive decontamination, the use of sucralfate for stress ulcer prophylaxis, semirecumbent positioning, and several other means of prevention are currently under investigation.

Abbreviations used in Chapter 29

AR = antibiotic response
ARDS = adult respiratory distress syndrome
BAL = bronchoalveolar lavage
BBS = blind bronchial sampling
CAP = community-acquired pneumonia
CDC = Centers for Disease Control
CFU = colony-forming units
CPIS = Clinical Pulmonary Infection Score
FiO_2 = fraction of inspired oxygen
GNRs = gram-negative rods
GPC = gram-positive cocci
H_2 = $histamine_2$ receptor
ICU = intensive care unit
LRT = lower respiratory tract
MRSA = methicillin-resistant *Staphylococcus aureus*
NNIS = National Nosocomial Infections Surveillance System
NP = nosocomial pneumonia
NPV = negative predictive value
PaO_2 = partial pressure of oxygen in arterial blood
PM-BAL = protected mini-bronchoalveolar lavage
PPV = positive predictive value
PSB = protected specimen brush

P-TPC = protected telescoping plugged catheter
TPC = telescoping plugged catheter
VAP = ventilator-associated pneumonia
vs. = versus
WBC = white blood cells

References

1. A'Court. Nosocomial pneumonia in the intensive care unit: mechanisms and significance. *Thorax* 1992;47:465. Review.
2. Al-Ujayli. Pneumonia due to *Staphylococcus aureus* infection. *Clin Chest Med* 1995; 16:111.
3. Andrews. Diagnosis of nosocomial bacterial pneumonia in acute, diffuse, lung injury. *Chest* 1981;80:254.
4. Baker. Decision making in nosocomial pneumonia: an analytic approach to the interpretation of quantitative cultures. *Chest* 1995;107:85.
5. Bartlett. Bacteriology of hospital-acquired pneumonia. *Arch Intern Med* 1986; 146:868.
6. Bassin. Prevention of ventilator-associated pneumonia: an attainable goal? *Clin* Chest Med 1995;16:195.
7. Bell. Multiple organ system failure and infection in adult respiratory distress syndrome. *Ann Intern Med* 1983;99:293.
8. Ben-Menachem. Prophylaxis for stress-related gastric hemorrhage in the medical intensive care unit: a randomized, controlled, single blind study. *Ann Intern Med* 1994;121:568.
9. Boden. Endobronchial pH: relevance to aminoglycoside activity in gram-negative bacillary pneumonia. *Am Rev Respir Dis* 1983;127:39.
10. Bonten. The stomach is not a source for colonization of the upper respiratory tract and pneumonia in ICU patients. *Chest* 1994;105:878.
11. Bonten. The role of intragastric acidity and stress ulcer prophylaxis on colonization and infection in mechanically ventilated ICU patients: a stratified, randomized, double-blind study of sucralfate versus antacids. *Am J Respir Crit Care Med* 1995;152:1825.
12. Brown. Double-blind study of endotracheal tobramycin in the treatment of gram-negative bacterial pneumonia. *Antimicrob Agents Chemother* 1990;34:269.
13. Bryan. Bacteremic nosocomial pneumonia: analysis of 172 episodes from a single metropolitan area. *Am Rev Respir Dis* 1984;129:668.
14. Celis. Nosocomial pneumonia: a multivariate analysis of risk and prognosis. *Chest* 1988;93:318.
15. Centers for Disease Control. Public health focus: surveillance, prevention, and control of nosocomial infection. *MMWR Morb Mortal Wkly Rep* 1992;41:783.
16. Centers for Disease Control. CDC definitions of nosocomial infections, 1988. *Am Rev Respir Dis* 1989;139:1058.
17. Center for Disease Control. CDC guideline for prevention of nosocomial pneumonia. *Infect Control Hosp Epidemiol* 1994;15:587.
18. Chastre. Diagnosis of nosocomial pneumonia in intubated patients undergoing ventilation: comparison of the usefulness of bronchoalveolar lavage and the protected specimen brush. *Am J Med* 1988;85:45.
19. Chastre. Quantification of BAL cells containing intracellular bacteria rapidly identifies ventilated patients with nosocomial pneumonia. *Chest* 1989;95:191S.
20. Chastre. Prospective evaluation of the protected specimen brush for the diagnosis of pulmonary infections in ventilated patients. *Am Rev Respir Dis* 1984;130:924.
21. Chastre. Invasive diagnostic testing should be routinely used to manage ventilated patients with suspected pneumonia. *Am J Respir Crit Care Med* 1994;150: 570.
22. Cockerill. Today's role for selective decontamination of the digestive tract: Can

antibiotic prophylaxis prevent nosocomial infection? *Journal of Critical Illness* 1994;9:486.

23. Cook. Nosocomial pneumonia and the role of gastric pH: a meta-analysis. *Chest* 1991;100:7.
24. Craven. Epidemiology of nosocomial pneumonia: new perspectives on an old disease. *Chest* 1995;108:1S. Review.
25. Craven. Contaminated condensate in mechanical ventilator circuits: a risk factor for nosocomial pneumonia. *Am Rev Respir Dis* 1984;129:625.
26. Craven. Risk factors for pneumonia and fatality in patients receiving continuous mechanical ventilation. *Am Rev Respir Dis* 1986;133:792.
27. Dal Nogare. Nosocomial pneumonia in the medical and surgical patient: risk factors and primary management. *Med Clin North Am* 1994;78:1081. Review.
28. Dotson. The effect of antibiotic therapy on recovery of intracellular bacteria from bronchoalveolar lavage in suspected ventilator-associated nosocomial pneumonia. *Chest* 1993;103:541.
29. Dreyfuss. Clinical significance of borderline quantitative protected brush specimen culture results. *Am Rev Respir Dis* 1993;147:946.
30. Driks. Nosocomial pneumonia in intubated patients given sucralfate as compared with antacids or histamine type 2 blockers: the role of gastric colonization. *N Engl J Med* 1987;317:1376.
31. DuMoulin. Aspiration of gastric bacteria in antacid-treated patients: a frequent cause of postoperative colonisation of the airway. *Lancet* 1982;i:242.
32. Dunn. Ventilator-associated pneumonia caused by *Pseudomonas* infection. *Clin* Chest Med 1995;16:95.
33. Elpern. Incidence of aspiration in tracheally intubated patients. *Heart Lung* 1987; 16:527.
34. Fagon. Nosocomial pneumonia in ventilated patients: a cohort study evaluating attributable mortality and hospital stay. *Am J Med* 1993;94:281.
35. Fagon. Nosocomial pneumonia in patients receiving continuous mechanical ventilation. Prospective analysis of 52 episodes with use of a protected specimen brush and quantitative culture techniques. *Am Rev Respir Dis* 1989;139:877.
36. Fagon. Evaluation of clinical judgment in the identification and treatment of nosocomial pneumonia in ventilated patients. *Chest* 1993;103:547.
37. Fagon. Detection of nosocomial lung infection in ventilated patients: use of a protected specimen brush and quantitative culture techniques in 147 patients. *Am Rev Respir Dis* 1988;138:110.
38. Felmingham. Antibiotic resistance: Do we need new therapeutic approaches? *Chest* 1995;108:70S.
39. Ferrer. Utility of selective digestive decontamination in mechanically ventilated patients. *Ann Intern Med* 1994;120:389.
40. Fiel. Aerosol delivery of antibiotics to the lower airways of patients with cystic fibrosis. *Chest* 1995;107:61S.
41. Fink. Treatment of severe pneumonia in hospitalized patients: results of a multicenter, randomized, double-blind trial comparing intravenous ciprofloxacin with imipenem-cilastatin. *Antimicrob Agents Chemother* 1994;38:547.
42. Garrard. The diagnosis of pneumonia in the critically ill. *Chest* 1995;108:17S.
43. Gastinne. A controlled trial in intensive care units of selective decontamination of the digestive tract with nonabsorbable antibiotics. *N Engl J Med* 1992;326:594.
44. George. Epidemiology of nosocomial pneumonia in intensive care unit patients. *Clin* Chest Med 1995;16:29. Review.
45. Griffin. New approaches in the diagnosis of nosocomial pneumonia. *Med Clin North Am* 1994;78:1091. Review.
46. Gross. Deaths from nosocomial infections: experience in a university hospital and a community hospital. *Am J Med* 1980;68:219.
47. Guerin. Nosocomial bacteremia and sinusitis in nasotracheally intubated patients in intensive care. *Rev Infect Dis* 1988;10:1226.
48. Haley. Nosocomial infections in U.S. hospitals, 1975–1976: estimated frequency by selected characteristics of patients. *Am J Med* 1981;70:947.

49. Hanson. Risk factors for nosocomial pneumonia in the elderly. *Am J Med* 1992;92:161.
50. Heyland. Effect of acidified enteral feedings on gastric colonization in the critically ill patient. *Crit Care Med* 1992;20:1388.
51. Holladay. Nosocomial viral pneumonia in the intensive care unit. *Clin* Chest Med 1995;16:121.
52. Holzapfel. Influence of long-term oro- or nasotracheal intubation on nosocomial maxillary sinusitis and pneumonia: results of a prospective, randomized, clinical trial. *Crit Care Med* 1993;21:1132.
53. Horan. Nosocomial infection surveillance. *MMWR Morb Mortal Wkly Rep* 1986;35(1SS):17SS.
54. Huxley. Pharyngeal aspiration in normal adults and patients with depressed consciousness. *Am J Med* 1978;64:564.
55. Ibanez. Gastroesophageal reflux and aspiration of gastric contents during nasogastric feeding: the effect of posture. *Intensive Care Med* 1988;14(s2):296. Abstract.
56. Inglis. Tracheal tube biofilm as a source of bacterial colonization of the lung. *J Clin Microb* 1989;27:2014.
57. Jimenez. Incidence and etiology of pneumonia acquired during mechanical ventilation. *Crit Care Med* 1989;17:882.
58. Johanson. Changing pharyngeal bacterial flora of hospitalized patients: emergence of gram-negative bacilli. *N Engl J Med* 1969;281:1137.
59. Johanson. Bacterial adherence to epithelial cells in bacillary colonization of the respiratory tract. *Am Rev Respir Dis* 1980;121:55.
60. Johanson. Nosocomial respiratory infections with gram-negative bacilli: the significance of colonization of the respiratory tract. *Ann Intern Med* 1972;77:701.
61. Johanson. Bacteriologic diagnosis of nosocomial pneumonia following prolonged mechanical ventilation. *Am Rev Respir Dis* 1988;137:259.
62. Joshi. A predictive risk index for nosocomial pneumonia in the intensive care unit. *Am J Med* 1992;93:135.
63. Kahn. Diagnosing bacterial respiratory infection by bronchoalveolar lavage. *J Infect Dis* 1987;155:862.
64. Kirby. Legionnaires' disease: report of sixty-five nosocomially acquired cases and review of the literature. *Medicine (Baltimore)* 1980;59:188.
65. Kollef. Ventilator-associated pneumonia: a multivariate analysis. *JAMA* 1993;270:1965.
66. Kollef. The safety and diagnostic accuracy of minibronchoalveolar lavage in patients with suspected ventilator-associated pneumonia. *Ann Intern Med* 1995;122:743.
67. Kollef. Antibiotic use and antibiotic resistance in the intensive care unit: Are we curing or creating disease? *Heart Lung* 1994;23:363.
68. LaForce. Human oral defenses against gram-negative rods. *Am Rev Respir Dis* 1976;114:929.
69. Lambert. Comparison of tracheal aspirates and protected brush catheter specimens for identifying pathogenic bacteria in mechanically ventilated patients. *Am J Med Sci* 1989;297:377.
70. Langer. Long-term respiratory support and risk of pneumonia in critically ill patients. *Am Rev Respir Dis* 1989;140:302.
71. Leu. Hospital-acquired pneumonia: attributable mortality and morbidity. *Am J Epidemiol* 1989;129:1258.
72. Levine. The impact of tracheal intubation on host defenses and risks for nosocomial pneumonia. *Clin Chest Med* 1991;12:523.
73. Lowenkron. Definition and evaluation of the resolution of nosocomial pneumonia. *Semin Respir Infect* 1992;7:271.
74. Lynch. Nosocomial pneumonia in the ICU: current treatment strategies. The pros and cons of monotherapy versus combination regimens. *Journal of Critical Illness* 1995;10:332.
75. Lynch. Nosocomial pneumonia: Which agent(s) to use? *J Respir Dis* 1992;13:1123.
76. Mandell. Antibiotics for pneumonia therapy. *Med Clin North Am* 1994;78:997.

77. Mandell. Initial antimicrobial treatment of hospital acquired pneumonia in adults: a conference report. *Can J Infect Dis* 1993;4:317.
78. Marquette. Diagnostic efficiency of endotracheal aspirates with quantitative bacterial cultures in intubated patients with suspected pneumonia. *Am Rev Respir Dis* 1993;148:138.
79. Martin. The relationship between malnutrition and lung infection. *Clin Chest Med* 1987;8:359. Review.
80. Meduri. Diagnosis and differential diagnosis of ventilator-associated pneumonia. *Clin Chest Med* 1995;16:61. Review.
81. Meduri. The standardization of bronchoscopic techniques for ventilator-associated pneumonia. *Chest* 1992;102:557S.
82. Meduri. Ventilator-associated pneumonia in patients with respiratory failure: a diagnostic approach. *Chest* 1990;97:1208.
83. Meduri. Protected bronchoalveolar lavage: a new bronchoscopic technique to retrieve uncontaminated distal airway secretions. *Am Rev Respir Dis* 1991;143:855.
84. Mier. Is penicillin G an adequate initial treatment for aspiration pneumonia? A prospective evaluation using a protected specimen brush and quantitative cultures. *Intensive Care Med* 1993;19:279.
85. Montravers. Follow up protected specimen brushes to assess treatment in nosocomial pneumonia. *Am Rev Respir Dis* 1993;147:38.
86. Niederman. An approach to empiric therapy of nosocomial pneumonia. *Med Clin North Am* 1994;78:1123.
87. Niederman. Invasive diagnostic testing is not needed routinely to manage suspected ventilator-associated pneumonia. *Am J Respir Crit Care Med* 1994;150:565.
88. Papazian. Bronchoscopic or blind sampling techniques for the diagnosis of ventilator-associated pneumonia. *Am J Respir Crit Care Med* 1995;152:1982.
89. Pham. Diagnosis of nosocomial pneumonia in mechanically ventilated patients: comparison of a plugged telescoping catheter with the protected specimen brush. *Am Rev Respir Dis* 1991;143:1055.
90. Pingleton. Patient selection for clinical investigation of ventilator-associated pneumonia: criteria for evaluating diagnostic techniques. *Chest* 1992;102(Suppl 1):553S.
91. Pingleton. Enteral nutrition in patients receiving mechanical ventilation: multiple sources of tracheal colonization include the stomach. *Am J Med* 1986;80:827.
92. Prod'hom. Nosocomial pneumonia in mechanically ventilated patients receiving antacid, ranitidine, or sucralfate as prophylaxis for stress ulcer. *Ann Intern Med* 1994;120:653.
93. Pugin. Diagnosis of ventilator-associated pneumonia by bacteriologic analysis of bronchoscopic and nonbronchoscopic "blind" bronchoalveolar lavage fluid. *Am Rev Respir Dis* 1991;143:1121.
94. Pugin. Oropharyngeal decontamination decreases incidence of ventilator-associated pneumonia: a randomized, placebo-controlled, double-blind clinical trial. *JAMA* 1991;265:2704.
95. Rello. Incidence, etiology, and outcome of nosocomial pneumonia in mechanically ventilated patients. *Chest* 1991;100:439.
96. Rello. Pneumonia due to *Haemophilus influenzae* among mechanically ventilated patients: incidence, outcome, and risk factors. *Chest* 1992;102:1562.
97. Rello. Impact of previous antimicrobial therapy on the etiology and outcome of ventilator-associated pneumonia. *Chest* 1993;104:1230.
98. Rello. Risk factors for *Staphylococcus aureus* nosocomial pneumonia in critically ill patients. *Am Rev Respir Dis* 1990;142:1320.
99. Rouby. Nosocomial bronchopneumonia in the critically ill: histologic and bacteriologic aspects. *Am Rev Respir Dis* 1992;146:1059.
100. Sahn. Continuous lateral rotational therapy and nosocomial pneumonia. *Chest* 1991; 99:1263.
101. Salata. Diagnosis of nosocomial pneumonia in intubated intensive care unit patients. *Am Rev Respir Dis* 1987;135:426.
102. Scheld. Nosocomial pneumonia: pathogenesis and recent advances in diagnosis and therapy. *Rev Infect Dis* 1991;13(Suppl 9):S743. Review.

103. Simms. Role of gastric colonization in the development of pneumonia in critically ill trauma patients: results of a prospective randomized trial. *J Trauma* 1991; 31:531.
104. Skerrett. Host defenses against respiratory infection. *Med Clin North Am* 1994; 78:941.
105. Torres. Gastric and pharyngeal flora in nosocomial pneumonia acquired during mechanical ventilation. *Am Rev Respir Dis* 1993;148:352.
106. Torres. Incidence, risk, and prognosis factors of nosocomial pneumonia in mechanically ventilated patients. *Am Rev Respir Dis* 1990;142;523.
107. Torres. Validation of different techniques for the diagnosis of ventilator-associated pneumonia: comparison with immediate postmortem pulmonary biopsy. *Am J Crit Care Med* 1994;149:324.
108. Torres. Diagnostic value of telescoping plugged catheters in mechanically ventilated patients with bacterial pneumonia using the Metras catheter. *Am Rev Respir Dis* 1988;138:117.
109. Torres. Specificity of endotracheal aspiration, protected specimen brush, and bronchoalveolar lavage in mechanically ventilated patients. *Am Rev Respir Dis* 1993;147:952.
110. Torres. Diagnostic value of quantitative cultures of bronchoalveolar lavage and telescoping plugged catheters in mechanically ventilated patients with bacterial pneumonia. *Am Rev Respir Dis* 1989;140:306.
111. Torres. Pulmonary aspiration of gastric contents in patients receiving mechanical ventilation: the effect of body position. *Ann Intern Med* 1992;116:540.
112. Tryba. Prophylaxis of stress ulcer bleeding: a meta-analysis. *J Clin Gastroenterol* 1991;13(Suppl 2):S44.
113. Valles. Continuous aspiration of subglottic secretions in preventing ventilator-associated pneumonia. *Ann Intern Med* 1995;122:179.
114. Valcke. Penetration of netilmicin in the lower respiratory tract after once-daily dosing. *Chest* 1992;101:1028.
115. Valenti. Nosocomial viral infections: epidemiology and significance. *Infect Control* 1980;1:33.
116. Vandenbrouke-Grauls. Effects of selective decontamination of the digestive tract on respiratory tract infections and mortality in the intensive care unit. *Lancet* 1991;338:859.
117. Wunderlink. The radiologic diagnosis of autopsy-proven ventilator-associated pneumonia. *Chest* 1992;101:458.
118. Wunderlink. Ventilator-associated pneumonia: failure to respond to antibiotic therapy. *Clin Chest Med* 1995;16:173.
119. Wunderlink. Methodology for clinical investigation of ventilator-associated pneumonia: epidemiology and therapeutic intervention. *Chest* 1991;102:580S.

30 Spontaneous Bacterial Peritonitis

Burton W. Lee and
Morton N. Swartz

A. Introduction

1. In a 1992 review of the literature by Garcia-Tsao, the prevalence of spontaneous bacterial peritonitis (SBP) was estimated to be about 19% in cirrhotic patients with ascites (12). It is a serious illness; the case fatality rate remains 36% to 70% despite prompt diagnosis and therapy (11,20,32,41). Furthermore, 69% of patients who recover from SBP have a recurrence within 1 year (42).
2. **Definitions (see Table 30-1)**
   a. **Spontaneous Bacterial Peritonitis**—SBP is a bacterial infection of preexisting ascitic fluid (AF) in the absence of an obvious intraabdominal source. In adults, SBP occurs most commonly in association with cirrhosis. SBP that occurs in association with nephrotic syndrome and ascites is mainly, although not exclusively, a pediatric problem. The discussion in this chapter focuses primarily on patients with cirrhosis and ascites. In a strict sense, SBP is characterized by neutrocytic ascites and a positive AF culture. Neutrocytic ascites is usually defined as >250 to 500 neutrophils per microliter of AF.
   b. **Culture-Negative Neutrocytic Ascites**—A variant of culture-positive SBP is culture-negative neutrocytic ascites (CNNA). In CNNA, the AF culture is negative for organisms despite the presence of neutrocytic ascites. CNNA accounts for 18% to 35% of patients with SBP (20,21,32,41). In this chapter, SBP refers to both culture-positive SBP and CNNA unless otherwise specified.
   c. **Nonneutrocytic Bacterascites**—Nonneutrocytic bacterascites (NNBA) is a controversial entity characterized by positive AF culture of a single organism in the absence of neutrocytic ascites. It is unclear whether NNBA represents early or resolving SBP or a "stalemate" between the pathogen and the host. Unlike CNNA, NNBA is not included in most definitions of SBP.
   d. **Secondary Peritonitis**—Secondary peritonitis refers to peritonitis that is associated with an intraabdominal abscess or a perforated viscus. It may occur as a complication of peptic ulcer disease, gall bladder disease, appendicitis, infectious enterocolitis, inflammatory bowel disease, diverticulitis, bowel malignancy, abdominal or pelvic surgery, or trauma. Peritonitis also affects about 60% of peritoneal dialysis patients during the first year of dialysis (8). It is a leading cause of peritoneal dialysis failure. Patients with secondary peritonitis or peritoneal dialysis catheter-associated peritonitis are traditionally considered separately from those with SBP.

Table 30-1 Types of peritonitis

	Neutrocytic Ascites?	Positive Ascites Culture?
Culture-positive spontaneous bacterial peritonitis	Yes	Yes
Culture-negative neutrocytic ascites	Yes	No
Nonneutrocytic bacterascites	No	Yes

3. Culture-Positive Spontaneous Bacterial Peritonitis

a. Etiology—Aerobic gram-negative rods, followed by gram-positive cocci, are the most common causes of culture-positive SBP. Anaerobes are relatively rare, accounting for <5% in most series. In almost all cases, a single organism is responsible for the infection. The estimated prevalence of various etiologic organisms in some of the reviews are summarized in the Table 30-2 (4,11,42).

b. Clinical Manifestations—The reported symptoms and signs of SBP are summarized in Table 30-3 (3,33,41).

4. Culture-Negative Neutrocytic Ascites

a. There is now good evidence that CNNA is a variant form of bacterial peritonitis that requires antibiotic treatment. Among the patients who died

Table 30-2 Microbial etiology of culture-positive SBP

	Wilcox 1987 (44) (N=253)	Garcia-Tsao 1992 (12) (N=746)	Bhuva 1994 (4) (N=263)
Study design	Literature review of 15 studies of 5 or more patients with culture-positive SBP*	Literature review of 27 studies of 10 or more patients with culture-positive SBP*	Literature review of 6 studies of patients with culture-positive SBP*
Gram-negative bacilli			
Escherichia coli	47%	47%	46%
Klebsiella	11%	13%	9%
Other	11%	13%	8%
Total	69%	72%	63%
Gram-positive cocci			
Pneumococcus	8%	7%	30%
Other streptococci	13%	12%	
Staphylococci	4%	4%	<6%
Enterococcus	5%	5%	?
Total	30%	29%	–
Anaerobes	5%	5%	<1%
Polymicrobial	8%	8%	?

*The data from some of the studies are included in more than one review.

Table 30-3 Major symptoms and signs of SBP

	Terg 1992 (41)	Runyon 1991 (33)	Ariza 1991 (3)
Subjects	64 patients with CNNA or culture-positive SBP	90 patients with CNNA or culture-positive SBP	52 episodes of gram-negative rod SBP
Fever	41%	68%	83%
Abdominal pain	45%	57%	65%
Rebound tenderness	—	9%	42%
Ileus	—	11%	—
Confusion or encephalopathy	36%	49%	46%
Positive ascitic fluid culture	56%	68%	85%
Positive blood culture	44%	29%	61%
In-hospital death rate	40%	38%	50%

with CNNA in one study, 78% had fever, positive blood culture, or persistent neutrocytic ascites at the time of death (31). None of the AF cultures for tuberculosis or fungus was positive. Among the patients who had repeat paracentesis, all had a decline in AF neutrophil count with antibiotic therapy. Similarly, all patients who were initially febrile defervesced with treatment. CNNA is thought to represent false-negative cases of culture-positive SBP. Alternatively, it may represent early or resolving SBP (4,12, 44). The incidence of CNNA may decline in the future as culture techniques improve (5,7,29,35,38).

b. Clinical Features of CNNA Versus Culture-Positive SBP—Several studies compared the clinical course of culture-positive SBP versus CNNA (11,20,32,41). In general, the clinical presentation, laboratory abnormalities, and AF characteristics were similar between the two groups. However, the SBP patients were more likely to have positive blood cultures than CNNA patients. Representative studies by Runyon and Terg are summarized in Table 30-4 (32,41).

c. Some studies have suggested that the prognosis is better for patients with CNNA than for those with culture-positive SBP. In Pelletier's comparison of 38 patients with culture-positive SBP versus 15 patients with CNNA, the 1-month mortality rates were 50% and 20%, respectively (20). A more favorable outcome with CNNA was also reported by Fong (11). However, other studies did not confirm this observation (32,41,43).

5. Nonneutrocytic Bacterascites

a. Asymptomatic NNBA—In general, asymptomatic patients with NNBA do not require empiric antibiotic therapy. Pelletier compared 36 patients with SBP versus 22 patients with asymptomatic NNBA. NNBA was defined as positive AF culture with an AF neutrophil count <250 cells/µl. None of the patients with asymptomatic NNBA had fever, chills, abdominal pain, or abdominal tenderness. Fifty-four percent of asymptomatic NNBA patients did not receive antibiotic therapy. Blood culture bottles were inoculated with AF at the bedside (19) (see Table 30-5).

(1) Patients with asymptomatic NNBA tended to have less advanced liver disease than those with SBP.

Table 30-4 Clinical and laboratory features of CNNA vs. culture-positive SBP

Reference and Study Design	Runyon (32)—Retrospective review of all cases of peritonitis at one hospital of over an 8-y period. Blood cuture bottles were not inoculated with AF at the bedside. CNNA patients had AF neutrophil count >500 cells/µl, negative AF culture, no prior history of antibiotic therapy, and no intra-abdominal source of infection.			Terg (41)—Retrospective review of all cases of peritonitis at two hospitals over a 7-y period. Blood culture bottles were inoculated with AF at the bedside. CNNA patients had AF neutrophil count >250 cells/µl, negative AF culture, no prior history of antibiotic therapy, and no intraabdominal source of infection.		
	CNNA (N=18)	**SBP (N=33)**	***P***	**CNNA (N=28)**	**SBP (N=36)**	***P***
Fever	50%	58%	NS	36%	44%	NS
Abdominal Pain	72%	58%	NS	43%	47%	NS
Encephalopathy	61%	73%	NS	32%	39%	NS
Positive blood culture	33%	52%	?	11%	71%	<0.01
Mean AF neutrophil count (cells/µl)	5100	5200	NS	3215	2872	NS
In-hospital mortality	50%	70%	NS	46%	36%	NS
12-mo mortality	—	—	—	69%	68%	NS
Risk of recurrent SBP	—	—	—	34%	33%	NS

(2) Only 13.6% of patients with asymptomatic NNBA developed clinical peritonitis during the study. Even among the 12 patients who did not receive antibiotic therapy, no patient developed peritonitis.

(3) The mortality rate was significantly lower for patients with asymptomatic NNBA.

b. **Symptomatic NNBA**—In contrast to asymptomatic patients, those with symptomatic NNBA should be treated with empiric antibiotics. Runyon reported a series of 21 patients with untreated NNBA who had a second paracentesis. Bacterascites resolved spontaneously in 62% of these patients, and 38% progressed to SBP. The only clinical factor predictive of progression to SBP was the presence or absence of symptoms. For example, all patients who progressed to SBP were symptomatic at the time of initial paracentesis. In contrast, 54% of patients with spontaneously resolved bacterascites were asymptomatic at the time of initial paracentesis. Therefore, the risk of progression to SBP was 57% for symptomatic patients and 0% for asymptomatic patients in this study (27). However, this retrospective observation awaits further confirmation.

B. **Risk Factors for SBP**—Prospective studies have identified numerous risk factors for SBP, including low AF opsonic activity, low AF complement activity, low AF protein, high serum bilirubin, high prothrombin time, low serum albumin, recent gastrointestinal hemorrhage, and hepatic encephalopathy (2,18,25,26,40,42). In general, these risk factors fall into two categories: markers of low AF opsonic activity (AF protein concentration, AF complement activity) and markers of poor hepatic function (bilirubin, prothrombin time, serum albumin, gastrointestinal bleeding, and hepatic encephalopathy) (2,25,26,34,36,40). The study by Andreu is described here for illustration. This prospective study involved 110 cirrhotic patients with sterile ascites who were observed for an average of 46 weeks for development of SBP (2). Patients with bilirubin >15 mg/dl, creatinine >3 mg/dl, platelet count <40,000 per microliter, known malignancy, human immunodeficiency virus infection, or NNBA were excluded. Serum samples were analyzed for liver function, renal function, complete blood count, protein, complement activity, and immunoglobulin levels. AF samples were analyzed for protein, pH, cell count, cytology, culture, complement activity, immunoglobulin levels, and opsonic activity.

1. Overall, 25% of the patients developed SBP. The 1-year all-cause mortality rates were 62% and 34% for patients with and without SBP, respectively. Multivariate analysis revealed low AF opsonic activity, low serum albumin, high prothrombin time, and high serum bilirubin as predictors of SBP. The single best predictor was low AF opsonic activity. Patients with low opsonic activity had a 35% risk of developing SBP by 6 months, compared with 6% for patients with high opsonic activity (P=0.0001). The AF protein concentration positively correlated with the AF opsonic activity.
2. When the multivariate analysis was limited to only those variables that are commonly used in clinical practice, high serum bilirubin (>2.5 mg/dl) and low AF protein (<1 g/dl) were the best independent predictors of SBP (see Table 30–6).

Table 30-5 Clinical and laboratory features of asymptomatic NNBA vs. SBP (19)

	Asymptomatic NNBA (N=22)	SBP (N=36)	*P*
Child–Pugh score	10.9	12.3	0.002
Ascitic neutrophil count (cells/μl)	30	6600	0.001
Gram-negative rod infection	50%	73%	NS
Gram-positive bacterial infection	50%	27%	NS
1-mo mortality rate	27%	55%	<0.05

Table 30-6 Multivariate predictors of SBP (2)

	AF Protein <1 g/dl (N=55)	AF Protein >1 g/dl (N=55)	*P*	Serum Bilirubin <2.5 mg/dl (N=56)	Serum Bilirubin >2.5 mg/dl (N=54)	*P*
6-mo risk of SBP	32%	7%	0.0035	11%	32%	0.0026

C. Diagnosis

1. **SBP Versus Sterile Ascites**—Although gram-stained smears of AF are positive only in a minority of cases of SBP, a positive result can aid in the initial selection of antibiotics. AF cultures are more helpful, but they are negative in 18% to 35% of patients with SBP (20,21,32,41). Furthermore, the results become available only after 1 to 2 days of laboratory turnaround time. Therefore, strict reliance on culture results would cause high false-negative rates as well as unacceptable delays in treatment. In order to overcome this problem, many investigators have evaluated other parameters that allow rapid diagnosis of SBP, including AF pH, arterial-AF pH gap, AF lactate concentration, and AF neutrophil count (6,13,15,17,22, 28,31,37,45). The parameter that has consistently emerged as the single best predictor of SBP is the AF neutrophil count. The value of the AF lactate level or the arterial-AF pH gap is less certain (1,12,24,28,37). A study by Runyon is described here for illustration. This is the largest prospective study to date, involving 175 patients with 206 AF samples. Patients hospitalized with ascites underwent routine paracentesis at admission. Paracentesis was repeated if the patient developed symptoms or signs suggestive of infection. Blood culture bottles were inoculated with AF at the bedside. Based on the results of AF analysis, patients were divided into one of the following categories: sterile ascites, SBP, CNNA, NNBA, secondary peritonitis, tuberculous peritonitis, cardiac ascites, ascites related to peritoneal malignancy, and ascites related to hepatocellular carcinoma (28).
   a. **AF pH and Arterial-AF pH Gap**—Compared to patients with sterile ascites, those with SBP or secondary peritonitis had significantly decreased AF pH and elevated arterial-AF pH gap. The average AF pH values were 7.47, 7.35, and 7.07 for patients with sterile ascites, SBP, and secondary peritonitis, respectively. The mean pH gaps were 0.02, 0.10, and 0.53, respectively. Although these differences were statistically significant, the pH (<7.35) and the pH gap (>0.10) were not clinically useful because their sensitivities for SBP were only 43% and 32%, respectively.
   b. **AF Lactate**—Compared to patients with sterile ascites, those with SBP or NNBA had significantly elevated AF lactate levels. The average AF lactate levels were 14.3, 35.5, and 26.0 mg/dl for patients with sterile ascites, SBP, and NNBA, respectively. Again, these differences were statistically significant, but the AF lactate level (>32 mg/dl) was not clinically useful because its sensitivity for SBP was only 36%.
   c. **AF Neutrophil Count**—The single best diagnostic criterion for SBP was an AF neutrophil count >250 cells/μl. The sensitivity and specificity of this criterion for SBP were 100% and 81%, respectively. If a cutoff of 500 cells/μl is used, the sensitivity and specificity are 86% and 85%, respectively. However, these high sensitivities are not surprising because, by definition, patients with SBP had to have neutrocytic ascites.
   d. In a review of the literature by Garcia-Tsao, the sensitivity and specificity of the AF neutrophil count (>250 cells/μl) for SBP were 84% and 93%, respectively. In comparison, these values for AF lactate level (>25 to 35 mg/dl) were 58% and 93%, respectively, and for arterial-AF pH gap (>0.10) they were 55% and 96%, respectively (12). Therefore, the single most useful diagnostic criterion for SBP remains the AF neutrophil count.

2. **SBP Versus Intraperitoneal Malignancy or Bleeding**—The utility of AF analysis decreases if there is intraperitoneal malignancy or bleeding. In a study by Yang, patients with peritoneal metastasis or intraperitoneal bleeding could not be reliably distinguished from those with SBP by the traditional criteria (45). This prospective study divided 109 consecutive patients with ascites into multiple subgroups: normal sterile ascites (42 patients), CNNA (6 patients), sterile ascites with systemic infection (8 patients), culture-positive SBP (10 patients), hepatocellular carcinoma with intraperitoneal bleeding (10 patients), hepatocellular carcinoma without bleeding (16 patients), cancer with peritoneal metastasis (11 patients), and cancer with liver metastasis (6 patients). The AF lactate concentration, arterial-AF pH gap, and AF neutrophil count were analyzed for each subgroup.
   - **a.** An average AF neutrophil count >500 cells/μl was associated with hepatocellular carcinoma with intraperitoneal bleeding (mean, 1057 cells/μl), cancer with peritoneal metastasis (mean, 868 cells/μl), CNNA (mean, 2716 cells/μl), and culture-positive SBP (mean, 9522 cells/μl).
   - **b.** The average arterial-AF pH gaps were similar for hepatocellular carcinoma with intraperitoneal bleeding (mean, 0.082), cancer with peritoneal metastasis (mean, 0.082), and culture-positive SBP (mean, 0.101).
   - **c.** An average AF lactate concentration >25 mg/dl was associated with the presence of hepatocellular carcinoma with intraperitoneal bleeding (mean, 43 mg/dl), cancer with peritoneal metastasis (mean, 34 mg/dl), sterile ascites with systemic infection (mean, 52 mg/dl), and culture-positive SBP (mean, 37 mg/dl).
3. **SBP Versus Secondary Peritonitis**—A retrospective study suggested that secondary peritonitis may be distinguished from SBP by the concentration of glucose, lactate dehydrogenase (LDH), and total protein in the AF. This study involved 33 cases of SBP, 6 of secondary peritonitis, and 20 of sterile ascites. The symptoms, signs, and AF characteristics were compared (31) (see Table 30-7).
   - **a.** The average AF neutrophil count was statistically similar between the patients with SBP (5200 cells/μl) and those with secondary peritonitis (8300 cells/μl). In addition, the clinical signs and symptoms did not differ significantly between these two groups. However, polymicrobial infection was present in 100% of patients with secondary peritonitis, compared with 12% of SBP patients ($P<0.001$).
   - **b.** The AF concentrations of LDH, protein, and glucose were significantly different in patients with secondary peritonitis, compared with those with SBP. All 6 patients with secondary peritonitis met at least two of the following three criteria: AF glucose <50 mg/dl, AF protein >1 g/dl, and AF LDH >225 mU/ml. In comparison, only 6% of SBP patients met two or more of these criteria.
4. Numerous studies have demonstrated that the sensitivity of AF culture can be increased by bedside inoculation of blood culture bottles (5,7,29,35,38). The study by Castellote is described for illustration. Over a 21-month period, the AFs of 70 consecutive patients with SBP were cultured by bedside inoculation of blood culture bottles and also by the conventional method. The conventional

Table 30-7 Ascitic fluid characteristics of secondary peritonitis vs. SBP (31)

	Secondary Peritonitis (N=6)	SBP (N=33)	*P*
Mean AF protein	2.5 g/dl	0.8 g/dl	<0.001
Mean AF glucose	36 mg/dl	128 mg/dl	<0.005
Mean AF LDH	847 mU/μl	173 mU/μl	<0.001

method involved centrifugation of 10 ml of AF and inoculation of the sediment into various culture media (7).

a. The blood culture bottles inoculated with AF showed growth in 77% of patients, compared with 57% by the conventional method (P=0.0001). No patient had a positive culture by the conventional method only, but 14 patients had a positive culture by the bedside inoculation method only.

b. The isolated organism was resistant to the empiric antibiotic regimen in 4 of the 14 patients whose culture was positive by bedside inoculation only. Therefore, whenever possible, AF should be inoculated into blood culture bottles at the bedside at the time of paracentesis.

D. Empiric Antibiotic Therapy for SBP

1. Traditionally, ampicillin plus an aminoglycoside was recommended for treatment of SBP (44). However, because of the potential nephrotoxicity associated with that regimen, monotherapy with a third-generation cephalosporin (*e.g.*, cefotaxime) is now the treatment of choice (4,12). In an uncontrolled series of 213 consecutive episodes of SBP treated with cefotaxime, infection was successfully eradicated in 77% (43). In the only randomized comparison to date, Felisart found that cefotaxime was more effective than the combination of ampicillin plus tobramycin (10). That study involved 73 consecutive cirrhotic patients with severe bacterial infections, 83% of whom had CNNA or culture-positive SBP. Patients allergic to β-lactam drugs or aminoglycosides were excluded. The infection was considered cured if all clinical and laboratory manifestations of the infection disappeared and if the repeat AF culture 2 days after cessation of antibiotics remained negative.

   a. Infection was cured in only 56% of patients treated with the combination of ampicillin plus tobramycin, compared with 85% of those treated with cefotaxime (P<0.02). However, there was no difference in mortality between the two groups during the study.

   b. Treatment-related nephrotoxicity occurred in 7% of patients treated with the combination of ampicillin plus tobramycin but in none of those treated with cefotaxime (P=NS). The overall risk of nephrotoxicity was not different between the two groups.

2. An alternative to a third-generation cephalosporin drug may be amoxicillin-clavulanic acid. Grange reported the results of a prospective, uncontrolled study of amoxicillin (1 g IV q 6 hours for 14 days) plus clavulanic acid (0.2 g IV q 6 hours for 14 days) in 23 patients with 27 episodes of culture-positive SBP or CNNA. Infection was successfully treated in 85% of patients (16). However, a randomized, controlled comparison with cefotaxime would be of interest. Furthermore, the IV form of this drug is not yet available in United States. Ampicillin-sulbactam or ticarcillin-clavulanic acid may be reasonable substitutes.

3. Monotherapy with aztreonam has been tested for patients with documented gram-negative SBP, but the risk of gram-positive bacterial superinfection was found to be higher with aztreonam than with cefotaxime. Streptococcal superinfections occurred in 14.2% of patients treated with aztreonam but in none of those treated with cefotaxime. The risk of relapse and the rate of mortality were similar between the two groups (3).

4. **Duration of Antibiotic Therapy**

   a. **Short Versus Long Therapy**—Traditionally, the duration of antibiotic therapy for SBP was 10 to 14 days. Recently, 5 days of therapy has been shown to be equally as effective as 10 days. In a prospective randomized controlled trial, Runyon compared 5 days versus 10 days of cefotaxime (2 g IV q 8 hours) in 90 patients with culture-positive SBP or CNNA. Patients were well matched in terms of clinical and laboratory characteristics at the time of enrollment. Patients with secondary peritonitis, peritoneal carcinomatosis, intraperitoneal bleeding, pancreatitis, or tuberculous peritonitis were excluded. Relapse was defined as reoccurrence of SBP caused by the same organism (identical genus and species) that caused the initial infection. Reinfection was defined as reoccurrence of SBP caused by an organism different from the one that caused the initial infection (33).

(1) There were no significant differences in infection-related mortality, overall mortality, or bacteriologic cure rate. The need for additional antibiotics, rate of relapse, rate of reinfection, and risk of side effects were also similar between the two groups.

(2) Patients treated with 5 days of cefotaxime had an average length of hospital stay of 37 days, compared with 50 days for those receiving 10 days of therapy (*P*=NS). The average cost of antibiotic therapy was $259 per patient with 5-day therapy and $486 per patient with 10-day therapy.

b. Response of the Ascitic Fluid Neutrophil Count to Treatment—The response of the AF neutrophil count to treatment may be an alternative guide for optimal duration of therapy. In a nonrandomized study, Fong prospectively compared "empiric duration" of therapy versus duration guided by the response of the AF neutrophil count to treatment. Ten patients treated for empiric duration received an average of 9.6 days of antibiotic therapy (range, 5 to 14 days); the criteria used to determine this duration were not specified. Twenty-three patients were treated until the AF neutrophil count dropped to <250 cells/µl. The mean Child-Pugh scores were comparable between the two groups. All patients had culture-positive SBP or CNNA. Those with pancreatitis, secondary peritonitis, tuberculous or fungal peritonitis, cardiac ascites, or peritoneal carcinomatosis were excluded (11).

(1) The average duration of antibiotics in the empiric group was 9.6 days, compared with 4.8 days in the neutrophil count group (*P*<0.01). There were no significant differences between the two groups in rate of mortality or risk of recurrent SBP during hospitalization.

(2) In addition, the response of the AF neutrophil count to treatment provided prognostic information. Nineteen patients who survived the infection had an average decrease of 92% in the AF neutrophil count at 48 hours, compared with a 66% decrease for the 11 patients who died.

E. Prognostic Factors

1. Toledo recently identified six factors predictive of in-hospital death in 185 consecutive patients with 213 episodes of SBP. All patients were treated initially with cefotaxime. Cefotaxime successfully eradicated the infection in 77% of patients. The in-hospital mortality rate was 38%. Fifty-one clinical and laboratory variables measured at the time of diagnosis were examined for their relation to survival (43).

a. In a multivariate analysis, four quantitative factors were predictive of in-hospital death: elevated blood urea nitrogen (BUN), elevated serum aspartate aminotransferase (AST), older age, and higher Child-Pugh score. The most powerful independent predictors of death in this study were the BUN and the AST levels. Patients who died had an average BUN of 45 mg/dl and an average AST of 150 U/L, compared with 27 mg/dl and 67 U/L, respectively, for those who survived.

b. The multivariate analysis also identified two qualitative factors predictive of in-hospital death: presence of ileus and hospital-acquired SBP. Patients with an ileus had a 30% survival rate, compared with 63% for those without ileus (*P*=0.041). Similarly, 50% of patients with hospital-acquired SBP survived, compared with 73% of those with community-acquired SBP (*P*=0.001).

c. None of the microbiologic features (*e.g.*, positive versus negative AF culture, species of the isolated organism) correlated with the survival rate.

F. Prophylaxis Against SBP

1. Because the case-fatality rate for SBP is 36% to 70% despite prompt diagnosis and therapy (11,20,32,41), some authors have advocated prophylactic therapy for those at high risk for development of SBP (14,23,39).

a. Hospitalized Patients with Gastrointestinal Hemorrhage—In a study by Rimola, oral, nonabsorbable antibiotics given prophylactically decreased the risk of infection in cirrhotic patients with gastrointestinal hemorrhage. The overall risk of infection was 16% for patients given prophylaxis (gentamicin plus vancomycin plus nystatin or neomycin plus colistin plus nystatin), compared with 35% for those not given prophylaxis. However, there was no difference in survival (23).

b. Hospitalized Patients with Low AF Protein Concentration

(1) In a prospective randomized controlled trial, Soriano compared norfloxacin (400 mg PO daily) versus no treatment in 63 consecutive cirrhotic patients with low AF protein (<1.5 g/dl). No patient had a positive AF culture or AF neutrophil count >500 cells/μl at the time of admission; 94% had not had a prior episode of SBP. Prophylaxis was continued for the duration of hospitalization (39). As shown in Table 30-8, the overall risk of infection, risk of SBP, and risk of gram-negative infection were all significantly reduced with norfloxacin. The risk of death during hospitalization was also lower with norfloxacin, but the difference was not statistically significant.

(2) In a similar randomized study involving 60 cirrhotic patients with low AF protein (<1.5 g/dl), ciprofloxacin (750 mg PO once per week for 6 months) was significantly better than placebo in reducing the risk of SBP (3.6% versus 22%, $P<0.05$) (23a). In addition, the duration of hospitalization was also lower in the ciprofloxacin group (9.3 days versus 17.6 days, $P<0.05$).

c. Secondary Prophylaxis—Because the 1-year risk of recurrent infection in patients surviving an episode of SBP may be as high as 69%, prophylaxis has also been tested in this group. Gines compared norfloxacin (400 mg PO daily) versus placebo in 80 cirrhotic patients who had survived an episode of SBP. Patients were monitored as outpatients monthly for 3 months, then bimonthly. Average duration of follow-up was 6.4 months (14). (see Table 30-9).

(1) The risk of recurrent SBP was significantly lower in patients treated with norfloxacin. Only 1 patient in the norfloxacin group developed gram-negative rod SBP; this patient was noncompliant with the drug regimen.

(2) There was no significant difference in survival.

d. All of these studies showed that prophylactic antibiotics can decrease the rate of SBP in high-risk patients. However, no study has shown a statistically significant survival benefit. Because there is significant concern over the emergence of drug-resistant organisms, some authors do not recom-

Table 30-8 Norfloxacin vs. control in cirrhotics with low AF protein (39)

	Norfloxacin (N=32)	Control (N=31)	*P*
Overall risk of infection	3%	42%	<0.005
Risk of SBP	0%	22%	<0.05
Risk of gram-negative rod infection	0%	29%	<0.001
Risk of death	6%	16%	NS

Table 30-9 Norfloxacin vs. control for secondary prophylaxis of SBP (14)

	Norfloxacin (N=40)	Control (N=40)	*P*
Risk of SBP	12%	35%	0.014
Risk of gram-negative rod SBP	3%	25%	0.0029
Risk of death	17%	25%	NS

mend routine prophylaxis until a clear survival advantage can be demonstrated (9,12).

2. **Diuresis**—There is some evidence that diuretics may decrease the risk of SBP. Runyon has demonstrated that diuresis can increase the protein concentration and the opsonic activity of the AF (30,34,36). Because these factors correlate with the risk of developing SBP, diuresis may protect against peritonitis. In a nonrandomized study involving 28 patients with SBP, no patient who was diuresed effectively developed recurrent SBP. In contrast, 29% of those who could not be diuresed developed recurrent SBP. However, the difference was not statistically significant (30).

G. Summary

1. SBP is a serious infection that affects about 19% of cirrhotic patients with ascites. Despite prompt diagnosis and therapy, the case-fatality rate ranges from 36% to 70%. Furthermore, about 69% of patients who survive an index episode suffer a second episode within 1 year. The best predictor for development of SBP is AF protein concentration <1 g/dl, which appears to be a marker for low opsonic activity of the AF.
2. Diagnosis of SBP can usually be established by AF analysis. If the AF neutrophil count is >250 to 500 cells/µl, empiric antibiotic therapy should be started. False-positive causes of elevated ascitic neutrophil count should be considered, including secondary peritonitis, pancreatitis, intraperitoneal bleeding, and peritoneal metastasis. For improved diagnostic yield, blood culture bottles should be inoculated with AF at the bedside. The AF cultures are usually positive, but CNNA accounts for 18% to 35% of SBP in most series.
3. The treatment of choice for SBP is a third-generation cephalosporin such as cefotaxime. Alternatives include amoxicillin-clavulanic acid, ampicillin-sulbactam, or ticarcillin-clavulanic acid. Monotherapy with aztreonam is suboptimal because it lacks coverage for gram-positive bacteria. The combination of ampicillin plus an aminoglycoside has fallen out of favor because of potential nephrotoxicity; in one study, it was also less effective than cefotaxime.
4. The role of prophylactic antibiotics remain controversial. Some authors advocate the use of prophylactic antibiotics for high-risk patients, including those hospitalized with low-protein ascites, decompensated liver disease, or gastrointestinal hemorrhage. Prophylaxis has also been recommended for patients surviving an index episode of SBP. For both primary and secondary prophylaxis, norfloxacin significantly decreased the risk of first or recurrent SBP in these patients; however, no statistically significant survival benefit was demonstrated. In the absence of survival benefit, some experts discourage routine prophylaxis because of concern about the emergence of resistant organisms.

Abbreviations used in Chapter 30

AF = ascitic fluid
AST = aspartate aminotransferase
BUN = blood urea nitrogen
CNNA = culture-negative neutrocytic ascites
IV = intravenous
LDH = lactate dehydrogenase
NNBA = nonneutrocytic bacterascites
NS = not significant
P = probability value
PO = per os
q = every
SBP = spontaneous bacterial peritonitis

References

1. Albillos. Ascitic fluid polymorphonuclear cell count and serum to ascites albumin gradient in the diagnosis of bacterial peritonitis. *Gastroenterology* 1990;1990:134.
2. Andreu. Risk factors for spontaneous bacterial peritonitis in cirrhotic patients with ascites. *Gastroenterology* 1993;104:1133.
3. Ariza. Evaluation of aztreonam in the treatment of spontaneous bacterial peritonitis in patients with cirrhosis. *Hepatology* 1986;6:906.
4. Bhuva. Spontaneous bacterial peritonitis: an update on evaluation, management, and prevention. *Am J Med* 1994;97:169. Review.
5. Bobadilla. Improved method for bacteriological diagnosis of spontaneous bacterial peritonitis. *J Clin Microbiol* 1989;27:2145.
6. Brook. Measurement of lactate in ascitic fluid: an aid in the diagnosis of peritonitis with particular relevance to spontaneous bacterial peritonitis of the cirrhotic. *Dig Dis Sci* 1981;26:1089.
7. Castellote. Comparison of two ascitic fluid culture methods in cirrhotic patients with spontaneous bacterial peritonitis. *Am J Gastroenterol* 1990;85:1605.
8. Corey. An approach to the statistical analysis of peritonitis data from patients on CAPD. *Perit Dial Bull* 1981;1(Suppl):29.
9. Dupeyron. Rapid emergence of quinolone resistance in cirrhotic patients treated with norfloxacin to prevent spontaneous bacterial peritonitis. *Antimicrob Agents Chemother* 1994;38:340.
10. Felisart. Cefotaxime is more effective than is ampicillin-tobramycin in cirrhotics with severe infections. *Hepatology* 1985;5:457.
11. Fong. Polymorphonuclear cell count response and duration of antibiotic therapy in spontaneous bacterial peritonitis. *Hepatology* 1989;9:423.
12. Garcia-Tsao. Spontaneous bacterial peritonitis. *Gastroenterol Clin North Am* 1992; 21:257. Review.
13. Garcia-Tsao. The diagnosis of bacterial peritonitis: comparison of pH, lactate concentration and leukocyte count. *Hepatology* 1985;5:91.
14. Gines. Norfloxacin prevents spontaneous bacterial peritonitis recurrence in cirrhosis: results of a double-blind, placebo-controlled trial. *Hepatology* 1990;12(4 Pt 1):716.
15. Gitlin. The pH of ascitic fluid in the diagnosis of spontaneous bacterial peritonitis in alcoholic cirrhosis. *Hepatology* 1982;2:408.
16. Grange. Amoxicillin-clavulanic acid therapy of spontaneous bacterial peritonitis: a prospective study of twenty-seven cases in cirrhotic patients. *Hepatology* 1990;11: 360.
17. Guyton. The rapid determination of ascitic fluid L-lactate for the diagnosis of spontaneous bacterial peritonitis. Am J *Gastroenterology* 1983;78:231.
18. Llach. Incidence and predictive factors of first episode of spontaneous bacterial peritonitis in cirrhosis with ascites: relevance of ascitic fluid protein concentration. *Hepatology* 1992;16:724.
19. Pelletier. Asymptomatic bacterascites: is it spontaneous bacterial peritonitis? *Hepatology* 1991;14:112.
20. Pelletier. Culture-negative neutrocytic ascites: a less severe variant of spontaneous bacterial peritonitis. *J Hepatol* 1990;10:327.
21. Pinzello. Spontaneous bacterial peritonitis: a prospective investigation in predominantly nonalcoholic cirrhotic patients. *Hepatology* 1983;3:545.
22. Pinzello. Is the acidity of ascitic fluid a reliable index in making the presumptive diagnosis of spontaneous bacterial peritonitis? *Hepatology* 1986;6:244.
23. Rimola. Oral, nonabsorbable antibiotics prevent infection in cirrhotics with gastrointestinal hemorrhage. *Hepatology* 1985;5:463.

23a. Rolachon. Ciprofloxacin and long-term prevention of spontaneous bacterial peritonitis: results of a prospective controlled trial. *Hepatology* 1995;22:1171.

24. Runyon. Care of patients with ascites. *N Engl J Med* 1994;330:337.
25. Runyon. Low-protein-concentration ascitic fluid is predisposed to spontaneous bacterial peritonitis. *Gastroenterology* 1986;91:1343.

26. Runyon. Patients with deficient ascitic fluid opsonic activity are predisposed to spontaneous bacterial peritonitis. *Hepatology* 1988;8:632. Published erratum appears in *Hepatology* 1988;8:1184.
27. Runyon. Monomicrobial nonneutrocytic bacterascites: a variant of spontaneous bacterial peritonitis. *Hepatology* 1990;12(4 Pt 1):710.
28. Runyon. Ascitic fluid pH and lactate: insensitive and nonspecific tests in detecting ascitic fluid infection. *Hepatology* 1991;13:929.
29. Runyon. Bedside inoculation of blood culture bottles with ascitic fluid is superior to delayed inoculation in the detection of spontaneous bacterial peritonitis. *J Clin Microbiol* 1990;28:2811.
30. Runyon. Diuresis increases ascitic fluid opsonic activity in patients who survive spontaneous bacterial peritonitis. *J Hepatol* 1992;14:249.
31. Runyon. Ascitic fluid analysis in the differentiation of spontaneous bacterial peritonitis from gastrointestinal tract perforation into ascitic fluid. *Hepatology* 1984; 4:447.
32. Runyon. Culture-negative neutrocytic ascites: a variant of spontaneous bacterial peritonitis. *Hepatology* 1984;4:1209.
33. Runyon. Short-course versus long-course antibiotic treatment of spontaneous bacterial peritonitis: a randomized controlled study of 100 patients. (See Comments.) *Gastroenterology* 1991;100:1737.
34. Runyon. Opsonic activity of human ascitic fluid: a potentially important protective mechanism against spontaneous bacterial peritonitis. *Hepatology* 1985;5:634.
35. Runyon. Inoculation of blood culture bottles with ascitic fluid: improved detection of spontaneous bacterial peritonitis. *Arch Intern Med* 1987;147:73.
36. Runyon. Diuresis of cirrhotic ascites increases its opsonic activity and may help prevent spontaneous bacterial peritonitis. *Hepatology* 1986;6:396.
37. Scemama. Ascitic fluid pH in alcoholic cirrhosis: a reevaluation of its use in the diagnosis of spontaneous bacterial peritonitis. Gut 1985;26:332.
38. Siersema. Blood culture bottles are superior to lysis-centrifugation tubes for bacteriological diagnosis of spontaneous bacterial peritonitis. *J Clin Microbiol* 1992; 30:667.
39. Soriano. Selective intestinal decontamination prevents spontaneous bacterial peritonitis. *Gastroenterology* 1991;100:477.
40. Such. Low C3 in cirrhotic ascites predisposes to spontaneous bacterial peritonitis. *J Hepatol* 1988;6:80.
41. Terg. Analysis of clinical course and prognosis of culture-positive spontaneous bacterial peritonitis and neutrocytic ascites: evidence of the same disease. *Dig Dis Sci* 1992;37:1499.
42. Tito. Recurrence of spontaneous bacterial peritonitis in cirrhosis: frequency and predictive factors. *Hepatology* 1988;8:27.
43. Toledo. Spontaneous bacterial peritonitis in cirrhosis: predictive factors of infection resolution and survival in patients treated with cefotaxime. *Hepatology* 1993; 17:251.
44. Wilcox. Spontaneous bacterial peritonitis: a review of pathogenesis, diagnosis, and treatment. *Medicine (Baltimore)* 1987;66:447. Review.
45. Yang. White count, pH and lactate in ascites in the diagnosis of spontaneous bacterial peritonitis. *Hepatology* 1985;5:85.

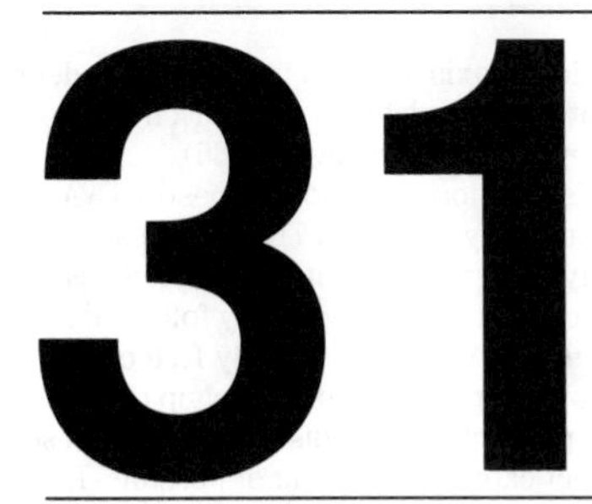

Ischemic Stroke and Transient Ischemic Attack: Overview and Acute Treatment

Will P. Schmitt, Burton W. Lee, and Walter J. Koroshetz

A. Introduction

1. Each year in the United States, about 500,000 people experience new strokes. Stroke is the third leading cause of death, accounting for 150,000 to 175,000 deaths per year (13,86,90). Among those who suffer new strokes, only 55% live longer than 6 months (11). However, in most industrialized countries, the mortality rate associated with stroke has been declining (12). Nevertheless, the burden of stroke on society is far greater than the simple mortality figures, because only one-half to two-thirds of the survivors of stroke regain their previous level of function by 6 months (11,12,80).
2. **Types of Cerebrovascular Accidents**—Because the terminology used to describe cerebrovascular accidents (CVAs) differs somewhat from author to author, the categories of CVAs as used in this book are defined here.
   - **a.** CVAs may be divided into two categories: hemorrhagic and ischemic stroke. The focus of Chapters 31 and 32 is limited to transient ischemic attacks (TIAs) and ischemic strokes. TIA is arbitrarily defined as transient loss of brain function lasting <24 hours, localized to a part of the brain supplied by a particular cerebrovascular system, and not attributable to a cause other than ischemia. Ischemic stroke is defined as loss of brain function persisting >24 hours, caused by insufficient blood flow in a particular vascular territory (85). Injuries to the brain resulting from infection, tumor, or subdural hematoma are excluded from these definitions.
   - **b.** If complete neurologic recovery occurs within 3 weeks (but takes >24 hours), stroke is sometimes termed "reversible ischemic neurologic deficit." If there is little or no functional disability at 1 to 3 months after the initial event, it is considered a minor stroke. An event that causes extensive neurologic damage without significant functional recovery is considered a major stroke. In most cases, these determinations are made only retrospectively.
   - **c.** Ischemic strokes may also be classified according to the pathophysiologic mechanism involved: thrombosis or embolism. Thrombotic strokes may occur as a result of large artery stenosis, small vessel disease (lacunes), or venous disease. In some cases, large vessel occlusive disease (with or without episodes of systemic hypotension) can lead to a low-flow state, especially in a border zone between two vascular territories, causing so-called watershed infarcts. The heart is the most common source of embolism, but artery-to-artery embolism from the aorta, the carotid artery, or other large vessels may occur. A paradoxical venous source of embolism from a patent foramen ovale (PFO) is also possible. In patients with internal carotid artery disease, thrombosis at the site of stenosis and embolism to a distal cerebral artery may both play important roles in causing strokes.
   - **d.** Finally, CVAs may be divided according to the vascular territory involved: anterior versus posterior circulation CVAs. Anterior CVAs are characterized by focal unilateral weakness, sensory deficits, dysarthria, or aphasia if the stroke involves the dominant hemisphere and neglect if the stroke involves the nondominant hemisphere. Transient monocular blindness is a common warning symptom of internal carotid artery disease. Bilateral

symptoms, vertigo, double vision, ataxia, dysphagia, tinnitus, or depressed level of consciousness are not characteristic of anterior circulation CVAs but may be suggestive of posterior circulation events (85).

e. Table 31-1 summarizes the distribution of various types of CVAs in two large studies. One study prospectively evaluated 713 stroke patients hospitalized at one of four university centers, all of whom were registered in the Stroke Data Bank (45). The second study prospectively followed 5734 individuals from the general population who were initially free of stroke, 472 of whom later developed CVAs during 10 years of follow-up (89).

f. Because stroke may be an end product of many disease processes, segregation of strokes into their correct category is often not possible. Even after careful evaluation, no clear cause may be apparent in up to 24% of patients with acute ischemic strokes (45). Therefore, evaluation of potential therapies for a particular type of acute stroke has been difficult; this in part explains the relative paucity of reliable data in this area.

B. Risk Factors for Stroke (50)—Based on the prospectively derived data from the Physicians Health Study, the rate of stroke was 0.18 events per 100 patient-years among asymptomatic, healthy male physicians who were assigned to the placebo arm (76). However, the presence of other comorbid conditions (*e.g.*, hypertension, atrial fibrillation [AF], valvular heart disease) can substantially increase this risk. The major risk factors for stroke are presented in the following sections, and the specific strategies for prevention of stroke in these populations are discussed in Chapter 32.

1. Epidemiologic Risk Factors for Stroke

a. Age—The incidence of stroke increases exponentially with age. An octogenarian has 100 times the risk of stroke of a 30-year-old person. The cumulative lifetime risk of stroke is 3% by age 65 and increases to 33% by age 90 (13).

b. Alcohol—Moderate consumption of alcohol has been associated with a decrease in the incidence of nonhemorrhagic stroke. According to data from case-controlled studies, lifetime teetotalers have an estimated twofold increase in the risk of stroke (29,75). On the other hand, heavy consumption of alcohol (>200 g or 25 drinks per week) is associated with a fourfold increase in the risk of stroke. Drinking at any level appears to increase the risk of hemorrhagic stroke (75).

c. Social Factors—In cross-cultural studies in Great Britain and the United States, Afro-American and Afro-Caribbean subjects appear to have an increased risk of stroke, independent of blood pressure or lipid levels. This association also holds true for socioeconomic status—that is, the lower the socioeconomic status, the higher the risk of stroke (13).

2. Risk Factors for Atherosclerosis and the Risk of Stroke

a. Hypertension—On a population basis, hypertension is probably the most

Table 31-1 Distribution of various types of cerebrovascular accidents

	Data From the Stroke Data Bank (45) (N=713)	Population-Based Data (89) (N=472)
TIA	11%	22.5%
Stroke	89%	76.0%
Hemorrhagic stroke	33%	9.3%
Intracerebral hemorrhage	16%	4.4%
Subarachnoid hemorrhage	17%	4.9%
Ischemic stroke	56%	66.7%
Thrombotic stroke	36%	44.5%
Embolic stroke	20%	22.2%

important modifiable risk factor for stroke. Both diastolic and isolated systolic hypertension contribute to the risk of stroke (5,49). In a metaanalysis of nine major observational studies involving 420,000 patients (96% male), the risk of stroke doubled with each 10 mm Hg increment of diastolic blood pressure above 76 mm Hg. An increase in the risk of stroke with lower blood pressures, the so-called "J-curve" phenomenon, was not observed in the study (49).

b. **Hyperlipidemia**—In the Multiple Risk Factor Intervention Trial, patients with total cholesterol levels >280 mg/dl had a 2.6 times higher risk of death from nonhemorrhagic stroke than patients with lower levels of cholesterol. On the other hand, patients with serum cholesterol levels <160 mg/dl had a twofold to threefold increase in the risk of hemorrhagic stroke. The reason for the latter association is not clear, but alcoholism or cancer may have been confounding variables, responsible for both low serum cholesterol levels and increased risk of hemorrhage (38).

c. **Smoking**—In the Multiple Risk Factor Intervention Trial, the participants who died of stroke were twice as likely to have been smokers (38).

d. **Diabetes Mellitus**—In the Honolulu Heart Study, after controlling for lipids and hypertension, Japanese-American men with diabetes mellitus had a twofold to threefold increase in the risk of stroke (16).

3. **Atrial Fibrillation and the Risk of Stroke**—See Chapter 1 for more details.

   a. Most patients with AF have a significantly increased risk of embolic stroke. Patients with AF caused by rheumatic heart disease have a 17-fold higher risk of stroke than the general population (41). Patients with nonrheumatic AF (NRAF) are also at high risk of stroke. In the Framingham Heart Study, after adjusting for the presence of other risk factors, the risk of stroke was five times higher in patients with NRAF (87).

   b. However, the risk of stroke is not uniform in patients with NRAF. In an analysis of the pooled data from five randomized trials of anticoagulant therapy in patients with NRAF, the independent risk factors for stroke were hypertension, diabetes mellitus, and age >65 years (3). In another study, patients with a prior history of arterial thromboembolism, hypertension, or congestive heart failure and those with an enlarged left atrium or left ventricular dysfunction on echocardiography were at particularly high risk for stroke (73,74).

   c. For patients with AF but none of these risk factors, the annual risk of stroke is <2.5% (25,43). Patients with AF but no clinical evidence of cardiac disease, so-called lone AF, have a particularly low risk of stroke. In a report from the Mayo clinic, the risk of stroke was only 0.35 events per 100 person-years among 97 patients with lone AF (43). In that study, the definition of lone AF was very strict, excluding all patients with coronary artery disease, hyperthyroidism, valvular heart disease, mitral valve prolapse, congestive heart failure, cardiomyopathy, chronic obstructive pulmonary disease, cardiomegaly on chest radiographic film, hypertension, diabetes mellitus, or age >60 years. Only 2.7% of patients with AF fulfilled this strict definition of lone AF.

4. **Myocardial Infarction and the Risk of Stroke**

   a. The risk of stroke appears to increase in the period after myocardial infarction (MI), probably because of thrombus that forms in the infarcted, akinetic or dyskinetic regions of the heart. Without the use of early anticoagulation or aspirin therapy, the incidence of stroke is about 2.5% during the first 2 to 4 weeks after MI (19). Earlier studies suggested that the risk of stroke is higher with anterior MIs than inferior MIs, about 6% versus 1%, respectively (19). However, in a retrospective multivariate analysis involving 2500 patients with acute MI, the 2-year risk of stroke or TIA did not vary with the location of the infarct. In both groups, the incidence of CVA was 3% to 4% (8). About 50% of post-MI strokes occur within the first week after the event, and another 25% occur during the second week. The rate of stroke usually declines after the first 3 months, but the risk may remain high if the patient has other predisposing factors such as low ejection fraction, ventricular aneurysm, apical thrombus, AF, or valvular heart disease (36).

b. Post-MI patients with a left ventricular thrombus (LVT) have a higher risk of embolism than those without LVT. For example, in one prospective study involving 150 consecutive patients during the peri-MI period, the risk of systemic embolism was 27% in those with an echocardiographically identified LVT, compared with 2% in those without an LVT (39). LVT tends to form in areas of abnormal ventricular wall motion. Consequently, LVT is more often associated with anterior MIs than with inferior MIs. An aggregate of small studies suggest that LVT develops in about 40% of anterior MIs. Most intracardiac thrombi develop within the first 2 weeks after an MI (19).

5. **Congestive Heart Failure and the Risk of Stroke**—Although the data are scanty, congestive heart failure appears to be an independent risk factor for stroke. In Fuster's retrospective analysis of 104 patients with dilated cardiomyopathy, a thromboembolic complication developed in 18% of the non-anticoagulated patients during mean follow-up of 11 years (26). More recent data suggest that patients with dilated cardiomyopathy who are in sinus rhythm have a 2.0% to 3.5% annual risk of stroke (4). This risk appears to be relatively constant over time. Compared with the clots that are found in post-MI patients, LVT detected in patients with dilated cardiomyopathy may be smaller in size (4).

6. **Carotid Artery Disease and the Risk of Stroke**

a. Approximately 15% of all strokes are caused by atherosclerotic disease of the carotid arteries (62,86). As shown in Table 31-2, the prevalence of significant carotid artery disease (defined as >75% stenosis) varies from 1.2% in asymptomatic patients without bruits to 60% in those who have had a stroke ipsilateral to the side with the bruit (91).

b. Among asymptomatic patients, the incidence of carotid artery bruits increases with age from 3.5% among persons 44 to 55 years old to 7.0% among those 65 to 79 years old (34,88). The presence of bruits is an independent risk factor for stroke as well as a general indicator of atherosclerosis. Patients with carotid bruits have a twofold increase in the risk of MI, a two to three times higher risk of stroke, and a 1.5- to 2-fold increase in the risk of death (88). The presence of bruit is a risk factor for CVAs on either side, not merely the CVAs attributable to the side with the bruit (34). In the Framingham study, patients with bruits had a 12% risk of stroke over 8 years, but fewer than half of these events occurred on the side with the bruits (86).

c. In both symptomatic and asymptomatic patients, the risk of stroke increases with the degree of carotid artery stenosis. For example, in one study in which 10 episodes of stroke or TIA occurred among 167 patients with asymptomatic bruits, 9 of the 10 patients had >80% carotid artery stenosis. Patients who had progression of their stenosis during follow-up were at particularly high risk of subsequent stroke, TIA, or asymptomatic carotid occlusion (68). Furthermore, in a subgroup analysis of the data from the North American Symptomatic Carotid Endarterectomy Trial, the 2-year risk of stroke among med-

Table 31-2 Prevalence of carotid artery disease in various populations (91)

	Patients With Stroke and Bruits (N=66)	Patients With Anterior TIA and Bruits (N=222)	Asymptomatic Patients with Bruits (N=500)	Asymptomatic Patients Without Bruits (N=500)
Mean age	70	69	64	66
Number (%) of patients with > 75% carotid artery stenosis	40 (60%)	96 (43%)	85 (17%)	6 (1.2%)

ically managed patients with an ipsilateral TIA or small stroke was 35% for those with 90% to 99% carotid stenosis, compared with 20% for those with 70% to 79% carotid stenosis (58). In contrast, in the European Carotid Surgery Trial, the 2-year risk of stroke was only 1.3% among medically managed symptomatic patients with 0% to 29% carotid stenosis (24). Once a patient with carotid artery disease has had a stroke or TIA, the risk of recurrent stroke becomes even higher. About 35% to 40% of patients with carotid artery disease and a history of anterior circulation TIA suffer a stroke within 4 years (48,88).

7. **Patent Foramen Ovale and the Risk of Stroke**—PFO is present in a disproportionate number of young patients with unexplained strokes. In case-control studies, patients with unexplained strokes were four times more likely to have a PFO than normal control patients or patients with a stroke with an identifiable cause. In one study involving 42 patients with clinically suspected thromboembolism and echocardiographically demonstrated PFO, 57% had deep venous thrombosis (DVT) on venogram. In most cases, the DVTs were not clinically apparent before venography (46,78,84).
8. **Prosthetic Heart Valves and the Risk of Stroke**
   a. **Mechanical Prosthetic Valves**—In a review of the literature by Stein, the rate of thromboembolism in patients with mechanical heart valves when no long-term anticoagulant or antiplatelet therapy was used ranged from 12 to 75 events per 100 patient-years (77). With long-term anticoagulation, this risk was reduced to 0 to 4.6 events per 100 patient-years for tilting-disk (St. Jude or Björk-Shiley) valves and 1.8 to 15.5 events per 100 patient-years for ball-and-cage valves (77). The risk of thromboembolism appears to be higher for prosthetic mitral valves than for aortic valves. In one report, when no anticoagulant or antiplatelet therapy was used, the rate of thromboembolism associated with the St. Jude aortic valve was 12.4 events per 100 patient-years, compared with 22.2 events per 100 patient-years when the valves were in the mitral position (6).
   b. **Bioprosthetic Valves**—For the first few weeks after surgery, patients with bioprosthetic valves are at an increased risk of thromboembolism if no antiplatelet or anticoagulant therapy is used. Estimates of this risk have been as high as 67% to 80% in some series (33,37,60). Beyond the first few months, however, the risk of thromboembolism with a bioprosthetic valve is generally much less than that with a mechanical valve. In the review of the literature by Stein, when no anticoagulant or antiplatelet therapy was used, the estimated risk of thromboembolism with bioprosthetic aortic valves ranged from 0.2 to 2.9 events per 100 patient-years (77). This estimate assumed that the patient was anticoagulated postoperatively for the first 6 to 12 weeks. Similar rates of thromboembolism have been quoted for patients with a bioprosthetic mitral valve (20).
9. **Aortic Arch Atherosclerosis and the Risk of Stroke**—In a case-control study, as measured by transesophageal echocardiography (TEE), patients with atherosclerotic plaques of >4 mm thickness in the ascending aorta were nine times more likely to suffer from stroke than age-matched controls. These plaques may be an important source of stroke in patients without other identifiable risk factors (1).
10. **Mitral Valve Prolapse and the Risk of Stroke**—Mitral valve prolapse has been linked to strokes, especially TIAs and ocular strokes. However, mitral valve prolapse is a common condition that affects 4% to 5% of the US population, so the true risk of stroke in patients with this condition has been difficult to ascertain. Best estimates of the absolute risk of stroke in all persons with mitral valve prolapse range from 1 in 6000 to 1 in 11,000 per year (18,47). Subgroups of patients who are male, who are older, or who have thickened leaflets with associated mitral regurgitation or mitral annulus abnormalities appear to have the highest risks (18). On the other hand, most patients with mitral valve prolapse, especially young women, lack these features and probably do not have an increased risk of stroke.
11. **Mitral Annular Calcification and the Risk of Stroke**—In an analysis of the

data from the Framingham study, elderly patients with mitral annular calcifications were two times more likely to have a stroke during 8 years of follow-up than control patients without this finding. There appeared to be a linear relation between the degree of calcification and the relative risk of stroke (7).

12. **Prior History of Stroke or TIA and the Risk of Recurrent Stroke**—In patients who have had a previous stroke or TIA, the risk of recurrent stroke is about 12% during the first year if left untreated. Beyond that time, the risk remains at about 7% per year. This corresponds to a sevenfold increase in the risk of stroke, compared with the general population. The rate of recurrent stroke after a TIA appears to be similar to the risk after a completed stroke. However, after a retinal stroke, the risk of recurrence appears to be lower, compared with other types of stroke (83). Among the 1273 patients with ischemic cerebral infarction who were registered in the Stroke Data Bank, the 30-day and 2-year cumulative risks of recurrent stroke were 3.3% and 14.1%, respectively (35,70). Patients with recurrent stroke within 30 days of the index event had a 20% case-fatality rate, compared with a rate of 7.4% among those without recurrence (70).

C. Initial Evaluation of a Patient with Stroke (15)

1. The major goals during the initial evaluation of a patient with acute stroke are to stabilize the patient, to clinically and radiologically classify the type of stroke (*e.g.*, hemorrhagic versus ischemic, embolic versus nonembolic, anterior versus posterior circulation), and to limit the extent of neuronal injury. A careful history and physical examination should be performed, including a thorough neurologic examination. Intravenous access should be established, and routine laboratory analysis should include chest film, electrocardiogram (ECG), complete blood count, creatinine, coagulation studies, electrolytes, glucose, and toxin screen, if indicated. Endotracheal intubation should be considered if the patient is susceptible to aspiration.
2. Computed tomography (CT) scan of the head should be performed as soon as possible to rule out an intracranial hemorrhage. Subtle changes may be detected within hours of an acute infarct, but the full extent of the damage may not be apparent on the CT scan for several days. Therefore, it is common practice to perform a second head CT evaluation 2 to 3 days after the initial event. Furthermore, the brainstem structures are poorly visualized with CT. Magnetic resonance imaging is more useful than CT for evaluation of the brainstem structures and is often able to detect ischemic injury in its acute phase (22).
3. Carotid noninvasive studies should be performed in patients who present with suspected CVAs attributable to the anterior circulation. In those who present with anterior circulation TIAs, about half have ipsilateral carotid stenosis of >75%. Between 10% and 15% of frank strokes are attributable to carotid artery disease (62,86). In a study that used conventional angiography as the gold standard, there was no significant difference in the sensitivity or specificity of carotid noninvasive studies and magnetic resonance angiography (MRA) for identification of carotid artery stenosis of >70%. However, both techniques tended to overestimate the degree of stenosis, compared with conventional angiography, and carotid noninvasive studies were more likely to misdiagnose a completely occluded artery than was MRA (54).
4. Echocardiography should be performed in patients who have a history of cardiac disease or abnormal ECGs. It should also be considered in those who are at risk for endocarditis. Echocardiography may reveal an embolic source in 10% to 30% of these patients. However, echocardiography is positive in fewer than 2% of patients who have normal ECGs and no history of cardiac disease. In younger patients with CVAs but no identifiable risk factors for stroke, addition of an agitated saline contrast study to the standard echocardiogram may be useful in detecting the presence of a PFO (9,19). TEE is more sensitive than transthoracic echocardiography, especially for detecting plaques in the aortic arch or atrial thrombi (1,4). However, it is more invasive and is cumbersome to perform.
5. The yield of a 24-hour Holter monitor is low in patients with no prior history of

arrhythmia. Only about 2% of such patients are found to have an occult arrhythmia on Holter monitoring that would potentially explain the embolic event (19,21,44). Evidence of paroxysmal AF, however, has major therapeutic implications for prevention of future strokes.

6. In up to 20% of strokes, more than one plausible cause may be found. For example, in one study, 19% of patients with TIAs had potential sources from the carotid artery as well as the heart (9). On the other hand, despite careful investigation, no clear source may be identified in up to 25% percent of strokes. Transcranial Doppler study or TEE may be useful in some of these patients. However, the additional utility of these techniques has not been rigorously studied (5,45).
7. Transcranial Doppler study and MRA are useful noninvasive tools for detecting intravascular stenosis caused by atherosclerosis, angiitis, or Moya-Moya disease. MRA can also detect carotid or vertebral artery dissection. Currently, cerebral angiography gives the most definitive information about the vascular anatomy, including the state of collateral circulation through the circle of Willis. It is often necessary to document the severity and precise location of internal carotid, intracranial, and vertebrobasilar stenoses and to detect cerebral angiitis, vascular malformations, aneurysms, or Moya-Moya disease. Because it is an invasive procedure, angiography carries the risk of procedure-related stroke, contrast-related congestive heart failure or renal failure, and complications from arterial puncture.

D. Acute Medical Management of Ischemic Stroke—Acute medical management of ischemic stroke is aimed at limiting the extent of further neuronal injury. Antiplatelet agents and heparin are being used in some centers in an attempt to decrease the risk of recurrent embolism or the rate of clot extension, or both. Thrombolytic drugs are being tested with the goal of rapid restoration of cerebral blood flow to ischemic tissue. Nimodipine, a calcium channel blocker with good brain penetration, has been tested with the hope of increasing cerebral blood flow and offering cytoprotection to ischemic brain tissue. Although there are ample data in support of various interventions that prevent stroke, the data in support of any intervention for treatment of acute stroke are relatively scarce. A major problem is the absence of well-designed, controlled trials of adequate size. If the 1-month mortality rate after acute stroke is assumed to be 10%, >10,000 patients are needed in a trial to demonstrate a 15% mortality benefit from an intervention. However, <2000 patients had been enrolled as of 1994 in various antiplatelet or anticoagulant trials for acute stroke. Therefore, it is still unknown whether the various agents are effective for acute stroke (72). Consequently, management strategies for acute stroke differ widely from center to center (51,72).

1. Antiplatelet Agents and Heparin

a. There are no data from well-designed studies to suggest that antiplatelet agents (*e.g.*, aspirin, ticlopidine) are effective in treatment of patients with acute stroke (72). Similarly, although unfractionated heparin is used in some centers for selected patients with ischemic stroke, it has never convincingly improved mortality or morbidity in a randomized trial. In theory, heparin may limit progression of thrombosis or decrease the risk of recurrent embolism, thereby limiting morbidity and improving survival. In addition, it may decrease the risk of DVT and pulmonary embolism in patients with acute stroke. However, there is concern that heparin may participate in the conversion of some bland infarcts into hemorrhagic ones or minimally hemorrhagic infarcts into frank hematomas. Patients with large infarcts, uncontrolled hypertension, or embolic stroke may be at increased risk for hemorrhage compared with patients without these conditions. Therefore, some authors recommend that anticoagulation should be avoided in these patients, whereas others contend that heparin should not be used in any patient with ischemic stroke (17,64). Still others assert that heparin should be used in most patients with acute ischemic stroke and that a randomized comparison with placebo is unethical (71). Nevertheless, most agree that heparin is important in the treatment of stroke caused by basilar artery stenosis. Heparin may also help prevent complete occlusion of a very stenotic carotid artery. In addition, heparin is standard therapy for acute carotid or vertebral artery dissection in adults. Given such controversy, the completion of the International Stroke Trial, which will compare heparin, aspirin, and placebo in patients with acute ischemic stroke, is much awaited.

b. In the meanwhile, two prospective randomized controlled trials (PRCTs) have evaluated the efficacy and safety of IV unfractionated heparin for acute stroke in the post-CT era; these are described in the following sections (17,23).

(1) Heparin for Embolic Stroke—In a nonblinded fashion, one study compared immediate versus delayed anticoagulation in patients with embolic stroke whose neurologic deficits lasted >24 hours. The study involved 45 patients with abrupt, focal brain infarction and a history of one of the following: rheumatic heart disease, AF, congestive heart failure, recent MI, left ventricular aneurysm, or nonorganic prosthetic valves. All patients were enrolled within 48 hours of the event and were observed for 14 days. At the time of enrollment, chest film, ECG, contrast CT scan of the head, coagulation tests, stool guaiac test, and other routine laboratory tests were performed for all patients. The study excluded patients with intracranial hemorrhage, gastrointestinal bleeding, history of peptic ulcer disease, persistent hypertension >180/115 mm Hg, septic embolism, and those being treated with warfarin who had a prothrombin time >1.5 times control. Immediate anticoagulation (5000 to 10,000 U as a bolus of IV heparin, followed by a continuous infusion to maintain partial thromboplastin time at 1.5 to 2.5 times control) was compared with delayed anticoagulation (no anticoagulation for the first 10 days). Antiplatelet therapy was not allowed (17) (see Table 31-3).

(a) The study was terminated before statistically significant outcomes were achieved. However, there was a trend toward fewer deaths and a lower rate of recurrent brain embolisms with heparin. Interestingly, the risk of hemorrhagic transformation of bland infarcts was also nonsignificantly lower with anticoagulation.

(b) There were no major complications associated with immediate anticoagulation. Two patients in the delayed anticoagulation group, both of whom had large infarcts on initial CT, suffered hemorrhagic transformation of bland infarcts. In addition, DVT occurred in one non-anticoagulated patient, whereas no DVTs occurred in anticoagulated patients.

(c) The obvious weakness in the study is the small size. In addition, fewer patients in the immediate anticoagulation group had large infarcts on initial CT scan (*P*=NS), which may have biased the study in favor of this group.

(2) Heparin for Nonembolic Ischemic Stroke—In a double-blind fash-

Table 31-3 Immediate vs. delayed anticoagulation in acute embolic stroke (17)

	Immediate Anticoagulation (N=24)	Delayed Anticoagulation (N=21)	*P*
Large infarct	20.8%	38.1%	NS
Transformation into hemorrhagic infarction	0%	9.5%	NS
Recurrent embolism	0%	9.5%	NS
Death	0%	9.5%	NS
DVT	0%	4.8%	NS

ion, another study compared heparin (started within 48 hours of onset of symptoms and adjusted to maintain partial thromboplastin time between 50 and 70 seconds for 7 days) versus placebo in 225 patients with nonembolic ischemic stroke. Patients with hemorrhagic infarction, previous neurologic deficits, recent MI, valvular heart disease, diastolic blood pressure >110 mm Hg, or contraindications to heparin therapy were excluded. In addition, patients who were not fully conscious, those who had severe deficits based on a predetermined scale, and those with evidence of stroke progression within 1 hour before enrollment were excluded. Except for the 5 patients with lone AF, patients with AF were also excluded (23) (see Table 31-4).

(a) Heparin failed to improve any meaningful clinical outcome in this population. The rate of neurologic improvement by day 7 was similar in the two groups. In addition, there were no significant differences in the rate of stroke progression or in the levels of neurologic function at day 7, 3 months, and 1 year.

(b) There was no significant difference in the mortality rate at day 7. However, by 1 year, significantly more patients assigned to heparin had died. The reason for the excess deaths is unknown. Because most of the deaths occurred between 3 months and 1 year after randomization, the excess deaths appeared to be unrelated to treatment. On the other hand, the poorer outcome in the heparin group may be an indicator of uneven randomization, which may have biased the study in favor of placebo.

c. Although the role of IV heparin for acute treatment of stroke remains controversial, several randomized studies have reported that heparin decreases the risk of DVTs in patients with acute stroke (53,67,81). Usually, the clot is found in the paralyzed limb (57,82). According to a metaanalysis of all randomized trials evaluating the efficacy of heparin for prevention of DVT in patients with acute stroke, there was a 79% reduction in the risk of DVT ($P<0.00001$) and a 58% reduction in the risk of pulmonary embolism (P=NS) with heparin (72). However, because low-dose subcutaneous heparin is sufficient for reducing the risk of DVT, full-dose IV heparin is probably unnecessary if administered solely for this purpose.

d. Low-Molecular-Weight Heparin—The results of a recent PRCT suggest that a low-molecular-weight heparin, nadroparin, may improve outcome in patients with acute ischemic stroke. The study randomized 306 acute stroke patients to high-dose nadroparin (4100 IU BID SC), low-dose nadroparin (4100 IU QD SC), or placebo for 10 days. Aspirin was not started until day 11 in any group. At 6 months, there were no differences in mortality among the three groups, but fewer patients in the high-dose nadroparin group had "poor" outcome, defined prospectively as death or dependency with respect to activities of daily living ($P<0.005$); 45% of the patients in the high-dose group had poor outcome compared to 52% and 65% of the patients in the low-dose and placebo groups, respectively (42a).

2. Thrombolysis—Unlike heparin, thrombolytic agents can actively dissolve clot and rapidly restore the patency of an occluded vessel. In theory, if administered before irreversible damage occurs, thrombolytic agents may limit the extent of infarction in patients with acute ischemic stroke. Early pilot studies have been

Table 31-4 Heparin vs. placebo in acute nonembolic stroke (23)

	Heparin (N=112)	Placebo (N=113)	*P*
Neurologic improvement by day 7	26.6%	24.3%	NS
Stroke progression during therapy	17.0%	19.5%	NS
7-d mortality rate	1.8%	0.9%	NS
1-y mortality rate	15.2%	7.1%	<0.05

encouraging (14,31). However, hemorrhagic transformation of bland infarct has been reported in as many as 53% of patients given IV tissue plasminogen activator (tPA), compared with 42% of those given placebo (55). If given in doses >0.95 mg/kg or if initiated >6 hours from the onset of symptoms, tPA may be associated with a high risk of intracranial or systemic hemorrhage (14,69). For maximal benefit and safety, some studies suggest that tPA should be given within 90 minutes of onset of symptoms (14,32). The results of recent PRCTs comparing thrombolytic therapy to placebo are conflicting.

a. When administered within 180 minutes of symptom onset, tPA (0.9 mg/kg) was superior to placebo in terms of reducing neurologic and functional deficits at 3 months; patients treated with tPA were 30% more likely to have minimal or no disability at 3 months compared to those treated with placebo. On the other hand, the rates of symptomatic intracerebral hemorrhage were higher with tPA than with placebo (6.4% vs. 0.6%, $P<0.001$). The 3-month mortality rates were statistically similar between the two groups (17% with tPA and 21% with placebo) (56a). One criticism of this study is that the placebo group did not receive aspirin or heparin. It is also unclear whether patients can routinely be evaluated and given tPA within 3 hours of symptom-onset under noninvestigational settings.

b. In a PRCT of 622 patients with acute ischemic stroke, patients were randomized in a 2-by-2 factorial design to receive streptokinase alone (1.5 million units), aspirin alone (300 mg/day), both, or neither within 6 hours of symptom-onset. Patients who received streptokinase (either alone or with aspirin) had a significantly higher 10-day mortality rate (OR 2.7; 95% CI (1.7-4.3)) compared to control patients. The 6-month mortality rate for patients treated with both streptokinase and aspirin was 44% compared to 29% for patients treated with placebo ($P<0.01$). Interestingly, while more patients died in the thrombolytic arm, those who survived had lower rates of disability; at 6 months, 20% of patients treated with both streptokinase and aspirin were disabled compared to 39% of the patients treated with placebo ($P<0.001$) (94).

c. It appears that thrombolytic therapy can limit the amount of ischemic injury due to an acute stroke but at the cost of significant short-term mortality and increased risk of bleeding. Furthermore, given the need to treat patients within few hours of symptom-onset, it is not clear how widely thrombolytic therapy can be applied. It is also unclear how thrombolytic therapy compares with standard or low-molecular-weight heparin (with or without aspirin). More studies are needed to determine the precise role of thrombolytic therapy for management of acute ischemic strokes.

3. **Blood Pressure Control**—No well-designed trials have evaluated the role of blood pressure control in patients with acute stroke. However, there are some data to suggest that aggressive treatment of hypertension may significantly decrease cerebral blood flow. In addition, at least in one study, the probability of early stroke progression was inversely related to the systolic blood pressure on admission. With each 20 mm Hg increase in the systolic blood pressure, the relative risk of early stroke progression decreased by a factor of 0.66 ($P=0.0003$) (40). Therefore, in the setting of acute stroke, many neurologists treat hypertension only if the diastolic blood pressure becomes excessive (*i.e.*, >110 to 120 mm Hg) (79).
4. **Nimodipine**—Nimodipine has been shown in randomized trials to decrease the subsequent rate of cerebral infarction in patients with subarachnoid hemorrhage. It has also been shown to reduce the rate of other adverse events such as death, vegetative state, or severe disability (30,56,59,63,65,66). However, the role of nimodipine in patients with acute ischemic stroke has been less clear. Some studies found that nimodipine, compared with placebo, improved the neurologic outcome and reduced the mortality rate in patients with acute ischemic stroke (27,61). However, other studies failed to confirm these findings (2, 10,52), and in some cases nimodipine was associated with a higher mortality rate (42) or delayed neurologic recovery (80) when compared with placebo. Some investigators have suggested that the benefit of nimodipine therapy may

be limited to men, patients with moderate to severe neurologic deficits, those treated within 24 hours of the onset of symptoms, or those older than 65 years of age (2,10,27,28,52,61). Still others found no benefit to nimodipine therapy even when patient randomization was stratified by severity of stroke, time of onset of therapy, and age (42). Representative studies are described here.

a. Study Demonstrating Improved Outcome with Nimodipine—In a double-blind PRCT involving 186 patients with acute ischemic stroke, Gelmers compared nimodipine (30 mg q 6 hours for 28 days, started within 24 hours of the onset of symptoms) versus placebo. All patients received subcutaneous heparin for prevention of DVT and depolymerized low-molecular-weight dextran for treatment of acute stroke. Patients with intracranial hemorrhage or complicated migraine were excluded. Concurrent therapy with other calcium channel blockers was not permitted (27).

(1) There was a significant improvement in survival with nimodipine. During the 4-week treatment period, 8.6% of patients treated with nimodipine died, compared with 20.4% of patients treated with placebo ($P<0.05$).

(2) Neurologic recovery, as measured on a standardized scale, was also superior with nimodipine at 4 weeks ($P=0.01$).

(3) Subgroup analysis revealed that the mortality and morbidity benefit may be limited to men and those with moderate to severe neurologic deficits at the time of enrollment.

(4) One criticism of this study was that the 4-week follow-up period was too short for determining meaningful end points in patients with stroke. Furthermore, a mortality benefit may be less meaningful if it results in more patients surviving with severe neurologic deficits (80).

b. Study Demonstrating Potential Benefit Only for a Subgroup of Patients Treated Early—In a double-blind study, the American Nimodipine Study Group randomly assigned 1064 patients with acute ischemic stroke to one of four regimens for 21 days: placebo, 60 mg/day of nimodipine, 120 mg/day of nimodipine, or 240 mg/day of nimodipine. All patients were treated within 48 hours of onset of symptoms. Those with neurologic dysfunction caused by intracranial hemorrhage, tumor, infection, trauma, or nonischemic brain disorders were excluded. Patients with embolic strokes were anticoagulated (2).

(1) With any dose of nimodipine therapy, there was no significant benefit in terms of 6-month rate of survival, recurrent stroke, stroke progression, or functional recovery compared with placebo.

(2) In preplanned subgroup analysis, patients who were treated within 18 hours of onset of symptoms with 120 mg/day of nimodipine were less likely to have worsening neurologic function on day 4 than patients treated with placebo (18.6% versus 29.2%, respectively). In addition, patients whose initial CT scans did not reveal an infarction were more likely to benefit from nimodipine therapy than patients whose initial CT scans were positive for infarction. These observations are consistent with the hypothesis that nimodipine may improve outcome when the cerebral tissue has not yet suffered irreversible infarction.

c. Study Demonstrating No Significant Benefit to Nimodipine Therapy—British investigators compared nimodipine (40 mg TID for 21 days) versus placebo in a much larger trial involving 1215 patients with acute ischemic stroke. Patients were treated within 48 hours of onset of symptoms. The primary end point of the study was functional independence at 6 months, defined by a predetermined standardized scale. This end point was chosen because the authors believed that a mortality benefit is less meaningful if it merely causes more patients to survive with severe neurologic deficits. All patients were functionally independent before the event and were conscious and able to swallow at the time of enrollment. CT scan was not required before enrollment in this study.

(1) At 6 months, there was no significant difference in the percent of patients functioning independently. Fifty-five percent of patients who received nimodipine were independent, compared with 58% of patients receiving placebo.

(2) Similarly, the overall functional assessment scores, as measured on predetermined standardized scales, were similar between the two groups at 6 months. In fact, there was a modest delay in neurologic recovery with nimodipine at 3 weeks.

(3) There was a slight trend toward higher mortality with nimodipine at 6 months (15.1% versus 12.4%), but the difference was not statistically significant.

(4) No benefit to nimodipine therapy was found even when the analysis was limited to the 441 patients who were treated within 24 hours of onset of symptoms.

F. Conclusions

1. The major goals during the initial evaluation of a patient with acute stroke are to stabilize the patient, to clinically and radiologically classify the type of stroke (*e.g.*, hemorrhagic versus ischemic, embolic versus nonembolic, anterior versus posterior circulation), and to limit the extent of neuronal injury. CT scan of the head should be performed as soon as possible to rule out an intracranial hemorrhage. Subtle changes may be detected within hours of an acute infarct, but the full extent of the damage may not be apparent on CT scan for several days. Therefore, it is common practice to perform a second head CT evaluation within 2 to 3 days after the initial event. Carotid noninvasive studies should be performed in patients who present with suspected stroke or TIA attributable to the anterior circulation. Transcranial Doppler study or MRA should be considered for patients with stroke or TIA attributable to the posterior circulation. Echo cardiography should be performed in patients who have a history of cardiac disease or abnormal ECGs. In younger patients with CVAs but no identifiable risk factors for stroke, addition of an agitated saline contrast study to the standard echocardiogram may be useful to detect the presence of a PFO. The diagnostic yield of a 24-hour Holter monitor is low in patients with no prior history of arrhythmia. In up to 20% of strokes, more than one plausible mechanism may be found. On the other hand, despite careful investigation, no clear source is identified in up to 25% percent of strokes.
2. Although there are ample data in support of various interventions that prevent stroke, the data in support of any intervention for treatment of acute stroke are relatively scarce. A major problem has been the paucity of well-designed, controlled trials of adequate size. Consequently, management strategies for acute stroke differ widely from center to center.
3. There are no data from well-designed studies to suggest that antiplatelet agents (*e.g.*, aspirin, ticlopidine) are effective in treatment of patients with acute stroke. Similarly, although unfractionated heparin is used in some centers for treatment of selected patients with ischemic stroke, it has not convincingly improved mortality or morbidity in randomized trials. In a small randomized trial involving 45 patients with embolic strokes, there was a nonsignificant trend toward fewer deaths, recurrent brain embolisms, and hemorrhagic transformations of bland infarcts with immediate anticoagulation. If this small study is taken at face value, heparin may offer some benefit for patients with embolic stroke, although confirmation from a larger, well-designed trial is necessary. However, in a double-blind PRCT involving 215 patients with nonembolic ischemic strokes, immediate anticoagulation did not improve any important clinical outcome. If this study is taken at face value, immediate anticoagulation does not appear to offer any benefit for patients with nonembolic ischemic strokes. The International Stroke Trial, which compares heparin, aspirin, or placebo in patients with acute ischemic stroke, may answer these questions more definitively. The results of a recent PRCT suggest that low-molecular-weight heparin may improve outcome in patients with acute ischemic stroke, but further studies are needed.
4. Nimodipine, a calcium channel blocker with good brain penetration, decreases

the subsequent rate of cerebral infarction in patients with subarachnoid hemorrhage. It also reduces the risk of other adverse events such as death, vegetative state, or severe disability. However, the role of nimodipine therapy in patients with acute ischemic stroke is less clear. In some studies, nimodipine improved the neurologic outcome and reduced the mortality rate compared with placebo. However, later studies failed to confirm these findings, and in some cases nimodipine was associated with a higher mortality rate or delayed neurologic recovery, compared with placebo. Some investigators have suggested that the benefit of nimodipine therapy may be limited to men, patients with moderate to severe neurologic deficits, those being treated within 12 to 24 hours of the onset of symptoms, or those older than 65 years of age. Still others found no benefit to nimodipine therapy even when the patient randomization process was stratified by severity of stroke, onset of therapy, and age of the patient.

5. Thrombolytic drugs can actively dissolve clot and rapidly restore the patency of an occluded vessel. In theory, if a thrombolytic drug is given before irreversible damage occurs, it may limit the extent of infraction in patients with acute ischemic stroke. Early studies show that thrombolytic therapy may limit the amount of ischemic injury due to an acute stroke but perhaps at the cost of significant short-term mortality and increased risk of bleeding. Studies comparing tPA to aspirin and/or heparin are needed to futher delineate the role of thrombolytic therapy in management of acute ischemic stroke.

Abbreviations used in Chapter 31

AF = atrial fibrillation
CT = computed tomography
CVA = cerebrovascular accident
DVT = deep venous thrombosis
ECG = electrocardiogram
IV = intravenous
LVT = left ventricular thrombus
MI = myocardial infarction
MRA = magnetic resonance angiography
N = number of patients in population
NRAF = nonrheumatic atrial fibrillation
P = probability value
PFO = patent foramen ovale
PRCT = prospective randomized controlled trial
q = every
TEE = transesophageal echocardiography
TIA = transient ischemic attack
TID = three times daily
tPA = tissue plasminogen activator

References

1. Amarenco. Atherosclerotic disease of the aortic arch and the risk of ischemic stroke. *N Engl J Med* 1994;331:1474.
2. American Nimodipine Study Group. Clinical trial of nimodipine in acute ischemic stroke. *Stroke* 1992;23:3.
3. Atrial Fibrillation Investigators. Risk factors for stroke and efficacy of antithrombotic therapy in atrial fibrillation. *Arch Intern Med* 1994;154:1449.
4. Baker. Management of heart failure IV: anticoagulation for patients with heart failure due to left ventricular systolic dysfunction. *JAMA* 1994;20:1614.

5. Barnett. *Pathophysiology, Diagnosis and Management: Stroke*, vol 1. New York: Churchill Livingstone, 1986:283.
6. Baudet. A 5 1/2 year experience with the St. Jude medical cardiac valve prosthesis. *J Thoracic Cardiovasc Surg* 1985;90:137.
7. Benjamin. Mitral annular calcification and the risk of stroke in an elderly cohort. *N Engl J Med* 1992;327:374.
8. Bodenheim. Relation between myocardial infarction and stroke. *J Am Coll Cardiol* 1994;24:61.
9. Bogousslavsky. Cardiac and arterial lesions in carotid transient ischemic attacks. *Arch Neurol* 1987;43:223.
10. Bogousslavsky. Double-blind study of nimodipine in non-severe stroke. *Eur Neurol* 1990;30:23.
11. Bonita. Event, incidence and case-fatality rates of cerebrovascular disease in Auckland, New Zealand. *Am J Epidemiol* 1984;120:236.
12. Bonita. International trends in stroke mortality: 1970–1985. *Stroke* 1990;32:989.
13. Bonita. Epidemiology of stroke. *Lancet* 1992;339:342.
14. Brott. Urgent therapy for stroke: part I. Pilot study of tissue plasminogen activator administered within 90 minutes. *Stroke* 1992;23:632.
15. Brown. Transient ischemic attack and minor ischemic stroke: an algorithm for evaluation and treatment. *Mayo Clin Proc* 1994;69:1027.
16. Burchfiel. Glucose intolerance and 22-year stroke incidence: the Honolulu heart program. *Stroke* 1994;25:951.
17. Cerebral Embolism Study Group. Immediate anticoagulation of embolic stroke: a randomized trial. *Stroke* 1983;14:668.
18. Cerebral Embolism Task Force. Cardiogenic brain embolism. *Arch Neurol* 1986;43:71.
19. Cerebral Embolism Task Force. Cardiogenic brain embolism: the second report of the Cerebral Embolism Task Force. *Arch Neurol* 1989;46:727.
20. Cohn. Early and late risk of mitral valve replacement. *J Thorac Cardiovasc Surg* 1985;90:872.
21. Come. Roles of echocardiography and arrhythmia monitoring in the evaluation of patients with suspected systemic embolism. *Ann Neurol* 1983,;13:527.
22. Donnan. Investigation of patients with stroke and TIA. *Lancet* 1992;339:473.
23. Duke. Intravenous heparin for the prevention of stroke progression in acute partial stable stroke. *Ann Intern Med* 1986;105:825.
24. European Carotid Surgery Trialists' Collaborative Group. MRC European Carotid Surgery Trial: interim results for symptomatic patients with severe (70–99%) or mild (0–29%) carotid stenosis. *Lancet* 1991;337:1235.
25. Ezekowitz. Warfarin in the prevention of stroke associated with nonrheumatic atrial fibrillation. *N Engl J Med* 1992;327:1406.
26. Fuster. The natural history of idiopathic dilated cardiomyopathy. *Am J Cardiol* 1981; 47:525.
27. Gelmers. A controlled trial of nimodipine in acute ischemic stroke. *N Engl J Med* 1988;318:203.
28. Gelmers. Effect of nimodipine on acute ischemic stroke: pooled results from five randomized trials. *Stroke* 1990;21(Suppl):IV81.
29. Gill. Stroke and alcohol consumption. *N Engl J Med* 1986;315:1041.
30. Grotenhuis. Prevention of symptomatic vasospasm after SAH by constant venous infusion of nimodipine. *Neurol Res* 1986;8:243.
31. Haley. Pilot randomized trial of tissue plasminogen activator in acute ischemic stroke. *Stroke* 1993;24:100.
32. Haley. Urgent therapy for stroke: part II. Pilot study of tissue plasminogen activator administered 91–180 minutes from onset. *Stroke* 1992;23:641.
33. Hetzer. Thromboembolism and anticoagulation after isolated mitral valve replacement with porcine heterografts. In: Cohn, ed. *Proceedings, Second International Symposium on Cardiac Bioprosthesis*. New York: Yorke Medical Books, 1982:170.
34. Heyman. Risk of stroke in asymptomatic persons with cervical bruits: a population study in Evans County, Georgia. *N Engl J Med* 1980;302:838.
35. Hier. Stroke recurrence within 2 years after ischemic infarction. *Stroke* 1991;22: 155.

36. Holmberg. Strategies for preventing an initial cardioembolic stroke. *Journal of Critical Illness* 1993;8:895.
37. Ionescu. Clinical durability of the pericardial xenograft valve: ten years experience with mitral replacement. *Ann Thorac Surg* 1982;34:265.
38. Iso. Serum cholesterol levels and six-year mortality from stroke in 350,977 men screened for the Multiple Risk Factor Intervention Trial. *New Engl J Med* 1989;320:904.
39. Johannessen. Risk factors for embolisation in patients with left ventricular thrombi and acute myocardial infarction. *Br Heart J* 1988;60:104.
40. Jorgenson. Effect of blood pressure and diabetes on stroke in progression. *Lancet* 1994;344:156.
41. Kannel. Epidemiologic features of chronic atrial fibrillation: the Framingham study. *New Engl J Med* 1982;306:1018.
42. Kaste. A randomized, double-blind, placebo-controlled trial of nimodipine in acute ischemic hemispheric stroke. *Stroke* 1994;25:1348.
42a. Kay. Low-molecular-weight heparin for the treatment of acute ischemic stroke. *New Engl J Med* 1995;331:1588.
43. Kopecky. The natural history of lone atrial fibrillation: a population-based study over three decades. *New Engl J Med* 1987;317:669.
44. Koudstaal. Holter monitoring in patients with transient and focal ischemic attacks of the brain. *Stroke* 1986;17:192.
45. Kunitz. The pilot stroke data bank: definition, design and data. *Stroke* 1984;15:740.
46. Lechat. Prevalence of patent foramen ovale in patients with stroke. *New Engl J Med* 1988;318:1148.
47. Levine. Antithrombotic therapy in valvular heart disease. *Chest* 1992;4S:434S.
48. Levy. Carotid endarterectomy: when and why. *JAMA* 1991;266:3332.
49. MacMahon. Blood pressure, stroke, and coronary heart disease: part 1. Prolonged differences in blood pressure: prospective observational studies corrected for the regression dilution bias. *Lancet* 1990;335:765.
50. Marmot. Primary prevention of stroke. *Lancet* 1992;339:344.
51. Marsh. Use of antithrombotic drugs in the treatment of acute ischaemic stroke: a survey of neurologists in practice in the United States. *Neurology* 1989;39:1631.
52. Martinez-Vila. Placebo-controlled trial of nimodipine in the treatment of acute ischemic cerebral infarction. *Stroke* 1990;21:1023.
52a. MAST-I Group. Randomized controlled trial of streptokinase, aspirin, and combination of both in treatment of acute ischaemic stroke. *Lancet* 1995;346:1509.
53. McCarthy. Low dose heparin as a prophylaxis against deep-vein thrombosis after acute stroke. *Lancet* 1977;2:800.
54. Mittl. Blinded-reader comparison of magnetic resonance angiography and duplex ultrasonography for carotid bifurcation stenosis. *Stroke* 1994;25:4.
55. Mori. Double-blind, placebo-controlled trial of recombinant tissue plasminogen activator (rt-PA) in acute carotid stroke. *Neurology* 1991;41:347. Abstract.
56. Neil-Dwyer. Early intervention with nimodipine in subarachnoid haemorrhage. *Eur Heart J* 1987;8(Suppl K):41.
56a. NINDS rt-PA Stroke Study Group. Tissue plasminogen activator for acute ischemic stroke. *New Engl J Med* 1995;333:1581.
57. Noel. Atrial fibrillation as a risk factor for deep venous thrombosis and pulmonary emboli in stroke patients. *Stroke* 1991;22:760.
58. North American Symptomatic Carotid Endarterectomy Trial Collaborators. Beneficial effect of carotid endarterectomy in symptomatic patients with high-grade carotid stenosis. *New Engl J Med* 1991;325:445.
59. Ohman. Long-term effects of nimodipine on cerebral infarcts and outcome after aneurysmal subarachnoid hemorrhage and surgery. *J Neurosurg* 1991;74:8.
60. Oyer. Valve replacement with the Starr-Edwards and Hancock prostheses: comparative analysis of late morbidity and mortality. *Ann Surg* 1977;186:301.
61. Paci. Nimodipine in acute ischemic stroke: a double-blind controlled study. *Acta Neurol Scand* 1989;80:282.
62. Pessin. Clinical and angiographic features of carotid transient ischemic attacks. *N Engl J Med* 1977;296:358.

63. Petruk. Nimodipine treatment in poor-grade aneurysm patients: results of a multicenter double-blind placebo-controlled trial. *J Neurosurg* 1988;68:505.
64. Phillips. An alternative view of heparin anticoagulation in acute focal brain ischemia. *Stroke* 1989;20:295.
65. Pickard. Effect of oral nimodipine on cerebral infarction and outcome after subarachnoid hemorrhage: British Aneurysm Nimodipine Trial. *Br Med J* 1989;298:636.
66. Popovic. Experience with nimodipine in aneurysmal subarachnoid haemorrhage. *Med J Aust* 1993;158:91.
67. Prins. Prophylaxis of deep venous thrombosis with a low-molecular weight heparin (Kabi 2165/Fragmin) in stroke patients. *Haemostasis* 1989;19:245.
68. Roederer. The natural history of carotid disease in asymptomatic patients with cervical bruits. *Stroke* 1984;15:605.
69. rt-PA Acute Stroke Study Group. An open safety/efficacy trial of rt-PA in acute thromboembolic stroke: final report. *Stroke* 1991;22:153. Abstract.
70. Sacco. Determinants of early recurrence of cerebral infarction: The Stroke Data Bank. *Stroke* 1989;20:983.
71. Sage. The use and overuse of heparin in therapeutic trials. *Arch Neurol* 1985;42:315.
72. Sandercock. Antithrombotic therapy in acute ischaemic stroke: an overview of the completed randomised trials. *J Neurol Neurosurg Psychiatry* 1993;56:17.
73. SPAF Investigators. Predictors of thromboembolism in atrial fibrillation: I. Clinical features of patients at risk. *Ann Intern Med* 1992;116:1.
74. SPAF Investigators. Predictors of thromboembolism in atrial fibrillation: II. Echocardiographic features of patients at risk. *Ann Intern Med* 1992;116:6.
75. Stampfer. A prospective study of moderate alcohol consumption and the risk of coronary artery disease and stroke in women. *N Engl J Med* 1988;319:267.
76. Steering Committee of the Physicians' Health Study Research Group. Final report on the aspirin component of the ongoing Physicians' Health Study. *N Engl J Med* 1989;321:129.
77. Stein. Antithrombotic therapy in patients with mechanical and biological prosthetic heart valves. *Chest* 1992;102:445S.
78. Stollberger. The prevalence of deep venous thrombosis in patients with suspected paradoxical embolism. *Ann Intern Med* 1993;119:461.
79. Strandgaard. Autoregulation of cerebral blood flow in hypertensive patients. *Circulation* 1976;53:720.
80. Trust Study Group. Randomised, double-blind, placebo-controlled trial of nimodipine in acute stroke. *Lancet* 1990;336:1205.
81. Turpie. Double-blind randomised trial of Org 10172 low-molecular-weight heparinoid in prevention of deep-vein thrombosis in thrombotic stroke. *Lancet* 1987;1:523.
82. Warlow. Deep venous thrombosis of the legs after strokes: part I. Incidence and predisposing factors. *Br Med J* 1976;1:1178.
83. Warlow. Secondary prevention of stroke. *Lancet* 1992;339:724.
84. Webster. Patent foramen ovale in young stroke patients. *Lancet* 1988:11.
85. WHO MONICA Project Principal Investigators. The World Health Organization MONICA (monitoring trends and determinants in cardiovascular disease): a major international collaboration. *J Clin Epidemiol* 1988;41:105.
86. Wolf. Epidemiology of cerebrovascular disease. In: Russell, ed. *Vascular Disease of the Central Nervous System*. New York: Churchill Livingstone, 1983:3.
87. Wolf. Atrial fibrillation as an independent risk factor for stroke: the Framingham Study. *Stroke* 1991;22:983.
88. Wolf. Asymptomatic carotid bruit and risk of stroke. *JAMA* 1981;245:1442.
89. Wolf. Probability of stroke: a risk profile from the Framingham study. *Stroke* 1991;22:312.
90. Wolf. Epidemiology of strokes in North America. In: Barnett, ed. *Stroke: Pathophysiology, Diagnosis, and Management*, vol 1. New York: Churchill Livingstone, 1986:19.
91. Zhu. Role of carotid stenosis in ischemic stroke. *Stroke* 1990;21:1131.

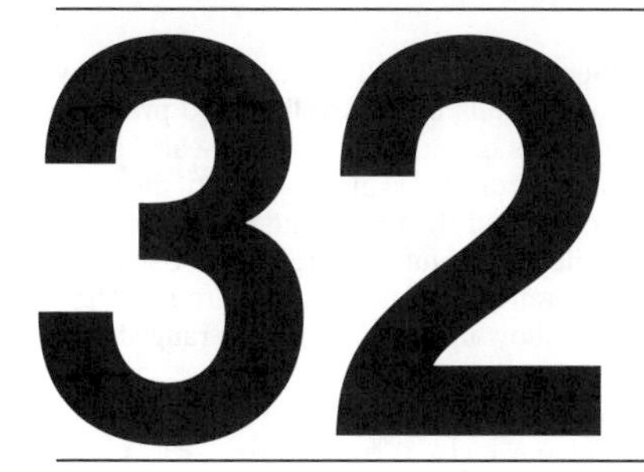

Prevention of Ischemic Stroke and Transient Ischemic Attack

Will P. Schmitt, Burton W. Lee, and Walter J. Koroshetz

A. Prevention of Stroke in Asymptomatic Healthy Individuals—Two large randomized trials demonstrated that regular use of aspirin does not reduce the risk of stroke in asymptomatic healthy people (52,61). The Physicians' Health Study, the larger of the two trials, is described here for illustration. This double-blind prospective randomized controlled trial (PRCT) randomly assigned 22,071 healthy male physicians to one of four groups using a two-by-two design: aspirin (325 mg QOD) plus β-carotene, aspirin plus placebo, β-carotene plus placebo, or double placebo. The average length of follow-up was 60.2 months. The percentages of subjects with diastolic blood pressures >90 mm Hg, systolic blood pressures >150 mm Hg, and serum cholesterol levels >210 mg/dl were 9.1%, 3.9%, and 18.3%, respectively. About half of the subjects were past or current smokers, and 2.4% had diabetes mellitus (61) (see Table 32-1).

1. Aspirin did not reduce the risk of stroke or any category of stroke. In fact, hemorrhagic strokes occurred almost twice as often with aspirin as with placebo, but the difference was not statistically significant ($P=0.06$). On the other hand, the risk of myocardial infarction (MI) was significantly reduced, by 44% ($P<0.00001$).
2. There was no significant difference in the rate of overall death or cardiovascular death between the two groups. However, the combined risk of MI, stroke, or cardiovascular death was significantly lower with aspirin than with placebo ($P=0.01$).
3. Bleeding episodes that required blood transfusions were uncommon in both groups but did occur more often in patients taking aspirin than those taking placebo (48 versus 28 events; $P=0.02$).

B. Prevention of Stroke in Patients with Hypertension

1. **Treatment of Diastolic Hypertension**—Several large studies demonstrated that antihypertensive therapy significantly decreases the risk of stroke in patients with diastolic hypertension (19,38,44). Collins conducted a metaanalysis of 14 unconfounded PRCTs that evaluated the efficacy of antihypertensive

Table 32-1 Aspirin for stroke prevention in asymptomatic healthy subjects (61)

	Aspirin* (N=11,037)	Placebo* (N=11,034)	*P*
MIs	254.8	439.7	<0.00001
All strokes	217.7	179.4	NS
Ischemic strokes	166.5	150.1	NS
Hemorrhagic strokes	42.1	22.0	NS
All deaths	395.3	413.7	NS
Cardiovascular deaths	147.6	151.3	NS
Cardiovascular death, nonfatal MI, or nonfatal stroke	559.3	674.4	0.01

*Events per 100,000 person-years.

therapy in a total of 36,908 patients with mild to moderate diastolic hypertension. Most of the patients in the analysis had diastolic blood pressures ≤110 mm Hg. In general, most of the trials employed a "stepped-care" approach to therapy, by which the dose of the first drug was increased until the target blood pressure of 90 mm Hg was reached, and then a second drug was added if the first drug was not successful at its maximum tolerated dose. Usually the first-line drug was a diuretic, but propranolol, atenolol, or reserpine were used in some cases. The mean length of follow-up was 5 years but ranged from 1.5 to 7.0 years (17) (see Table 32-2).

- **a.** With an average decrease in diastolic blood pressure of 5 to 6 mm Hg, the risk of stroke significantly decreased by 42% after 2 to 3 years of antihypertensive therapy (95% CI, 33% to 50%). Both the risks of fatal and nonfatal strokes were reduced.
- **b.** Most of the individual trials did not demonstrate a statistically significant reduction in coronary heart disease events. However, in the metaanalysis, antihypertensive therapy significantly decreased the risk of these events, by 14% (95% CI, 4% to 22%). It also significantly reduced the rates of vascular death and death from any cause.
- **c.** It is assumed, but not proven, that the newer antihypertensive agents such as calcium channel blockers or angiotensin-converting enzyme inhibitors are effective as the agents used in these trials.

2. Treatment of Isolated Systolic Hypertension—As demonstrated in the Systolic Hypertension in the Elderly Program (SHEP) study, treatment of isolated systolic hypertension also decreases the risk of stroke. This double-blind PRCT randomly assigned 4736 elderly patients to receive either placebo or stepped-care antihypertensive treatment. All patients had a systolic blood pressure ≥160 mm Hg but a diastolic blood pressure ≤90 mm Hg. The first-line drug was chlorthalidone or matching placebo. Atenolol or matching placebo was added for patients refractory to chlorthalidone. The average age of the patients was 71.6 years; 14% were black, and 57% were women. The mean length of follow-up was 4.5 years (59) (see Table 32-3).

- **a.** Antihypertensive therapy significantly reduced the rate of stroke in patients with isolated systolic hypertension. For every 100 patients treated for 5 years, three strokes were prevented. This benefit is noteworthy given the fact that 35% of the patients assigned to placebo were taking antihypertensive medications. As described later, the risk of MI was also reduced with antihypertensive therapy.
- **b.** Overall, for every 100 patients treated for 5 years, 55 major cardiovascular events were prevented with antihypertensive therapy. The combined end point of nonfatal MI or death from coronary artery disease was reduced by 27% with antihypertensive therapy.
- **c.** However, the risks of death from stroke, cardiovascular cause, or any cause were not statistically different in the two groups.

Table 32-2 Treatment of diastolic hypertension for stroke prevention (17)

	Allocation to Treatment (N=18,487)	Allocation to Control (N=18,407)	*P*
Fatal strokes	87	160	<0.0001
All strokes	289	484	<0.0001
Fatal coronary heart disease	316	356	NS
All coronary heart disease	671	771	<0.01
Vascular deaths	489	613	<0.0002
All deaths	885	1014	<0.003

Table 32-3 Treatment of isolated systolic hypertension for stroke prevention (59)

	Active Treatment (N=2365)	Placebo (N=2371)	Relative Risk	95% Confidence Interval
Decrease in blood pressure during the trial (systolic/diastolic)	26/9 mm Hg	15/4 mm Hg	—	—
Stroke	96	149	0.63	0.49–0.82
MI	50	74	0.67	0.47–0.96
Deaths due to stroke	10	14	0.71	0.31–1.59
Cardiovascular deaths	90	112	0.80	0.60–1.05
Total deaths	213	242	0.87	0.73–1.05
All cardiovascular events	289	414	0.68	0.58–0.79
Nonfatal MI or death from coronary artery disease	104	141	0.73	0.57–0.94

C. Prevention of Stroke in Patients with Chronic Stable Angina Pectoris—Prophylactic therapy with aspirin is associated with an increased risk of stroke in patients with chronic stable angina pectoris. As part of the Physicians' Health Study, 333 male physicians with a history of chronic stable angina pectoris were randomly assigned to receive either aspirin (325 mg QOD) or placebo. None of the patients had a prior history of stroke, transient ischemic attack (TIA), or MI. Patients were observed for an average of 60.2 months. Other details of the study were described previously (54) (see Table 32-4).

1. After controlling for other cardiovascular risk factors in a proportional hazards model, aspirin therapy significantly reduced the risk of MI, by 87%. MI occurred in 3.9% of patients receiving aspirin, compared with 12.9% of patients receiving placebo ($P<0.001$).
2. However, the risk of stroke was significantly higher with aspirin therapy. Stroke occurred in 6.2% of patients receiving aspirin, compared with 1.3% of those receiving placebo ($P=0.02$).
3. The overall risk of death was lower with aspirin therapy, but the difference was not statistically significant. A total of 3.9% of patients receiving aspirin died, compared with 7.1% of those receiving placebo.

D. Prevention of Stroke in Patients with Myocardial Infarction

1. Prevention of Stroke in the Acute Phase of MI

a. Antiplatelet Agents—The International Study of Infarct Survival (ISIS-2) study randomly assigned 17,187 patients suspected of having an acute MI to one of four groups in a two-by-two design: aspirin (160 mg/day started in the emergency room and continued for 1 month) plus placebo, streptokinase (1.5 million U over 1 hour) plus placebo, aspirin plus streptokinase, or double placebo. All patients were enrolled within 24 hours of onset of chest pain (40) (see Table 32-5).

Table 32-4 Aspirin for stroke prevention in chronic stable angina pectoris (54)

	Aspirin (N=178)	Placebo (N=155)	*P*
MI	3.9%	12.9%	<0.0001
Stroke	6.2%	1.3%	0.02
Overall mortality	3.9%	7.1%	NS

(1) Aspirin significantly decreased the risk of subsequent MI, from 3.3% to 1.8%, and the rate of vascular mortality, from 11.8% to 9.4%.

(2) Aspirin also reduced the rate of stroke, from 0.9% to 0.5%, during the 5-week follow-up period.

b. **Anticoagulation**—According to the Second Report of the Cerebral Embolism Task Force, an aggregate of all randomized trials of heparin versus control in patients with acute MI suggested that anticoagulation decreases the risk of left ventricular thrombus (LVT) formation by about 60%. With the early use of heparin, the rate of LVT formation decreased from 19.8% to 8.0% (14). The risk of stroke also declined with anticoagulation, by about 60% (2.8% with control versus 1.1% with heparin), but this trend could not be statistically confirmed because of the insufficient number of embolic events in these studies. (See the section on intracardiac thrombus for further discussion.)

2. Prevention of Stroke in Patients Surviving the Acute Phase of MI

a. **Antiplatelet Agents**—The Antiplatelet Trialists' Collaboration recently published a metaanalysis of all randomized trials that evaluated the role of antiplatelet agents for prevention of stroke, MI, or death in various categories of patients. Collectively in various trials, 19,791 post-MI patients were randomly assigned to receive either control or antiplatelet therapy for one or more months. Most of the studies used aspirin, although some studies used sulphinpyrazone or the combination of aspirin plus dipyridamole. The mean duration of therapy was 27 months (3) (see Table 32-6).

(1) Antiplatelet therapy prevented 6 nonfatal strokes and 13 vascular deaths per 1000 post-MI patients treated. It also prevented 18 recurrent MIs and 36 vascular events (MI, stroke, or vascular death) per 1000 patients treated.

(2) Most of these patients received a relatively high dose of aspirin, in the range of 500 to 1000 mg/day. When the data from the trials comparing 75 to 325 mg versus 500 to 1500 mg of aspirin were pooled for metaanalysis, the lower doses appeared to be equally as effective as the higher doses. However, because of the relatively low number of vascular events in this comparison, small differences in efficacy could not be ruled out (3).

b. **Anticoagulation**—Two large PRCTs involving post-MI patients have demonstrated a significant reduction in the risk of stroke with anticoagulation. The major features of these two studies are summarized in the following sections (2,60).

(1) The Warfarin Reinfarction Study (WARIS) was a double-blind PRCT involving 1214 survivors of MI. The study compared warfarin (started at the time of discharge with an INR goal of 2.8 to 4.8) versus placebo. Patients on antiplatelet therapy and those with a history of peptic ulcer disease or bleeding diathesis were excluded from the study. The average length of follow-up was 37 months. An intention-to-treat analysis was used (60) (see Table 32-7).

Table 32-5 Aspirin for stroke prevention in the acute phase of MI (40)

	Aspirin (N=8587)	Placebo (N=8600)	*P*
All strokes	0.5%	0.9%	<0.01
Recurrent MI	1.8%	3.3%	<0.00001
5-wk vascular mortality rate	9.4%	11.8%	<0.00001
Risk of bleeding requiring blood transfusion	0.4%	0.4%	NS

(a) Compared with placebo, anticoagulation therapy significantly decreased the risks of stroke, recurrent MI, and death, by 55%, 34%, and 24%, respectively.

(b) However, five intracranial and eight nonintracranial major bleeding episodes were associated with warfarin, for an overall risk of major bleeding of 0.6% per year.

(2) Another double-blind PRCT, the Anticoagulants in the Secondary Prevention of Events in Coronary Thrombosis (ASPECT) trial, compared nicoumalone or phenprocoumon (started within 6 weeks of discharge with INR goal of 2.8 to 4.8) versus placebo among 3404 survivors of MI. The use of other antithrombotic drugs was discouraged. An intention-to-treat analysis was used (2) (see Table 32-8).

(a) The rate of all cerebrovascular events (cerebral infarctions, intracranial hemorrhages, TIAs, and unspecified strokes) was significantly reduced, from 3.6% to 2.2%, with anticoagulant therapy. The rate of cerebral infarctions was reduced from 2.5% to 0.9% and the rate of recurrent MI from 14.2% to 6.7%.

(b) However, there was no significant difference in survival, and there was an increase in the rate of intracranial bleeding from 0.1% to 1.0% with anticoagulation.

Table 32-6 Antiplatelet agents for stroke prevention in post-MI patients (3)

	Antiplatelet Therapy (N=9877)	Placebo (N=9914)	Reduction in No. Events per 1000 Patients Treated	*P*
MI, stroke, or vascular death	13.5%	17.1%	36	<0.00001
Nonfatal MI	4.7%	6.5%	18	<0.00001
Nonfatal stroke	1.0%	1.5%	6	0.0005
Vascular death	8.1%	9.4%	13	<0.005
Death from any cause	9.2%	10.4%	12	0.02

Table 32-7 WARIS: anticoagulants for stroke prevention in post-MI patients (60)

	Placebo (N=607)	Warfarin (N=607)	*P*
Cerebrovascular events	7.2%	3.3%	0.0015
Recurrent MI	20.4%	13.5%	0.0007
Overall mortality	20.3%	15.5%	0.027
Intracranial hemorrhage	0%	1.0%	NS
Major bleeding	0%	2.1%	<0.05

Table 32-8 ASPECT: anticoagulants for stroke prevention in post-MI patients (2)

	Placebo (N=1704)	Anticoagulation (N=1700)	*P*
Cerebrovascular events	3.6%	2.2%	<0.05
Recurrent MI	14.2%	6.7%	<0.05
Overall mortality	11.1%	10.0%	NS
Intracranial hemorrhage	0.1%	1.0%	?
Major bleeding	1.1%	4.3%	<0.05

(3) In summary, anticoagulation appears to be effective for preventing strokes in post-MI patients, but at the cost of increased risk of hemorrhage. However, the target INR was relatively high in each of these trials, and the risk of hemorrhagic complications might have been lower had the trials used an INR goal of 2.0 to 3.0 instead. Regardless, the critical question is whether warfarin has significant advantages over aspirin for long-term treatment of post-MI patients or whether there is additive benefit if it is combined with aspirin. Studies are currently underway that specifically investigate these strategies in post-MI patients, comparing anticoagulation versus aspirin and low- versus high-intensity anticoagulation.

3. Prevention of Stroke in Post-MI Patients with an Intracardiac Thrombus

a. As long as there are no contraindications to anticoagulation, one approach to reducing the risk of stroke in post-MI patients is to anticoagulate all patients with acute anterior MIs in order to prevent the formation of thrombus in the first place. As discussed previously, this strategy may decrease the risk of thrombus formation by as much as 60% (14). The optimal dose, duration, or route of administration of heparin is not known, but 12,500 U q 12 hours of subcutaneous heparin was more effective in preventing the formation of LVT than 5000 U q 12 hours (11% versus 38% respectively; $P=0.0004$) (70). If a subsequent echocardiogram reveals a significant wall motion abnormality or an LVT, chronic anticoagulation with warfarin may be continued for 3 to 6 months.

b. An alternative strategy for reducing the risk of stroke in post-MI patients is to anticoagulate only those patients with an LVT identified on screening echocardiography. However, there is no consensus as to when and which post-MI patients should be screened for LVT. Screening within 48 hours of an MI may be too soon to detect many thrombi, but screening at a later time may miss some opportunities for intervention, because embolization sometimes occurs synchronously with the development of a thrombus. In a pooled analysis of the available data by the Cerebral Embolism Task Force, the risk of systemic embolization within 1 month of acute MI was 12% among 116 non-anticoagulated patients with LVT, compared with 10% among 124 patients with LVT who were promptly anticoagulated. Therefore, initiation of anticoagulation after the detection of LVT does not appear to necessarily reduce the risk of stroke. However, if those initially anticoagulated only with warfarin (40 out of 124 patients) are excluded from the analysis, the risk of systemic embolization was 2% among the 84 patients treated with heparin (14). Still another approach is to screen all patients with echocardiography and to anticoagulate those with ventricular aneurysms or wall motion abnormalities, whether or not an LVT is present. Given the available data, these strategies all appear to be reasonable, but none has been convincingly validated in a clinical trial.

c. Even fewer data are available regarding the optimal management of LVTs that are temporally removed from an acute MI. In one study involving 57 patients with echocardiographically detected LVT at a mean of 32 months after an acute MI, the risk of embolism was about 5.5% per year (63). In a small randomized trial involving 34 patients with echocardiographically detected LVT at a mean of 4 weeks from an acute MI, LVT resolved in 88% of anticoagulated patients, compared with 24% of non-anticoagulated patients. No embolic episodes occurred in either group (69).

E. Prevention of Stroke in Patients with Nonischemic Dilated Cardiomyopathy—The role of anticoagulation for prevention of stroke in patients with dilated cardiomyopathy is controversial. To date, there have been no PRCTs that attempted to answer this question. However, there are suggestive data from small retrospective studies that warfarin may reduce the risk of embolic stroke in this population. For example, in a retrospective analysis of 104 patients with dilated cardiomyopathy, no embolic events occurred among the anticoagulated patients, compared with 19 embolic events among non-anticoagulated patients (30). In particular, patients with atrial fibrillation (AF) or ejection fraction <30% appeared to benefit most from anticoagulation. PRCTs are clearly needed in this area (7,27).

F. Prevention of Stroke in Patients with Hyperlipidemia—There are conflicting data on the effectiveness of lipid-lowering therapy for prevention of stroke. In the Helsinki Heart Study, which randomly assigned 4081 asymptomatic middle-aged men to receive either placebo or gemfibrozil for 5 years, the risk of stroke was not significantly different in the two groups (29). Furthermore, in a recent metaanalysis of trials of lipid-lowering therapies, there was no significant reduction in the rate of stroke, although the mean duration of follow-up was only 5.5 years (5). However, in a recent post-hoc analysis of the Scandinavian Simvastatin Survival Study, in which 4500 patients with known coronary artery disease were randomly assigned to receive either simvastatin or placebo, simvastatin reduced the combined rate of fatal and nonfatal cerebrovascular events by 30% ($P=0.024$) (58).

G. Prevention of Stroke in Patients with Atrial Fibrillation—AF is a potent risk factor for cardioembolic stroke. Compared with the general population, the risk of stroke is fivefold higher for patients with nonrheumatic AF and 17-fold higher for those with rheumatic heart disease and AF (41,74,75). Based on the results of several large PRCTs, anticoagulation is now recommended for most patients with AF for prevention of stroke (10,18,23,25,51,64,65). For the purpose of discussion, it is useful to group patients with AF according to their risk of thromboembolism—that is, valvular (rheumatic) AF, nonvalvular (nonrheumatic) AF, and lone AF. (See Chapter 1 for a more complete discussion of this topic.)

1. **Valvular AF**—Despite the lack of PRCTs, long-term anticoagulation has become a standard therapy for patients with valvular AF because of the relatively high risk of thromboembolism. In Szekely's retrospective study involving 754 patients with rheumatic heart disease, a thromboembolic complication occurred in 22.3% of the patients in AF, compared with 3.8% of the patients in sinus rhythm. Among those patients in AF, two thromboembolic events were observed in 30 anticoagulated patients, compared with 34 events in 98 non-anticoagulated patients. Furthermore, once a thromboembolic complication occurred, the risk of recurrence was 3.4% with anticoagulation and 9.6% without anticoagulation (68).
2. **Lone AF**—Lone AF usually refers to AF that occurs in patients without clinical heart disease. In a report from the Mayo Clinic, the risk of stroke in patients with lone AF (0.35 events per 100 person-years among 97 patients) did not differ from the risk in the general population (42). Lone AF was strictly defined in this study, which excluded all patients with coronary artery disease, hyperthyroidism, valvular heart disease (including mitral valve prolapse), congestive heart failure, cardiomyopathy, chronic obstructive pulmonary disease, cardiomegaly on chest radiographic film, hypertension, diabetes mellitus, or age >60 years. Only 2.7% of the patients with AF fulfilled the strict criteria of lone AF. If lone AF is defined as outlined in the Mayo Clinic study, prophylactic anticoagulation does not appear to be necessary. However, in another study, which used a less stringent definition of lone AF, the age-adjusted risk of stroke was 28.2%, compared with a risk of 6.8% among the age- and sex-matched control patients without AF. (11)
3. **Nonrheumatic Atrial Fibrillation**—Until recently, the value of prophylactic therapy against stroke in patients with nonrheumatic atrial fibrillation (NRAF) was controversial. However, several large PRCTs have clarified this issue (10, 18,23,26,51,64,65).
   a. **Coumadin**
      (1) Six studies compared Coumadin (warfarin) versus placebo or no treatment (10,18,23,25,51,64). One study was a secondary prevention trial (23), and the rest were studies of primary prevention.
      (2) Five of these six studies found that warfarin significantly decreased the risk of stroke, compared with placebo or no treatment. The average risk reduction ranged from 60% to 86% (10,23,25,51,64). The sixth study also favored warfarin, but the 37% reduction in the risk of stroke was not statistically significant (18).

(3) The risk of hemorrhage leading to death, hospitalization, or transfusion was not significantly different between the warfarin and control groups (10,23,51,64). Not surprisingly, however, the risk of less severe bleeding episodes was substantially higher with warfarin (10,23,51).

b. Aspirin

(1) Four PRCTs evaluated the role of aspirin in prevention of stroke in patients with NRAF (23,51,64,65). One study was a secondary prevention trial (23), and the rest were studies of primary prevention.

(2) Among the three studies that compared aspirin versus placebo or no therapy (23,51,64), only one (64) showed a significant reduction in the risk of stroke with aspirin. In this study, 325 mg/day of aspirin reduced the risk of stroke or systemic embolism by 42%, compared with placebo.

(3) The fourth study directly compared aspirin versus warfarin in patients with NRAF (65). There was a statistically nonsignificant 32% reduction in the risk of stroke with warfarin. When the data from these studies were pooled for metaanalysis, there was a 49% reduction in the risk of stroke with warfarin compared to aspirin (1,6).

c. Predicting the Risk of Stroke for a Patient with NRAF—In a collaborative analysis of the pooled data from five randomized trials (10,18,25, 51,64), the best independent predictors of stroke were older age, previous stroke or TIA, hypertension, and diabetes mellitus (6). A history of MI, congestive heart failure, or angina was also important, but these conditions were not independently predictive in multivariate analysis. The incidences of stroke for various combinations of risk factors are summarized in the following sections.

(1) For patients <65 years old with one or more independent predictors of stroke (hypertension, diabetes mellitus, or previous stroke or TIA), the annual incidence of stroke was 4.9%. The annual incidence was 5.7% for similar patients between 65 and 75 years old, and 8.1% for those ≥75 years of age. Warfarin reduced the risk of stroke in all of these subgroups.

(2) For patients <65 years old without any of these independent predictors, the annual incidence of stroke was only 1.0%. The annual incidence was 4.3% for similar patients between 65 and 75 years old, and 3.5% for those ≥75 years of age. Warfarin reduced the risk of stroke in the two older subgroups but not in patients younger than 65 years of age.

(3) Patients with lone AF had very low rates of stroke. The annual incidence of stroke was 0% among untreated patients <60 years old without hypertension, diabetes mellitus, previous stroke, TIA, congestive heart failure, angina, or MI. The annual incidences were 1.6%, 2.1%, and 3.0% for patients with lone AF in their 60s, in their 70s, and older than 80 years, respectively.

(4) Based on these results, anticoagulation is recommended for most patients with nonvalvular AF. However, it does not appear to be necessary for patients <65 years of age who do not have a history of diabetes mellitus, hypertension, previous stroke, or TIA. Similarly, patients with lone AF who are <60 or 70 years old also may not need anticoagulation. Aspirin may be preferred to warfarin for these low-risk patients.

H. Prevention of Stroke in Patients with Prosthetic Heart Valves

1. Mechanical Heart Valves—In a review of the literature by Stein, when no long-term anticoagulant or antiplatelet therapy was used, the rate of thromboembolism in patients with mechanical heart valves ranged from 12 to 75 events per 100 patient-years (62). In the same review, long-term anticoagulation reduced the risk of thromboembolism to between 0 and 4.6 events per 100 patient-years for tilting (St. Jude or Björk-Shiley) disk valves and between 1.8 and 15.5 events per 100 patient-years for ball-and-cage valves (62). Prosthetic mitral valves appear to be associated with a higher risk of thromboembolism than prosthetic aortic valves. For example, in one report, when no anticoagulant or antiplatelet therapy was used, the rate of thromboembolism associated with the St. Jude aortic valves was 12.4 events per 100 patient-years, compared with 22.2 events per 100 patient-years with St. Jude mitral valves (9).

a. Level of Anticoagulation—When used for prevention of thromboembolic complications in patients with prosthetic heart valves, a moderate level of anticoagulation appears to be as effective as, and safer than, higher levels of anticoagulation. In a PRCT by Saour, 258 patients with various mechanical prosthetic heart valves were randomly assigned to receive either low-intensity anticoagulation (INR goal of 2.65) or high-intensity anticoagulation (INR goal of 9). Mean follow-up was 3.5 years (57).

(1) There was no significant difference in the rate of embolic events between the two groups. In the low-intensity group, there were 4.0 events per 100 patient-years, compared with 3.7 events per 100 patient-years in the high-intensity group. More than half of the embolic events occurred when the INR was less than 2.0.

(2) Bleeding complications were more common with high-intensity therapy. There were 2.1 major bleeding events per 100 patient-years (including two fatal intracranial bleeding episodes) in the high-intensity group, compared with 0.9 events per 100 patient-years in the low-intensity group (*P*=NS). In addition, there were 5.2 minor bleeding events per 100 patient-years in the low-intensity anticoagulation group, compared with 10.1 events per 100 patient-years in the high-intensity group ($p < 0.001$).

(3) Therefore, the current recommendations are to anticoagulate patients with prosthetic heart valves, with an INR goal of 2.5 to 3.5 (62).

b. Anticoagulant Versus Antiplatelet Therapy

(1) Prosthetic Mitral Valves—For most patients with mechanical heart valves, anticoagulation with warfarin is preferred to antiplatelet therapy, particularly if the valve is in the mitral position. The following study by Mok illustrates this point (45). In a PRCT, warfarin (target prothrombin time ratio [PTR] of 1.8 to 2.5) was compared with dipyridamole (150 to 225 mg/day) plus aspirin (650 to 990 mg/day) in patients with Starr-Edwards ball valves or Björk-Shiley disk valves. As demonstrated in Table 32-9, warfarin was superior to antiplatelet therapy for prevention of thromboembolic complications. In a subgroup analysis, this difference was most notable for patients with prosthetic mitral valves.

(2) Prosthetic Aortic Valves—As discussed previously, the risk of thromboembolism appears to be lower with prosthetic aortic valves than with mitral valves. This observation has led some investigators to use antiplatelet therapy alone for patients with prosthetic valves in the aortic position. Indeed, in the study just described, antiplatelet therapy

Table 32-9 Stroke prevention in patients with mechanical heart valves (45)

	Antiplatelet Therapy	Warfarin	*P*
Overall rate of thromboembolic events*	9.8	2.2	0.004
Rate of thromboembolic events in patients with prosthetic mitral valves*	12.4	1.9	0.005
Rate of thromboembolic events in patients with the prosthetic aortic valves*	3.8	3.6	NS

*per 100 patient-years

was as effective as anticoagulant therapy in patients with prosthetic aortic valves but not in those with prosthetic mitral valves (45). A few small studies further support this observation. In one uncontrolled study, 52 patients with single St. Jude aortic valve replacement were given antiplatelet therapy and observed for a total of 123 patient-years. The rate of thromboembolic complications was 2.1 events per 100 patient-years, a risk similar to that reported with anticoagulant therapy in most series. Local thrombus formation and subsequent malfunction of the valves accounted for all of the complications (53). In another nonrandomized study involving 83 patients with St. Jude aortic valve replacement, there were no significant differences in the rates of death or nonfatal complications between patients treated with anticoagulant therapy and those given antiplatelet therapy (34). Nevertheless, given the small size of these studies and the potential confounding problems associated with nonrandomized or uncontrolled reports, antiplatelet therapy is probably best reserved for those patients who have strong contraindications to long-term anticoagulation (62).

c. Combination of Anticoagulant and Antiplatelet Therapy—Whether the combination of anticoagulant plus antiplatelet therapy is superior to anticoagulant therapy alone for the prevention of thromboembolic complications in patients with prosthetic heart valves is still a matter of debate. Representative studies are described here.

(1) In a double-blind PRCT involving 370 patients with mechanical or bioprosthetic prosthetic heart valves, Turpie found that the addition of aspirin (100 mg/day) to warfarin (INR 3.0 to 4.5) markedly decreased the risk of thromboembolic events, compared with warfarin alone (71). The rate of thromboembolism was 1.6 events per 100 patient-years with the combination of aspirin plus warfarin, compared with 4.7 events per 100 patient-years with warfarin alone ($P<0.001$). Although there was no significant difference in the rate of major hemorrhagic events, there was a moderate increase in the risk of all hemorrhagic events with the combination therapy (35% versus 22%). The results of this study should be viewed with some caution, because the rate of 4.7 thromboembolisms per 100 patient-years with warfarin is higher than rates found in other trials. This suggests that, at least in part, the observed benefit of aspirin may have resulted from an excess of thromboembolic events in the warfarin group (see Table 32-10).

(2) In a PRCT involving 92 patients with Starr-Edwards valves, the addition of dipyridamole (400 mg/day) to warfarin was superior to the use of warfarin alone (PTR of 1.9 to 2.3) for decreasing the risk of thromboembolic events (66). There were 2.2 thromboembolic events per 100 patient-years with the combination of dipyridamole plus warfarin, compared with 15.5 events per 100 patient-years with warfarin alone.

(3) In contrast to the two studies just discussed, Chesebro's randomized trial comparing dipyridamole (400 mg/day) plus warfarin, aspirin (500

Table 32-10 Warfarin with and without aspirin for prosthetic heart valves (71)

	Aspirin Plus Warfarin (N=186)	Warfarin Alone (N=184)	*P*
Rate of thromboembolisms per 100 patient-years	1.6	4.7	0.0003
Total hemorrhagic events (annual event rate)	35%	22%	0.02
Major hemorrhagic events (annual event rate)	8.5%	6.6%	NS

mg/day) plus warfarin, or warfarin alone (PTR of 1.5 to 2.5) in patients with mechanical heart valves failed to demonstrate any benefit with the addition of either antiplatelet agent to warfarin (15). The rates of thromboembolism were 1.2, 0.5, and 1.8 events per 100 patient-years with warfarin alone, warfarin plus dipyridamole, and warfarin plus aspirin, respectively. These rates were not statistically different from one another. However, there was a statistically significant excess of bleeding complications with the combination of aspirin plus warfarin, compared with warfarin alone (6.6 versus 1.8 events per 100 patient-years; $P<0.001$).

2. Bioprosthetic Heart Valves

a. For the first few weeks after surgery, patients with a bioprosthetic valve are at increased risk of thromboembolism if no antiplatelet or anticoagulant therapy is used. The estimate of this risk has been as high as 67% to 80% in some series (36,39,50). Therefore, most authors recommend that all recipients of a bioprosthetic valve be anticoagulated for the first 3 months, with an INR goal of 2.0 to 3.0 (62).

b. Beyond the first few months, however, the risk of thromboembolism with a bioprosthetic valve is generally much less than with a mechanical valve. In the review of the literature by Stein, when no anticoagulant or antiplatelet therapy was used, the estimated risk of thromboembolism with bioprosthetic aortic valves ranged from 0.2 to 2.9 events per 100 patient-years (62). This estimate assumed that patients were anticoagulated postoperatively for the first 6 to 12 weeks and remained in sinus rhythm. Similar rates of thromboembolism have been quoted for patients with bioprosthetic mitral valves (16).

c. Given such low rates of thromboembolic complications among patients with bioprosthetic valves, it is not clear what type of prophylactic therapy is necessary, if any. In two studies in which a total of 445 patients with bioprosthetic valves were simply monitored for 2 to 3 years with aspirin therapy alone, no thromboembolic events were observed (47,48). To date, no PRCT of adequate size has evaluated the efficacy of anticoagulant or antiplatelet therapy in patients with bioprosthetic valves. Given the available data, aspirin (325 mg/day) alone may be sufficient prophylaxis for patients with bioprosthetic valves who are otherwise at low risk for thromboembolism. For those with factors placing them at higher risk for thromboembolism (*e.g.*, AF, dilated left atrium, intracardiac thrombus, prior history of thromboembolism), long-term anticoagulation with warfarin should be used (62).

3. In summary, all patients with mechanical prosthetic valves should be treated with long-term anticoagulation, with an INR goal of 2.5 to 3.5. Some but not all studies suggest that the combination of antiplatelet therapy plus warfarin offers additional protection against thromboembolism, compared with warfarin alone. However, this combination therapy may increase the risk of bleeding complications. All patients with bioprosthetic valves should be anticoagulated for the first 3 months, particularly if the valve is in the mitral position. Beyond this period, long-term therapy with aspirin may be sufficient for low-risk patients.

I. Prevention of Stroke in Patients with Carotid Artery Stenosis

1. Carotid Endarterectomy for Secondary Prevention

a. Symptomatic Patients with Severe Carotid Artery Disease—Three major PRCTs compared carotid endarterectomy (CEA) versus medical therapy for prevention of stroke in symptomatic patients with carotid artery disease (24,43,46). Two of these studies, the European Carotid Surgery Trial (ECST) and the North American Symptomatic Carotid Endarterectomy Trial (NASCET), clearly demonstrated that CEA is superior to aspirin for symptomatic patients with severe (70% to 99%) carotid artery stenosis (24, 46). The third study, the Veterans Affairs (VA) Cooperative Study, also favored CEA but was stopped early when the results of the ECST and

NASCET were released (43). The NASCET study is described here for illustration. In this PRCT, patients who had suffered a TIA or minor stroke (within the preceding 120 days) with ipsilateral carotid artery stenosis (30% to 99% by angiography) were randomly assigned to receive either medical therapy (usually 1300 mg/day of aspirin plus antihypertensive, antilipid, or antidiabetic therapy as indicated) or CEA plus medical therapy. Patients were divided into one of two predetermined strata: moderate stenosis (30% to 69%) and severe stenosis (70% to 99%). The average age of the subjects was 66 years, and 69% were men. After a mean follow-up of 18 months, the study was terminated early for patients with severe stenosis because CEA plus medical therapy was clearly superior to medical therapy alone for this group. At the termination of the study, 662 patients with severe carotid artery stenosis had been randomly assigned to treatment, and no patient was lost to follow-up (46) (see Table 32-11).

(1) The cumulative 2-year rate of any ipsilateral stroke was significantly reduced from 26% with medical therapy to 9% with CEA. Similarly, CEA significantly reduced the risks of all strokes, stroke or death, major ipsilateral stroke, all major strokes, and major stroke or death.

(2) A secondary analysis of the data revealed that, with increasing severity of stenosis, CEA offered greater reductions in the risk of stroke. For example, the absolute risk reduction of ipsilateral stroke with CEA was 26% for those with 90% to 99% stenosis, 18% for those with 80% to 89% stenosis, and 12% for those with 70% to 79% stenosis.

(3) The rate of perioperative complications in this trial was low, 2.1% for major stroke or death. During the same period, the rate of major stroke or death among medically managed patients was 0.9%. However, such favorable rates of complications may not apply in centers with less experienced surgeons. All patients in this study underwent contrast angiography, which introduced an angiography-related stroke risk of 0.5% to 1.0%. If CEA is performed based on the results of magnetic resonance angiography rather than conventional angiography, the risk-benefit ratio of CEA may become even more favorable.

(4) The patients in this study were relatively young and healthy. Patients older than 80 years of age and those whose life expectancy was <5 years were excluded from the trial. In addition, those with AF, valvular heart disease, or recent MI were also excluded. Therefore, it is unclear whether the findings of this study can be generalized to less selected populations.

b. Symptomatic Patients with Moderate Carotid Artery Stenosis—The role of CEA for symptomatic patients with moderate (30% to 69%) carotid artery stenosis is not yet known. Both the NASCET and the ECST have continuing study arms that may eventually answer this question.

c. Symptomatic Patients with Mild Carotid Artery Stenosis—The ECST has demonstrated that CEA is not indicated for patients with mild (0% to 29%) carotid artery stenosis. In one arm of the study, 374 symptomatic patients with mild carotid artery stenosis were randomly assigned to receive either CEA plus medical therapy or medical therapy alone. Medical therapy consisted of aspirin, treatment of hypertension, and advice to quit smok-

Table 32-11 CEA for symptomatic severe carotid artery disease (46)

	Medical Therapy (N=331)	CEA (N=328)	*P*
Any ipsilateral stroke	26.0%	9.0%	<0.001
Any major or fatal stroke	13.1%	3.7%	<0.001
Any stroke or death	32.3%	15.8%	<0.001

ing. All patients had had a mild stroke or TIA attributable to the carotid lesion within 6 months of enrollment into the study (24).

(1) After a mean follow-up of 2.7 years, there was no significant difference in the rate of ipsilateral stroke between the two groups. In fact, only 1.3% of patients assigned to medical therapy suffered an ipsilateral stroke.

(2) Furthermore, only 22% of the subsequent strokes occurred ipsilateral to the stenotic artery. In contrast, in the severe stenosis arm of the NASCET, 95% of the strokes occurred ipsilateral to the stenotic artery (46). These observations suggest that mild carotid stenosis is less likely to be the cause of future strokes than severe carotid stenosis. Therefore, it is unlikely that CEA would offer additional reduction in the risk of ipsilateral stroke.

2. CEA for Asymptomatic Patients with Significant Carotid Stenosis—The role of prophylactic CEA for patients with asymptomatic carotid artery stenosis is controversial (4,13,37). The Carotid Artery Stenosis with Asymptomatic Narrowing: Operation vs. Aspirin Study (CASANOVA) study failed to demonstrate any benefit of CEA for this population (13). However, the validity of this conclusion has been questioned because of the small sample size, large percent of patients crossing over to the other treatment arm, and complicated study design, all of which make the interpretation of the data difficult (22). The other two trials, the VA study and the Asymptomatic Carotid Atherosclerosis Study (ACAS) study, are described here.

a. The VA study randomly assigned 444 patients with asymptomatic carotid artery stenosis (>50% by angiography) to receive either CEA plus medical therapy or medical therapy alone (including 650 mg of aspirin BID). None of the patients had ipsilateral neurologic symptoms attributable to the carotid stenosis, but some had neurologic symptoms attributable to the contralateral carotid artery. Two thirds of the patients had an asymptomatic bruit discovered during routine physical examination, and the rest had the stenosis detected after receiving a CEA on the contralateral side. The mean age was 64.5 years, and all patients were male. Patients with poor overall health, previous stroke, or life expectancy <5 years were excluded from the study, as were those who were intolerant to aspirin. The mean length of follow-up was 47.9 months. An intention-to-treat analysis was used (37).

(1) In the CEA group, the 30-day postoperative mortality was 1.9%. Another 2.4% suffered nonfatal strokes after surgery and 0.4% after angiography. Therefore, the risk of permanent stroke or death within 30 days of randomization was 4.7% with CEA. In comparison, the risk of permanent stroke or death was only 0.9% with medical therapy.

(2) With CEA, there was a significant reduction in the combined risk of ipsilateral TIA, transmonocular blindness (TMB), or stroke, from 20.6% to 8.0% ($P<0.001$), and in the combined risk of all TIA, TMB, or stroke, from 24.5% to 12.8% ($P<0.002$).

(3) However, the value of prevention of TIA or TMB at the cost of perioperative stroke or death has been questioned (8). In fact, when TIA and TMB are eliminated as end points, there was no significant difference in the rate of strokes (8.6% with surgery versus 12.4% with medical therapy), in the rate of death from any cause (32.7% versus 31.8%), or in the combined rate of stroke or death (41.2% versus 44.2%).

(4) This study has been criticized for many reasons. About a third of the patients in both groups died during the study, mostly as a result of cardiac disease. As the authors of the study have argued, in the presence of such high mortality rates from other causes, measurement of differences in less frequent events such as strokes may be difficult. In addition, the rate of neurologic events for patients with moderate stenosis (50% to 75%) was not different from the rate for those with severe stenosis (76% to 99%), which conflicts with the data from the NASCET and other studies. This discrepancy raises concern that the study may have lacked statistical power to observe important differences in outcome due to type II error (8).

b. In the ACAS trial, 1662 asymptomatic patients with carotid artery disease (>60% stenosis by angiography or by noninvasive measures) were randomly assigned to receive either CEA or medical management (*i.e.*, risk factor modifications and aspirin 325 mg/day). A third of the patients were women, half were between 60 and 69 years of age, and 37% were between 70 and 79 years of age. The median length of follow-up was 2.7 years. Patients with a prior history of TIA, stroke, or CEA of the randomized artery were excluded, as were those with AF, unstable angina, severe diabetes, or uncontrolled hypertension. Patients with poor life expectancy and age >79 years were also excluded (24a) (see Table 32-12).

(1) The study was terminated early, after a significant benefit was demonstrated with surgery. The rate of stroke was 4.8% in patients receiving CEA, compared with 10.6% in those receiving medical treatment, a relative risk reduction of 55% (95% CI, 23% to 73% by Kaplan–Meier analysis). Similarly, the risk of ipsilateral stroke, any perioperative stroke, or death was 5.1% with CEA compared to 11.0% with medical therapy (P=0.004).

(2) However, subgroup analysis suggests that the benefit of CEA in asymptomatic individuals may be confined to men. The relative reduction in the rate of stroke with CEA was 69% for men but only 16% for women. In addition, CEA did not decrease the risk of major disabling stroke.

(3) The perioperative rate of stroke or death was only 3.5%, 1.2% attributable to the angiogram and 2.3% to the CEA itself. However, these low complication rates may not apply in centers with less experienced surgeons.

3. Summary of the Role of CEA for Prevention of Stroke

a. CEA is clearly indicated for patients with severe carotid artery disease (70% to 99% stenosis) who have had a TIA, an episode of TMB, or a small stroke attributable to the carotid lesion.

b. However, CEA is not beneficial for patients with mild carotid artery stenosis (0% to 29%), and its efficacy for those with moderate stenosis (30% to 69%) is still being evaluated. In addition, the benefit of CEA may be realized only in centers where technical proficiency with the operation is high and the combined mortality and morbidity is low. Furthermore, because these trials included relatively few women and excluded patients >80 years of age as well as those with AF, it is unclear whether the benefit of CEA can be extended to these patients.

c. CEA may also be effective in decreasing the risk of stroke in patients with asymptomatic carotid artery disease (>60% stenosis). However, the benefit of CEA may be limited to men, and CEA may not decrease the risk of major disabling strokes.

Table 32-12 CEA for asymptomatic severe carotid artery disease (24a)

	Medical Therapy (N=233)	CEA (N=211)	*P*
Ipsilateral TIA, TMB, or stroke	20.6%	8.0%	<0.001
All TIA, TMB, or stroke	24.5%	12.8%	<0.002
All strokes	12.4%	8.6%	NS
Any stroke or death	44.2%	41.2%	NS
Perioperative stroke or death	0.9%	4.7%	NS

J. Secondary Prevention of Other Types of Stroke—As discussed previously, patients who have had an embolic stroke usually require anticoagulation directed at the specific source of embolism (*e.g.*, AF, LVT, MI), and those with stroke or TIA and significant ipsilateral carotid artery stenosis should be evaluated for carotid endarterectomy. The options for secondary prevention of stroke in patients with less well-classified ischemic stroke or TIA are presented in the following sections.

1. Aspirin for Secondary Prevention of Stroke

a. Efficacy of Aspirin—The Antiplatelet Trialists' Collaboration published a metaanalysis of all randomized trials that evaluated the role of antiplatelet agents for prevention of stroke, MI, or death in various categories of patients. Collectively in various PRCTs, 11,707 patients with stroke or TIA were randomly assigned to receive either antiplatelet therapy or control. Most of the studies used aspirin (300 to 1500 mg/day), although some studies used sulphinpyrazone or the combination of aspirin plus dipyridamole. The mean duration of therapy was 33 months (3) (see Table 32-13).

(1) With antiplatelet therapy, there was a 23% odds reduction in the risk of recurrent nonfatal stroke (from 10.2% to 8.2%), 36% odds reduction in the risk of nonfatal MI (from 2.9% to 1.9%), and a 16% odds reduction in the risk of death from any cause (from 13.3% to 11.6%).

(2) Overall, there was a 22% odds reduction in the risk of all vascular events (*i.e.*, MI, stroke, vascular death).

(3) The benefits of aspirin were observed for men as well as women and for middle-aged as well as elderly patients.

b. Optimal Dose of Aspirin—Although aspirin has become a well-accepted therapy for secondary prevention of stroke, the optimal dose is still a subject of much interest and controversy. To date, three major trials have tested the efficacy of low-dose aspirin (30 to 300 mg/day) for secondary prevention of stroke.

(1) In the United Kingdom Transient Ischaemic Attack (UK-TIA) study, 2435 patients with minor ischemic stroke or TIA were randomly assigned to one of three groups: high-dose aspirin (1200 mg/day), moderate-dose aspirin (300 mg/day), or placebo. Patients were treated for a mean of 4 years. When the two aspirin groups were combined and compared with the placebo group, there was a 15% reduction in the odds of suffering a nonfatal MI, nonfatal major stroke, or death (P=0.01). There were no statistically significant differences in outcome between the two aspirin groups except for an increased risk of gastrotoxicity with the higher dose (72,73).

(2) In the Dutch TIA study, 3131 patients with minor strokes or TIAs were randomly assigned in a double-blind fashion to receive either moderate-dose (283 mg/day) or low-dose (30 mg/day) aspirin. During mean follow-up of 2.6 years, there was no significant difference between the two aspirin doses in the risk of death or in the rate of vascular events (nonfatal MI, nonfatal stroke, and vascular death) (20).

Table 32-13 Antiplatelet agents for secondary stroke prevention (3)

	Antiplatelet Therapy (N=5837)	Control (N=5870)	*P*
Nonfatal stroke	8.2%	10.2%	<0.0005
Nonfatal MI	1.9%	2.9%	<0.001
Death due to any cause	11.6%	13.3%	<0.01
All vascular events (MI, stroke, vascular death)	18.4%	22.2%	<0.00001

(3) In the Swedish Aspirin Low-Dose Trial (SALT), 1360 patients with minor strokes or TIAs were randomly assigned to receive either aspirin (75 mg/day) or placebo. During a median follow-up of 32 months, there was an 18% reduction in the risk of stroke or death (P=0.02) (56).

(4) Based on these studies, 30 to 300 mg/day of aspirin appears to be effective for secondary prevention of stroke and to be equivalent to 1200 mg/day. However, the two aspirin groups had to be combined to demonstrate a statistically significant benefit over placebo in the UK-TIA study, because there were not enough events in the aspirin groups individually. Therefore, the study may have had insufficient power to exclude significant differences between the two aspirin groups (21).

2. **Ticlopidine for Secondary Prevention of Stroke**—Ticlopidine is a relatively new antiplatelet agent that blocks platelet aggregation mediated by the adenosine diphosphate pathway (28). It appears to be effective for secondary prevention of stroke, although its adverse-effects profile limits the enthusiasm for its use.

a. **Ticlopidine Versus Placebo**—In a double-blind PRCT, 1072 patients who had had a recent thromboembolic ischemic stroke were randomly assigned to receive either ticlopidine (250 mg BID) or placebo and were observed for a mean of 24 months. Patients were enrolled within 1 week to 4 months from the stroke. Only those patients with at least some residual neurologic deficits were enrolled, but bedridden patients were excluded. The findings were presented in various ways, but the results of the intention-to-treat analysis are presented below (32) (see Table 32-14).

(1) There was a 23.3% reduction in the risk of all vascular events (MI, stroke, and vascular death) for ticlopidine, compared with placebo (P=0.02). Furthermore, there was a statistically nonsignificant 20.5% reduction in the risk of all strokes (fatal and nonfatal) with ticlopidine.

(2) Adverse effects of ticlopidine included neutropenia (2.1%), rash (14.9%), diarrhea (21.5%), bleeding (6.5%), and abnormal liver function (4.4%). Overall, 54% of patients on ticlopidine reported adverse experiences, compared with 34% of those on placebo.

(3) Unlike most of the other secondary stroke prevention trials which involved patients with TIAs and minor strokes, most of the patients in this ticlopidine study had major strokes. In the Swedish Cooperative Study, the only other trial that has tested antiplatelet agents among patients with major strokes, aspirin did not significantly reduce the rate of future strokes or other vascular events (67). A direct comparison between aspirin and ticlopidine would be of interest in order to test whether ticlopidine is more effective than aspirin for secondary prevention of vascular events after a major stroke.

b. **Ticlopidine Versus Aspirin**—In a double-blind PRCT involving 3069 patients with TIAs, reversible ischemic neurologic deficit, or minor strokes (the Ticlopidine Aspirin Stroke Study [TASS]), ticlopidine (250 mg BID) was directly compared to aspirin (650 mg BID). Other antiplatelet or anticoagulant agents were not permitted during the study. Patients with embolic strokes, gastrointestinal bleeding, hematologic disorders, cancer, or peptic

Table 32-14 Ticlopidine vs. placebo for secondary stroke prevention (32)

	Ticlopidine* (N=525)	Placebo* (N=528)	P
All vascular events (MI, stroke, vascular death)	11.3	14.8	0.020
All strokes (fatal and nonfatal)	8.5%	10.7%	NS

*Events per 100 patient-years.

ulcer disease were excluded. Patients were observed for 2 to 6 years (35) (see Table 32-15).

(1) Ticlopidine was superior to aspirin in decreasing the rate of fatal and nonfatal strokes (21% risk reduction) and the combined rate of death or nonfatal stroke (12% risk reduction). Modest advantages of ticlopidine were observed in both sexes.

(2) Once again, side effects were common with ticlopidine and included diarrhea (20%), dyspepsia (13%), rash (12%), hemorrhage (9%), urticaria (2%), and severe neutropenia (0.9%). In addition, compared with the mean pretreatment level, the mean serum cholesterol value increased by 9% with ticlopidine. Overall, 20.9% of patients receiving ticlopidine experienced adverse effects leading to termination of therapy, compared with 14.5% of patients receiving aspirin ($P<0.05$).

(3) In a subgroup analysis of the same data, some populations appeared to benefit more from ticlopidine than others. These groups included patients with vertebrobasilar symptoms, those with diffuse atherosclerotic disease rather than high-grade carotid stenosis, those with persistent symptoms while receiving aspirin or anticoagulant therapy, and women. On the other hand, patients with high-grade carotid stenosis derived more benefit from aspirin than from ticlopidine (33). However, these findings require further validation.

c. Based on these studies, ticlopidine appears to be effective for secondary prevention of stroke. It also appears to have modest advantages over aspirin. However, its high cost and the poor side-effects profile sway most clinicians from using it routinely. Ticlodipine may best be reserved for those patients who have failed or are intolerant to aspirin therapy. If it is used, patients should be counseled and monitored carefully for development of neutropenia.

3. Warfarin for Secondary Prevention of Stroke

a. In general, long-term anticoagulation is indicated for patients who have had an embolic stroke (*i.e.*, due to AF) in order to prevent its recurrence. However, for patients who have had other types of stroke (*e.g.*, stroke of unknown origin, lacunar stroke, stroke caused by middle cerebral artery (MCA) stenosis) or TIA, the role of long-term anticoagulation is less certain. Among the three randomized studies that have addressed this issue since CT scans became routinely available, none demonstrated a significant benefit of anticoagulation over antiplatelet therapy (12,31,49). These studies are small, ranging in size from 125 to 141 patients. The length of follow-up ranged from 12 to 24 months, and the intensity of anticoagulation varied from INR of 2.0 to 4.0. Two of the studies compared anticoagulation versus aspirin plus dipyridamole (12,49), and the third compared anticoagulation versus aspirin (31). Although anticoagulation was not superior to antiplatelet therapy, the small number of clinical outcome events in these studies raises the possibility of type II error. However, as shown in Table 32-16, even when the results of these three trials were combined, there were no significant differences in the rates of stroke, stroke or death, or intracranial

Table 32-15 Ticlopidine vs. aspirin for secondary stroke prevention (35)

	Ticlopidine* (N=1529)	Aspirin* (N=1540)	*P*
Rate of nonfatal stroke or death from any cause at 3 y	17%	19%	0.048
Rate of all strokes (fatal and nonfatal) at 3 y	10%	13%	0.024

*Events per 100 patient-years.

hemorrhage (55). Currently, a large PRCT comparing warfarin versus aspirin is underway to better address this important issue.

b. For now, the best available evidence does not suggest that anticoagulation is superior to aspirin for secondary prophylaxis of stroke in patients with stroke or TIA not related to AF. In practice, warfarin is often used for patients with severe vertebrobasilar stenosis, for those who experience persistent symptoms attributable to cerebrovascular disease despite antiplatelet therapy, and for nonsurgical candidates with symptomatic carotid artery stenosis. However, there are no data from randomized controlled studies to support or refute these strategies (55).

K. Summary

1. **Asymptomatic Healthy Patients**—Although aspirin decreases the risk of MI, it does not reduce the risk of stroke. In fact, the risk of stroke, particularly hemorrhagic stroke, appears to be higher with aspirin therapy.
2. **Patients with Hypertension**—Antihypertensive therapy decreases the risk of stroke in patients with diastolic hypertension or isolated systolic hypertension. With an average decrease in the diastolic blood pressure of 5 to 6 mm Hg, the risk of stroke decreased by 42% after 2 to 3 years of antihypertensive therapy.
3. **Patients with Chronic Stable Angina**—Although aspirin decreased the risk of MI, it increased the risk of stroke in patients with chronic stable angina.
4. **Patients with Myocardial Infarction**—In the acute phase of MI, aspirin decreased the risk of stroke, recurrent MI, and vascular death. Early use of heparin appears to decrease the rate of LVT formation and may also decrease the rate of stroke. However, further studies are needed in this area. In post-MI patients (nonacute phase of MI), both aspirin and warfarin reduced the rate of stroke and recurrent MI. However, warfarin increased the risk of bleeding complications, including intracranial hemorrhage. Because the target INRs used in these trials were relatively high, it is unknown whether lower-intensity anticoagulation would have decreased the risk of major bleeding. In addition, it is unknown whether warfarin or warfarin plus aspirin is superior to aspirin alone in terms of overall efficacy and safety, and further studies are needed.
5. **Prevention of Stroke in Patients with Atrial Fibrillation**—In general, patients with AF and valvular heart disease require chronic anticoagulation. Most patients with NRAF also benefit from anticoagulation. However, anticoagulation is probably not necessary for patients <65 years of age who do not have a history hypertension, diabetes mellitus, or previous stroke or TIA. Aspirin may be sufficient for these patients. Similarly, patients with lone AF who are <60 or 70 years of age probably do not require anticoagulation.
6. **Patients with Prosthetic Heart Valves**—All patients with mechanical prosthetic valves should be treated with long-term anticoagulation with an INR goal of 2.5 to 3.5. Based on the available data, it is unclear whether the combination of antiplatelet therapy plus warfarin offers additional protection against thromboembolism compared with warfarin alone. All patients with bioprosthetic valves should be anticoagulated for the first 3 months, particularly if the valve is in the mitral position. Beyond this period, long-term therapy with aspirin may be sufficient for low-risk patients.
7. **Patients with Carotid Artery Stenosis**—CEA is clearly indicated for patients

Table 32-16 Anticoagulant vs. antiplatelet therapy in nonembolic stroke (55)

	Anticoagulation	Antiplatelet Therapy
Total no. of patient-years	384	409
Stroke*	2.6	3.2
Stroke or death*	5.2	5.9
Intracranial hemorrhage*	0.3	0.7

*Events per 100 patient-years.

with severe carotid artery disease (70% to 99% stenosis) who have had a TIA, an episode of TMB, or a small stroke attributable to the carotid lesion. However, CEA is not beneficial for patients with mild carotid artery stenosis (0% to 29%), and its efficacy for those with moderate carotid artery stenosis (30% to 69%) is still being evaluated. Because these trials randomized relatively few women and excluded patients >80 years old as well as those with AF, it is unclear whether the benefit of CEA can be extended to these patients. The role of CEA for asymptomatic patients with carotid artery disease is controversial (73a). According to the ACAS trial CEA was effective in decreasing the risk of stroke in asymptomatic patients with >60% stenosis of the carotid artery. However, CEA did not decrease the risk of major disabling stroke, or death. There may be subgroups of patients with asymptomatic carotid stenoses who derive more benefit from CEA, but this has yet to be proven.

8. **Patients with Other Types of Ischemic Stroke or TIA**—Aspirin clearly offers some benefit in secondary prevention of stroke in patients with a prior history of non–AF-related ischemic stroke or TIA. However, the benefit of aspirin has been demonstrated only in patients with minor strokes or TIAs. In one trial involving patients with major strokes, aspirin was not superior to placebo for secondary stroke prevention. On the other hand, ticlopidine was clearly superior to placebo in patients with major strokes. Therefore, a direct comparison of ticlopidine versus aspirin in patients with major strokes would be of interest. Ticlopidine was also marginally superior to aspirin in patients with minor stroke or TIA. However, its high cost and the poor side-effects profile limit the enthusiasm for its use. Finally, a large multicenter PRCT is underway to compare warfarin versus aspirin in patients with stroke not related to AF or severe carotid stenosis.

Abbreviations used in Chapter 32

ACAS = Asymptomatic Carotid Atherosclerosis Study
AF = atrial fibrillation
BID = twice daily
CEA = carotid endarterectomy
CI = confidence interval
ECST = European Carotid Surgery Trial
INR = international normalized ratio
LVT = left ventricular thrombus
MI = myocardial infarction
N = number of patients in population
NASCET = North American Symptomatic Carotid Endarterectomy Trial
NRAF = nonrheumatic atrial fibrillation
NS = not statistically significant
P = probability value
PRCT = prospective randomized controlled trial
PTR = prothrombin time ratio
q = every
QOD = every other day
TIA = transient ischemic attack
TMB = transmonocular blindness
VA = Veterans Administration
vs. = versus

References

1. Albers. Atrial fibrillation and stroke: three new studies, three remaining questions. *Arch Intern Med* 1994;154:1443.

2. Anticoagulation in the Secondary Prevention of Events in Coronary Thrombosis (ASPECT) Research Group. Effect of long-term oral anticoagulant treatment on mortality and cardiovascular morbidity after myocardial infarction. *Lancet* 1994; 343:499.
3. Antiplatelet Trialists' Collaboration. Collaborative overview of randomised trials of antiplatelet therapy: I. Prevention of death, myocardial infarction, and stroke by prolonged antiplatelet therapy in various categories of patients. *Br Med J* 1994; 308:81.
4. Asymptomatic Carotid Atherosclerosis Study Group. Study design for randomized prospective trial of carotid endarterectomy for asymptomatic atherosclerosis. *Stroke* 1989;20:844.
5. Atkins. Cholesterol reduction and the risk for stroke in men: a meta-analysis of randomized, controlled trials. *Ann Intern Med* 1993;119:136.
6. Atrial Fibrillation Investigators. Risk factors for stroke and efficacy of antithrombotic therapy in atrial fibrillation. *Arch Intern Med* 1994;154:1449.
7. Baker. Management of heart failure: IV. Anticoagulation for patients with heart failure due to left ventricular systolic dysfunction. *JAMA* 1994;20:1614.
8. Barnett. Carotid endarterectomy for asymptomatic carotid stenosis. *N Engl J Med* 1993;328:276.
9. Baudet. A 5 1/2 year experience with the St. Jude medical cardiac valve prosthesis. *J Thorac Cardiovasc Surg* 1985;90:137.
10. Boston Area Anticoagulation Trial for Atrial Fibrillation Investigators. The effect of low-dose warfarin on the risk of stroke in patients with nonrheumatic atrial fibrillation. *N Engl J Med* 1990;323:1505.
11. Brand. Characteristics and prognosis of lone atrial fibrillation: 30 year follow-up in the Framingham study. *JAMA* 1985;254:3449.
12. Buren. Treatment program and comparison between anticoagulants and platelet aggregation inhibitors after transient ischemic attack. *Stroke* 1981;12:578.
13. CASANOVA Study Group. Carotid surgery versus medical therapy in asymptomatic carotid stenosis. *Stroke* 1991;22:1229.
14. Cerebral Embolism Task Force. Cardiogenic brain embolism. The second report of the cerebral embolism task force. *Arch Neurol* 1989;46:727.
15. Chesebro. Trial of combined warfarin plus dipyridamole or aspirin therapy in prosthetic heart valve replacement: danger of aspirin compared with dipyridamole. *Am J Cardiol* 1983;51:1537.
16. Cohn. Early and late risk of mitral valve replacement. *J Thorac Cardiovasc Surg* 1985;90:872.
17. Collins. Blood pressure, stroke, and coronary heart disease: part 2. Short term reductions in blood pressure: overview of randomised drug trials in the epidemiologic context. *Lancet* 1990;335:827.
18. Connolly. Canadian atrial fibrillation anticoagulation study. *J Am Coll Cardiol* 1991; 18:349.
19. Coope. Randomised trial of treatment of hypertension in the elderly in primary care. *Br Med J* 1986;293:1145.
20. Dutch TIA Trial Study Group. A comparison of two doses of aspirin (30 mg vs. 283 mg a day) in patients after a transient ischemic attack or minor ischemic stroke. *N Engl J Med* 1991;325:1261.
21. Dyken. Low-dose aspirin and stroke. *Stroke* 1992;23:1395.
22. Easton. Carotid endarterectomy: trials and tribulations. *Ann Neurol* 1994;35:5.
23. European Atrial Fibrillation Trial Study Group. Secondary prevention in nonrheumatic atrial fibrillation after transient ischaemic attack or minor stroke. *Lancet* 1993;342:1255.
24. European Carotid Surgery Trialists' Collaborative Group. MRC European Carotid Surgery Trial: interim results for symptomatic patients with severe (70-99%) or mild (0-29%) carotid stenosis. *Lancet* 1991;337:1235.

24a. Executive Committee for the Asymptomatic Carotid Atherosclerosis Study. Endarterectomy for asymptomatic carotid stenosis. *JAMA* 1995;273:1421.

25. Ezekowitz. Warfarin in the prevention of stroke associated with nonrheumatic atrial fibrillation. *N Engl J Med* 1992;327:1406.

26. Ezekowitz. VA cooperative study of warfarin in the prevention of stroke associated with nonrheumatic atrial fibrillation. *N Engl J Med* 1992;327:1406.
27. Falk. A plea for a clinical trial of anticoagulation in dilated cardiomyopathy. *Am J Cardiol* 1990;65:914.
28. Feliste. Broad spectrum anti-platelet activity of ticlopidine and PCR 4099 involves the suppression of the effects of released ADP. *Thromb Res* 1987;48:403.
29. Frick. Helsinki Heart Study: primary prevention trial with gemfibrozil in middle-aged men with dyslipidemia. Safety of treatment, changes in risk factors and incidence of coronary heart disease. *N Engl J Med* 1987;317:1237.
30. Fuster. The natural history of idiopathic dilated cardiomyopathy. *Am J Cardiol* 1981;47:525.
31. Garde. Treatment after transient ischemic attacks: a comparison between anticoagulant drug and inhibition of platelet aggregation. *Stroke* 1983;14:677.
32. Gent. The Canadian American Ticlopidine Study (CATS) in thromboembolic stroke. *Lancet* 1989;1:1215.
33. Grotta. Prevention of stroke with ticlopidine: Who benefits most? *Neurology* 1992;42:111.
34. Hartz. Comparative study of warfarin versus antiplatelet therapy in patients with a St. Jude Medical valve in the aortic position. *J Thorac Cardiovasc Surg* 1986;92:684.
35. Hass. A randomized trial comparing ticlopidine hydrochloride with aspirin for the prevention of stroke in high-risk patients. *N Engl J Med* 1989;321:501.
36. Hetzer. Thromboembolism and anticoagulation after isolated mitral valve replacement with porcine heterografts. In: Cohn, ed. *Proceedings, Second International Symposium on Cardiac Bioprosthesis*. New York: Yorke Medical Books, 1982:170.
37. Hobson. Efficacy of carotid endarterectomy for asymptomatic carotid stenosis. *N Engl J Med* 1993;328:221.
38. Hypertension Detection and Follow-up Program Cooperative Group. Five-year findings of the Hypertension Detection and Follow-up Program: III. Reduction in stroke incidence among persons with high blood pressure. *JAMA* 1982;247:633.
39. Ionescu. Clinical durability of the pericardial xenograft valve: ten years experience with mitral replacement. *Ann Thorac Surg* 1982;34:265.
40. ISIS-2 (Second International Study of Infarct Survival) Collaborative Group. Randomised trial of intravenous streptokinase, oral aspirin, both, or neither among 17,187 cases of suspected acute myocardial infarction: ISIS-2. *Lancet* 1988;2:349.
41. Kannel. Epidemiologic features of chronic atrial fibrillation: the Framingham study. *N Engl J Med* 1982;306:1018.
42. Kopecky. The natural history of lone atrial fibrillation: a population-based study over three decades. *N Engl J Med* 1987;317:669.
43. Mayberg. Carotid endarterectomy and prevention of cerebral ischemia in symptomatic carotid stenosis. *JAMA* 1991;266:3289.
44. Medical Research Council Working Party. MRC trial of treatment of mild hypertension: principal results. *Br Med J* 1985;291:97.
45. Mok. Warfarin versus dipyridamole-aspirin and pentoxyfylline-aspirin for the prevention of prosthetic heart valve thromboembolism: a prospective randomized clinical trial. *Circulation* 1985;72:1059.
46. North American Symptomatic Carotid Endarterectomy Trial Collaborators. Beneficial effect of carotid endarterectomy in symptomatic patients with high-grade carotid stenosis. *N Engl J Med* 1991;325:445.
47. Nunez. Aspirin or Coumadin as the drug of choice for valve replacement with porcine bioprosthesis. *Ann Thorac Surg* 1982;33:354.
48. Nunez. Prevention of thromboembolism using aspirin after mitral valve replacement with porcine bioprosthesis. *Ann Thorac Surg* 1984;37:84.
49. Olsson. Anticoagulant vs. antiplatelet therapy as prophylactic against cerebral infarction in transient ischemic attacks. *Stroke* 1980;11:4.
50. Oyer. Valve replacement with the Starr-Edwards and Hancock prostheses: comparative analysis of late morbidity and mortality. *Ann Surg* 1977;186:301.
51. Petersen. Placebo-controlled, randomized trial of warfarin and aspirin for prevention of thromboembolic complications in chronic atrial fibrillation: The Copenhagen AFASAK study. *Lancet* 1989;1:175.

52. Peto. Randomised trial of prophylactic daily aspirin in British male doctors. *Br Med J* 1989;296:313.
53. Ribeiro. Antiplatelet drugs and the incidence of thromboembolic complications of the St. Jude Medical aortic prosthesis in patients with rheumatic heart disease. *J Thorac Cardiovasc Surg* 1986;91:92.
54. Ridker. Low-dose aspirin therapy for chronic stable angina: a randomized, placebo-controlled clinical trial. *Ann Intern Med* 1991;114:835.
55. Rothrock. Antithrombotic therapy in cerebrovascular disease. *Ann Intern Med* 1991; 115:885.
56. SALT Collaborative Group. Swedish Aspirin Low-Dose Trial (SALT) of 75 mg aspirin as secondary prophylaxis after cerebrovascular ischaemic events. *Lancet* 1991; 338:1345.
57. Saour. Trial of different intensities of anticoagulation therapy in patients with substitute heart valves. *N Engl J Med* 1990;322:428.
58. Scandinavian Simvastatin Survival Study Group. Randomized trial of cholesterol lowering in 4444 patients with coronary heart disease: the Scandinavian Simvastatin Survival Study (4S). *Lancet* 1994;334:1383.
59. SHEP Cooperative Research Group. Prevention of stroke by antihypertensive drug treatment in older persons with isolated systolic hypertension: final results of the Systolic Hypertension in the Elderly Program (SHEP). *JAMA* 1991;265:3255.
60. Smith. The effect of warfarin on mortality and reinfarction after myocardial infarction. *N Engl J Med* 1990;323:147.
61. Steering Committee of the Physicians' Health Study Research Group. Final report on the aspirin component of the ongoing Physicians' Health Study. *N Engl J Med* 1989;321:129.
62. Stein. Antithrombotic therapy in patients with mechanical and biological prosthetic heart valves. *Chest* 1992;102(4S):445S.
63. Stratton. Increased embolic risk in patients with left ventricular thrombi. *Circulation* 1987;75:1004.
64. Stroke Prevention in Atrial Fibrillation Investigators. The stroke prevention in atrial fibrillation study: final results. *Circulation* 1991;84:527.
65. Stroke Prevention in Atrial Fibrillation Investigators. Warfarin versus aspirin for prevention of thromboembolism in atrial fibrillation: Stroke Prevention in Atrial Fibrillation II Study. *Lancet* 1994;343:687.
66. Sullivan. Effect of dipyridamole on the incidence of arterial emboli after cardiac valve replacement. *Circulation* 1969;39-40(Supplement 1):I.
67. Swedish Cooperative Study Group. High dose aspirin after cerebral infarction. *Stroke* 1987;18:325.
68. Szekely. Systemic embolism and anticoagulant prophylaxis in rheumatic heart disease. *Br Med J* 1964;1:1209.
69. Tramarin. Two-dimensional echocardiographic assessment of anticoagulant therapy in left ventricular thrombosis early after acute myocardial infarction. *Eur Heart J* 1986;7:482.
70. Turpie. Comparison of high-dose with low-dose subcutaneous heparin to prevent left ventricular mural thrombosis in patients with acute transmural anterior myocardial infarction. *N Engl J Med* 1989;320:352.
71. Turpie. Reduction in mortality by adding aspirin (100 mg) to oral anticoagulants in patients with heart valve replacement. *J Am Coll Cardiol* 1992;19(Supplement A):103A. Abstract.
72. UK-TIA Study Group. United Kingdom Transient Ischaemic Attack (UK-TIA) aspirin trial: interim results. *Br Med J* 1988;296:316.
73. UK-TIA Study Group. The United Kingdom Transient Ischaemic Attack (UK-TIA) aspirin trial: final results. *J Neurol Neurosurg Psychiatry* 1991;54:1044.
73a. Warlow. Endarterectomy for asymptomatic carotid stenosis? *Lancet* 1995;345:1254.
74. Wolf. Atrial fibrillation as an independent risk factor for stroke: the Framingham Study. *Stroke* 1991;22:983.
75. Wolf. Probability of stroke: a risk profile from the Framingham Study. *Stroke* 1991; 22:312.

33 Alcohol Withdrawal Syndrome

Burton W. Lee and
Walter J. Koroshetz

A. Introduction

1. Each year, 1.2 million Americans are hospitalized with problems related to alcohol abuse. Among these patients, about 5% develop delirium tremens (DT) and countless more experience symptoms of minor withdrawal. Mortality associated with DT have been reported to be about 20% in the past, but with better therapeutic and supportive measures, it has been reduced to as low as 1% in more recent reports (10,12).
2. The exact mechanism of withdrawal is not known, but the most widely accepted view is the Kalant model. This model proposes that with chronic alcohol abuse, the body adapts to the depressant effect of alcohol on the central nervous system with a compensatory increase in neuronal activity. Consequently, with abrupt withdrawal of alcohol, the body predominantly experiences the unopposed neuronal activity, which is characterized by tremor, fever, tachycardia, hypertension, hallucinations, seizures, agitation, irritability, or delirium. The pattern of withdrawal is often stereotypical in an individual patient (12).
3. **Pharmacology of Alcohol**
   a. **Toxicity**—Alcohol toxicity depends on many factors, including the total dose, the pattern of use, the presence or absence of food in the stomach, the presence or absence of other drugs in the body, the patient's underlying medical and physical state, and the level of tolerance to alcohol. Unlike opiates or benzodiazepines, there is no specific antagonist that can reverse the toxic effects of alcohol. It is a general sedative that acts on the lipid bulk phase of cell membranes; at toxic levels, alcohol also blocks the *N*-methyl-D-aspartate–type glutamate receptors. The median lethal dose is approximately 5000 mg/L, but there is great individual variability. Most of the deaths are attributable to respiratory depression (9).
   b. **Metabolism**—A normal 70-kg man can metabolize about 10 g of ethanol per hour, which is equivalent to about 1 can of beer per hour. A nonalcoholic person can clear alcohol from a blood level of 4000 mg/L to zero in about 20 hours. An alcoholic person can clear it significantly faster (9). Because alcohol is rapidly absorbed from the gastrointestinal tract, gastric lavage or activated charcoal is of little value. Furthermore, there are no clinically useful agents that hasten the metabolism of alcohol. However, hemodialysis may be useful in extreme cases (9).

B. Clinical Manifestations

1. **Early or Minor Withdrawal Syndrome**—Early withdrawal symptoms occur in about 80% of chronic alcoholic patients who abruptly abstain from drinking (13). Symptoms start about 8 hours from abstinence and peak in severity at 24 to 36 hours. Clinical features include tachycardia, hypertension, fever, tremor, sweats, nausea, vomiting, agitation, irritability, vigilance, anxiety, and craving for alcohol (12).
2. **Alcoholic Hallucinosis**—Alcoholic hallucinosis occurs in about 18% of chronic alcoholic patients who abruptly abstain from drinking (13). Symptoms start about 24 hours from abstinence and end by day 2 or 3. Hallucinations are

more often visual than auditory. The presence or absence of hallucinosis does not predict the likelihood of progressing to DT. Patients have an intact sensorium at this stage (12).

3. **Alcohol Withdrawal Seizures**—Seizures occur in about 23% of chronic alcoholic patients who abruptly abstain from drinking. This risk is higher if the patient has a prior history of idiopathic or withdrawal seizures (13). Seizures may begin about 12 hours from abstinence, and the likelihood of seizure peaks at about 24 hours. Withdrawal seizures tend to be generalized and tonic-clonic. Usually there is one convulsion or a rapid burst of several convulsions. Only 3% progress to status epilepticus (12). Therefore, repeat seizures should prompt an investigation of other potential causes.
4. **Delirium Tremens**—DT occurs in about 5% of chronic alcoholic patients who abruptly abstain from drinking (13). This syndrome is restricted to patients who have a long and intense history of alcohol abuse. Consequently, it is uncommon in patients <30 years old. The risk of DT is higher if there is a prior history of major withdrawal. DT begins about 48 hours from abstinence but can start up to 14 days later. Once the syndrome begins, most episodes resolve within 72 hours. In general, alcohol withdrawal syndrome includes delirium, hallucination, hyperactivity, agitation, hypertension, tachycardia, fever, tremor, and sweats. Before DT can be diagnosed, other conditions that can mimic DT should be ruled out. These include sepsis, meningitis, hypoxia, seizure, hypoglycemia, thiamine deficiency, toxic ingestion, and subdural hematoma (12).
5. **Other Complications**
   a. **Wernicke's Encephalopathy**—Wernicke's syndrome is characterized by the clinical triad of ataxia, ocular dysfunction (ophthalmoplegia, nystagmus), and cognitive impairment. The neurologic deficits are reversible if treated early but become permanent if treatment is delayed, leading to encephalopathy, coma, and death. This syndrome is caused by thiamine deficiency and may be precipitated by administration of IV dextrose in poorly nourished patients. Timely administration of thiamine can rapidly reverse these symptoms. Thiamine should be given before infusion of dextrose for patients at risk for this syndrome (12).
   b. **Korsakoff's Syndrome**—This syndrome is a chronic state characterized by severe memory impairment that is out of proportion to other cognitive dysfunction. These patients are alert and have an intact sensorium but often confabulate. This syndrome is also caused by thiamine deficiency. It can follow an attack of Wernicke's syndrome or occur independently (12). The Wernicke–Korsakoff syndrome is also observed in other groups of poorly nourished patients with cancer or digestive disorders.

C. Management

1. **General Approach To Alcohol Withdrawal** (9,12)
   a. As with any other acutely ill patient, a careful history and physical examination should be performed. Information regarding the amount and pattern of alcohol use, the reasons for abstinence, and the prior history of seizures, Wernicke's encephalopathy, or DT should be ascertained. The vital signs, respiratory status, complete neurologic examination, and stool guaiac examination should also be noted. Trauma with subdural hematoma, pneumonia, sepsis, meningitis, metabolic acidosis and other serious concomitant conditions should carefully be excluded, because they are not uncommon in this patient population. Laboratory evaluation should include electrolytes, creatinine, glucose, amylase, magnesium, phosphate, liver function tests, creatine phosphokinase, complete blood count, prothrombin time, toxin screen, and chest film.
   b. The patient should be placed in a quiet, well-lighted room, and physical restraints should be avoided if possible. Parenteral thiamine should be given as soon as possible and before administration of IV fluids containing dextrose. Most clinicians also give multivitamins and folate. There is little support for this in the literature, but the practice is inexpensive and harmless.

2. More than 135 drugs and drug combinations have been reported in the literature for treatment of alcohol withdrawal. However, only a few have been shown to be useful in controlled studies (9). Because most of these studies were small in size and poor in quality, firm conclusions are not possible (12).
   a. **Alcohol**—The use of alcohol to prevent alcohol withdrawal makes pharmacologic sense. However, it is not popular in clinical practice, because alcohol has a short half-life and therefore requires frequent administration. It may also perpetuate the existing metabolic abnormalities. Furthermore, there is concern that it may promote the acceptance of alcohol (9,12).
   b. **Benzodiazepines**
      (1) Kaim studied the role of chlordiazepoxide for treatment of alcohol withdrawal in a prospective randomized controlled trial (PRCT) involving 537 veterans. All patients had at least 2 weeks of heavy alcohol use or were found to be withdrawing from alcohol during an admission for another medical problem. All were required to have at least four of the following eight features: (a) anorexia, nausea, or vomiting; (b) sweats; (c) insomnia; (d) tremor; (e) irritability; (f) apprehension; (g) depression; and (h) clouded sensorium. Patients currently in DT and those with a history of epilepsy were excluded. The study compared five treatment groups as shown in Table 33-1 (3).
         (a) Chlordiazepoxide was superior to placebo, hydroxyzine, chlorpromazine, or thiamine in decreasing the risk of DT or seizures. However, no statistical calculations were reported (see Table 33-2).
         (b) Most patients improved rapidly and did not progress to seizures or DT. This was true even in the placebo group.
      (2) Chlordiazepoxide is the best studied benzodiazepine and should be the drug of choice in most cases. However, oxazepam or lorazepam may be used in patients with severe liver dysfunction. In patients who have already developed DT, diazepam (5 to 10 mg IV q 5 minutes) may be used until the patient is calm but awake. Except for lorazepam, IM administration of benzodiazepines should be avoided because of erratic absorption. Typical recommended doses of the commonly used benzodiazepines are listed in Table 33-3. Each day, the drug should be tapered by 25% of the original dose.
      (3) Alternatively, benzodiazepines may be administered following an individualized, symptom-triggered dosing schedule. Saitz compared a fixed-dosing regimen of chlordiazepoxide versus a symptom-triggered regimen in 101 patients admitted for alcohol withdrawal to a Veterans Affairs hospital. Patients with a prior history of seizures and those who were using or withdrawing from opiates, benzodiazepines, barbiturates, clonidine, or β-blockers were excluded. The severity of withdrawal was measured with the use of a revised version of the Clinical Institute Withdrawal Assessment for Alcohol (CIWA-Ar) scale, which measures the severity of nausea, tremor, autonomic hyperactivity, anxiety, agitation, headache, disorientation, and tactile, visual, auditory disturbances. A

Table 33-1 Summary of the five treatment regimens compared in Kaim's PRCT (3)

Group	IM medication	PO medication
Chlordiazepoxide	Chlordiazepoxide 50 mg IM q 6 h	Placebo PO q 6 h
Chlorpromazine	Placebo IM q 6 h	Chlorpromazine 100 mg PO q 6 h
Hydroxyzine	Hydroxyzine 100 mg IM q 6 h	Placebo PO q 6 h
Thiamine	Thiamine 100 mg IM q 6 h	Placebo PO q 6 h
Placebo	Placebo IM q 6 h	Placebo PO q 6 h

Table 33-2 Results of Kaim's study (3)

	Chlordiazepoxide (N=103)	Hydroxyzine (N=103)	Chlorpromazine (N=98)	Thiamine (N=103)	Placebo (N=130)	*P*
Patients who requested discharge or left AMA	11%	2%	9%	9%	5%	?
Patients whose symptoms or signs worsened despite therapy	1%	3%	2%	6%	2%	?
DTs	1%	4%	7%	4%	6%	?
Seizures	1%	8%	12%	7%	7%	?
DTs or seizures	2%	10%	16%	11%	12%	?

specially trained nurse assessed the vital signs, level of alertness, and CIWA-Ar score at baseline, every 8 hours, and 1 hour after each dose of medication. Physicians, nurses, and subjects were blinded to the treatment assignment. Patients assigned to the fixed-dosed regimen received 50 mg of chlordiazepoxide every 6 hours for four doses, followed by 25 mg every 6 hours for eight doses. In addition, 25 to 100 mg of chlordiazepoxide every hour was given PRN when the CIWA-Ar score exceeded 8. Patients assigned to the symptom-triggered regimen received doses of identical placebo plus 25 to 100 mg of chlordiazepoxide every 1 hour PRN when the CIWA-Ar score exceeded 8. (7)

(a) Patients assigned to the fixed-dosing regimen received a mean total dose of 425 mg of chlordiazepoxide over a mean duration of 68 hours. In contrast, those assigned to the symptom-triggered regimen received a mean total dose of 100 mg of chlordiazepoxide over a mean duration of 9 hours. These differences were both statistically significant ($P<0.001$).

(b) Despite shorter courses of therapy and the use of smaller amounts of medications, patients assigned to the symptom-triggered regimen had outcomes similar to those of patients assigned to the fixed-dosing regimen. Specifically, there were no significant differences in the rates of DT, hallucinations, seizures, or readmissions. In addition, the peak CIWA-Ar scores were also similar in the two groups.

(c) However, it is unclear whether these finding can be generalized to women, because all but one subject in the study were men. Furthermore, patients with a prior history seizures were excluded from the study. Finally, a symptom-triggered dosing regimen may be less successful at centers where the nurses and physicians are not familiar with the CIWA-Ar or another comparable scale.

c. β-Blockers—Kraus compared atenolol (0 mg for heart rate <50 bpm, 50 mg QD for heart rate of 50 to 80 bpm, 100 mg QD for heart rate >80 bpm) versus placebo in a double-blind PRCT of 120 chronic alcoholic patients between the ages of 16 and 65 years. The study excluded combative patients and those who had had a seizure during the current admission. Patients with a history of polysubstance abuse, insulin-dependent diabetes mellitus, chronic obstructive pulmonary disease, asthma, or hypertension were also excluded. Oxazepam was given as needed, but no benzodiazepine was administered on a round-the-clock basis. The percentages of patients with normal vital signs (blood pressure, heart rate, temperature), normal clinical features (tremor, seizures, level of consciousness), and normal behavioral features (anxiety, agitation, hallucination) were recorded (5).

(1) Atenolol was superior to placebo in normalizing the vital signs. However, there were no differences in the percentage of patients with normal clinical features or normal behavioral features (see Table 33-4).

(2) Atenolol-treated patients required less oxazepam and had shorter length of hospital stay (see Table 33-5).

Table 33-3 Commonly used benzodiazepines for treatment of alcohol withdrawal

	Typical dose	Route	Half-life
Chlordiazepoxide	25–100 mg q 6 h	PO	50–100 h
Diazepam	5–20 mg q 6 h	PO/IV	30–60 h
Lorazepam	1–2 mg q 4 h	PO/IV/IM	10–20 h
Oxazepam	15–30 mg q 4 h	PO	5–10 h

Table 33-4 Kraus' PRCT of atenolol vs. placebo: general outcome (5)

	% With Normal Vital Signs			% With Normal Clinical Features			% With Normal Behavioral Features		
	Atenolol (N=61)	Placebo (N=59)	*P*	Atenolol (N=61)	Placebo (N=59)	*P*	Atenolol (N=61)	Placebo (N=59)	*P*
Day 1	54%	20%	<0.001	64%	52%	NS	41%	51%	NS
Day 3	48%	32%	?	70%	61%	NS	59%	63%	NS
Day 5	84%	56%	?	90%	81%	NS	87%	73%	NS
Day 7	97%	83%	?	97%	86%	NS	98%	88%	NS

Table 33-5 Kraus' PRCT: effect on oxazepam-requirement and length-of-stay (5)

	Atenolol (N=61)	Placebo (N=59)	*P*
Average daily dose of oxazepam (mg)			
Day 1	58	81	<0.001
Day 3	36	65	<0.001
Day 5	15	65	<0.001
Day 7	0	71	<0.001
Length of hospital stay (d)	4.4	5.1	<0.02

(3) Among patients with an abnormal feature on day 0, atenolol significantly improved the likelihood of having that feature normalized on subsequent days. However, patients with all normal features on day 0 did not benefit from atenolol (see Table 33-6).

(4) In summary, atenolol shortened the length of hospital stay by 0.7 days, decreased the need for benzodiazepines, and normalized vital signs faster than placebo. Although these results were statistically significant, the clinical significance of these benefits is less clear. It is uncertain whether atenolol would offer any additional benefit for patients being treated with round-the-clock benzodiazepine.

d. Clonidine—In a PRCT of 61 chronic alcoholic patients, Baumgartner compared clonidine (0.2 mg) versus chlordiazepoxide (50 mg) according to the following schedule: one dose of clonidine or chlordiazepoxide on day 1, three doses on day 2, two doses on day 3, and one dose on day 4. No other medications were permitted. Patients with a history of seizures and those using prescription or illicit drugs were excluded. The outcome measures in-

Table 33-6 Kraus' PRCT: outcome in patients with abnormal features on day 0 (5)

	% With Normal Vital Signs Who Were Abnormal On Day 0			% With Normal Clinical Features Who Were Abnormal On Day 0			% With Normal Behavioral Features Who Were Abnormal On Day 0		
	Atenolol (N=50)	Placebo (N=51)	*P*	Atenolol (N=33)	Placebo (N=32)	*P*	Atenolol (N=43)	Placebo (N=40)	*P*
Day 1	24%	6%	<0.001	16%	9%	<0.05	12%	15%	NS
Day 3	20%	12%	<0.05	18%	12%	<0.05	23%	11%	<0.05
Day 5	41%	28%	<0.05	29%	23%	<0.05	36%	24%	<0.05
Day 7	48%	41%	NS	32%	25%	<0.05	42%	34%	<0.05

cluded an assessment of the patient's physiologic status using the Alcohol Withdrawal Scale (AWS), the patient's psychological status using the Cognitive Capacity Screening Examination (CCSE), and the patient's subjective status using the Alcohol Withdrawal Self-Rating Scale of Symptom Severity (SRS) (1) (see Table 33-7).

(1) Clonidine was superior to chlordiazepoxide in improving the heart rate, the systolic blood pressure, and the mean AWS score.

(2) There was no difference in regard to diaphoresis, restlessness, tremor, CCSE score, SRS score, or the rate of adverse reactions.

(3) The authors argued that clonidine is superior to chlordiazepoxide because it better controlled physiologic withdrawal parameters and because it has less potential for abuse. However, the route of administration of chlordiazepoxide was not specified. Because IM injections of benzodiazepines can be associated with erratic absorption, this study may have been biased in favor of clonidine.

e. Barbiturates—In a PRCT of 109 chronic alcoholic patients with withdrawal symptoms, Kramp compared barbital (500 mg PO q 30 minutes) plus IM placebo versus diazepam (20 mg IM q 30 minutes) plus oral placebo. A maximum of 10 doses in the first 24 hours and 6 doses in the second 24 hours was permitted; thereafter, doses were given every 6 hours. Patients were categorized as grade 1 (tremor only), grade 2 (tremor and hallucinations), or grade 3 (tremor, hallucinations, and disorientation). Patients taking psychoactive drugs and those with a positive toxin screen for alcohol were excluded (4) (see Table 33-8).

(1) Barbital was superior to diazepam for grade 3 patients but not for grade 1 or grade 2 patients.

(2) However, because IM injections of diazepam may be erratically absorbed, the study may have been biased in favor of barbital. In addition, the trial's small sample size, its use of subgroup analysis, and the subjective end point of "satisfactory treatment" detract from its validity.

f. Paraldehyde—Paraldehyde was once the drug of choice for alcohol withdrawal. However, it has fallen out of favor because it is difficult to administer. It cannot be given intravenously, IM shots are very painful, and it can cause severe local reactions. Oral or rectal administration may be impractical for agitated patients. It is also malodorous and hepatotoxic, and it can cause metabolic acidosis. Studies comparing paraldehyde with benzodi-

Table 33-7 PRCT of clonidine vs. chlordiazepoxide (1)

	Clonidine (N=26)	Chlordiazepoxide (N=21)	*P*
Posttreatment AWS score	4.0	5.3	<0.02
Posttreatment sitting systolic blood pressure	113 mm Hg	123 mm Hg	<0.01
Posttreatment heart rate	77.1 bpm	87.8 bpm	<0.001

Table 33-8 PRCT of diazepam vs. barbital (4)

		% of Patients Satisfactorily Treated		
	N	Grade 1	Grade 2	Grade 3
Diazepam	44	91%	88%	46%
Barbital	47	79%	73%	88%
P	—	NS	NS	<0.05

azepines in the treatment of alcohol withdrawal have shown conflicting results (2,11).

3. Antiseizure Medications

a. Patients with a Prior History of Adult-Onset Seizures—Sampliner compared phenytoin (100 mg TID for 5 days) versus placebo in a PRCT of 136 chronic alcoholic patients who had been drinking heavily for 4 weeks before admission. All had a history of seizures (idiopathic or withdrawal), but none was taking any antiseizure medication for 2 weeks before admission. All patients received chlordiazepoxide as needed. The study was blind for the patients, nurses, and house officers but not to the investigators (8) (see Table 33-9).

(1) Dilantin was better than placebo for prevention of withdrawal seizures (P=0.005).

(2) Patients were not loaded with phenytoin in this study. Theoretically, it can take 5 to 15 days to achieve a therapeutic phenytoin level without a loading dose. The average serum level in these patients was 3 to 4 mg/ml, which is lower than the recommended level of about 10 mg/ml. This observation suggests that withdrawal seizures may be more responsive to phenytoin than idiopathic seizures.

b. Patients with No Prior History of Seizures—In low-risk patients, the available data do not support the routine use of seizure prophylaxis.

(1) Sampliner's study also retrospectively examined 2200 chronic alcoholic patients who either had no history of seizures (97%) or were currently being treated for a history of seizures (3%). The risk of seizures was only 0.18% in this population during alcohol withdrawal (8).

(2) Rothstein compared phenytoin (200 mg PO BID) versus no therapy in a PRCT of 200 chronic alcoholic patients who drank at least 480 ml of "hard" liquor per day for 5 days before admission. Study excluded patients with any prior history of phenytoin use and those with a history of seizures within 2 weeks of admission. All patients received thiamine daily and chlordiazepoxide as needed (6). Chlordiazepoxide was just as effective as phenytoin plus chlordiazepoxide in preventing seizures (see Table 33-10).

D. Summary

1. Benzodiazepines remain the therapy of choice in most patients with alcohol withdrawal. The largest study to date showed benzodiazepines to be superior to placebo in decreasing the risk of DT or seizures.

a. The best studied drug is chlordiazepoxide. In patients with severe hepatic dysfunction, oxazepam or lorazepam may be substituted. In patients actively experiencing DT, diazepam (5 to 10 mg q 5 minutes IV) may be used

Table 33-9 PRCT of phenytoin vs. placebo in high-risk patients (8)

	Placebo (N=66)	Dilantin (N=70)	*P*
Seizures during days 1–5	16.7%	0%	0.005
Any seizure during hospitalization	16.7%	2.9%	0.005

Table 33-10 PRCT of phenytoin vs. placebo in low-risk patients (6)

	Control (N=100)	Dilantin (N=100)	*P*
Seizures	0	0	NS
DTs	4%	5%	NS
Deaths	0	0	NS

until the patient is calm but awake. Then 5 to 10 mg of diazepam may be repeated every 1 to 6 hours as needed.

   b. Currently, a round-the-clock dosing regimen is most commonly used. Typically, 25 to 100 mg of chlordiazepoxide is initially given every 6 hours, and subsequent doses are tapered by 25% of the original dose each day. However, in a recent trial, a symptom-triggered dosing regimen resulted in shorter duration of therapy and use of fewer milligrams of chlordiazepoxide, compared with a predetermined, fixed-dosing regimen.

2. Some studies have shown β-blockers, clonidine, paraldehyde, or barbiturates to be equal to or better than benzodiazepines in treatment of alcohol withdrawal (see Table 33-11). In general, these studies can be criticized for their small size, poor study design, ill-defined end points, and use of intramuscular rather than intravenous or oral administration of benzodiazepines. As better studies become available, some of these agents may prove to be reasonable alternatives to benzodiazepines.

3. Seizure Prophylaxis

   a. Low-Risk Patients—In patients without a prior history of seizures, the risk of withdrawal seizures is extremely low with benzodiazepine therapy alone. Therefore, prophylactic use of phenytoin does not appear to be necessary in this population.

   b. High-Risk Patients—In patients with a prior history of seizures, the risk of withdrawal seizures is substantial with benzodiazepine therapy alone. Phenytoin (100 mg PO TID with or without a loading dose of 1 g IV) can significantly decrease this risk.

Table 33-11 Non-benzodiazepine treatment options for alcohol withdrawal

	Dose
Atenolol	25–100 mg PO QD titrated to the heart rate
Clonidine	0.2 mg PO times 1 dose on day 1, 3 doses on day 2, 2 doses on day 3, and 1 dose on day 4
Paraldehyde	10 ml PO, PR, or IM q 2–4 h
Barbital	500 mg PO q 30 min up to 10 doses on day 1, up to 6 doses on day 2, then q 6 h

Abbreviations used in Chapter 33

AMA = against medical advice
AWS = Alcohol Withdrawal Scale
BID = twice daily
bpm = beats per minute
CCSE = Cognitive Capacity Screening Examination
CIWA-Ar scale = Clinical Institute Withdrawal Assessment for Alcohol, Revised
DT = delirium tremens
IM = intramuscular
IV = intravenous
N = number of patients
P = probability value
PO = per os
PR = per rectum
PRCT = prospective randomized controlled trial
PRN = as needed
q = every
QD = once daily

SRS = Alcohol Withdrawal Self-Rating Scale of Symptom Severity
TID = three times daily
vs. = versus

References

1. Baumgartner. Clonidine vs. chlordiazepoxide in the management of acute alcohol withdrawal syndrome. *Arch Intern Med* 1987;147:1223.
2. Golbert. Comparative evaluation of treatments of alcohol withdrawal syndromes. *JAMA* 1967;201:113.
3. Kaim. Treatment of the acute alcohol withdrawal states: a comparison of four drugs. *Am J Psychiatry* 1969;125:1640.
4. Kramp. Delirium tremens: a double blind comparison of diazepam and barbital treatment. *Acta Psychiatr Scand* 1978;58:174.
5. Kraus. Randomized clinical trial of atenolol in patients with alcohol withdrawal. *N Engl J Med* 1985;313:905.
6. Rothstein. Prevention of alcohol withdrawal seizures: the roles of diphenylhydantoin and chlordiazepoxide. *Am J Psychiatry* 1973; 130:1381.
7. Saitz. Individualized treatment for alcohol withdrawal: a randomized double-blind controlled trial. *JAMA* 1994;272:519.
8. Sampliner. Diphenylhydantoin control of alcohol withdrawal seizures: results of a controlled study. *JAMA* 1974;230:1430.
9. Sellers. Alcohol intoxication and withdrawal. *N Engl J Med* 1976;294:757.
10. Tavel. A critical analysis of mortality associated with delirium tremens: review of 39 fatalities in a nine-year period. *Am J Med Sci* 1961;242:18.
11. Thompson. Diazepam and paraldehyde for treatment of severe delirium tremens: a controlled trial. *Ann Intern Med* 1975;82:175.
12. Turner. Alcohol withdrawal syndromes: a review of pathophysiology, clinical presentation, and treatment. *J Gen Intern Med* 1989;4:432.
13. Victor. Effect of alcohol on the nervous system. *Res Publ Assoc Res Nerv Ment Dis* 1953;32:526.

34 Syncope: Diagnosis and Management

John J. Lepore and
Patrick T. O'Gara

A. Introduction

1. **Definition**—Syncope can be defined as sudden, transient loss of consciousness and postural tone without residual neurologic deficits and not requiring medical resuscitation. Using these criteria, clinical events not considered to be syncope include stroke, shock, coma, and sudden cardiac death. Most investigators also exclude seizures and psychiatric disorders such as panic attacks, conversion disorders, and somatization.
2. **Epidemiology**—Syncope is a common problem, accounting for an estimated 3% of emergency department visits and 1% of hospital admissions (11,26,28). Among 2336 men and 2873 women (30 to 62 years old at the time of entry) who were monitored for 26 years in the Framingham study, 3% of men and 3.5% of women reported at least one syncopal event (47). In a prospective evaluation of 711 nursing home patients (mean age, 87 years), there was a 6% annual and a 23% lifetime incidence of syncope (38).

B. Causes of Syncope

Causes of Syncope—The fundamental pathophysiologic mechanism for syncope is transient interruption of cerebral perfusion. Approximately 10 seconds of hypoperfusion is necessary to cause syncope. There are two principal mechanisms by which cerebral hypoperfusion occurs: a sudden loss of peripheral vascular tone or a sudden decline in cardiac output. A wide variety of conditions cause syncope by these mechanisms.

1. **Cardiac Syncope**—Major cardiac causes of syncope are summarized in Table 34-1.
   a. **Mechanical**—Mechanical cardiac causes of syncope interfere directly with the pump function of the heart by anatomic obstruction of the normal cardiopulmonary circuit, by direct myocardial damage, or by extrinsic compression of the cardiac chambers.
      (1) **Obstruction of Left-sided Cardiac Blood Flow**
         (a) **Aortic Stenosis (AS)**—Syncope is usually a late manifestation of AS, and it typically occurs after the development of angina. A

Table 34-1 Major causes of cardiac syncope

Mechanical causes of cardiac syncope	Electrical causes of cardiac syncope	Miscellaneous
Aortic stenosis	Bradyarrhythmias	Aortic dissection
Other valvular stenoses	Heart block	Hypovolemia
Hypertrophic cardiomyopathy	Supraventricular tachycardia	
Atrial myxoma	Ventricular tachycardia	
Pulmonary hypertension	Ventricular fibrillation	
Pulmonary embolus	Pacemaker failure	
Massive MI		
Cardiac tamponade		

characteristic feature of syncope related to AS is its association with exertion. With severe AS, a fixed aortic valve obstruction results in a fixed maximum cardiac output. When significant vasodilatation occurs with exercise, the appropriate increase in cardiac output cannot be achieved and syncope may occur.

(b) **Hypertrophic Cardiomyopathy (HCM)**—The hypertrophic myocardial tissue in HCM may cause dynamic obstruction to left ventricular outflow in the form of subvalvular aortic stenosis. As with valvular AS, syncope in HCM is often exertional, but postexertional syncope is more common. Conditions that impede ventricular filling, such as tachycardia or hypovolemia, can exacerbate the outflow obstruction and make syncope more likely. However, more important mechanisms for syncope in patients with HCM are ventricular arrhythmia and poorly tolerated atrial fibrillation.

(c) **Mitral Stenosis (MS)**—The pathophysiology of syncope in MS is similar to that in AS, but it occurs less commonly. It is also typically associated with exertion. Rapid atrial fibrillation and cerebral embolism are other potential mechanisms of syncope in patients with MS.

(d) **Miscellaneous Conditions**—Left atrial myxoma or other cardiac tumors can cause syncope by obstruction of left ventricular filling. In patients with prosthetic heart valves, inadequate anticoagulation or a hypercoagulable state can promote thrombosis of the valves, although rarely to a degree that results in syncope.

(2) **Obstruction of Right-sided Cardiac Blood Flow**—The mechanism of syncope in these disorders is similar to that of AS, except that the generation of adequate cardiac output is limited by obstruction to blood flow through the right side of the heart and/or the pulmonary arterial tree. Examples include pulmonic stenosis, pulmonary hypertension, massive pulmonary embolus, tricuspid stenosis, and right atrial myxoma.

(3) **Pump Failure**—In patients with an acute myocardial infarction (MI), the amount of infarcted myocardium can be large enough to cause syncope through pump failure, although the clinical presentation in this situation is more likely to be cardiogenic shock than classic syncope. The more common mechanisms for syncope related to MI are bradycardia, heart block, and ventricular arrhythmias, especially ventricular tachycardia (VT) or fibrillation.

(4) **Cardiac Tamponade**—With tamponade, fluid in the pericardial space causes extrinsic compression of the cardiac chambers and impairs cardiac output. As with HCM, hypovolemia, tachycardia, or exertion can increase the risk of syncope.

b. Electrical

(1) Bradyarrhythmia

(a) **Sinus Node Dysfunction**—Sinus bradycardia or pauses can occur in association with conduction system disease, ischemic heart disease, or drug toxicity. In the setting of sick sinus syndrome (brady-tachy syndrome), it may be difficult to determine whether syncope occurred because of the sinus node dysfunction or because of the supraventricular tachycardia (SVT).

(b) **Atrioventricular (AV) Block**—Although first-degree AV block and Mobitz type I second-degree AV block are extremely well tolerated, Mobitz type II second-degree or third-degree AV block can cause syncope if the ventricular rate is inadequate.

(2) Tachyarrhythmia

(a) **Atrial Fibrillation and Atrial Flutter**—With the loss of active atrial contribution to ventricular filling and the shortening of diastole caused by tachycardia, cardiac output may fall to such an extent as to cause syncope, particularly in patients with marginal baseline cardiac function. In such patients, restoration of sinus rhythm may improve the cardiac output and prevent syncope.

(b) **Paroxysmal SVT and Other Atrial Tachycardias**—Organized atrial activity is maintained, but syncope may occur at very high ventricular rates. It is important to exclude Wolff-Parkinson-White (WPW) syndrome in a young patient who presents with syncope and SVT.

(c) **Ventricular Tachycardia**—This arrhythmia is poorly tolerated when sustained and usually results in syncope. In the setting of a relatively slow rate or in a young, otherwise healthy patient, it can sometimes be tolerated for extended periods.

(d) **Ventricular Fibrillation**—Loss of organized ventricular electrical and mechanical activity results in cessation of cardiac output. Therefore, ventricular fibrillation universally causes loss of consciousness.

(3) **Pacemaker Failure**—In patients with a pacemaker, failure of sensing or pacing by the pacemaker can cause syncope.

(4) **Aortic Dissection**—Syncope can result from aortic dissection by several mechanisms, including cardiac tamponade from hemopericardium, ischemic arrhythmia or pump failure from coronary artery dissection, or hypovolemia from blood loss. Dissection into the cerebral vessels can also result in stroke or seizure.

2. **Neurologic Syncope (see Table 34-2)**

a. **Neurocardiogenic syncope** (NCS), more commonly known as vasovagal syncope, consists of neurally mediated bradycardia or loss of peripheral vascular resistance, which results in a sudden loss of blood pressure and cerebral hypoperfusion. Syncope occurs characteristically during a stressful, painful, or emotional situation and usually with the patient in the upright position. The episodes are often preceded by a prodrome of nausea, pallor, diaphoresis, and blurred vision. The proposed pathophysiologic mechanism involves a reflex arc. The afferent limb begins with a reduced preload in the upright position, which causes adrenergic stimulation and enhanced ventricular contraction. Ventricular C-fiber mechanoreceptors are stimulated by the increased intracavitary pressures and complete the afferent loop to the brainstem. The efferent limb consists of an increased vagal inhibitory tone at the sinoatrial and AV nodes and a decreased sympathetic tone in the heart and the peripheral vasculature. Syncope results from inappropriate bradycardia and decreased vascular tone at a time when there is an increased demand for cardiac output. Patients with predominantly bradycardia are said to have a cardioinhibitory response, whereas patients with predominantly hypotension are said to have a vasodepressor response (1).

b. **Situational Syncope**—In some patients, NCS can occur in specific and reproducible circumstances such as micturition, coughing, deglutition, Valsalva maneuver, sneezing, medical instrumentation, or diving. These patients have exaggerated vasodepressor or cardioinhibitory autonomic reflexes during these activities that may predispose them to syncope.

c. **Carotid Sinus Hypersensitivity**—Patients with this disorder experience syncope with head turning, shaving, or wearing shirts with tight collars. The mechanism for syncope involves hypersensitivity of the carotid baro-

Table 34-2 Major neurologic causes of syncope

Major neurologic causes of syncope
Neurocardiogenic syncope
Situational syncope
Carotid hypersensitivity
Orthostatic hypotension
Cerebrovascular insufficiency
Seizure

receptors, which participates in a reflex arc involving cardioinhibitory and vasodepressor limbs similar to those in NCS.

d. **Orthostatic Hypotension**—This condition should be considered in all patients with syncope. Orthostatic hypotension can result from hypovolemia, autonomic insufficiency (*e.g.*, diabetes mellitus, multiple sclerosis, amyloidosis, Parkinson's disease, alcoholism), or drug toxicity. In older patients, orthostatic hypotension is often found concomitantly with other causes of syncope (38).

e. **Cerebrovascular Insufficiency**

(1) **Anterior Circulation**—Carotid artery stenosis is a very rare cause of syncope (39), but it can occur in the setting of severe bilateral disease or with concomitant stenoses in the circle of Willis or the posterior circulation. Carotid stenoses can, however, lower the threshold for syncope in patients with other causes of cerebral hypoperfusion.

(2) **Posterior Circulation**—Vertebrobasilar insufficiency is also a very rare cause of syncope and, when present, should be associated with symptoms of brainstem dysfunction such as vertigo, ataxia, dysarthria, or diplopia (39).

(3) **Subclavian Steal Syndrome**—This phenomenon occurs when stenosis exists in the subclavian artery at a site proximal to the origin of the vertebral artery. With excessive arm exercise (on the side of the stenosis), syncope may occur as a result of retrograde blood flow from the ipsilateral vertebral artery to the arm. Asymmetric pulses in the arms may be a clue to this cause of syncope.

f. **Seizures**—Although not traditionally considered a form of syncope, seizures can mimic many features of syncope, and in some circumstances it may be difficult to distinguish between these conditions. A witness to the syncopal event is invaluable in this setting. The presence of a postictal state, Todd's paresis, urinary incontinence, or oropharyngeal trauma supports the diagnosis of seizures.

3. **Miscellaneous Causes**

a. **Drugs and Toxins**—Because a wide variety of drugs and toxins can cause syncope, a thorough history of medication use and toxin exposure is essential. Some of the drugs that are commonly implicated as a cause of syncope are listed in Table 34-3.

b. **Metabolic**—Although metabolic derangements associated with syncope of-

Table 34-3 Drugs and toxins associated with syncope

Class of Drug or Toxin	Mechanism of Syncope
Antihypertensives	
Vasodilators	Orthostatic hypotension
ACE inhibitors	
Nitrates	
Hydralazine	
β-Blockers	Bradycardia, heart block
Calcium channel blockers	Bradycardia, heart block
Digoxin	Tachyarrhythmia, bradyarrhythmia, heart block
Diuretics	Volume depletion, hypokalemia-induced arrhythmia
Macrolide antibiotics	QT prolongation and VT
Phenothiazines	QT prolongation and VT
Antihistamines	QT prolongation and VT
Antiarrhythmic agents	Proarrhythmic effects
Amphetamines, cocaine	Tachyarrhythmia
Insulin	Hypoglycemia
Alcohol	Autonomic failure
	Withdrawal seizure

ten occur in the setting of concomitant cardiac or neurologic disease, there are several primary metabolic causes of syncope. These are summarized in Table 34-4.

4. **Incidence of Syncope from Various Causes**—In the literature, the reported proportion of syncope resulting from a given cause differs significantly from study to study (11,16,17,25,31,38,40,48). Variations in the inclusion criteria, the definitions of syncope, and the extent of diagnostic evaluation probably account for these differences. In most studies, the cause of the syncopal event could not be explained in about 40% of patients despite a thorough diagnostic evaluation. NCS (1% to 37%), cardiac syncope (4% to 36%), orthostasis (4% to 10%), and situational syncope (1% to 10%) accounted for most of the events with known causes. The major findings of each study are summarized in Table 34-5. A more detailed discussion of the representative studies follows.
   a. The largest series, reported by Kapoor in 1990 (31), included 433 cases of syncope identified prospectively over a 3-year period. The mean age of the patients was 56 years. The cause of syncope could not be determined in 179 cases (41%). A cardiac cause accounted for 25% of the cases. The most common specific causes were VT (11%), orthostatic hypotension (10%), situational syncope (8%), NCS (8%), and sick sinus syndrome (3%).
   b. In a retrospective review of all patients presenting to an emergency department during a 1-year period, Day identified 198 patients with "transient loss of consciousness" (11). In contrast to the Kapoor study (31), the cause of syncope was unknown in only 13% of the cases and cardiac syncope accounted for only 9% of the cases. The most common causes of transient loss of consciousness were vasovagal events (29%), new seizures (29%), and psychiatric conditions (7%). The discrepancy of findings between Day's and Kapoor's studies may have resulted from a younger patient population (average age, 44 years) and the inclusion of seizures and psychiatric diseases in the definition of syncope in the Day's study.
   c. In a similar study of 170 patients presenting to an emergency department, Martin (40) found a relatively high incidence of vasovagal syncope (37%) and a low incidence of cardiac syncope (4%). The mean age of patients with cardiac syncope (62 years) was considerably higher than that of patients with vasovagal syncope (36 years).
   d. Over a 1-year period, Silverstein (48) studied 108 consecutive patients admitted to a medical intensive care unit with syncope. Cardiac syncope accounted for 36% of the cases. The high proportion of cardiac causes of syncope undoubtedly reflected the selected patient population admitted to an intensive care unit.
   e. In a prospective evaluation of 711 nursing home patients (mean age, 87 years), Lipsitz (38) found that 81% of patients with syncope had two or more conditions that may have contributed to the syncopal event. This study emphasizes the point that identification of one potential cause of syncope should not necessarily end the diagnostic evaluation, particularly in the elderly patient.

C. **Establishing the Cause of Syncope**—Despite an extensive evaluation, a specific cause of syncope could not be determined about 40% of the time in the large case series described (11,16,17,25,31,38,40,48). When a diagnosis was made, the history and the physical examination established the diagnosis in 55% to 85% of the cases (11,17,25,30,31,40,48). In the largest of these studies, which included 433 cases of

Table 34-4 Major metabolic causes of syncope

Metabolic Disorder	Mechanism of Syncope
Hypoglycemia	Neuroglycopenia
Hypoxemia	Cerebral hypoxemia
Hyperventilation	Cerebral vasoconstriction

Table 34-5 Causes of syncope in various studies

	Day (11) (N=198)	Engle (16) (N=176)	Engle (17) (N=100)	Kapoor (25) (N=204)	Kapoor (31) (N=433)	Lipsitz (38) (N=67)	Martin (40) (N=170)	Silverstein (48) (N=108)
Vasovagal syncope	29%	36%	18%	4%	8%	4%	37%	1%
Seizure	29%	1%	4%	1%	2%	4%	9%	—
Cardiac syncope								
Mechanical	4%	2%	6%	6%	4%	16%	1%	9%
Electrical	5%	7%	14%	20%	21%	5%	3%	27%
Drug-related syncope	7%	4%	1%	3%	2%	12%	2%	4%
Psychiatric causes	5%	1%	2%	—	1%	—	1%	—
Orthostasis	4%	6%	9%	7%	10%	10%	8%	4%
Situational syncope	1%	3%	2%	7%	8%	10%	2%	1%
Miscellaneous causes	6%	2%	5%	4%	3%	8%	—	7%
Unexplained syncope	13%	39%	39%	48%	41%	31%	38%	47%

syncope (31), the history and the physical examination revealed the cause in 55% of the 254 cases in which a specific diagnosis was made. The most common diagnoses made in this manner were orthostatic hypotension (31%), situational syncope (26%), and vasovagal syncope (25%). In addition, further evaluation based on the clues obtained in the history and the physical examination can significantly increase the diagnostic yield of each test. In Kapoor's series (31), further diagnostic testing identified the cause of syncope in an additional 114 patients (26%). The most useful diagnostic tests were prolonged electrocardiographic (ECG) monitoring (54 diagnoses), ECG or rhythm strip (30 diagnoses), cardiac catheterization (11 diagnoses), and electrophysiologic studies (EPS; 7 diagnoses). NCS and psychiatric conditions probably account for a large proportion of the unexplained syncopal events (30). Upright tilt table testing (see later discussion) is a promising approach for diagnosing NCS. Psychiatric conditions in which syncope can be part of the clinical spectrum include panic disorder, major depression, and somatization disorder (37).

1. **History**—A complete evaluation should include a thorough review of the precipitating factors, associated symptoms and signs, past medical history, medication history, and family history. In general, a very detailed step-by-step description of the entire event should be taken from the patient and from all available witnesses. A history of prior syncopal events, recent surgery, or relevant cardiac or neurologic disease should be noted.
   a. **Precipitating Factors**
      (1) **Exertion**—Exertional syncope is characteristic of AS or HCM. Classically, syncope associated with HCM occurs in the recovery phase of exercise, when vasodilatation and hyperdynamic state are maximal. Syncope with exercise may also occur with mitral stenosis, other valvular heart diseases, or various causes of pulmonary hypertension or reduced cardiac output. Exertional syncope in the setting of dyspnea or chest pain suggests ischemic ventricular arrhythmia.
      (2) **Position**—Syncope on arising from the recumbent or seated position strongly suggests orthostatic hypotension.
      (3) **Neck or Arm Movement**—Syncope associated with head turning, shaving, or wearing a shirt with a tight collar suggests carotid sinus hypersensitivity. Subclavian steal syndrome is suggested when syncope occurs with exertion of one arm but not the other.
      (4) **Specific Situations**—Cough, micturition, defecation, swallowing, and laughing have all been associated with situational syncope. Fear, pain, medical instrumentation, and emotional stress are characteristic settings for vasovagal syncope.
   b. **Associated Symptoms or Signs**—Prodromal symptoms such as diaphoresis, nausea, and blurred vision are characteristic of vasovagal syncope. The presence of a postictal state, urinary incontinence, prodromal aura, or repetitive movements favors the diagnosis of seizure as opposed to syncope. A history of thirst, diarrhea, vomiting, polyuria, or gastrointestinal bleeding suggests volume depletion as the cause of orthostatic syncope. Very sudden onset of syncope without warning, significant traumatic injury incurred during the event, and prompt, complete recovery of consciousness suggest ventricular arrhythmia as the cause of syncope. For example, in one study involving 170 patients presenting to an emergency department with syncope, the duration of the symptomatic warning period in patients with cardiac syncope was ≤10 seconds, compared with ≥10 seconds for vasovagal syncope (40).
   c. **Medications**—In addition to obtaining a current list of medications, it is important to investigate patient compliance, proper understanding of the dosing regimen, recent changes in medications, and recent refills. In some cases, a drug challenge under carefully monitored settings may confirm the diagnosis of drug-induced syncope.
   d. **Family History**—A strong family history of syncope, particularly in a young person, is worrisome because it suggests a cardiac cause of syncope such as HCM, long QT syndrome, WPW syndrome, or premature coronary artery disease.

2. **Physical Examination**
   a. **Orthostatic Vital Signs**—In elderly patients, an orthostatic decrease in the systolic blood pressure by ≥20 mm Hg has been associated with increased risks of falling, syncope, and death (3). The patient should be in the standing position for at least 2 minutes before the blood pressure is measured. In order for the syncopal event to be attributed to orthostasis, the patient should be symptomatic during the maneuver, because up to 20% of otherwise healthy elderly patients have orthostatic hypotension (30).
   b. **Carotid Sinus Massage**—This maneuver is performed by applying moderate pressure to one carotid artery during continuous ECG monitoring. However, this maneuver should be avoided in patients with carotid bruits. The duration of the massage should not exceed 5 to 10 seconds, and carotid flow should not be interrupted completely (51). A positive response can be either cardioinhibitory (sinus pause of >3 seconds) or vasodepressor (a decrease in blood pressure of >50 mm Hg). In contrast to orthostatic hypotension, a diagnosis of carotid sinus hypersensitivity can be made even when symptoms are not duplicated during the maneuver (52). The carotid arteries should also be evaluated for the intensity and the timing of upstroke and for bruits, which could suggest the presence of AS or carotid artery disease.
   c. **Cardiac Examination**—A complete cardiac examination is important. In particular, the rhythm, the rate, and the presence or absence of murmurs should be noted. Evidence of left ventricular hypertrophy (fourth heart sound, left ventricular heave) or ventricular dysfunction (third heart sound, laterally displaced cardiac impulse, rales, distended neck veins, peripheral edema) should be sought.
   d. **Neurologic Examination**—A careful neurologic examination is important to exclude focal abnormalities that may suggest the presence of stroke or other central nervous system lesions warranting further investigation.
   e. **Miscellaneous**—Vascular pulses should be examined for evidence of carotid artery disease, aortic dissection, aortic aneurysm, or subclavian steal. In appropriate settings, a rectal examination with stool guaiac testing is important to exclude gastrointestinal bleeding as a cause of syncope.
3. **Diagnostic Testing**
   a. **Electrocardiogram**—The ECG is an essential component of the syncope work-up. Abnormalities that suggest a cardiac cause of syncope include bradycardia or sinus pauses, conduction system disease (AV block, bundle branch block), evidence of structural heart disease (atrial or ventricular hypertrophy, ventricular aneurysm), ischemic heart disease (old or new MI, myocardial ischemia), drug toxicity (digoxin effect, prolonged QT interval), atrial or ventricular tachyarrhythmia, and clues suggesting arrhythmia (ectopic atrial or ventricular beats, prolonged QT interval, bypass tract of WPW). Although the ECG is abnormal in as many as 50% of patients with syncope (31), it definitively identifies the cause of syncope in only 2% to 11% of cases (11,17,25,31,40,48). In the 433 patients with syncope evaluated by Kapoor (31), 206 (48%) had an abnormal ECG. However, the ECG abnormality identified the cause of syncope in only 30 patients (7%). The diagnostic ECG findings included symptomatic bradycardia or VT (9 patients), sinus pauses (6 patients), acute MI (5 patients), third-degree AV block (4 patients), symptomatic SVT (4 patients), and pacemaker failure (2 patients). The ECG abnormality was not diagnostic of the cause of syncope in the remaining 176 patients. The abnormal but nondiagnostic ECG findings included old MI (58 patients), left ventricular hypertrophy (40 patients), left axis deviation (37 patients), and bifascicular block (22 patients).
   b. **Echocardiography**—An echocardiogram is useful when structural heart disease is suspected based on the history, physical examination, chest film, or ECG. The echocardiographic findings that may suggest a cause of syncope include valvular heart disease, hypertrophic cardiomyopathy, pulmonary hypertension, cardiac tamponade, and intracardiac mass. Regional

wall motion abnormality, reduced left ventricular function, and cardiac chamber enlargement are nonspecific findings but may increase the suspicion for arrhythmia as the cause of syncope in appropriate settings.

c. Prolonged ECG (Holter) Monitoring—This test is targeted for patients in whom there is a strong clinical suspicion for an arrhythmic cause of syncope, but in whom an arrhythmia is not identified on the initial ECG (15,21,28).

(1) Diagnostic Yield

(a) As with the ECG, the results of 24-hour Holter monitoring are frequently abnormal in patients presenting with syncope, but only rarely does the abnormality actually identify the cause of syncope. In an analysis of nine studies evaluating the diagnostic efficacy of prolonged ECG monitoring for syncope (total of 2612 patients), Kapoor (28) pointed out that 17% of patients had significant arrhythmia during monitoring but only 4% had symptoms reminiscent of the syncopal episode associated with the arrhythmia (see Table 34-6).

(b) In the largest study reported to date, Gibson (21) identified 1512 patients over a 5-year period who were referred to an outpatient 24-hour ECG monitoring center for evaluation of syncope. A significant arrhythmia likely to result in syncope (*i.e.*, high-grade AV block or VT) was found in 131 patients (9%), but only 6 of these patients reported symptoms at the time of the noted arrhythmia. In addition, of the 1004 patients who were older than 60 years of age, 32 (3%) met the criteria for sick sinus syndrome but only 2 had symptoms corresponding to the noted abnormality (see Table 34-7).

(c) In the same study, although 15 patients had syncope and 240 had presyncope during monitoring, arrhythmia was detected in only 30 (12%) of the symptomatic patients (21) (see Table 34-8).

Table 34-6 Correlation of symptoms and arrhythmia on 24-hour HM (28)

Patients with symptoms		Patients without symptoms	
Arrhythmia 4%	No Arrhythmia 17%	Arrhythmia 13%	No Arrhythmia 69%

Table 34-7 Correlation of symptoms and abnormal findings on 24-hour HM (21)

	N	Syncope or presyncope
High-grade AV block or VT (all age groups)	131	6 (5%)
Sick sinus syndrome (patients >60 y)	32	2 (6%)

Table 34-8 Correlation of symptoms and arrhythmia on 24-hour HM (21)

Symptom	N	Associated arrhythmia	No associated arrhythmia
Syncope	15	7	8
Presyncope	240	23	217
Total	255	30	225

(d) The positive diagnostic yield of symptomatic arrhythmia in the patients monitored was therefore only 2% (30 of 1512). The authors noted that the test may be considered more useful as a negative diagnostic clue, since 15% (225 of 1512) experienced syncope or presyncope without any arrhythmia noted on the monitor, thereby excluding arrhythmia as the cause of their syncope.

(2) Duration of Monitoring—A prospective evaluation by Bass (5) indicated that the diagnostic yield can be increased with an additional 24 hours of ECG monitoring if an arrhythmic cause of syncope is not identified in the first 24 hours. However, a third 24-hour period did not significantly increase the yield of the test. This study evaluated 95 consecutive patients whose syncopal episode remained unexplained despite a careful review of history, physical examination, and ECG. Each patient underwent three serial 24-hour ECG recordings. A major abnormality was noted in 15% of the patients during the first 24-hour recording, and in another 11% during the second 24-hour study. During the third 24-hour study, only 3 (4%) patients had major abnormalities. A limitation of this study is that only 1 of the many patients with a major ECG abnormality had associated symptoms during monitoring. The significance of finding asymptomatic arrhythmias during 24-hour monitoring remains unclear; there has been no well-designed study that demonstrates that treatment of these patients decreases the risk of future syncope.

(3) Prognostic Clues—Despite the low positive diagnostic yield, Holter monitoring can provide useful prognostic data in patients with syncope even if the exact cause is not identified. For example, in a series of 235 patients with syncope of unknown cause who were observed for a mean of 24 months (33), patients with frequent ventricular ectopy or VT on 24-hour ECG monitoring had a higher risk of death, including sudden cardiac death, than patients with rare ventricular ectopy. In Cox regression analysis, the hazard ratio for frequent premature ventricular contractions was 3.7 for overall mortality and 14.9 for sudden cardiac death. In addition, sinus pause (>2 seconds) was an independent risk factor for overall mortality (hazard ratio, 3.3). The authors concluded that patients with complex ventricular ectopy or prolonged sinus pauses on Holter monitoring should be considered for EPS, cardiac stress testing, or cardiac catheterization (see Table 34-9).

d. Loop Event Recorder—Like the Holter monitor, the loop event recorder continuously monitors a patient's cardiac rhythm. However, it does not store the rhythm in memory unless it is activated by a patient who experiences symptoms compatible with syncope or presyncope. It is capable of storing several minutes of the cardiac rhythm before being activated, so that the rhythm preceding or accompanying the symptomatic event can be recorded. The goal is to identify arrhythmias in patients with recurrent syncope whose Holter monitor results are nondiagnostic. However, because the rate of recurrence for syncope may be as low as 16% at 6 months according to one study (27), the additional yield of loop recording is also low.

Table 34-9 Prognostic significance of abnormal findings on 24-hour HM (33)

	Outcome At 2 Y	
Holter abnormality	Sudden death	Overall mortality
VT	18.7% (*P*<0.0001)	36.5% (*P*<0.00001)
Frequent or paired PVCs	18.2% (*P*<0.001)	28.3% (*P*<0.003)
Rare PVCs	4.0%	10.8%

Linzer (36) prospectively evaluated the diagnostic yield of 1 month of loop recording in 57 patients whose syncope remained unexplained after Holter monitoring. Of the 32 patients who developed subsequent symptoms (syncope or near syncope), the event was successfully recorded in 14 patients; 7 had an associated cardiac arrhythmia, but 7 had a normal recording. The positive diagnostic yield was therefore 12% (7 of 57).

e. **Signal-Averaged Electrocardiogram (SA-ECG)**—When VT is highly suspected in a patient with recurrent syncope, SA-ECG may be useful if the ECG and the Holter monitoring results are nondiagnostic. A computer-enhanced high-resolution ECG is used to detect low-amplitude, delayed potentials in the terminal portion of the QRS complex. These delayed potentials are thought to represent delayed depolarization in areas of ventricular scar and are associated with an increased risk for VT. SA-ECG has been used to screen for inducible VT (12,42,44). Gang performed SA-ECG and EPS in 24 patients with syncope of unknown cause (20). Of 9 patients with sustained VT (8 inducible at EPS and 1 spontaneous), 8 had positive SA-ECG (89% sensitivity). Of the remaining 15 patients without sustained VT, none had a positive SA-ECG (100% specificity). In a similar prospective study, Winters (54) evaluated 34 patients with syncope of unknown origin and normal results on Holter monitoring. During EPS, 12 patients had inducible VT. An abnormally low root-mean-square voltage of the terminal 40 msec of the QRS complex on the SA-EKG had the highest sensitivity (82%) and specificity (91%) for detection of inducible VT. About 30% to 40% of the patients in these two studies had coronary artery disease, but the distribution of these patients in the inducible and noninducible groups was not clearly specified. It is not known whether SA-ECG would be any more useful for predicting inducible VT in the subset of patients with syncope and coronary artery disease. Further studies are needed before SA-ECG can be recommended for routine use.

f. **Exercise Stress Testing**—The role of exercise stress testing for evaluation of syncope is limited. When the diagnostic yield of 24-hour Holter monitoring was compared with the results of exercise stress testing in 119 patients with syncope, arrhythmias that could account for syncope were found in 63 patients by Holter monitoring alone, in 10 patients by both studies, but in only 3 patients by exercise testing alone (7). Nonetheless, if significant cardiac ischemia is clinically suspected, diagnosis and risk stratification of coronary artery disease should be pursued by exercise testing or coronary angiography.

g. **Cardiac Catheterization**—Cardiac catheterization is not a routine component of the syncope workup. However, it is valuable when noninvasive tests such as echocardiography, exercise stress testing, or 24-hour Holter monitoring suggest the presence of significant pulmonary hypertension, ischemic heart disease, valvular heart disease, or other structural heart disease as the cause of syncope.

h. **Electrophysiologic Studies**

(1) **General Techniques and Applications**—Electrophysiologic evaluation involves cardiac catheterization with specialized catheters that can administer electrical impulses and record electrical activity. During EPS, spontaneous cardiac arrhythmias can be detected; cardiac arrhythmias can be induced by programmed electrical stimulation; a specific anatomic focus of arrhythmia can be identified and sometimes ablated; and the function of the sinoatrial node, the AV node, and the conduction system can be evaluated (14). Although there are no universally accepted indications for EPS, there are some predictors of a positive or a negative EPS which can guide the clinician's decision in each case.

(2) **Predictors of Outcome of EPS**—In a study specifically designed to identify the predictors of outcome of EPS, 104 patients with unexplained syncope underwent EPS (34). Thirty-one patients had a posi-

tive finding that could account for the initial syncopal episode, but 73 patients had a negative test. In univariate analysis, depressed left ventricular function, bundle branch block, history of coronary artery disease, and previous MI were the strongest predictors of a positive test. In contrast, normal left ventricular function, absence of structural heart disease, and normal ECG were the strongest predictors of a negative test. These findings are summarized in Table 34-10.

(3) **Diagnostic Yield in Patients with Syncope**—The diagnostic yield of EPS for evaluation of syncope depends to a large extent on the definition of a positive test. Sustained inducible monomorphic VT, sinus recovery time >3 seconds, infranodal block induced by pacing, and inducible symptomatic SVT are generally accepted as positive findings that may account for the initial syncopal event. Kapoor (30) reviewed the results of 11 studies evaluating the role of EPS in unexplained syncope. In a total of 844 patients, abnormal results were obtained in an average of 51% (range, 18% to 75%) and included inducible VT (45%), abnormal conduction system disease (28%), and inducible symptomatic SVT (22%). Five percent of patients had hypervagotonia or carotid sinus hypersensitivity. However, for several important reasons (13,30,41), identification of an abnormality during EPS cannot be equated with conclusively finding the actual cause of syncope. For example, SVT, atrial fibrillation, and atrial flutter are frequently induced with atrial pacing even in patients without syncopal symptoms. Furthermore, although inducible sustained monomorphic VT is highly suggestive of spontaneous VT as the cause of syncope, inducible polymorphic VT or nonsustained VT are nonspecific and can result from aggressive ventricular stimulation even in normal patients. Finally, measures of sinus node function such as sinus node recovery time and sinoatrial conduction time are not sensitive for sinus node dysfunction. Measures of AV conduction depend on the autonomic tone, which can be highly variable even among normal subjects. A reasonable approach is to assign a particular EPS abnormality as the cause of syncope only if compatible symptoms are reproduced at the time the abnormality is recorded.

(4) **Prognostic Significance**—Diagnosis of the cause of syncope by EPS has important implications for prognosis and treatment (4,35). Many studies have confirmed a significantly poorer outcome for patients with abnormal results on EPS. Bass (4) retrospectively studied a cohort of 70 patients who underwent EPS for unexplained syncope. The 3-year mortality rate and the rate of sudden cardiac death were significantly higher in the 37 patients with an abnormal test than in the 33 patients with a normal test (see Table 34-11).

Table 34-10 Predictors of positive and negative EPS outcomes (34)

	Positive EPS (%)	Negative EPS (%)	*P*	Relative risk for Positive EPS
Ejection fraction <40%	65	3	<0.00001	64.5
Bundle branch block	68	5	<0.00003	49.0
Coronary artery disease	74	16	<0.00003	18.2
Previous MI	55	8	<0.00006	13.5
Injury during syncope	29	8	<0.01	4.5
Ejection fraction >40%	35	97	<0.00001	0.02
No structural heart disease	3	63	<0.00001	0.02
Normal ECG	6	67	<0.0001	0.03
No VEA on Holter monitoring	0	34	<0.0001	—
Syncope >5 min	0	24	<0.0008	—

(5) Treatment—When arrhythmia or conduction abnormality is determined to be the cause of syncope, treatment options include antiarrhythmic medications, permanent pacemaker, automatic implantable cardiac defibrillator, and radiofrequency catheter ablation. The specific indications for these interventions remain controversial and are areas of active investigation.

i. Upright Tilt Table Testing

(1) Testing Protocol—The tilt table test is intended to be a provocative test for NCS. The patient is placed in a supine position on a tilt table that has a firm foot board. The table is then brought suddenly to an upright position (usually 60°), where it is maintained for 45 to 60 minutes with continuous heart rate and blood pressure monitoring. A positive response consists of presyncope or syncope associated with bradycardia or hypotension. To increase the sensitivity of the test, some centers also use isoproterenol (2), which causes forceful ventricular contraction and augments stimulation of the ventricular C fibers during the tilt maneuver. If a positive response is not obtained with the usual protocol, the patient is brought back to the supine position, and the protocol may be repeated with escalating doses of isoproterenol until a positive response or a dose-limiting side effect (typically tachycardia) is encountered (19). Although numerous studies have evaluated the role of upright tilt table testing in the diagnosis of syncope, meaningful comparisons between them are difficult because of the differences in the protocol used (degree of tilt, duration of upright position), the environmental factors in the testing laboratory (temperature, noise, time of day), the dose of isoproterenol used, the method of blood pressure monitoring (invasive versus noninvasive), and whether or not patients fasted overnight (19,29,50).

(2) Diagnostic Utility—In a review of 23 studies using upright tilt testing for evaluation of patients with unexplained syncope (14 with and 9 without isoproterenol), an average of 66% (range, 39% to 87%) of patients in the studies with isoproterenol and 50% (range, 26% to 90%) of those in the studies without isoproterenol had positive tilt table tests (29). However, the sensitivity and specificity of the test are difficult to determine because of the lack of a gold standard test for NCS and the lack of a consensus on what constitutes an abnormal test (9,32,53).

(3) Clinical Application—For patients with NCS, several treatment options are available (see later discussion). Some studies (23,49) found that repeat tilt testing can be useful to determine the efficacy of a pharmacologic intervention. Others found that the test was not adequately reproducible for this purpose. When Brooks tested 109 patients with unexplained syncope with passive tilt testing on two consecutive days, the results of the first test differed from those of the second in 37% of patients (8). Therefore, the role of tilt table testing in the evaluation of unexplained syncope remains investigational.

j. Head Computed Tomography or Magnetic Resonance Imaging—Imaging studies of the head and brain are most useful for diagnosing stroke, intracerebral bleed, or intracerebral mass. These conditions are almost always associated with a focal neurologic finding or other specific clues, such as a

Table 34-11 Prognostic significance of abnormal EPS findings (4)

	Normal EPS (N=33)	Abnormal EPS (N=37)	*P*
3-Y mortality	15%	61%	<0.001
3-Y sudden cardiac death	9%	48%	<0.002

history of head trauma, focal neurologic complaint, headache, known cerebrovascular disease, or seizure. If one or more of these clues is present in a patient with syncope, an imaging study is indicated. However, because the yield of these studies is low in the absence of specific clues, they should be avoided for routine evaluation of syncope. For example, in a series of 433 patients with syncope, the head computed tomography scan was abnormal in 39 of 134 patients scanned, but in no case was the cause of syncope identified by this study (31). The abnormal findings included cerebral atrophy (19 patients), old stroke (12 patients), subdural bleeding from trauma incurred with the syncopal event (5 patients), newly diagnosed sellar mass (2 patients), and meningioma (1 patient). The latter 3 patients had other explanations for their syncope.

k. **Electroencephalogram (EEG)**—The EEG is important for evaluation of seizure but not syncope. For evaluation of patients with transient loss of consciousness, the diagnostic yield of the EEG is very low unless the history or physical examination strongly suggests seizure as the cause of syncope. Davis (10) reviewed all EEG results from a single hospital over a 2-year period. Although EEG findings were abnormal in 15 of the 99 patients referred for evaluation of presyncope, syncope, or complaints similar to syncope, the noted abnormality was diagnostic of seizure in only 1 patient. The nondiagnostic abnormalities included generalized slowing (11 patients) and focal slowing (3 patients). Therefore, the EEG should not be a routine part of the syncope evaluation but should be reserved for those in whom a seizure disorder is strongly suspected.

l. **Cerebrovascular Studies**—Isolated syncope is a rare presentation of cerebrovascular disease. Therefore, evaluation of the anterior or posterior cerebral circulation by ultrasound, magnetic resonance angiography, or contrast angiography should not be a routine part of syncope evaluation.

D. Treatment

1. **Cardiac Syncope**—The treatment of cardiac syncope is specific to the exact cause. Valvular heart disease can be treated by surgery or catheter-based techniques. Cardiac arrhythmia may be managed medically, with radiofrequency catheter ablation, or by insertion of an automatic implantable cardiac defibrillator. Ischemia may be treated medically or by various revascularization techniques. Heart block or sinus node dysfunction may be treated with implantation of a permanent pacemaker. A complete discussion of these therapeutic options is beyond the scope of this chapter.

2. **Neurocardiogenic Syncope**—The increasing awareness of NCS as a major cause of syncope has led to several recent advances in therapy.

   a. **Drug Therapy**—The feature common to the various drugs used in treatment of NCS is that they interfere with the NCS reflex arc by decreasing ventricular inotropy, inhibiting activation of myocardial C fibers, interfering with the cholinergic input to the AV node, blocking adenosine- or serotonin-mediated hypotension and bradycardia, or directly stimulating peripheral α-receptors (2,22,23,24,43,45,49) (see Table 34-12).

   b. **Pacemaker**—Sequential AV pacing is an attractive theoretical therapeutic option for NCS, particularly in patients with predominantly cardioin-

Table 34-12 Drug therapy for neurocardiogenic syncope

Drug	Proposed mechanism	Reference
β-Blockers	Inhibition of C fibers, negative inotropy	(23), (49)
Disopyramide	Anticholinergic effect, negative inotropy	(43)
Theophylline	Adenosine receptor blockade	(45)
Fluoxetine	Decreased postsynaptic serotonin transmission	(22)
Ephedrine	α-sympathetic agonism	(24)

hibitory responses (6). In a small study of 10 patients with reproducible syncope on passive tilt testing, Fitzpatrick (18) found that as many as 85% of syncopal events could be aborted with sequential AV pacing in patients with NCS. In a similar study with longer follow-up (average, 50 months) involving 37 patients with predominantly cardioinhibitory response on tilt testing, dual-chamber pacing alleviated symptoms in 89% and eliminated symptoms in 27% (46). In contrast, in a direct comparison of drug therapy (metoprolol, theophylline, or disopyramide) versus sequential AV pacing in 22 patients with syncope inducible by upright tilt testing, Sra (49) demonstrated that 94% of patients treated with drug therapy were symptom free at a median follow-up of 16 months, whereas all patients treated with pacing experienced either recurrent syncope or persistent symptoms at tilt testing. Large randomized, well-designed trials are needed to clarify the roles of various drugs and of pacing in patients with NCS.

c. **Volume Expansion**—Prevention of a hypovolemic state can theoretically limit orthostatic pooling of blood in the lower body, thereby avoiding reflex tachycardia and inotropy and preventing the reflex arc from being initiated. This has been addressed clinically with dietary salt supplements, high fluid intake, and adrenocorticoid therapy (*e.g.*, fludrocortisone).

E. Prognosis

1. **Mortality and Sudden Death**—Establishing the cause of syncope is obviously important for therapy, but it is also helpful for prognosis. Numerous studies report a significant increase in the risk of overall mortality and the rate of sudden cardiac death in patients with cardiac syncope, compared with those with noncardiac syncope. The overall 1-year mortality rate ranged from 18% to 33% for cardiac syncope, compared with 0% to 12% for noncardiac or unexplained syncope (11,17,25,31,40,48). In the largest series, involving 433 patients with syncope observed for a mean of 40 months, the overall actuarial 5-year mortality rate was 34% and the rate of sudden death was 14% (31) (see Table 34-13) . Patients with cardiac syncope had a statistically significant increase in the risk of overall mortality and in the rate of sudden death, compared with those with noncardiac syncope. In Cox regression analysis, cardiac syncope was an independent predictor of mortality (hazard ratio, 2.2).
2. **Rate of Recurrence**—Recurrence of syncope is common and does not appear to be a predictor of mortality. Of 433 patients observed for a mean of 30 months, syncope recurred in 34% (27). The rates of recurrence in cardiac, noncardiac, and unexplained syncope were statistically similar at 34%, 36%, and 43%, respectively. In Cox regression analysis, recurrence of syncope was not a predictor of mortality (RR, 0.9; 95% CI, 0.5 to 1.6) or of sudden death (RR, 0.5; 95% CI, 0.2 to 1.5).

F. Conclusions

1. Syncope is a common clinical event. Cardiac syncope and vasovagal syncope are the most common diagnoses made, but a diagnosis cannot be assigned in approximately 40% of the cases.
2. Diagnostic evaluation should be individualized for each patient. The history and physical examination can identify the cause of syncope in >50% of cases, and specific tests directed by the history and physical examination can identify the cause in another 25%. Echocardiography, cardiac catheterization, head computed tomography, magnetic resonance imaging, EEG, and cerebrovascu-

Table 34-13 Prognostic significance of cardiac versus noncardiac syncope (31)

	Cause of Syncope		
Outcome	Cardiac	Noncardiac	Unknown
5-Y cumulative mortality rate	51%	30% ($P<0.00001$)	24% ($P<0.00001$)
5-Y sudden death rate	33%	5% ($P<0.00001$)	9% ($P<0.00001$)

lar studies should not be routinely ordered unless there is a specific indication for these tests.

3. However, an aggressive and thorough workup is warranted, especially when a cardiac cause is suspected. The diagnostic yield of the standard ECG is low, and the yield is increased only to a limited extent by prolonged ECG monitoring. The loop event recorder also has had limited success in diagnosing the cause of recurrent syncope. EPS can identify abnormalities in about 50% of patients with unexplained syncope and structural heart disease, but the identified abnormality cannot always be assumed to be the actual cause of syncope. Upright tilt table testing is intended to be a provocative test for NCS, but its role in the evaluation of unexplained syncope remains investigational. Refinement of the diagnostic criteria used in EPS and upright tilt table testing will be an important advance.
4. Compared to patients with noncardiac or unexplained syncope, those with a cardiac cause have a significantly worse prognosis. Therefore, an important goal in the evaluation of patients with syncope is to exclude cardiac syncope. Syncope recurs commonly, but recurrence is not necessarily associated with a worse prognosis.
5. Treatment of syncope is directed toward the specific cardiac, neurologic, or metabolic cause. Large-scale clinical trials evaluating the efficacy of various therapies for patients with syncope will also be an important advance.

Abbreviations used in Chapter 34

ACE = angiotensin-converting enzyme
AS = aortic stenosis
AV = atrioventricular
CI = confidence interval
ECG = electrocardiogram
EEG = electroencephalogram
EPS = electrophysiologic studies
HCM = hypertrophic cardiomyopathy
MI = myocardial infarction
MS = mitral stenosis
NCS = Neurocardiogenic syncope
PVC = premature ventricular contraction
RR = relative risk
SA-ECG = signal-averaged electrocardiogram
SVT = supraventricular tachycardia
VEA = ventricular ectopic activity
VT = ventricular tachycardia
WPW = Wolff-Parkinson-White syndrome

References

1. Abboud. Neurocardiogenic syncope. *N Engl J Med* 1993;328:1117.
2. Almquist. Provocation of bradycardia and hypotension by isoproterenol and upright posture in patients with unexplained syncope. *N Engl J Med* 1989;320:346.
3. Atkins. Syncope and orthostatic hypotension. *Am J Med* 1992;91:179.
4. Bass. Long-term prognosis of patients undergoing electrophysiologic studies for syncope of unknown origin. *Am J Cardiol* 1988;62:1186.
5. Bass. The duration of Holter monitoring in patients with syncope: is 24 hours enough? *Arch Intern Med* 1990;150:1073.

6. Benditt. Cardiac pacing for prevention of recurrent vasovagal syncope. *Ann Intern Med* 1995;122:204. Review.
7. Boudoulas. Superiority of 24-hour outpatient monitoring over multi-stage exercise testing for the evaluation of syncope. *J Electrocardiol* 1979;12:103.
8. Brooks. Prospective evaluation of day-to-day reproducibility of upright tilt table testing in unexplained syncope. *Am J Cardiol* 1993;71:1289.
9. Calkins. Comparison of responses to isoproterenol and epinephrine during head-up tilt in suspected vasodepressor syncope. *Am J Cardiol* 1991;67:207.
10. Davis. Electroencephalography should not be routine in the evaluation of syncope in adults. *Arch Intern Med* 1990;150:2027.
11. Day. Evaluation and outcome of emergency room patients with transient loss of consciousness. *Am J Med* 1982;73:15.
12. Denniss. Prognostic significance of ventricular tachycardia and fibrillation induced at programmed stimulation and delayed potentials detected on the signal-averaged electrocardiograms of survivors of acute myocardial infarction. *Circulation* 1986;74:731.
13. DiMarco. Electrophysiologic studies in patients with unexplained syncope. *Circulation* 1987;75(Suppl III):140. Review.
14. DiMarco. Intracardiac electrophysiology techniques in recurrent syncope of unknown cause. *Ann Intern Med* 1981;95:542.
15. DiMarco. Use of ambulatory electrocardiographic (Holter) monitoring. *Ann Intern Med* 1986;113:53. Review.
16. Eagle. Evaluation of prognostic classifications for patients with syncope. *Am J Med* 1985;79:455.
17. Eagle. The impact of diagnostic tests in evaluating patients with syncope. *Yale J Biol Med* 1983;56:1.
18. Fitzpatrick. Dual-chamber pacing aborts vasovagal syncope induced by head-up 60-degree tilt. *Pacing Clin Electrophysiol* 1991;14:13.
19. Fitzpatrick. Methodology of head-up tilt testing in patients with unexplained syncope. *J Am Coll Cardiol* 1991;17:125.
20. Gang. Detection of late potentials on the surface electrocardiogram in unexplained syncope. *Am J Cardiol* 1986;58:1014.
21. Gibson. Diagnostic efficacy of 24-hour electrocardiographic monitoring for syncope. *Am J Cardiol* 1984;53:1013.
22. Grubb. Usefulness of fluoxetine hydrochloride for prevention of resistant upright tilt induced syncope. *Pacing Clin Electrophysiol* 1993;16:458.
23. Grubb. Utility of upright tilt table testing in the evaluation and management of syncope of unknown origin. *Am J Med* 1991;90:6.
24. Janosik. Efficacy of oral ephedrine sulfate in preventing neurocardiogenic syncope. *Circulation* 1991;84 (Suppl II):234. Abstract.
25. Kapoor. A prospective evaluation and follow-up of patients with syncope. *N Engl J Med* 1983;309:197.
26. Kapoor. Diagnosis and natural history of syncope and the role of invasive electrophysiologic testing. *Am J Cardiol* 1989;63:730. Review.
27. Kapoor. Diagnostic and prognostic implications of recurrences in patients with syncope. *Am J Med* 1987;83:700.
28. Kapoor. Diagnostic evaluation of syncope. *Am J Med* 1991;90:91. Review.
29. Kapoor. Evaluating unexplained syncope with upright tilt testing. *Cleve Clin J Med* 1995;62:305. Review.
30. Kapoor. Evaluation and management of the patient with syncope. *JAMA* 1992; 268:2553. Review.
31. Kapoor. Evaluation and outcome of patients with syncope. *Medicine (Baltimore)* 1990;69:160.
32. Kapoor. Evaluation of upright tilt testing with isoproterenol: a non-specific test. *Ann Intern Med* 1992;116:358.
33. Kapoor. Prolonged electrocardiographic monitoring in patients with syncope: importance of frequent or repetitive ventricular ectopy. *Am J Med* 1987;82:20.
34. Krol. Electrophysiologic testing in patients with unexplained syncope: clinical and noninvasive predictors of outcome. *J Am Coll Cardiol* 1987;10:358.

35. Kushner. Natural history of patients with unexplained syncope and a non-diagnostic electrophysiologic study. *J Am Coll Cardiol* 1989;14:391.
36. Linzer. Incremental diagnostic yield of loop electrocardiographic recorders in unexplained syncope. *Am J Cardiol* 1990;66:214.
37. Linzer. Psychiatric syncope. *Psychosomatics* 1990;31:181.
38. Lipsitz. Syncope in an elderly, institutionalized population: prevalence, incidence, and associated risk. *Q J Med* 1985;55:45.
39. Manolis. Syncope: current diagnostic evaluation and management. *Ann Intern Med* 1990;112:850. Review.
40. Martin. Prospective evaluation of syncope. *Ann Emerg Med* 1984;13:499.
41. McAnulty. Syncope of unknown origin: the role of electrophysiologic studies. *Circulation* 1987;75(Suppl III):144. Review.
42. Mehta. Significance of signal-averaged electrocardiography in relation to endomyocardial biopsy and ventricular stimulation studies in patients with ventricular tachycardia without apparent heart disease. *J Am Coll Cardiol* 1989;14:372.
43. Milstein. Usefulness of disopyramide for prevention of upright tilt-induced hypotension-bradycardia. *Am J Cardiol* 1990;65:1339.
44. Nalos. The signal-averaged electrocardiogram as a screening test for inducibility of sustained ventricular tachycardia in high risk patients: a prospective study. *J Am Coll Cardiol* 1987;9:539.
45. Nelson. The autonomic and hemodynamic effects of oral theophylline in patients with vasodepressor syncope. *Arch Intern Med* 1991;151:2425.
46. Peterson. Permanent pacing for cardioinhibitory malignant vasovagal syndrome. *Br Heart J* 1994;71:274.
47. Savage. Epidemiologic features of isolated syncope: the Framingham Study. *Stroke* 1985;16:626.
48. Silverstein. Patients with syncope admitted to medical intensive care units. *JAMA* 1982;248:1185.
49. Sra. Comparison of cardiac pacing with drug therapy in the treatment of neurocardiogenic (vasovagal) syncope with bradycardia or asystole. *N Engl J Med* 1993; 328:1085.
50. Sra. Unexplained syncope evaluated by electrophysiologic studies and head-up tilt testing. *Ann Intern Med* 1991;114:1013.
51. Steinberg. Use of the signal-averaged electrocardiogram for predicting inducible ventricular tachycardia in patients with unexplained syncope: relation to clinical variables in a multivariate analysis. *J Am Coll Cardiol* 1994;23:99.
52. Strasberg. Carotid sinus hypersensitivity and the carotid sinus syndrome. *Prog Cardiovasc Dis* 1989;31:379.
53. Waxman. Isoproterenol induction of vasodepressor-type reaction in vasodepressor-prone persons. *Am J Cardiol* 1989;63:58.
54. Winters. Signal averaging of the surface QRS complex predicts inducibility of ventricular tachycardia in patients with syncope of unknown origin: a prospective study. *J Am Coll Cardiol* 1987;10:775.

Subject Index

Locators followed by *f* indicate figures.
Locators followed by *t* indicate tables.

F

H